HUMAN PATHOLOGY

BY

HOWARD T. KARSNER, M.D.

Professor of Pathology
Western Reserve University, Cleveland, Ohio

460 Illustrations in Black and White
and 24 Subjects in Color on 16 Plates

SIXTH EDITION
COMPLETELY REVISED AND RESET

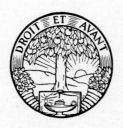

Philadelphia   Montreal   London

J. B. LIPPINCOTT COMPANY

TO MY WIFE

Preface to the Sixth Edition

The preparation of this edition has permitted simplification and clarification of the text, inclusion of new material to make it comprehensive and modern, and provision of new and improved illustrations. In order to avoid increase in size of the volume, certain discussions have been shortened and topics not strictly germane to the subject of pathology have been omitted. The fact that the book has been entirely reset indicates the extent of the revision. About half the text has been rewritten and certain parts have been rearranged. Advantage has been taken of the opportunity to modernize the format. The shortened lines provided by the printing of two columns to the page should facilitate reading and study.

A section on vitamin deficiencies has been included in the first chapter. The discussion of disturbances of circulation covers modern views on edema and on shock. The chapter on principles of infectious diseases has been enlarged to include examples of diseases due to protozoa, spirochetal organisms, rickettsiae and viruses. The material on infectious granulomata has been reclassified and a section on sarcoidosis added. The chapter on tumors has been largely rewritten to incorporate the results of recent research.

In the chapters on systemic pathology, the subject of endocarditis has been reorientated, that of anemias has been rearranged in accord with current conceptions of hematology, the modern views on pneumonia and pneumonitis have been included, cirrhosis of the liver is presented in the light of the newer studies of dietary alterations, and pyelonephritis is discussed with appropriate attention to its functional significance. Tumors of the gonads are now discussed in relation to their associated endocrine disturbances. The chapter on ductless glands has been brought into line with prevailing views on endocrinology, with especial reference to tumors of these organs. The material on tumors of bones and of synovia has been rewritten. The chapter on nervous system has been modernized, especially in reference to viral diseases. Many other changes have been made throughout the book.

A textbook of pathology should not be a mere catalogue of morbid anatomy. A knowledge of morphologic changes is fundamental to a comprehension of the subject, but must be expanded by a co-ordination of the physiologic and biochemical implications of altered structure. Furthermore, the functional disturbances should be interpreted in terms of clinical manifestations. To this end, disease and its effects in the living patient have been correlated as closely as is consistent with the primary objectives of the book.

As heretofore, illustrations are used to supplement the text rather than to replace it. Well over a hundred new illustrations have been provided, most in half-tone reproduction and some in color. Many are photomicrographs, reproduced in a size adequate for a comprehension of what is seen under the microscope. The photographs and photomicrographs largely replace the older and less instructive drawings. Many of the legends have been revised in order that they may be clearly explanatory.

Since the history of pathology is now presented in excellent books and articles, the list of references has been changed so as to delete those to the older literature and to include articles and reviews especially valuable for supplementary reading. The new references are almost entirely to articles in English and it is hoped that the student will be stimulated thereby to enlarge his horizon. Without materially increasing the total number, 680 new references have been inserted. At the suggestion of the publishers, the bibliographic style has been changed so as to follow in a general way that of Biological Abstracts.

Grateful acknowledgment is made to those whose use of previous editions has necessitated the preparation of this sixth edition. The author is deeply indebted to numerous associates for their interest and help. Dr. Simon Koletsky has given time, energy and initiative to critical reading of the manuscript. Major William B. Wartman, now overseas, and Dr. Thomas C. Laipply have aided significantly in the selection and preparation of the illustrations. Dr. Horace K. Giffen has helped with the illustrations and has carefully checked the galley proofs and references. Dr. Thomas J. Hill has revised the material on teeth. Other members of the staff in Pathology have given many valuable suggestions. Dr. R. F. Parker and Dr. R. W. Heinle, of the Department of Medicine, have given guidance in preparation of the material on viral diseases and on hematology. As heretofore, Dr. Harry Goldblatt has supervised the arrangement of the index.

As in previous editions, the manuscript has been typed by Miss Catherine E. Lennon. It is only just to say that her keen interest and unflagging energy have contributed vastly more than the transfer of illegible handwriting to the typed sheet. Miss Mary Johnstone, editorial assistant to the publishers, has given meticulously careful attention to arrangement and clarification of the text. Miss Ada L. Floyd and her assistants in the Cleveland Medical Library have given much time and valuable attention to corrections of the bibliography. Miss Theodora Bergsland, Mr. B. W. Brownlow and Miss Bessie L. Strong, of the Division of Illustration of the Institute of Pathology, have been devoted and precise in their work. It is a pleasure to make these acknowledgments. To say that the author is deeply grateful is a gross understatement of his sense of appreciation.

HOWARD T. KARSNER

PREFACE TO THE FIRST EDITION

THE history of pathology shows a gradual evolution from a subject based almost entirely on morphology to one so comprehensive that as H. R. Dean says, "to the pathologist—all medical things are pathology." From this point of view clinical medicine is applied pathology. At any rate, pathology is no longer merely the study of morbid form, although no evolution or development can divorce from it the fundamental importance of pathological anatomy. The purpose of this book is to present the morphological alterations incident to disease, in the light of modern views as to their functional significance. The subject matter is confined to human pathology, since the work is designed for students and practitioners of medicine, but general biology has been called upon to furnish data relevant to the origin, course and natural history of disease as it affects man. The features of morbid anatomy and histology are studied objectively and are looked upon as established facts. At the present time, explanations of disease and interpretations of its phenomena are often hypothetical and the attempt is made in the discussions to distinguish clearly between fact and theory. A working knowledge of normal anatomy and physiology and of bacteriology is prerequisite to a comprehension of pathology. These subjects are correlated with the processes and products of disease and, with the more important topics, the whole concept is employed as a basis for a brief introduction to the clinic. In summary this is a textbook of pathological anatomy and histology, related to the broader functional aspects of disease.

A textbook is only an introduction to the essentials of a subject. References may be given to the literature, but, in view of the rapid advances of biological and medical research, only by observation, investigation and well directed reading can the subject matter be kept abreast of the times. An important part of education is acquaintance with the names of those who have furnished its heritage. In the earlier chapters the names of investigators are given in the text infrequently and the student can get the references from the list at the end of each chapter. Later, however, as greater familiarity with the subject is assumed, the names are inserted more freely. In so far as possible references are made to journals easily accessible and in the English language. The bibliography is in no sense complete, but is so selected that by its use an introduction to the literature of pathology may be gained. The mode of reference is in general accord with that of the American Medical Association.

The conventional division into general and special pathology has been adopted as the result of a long teaching experience. It is believed that this arrangement is in harmony with the position of pathology in the medical curriculum and best serves to present the subject as an introduction to, and a basis for, the clinical branches. For the advanced student and the practitioner it affords convenience of reference.

At the beginning of each chapter in general pathology the factual material is arranged in tabular form so as to give each topic its relative associations in the entire subject. This is regarded as of distinct pedagogic importance and in our experience has established its value. It may also serve as the basis of the problem method in the teaching of pathology, but before problems can be set it seems essential to provide a background of major and minor premises in the mind of the student.

Many of the illustrations were made under the direction of Doctor Simon Flexner for a book on pathology which he proposed to write. Manifold duties prevented him from completing a manuscript and the illustrations have been turned over to the author, who cordially acknowledges his gratitude. Thanks are due the Surgeon General of the Army and Major James F. Coupal for the use of photographs made at the Army Medical Museum, Washington, D.C. Other illustrations have been made from a rich material provided by association with several hospitals in this and other cities. The entire list of illustrations has been carefully selected and limited. Their purpose is to clarify the text rather than to provide a pictorial atlas.

It is a pleasure to express grateful appreciation of aid rendered by numerous friends. Maurice L. Richardson, M.D., Benjamin S. Kline, M.D., and Harry Goldblatt, M.D., have given freely of their time in criticism of the manuscript. Miss Catherine E. Lennon, who has prepared the index and repeatedly typed the manuscript, has been an invaluable and faithful assistant. Mr. J. C. Harding, Librarian of the Cleveland Medical Library, has kindly checked the references. The drawings have been made by Mr. Louis Schmidt and Mr. E. F. Faber. Several friends, notably Wade H. Brown, M.D., Louise Pearce, M.D., and Stanley Cobb, M.D., authorities in their fields, have criticized certain parts of the manuscript. The author absolves all of these from responsibility for statements in the text but extends his warmest thanks for their interest and help.

HOWARD T. KARSNER.

CLEVELAND, OHIO.

Contents

PART ONE : GENERAL PATHOLOGY

PART TWO : SYSTEMIC PATHOLOGY

CONTENTS

PART ONE

GENERAL PATHOLOGY

CONTENTS

1

General Phenomena of Disease

INTRODUCTION

The term "pathology" is derived from the Greek words *pathos* and *logos*, which are freely and perhaps loosely interpreted to mean respectively suffering or disease and study or science. The definition of pathology as the study of disease gives a somewhat vague impression of the field covered. The scope of the subject may be clarified by an outline of the duties of the professional pathologist in a hospital. He performs autopsies and makes diagnoses of the conditions disclosed. He examines specimens removed at surgical operation and his opinion is often of use in management of the patient's disease. In his hospital routine, he is usually responsible for clinical bacteriology and immunology. He may be called upon to make blood counts, urinalyses, chemical examination of the blood, study gastric contents and other fluids. He may prepare vaccines and immune sera and be called into consultation on treatment of tumors and other diseases. He spends most of his time in the laboratory, but his work is closely related to living patients. Even the autopsy yields information of importance to surviving relatives, serves to appraise diagnostic methods and treatment, and furnishes most important information for the advancement of medical knowledge. Thus pathology covers the causes, processes and effects of disease, and in a limited way some of the treatment.

Disease means loss of health and health is that state of the body in which there is complete harmony with the environment, both external and internal. The term applies especially to acquired disruptions of harmony with the environment but is not usually used in connection with congenital anomalies. Pathologic anatomy is the study of the changes in structure of diseased organs and tissues. It is necessary and basic to an understanding of disease in the living patient. The accompanying alterations of function, or pathologic physiology and biochemistry, must be closely correlated with changes in structure if there is to be any clear conception of disease as a whole, its causes, processes, prevention and treatment. Pathology uses the methods developed by other sciences, but often modified to suit its particular purposes. Thus the autopsy is a modified dissection, the microscopic technic is like that of the histologist, the methods of bacteriology adapted to pathogenic organisms and so on. Physiologic and other types of experiment are conducted to clarify the causes and processes of disease. Statistical methods are employed for the analysis of collected data. In order to progress satisfactorily, the student should have a working knowledge of embryology, cytology, histology, anatomy, physiology, biochemistry, bacteriology, protozoology and immunology.

The history of the development of pathology is closely interrelated with that of medicine as a whole. The knowledge of today is a summation of centuries of study. From our scientific forbears we have a proud heritage; to them we owe a great debt. The story of pathology has been well told by Krumbhaar.

CAUSES OF DISEASE

The study of the causes of disease is called etiology, and forms an important basis for all work in preventive, diagnostic and

3

curative medicine. Causes may be classified in a variety of ways, such as point of origin within or without the body, and the nature of the agent whether physical, chemical, mechanical, bacterial, or animal; but the most important classes are predisposing and exciting. Predisposing, remote, distant or preparatory causes are those which produce a tendency to acquire disease or prepare the body for the action of the direct cause. Exciting, proximate, determining, immediate or direct causes are those which incite the actual disease processes. Any cause may be classified as general, when it affects large numbers; individual, when it operates on a single organism; or special, when it leads to a special type of disease. Our brief discussion will proceed on the basis of this last classification including in each group the predisposing and direct action of the factors discussed.

General Causes

General causes are concerned especially with the environment, such as temperature, air, water, soil, etc.

Temperature. Man, being a warm-blooded animal, has a practically constant normal body temperature maintained by the mechanism of thermotaxis, which operates to preserve the level of body temperature in the face of changing environmental temperature. Extremes are better met if the air be relatively dry.

HIGH TEMPERATURES, be they natural, produced in fever cabinets, or caused otherwise, may result in heat exhaustion or heat stroke. Great elevation of body temperature and its associated effects (as discussed in the chapter on Infectious Diseases), unconsciousness (coma) and sometimes death occur. The coma is probably due to edema of the brain, sometimes associated with tiny hemorrhages, called petechiae. Similar petechiae may occur elsewhere in the body. Wilson describes hemorrhage under the endocardium of the left ventricle especially in the region of the bundle of His, to which he attaches great significance. Rigor mortis is said to set in early and putrefaction to come on rapidly. The work of Murphy and his colleagues indicates that dry heat increases the number of lymphocytes in the blood and augments resistance to tuberculosis and to experimentally transplantable tumors; this has not been applied directly to man.

Local burns are caused by dry and moist heat, such as hot irons and scalding water, by roentgen rays, radium, electricity, caustics and war gases (e.g., mustard gas). Some of these have special features, but burns due to heat are generally divided into three degrees: first degree, with redness of the skin or erythema; second degree, with blisters; and third degree, with actual destruction of tissues. Deforming scars often follow extensive third degree burns. If burns of second and third degrees are extensive, shock with its hemoconcentration and other manifestations may ensue. Shock is discussed in the chapter on General Disturbances of Circulation. Infection of the burned surface may add to the hazards of the condition. Hemoconcentration has various physiologic effects, including fall of blood pressure and decreased renal output. Organs show hyperemia and degenerations. That poisons are generated in the destroyed tissues is controversial. At any rate, marked mid-zonal necrosis of the lobules of the liver is common and some patients develop ulcer of the duodenum, the so-called Curling's ulcer. (See Pack and Davis.) Extremes of heat and cold produce depression of general activity and cold may lead to crowding in ill-ventilated places thus increasing exposure to infections.

COLD. The effects of cold may be general or local. Extreme coldness of the environment may produce death. After a preliminary feeling of excitement, the skin may become either livid or pallid, the person becomes sleepy, sinks into coma and dies. The autopsy reveals nothing that is diagnostic. Colds and pneumonia may follow chilling, but these are infectious diseases not caused by the chill. It may well be that in these instances, internal hyperemia secondary to the peripheral vasoconstriction favors the growth of infective organisms (Mudd et al.). Local effects are seen in chilblains and in necrosis of fingers, toes, external ears and nose. In chilblains, the parts become blue, swollen and painful. This subsides but subsequent exposures are likely to bring on renewed attacks. The cause of necrosis (local death) of these parts is not altogether clear. It may perhaps be due to prolonged vasoconstriction with deprivation of blood flow;

this is more likely to occur if there is preceding disease of the blood vessels (Theis). Shunting of the circulation through the neuro-myoarterial structures of the skin, the subcutaneous glomi, has been suggested as a factor, but this is not proved. The formation of crystals of ice in the cells, when it occurs, leads to destruction of nucleus and cytoplasm. The therapeutic use of cold packs for hyperemia and inflammation leads to reduction of local temperature by vasoconstriction. It is also established experimentally that cold can depress the metabolism and multiplication of cells. These facts have been applied to the treatment of malignant tumors by the application of cold in such degree that local and general body temperature are reduced markedly and a sort of hibernation is effected for several days at a time. It is not yet possible to appraise the value of this form of treatment.

CLIMATE deals particularly with heat, cold and humidity, the last emphasizing the effects of the former. Sayres and Harrington find that high temperature reduces capacity for work, but is less effective if the humidity be low. Movement of the air tends to counteract the ill effects of high humidity except when external temperatures are above 37° C. Warm climates favor the multiplication of certain of the insect vectors of disease and in warm regions there is often careless disposal of excreta. The summer season, for a variety of reasons, predisposes to diseases of the intestinal canal, and winter to diseases of the respiratory tract, rickets, etc. Thus a hyperemic intestinal canal may be a favorable field for infection by bacteria which flourish on summer foods.

By the study of incidence of disease and meteorologic changes, Petersen and his associates have shown a certain correlation between disease and seasons and changes in the weather. These may determine changes in acid-base balance, basal metabolic rate, oxidation, hydration, cellular permeability and rhythms of blood constituents. That disease is actually caused in this manner is open to doubt, but it is likely that direct causes may act readily, that the course of existent disease may be modified and that hereditary dispositional and constitutional tendencies may be brought into relief.

Light and Electricity. It is well known that light is of importance to the maintenance of health. It is not altogether clear whether these effects are due to long wave lengths or short wave lengths and it is also probable that other influences operate simultaneously. Brown, Pearce and Van Allen show that diffuse sunlight is one of the factors which maintains mass relationships of organs and functional activity.

There are different wave lengths of light. The longer wave lengths, in the infra-red part of the spectrum, can warm the tissues but play little part in disease otherwise. The shorter wave lengths are of great importance. The general effects of light are discussed by Clark and by Bovie.

ROENTGEN RAYS AND RADIUM. The progressive advances in production of radiations, since the discovery of roentgen rays, the isolation of various rays for study, the difficulty of establishing units of dosage and the uncertainty of biologic reactions have resulted in accumulation of data that cannot be precisely evaluated. The following summary of our present information is general and subject to change as exact observations are contributed.

Excessive irradiation produces effects upon the body which may be acute or chronic, local or general. Important general effects including especially prostration and gastro-intestinal disturbances may follow massive and deep irradiation, after a latent period of several days. The severity is generally greater following roentgen ray than radium exposures, especially those to the abdomen. The available evidence incriminates protein disintegration products, particularly proteose. Intestinal ulceration occurs in experimental animals but is not constant in man. Protein metabolism is increased, and although variable the blood sugar is generally increased. Blood and urine chlorides are reduced.

Local effects upon the skin appear to be due largely to soft rays. Erythema appears in from a few days to about three weeks. Degeneration and destruction of the basal cells of the epiderm, followed by flattening of the papillae, and degeneration of sweat glands, sebaceous glands and hair follicles with depilation may be observed. Repeated exposures may cause hyperkeratinization, acanthosis and indolent ulcers. Squamous-cell cancers may develop with or without preceding ulcers. This is especially true upon the fingers and the dorsum of the hand.

Experimentally a lymphocytosis may occur, the only real evidence of a stimulating effect of irradiation upon cells, and although Wood and others disagree, Murphy attributes resistance to cancer in part to this change. Roentgen ray workers may show a leukopenia, especially of the polymorphonuclear neutrophils. Conversely leukemia has been attributed to repeated exposure. Profound anemia of aplastic type is also thought to be due to roentgen rays (Wegelin). There is no doubt that radium may produce a similar anemia. This has been observed frequently in painters of luminous dials. Radioactive substances accumulate permanently in the body and, from a position in the reticulo-endothelial system of the bone marrow, exhaust the hematogenic tissues. The bone may be rarified and fractured. Bone sarcoma may occur presumably due to the continued action of alpha rays not screened out by the skin (*see* Martland).

Viscera may be injured by deep roentgen ray therapy and by radium. Parenchymal degenerations may be followed by necrosis because of direct injury, vascular thrombosis and fibrosis. Intestinal ulceration, in this category, may be complicated by dense peritoneal adhesions. A genuine chronic nephritis has been produced in animals and has been reported in man. Injury to the myocardium is variable. The gonads are especially sensitive. Degeneration of spermatogenic cells is followed by their death and disappearance. The Sertoli cells may become swollen and proliferate; the interstitial cells are not affected. The graafian follicles of the ovary disappear but there is little or no effect upon corpora lutea or supporting tissues.

In the treatment of tumors, the short penetrating rays are of especial importance. The "law" of Bergonié and Tribondeau, that immature and dividing cells are destroyed more readily by irradiation than are mature cells, is applied in determining radiosensitivity of tumors. Application of this law is not without exception and Ewing points out that other factors such as situation, accessibility, vascularity, infection, general health, etc., may play an important part.

According to Failla, the ionization in the cell produced by irradiation leads first to swelling of the cell; this becomes more marked for several days and then many of the cells die. The swelling is due to imbibition of water, but the intracellular changes which elevate the osmotic pressure have not yet been determined. The blood vessels subsequently show proliferation of endothelium, thrombosis and occluding fibrosis, which interferes with nutrition and leads to necrosis. Inflammatory reactions, with phagocytosis of destroyed tissues and cells, ultimately leads to scar formation.

Experimentally, nuclear effects in germ cells, with disturbance of genes, may produce serious effects upon progeny (Muller, Weinstein, Curtis). In tissue cultures small doses depress mitosis temporarily and large doses for longer duration (Kemp and Juul). The biologic effects of neutrons have not yet been fully studied, but it can be said that in inhibition of growth, influence upon ova, production of chromosomal abnormalities, inhibition of mitosis, lethal effects on bacteria and destructive effects on certain tumors, as demonstrated in various species, neutrons developed from the cyclotron are considerably more effective per unit of ionization than are roentgen rays (Axelrod, Aebersold and Lawrence). Investigations in this direction are being actively pursued.

Radium is bactericidal, principally by the action of beta rays, but roentgen rays are not definitely bactericidal except in the presence of fluorescence (Newcomer). Short wave-length rays produce deterioration of immune bodies in vitro. The reader is referred to comprehensive articles by Colwell and Russ, by Warren and by Rolleston.

SHORT-WAVE-LENGTH RAYS. Various claims, often not too well established, are made for ultraviolet light. They are said to increase metabolism, to increase resistance to infection and to be bactericidal. It is well established, however, that short waves in the ultraviolet region favor the retention of calcium and phosphorus and are of use in the prevention and cure of rickets, a disease described in the chapter on Organs of Locomotion. This applies to sunlight and artificial sources of light. The immediate effects of sunlight depend upon the short waves, which cause the redness of hyperemia, sometimes with actual blistering due to slight inflammation. The subsequent tan color of sunburn is due to movement of pigment from the basal layer to upper layers of the epidermis. Only when exposure is prolonged is there an actual increase in the amount of cutaneous pigment. In people who are naturally especially sensitive, sunlight may produce outspoken inflammation. Exposure may be important in susceptible persons because of the disease known as xeroderma pigmentosa, which occurs in younger age groups and may be followed by carcinoma of the skin. It is thought that sunlight may produce carcinoma of the skin in occupations where exposure is prolonged, as in farming; but as concerns fishermen, the common cancer of the lip is probably due to tar used in mending nets. Experimentally, ultraviolet light can produce cutaneous tumors in animals. The presence of large amounts of porphyrins may sensitize the skin to light. Porphyria is probably a hereditary condition in man and certain animals and leads to this photosensitization, but the subject is not yet fully clarified as indicated in Chap. 2. Blum's exposition of sunlight and disease is recommended.

ELECTRIC SHOCK. Deaths from accidental electric shock occur especially in warm months because the moisture of the skin provides reduced resistance to currents at points of contact and ground. Voltage is more important than type of current. It is customary to speak of low-tension currents such as those used in household appliances and lighting, usually 110 and 220 volts, and of high-tension currents such as are used in industry, overhead transmission lines, underground cables, third rails, etc., in which the voltage ranges from about 600 to several thousand volts. High-tension lines and many low-tension lines carry alternating current. This is therefore a more frequent cause of shock than is direct current. The current passes through the body, including the bones, in the shortest line from contact to contact, as it would pass through a structureless gel.

With high-tension currents, death may be immediate or delayed. Low-tension currents kill at once or not at all. The cause of death is usually ventricular fibrillation, but death may occasionally result from respiratory failure. Experimentally, ventricular fibrillation is produced when the current acts in the last 0.05 to 0.06 seconds of systole; if it acts at other times during the cardiac cycle the fibrillation may be due to initiation of secondary stimuli that operate in that vulnerable period of systole.

Delayed death may be due to secondary shock, to the remote effects of burns, to infection of burned surfaces, or to the effects of falls or other trauma at the time of the accident. The body dead from the immediate effects of electric shock may show CURRENT MARKS at the points of contact, more so with high- than with low-tension currents. These are punctate, circular, elliptical or linear, slightly depressed, pale yellow marks, sometimes accompanied by blisters. Microscopically, there is a honeycombed appearance of the horny layer of the epidermis. These and deeper cells of the epidermis, often separated from one another and arranged in distorted whorls or spirals, may show elongation of cell body and nucleus. The epidermis and underlying corium may be fused together. The cells of sweat glands and hair follicles are often distorted and shrunken or needlelike. With high-tension currents especially, there may be surface burns, from first to third degree, due to the heat generated by the current or from burning of clothing. Also likely are hyperemia of the viscera, edema of the lungs, and petechiae of conjunctiva, pleura and pericardium. (See Jaffe; Halpern; Alexander and Weeks; Wegria and Wiggers.)

HIGH-FREQUENCY CURRENTS, so-called diathermy, are widely used in physical therapy. It is stated that short waves can injure tissues such as tumors and can kill bacteria, but it is generally agreed that the only proved effect of these high frequency oscillations is to produce heat in the tissues (Kovacs).

Sound is of little importance in pathology except as it may lead to, or increase the intensity of, psychoneuroses. It is said to induce deafness in such occupations as boiler making by producing a chronic fibrosis of the tympanic membrane.

Atmosphere is of importance particularly as concerns pressure, moisture, movements and composition. The optimum pressure for all functions is about 15 pounds to the square inch. Increases in pressure are well borne for short periods but fatigue appears early. The great danger is of sudden release of pressure, which may produce "caisson disease." Gases are under essentially the same pressure in the body as in the atmosphere, so that sudden release of pressure may produce bubbles in the body fluids and tissues. The bubbles are of greatest importance in the nervous system, where temporary or permanent disease of the tissue may occur. Low atmospheric pressures are observed at high altitudes and especially concern mountain dwellers and aviators. Schneider points out that although high altitudes condition low pressure, decreased temperature and humidity, increased sunshine and electrical alterations, "it is recognized that the controlling element in the physiological reactions is the diminished partial pressure of oxygen and the consequent imperfect aëration of the arterial blood." The acute symptoms, simulating drunkenness, due to sudden elevation or active exercise before acclimatization, are temporary and easily recovered from. Chronic anoxemia leads to ready fatigue, to an increase in the number of circulating erythrocytes, and although the point is controversial as yet, probably to reduced hydrogen-ion concentration of the blood. Exposure of cats and guinea pigs to atmospheres exceedingly low in oxygen leads to vascular degeneration in the brain, but this clears up readily. Prolonged or repeated exposures result in tiny hemorrhages from the injured vessels and consequent destruction of brain cells. The observations are not necessarily applicable to man (Thorner and Lewy). The moisture of atmosphere is of importance in that increased humidity often leads to ready fatigue and decreased bodily exercise. Humidity also favors bacterial growth. The presence of large bodies of water tends to equalize atmospheric temperatures. The movements of air are of importance in relation to chilling of the body surface and also in blowing insect carriers of disease over wider areas than they could otherwise travel.

THE COMPOSITION OF THE ATMOSPHERE other than as mentioned above concerns particulate content and gases. The particulate content of importance includes bacteria, either in dried form or in minute droplets of sputum or other secretion, protein dusts and inert dusts. Thus, infection may be directly transmitted in the air. Protein particles, such as pollens, epidermis and hairs of animals, may produce asthma, coryza and other reactions in those who are hypersensitive. Inert particles such as carbon, marble, iron, silica are considered in reference to diseases of the lungs in the chapter on Pigmentation. The normal gases of the atmosphere may vary in relative amounts and other gases may be present. The latter may be either harmless or directly injurious; for example carbon monoxide with its production of carbon monoxide hemoglobin, or nitrogen tetroxide (Wood) and other gases such as the war gases, which may directly cause or predispose to pulmonary inflammations. Numerous other lesions may be produced by atmospheric impurities and are important particularly in industrial medicine. Decrease of carbon dioxide is of little significance, but increases are important physiologically (Scott) and may lead to serious pathologic disturbances. Oxygen is present in the air in approximately optimum concentration, although wide ranges are possible with preservation of health. Martin, Loevenhart and Bunting find little change until oxygen is reduced to 12 per cent or less, when important pathologic changes occur. Experimentally, it has been found that long exposure to atmospheres containing 80 per cent or more oxygen induces a pneumonia (Karsner).

Huntington in an analysis of the geographic distribution of the influenza epidemics of 1918 points to the necessity for further study of how the human subject and the invading organisms are influenced by the atmosphere. Apparently only the weather is of significance in the variations in virulence of the epidemic in different localities.

Water, as it occurs in atmosphere, has been referred to. Water, as obtained for drinking and washing, as well as its availability for forestation and vegetable growth, generally is of the greatest importance in maintenance of health. Its capacity to carry the exciting causes of certain infectious diseases such as typhoid fever, cholera and dysentery are well known. Sedgwick and Mac-Nutt have observed that in several cities the purification of water has been followed not only by a decrease of water-borne diseases such as typhoid fever and diarrheas, but also of acute respiratory diseases and pulmonary tuberculosis. The death rate minus the typhoid component is generally decreased. The chemical composition of water may perhaps predispose to disease and there are claims that hard waters may lead to abnormal calcification in the body, but this is not proved. The relation of content of calcium and iodine to the development of goiter is discussed in the chapter on Ductless Glands.

From the material discussed above, it is apparent that the conditions under which man lives are of importance in the incidence and course of disease. Hygienic factors, such as housing, crowding, occupation, etc., are undoubtedly influential. The same is true of environment in the broad sense of ecology (Strong).

Individual Causes

Individual causes include age, sex, heredity, constitution, and such personal factors as food, clothing, occupation and psychic influences.

Age may be roughly divided into prenatal life, infancy, childhood, youth, early middle life, middle life and old age. Ballantyne and others discuss conditions of prenatal life, which include such factors as physical condition and nutrition of the mother, disturbances in placenta, fetal membranes and umbilical cord, abnormalities of embryonal and fetal development. At birth the infant is subjected to traumatic influences, to infection during labor and to sudden change in environment. In infancy, food offers important predisposing and direct causes of disease. Infections from the immediate family, more particularly the mother, may occur. The infant may possess certain factors of resistance to disease as exemplified in the presence of diphtheria antitoxin. In childhood such protection diminishes, and the child by its more independent life is subjected to changes in temperature, to contact with unclean surfaces and in school life to contacts with numerous sources of infection. In adolescence, sexual development interposes certain nervous factors and the danger of venereal disease. It is a period in which certain infectious diseases such as pulmonary tuberculosis and typhoid fever are likely to occur. In early middle life the individual has business, social and marital contacts which may lead to injurious mental stresses, indulgences of various kinds, exposure to traumatic injuries, and in women to the special stresses of pregnancy, puerperium, care of family, etc. In the later part of this period the incidence of tumors increases, extending through middle life up to the sixtieth year. Old age is complicated by the appearance of atrophic changes in the body and the clinical manifestations of these, as well as of fibrotic changes in blood vessels, heart, kidneys and other organs. Resistance to infections, particularly those of the respiratory tract, decreases.

Sex has an important influence upon disease as concerns organs especially developed in the two sexes, such as breast, uterus, prostate, gonads, etc. Many diseases not directly related to sex organs, are more frequent in males than females and comparatively few are more common in females. This appears to be due to an inherent vulnerability of males, not necessarily dependent upon differences in environment, occupation, habits and sex life (Allen).

Food is of importance not only as to quantity, but also as to quality, including balance, mineral and vitamin content. Adequate general nutrition is essential for growth, development and behavior. Variations include obesity at one extreme and emaciation at the other. Minerals are of importance in the building and maintenance of tissues, as for example blood (iron), bone (calcium), thyroid (iodine).

VITAMINS are essential to health. They vary considerably as to their chemical composition but either they or their precursors must be provided in the diet. Absorption of vitamins may be determined by other factors in the intestinal canal and in some instances the finished vitamin is synthesized in the body. Storage of vitamins is essential and varies with different vitamins. Inasmuch as the intake may be somewhat irregular, storage must be adequate. Vitamins may operate as catalyzers and influence oxidation-reduction phenomena. Although there are experimental demonstrations of injury due to excess intake of certain vitamins, this is only rarely observed in man. The principal disturbances in man are due to deficiency of the vitamins, the so-called avitaminoses.

Vitamin A deficiency results in wasting, and in the case of infants in retarded growth. Because of the absence of the antixerophthalmic factor, there may be disturbances in the eyes, especially in the form of small dry patches in the canthi, which are the result of hyperplasia and excessive cornification of the epithelium. This lesion may extend to the cornea and lead to its destruction. The skin may be scaly and the seat of furunculosis. Keratosis may plug hair follicles, tiny papules being formed. Several forms of dermatosis occur. Bleaching or loss of hair may be due to hyperplasia and hyperkeratinization of the hair follicles. In certain structures, particularly the trachea, the bronchi and the renal pelvis, the normal epithelium becomes transformed into a squamous epithelium, a process called metaplasia. Metaplasia may also occur in the larynx, the uterus, the tongue, the pancreas and the prostate. The night blindness that is common in avitaminosis A is evidently due to disturbances in the metabolism of visual purple. Degeneration of cells of the reticuloendothelial system is reported in animals. In experimental animals, the deficiency also causes metaplasia of the epithelium in the bronchi, urinary bladder and other sites, and great retardation of growth of bones without interference with growth of the central nervous system. (Wolbach and Bessey.)

Vitamin B₁ Deficiency. Vitamin B_1, or thiamin, is the one whose absence leads to beriberi, with its mild cardiac symptoms followed by edema, dyspepsia and then difficulty in locomotion. The principal lesion is found in the distal portions of the peripheral nerves. The cranial nerves below the seventh are only rarely affected. The nerves show no gross manifestations but microscopically there is vacuolar degeneration of the cells of Schwann, then fragmentation of the axis cylinders, followed by wallerian degeneration and the infiltration of lymphocytes into the nerve bundles. Examination of the heart grossly shows dilatation and hypertrophy, especially manifest in the right side. The weakness of the myocardium is indicated by a widespread passive hyperemia, together with edema. Various changes have been described microscopically in the myocardium but these alterations are not sufficiently constant to be pathognomonic. Other disturbances have been attributed to avitaminosis B_1, such as hypertrophy of the pylorus in adults and perhaps in infants, but this is not as yet firmly established.

Vitamin B₂ Complex Deficiencies. DEFICIENCIES OF RIBOFLAVIN, a member of the vitamin-B_2 complex, leads to eczematous inflammation of the scrotum, to glossitis, to stomatitis in the corners of the mouth, seborrhea in the nasolabial folds and follicular keratosis about the face. The eyes not infrequently show marked hyperemia about the margins of the cornea and this may be followed by growth of blood vessels into the cornea itself, said to be cured by administration of riboflavin. It is suggested that the Waterhouse-Friderichsen syndrome of meningitis, with purpura, adrenal hemorrhage, collapse and death may be related, because of adrenal hemorrhages in experimental riboflavin deficiency.

On pantothenic acid, another member of the group, information is almost entirely experimental, not yet applicable to disease in man.

Nicotinic-acid deficiency is apparently the principal cause of pellagra. In this the skin shows erythema, which microscopically is accompanied by hyperemia and edema of the papillae of the corium, and a deterioration of the loose connective tissue in the upper layer of the corium. This is followed by vesicular degeneration of the epidermis. The nervous lesions of pellagra are central rather than peripheral. Degeneration of the cortical cells of the brain, especially in the frontal lobe, is found and there may be myelin degeneration of tracts in the spinal cord.*

Biotin is presumably a member of the B complex. It is found widely in nature and is evidently essential to the life of the cell. It may perhaps play a part in the development of tumors, but its exact significance in human medicine is not known.

Vitamin-B deficiency is said to cause loss of color of the hair and this is attributed to a member of the complex, p-aminobenzoic acid. The clinical features of vitamin B deficiency are well covered by Sebrell.

Vitamin C, or ascorbic acid, deficiencies lead to the development of scurvy with its pallor, anemia, edema of the ankles, swelling of the gums, gingivitis and bleeding of the gums, together with falling out of teeth, and petechiae in the skin. Occurring in early life, there is disturbance of the development of bone, more fully described in the chapter on

Organs of Locomotion. During the development of teeth in children who are the victims of vitamin-C deficiency, the odontoblasts become shortened and separated from the dentine to produce a substance much like bone, surrounded by a thin shell of dentine. The bone of the jaw is likely to undergo rarefaction, so that teeth drop out. In the muscle of experimental animals there is a change resembling Zenker's hyaline necrosis of the muscle. In man, muscles that are especially subjected to stress show comparable changes together with hemorrhages. Noteworthy in the disease is fragility of capillaries but there is no proven anatomic basis for this. Presumably because vitamin-C deficiency has a retarding influence on growth of connective tissue and capillaries, it may delay the healing of wounds.

Vitamin-D deficiency leads to rickets and osteomalacia. Since vitamin D deals with the metabolism of calcium and phosphorus, adequate supplies of these minerals are necessary for its operation. The basis of vitamin D is ergosterol, which is a sterol found in the oils of fish and other animals. This is activated by irradiation and the most active component of the sterols so produced is calciferol. This is synthesized in the skin by the action of ultraviolet rays of daylight. In addition to deficiencies of ergosterol in the diet, rickets may be caused by other conditions. For example, in "renal rickets" there is an increased retention of phosphorus which in its turn leads to a low amount of calcium in the blood through some ill-understood mechanism. Obstruction to biliary outflow, especially congenital stenosis of the common bile duct, leads to a form of rickets presumably due to faulty absorption of fats and their contained vitamins or perhaps to disturbance in the liver itself. There are probably other conditions, not yet fully established, which lead to faulty absorption of vitamins or minerals with resultant rickets, as for example the rickets of celiac disease. Commonly there is hyperplasia of the parathyroid gland and hypoplasia of the teeth. In the chapter on Organs of Locomotion there is a description of the bony changes in rickets and in osteomalacia.

Vitamin E is the so-called fertility vitamin. In deficiencies in experimental male rats the spermatozoa come to lack motility without morphologic changes. Subsequently, however, there are peculiar degenerations in the testis resulting in ultimate fusion of spermatogenic cells to form large multinucleated giant cells. This is not true of mice. In female rats, the ovaries show no morphologic lesions and conception proceeds normally but the fetuses die and are resorbed. In the muscles of these animals there is waxy degeneration like that in Zenker's hyaline necrosis, together with slight hemorrhage. This change in the muscle has been found to be due to absence of vitamin E and probably to a second factor not yet known. (See Pappenheimer.)

The morphologic alterations in man have not been determined except that there has been one case in which the peculiar lesions of the testis have been identified. In the human female there are cases of habitual abortion, some of which are said to have been cured by the administration of the vitamin E in wheat-germ oil. The use of alpha tocopherol, purified vitamin E, in amyotrophic lateral sclerosis has not been firmly established.

Vitamin K includes a group of anti-hemorrhagic vitamins, but the natural vitamins are K_1 derived from alfalfa (green plants) and K_2 derived from putrefied fish meal. The essential chemical ingredient appears to be a quinone nucleus. According to Fieser, vitamin K_1 is 2-methyl-3-phytyl-1, 4-naphthaquinone, and K_2 probably the same with substitution of a difarnesyl chain in place of the phytyl chain. The vitamin can be synthesized by the action of bacteria, such as the colon bacillus, upon fish meal and can thus be prepared in the intestinal canal. Bile is essential to absorption of vitamin K, but synthetic products such as 2-methyl-1, 4-naphthaquinone, can be administered effectively by injection. This vitamin has to do with the maintenance of levels of prothrombin in the blood, and this is one reason why its absence leads to hemorrhages. In infants, the particular condition is hemorrhagic disease of the newborn, perhaps due to exhaustion of stores of vitamin K before intestinal bacterial activity can produce it or before it can be obtained in the food of the infant. In adults, the important condition leading to hemorrhage due to low prothrombin is obstructive jaundice, presumably because of lack of bile in the intestine. It is possible also that there is some dietary deficiency in adults which may produce the condition without either disease of the liver or jaundice. Several other vitamins have been discovered as the result of experimental work with animals, but their application to human disease is not established. (See Rose.)

Avitaminosis and Infections. The relation of avitaminosis to infections is not thoroughly understood. Nevertheless, in deficiencies of vitamin A, the metaplasia of the epithelium opens the way to infection, but it is possible that other factors may operate also. Scurvy is notoriously likely to be accompanied by infections but the mechanism has not been clearly established. In experimental animals the administration of ascorbic acid favors the development of immune bodies and appears to stimulate the formation of complement. As to the vitamin-B complex, experiments indicate an increased susceptibility to infection on the part of animals deficient in thiamin and of others deficient in riboflavin. This occurs in typhus fever in the rat, due to rickettsiae living within cells. Riboflavin deficiency with its decreased cellular oxidation may have a bearing on this lowered resistance to the disease. More complete discussion of the subject of vitamin deficiency is to be found in the book by Youmans and that by Eddy and Dalldorf.

AMINO ACIDS. In addition to their function as building blocks of proteins, certain of the amino acids appear to play a part in other metabolic processes. Experimental deficiency of tryptophane in rats leads to formation of cataracts, vascularization of the cornea, like that of riboflavin deficiency, alopecia, defective formation of dental enamel and other lesions (Albanese and Buschke). In human subjects, deficiency of argenine leads to great reduction of numbers of spermatozoa in semen, many of which are non-motile and the motility of the remainder much decreased. Addition of argenine to the diet results in full restoration. (Personal communication from L. Emmett Holt, Jr.) The fact that spermatozoa are rich in argenine may have a bearing on the matter.

Heredity. This term signifies the genetic relation between successive generations and more particularly the transmission of determinable characters through the germ plasm from one generation to another. It is important to distinguish between heredity, congenital faults of development, and intrauterine acquisition of disease. It is known that certain peculiarities of form are heritable, as, for example, webbed fingers and toes and extra digits (polydactylism), cleidocranial dysostosis (McCurdy and Baer) and synostosis (Davenport, Taylor and Nelson). Such may be direct from one generation to the next, or atavistic, skipping one or more generations. Functional defects, such as color blindness, may be heritable. To be regarded as a functional defect is the condition called hemophilia, which is transmitted by females but not exhibited by them. Morphologic characters are heritable and may be correlated with susceptibility to disease. The disposition to certain diseases appears to be familial and upon a hereditary basis. These include gout, obesity (Davenport), diabetes, asthma, eczema, angioneurotic edema and a number of nervous diseases. An interesting discussion is given by Macklin. Certain tumors, both benign and malignant, seem to be heritable, but as a rule the inherited factors concern susceptibility or resistance rather than the tumors themselves. This is discussed in the chapter on Tumors.

Disease may sometimes similarly affect several members of the same family. Such familial distribution is not necessarily an indication of heritability but may be due to the similarity of environment, food, habits, etc. The tendency to bear twins concerns dizygous twins, but the study of heredity of disease concerns especially monozygous twins. Various diseases may affect twins in the same manner, presumably because of the transmission of factors of resistance and infection (*see* Siemens). The occurrence of tumors of the same sort in twins is discussed in the chapter on Tumors.

CONGENITAL FAULTS in development include a wide variety of conditions from the simple marking of the body by umbilical cord to the most complex single and double monster formation.

INTRA-UTERINE ACQUISITION OF DISEASE, often called congenital disease, is best exemplified by syphilis, in which the fetus becomes diseased due to transfer of the causative organisms from the mother. Other infections can be similarly transferred. Toxic substances, the result of disease and introduced poisons, such as chloroform, produce degenerative changes in the fetus similar to those of the mother. Tuberculosis is only rarely of congenital or intra-uterine origin, most of the instances of early tuberculosis being due to postnatal acquisition of the disease. As has been indicated above, immune substances circulating in the maternal blood may also appear in that of the infant. Of impcrtance in this connection is the fact that erythroblastosis fetalis is now believed to be due to the inheritance by the fetus of RH factor from the father. The absorption of this factor from the fetus into the maternal blood stimulates the formation of an anti-RH factor. The transfer of this anti-RH factor to the fetus, which already has the RH factor in its corpuscles, leads to destruction of blood and consequently to erythroblastosis fetalis, with its anemia, hydrops and icterus, occurring singly or in combination. It will be seen that these phenomena are not hereditary in the true sense of the word. Racial susceptibilities and immunities are probably in part hereditary, due to the survival of the fit, and in part congenital; they are discussed fully in the text books of immunology.

CONSTITUTION AND DISPOSITION. The medicine of the ancients was so much confused by hypothetic and polemic discussions of constitution, disposition and temperament, that as modern biology with its exact observations developed, these topics apparently lost interest. Nevertheless a review by Hart includes a collection of more than 2000 references, principally in Continental languages.

Further work of importance includes that of Bauer, Naegeli, Crew, Draper, Stockard, Child, Davenport and others. Although the various terms employed by the increasing number of investigators are not yet fully clarified, constitution may be thought of as the sum of the morphologic and functional characters which control the individual in his relations with his environment. Some of these characters are hereditary, many are present at birth and some are acquired as the result of changes during the course of life. Draper bases constitution upon four "panels," anatomic, physiologic, psychologic and immunologic, all of which he believes to be interrelated. Barker refers to the variants as morphologic, exhibited as differences in build;

functional, manifested as differences in biochemical composition; and evolutive and involutive, characterized by differences in times of reaching developmental acme or in times of appearance of senescence. The morphologic panel or variant, or as it is frequently called, body type, is most available for study, and is generally constant throughout life, but even this may alter, especially as the result of lesions of ductless glands. The other panels or variants are probably distinctly less constant. Disposition in a general way signifies the expression of constitution in the reaction of the individual person or animal to stimuli which can produce disease. The term diathesis has the same general meaning, usually upon a chemical basis.

That many of the factors are heritable is undoubted. Davenport has catalogued sixty-nine human variants that are transmitted according to mendelian laws and among these must be many that have to do with constitution and disposition. Status asthenicus, status exudativus, status arthriticus and others seem to depend, in part at least, upon heritable factors. Status thymolymphaticus and status hypoplasticus appear to be related to abnormalities of the ductless glands, but it is conceivable that these very abnormalities may depend upon inheritance. Naegeli lays stress upon mutations, and the experimental alteration of genes by roentgen rays (Muller, Curtis) produces animals with structural changes that may well predispose to disease. These studies are suggestive rather than conclusive. It appears that those individuals with the asthenic habitus are especially susceptible to severe tuberculosis. A functional variant, or one in the physiologic panel, who metabolizes purines imperfectly may develop gout. The basis of these and other similar phenomena is, however, by no means well understood.

Wertheimer and Hesketh find it justifiable to assume a "certain correlation between morphological constitution, mental disease and personality." There are certain familial and hereditary, but not necessarily constitutional, organic nervous diseases which are discussed in the chapter on Nervous System. Draper's morphologic studies of constitution in relation to gastric ulcer, gallbladder disease and arthritis are of great interest but have been adversely criticized by Stockard and others. The study of experimental genetics clearly shows that genetic constitution plays a part in resistance and susceptibility to certain disease processes (Brown; Gowan; Aycock).

HORMONES. These products of the ductless glands have much to do with morphologic development of the body and behavior. The hormones act as stimulators and as catalyzers and coordinate many activities of the body. Some have been identified chemically, as for example thyroxin and the sex hormones. All appear to be necessary for life except those of the gonads. Overactivity, underactivity and perhaps alteration in the nature of the secretions produce physiologic and anatomic alterations of sufficient magnitude to justify calling them diseases. Coordination depends upon synergisms and antagonisms. The inhibitors fall into the category of chalones but it is possible experimentally to produce antihormones. These, however, have not yet been developed to a point where they are useful in human medicine. The influence of hormones is discussed further in subsequent chapters.

Special Causes

Special causes include the agents which give rise to special forms of disease and include physical, chemical and living agents. Among the physical agents, trauma has been much discussed. Generally speaking trauma causes local injury with its sequences, rather than disease. Chemical factors are significant in connection with local injuries and a variety of diseases such as gout and numerous intoxications. Living agents include the pathogenic bacteria and higher vegetable parasites and the pathogenic protozoan and metazoan parasites. There are certain diseases, such as influenza, common cold, poliomyelitis, smallpox, herpes simplex and others, caused by filterable viruses. These are discussed further in the chapter on Infectious Diseases. The interaction of parasite and host determines the nature and special manifestations of disease and is concerned with the aspects of virulence, resistance and immunity which are discussed in books on these subjects. Concomitance of two diseases, especially if they be of infectious origin, usually increases the severity of one or both, but the opposite effect may occasionally be observed (see Pearce).

An interesting discussion of the social and other implications of infectious diseases is given by Geddes Smith.

DISEASE

Disease may be acute, running a more or less regular or limited course, or chronic with an irregular, indefinite and usually progressive course. The regular course of acute disease may be continuous or periodic. The periodic form may be intermittent, when there are paroxysms of manifestations with intermissions during which the symptoms disappear although the disease is still present, or it may be remittent, when the symptoms are continuously present but show remissions during which symptoms are considerably ameliorated. A modification of the intermittent type of disease is the recurrent or relapsing type. Here the patient has a period of symptoms and apparently recovers only to be the victim of another similar attack. That true cure is effected in the interval is not always the case. Disease of this type may gradually become transformed into chronic disease, which is usually continuous, but may show some slight degree of periodicity. Among other classifications must be included that on the basis of severity. Thus, disease may be benign and of little importance to the patient, severe or intense. It may be fulminant or blasting with acute onset, short duration and early death. Malignant disease usually refers to malignant tumors, but is also applied to types of disease with serious symptoms, usually with destruction of tissue and fatal to the patient after a variable course.

Pathology

Although this term, as indicated in the definition, covers a wide field, this book deals principally with the alterations of form and function incident to disease. Pathology deals with biologic material and therefore with sequences of events or processes. Although the effects of disease are observed at given moments, such effects are to be regarded as a stage or stages in the natural history and evolution of the disease.

General pathology treats of disturbances which are common to the various tissues of the body. These disturbances are regarded broadly as retrogressive and progressive. The retrogressive changes include degenerations, infiltrations, abnormal pigmentary and mineral deposits, atrophy, necrosis, and certain circulatory disturbances. The progressive changes include hypertrophy, hyperplasia, tumor formation and certain aspects of inflammation.

Special or systemic pathology applies the laws of general pathology to the various organs and systems of the body and thus emphasizes the practical bearing upon individual diseases. It is important to remember, however, that disease of one organ or system is not infrequently reflected in disturbances of other organs and systems and these associations are of the utmost significance in the study of the living patient. It is also important to remember that disease is a process and that as it progresses there are changes from time to time. Each disease really has its own evolution and natural history.

REFERENCES

Albanese, A. A., and W. Buschke: Manifestations of Tryptophane Deficiency in Rats, Science, to appear in 1942.

Alexander, L., and A. W. Weeks: Electric Shock: Importance of Path, Distribution and Density of Current in Determining Symptoms and Pathology, Abst., Amer. Jour. Path., 17: 601, 1941.

Allen, E. V.: The Relationship of Sex to Disease, Ann. Int. Med., 7: 1000, 1934.

Axelrod, D., P. C. Aebersold, and J. H. Lawrence: Comparative Effects of Neutrons and X-rays on Three Tumors Irradiated in Vitro, Proc. Soc. Exp. Biol. & Med., 48: 251, 1941.

Aycock, W. L.: Constitutional Types and Susceptibility to Paralysis in Poliomyelitis, Amer. Jour. Med. Sci., 202: 456, 1941.

Ballantyne, J. W.: Manual of Antenatal Pathology and Hygiene, Edinburgh, 1902 and 1905.

Barker, Lewellys F.: The Relation of the Endocrine Glands to Heredity and Development, Science, 55: 685, 1922.

Bauer, J.: Konstitutionelle Disposition zu inneren Krankheiten, 3d ed. Berlin, 1924.

——: The Constitutional Principles in Clinical Medicine, Harvey Lectures, 1932-33, Baltimore, Williams & Wilkins, 28: 37, 1934.

Blum, H. F.: Photodynamic Action and Diseases Caused by Light, New York, Reinhold, 1941.

Bovie, W. T.: The Physiological Effects of Light Rays, Harvey Lectures, 1922-23, Philadelphia, Lippincott, 18: 72, 1924.

Brinkhous, K. M.: Plasma Prothrombin; Vitamin K, Medicine, 19: 329, 1940.

Brown, W. H.: Constitutional Variation and Susceptibility to Disease, Harvey Lectures, Baltimore, Williams & Wilkins, 24: 106, 1930.

Brown, W. H., L. Pearce, and C. M. Van Allen: Solar Energy, the Animal Organism and Susceptibility to Disease, Trans. Asso. Amer. Phys., 39: 351, 1924.

Child, C. M.: The General Relation between Susceptibility and Physiologic Condition, Arch. Int. Med., 32: 647, 1923.

Clark, J. H.: The Physiological Action of Light, Physiol. Rev., 2: 277, 1922.

Colwell, H. A., and S. Russ: Radium, X-Rays and the Living Cell, London, 1924.

Crew, F. A. E.: Organic Inheritance in Man, Edinburgh, 1927.

Curtis, W. C.: Old Problems and a New Technique, Science, 67: 141, 1928.

Davenport, C. B.: Heredity in Relation to Eugenics, New York, 1911. Body Build and Its Inheritance, Publication 329, Carnegie Institute of Washington, December, 1923.

——, H. L. Taylor, and L. A. Nelson: Radio-Ulnar Synostosis, Arch. Surg., 8: 705, 1924.

Doub, H. P., A. Bolliger, and F. W. Hartman: Immediate Metabolic Disturbances Following Deep Roentgen-ray Therapy, Jour. Amer. Med. Asso., 85: 1299, 1925.

Draper, G.: Human Constitution, A Consideration of Its Relationship to Disease, Philadelphia and London, 1924.

Eddy, W. H., and G. Dalldorf: The Avitaminoses. The Chemical, Clinical and Pathological Aspects of the Vitamin Deficiency Diseases, 2d ed., Baltimore, Williams and Wilkins, 1941.

Ewing, J.: Radiosensitivity, Radiology, 13: 313, 1929.

Failla, G.: Some Aspects of the Biological Effects of Ionizing Radiations, Amer. Jour. Roentgenol., 44: 649, 1940.

Fieser, L. F.: The Chemistry of Vitamin K, Ann. Int. Med., 15: 648, 1941.

Gowan, J. W.: Genetic Constitution as a Factor in Disease, Sigma Xi Quart., 23: 103, 1935.

Halpern, M., and G. Strassmann: Circumstances and Postmortem Findings, Especially Skin Lesions, in Accidental Electrocution, Abst., Amer. Jour. Path., 17: 592, 1941.

Hart: Konstitution und Disposition, Ergebn. Allg. Path. u. Path. Anat., 20(1): 1, 1922.

Huntington, E.: Causes of the Geographical Variations in the Influenza Epidemic of 1918 in the Cities of United States, Bull. National Research Council, 6: No. 34, 1923.

Hussey, R. G.: The Influence of X-rays on Properties of Blood, Jour. Gen. Physiol., 4: 511, 1922.

Jaffé, R. H.: Electropathology: A Review of the Pathologic Changes Produced by Electric Currents, Arch. Path. & Lab. Med., 5: 837, 1928.

Karsner, H. T.: The Pathological Effects of Atmospheres Rich in Oxygen, Jour. Exper. Med., 23: 149, 1916.

——, T. C. Shen, and S. A. Wahl: Studies of Uranium Poisoning; Influence of Light on Uranium Poisoning in Guinea Pigs, Jour. Med. Res., 43: 1, 1922.

Kemp, T., and J. Juul: Influence of Various Agents (X-Rays, Radium, Heat, Ether) upon Mitosis in Tissue Cultures, Acta Path. et Microbiol. Scand., 7: 279, 1930.

Kolodny, A.: Tissue Changes after Experimental Deep Roentgen Irradiation, Amer. Jour. Path., 1: 285, 1925.

Kovacs, R.: Short Wave Diathermy, Amer. Jour. Med. Sci., 200: 707, 1940.

Krumbhaar, E. B.: Pathology, being one of a series of primers on the history of medicine (Clio Medica), New York, Hoeber, 1937.

Lazarus-Barlow, W. S.: On the Histological Changes Produced in Certain Neoplastic and Normal Tissues in Man by the Gamma Rays of Radium, Reports of the Medical Research Council, No. 62, p. 21, 1922; On the Histological and Some Other Changes Produced in Animals by Exposure to the Gamma Rays of Radium, Ibid., No. 62, p. 33, 1922.

Macklin, M. T.: The Role of Heredity in Disease, Medicine, 14: 1, 1935.

Martin, H. G., A. S. Loevenhart, and C. H. Bunting: The Morphological Changes in the Tissues of the Rabbit as the Result of Reduced Oxidation, Jour. Exper. Med., 27: 399, 1918.

Martland, H. S.: Occupational Poisoning in Manufacture of Luminous Watch Dials, Jour. Amer. Med. Asso., 92: 466, 1929.

Mason, V. R., C. Courville, and E. Ziskind: The Porphyrins in Human Disease, Medicine, 12: 355, 1933.

Mathews, F. P.: Photosensitization and the Photodynamic Diseases of Man and the Lower Animals, Arch. Path., 23: 399, 1937.

Maximow, A. A.: Studies on the Changes Produced by Roentgen Rays in Inflamed Connective Tissue, Jour. Exper. Med., 37: 319, 1923.

McCurdy, I. J., and R. W. Baer: Hereditary Cleidocranial Dysostosis, Jour. Amer. Med. Asso., 81: 9, 1923.

Mudd, S., S. B. Grant, and A. Goldman: Etiology of Acute Inflammations of Nose, Pharynx and Tonsils, Jour. Lab. & Clin. Med., 6: 175, 253, 322, 1921.

Muller, H. J.: Artificial Transmutation of the Gene, Science, 66: 84, 1927.

Murphy, J. B.: The Lymphocyte in Resistance to Tissue Grafting, Malignant Disease, and Tuberculous Infection, Monograph No. 21, Rockefeller Inst. for Med. Research, 1926.

———, E. Sturm, and W. Nakahara: Series of Articles on Dry Heat and Lymphocytosis, Jour. Exper. Med., 29: 1, 17; 21; 25; 31; 35; 1919.

Naegeli, O.: Allgemeine Konstitutionslehre in naturwissenschaftlicher und medizinischer Betrachtung, Berlin, Springer, 1927.

Newcomer, H. S.: Bactericidal Fluorescence Excited by X-rays, Jour. Exper. Med., 26: 627, 1917.

Pack, G. T., and A. H. Davis: Burns, Philadelphia and London, Lippincott, 1930.

Packard, C.: The Susceptibility of Cells to Radium Radiations, Proc. Soc. Exp. Biol. & Med., 20: 226, 1923.

Pappenheimer, A. M.: Muscular Dystrophy in Mice on Vitamin E-Deficient Diet, Amer. Jour. Path., 18: 169, 1942.

Pearce, L.: Reciprocal Effects of Concomitant Infections, Jour. Exper. Med., 47: 611, 1928; 48: 125, 363, 1928.

Pearl, R.: The Biology of Death, Philadelphia and London, Lippincott, 1922.

Petersen, W. F.: Constitution and Disease, Physiol. Reviews, 12: 283, 1932.

Petersen, W. F., and M. E. Milliken: The Patient and the Weather. Vol. 4, Ann Arbor, Edwards, 1937.

Rolleston, H.: Critical Review. The Harmful Effects of Irradiation (X-Rays and Radium), Quart. Jour. Med., 24: 101, 1930.

Sayers, R. R., and B. Harrington: Physiological Effects of High Temperatures and Humidity With or Without Air Movement, Pub. Health Reports, 38: 1616, 1923.

Schneider, E. C.: Physiological Effects of Altitude, Physiol. Rev., 1: 631, 1921.

Scott, R. W.: Series of Articles on Carbon Dioxide in Blood, Amer. Jour. Physiol., 44: 196, 1917; Ibid., 47: 43, 1918; Proc. Soc. Exp. Biol. and Med., 17: 18, 1919; Arch. Int. Med., 26: 544, 1920.

Sebrell, W. H.: The Clinical Symptoms and Signs of Vitamin B Complex Deficiency, Ann. Int. Med., 15: 953, 1941.

Sedgwick, W. T., and J. S. MacNutt: On the Mills-Reincke Phenomenon and Hazen's Theorem, etc., Jour. Infect. Dis., 7: 489, 1910.

Sellards, A. W.: Investigations of Tropical Sunlight, etc., Jour. Med. Res., 38: 293, 1918-19.

Siemens, H. W.: Die Zwillingspathologie, Berlin, Springer, 1924.

Smith, G.: Plague on Us, New York, Commonwealth Fund, 1941.

Stockard, C. R.: Constitution and Type in Relation to Disease, Medicine, 5: 105, 1926.

Strong, R. P.: The Importance of Ecology in Relation to Disease, Science, 82: 307, 1935.

Theis, F. V.: Frostbite of Extremities. Clinical and Pathological Considerations in Its Diagnosis and Treatment, Arch. Phys. Ther., 21: 663, 1940.

Thorner, M. W., and F. H. Lewy: The Effects of Repeated Anoxia on the Brain. A histopathologic study, Jour. Amer. Med. Asso., 115: 1595, 1940.

Visher, S. S.: Climatic Laws, New York, 1924.

Warren, S. L.: The Physiological Effects of Roentgen Radiation upon Normal Body Tissues, Physiol. Rev., 8: 92, 1928.

Wegelin, C.: Zur pathologischen Anatomie der Röntgenanämie, Beitr. Path. Anat. u. Allg. Path., 84: 299, 1930.

Wégria, R., and C. J. Wiggers: Factors Determining the Production of Ventricular Fibrillation by Direct Currents (with a Note on Chronaxie), Amer. Jour. Physiol., 131: 104, 1940.

Weinstein, A.: The Production of Mutations and Rearrangement of Genes by X-Rays, Science, 67: 376, 1928.

Wertheimer, F. I., and F. E. Hesketh: The Significance of the Physical Constitution in Mental Disease, Medicine, 5: 375, 1926.

Wilson, G.: The Cardiopathology of Heatstroke, Jour. Amer. Med. Asso., 114: 557, 1940.

Wolbach, S. B.: The Pathological Histology of Chronic X-ray Dermatitis and Early X-ray Carcinoma, Jour. Med. Res., 21: 415, 1909.

———, and O. A. Bessey: Vitamin A Deficiency and the Nervous System, Arch. Path., 32: 689, 1941.

Wood, F. C.: Poisoning by Nitric Oxid Fumes, Arch. Int. Med., 10: 478, 1912. See also Delafield and Prudden's Textbook of Pathology, 13th ed., New York, Wood, 1925.

Youmans, J. B.: Nutritional Deficiencies. Diagnosis and Treatment, Philadelphia, Lippincott, 1941.

2

Pathologic Pigmentation

INTRODUCTION

Normally, pigments natural to the body take part in its metabolism. The functions of cutaneous pigments are not well understood, but the pigment of the choroid coat of the eye is important in vision, as is true also of the so-called visual purple. Hemoglobin is essential for the transport of oxygen and carbon dioxide and is a source of the bile pigments necessary for digestion and the absorption of fats and vitamin K. Certain cytochromes, the riboflavin of the vitamin-B_2 complex and others are important in oxidation-reduction mechanisms (Barron).

Pathologic pigmentation is either exogenous or endogenous. Endogenous pigmentation, pathologic in character, is due to increased amounts or abnormal position of natural pigments or may be a new pigment elaborated in the body. Exogenous pigmentation is due to pigments introduced from without. (See Oberndorfer.)

EXOGENOUS PIGMENTATION

Pigments enter the body from the surroundings in the form of particles or in solution. The particles may be in the inspired air, in foods and drugs, may be introduced by needles in tattooing or gain entrance by accidents such as the powder marks of explosions. Those taken in solution may be deposited by simple precipitation or as a result of chemical changes—for example, the combination of lead with hydrogen sulfide to form lead sulfide or combinations of silver to form a silver albuminate. Lipids may be aspirated into the lungs to produce lipid pneumonia but they more commonly enter in foods to form the pigment of fats, the lipochromes. Particulate matters are partially retained at the site of deposition and in part transferred to the neighboring lymph nodes either free in the lymphatic stream or ingested by phagocytosis in large mononuclear wandering cells. Some of the exogenous pigments, especially when deposited in the lungs, may have clinical importance because of disease incited by the pigment; others may be of only cosmetic importance and some are without effect.

Dusts in the Atmosphere

The dusts of the atmosphere may be classified as of inanimate origin including metallic and nonmetallic substances, and of animate origin including animal or vegetable substances. Most atmospheres contain a mixture of these elements, the proportionate and absolute amounts varying with the character of the environment.

Certain dusts are of no clinical significance because they produce little or no injury to the lungs. Others may produce enough disease of the lungs to reduce vital capacity and may predispose to and alter the course of infectious diseases of the lungs. Naturally, small particles are more likely to enter the lungs than large particles because the latter

17

remain suspended only a short time and are likely to be expelled from the nose and upper respiratory tract. Generally speaking, the particles are from about 1.2 to 12 micra in size, but Gardner has shown that size itself has no bearing on the effects on the tissues. The dust may be in the form of amorphous granules, spicules, crystals or occur as fibers with definite form such as hair, wool, cotton, etc. It is not likely that wool, hair or similar fibers do any harm, but Schilling claims that they may produce a disposition to bronchitis and emphysema.

The concentration of dusts in the atmosphere depends upon the environment and is different in the country, city streets, offices, shops, mines, etc. Determinations of the amount of dust in a given volume of air are subject to a large factor of error. Estimations vary between 0.2 gram and 3210 grams per million liters. A fair average for dusty atmospheres is probably in the neighborhood of 60 grams per million liters. Given an eight hour working day, about one million liters of air are respired in a year; yet a lifetime in such atmospheres results in accumulation in the lungs and peribronchial lymph nodes of much smaller amounts of dust than are found in the total volume of air respired.

Analyses have shown that the lungs of city dwellers contain from 0.19 to 2.72 grams of carbon, 0.04 to 0.69 gram of silica and 0.02 to 0.45 gram of calcium oxide per lung. The lungs of those resident in a smoky city contain about ten times as much carbon as those of residents of a nonindustrial town. Occupational accumulations have also been studied. The lungs of a chimney sweep have yielded 8 grams of carbon, and the lungs of miners of hard rock have contained as much as 4 grams of silica. Examinations of the lungs of knife grinders and iron miners have been demonstrated to contain great quantities of iron oxide. Ordinarily the amounts are much smaller even in lungs that appear to be fairly heavily pigmented on gross inspection. Long exposures are usually necessary before the disease is clinically manifest. Silicosis may produce symptoms after exposure of a year, but the usual minimum is from three to five years and the average is 12 or 13 years. Once established the disease is permanent even when the patient no longer works in the dusty atmosphere.

The amount of dust which reaches the lungs is relatively small, in the order of 4 to 24 per cent of that in the air. The hairs in the nose act as filters; some dust is deposited on the mucosa of nose, pharynx and bronchi and is moved outward by cilia and expelled with the secretions. Some is removed in the expired air and some is swallowed. Since the amount of pigment depends upon the quantity in the air and the duration of exposure, the lungs of children contain little or no pigment, those of city dwellers more than those in rural areas, while those of people in dusty occupations, such as mining, are likely to be deeply pigmented. Protective measures in these occupations are now effective in prevention.

Pneumonoconiosis

This term signifies the deposit of dust in the lungs together with the reaction of the tissues to the presence of the particles. The varieties are as different as the dusts, and they are named accordingly. The most important forms are anthrocosis (coal dust), silicosis (silicon dioxide), siderosis (iron dust), calcicosis (marble dust and absestosis and phytopneumonoconiosis (vegetable dusts). It has been claimed that the black opaque pigment of anthracosis is endogenous, but Taylor's studies indicate that it is exogenous and is soot. Although the distribution of the pigment varies as to its degree of wetting, it can be said that it is deposited in the atria and alveoli. Here it is ingested by large mononuclear wandering phagocytes derived from the septa and perhaps from transformed monocytes of the blood. The cells migrate to the lymphatics around the atria. Some die and liberate the pigment so that it is deposited in the lymphatics. Both pigment-laden cells and free pigment are transported to the bronchopulmonary and mediastinal lymph nodes. By deposit of pigment and consequent fibrosis, the lymph sinuses of the nodes may be blocked, so that lymph flow is reversed and added increments of pigment are carried to subpleural lymphatics. Rarely the lymph nodes, especially when tuberculous, may erode into pulmonary veins with subsequent deposit of small amounts in other organs, especially liver and spleen.

The physical character and the chemical composition of the pigment are the factors which determine reaction in the tissues. There are rare instances of aspiration of particles in such large amounts that acute inflammation, such as acute silicosis (Ritterhoff), ensues. Ordinarily the inflammation is so slight that it is unnoticed and is succeeded by growth of connective tissue, with consequent fibrosis of the lungs or lymph nodes. This is usually nodular in the lungs and becomes more and more marked as additional deposits take place. The fibrosis is slight in anthracosis, calcicosis and in most forms of

marked but sometimes significant lesions, especially if due to black iron oxide. Patients complain at first of cough and shortness of breath, but the fibrosis may so reduce the capillary bed of the lung as to lead to cardiac embarrassment with cyanosis and great disability. Associated acute infections or tuberculosis are common.

The pathologic anatomy of the pneumonoconioses is best illustrated by anthracosis. The other forms have special features but basically the condition is the same.

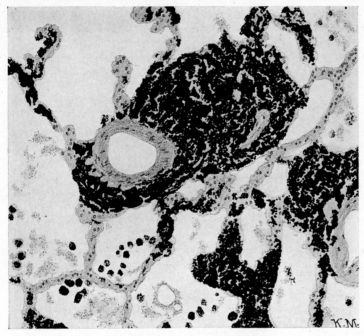

Anthracosis of the lung.

siderosis. Silica produces the most marked fibrosis and the nodules are peculiar in that there is a centrum of particles with rich reticulum, surrounded by a mass of hyalinized connective tissue in concentric whorls or basket-like pattern. The whole is usually well defined. Depending upon the size of the nodule, the roentgenologists divide silicosis into three degrees and a conglomerate form (Matz). In asbestosis, the fibrosis progresses more slowly. Peculiar to it are asbestos bodies, long slender cylinders with a transparent glistening capsule, composed of protein and a core of altered asbestos fiber containing the iron of the compound of silica, chrome iron and magnetite which is asbestos. The nodules are poorly defined. Siderosis produces less

Grossly, in the earlier stages the pigment is seen about the apex, the anterior border of the upper lobes and the posterior surface of both upper and lower lobes. The interlobar surfaces show little pigment. Later the outer surface is found to be pigmented in the position corresponding to the intercostal spaces. This becomes more marked and there is a network of pigmented lines corresponding to the subpleural lymphatics with accentuation at the junctions in the lymphatic lakes. Rarely the lung is a black mass with little distinction as to points of deposit. Often the pleural lymphatics stand out as opaque white or grayish white lines due to chronic lymphangitis.

Microscopically, this pigment is to be

found in the subpleural lymphatics, particularly where the vessels show their largest caliber, in the lymphatic lakes at the angular junction of alveoli and in the perivascular and peribronchial lymphatics. The pigment in these situations is principally within mononuclear cells whose nuclei frequently are obscured by the mass of pigment. As time goes on these cells may become elongated and appear as spindle cells; but in the ordinary sections cellular outline may not be distinguishable and the pigment appear to be in a fairly solid mass. Phagocytes containing pigment may remain in the alveoli for many years. Ordinarily, however, only few phago-

ally within mononuclear cells which occupy the sinuses and subsequently obscure and obliterate the follicles. Free pigment is more common in the lymph nodes than in the lungs.

Relation of Pneumoconiosis to Respiratory Diseases. The aspiration of dust may excite catarrh of the respiratory passages. If the dust be organic, as is the case with pollens, effluvia from animals, etc., and the individual be hypersensitive to such proteins, marked coryza and even asthma may develop. Earthy and metallic dusts may excite mild catarrhs of the upper respiratory passages. The more severe respiratory dis-

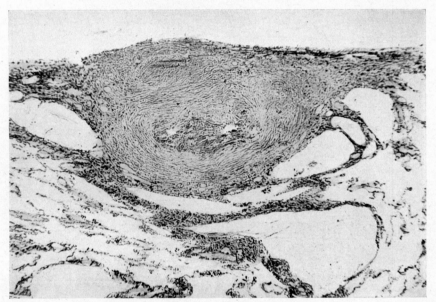

Nodular fibrosis in silicosis of human lung. Low power. Note concentric whorls of hyalinized connective tissue.

cytes are found in the alveoli except in the case of the hemosiderin of passive hyperemia. Only rarely is pigment free in the alveoli. Particles may occasionally be found in the connective tissues around lymphatics. Carbon is usually in the form of fine granules but it may be found as spicules. Iron is likely to be granular. Silica appears as spicules, which may be highly refractile (with Nicol prisms) and may be associated with sericite, a substance which has little or no significance (Cummins). The mediastinal lymph nodes exhibit pigmentation generally parallel in amount to that observed in the lungs but always in more concentrated form. This is usu-

eases to be considered in relation to pneumoconiosis include pulmonary tuberculosis and pneumonia. Marked pneumonoconiosis is a hazard to health. Silicosis is of especial importance in this connection because it is fairly common, but as far as effects on the lungs are concerned, the dusts of flint, slate, asbestos, carborundum, chalk, magnesium carbonate and perhaps other substances may produce significant lesions. The fibrosis in the lungs may be sufficient to interfere with function, but of the utmost importance is the influence of these pneumonoconioses on the bacterial diseases, tuberculosis and pneumonia. Evidence as to the relation of anthracosis and pulmonary tuberculosis is conflicting, but if there be a large component of silica to constitute anthracosilicosis or the silicosis be relatively pure, the associated fibrosis both promotes chronicity and favors the spread of the tuberculosis. If nodules continue to enlarge after exposure has ceased, there is associated tuberculosis, i.e., silicotuberculosis. Matz estimates that 75 per cent of silicotics die of pulmonary tuberculosis. Asbestosis favors the development and progress of tuberculosis, but whether this is due to its iron or silica is uncertain. Siderosis, if in the form of the red fibrotic lung, shows little tuberculosis, but, if in the form of the black lung of metal grinders and polishers, is prone to tuberculosis.

Pneumonia is thought to be especially frequent in victims of anthracosis. Haythorn is of the opinion that the anthracosis induces delayed resolution and organization, and believes this to be due to retarded lymph flow as the result of fibrosis of the lymphatics. Victims of silicosis are highly susceptible to pneumonia and the disease is likely to be atypical, with delayed resolution, organization, empyema and subsequent tuberculosis. There has been discussion of the possibility that silicosis may lead to primary carcinoma of the lung (bronchiogenic carcinoma) but Gardner's survey indicates that silicosis does not cause carcinoma. Papers of importance are those of Willis, of King and Belt, of Gardner, of Robertson, of Lanza, of Matz and of Sayers and Dreessen.

Certain amounts of the exogenous pigments introduced into the lungs are transported to the mediastinal lymph nodes, where the tissue reactions are much the same as in the lungs. Further transport occasionally occurs if, because of concomitant disease of the lymph nodes, especially tuberculosis, they break down so that the contents enter the pulmonary blood vessels, veins in particular. Anthracosis can be seen, even grossly, in liver and spleen, where it induces but little reaction. Silicosis of the spleen, however, may show nodules of fibrosis, like those of silicosis of the lungs.

The talcum powder which is used on rubber gloves may be deposited in the peritoneum, where it excites low-grade inflammation and ultimately fibrous adhesions. Foreign-body giant cells are found and there may

be tiny nodules, but the reaction to magnesium silicate, the material concerned here, is not so marked as is true in the lungs, where silicon dioxide operates. Granulomatous lesions of the stomach, with marked giant-cell formation, have been described, due to the hydrated aluminum silicate of kaolin (Cohn et al.).

Tattooing

Needles are used to introduce various pigments into the corium of the skin, such as lamp black, China or India ink, cinnabar, carmine, indigo, etc. The pigments, if not accompanied by infective organisms, produce only slight inflammation. Much of the pigment remains at the site, enclosed in clusters of mononuclear phagocytes. The pigment is in the form of opaque granules and the cells are often so crowded as to be indistinguishable. The phagocytes and free pigment are transported to the regional lymph nodes to be deposited first in the sinuses and then in

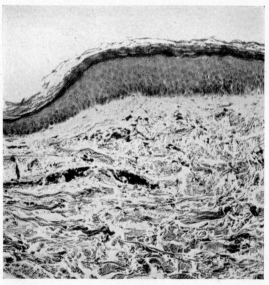

Tattooing of skin, showing pigment in the upper corium.

the substance of the nodes. Ultimately this results in fading of the tattoo, so that it often nearly disappears in the course of 10 or 15 years. Although there is little or no fibrosis in the corium, there is altered reaction to injury and in a general infection like syphilis, the cutaneous manifestations may be especially marked in the tattoo. Serious local infection may occur, but with modern methods of tattooing the introduction of syphilis is not so common as usually supposed (Rukstinat).

Argyria

Occasionally persons are seen who have an ashy gray color of the skin, almost corpse-like. It may be intensified to a pale

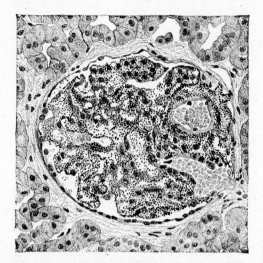

Argyria of human kidney, showing pigment granules in and about the endothelium of the glomerular capillaries.

blue color and may affect conjunctiva and mucous membranes. It is due to absorption of silver salts, taken internally or applied to the mucous membranes of the nose, but only when continued for a long time.

The deeper viscera may also be the seat of this pigmentation and in severe cases may show the ashen gray color grossly. Upon microscopic examination it is found that the pigment is deposited between rather than within cells, apparently occupying the cement substance, although Ohmori demonstrates that it is in the membrana propria. Upon fine examination of lightly pigmented blood vessels a network may be seen such as is the case in artificial staining with silver salts to demonstrate the outline of endothelial cells. In the skin, the pigment is found in the upper layers of the corium immediately under the epithelium and about the sweat and sebaceous glands. In the kidney, the pigment is found in the glomerular loops, between and about endothelial cells of these vessels, as well as in the connective tissue immediately surrounding the epithelium of the tubules in the

zone at the junction of cortex and pyramid. In the liver, the sinusoids, the smaller branches of the hepatic arterioles and of the portal veins may show the deposit, but it is not found in the glandular structure. In other organs, the same relative position of the pigment is found. The pigment is in the form of minute opaque granules. There is no evidence of direct irritation in the form of tissue reaction, nor is there good evidence of serious functional disturbance. (See Gettler, Rhoads and Weiss.)

Plumbism

Lead poisoning is common among those who work with this material. Apart from the symptoms of colic, peripheral paralyses and anemia, victims of this disease frequently show a deep blue pigmentation at the line of junction of the teeth and gums. The lead may be absorbed directly through the skin or enter the body through the nose or mouth in the form of dust either as a soluble or insoluble salt. In either case it circulates with the body fluids in the form of a soluble salt which on coming in contact with the hydrogen sulfide formed about the teeth, as the result of decomposition of food, leads to the formation of lead sulfide; this is deposited about the margin of the gums and produces the "blue line." Melanosis of the gum margins may also occur in lead workers. (See Aub, et al.)

Other metals may be deposited in the body but usually this occurs to such a slight extent that visible pigmentation is not observed. Following injection of salts of mercury, globules of metallic mercury may remain at the point of injection. Cases of bismuth poisoning have been reported in which pigmentation appears in the mucous membranes, particularly those of the colon and rectum.

Lipochromes

These pigments are naturally found in fat, corpus luteum, epithelium of seminal vesicle, epididymis, testis, ganglion cells and Kupffer cells of liver. They are various shades of yellow and are said to contain neutral fats and cholesterol. Most if not all the lipochromes, including carotenoid pigments, xanthophylls, anthocyanin, and flavon flower pigments, are exogenous and introduced in foods. The pigment of corpus luteum and of ganglion cells is identical with plant carotene. Palmer found that xanthophyll colors the egg yolk, body fat and blood serum of the fowl. The pigments themselves may fail to take fat stains and are usually finely dispersed and amorphous, except that they may be crystalline in the outer layers of the skin. The so-called lipofuscins, found in liver and muscle, are often thought of as waste pigments or even melanins originating in the body, but they are probably lipochromes which are often closely associated with melanins.

are derived in part from the blood pigment, yet bile pigments are so characteristic and under pathologic circumstances produce such striking changes that they deserve special and separate consideration. The melanins are found in the pigment of the hair, skin and choroid coat of the eye.

Blood Pigments

Hemoglobin is composed of a protein, globin, of basic nature probably allied to the histons, and a pigment presumably acid in nature called hemochromogen or hematin. In

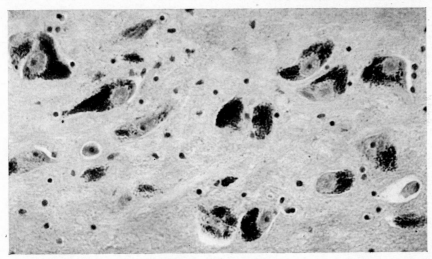

Pigmented ganglion cells.

The functions are not well known, except that carotene is a precursor of vitamin A. Excessive ingestion of the carotene-xanthophyll groups and of anthocyanine may result in pigmentation of skin, blood plasma and urine, but this recedes on correction of the diet. It is probable that the green color of chloroma, a rare tumor of myeloid origin, is due to lipochromes (Burgess).

ENDOGENOUS PIGMENTATION

The human body is provided normally with a variety of pigments which include blood pigments, bile pigments and melanins. The normal blood pigment is hemoglobin, which may be increased in amount in polycythemias and decreased in anemias. As a part of hematopoiesis, the hemoglobin undergoes a series of destructive and reconstructive changes. While it is true that bile pigments

spite of the fact that blood destruction and formation are constantly going on, hemoglobin is not normally present, at least not in demonstrable amounts, in the blood plasma or tissue fluids. Diseases associated with abnormally active blood destruction may be accompanied by the presence of considerable quantities of hemoglobin in the plasma, a condition termed hemoglobinemia. The kidney appears to have a fairly definite threshold for excretion of hemoglobin and if the amount in the blood exceed that amount contributed by about one-sixtieth of the total bulk of corpuscles, the pigment appears in the urine, hemoglobinuria. Postmortem examinations often show a red stain of the aorta, heart valves and other tissues as the result of destruction of blood corpuscles after death and the consequent liberation of hemoglobin. In all these instances the pigment is in dissolved form and the staining diffuse. Although not easily crystallizable, hemoglobin crystals, orange-yellow and irregularly acicular, may be found in decomposed blood especially after alcohol fixation, but probably never appear in this form during life. Hemoglobin itself is but slightly if at all toxic, and hemoglobinemia and hemoglobinuria probably add little to the seriousness of those diseases in which they appear: malaria, infectious and hemolytic jaundice, paroxysmal hemoglobinuria, hemolysis following transfusion, and other similar conditions.

Hemoglobin in solution in the plasma or within the red blood corpuscles may be transformed to methemoglobin, as seen in poisoning by coal-tar derivatives as well as by chlorates and by nitrobenzol. Bacteria may produce methemoglobin in vitro and in vivo, as has been demonstrated with the pneumococcus, *Streptococcus viridans* and other organisms. Nitrites formed in the intestine may be absorbed and produce methemoglobin. Hydrogen sulfide may likewise be absorbed and combine with hemoglobin to form sulfurmethemoglobin which is readily decomposed by weak acids to form methemoglobin. The green discoloration of the belly of cadavers is due in part to the formation of sulfurmethemoglobin. Methemoglobin stains tissues a chocolate-brown as compared with the bright red of hemoglobin staining. The blood and urine likewise exhibit a chocolate-brown color due to the presence of methemoglobin. Its positive identification depends upon spectroscopic examination.

Hemoglobin Derivatives. The metabolism of hemoglobin is not fully understood, but certain facts have been demonstrated which justify the setting up of a working hypothesis. The studies of Whipple and his associates upon experimental animals and man have been of especial value. The parent material within the body is a "pigment complex," without known composition. This may be derived from food proteins, especially liver and kidney, from body proteins and also from blood hemoglobin. It may give rise to blood hemoglobin, muscle hemoglobin and bile pigments. Inasmuch as it may be derived from and give rise to blood hemoglobin it is to be regarded as an intermediate in normal metabolism of this pigment in the body. If blood hemoglobin and muscle hemoglobin are interchangeable, pigment complex probably acts

in an intermediary capacity. The exact situation of these processes is not known but it is likely that the endothelial and other cells of liver, bone marrow and perhaps spleen, play an important part. It is further likely that the hemoglobin is furnished in completed form for the manufacture of erythrocytes.

These bile pigments may be derived directly from the pigment complex, from the blood hemoglobin and perhaps from the muscle hemoglobin. As demonstrated by Mann, this occurs principally in the bone marrow and spleen. It is possible, as proposed in the hypothesis of Addis, that bile pigment may be resynthesized into hemoglobin, but Whipple is convinced that after bile pigment gets into the intestine it is not resorbed. Its participation in hemoglobin metabolism, therefore, occurs entirely within the body. Urobilin and stercobilin are derived from bile pigments, the former by the activity of liver and bile passages and the latter by the activity of bacteria in the intestine. It seems unlikely that even although they have clinical diagnostic significance they play a part in metabolism of hemoglobin.

That the pigments observed in pathologic conditions, obviously derived from hemoglobin, are concerned in normal destruction and rebuilding of hemoglobin is open to question. Hematin has been found in blood of the splenic vein by Mann after introduction of hemoglobin in the artery. Iron is of considerable importance in blood metabolism and the iron-bearing pigment, hemosiderin, is commonly found pathologically, but its physiologic significance is not clear. Hematoidin, an iron-free fraction, is less common pathologically, but its resemblance to bilirubin suggests that it may take part in normal metabolism. The relation of the pigments seen in hemachromatosis and of some of the pigments of "wear and tear," of hemofuscin, the blood porphyrins, malarial pigment and others, to normal processes, if indeed any such relation exist, is still more obscure. The more important of the pathologic manifestations are considered in the following paragraphs.

Hematin occurs in the metabolism of hemoglobin and is essentially hemoglobin minus globin. Except for its appearance in large old blood clots, it is not commonly found. It has been reported in the blood in

chromium poisoning, malaria, pernicious anemia and forms of acute toxic hemolysis, congenital hematoporphyria and in poisoning by
certain of the war gases. In particulate form
it appears as amorphous, dark-brown, almost
black granules measuring but a few micra in
diameter. Brown, by an extensive series of
studies, is convinced that the pigmentation
resulting from malaria is hematin rather than
melanin as formerly believed.

The pigment of malaria may be found
in any part of the body but is particularly
prominent in the spleen and liver. The para-

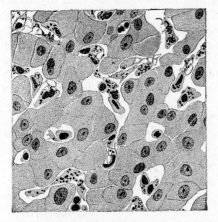

Malarial pigment in Kupffer cells of sinusoids of liver.

site of this disease lives in or upon the red
blood corpuscle and in the course of its development elaborates a pigment, presumably
from the hemoglobin of the corpuscle. When
the parasite undergoes its asexual division in
the human host, it breaks up into several
merozoites and the pigment is liberated into
the blood. The pigment is taken up by endothelial phagocytes, particularly of the liver
and spleen. If sufficiently marked the organs
may show a rich brown color grossly. Microscopically, the pigment is seen in the endothelial cells of the splenic pulp and occasionally lies free in the tissues. In the liver, it is
found in the lining endothelial cells of the
sinusoids and in the stellate Kupffer cells.
Similar but much less marked pigmentation
may be found in the vessels of the brain, intestine and other organs. The pigment is in
the form of minute opaque amorphous granules lying within the cytoplasm of the cells.
In severe cases of malaria the capillaries of
the brain and indeed of other organs may be

plugged by parasites containing pigment
granules. The pigment contains iron (Mayer),
as would be consistent with its identification
as hematin, but this iron content was formerly considered to indicate that the pigment is hemosiderin. On account of the difficulty of demonstrating the iron, others have
considered the pigment to be a melanin.
Schumm, however, has found hematin free
in the blood of malaria and Brown has not
only demonstrated that the pigment is hematin but states that an alkaline solution of
hematin will produce chills and fever in animals, closely resembling those symptoms of
malaria. Butterfield and Benedict could not
confirm this and maintain that the alkaline
menstruum produces slight fever regardless
of whether or not hematin is also present.
Hematin is further said to be toxic in that it
produces glomerular lesions in the kidney
and in massive doses produces a fall in blood
pressure.

It has been thought that hemosiderin
and hematoidin are derived from hematin,
but since hematin remains in the tissues a
long time without change it is more likely
that these two pigments are derived directly
from hemoglobin.

Hemosiderin. Both hemosiderin and
hematoidin are formed within cells, generally
of reticulo-endothelial origin, the former in
the course of about 24 hours and the latter
only after the lapse of several days (Muir
and Niven). It is apparently one of a group
of products containing iron which might be
placed in the inclusive term "cytosiderin"
(Menkin). The composition is not known
exactly but various studies indicate that
hemosiderin has not a fixed chemical formula.
The iron is in the form of ferric hydroxide,
probably colloidal, and it is in combination
with an organic substrate, presumably protein complexes. The iron is not firmly bound
as it is in hemoglobin. Ordinarily it can be
identified readily by use of the Perl test,
using potassium ferrocyanide and dilute hydrochloric acid, to produce Prussian blue.
Sometimes it is more firmly bound and must
be reduced by use of ammonium sulfide, as in
the Nishimura test which produces Turnbull
blue. Inasmuch as the iron of hemosiderin is
principally ferric, it is at least possible that
an oxidizing enzyme, probably but not necessarily intracellular, plays a part in the forma-

tion of hemosiderin. Hemosiderin is usually found in situations where oxygen is readily available, whereas hematoidin is likely to occur in necrotic and poorly oxygenated tissues.

Brown's studies indicated that hematin is not an intermediary in hemoglobin metabolism but Mann's observations reopen the question. The part played by hemosiderin in normal processes is also subject to discussion. The iron which is liberated by the destruction of hematin is not eliminated by the body in any considerable quantity and is apparently utilized in the formation of the new hemoglobin molecule, but that it does so through the formation of hemosiderin is not certain.

Hemosiderin is deposited particularly in the spleen and liver, apparently as a part of the normal activity of the body, since this

ity of destruction of the blood. As a result of this destruction the pigment is deposited in those particular parts of the tissue where the hyperemia is most marked.

In the liver, the pigment is to be found in the parenchymatous cells. Should the condition be simply the result of the normal wear and tear of hematopoiesis, only a few of the cells of the central part of the lobule are affected. If the condition be due to passive hyperemia, the same general situation of pigment is observed. In case of more extensive destruction of blood, such as occurs in pernicious anemia, all the cells of the lobule may be affected. In advanced cases, hemosiderin may also be found in the endothelial cells of the sinusoids. In the spleen, the pigment is found principally in the endothelial cells of the blood sinuses and in similar cells in the splenic pulp; not infrequently, how-

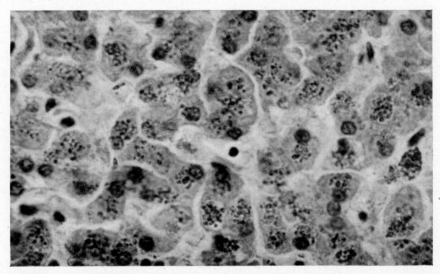

Hemosiderin in cells of the liver in pernicious anemia.

pigment is uniformly present in the liver and spleen of adult man and of many other animals. Pathologically, hemosiderin appears in these two organs and in other organs as the result of excessive blood destruction. This blood destruction occurs in various types of hemolytic anemia, most particularly in primary pernicious anemia. In these diseases the pigment deposit is especially rich in the liver and spleen. Passive hyperemia of various viscera is also an important cause of hemosiderin deposit. It is probable that the stagnation in the capillaries favors increased rapid-

ever, it is also found in the splenic pulp outside of cells. Hemosiderin pigmentation is sometimes observed in the kidney, more particularly, however, as the result of extensive blood destruction than of passive hyperemia. The pigment may be found in endothelial cells of the kidney, in the interstitial tissue and sometimes in the epithelial cells of the tubules. Occasionally, it may be excreted in the urine where it appears as granules either free or within phagocytic cells.

Hemosiderin pigmentation of the lung

PLATE I

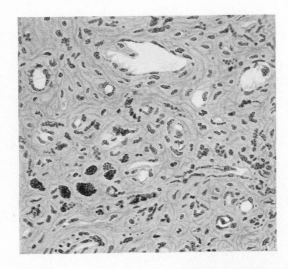

Granules of hemosiderin pigment in phagocytes. Taken from the margin of a focus of hemorrhage.

Hematoidin "burrs" in the necrotic portion of an old infarct.

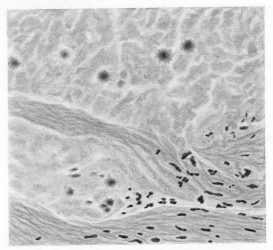

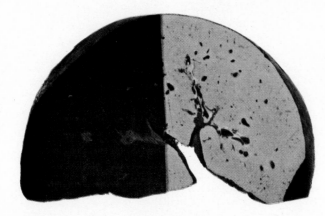

Kodachrome photograph of cross section of liver of hemochromatosis. The specimen was treated with dilute hydrochloric acid and potassium ferrocyanide (Perl's test for iron) and then a sliver cut away to show original brown color of specimen.

is found particularly in passive hyperemia of the organ, more especially that due to mitral stenosis. Under these conditions the pigment is practically entirely intracellular. These cells are probably endothelial cells which take up dead erythrocytes and in the course of time convert the hemoglobin into hemosiderin. Often the cells are found in large numbers within the pulmonary alveoli and also in the lymphatic spaces surrounding the bronchioles and blood vessels. A massive deposit of hemosiderin is likely to be found in the same situations in which anthracosis is found. In contradistinction to the "dust cells" which contain aspirated pigment, the cells

tissue leads to solution of the hemosiderin so that it is removed from the part by diffusion. Under ordinary conditions however, hemosiderin is relatively insoluble in normal body fluids and when deposited apparently remains in situ permanently. Widespread hemosiderosis occurs in hemochromatosis (to be discussed subsequently).

Hematoidin. The splitting of hemoglobin under pathological conditions yields an iron-free pigment called hematoidin, in addition to hemosiderin. It is frequently observed in old infarcts, particularly those of the spleen, but may occur in almost any dead tissue, which originally had a rich blood con-

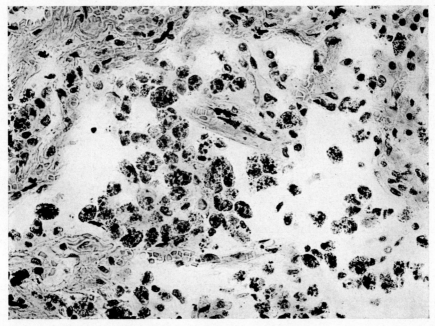

Hemosiderin in phagocytes of the lung.

containing hemosiderin are called "heart failure cells." Although fibrosis of the lung appears in connection with this condition, it is probable that the fibrosis depends rather upon the hyperemia than upon the presence of the pigment. In fact, there is little reason to believe that this pigment operates as an irritative foreign body in any situation.

In infarction hemorrhage is one of the primary occurrences. The subsequent destruction of the blood leads to hemosiderin formation in the margin of the infarct. This, however, is not likely to be permanent, because the acid formation due to the death of

tent. It is of orange-yellow or orange-red color by transmitted light and may be in amorphous granules, rhombic plates or more characteristically in sheaves of acicular crystals commonly referred to as "chestnut burrs." Microchemical tests for iron are negative, but concentrated mineral acids produce a series of color changes somewhat like those yielded by bile pigments. Ligation of a splenic vein in experimental animals is followed by a large deposit of hemosiderin which is considerably reduced in a few days but may reappear on restoration of the circulation. Oxygen must be concerned in this mechanism. In contrast, hematoidin occurs only in dead or dying tissue where the lack of oxygen and the changes associated therewith are probably of determining significance. Extensive blood destruction may be associated with the formation of excesses of both hematoidin and bilirubin. The color reactions to mineral acids are similar but not identical. Since bile is formed independently of the liver, the necessary participation of this organ in hematoidin formation is presumably excluded. Hueck considers that studies of this pigment show that it is not derived from hemosiderin but directly from hemoglobin and probably hemoglobin in solution. The color reactions to mineral acids may imply only a content of bile pigments or their derivatives. Formerly considered isomeric with bilirubin, hematoidin is now believed to have no fixed and definite formula and is probably a variable mixture of several closely related pigments, one of which may be bilirubin.

Porphyrins. Hemoglobin is a combination of protoporphyrin with iron and globin. From it are derived porphyrins of various orders. Increased output of porphyrins in urine and feces may occur in a variety of anemias, polycythemia, hemorrhage, deficiency diseases, infections and poisons, especially by coal-tar drugs. The urine may be of Burgundy-red color due to the presence of porphobilin and porphobilinogen. There are forms of acute and chronic porphyria of unknown cause. Congenital porphyria is a rare inborn fault of metabolism, probably inherited as a mendelian recessive, characterized by porphyrinuria, discoloration of skin and bones, due to impregnation by uroporphyrin I, and sensitivity to light in spring and summer. Dobriner and Rhoads think that there is an alteration of the normal ratio of formation of types I and III porphyrins with disproportionate synthesis of type I. (See also Nesbitt and Watkins.)

The sensitivity to light occurring in porphyria has long been thought to be manifested in such skin diseases as hydroa aestivale, but Blum is somewhat doubtful that here it is actually due to porphyrins. Although pigment in granular or crystalline form free or in combination with protoplasm may be found in tissues in porphyria, the principal changes are degenerations of nerve cells, myelin sheaths and axis cylinders in the spinal cord, nerves and sympathetic ganglia (Mason, Courville and Ziskind).

Hemofuscin. This is an iron-free pigment, deposited in fine yellowish-brown granules. It is found normally in the smooth muscle of the intestines and blood vessels. From only a slight amount in childhood, it increases until the subject is 30 or 40 years old and then decreases. The quantity depends on the nutritional state, the functional activity of the muscle and the age of the subject. It is probably not derived from the hemoglobin of the blood, but may perhaps be a product of myohemoglobin. It is not a lipochrome. Its main interest, pathologically, is its occurrence in hemochromatosis and in brown atrophy of heart and liver.

BROWN ATROPHY of the heart is considered here because the pigments concerned are probably derived from blood pigment.

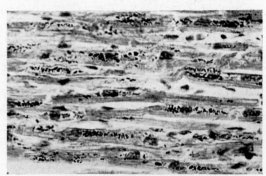

Brown atrophy of the heart.

Grossly, the heart is small, reduced in weight; the muscle is of dark brown color and the coronary vessels tortuous because they occupy a space shorter than normal. Microscopically, the fibers are reduced in diameter and length, the nuclei increased in number (Karsner, Saphir and Todd), and between their poles are bands of golden yellow or yellow-brown pigment granules. It has been thought that the increase in pigment is only relative because of the reduction in muscle volume, but it is probable that there is also an absolute increase in the amount of pigment. Although it was supposed to be, at least in part, ingested lipochrome, Connor was unable to extract lipochrome and identified it as a mixture of hemosiderin and hemofuscin.

Hemochromatosis. This is characterized by pigmentation of various organs, some of which are also fibrotic. Clinically, it exhibits the triad of hepatic enlargement, diabetes and pigmentation of the skin. There may be other associated endocrine disorders also, especially hypogonadism. It affects males far more often than females and occurs usually in early and late middle life. It is probably an inborn fault of metabolism of iron and perhaps of a property of mesoblastic tissues, especially those of liver and pancreas, which leads to excessive proliferation.

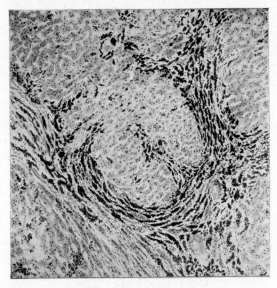

Hemochromatosis of the liver.

The diabetes is probably caused by involvement of the islets of Langerhans or the pituitary or both, the condition being called bronzed diabetes. In some cases the diabetes has not yet developed, but in many of these there is the diabetic type of glucose tolerance test. Diabetics show the condition in the proportion of one to every two or three thousand cases.

The organs most strikingly affected are liver and spleen, but in advanced cases hardly any organ escapes. The liver looks like that of Laennec cirrhosis except that it is diffusely yellowish brown in color. Microscopically the pigment is found in the markedly fibrotic portal spaces and also in the parenchymal cells. The pancreas is firm and of the same color. Sections show marked fibrosis and pigment in the connective tissues and acinar cells; often the islets are fibrous

and hyalinized. Fibrosis is not a conspicuous feature in the other pigmented organs. In the skin, the pigment is found principally in the upper corium, as well as in and around sweat glands and around capillaries. Biopsies are useful for diagnosis, but the iron can be identified in the living patient by intradermal injections of potassium ferrocyanide and dilute HCl (Fishback). The principal pigment is hemosiderin, but hemofuscin is also present in small quantities. Chemically the liver may contain 40 to 50 times the normal amount of iron and the pancreas even 100 times the normal. Except for the salivary glands, the other organs show no such marked increases. (See Sheldon.)

Melanotic Tumors. One of the commonest manifestations of pathologic pigmentation is the pigmented mole or nevus. This is a fault in development but may not appear until later life. There is a disturbance of arrangement in the cells that produce melanin, the melanoblasts. It is not a true tumor and is known as a hemartoma. Real tumors or neoplasms may develop from moles and from other regions in which pigmented cells exist naturally, as in the choroid coat of the eye and in the pia mater. Similar tumors are said to arise in the adrenal gland and in the rectum, and in the latter situation are probably due to misplacement of anal epithelium.

The term "melanoma" is loosely applied to moles and true tumors. It seems more desirable to designate the tumors as "melanoblastomas." Wherever the tumors arise they are highly malignant and are likely to be accompanied by many and widespread secondary growths or metastases, due to dissemination through lymphatics, blood vessels, or both. The original tumors are usually deeply pigmented and almost black. Metastases may be deeply, slightly or not pigmented in the gross. Microscopically, the tumor is richly cellular, the cells being of spindle form or rounded. The amount of pigment in the cytoplasm varies. Some cells are devoid of it and some may contain so many of the dark brown pigment granules that the nucleus is hidden. Pigment is occasionally deposited in tissues other than the tumors. The same general disturbance of pigment metabolism may lead to melanuria. In this condition the urine, when passed, is usually of normal color and either on standing or on the addition of oxidizing agents becomes of deep brown or brownish-black color. Sometimes it is dark colored when passed. It is assumed that melanin, as it circulates in the fluids of the body, is reduced, especially in the liver, to a colorless melanin, usually called melanogen. Oxidation restores the color. (Further discussion of these neoplasms is found in the chapter on Tumors.)

Melanins

Melanin pigments are the product of certain specialized cells found normally in the skin and hair follicles, the choroid coat of the eye and the pia mater, especially at the base of the brain. They can perhaps be elaborated by certain other cells, as those of heart muscle. These pigments have been classified as metabolic, indicating that they are produced by the metabolic activity of the cells, operating probably upon the proteins. Isolated melanins absorb the short rays of the spectrum and in life probably serve to protect against harmful effects of light. In milder degrees of sunburn, the melanin moves into the upper layers of the epidermis and in more marked tanning may be increased in amount. The fact that dark skins are more resistant to chemical irritants than light skins may possibly explain the low incidence of cancers of the skin in the dark races. Nevertheless, the pigmentation does not prevent penetration of light to the underlying tissues (Kinney).

It is impossible to speak of melanin as a single pigment because there are probably many varieties. The pigments are of large molecular size, insoluble in water and organic solvents and contain carbon, nitrogen, hydrogen and oxygen. According to Percival and Stewart, the melanins also contain certain amino-acids and the indole ring. The fact that there may be a positive pyrrhol reaction does not necessarily indicate a relation to blood pigment. Bloch's explanation of the formation of melanin is of great interest although not finally established. It was found that in certain plants tyrosinase may form a melanin from tyrosin, but this tyrosine-melanin is probably not identical with the melanin of animals. It was discovered that the first intermediate product in the formation of tyrosine-melanin is dihydroxyphenyl-alanine. Bloch noticed the resemblance of the formula of 3-4 DihydrOxyPhenylAlanine to that of epinephrine and simplified the term by calling it "dopa." He demonstrated that the melanoblasts of the skin can convert the colorless dopa into a dark insoluble melanin which he called dopa-melanin. This change was brought about by an oxidizing ferment called dopa-oxidase but the ferment acts only on dopa and not upon other substances such as pyrrhol, tryptophan, tyrosine or epinephrine. This method of observation is useful in identifying melanoblasts, as for example in pigmented moles and melanoblastoma. The oxidase is also present in the malpighian layer of the skin and in the choroid coat of the eye. Although 3-4 dihydroxyphenylalanine is not naturally present in the body, it is possible that the mother substance of melanin may give rise to pyrrhocatechin derivatives, among which are epinephrine and dopa. There has been much discussion concerning the presence of sulfur in melanin. Bloch maintains that sulfur and iron are accidental impurities. Ropshaw, however, affirms that sulfur is a natural part of melanin. He points out that cystein is present in the cytoplasm of cells within a more complex substance, glutathione, and that protamine is present in the nucleoprotein of the nucleus. Through cleavage, due to cell enzymes, these two bodies are freed and brought into contact. In the test tube, the mixture of these two substances produces a black precipitate. He suggests that this may be of importance in Addison's disease because of the fact that changes in sulfur metabolism are reported in this disease. It may be that vitamin-B complex is of some importance in melanin production, because its deficiency appears to be a cause of graying of the hair and this is especially true of deficiency of p-aminobenzoic acid, considered to be a member of the complex.

Addison's Disease. This is a syndrome in which occur pigmentation of the skin, loss of flesh and strength, rapid and weak cardiac action and low blood pressure, occasionally complicated by vomiting, nausea and other symptoms. The pigmentation of the skin is probably an increase in the amount of the normal pigment of that tissue. It may appear in patches distributed irregularly and often marked in those parts exposed to light and pressure, or it may be distributed diffusely over the body. It not uncommonly affects the mucous membranes of the mouth and, in the negro, this is often the only point at which the pigmentation can be demonstrated. The condition which causes Addison's disease is destruction of the adrenal gland. This may be due to tuberculosis of the gland, to cytotoxic suprarenal contraction, to tumors both primary and secondary, to amyloid and to other lesions. The significant part destroyed is the cortex. If there be damage to the medulla, it is probably secondary to the cortical disease. These lesions are discussed further in the chapter on Ductless Glands.

The pigment is known to be practically entirely melanin, the formation of which has been discussed already. In severe cases the presence of melanin similar to that seen in the melanuria of melanoblastoma is found in Addison's disease, and in other instances, crystals resembling hematoidin have been found in the pigmented parts.

Grossly, the pigmented skin and mucous membrane are of a bronze color resembling that seen after long exposure to the sun, but in this instance not limited to the exposed parts. Microscopically, the pigment is found in the malpighian cells of the epidermis, and in severe cases may be found in the upper layer of the corium in what are believed to be chromatophore cells. There is no reason to assume that the deposit of this pigment leads to reaction on the part of the tissue. The regional lymph nodes and the deeper tissues of the body do not show pigmentation.

Ochronosis. This rather rare condition exhibits pigmentation of cartilages, joint capsules, tendons, sometimes of the intima of blood vessels and of the epithelium of the kidney (Oppenheimer and Kline). There are usually no other symptoms and the patient's only complaint is the blue color of nose, ears and other places where the pigmented cartilage is seen through the skin. In some cases alkaptonuria appears, a condition in which the urine turns dark on exposure to air owing to the presence of homogentisic acid. In the earlier stages of the disease the pigmentation is diffuse but subsequently is found in the form of minute amorphous iron-free granules. The cause of the disease is unknown, but in one-fourth of the cases reported by Poulsen there was a history of prolonged dressing of wounds with phenol, producing the so-called exogenous ochronosis. According to Pick the pigment is formed from the effect of tyrosinase upon the aromatic groups of the protein molecule such as tyrosine and phenylalanine and related hydroxylized products. Thus it is in the general order of melanins. Similarly, the action of a like enzyme upon absorbed phenol leads to the same condition. Following a purely endogenous or exogenous origin, homogentisic acid may be produced from the aromatic groups and appear in the urine. Alkaptonuria is not a necessary part of ochronosis; it occurs in about half the cases and may appear independently of ochronosis.

Malarial Pigmentation. Many authorities consider that the pigment of malaria is a melanin, but Brown, in agreement with Carbone, considers it hematin or an immediate derivative since it contains iron and has the same solubilities and spectroscopic properties as hematin. Ewing also finds that malarial pigment behaves toward solvents as do the blood pigments. He is of the opinion, however, that there are several pigments found including that elaborated by the parasites as well as hematoidin and bilirubin or urobilin crystals or granules. In agreement with Brown, malarial pigment has been discussed with blood pigments.

Xanthomatosis

Included in this group are several conditions, the common feature of which is the deposit of neutral fats, cholesterol esters and phosphatides in nodular masses of distinctly yellow color. Slightly raised small yellow patches are frequent in the eyelids of older people, "xanthoma planum." Similar patches may be widespread, especially about the elbows, knees, palms of the hands and soles of the feet, "xanthoma tuberosum multiplex." Either of these may occur in diabetes, "xanthoma diabeticorum," or in icterus. Microscopically there is a collection of reticulo-endothelial cells, showing a finely vacuolated cytoplasm, which contains the lipoids. Foreign body giant cells about fatty acid crystals may be found. The nodules may become slightly or extensively fibrotic. Tumors of various kinds and inflamed tissues may contain xanthomatous foci. Visceral lesions occur and may be so grouped as to justify segregation into disease entities or syndromes. In this category is Christian-Schüller syndrome. Somewhat similar but involving other lipids are Niemann-Pick disease and Gaucher's disease. These conditions are discussed in the section on reticuloendothelial system in the chapter on the Hematopoietic System.

Bile Pigmentation

The pigment of bile is almost entirely bilirubin. This may be oxidized to the green pigment, biliverdin, a process which is much more pronounced and common in animals than in man. Animal bile is often green whereas normal human bile shows the brownish-yellow color of bilirubin. Examination of bile stones indicates that other pigments are present but these are probably the product of changes in bilirubin after having been deposited to form the calculi. Whipple found that bilirubin could be formed elsewhere than in the liver (*see* Rich). Mann and his collaborators demonstrated its production in the bone marrow and spleen and showed that the liver serves principally as an organ of excretion (*see also* Corr). Pathologically, the body may be pigmented by bile either as the result of obstruction to the outflow of bile or as the result of excessive formation of bile pigment with insufficient excretion. In local areas, bile pigment may be formed as the result of hemorrhage and therefore may pigment the surrounding tissue. Obstructive jaundice or obstructive icterus is due to occlusion of either the main bile duct or many of the smaller tributaries. Obstruction to the common duct is most commonly due to catarrhal inflammation of the lining but may also be due to the lodgment of gall stones, the contraction of cicatricial tissue, the pressure of tumors or enlarged lymph nodes, actual involvement by tumor growth and various forms of acute or chronic inflammation of the biliary passages. Sometimes inflammation may be of such a nature as not to compress the larger bile duct but may serve to occlude smaller bile passages. The involvement of the liver by tumors, rather primary than secondary, may also be so extensive as to produce jaundice. Obstruction to finer passages may be seen in chronic inflammatory processes in the liver itself, for example, in hypertrophic cirrhosis of the liver where there is an overgrowth of connective tissue between the liver cords. In the late stages of Laennec cirrhosis the same phenomenon may occur.

Jaundice as the result of excessive formation of bilirubin is usually due to great destruction of blood with much liberation of hematoidin. It is assumed in these circumstances that bilirubin is formed in such great excess that it cannot be excreted by the liver. It, therefore, accumulates in the blood and serves to pigment the tissues. Nevertheless, numerous observations have shown that not only is there an increase in bilirubin formation in these cases, but certain of them also show obstruction to the finer bile canals, not only those between the liver cells but also the very finest canals existing within the cytoplasm of the liver cells. Such obstruction may be due to swelling of the liver cells, or of the cells which line the bile capillaries and to plugging of the biliary passages by fibrin thrombi. It is now considered that the liver is an important seat of fibrinogen formation, and it seems possible that pathologic disturbances in this situation may lead to formation of small fibrin plugs. It has also been suggested that the poison which produces hemolysis may also serve to precipitate bile and that the small masses of bile precipitate may serve to plug finer vessels. Local formation of bile pigment may be seen in connection with bruises where, not infrequently, a greenish-yellow discoloration is observed. Hemorrhage into serous cavities such as the pleura and the meninges may, after a time, lead to the formation of bile pigment. In these situations hematoidin and other blood pigments are likely to be present also.

Pigmentation by bile is usually in the form of a diffuse coloration of cells and the pigment may be present in various secretions. It is seen externally in the skin and mucous membranes, particularly the conjunctiva. All the deep tissues may be pigmented including connective tissue and intercellular substance. After the bile in the blood reaches a certain concentration it also appears in the urine, and in extreme cases in the sputum and even other secretions. The pigment of the skin and conjunctiva is of deep brownish-yellow color and the same is true of the urine, but in the latter instance exposure to air may lead to sufficient oxidization to transform the bilirubin to biliverdin and change the color from brownish yellow to deep green. Examination of the blood shows that the plasma is also pigmented, and this phenomenon appears before pigmentation is observed in the skin or secretions. The concentration of pigment in the blood must reach about 1:50,000 before pigmentation of the urine appears. This concentration then constitutes the renal threshold value for bile pigment. Nevertheless, Blankenhorn is of the opinion that cases exist in which the pigment may appear in the skin and not in the urine, presumably because the bile is perhaps in some colloidal combination with protein so that it may be diffused into the skin but not be excreted through the kidney.

The bodies of those who have died recently and who had suffered from jaundice, the case of kidney disease when casts in the renal tubules may show the brown or green pigmentation. Usually the process of fixation, embedding and staining serves to oxidize the bilirubin so that it appears as the green biliverdin rather than the brownish-yellow bilirubin. In cases of obstructive jaundice that have been somewhat prolonged, the picture in the liver may be characteristic. In these circumstances precipitated bile pigment may be found in the form of amorphous masses in the bile ducts and in the bile capillaries. In the finer division of the bile capillaries the pigment may be found in irregularly stellate forms, due to the fact that the mass in the bile capillary is connected with that deposited in the intracellular biliary canaliculi. In the course of preparation of the tissue, the mass of bile pigment frequently shrinks, as do also the cells, and there is

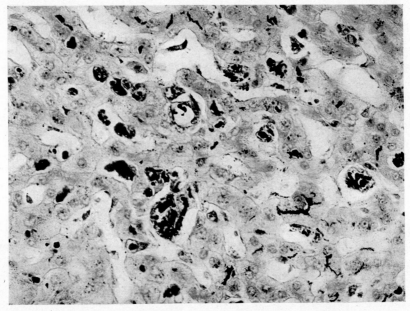

Bile pigmentation of the liver.

show a brownish-yellow pigmentation of the skin, the mucous membranes, the fat, and surfaces such as those of the heart valves and aorta, kidney and other viscera. After these organs have been exposed to the air for some time the color changes to a deep green. In practically all cases the pigmentation is deepest in the liver itself. In the majority of acute cases, histologic examination of the tissues shows little of the pigment except in

likely to be a small areola around the pigment between it and the surrounding cells. As has been mentioned above, in certain cases of jaundice due to destruction of blood, small fibrin clots and marked cloudy swelling of the parenchymatous cells of the liver may be found.

The effects of jaundice are both local and general. Functional disturbances in the liver occur with marked jaundice, especially if obstructive in type. Prolonged obstruction to outflow of bile, whether due to lesions in the extrahepatic ducts or widespread in the intrahepatic ducts, may lead ultimately to obstructive biliary cirrhosis. Horrall has shown that bile is poisonous to cells of the body and that this is due to the bile salts, especially the cholate portion. The principal effects are to be found in liver, kidney and heart. So-called liver death may be due to any of these, or combinations of them. The cardiac rate may be slowed, blood pressure decreased and cardiac arrhythmias may occur. Functional tests of hepatic functions may show depression and the detoxifying capacity is much reduced. Patients may also have the hepatorenal syndrome, in which renal insufficiency may go on to uremia. The lesion in the kidney is cholemic nephrosis. The tubular epithelium is degenerated and the lumina contain granular debris. Although the injury is probably due to the bile salts, bile pigment is found in the epithelial cells and tubular lumina. Thompson, Frazier and Ravdin point out that if there be no other antecedent renal disease, relief of the jaundice is followed by disappearance of the nephrosis. If the patient already have chronic disease of the kidneys, the nephrosis is less readily reversible. Bile salts also depress the nervous system with resultant unconsciousness and even transient paralyses.

Reduced resistance to infection is probably due to inhibition of the bactericidal properties of the blood by the bile salts. The tendency to hemorrhage in patients with jaundice is due to reduction in the level of prothrombin and this in turn is the result of inadequate absorption of vitamin K, the antihemorrhagic vitamin. The presence of bile in the intestine is necessary for absorption of vitamin K. Patients may be tided over acute episodes by injections of synthetic vitamin K, which increases the prothrombin of the blood.

Although experimental evidence shows that bile in itself is toxic, yet the disturbance of liver function by the obstruction of bile outflow, as well as by the direct toxic action of the bile upon the liver cells, must be considered. If the latter injury interfere with the detoxicating function of the liver, poisonous substances, which would otherwise be removed or destroyed, may accumulate and augment the disturbances produced by the jaundice.

Hemolytic Jaundice. In the course of many infectious diseases slight jaundice may appear, probably due to the destructive action of bacterial or other micro-organismal causes of disease upon red blood cells. Certainly many such organisms can and do produce hemotoxins. Certain forms of epidemic infectious jaundice are due to the *Spirochaeta icterohaemorrhagica*. In infancy, infection of the umbilical cord or its stump may lead to infective hemolytic jaundice. Icterus neonatorum, not infectious, occurs in the first few days of life and is associated with low levels of prothrombin due to the fact that stores of vitamin K are exhausted before they can be supplied in the infant's diet. Administration of vitamin K to the mother provides storage in the infant until it begins absorption in extra-uterine life.

HEMOLYTIC ICTERUS occurs in members of the same family and although often called congenital, the basic fault is probably hereditary. There is also an acquired form of the disease. Jaundice is usually moderate or slight and is associated especially with moderate secondary anemia and enlarged spleen. The erythrocytes are abnormally fragile, probably because many of them are somewhat spherical small cells. They are called microspherocytes. The spleen shows dilated vascular spaces and phagocytosis of red cells. Phagocytosis may also occur in the liver and in hyperplastic bone marrow. The jaundice is due to destruction of the red cells.

The influence of the spleen is not clearly understood and its enlargement appears to be due principally to the destruction of blood corpuscles; nevertheless, the removal of this organ is usually highly beneficial. The improvement is exhibited not only in the general clinical manifestations but also in the metabolism. The loss of nitrogen, calcium, magnesium, and iron as well as the increased excretion of uric acid, returns almost to normal level following operation. Further discussion is found in the chapter on Hematopoietic System.

DISSOCIATED JAUNDICE. The studies of Hoover and Blankenhorn have served to emphasize the importance of a condition known as "dissociated jaundice." This is particularly well exemplified in the hemolytic form of jaundice wherein the blood contains bile pigment but not bile salts. The term, however, applies to the presence of either bile salts, or bile pigment, without the other constituent. In cases of obstructive jaundice where both constituents would be present, the excretion by the kidney of bile salts may lead to a dissociated jaundice in which pigment only is present in the plasma. In case of hemolytic jaundice it seems likely that the dissociation is due to the fact that only bile pigment is formed in excess and gains access to the blood. This is advanced as an argument in favor of the idea that in such forms of jaundice the pigmentation may occur quite independently of any participation on the part of the liver. In any case the bile salts are more readily diffusible than are the pigments and are more easily secreted by the kidney.

REFERENCES

Addis, T.: A Working Hypothesis of Hemoglobin Pigment Metabolism, Arch. Int. Med., 15: 413, 1915.

Aub, J. C., L. T. Fairhall, A. S. Minot, and P. Reznikoff: Lead Poisoning, Medicine, 4: 1, 1925.

Barron, E. S. G.: Cellular Oxidation Systems, Physiol. Rev., 19: 184, 1939.

Belt, T. H.: The Pathology of Pneumonoconiosis. A Review, Amer. Jour. Med. Sci., 188: 418, 1934.

——: Silicosis of the Spleen: A Study of the Silicotic Nodule, Jour. Path. and Bact., 49: 39, 1939.

Blankenhorn, M. A.: The Bile Content of the Blood in Pernicious Anemia, Arch. Int. Med., 19: 344, 1917.

——: The Distribution of the Bile in Certain Types of Jaundice, Arch. Int. Med., 21: 282, 1918.

Bloch, B.: The Problem of Pigment Formation, Amer. Jour. Med. Sci., 177: 609, 1929; see also Jacobsen, C. C.: Melanin: A Review of Chemical Aspects of the Melanin Problem, Arch. Path., 17: 141, 391, 1934; Laidlaw, G.: Melanoma Studies. I. The Dopa Reaction in General Pathology, Amer. Jour. Path., 8: 477, 1932.

Blum, H. F.: Photodynamic Action and Diseases Caused by Light, New York, Reinhold, 1941.

Brown, W. H.: Series of Studies on Blood and Malarial Pigments, Jour. Exper. Med., 12: 623, 1910; 13: 290, 1911; 14: 612, 1911; 15: 579, 1912; 18: 96, 107, 1913. Arch. Int. Med., 12: 315, 1913.

Burgess, A. M.: Chloroma, Jour. Med. Res., 27: 133, 1913.

Cohn, A. L., A. S. White, and H. B. Weyrauch: Kaolin Granuloma of the Stomach, Jour. Amer. Med. Asso., 117: 2225, 1941.

Connor, C. L.: Studies on Lipochromes, Amer. Jour. Path., 4: 227, 235, 293, 1928.

Corr, P.: Histochemical Evidence Concerning the Site of the Formation of Bile Pigment, Arch. Path., 7: 84, 1929.

Cummins, S. L.: Sericite and Silica: Experimental Dust-Lesions in Rabbits, Brit. Jour. Exper. Path., 18: 395, 1937.

Dobriner, K., and C. P. Rhoads: The Porphyrins in Health and Disease, Physiol. Rev., 20: 416, 1940.

Drinker, C. K.: Modern Views Upon the Development of Lung Fibrosis, Jour. Indust. Hyg., 3: 295, 1922.

Fishback, H. R.: Clinical Demonstration of Iron in the Skin in Hemochromatosis, Jour. Lab. & Clin. Med., 25: 98, 1939.

Gardner, L. U.: Etiology of Pneumoconiosis, Jour. Amer. Med. Asso., 111: 1925, 1938.

——: The Pathology and Roentgenographic Manifestations of Pneumoconiosis, ibid., 114: 535, 1940.

Gettler, A. O., C. P. Rhoads, and S. Weiss: A Contribution to the Pathology of Generalized Argyria with a Discussion of the Fate of Silver in Human Body, Amer. Jour. Path., 3: 631, 1927.

Haythorn, S. R.: Unresolved Pneumonia Associated with Severe Anthracosis, Bull. Internat. Asso. Med. Museums, 7: 49, 1918.

——: Some Histological Evidences of the Disease Importance of Pulmonary Anthracosis, Jour. Med. Res., 29: 259, 1913-14.

Head, G. D., and R. A. Johnson: Carotinemia, Arch. Int. Med., 28: 268, 1921.

Hooper, C. W., and G. H. Whipple: Icterus. A Rapid Change of Hemoglobin to Bile Pigment in Pleural and Peritoneal Cavities, Jour. Exper. Med., 23: 137, 1916.

Hoover, C. F., and M. A. Blankenhorn: Dissociated Jaundice, Arch. Int. Med., 18: 289, 1916.

Horrall, O. H.: The Toxicity of Bile, Physiol. Rev., 11: 122, 1931.

Hueck, W.: Pigmentstudien, Beitr. Path. Anat. u. Allg. Path., 54: 68, 1912.

Karsner, H. T., O. Saphir, and T. W. Todd: The State of the Cardiac Muscle in Hypertrophy and Atrophy, Amer. Jour. Path., 1: 351, 1925.

King, E. J., and T. H. Belt: The Physiological and Pathological Aspects of Silica, Physiol. Rev., 18: 329, 1938.

Kinney, V. C.: Further Experiments in Light Penetration, etc., Amer. Jour. Electrotherap. and Radiol., 11: 201, 1922.

Lanza, A. J.: Silicosis and Asbestosis, Oxford Univ. Press, 1938.

Mallory, F. B., F. Parker, and R. N. Nye: Experimental Pigment Cirrhosis due to Copper and its Relation to Hemochromatosis, Jour. Med. Res., 42: 461, 1921-22.

Mann, F. C.: The Effects of Complete and Partial Removal of the Liver, Medicine, 6: 419, 1927.

Mason, V. R., C. Courville, and E. Ziskind: Porphyrins in Human Disease, Medicine, 12: 355, 1933.

Matz, P. B.: A Study of Silicosis, Amer. Jour. Med. Sci., 196: 548, 1938.

Menkin, V.: Experimental Siderosis. I. Arch. Path., 19: 53, 1935; —— and S. M. Talmadge: Experimental Siderosis. II. ibid., 19: 61, 1935.

Muir, R., and J. S. F. Niven: The Local Formation of Blood Pigments. Jour. Path. & Bact., 41: 183, 1935.

Nesbitt, S., and C. H. Watkins: Acute Porphyria, Amer. Jour. Med. Sci., 203: 74, 1942.

Oberndorfer, S.: Die pathologischen Pigmente, Ergebn. Allg. Path. u. Path. Anat., 19^2: 47, 1921.

Ohmori, D.: Bedeutung der Membrana Propria der Glomerulusschlingen in der Nierenpthologie, Virchow's Arch. Path. Anat., **234**: 53, 1921.

Opie, E. L.: A Case of Hemochromatosis, the Relation of Hemochromatosis to Bronzed Diabetes, Jour. Exper. Med., **4**: 279, 1899. ———: Diseases of the Pancreas, Philadelphia, Lippincott, 1903.

Oppenheimer, B. S., and B. S. Kline: Ochronosis, with a Study of an Additional Case, Arch. Int. Med., **29**: 732, 1922.

Palmer, L. S.: Carotinoids and Related Pigments, New York, 1922.

———, and H. L. Kempster: Relation of Plant Carotinoids to Growth, Fecundity and Reproduction of Fowls, Jour. Biol. Chem., **39**: 299, 1919.

Pearce, R. M., E. B. Krumbhaar, and C. H. Frazier: The Spleen and Anemia, Philadelphia, Lippincott, 1918.

Percival, G. H., and C. P. Stewart: Melanogenesis: A Review, Edinburgh Med. Jour., **37**: 497, 1930.

Permar, H. H.: The Development of the Mononuclear Phagocyte of the Lung, Jour. Med. Res., **42**: 147, 1921.

Rich, A. R.: The Formation of Bile Pigment. Physiol. Rev., **5**: 182, 1925.

Ritterhoff, R. J.: Acute Silicosis, Amer. Rev. Tuberc., **43**: 117, 1941.

Robertson, O. H.: Phagocytosis of Foreign Material in the Lung, Physiol. Rev., **21**: 112, 1941.

Ropshaw, H. J.: Melanogenesis with Special Reference to Sulfhydrils and Protamines, Amer. Jour. Physiol., **103**: 535, 1933.

Rous, P., and J. Oliver: Experimental Hemochromatosis, Jour. Exper. Med., **28**: 629, 1918; *see also* Trans. Asso. Amer. Phys., **33**: 133, 1918.

Rukstinat, G. J.: Tattoos: A Survey, with Special Reference to Tattoos and Scars as Indicators of Syphilis, Arch. Path., **31**: 640, 1941.

Sayers, R. R., and W. C. Dreessen: Asbestosis, Amer. Jour. Pub. Health, **29**: 205, 1939.

Schilling, K.: Ueber die schädlichen Einwirkungen des Baumwollstaubes auf die Atmungsorgane, Deutsch. Arch. Klin. Med., **146**: 163, 1925.

Schultze, K. W.: Zur Chemie des Hämosiderins, Beitr. Path. Anat. u. Allg. Path., **86**: 101, 1931.

Sheldon, J. H.: Hemochromatosis, London, Oxford University Press, 1935.

Sprunt, T. P.: Hemochromatosis, Arch. Int. Med., **8**: 75, 1911.

Taylor, F. A.: Pigment of Anthracosis, Proc. Soc. Exp. Biol. & Med., **48**: 70, 1941.

Thompson, L. L., W. D. Frazier, and I. S. Ravdin: The Renal Lesion in Obstructive Jaundice, Amer. Jour. Med. Sci., **199**: 305, 1940.

Wells, H. G.: Chemical Pathology, 5th ed. Philadelphia, Saunders, 1925.

———: Addison's Disease with Selective Destruction of the Suprarenal Cortex, Arch. Path., **10**: 499, 1930.

Whipple, G. H.: Pigment Metabolism and Regeneration of Hemoglobin in the Body, Arch. Int. Med., **29**: 711, 1922.

———, and C. W. Hooper: Hematogenous and Obstructive Icterus, Jour. Exper. Med., **17**: 593; 612, 1913.

Willis, H. S.: Pneumoconiosis and Tuberculosis, Medicine, **9**: 413, 1930.

3

Degenerations and Infiltrations

INTRODUCTION

The degenerations are characterized by changes in the cytoplasm, and sometimes also slight disturbances of the nucleus, which are indicative of deterioration of the cell. The infiltrations are alterations of the cell due to transport of materials from other situations and their accumulation within the cell. The two conditions are usually readily distinguishable, but this is not always true and there may be some overlapping. They are retrogressive processes, frequently encountered. Some have noteworthy clinical features and some are of interest principally to the pathologist.

CLOUDY SWELLING

Albuminous or Parenchymatous Degeneration

When death is due to infectious diseases or to other conditions in which the patient does not die abruptly, for example as the result of accident, autopsy discloses various degenerative changes. The most common and the least serious is cloudy swelling. This is found in what the pathologist calls parenchymatous cells, including glandular epithelium, muscle, endothelial cells and leukocytes. Upon gross examination, organs the seat of cloudy swelling are somewhat or even considerably enlarged, softer than usual, with a loss of normal luster and increase of opacity. In well-marked cases the organ resembles a parboiled animal organ. The swelling leads to tension of the capsule so that when the organ is cut the somewhat swollen substance bulges above the cut edge. The cross section is pale, soft and friable. If individual cells be teased out and examined fresh under the microscope, the cell is larger than normal, its outline not altogether distinct and the cytoplasm so granular that the nucleus is considerably obscured. If, however, a stained section be examined, the most important changes are increase in size of the cell and increase in granulation of the cytoplasm. In those organs limited by a capsule, the swelling of the cells may, by compression of their margins, make the outline somewhat more distinct than normal. In other instances, even in the stained preparation, the lack of definition of outline is apparent. Inasmuch as sectioning with the knife cuts through the cells, the hiding of the nucleus is not likely to be apparent in such material, especially when the nucleus is well stained. The granules, however, are coarser than the normal Altmann granules. In the later stages of cloudy swelling of the renal epithelium it is not unusual to note that the part of the cells nearest the lumen of the tubule has disappeared, and instead of finding the tubule almost completely blocked by the swollen cells, the lumen may be somewhat larger than normal and is outlined by a narrow rim of granular cells. As a rule, in cloudy swelling the nuclei show no definite change but in some instances a condensation of chromatin near

37

the nuclear membrane is observed. When shrinkage, fragmentation, or solution of the nuclei occurs, the condition is no longer cloudy swelling, for these nuclear changes indicate that cell death has occurred.

There is no close relation between the degree of cloudy swelling observed grossly and microscopically. It may seem to be slight grossly and prove to be marked microscopically. The converse is also true. Postmortem changes may resemble cloudy swelling so

ing of heart, liver, kidneys, and other parenchymatous organs. Poisons introduced from without also produce cloudy swelling, notably cantharidin, phosphorus and mercury. The use of these agents is an important means of producing experimental cloudy swelling. Since the earliest change demonstrable in parenchymatous cells following occlusion of an artery is cloudy swelling, reduction of nutrition and oxidation may be regarded as important causes. Similarly, gen-

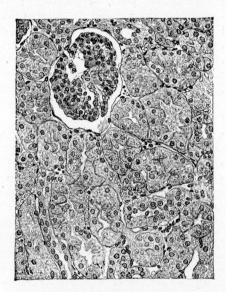 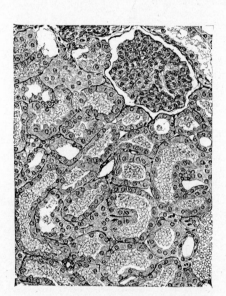

Cloudy swelling of the kidney. The illustration shows the earlier stage in which the cells are swollen, granular and in places occlude the lumen of the tubule. The illustration on the right shows a later stage in which part of the cytoplasm has disappeared, leaving a narrow rim of cells and albuminous granular precipitate in the lumina, representing precipitated protein of the urine.

closely that some have denied the existence of the latter. Nevertheless, autopsies on patients within a half hour of death and experimental production of cloudy swelling leave no doubt that it occurs. If doubt exists, the pathologist always inquires as to the possibility of conditions that might produce postmortem changes. These bring about marked cytoplasmic changes and also early changes in the nucleus and are accompanied by comparable changes in connective tissues and erythrocytes which are not subject to cloudy swelling.

The poisonous substances of infectious diseases are the most important causes of cloudy swelling. It is extremely rare that an autopsy on a patient dead of infectious disease fails to show well-marked cloudy swell-

eral starvation may lead to a moderate degree of the same change. Extensive surface burns are also complicated by cloudy swelling of the viscera, and it is highly probable that this is the result of concentration of body fluids rather than due to poisonous products of tissue destruction (Pack and Davis). Exposure to high temperatures also leads to cloudy swelling.

Overwork of an organ may possibly lead to cloudy swelling. It was shown early in the study of this condition that if one kidney be thrown out of function by ligating its artery or vein, the opposite organ when examined in the course of 12 to 24 hours, shows very definite swelling of its epithelium. If this occur following the surgical removal of a kidney in man, it is evanescent and followed quickly by recovery. It is probable that the process is one of excitation and depression of the cell in response to irritation, presumably brought about by the various causes enumerated above (Davidman and Dolley; Fricke, Groll and Meyer). Thus the process can be looked upon as a physiologic response to various stimuli. It is reversible in that it clears up readily upon removal of the cause. It may, however, progress to death of the cell, an irreversible state.

The basic facts of cloudy swelling are that organs and cells are enlarged due to imbibition of water and that the cytoplasm of cells shows increased granularity. That water is taken up is indicated by the fact that with an increase in the weight of the organ, there is reduction of specific gravity and a percentile decrease of dry weight. What causes the imbibition of water is not clear. Various injuries to cells may produce increased permeability (Lucké and McCutcheon) but there are probably underlying internal changes. The retrogressive nature of the process suggests that there is an alteration of hydrogen-ion concentration toward the acid side and the resultant acid-protein is hydrophilic. Protein cleavage is augmented as shown by increased amount of dialyzable N and amino-acids, but the total protein content is not altered. Thus there would be swelling of the cellular colloids and increased osmotic pressure. The imbibition of water disturbs the balance of colloids in the cell with aggregation of the protein molecules, appearance of granules and cloudiness of the cytoplasm. The granules are protein, since the xanthoproteic reaction is positive. They are not the result of heat coagulation because they are soluble in dilute acetic acid and dilute potassium hydrate. Although enlargement and enspherulation of mitochondria are the first response to cellular injury (Duthie), it is known by staining reactions that the granules of cloudy swelling are not composed of either mitochondria or Altmann granules. An indication of the disturbance of internal colloid balance is found in the presence of a few lipoid droplets. Identification of a few droplets of neutral fat indicates that the process has gone on in the direction of fatty degeneration. The phenomena of cloudy swelling include imbibition of water, condensation of protein aggregates, especially at the surface of the cell, with consequent cloudiness of the cytoplasm.

In different stages of the disease, patients who have infectious disease may show such manifestations as low blood pressure, albumin and casts in the urine and digestive disturbances. By comparison with the effects of experimental cloudy swelling, it is probable that these clinical features are due at least in part to cloudy swelling of the muscle of the heart and arteries, of the renal epithelium and of the parenchymal cells of digestive glands. When the underlying infectious disease subsides, these conditions usually clear up. With considerable severity or long duration or both, the cloudy swelling may progress to other changes of more importance such as fatty degeneration, or death of the cells involved.

HYDROPIC DEGENERATION

Cloudy swelling, as has been stated, exhibits imbibition of water, and hydropic degeneration differs only in degree. It is a term used conveniently to designate a condition in which the water is present in numerous droplets so as to dominate the picture of the cellular change. The same general causes operate to produce hydropic degeneration as noted in connection with cloudy swelling. Grossly, the organs have the same general appearance as is seen in cloudy swelling except that they may be softer and more friable.

Microscopically, small or large globules appear within the cytoplasm, rarely within the nucleus. In certain instances, particularly where the hydropic degeneration occurs in the neighborhood of inflammation, and in the earlier stages of central necrosis of the liver, it is possible to demonstrate small accumulations of fibrin within the globules, as Mallory has pointed out. This deposition probably results from the elaboration, in the cells themselves, of a fluid characteristic of inflammation. Fibrin separates out and the fluid which remains is serum. Hydropic degeneration is due to much the same causes as is cloudy swelling, but with greater response by the cell. It is also reversible upon removal of the cause, except that when fibrin is produced the injury may lead to death of the cell.

FATTY METAMORPHOSIS

Human fat contains the unsaturated oleic acid and the saturated palmitic and stearic acids. The combination of these to form the body fat differs in different parts of the body but in a general way is fairly constant. As age advances the oleic fat increases relatively in amount. The constitution of fat is also influenced by the diet. Under normal conditions much of the fat of the body is derived from that in the food, and if conditions be distinctly abnormal, the food fat may be in part reproduced in the fat storehouses of the body. For example, if a dog be starved and then fed with fat different from that of his own body, the subsequent accumulation of fat is similar to that in the food. In metabolic processes, carbohydrate is oxidized more readily than is fat. The fat is thus said to be protected so that it remains in the depots. Diets rich in carbohydrates may permit accumulations of fat in this manner as well as by synthesis of fat from carbohydrate, presumably through the influence of vitamin B_1. The body protein is protected primarily by consumption of carbohydrate and secondarily by utilization of fat. Protein may be utilized in normal body metabolism but only to a small degree. Fat accumulates in the body in what are called fat depots, but as Wells indicates these act as specialized tissues to store fat and give it up for the production of energy. The depots are connective tissues such as occur in the subcutaneous tissues, omentum, retroperitoneal tissues, grooves of the heart, etc. They are derived from primitive embryonal fat-organs. The liver also acts in the same specialized fashion. An example of this specialization is the fact that if skin and subcutaneous tissues of the abdominal wall be transplanted to the back of the hand, where there is ordinarily little fat, the new tissue retains its capacity to accumulate fat.

In mature fatty tissue, the fat is in large droplets, practically filling the cell. Usually the nucleus is pushed to one side and the cell takes on the "signet ring" form. In contrast, the cytoplasm of the immature fat cells contains numerous small globules; these cells may be found occasionally in adult fat and tumors of fatty tissues, the lipomas. Lipomas accumulate fat, but rarely if ever is it utilized for production of energy, even

though it does not appear to differ in chemical composition from normal fat. There is some relation between fat-organs and lymphatic apparatus and nerves, as noted below. Endocrine glands have some bearing on fat metabolism, as will also be outlined subsequently. That the fat-organs are endocrines themselves is not certain. Wells suggests that

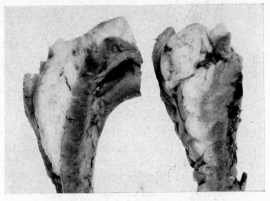

Cross section of upper portion of right ventricle of two hearts. Specimen at left shows sharp line of demarcation between subepicardial fat and myocardium. Specimen at right shows loss of demarcation because of fat infiltration into myocardium.

fat in the involuted thymus and in the adrenal cortex may perhaps store vitamins A and D. It is not to be forgotten that oxidation is essential to metabolism of fat.

The term fatty metamorphosis covers both fat infiltration and fatty degeneration, although it must be admitted that distinctions cannot always be made. Fat infiltration is either an increase in amount of fat already present or its appearance in abnormal situations. It refers to neutral fats. Ordinarily it leads to no great disturbance of function. In fatty degeneration, however, there is a degeneration of cells with appearance of neutral fats and often lipoids and their esters. In such organs as heart, liver and kidneys, it may impair function seriously.

Fat Infiltration

Except for the liver, this occurs only in the connective tissues which constitute fat-organs. The gross description varies with the organ involved. Thus, in the heart, the normal sharp line of distinction between subepicardial fat and myocardium, seen in the cross section, is obscured or obliterated and fat may extend more or less deeply into the myocardium. In the pancreas, the fat normally surrounding the organ extends down between the lobules. The liver of fat infiltration is usually large, pale yellow, with tense capsule and rounding of the anterior edge. It cuts with normal resistance and greases the

lobules. Characteristically, the liver shows signet-ring parenchymal cells, each containing a single large droplet of fat. This is marked in the periphery of the lobule and in advanced cases may extend practically throughout the lobule. This does not mean,

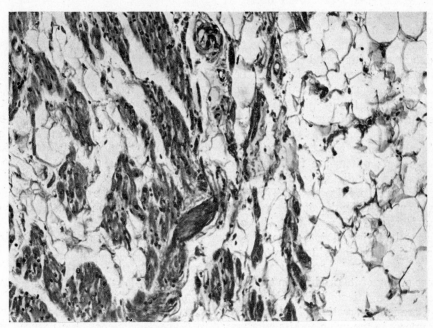

Fat infiltration of the heart. The fat appears between the atrophic muscle-fiber cells.

knife. The cross section is greasy and yellow, with little distinction of the lobules.

Microscopically, the heart shows fatty connective tissue between the groups of fiber

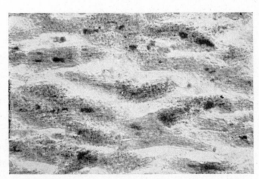

Fatty degeneration of the cardiac muscle stained with Sudan III. Note the stained droplets in the muscle-fiber cells.

cells of the myocardium; these are often atrophic. In the pancreas, the fatty connective tissue is found between lobules deep in the organ and may even extend into the

however, that cells with many small droplets do not occur. In other organs, fat infiltration occurs in the connective tissues and it is only in the liver that there is trouble in distinction between fat infiltration and fatty degeneration.

The explanation of why fat accumulates in the body to produce fat infiltration is not absolutely clear but in all likelihood vitamins, hormones and endocrine glands are important. Basically, of course, accumulation of fat means intake of a greater amount of food than is expended in the production of energy. It is known that the fat is in the form of neutral fat and that neutral fats in the diet are more favorable to the deposit of fat in the tissues than are the unsaturated glycerides. Obese people are likely to show fat infiltration of various organs, including the liver. In cases of inanition in both children and adults, fatty livers may be found, but on the basis of experimental observations it is said that vitamin B_1 must be adequate in amount. In tuberculous patients, fatty liver is not infrequent and it may be that this is due to the high caloric diet customary in the treatment. Probably, however, there must also be an adequate supply of vitamin B_1. Those who drink large amounts of beer and other malted beverages are often obese. It has been supposed that the alcohol, being readily oxidized, protects fats and permits their accumulation. It may also be true that alcohol depresses oxidation. Perhaps in consumption of large quantities of malted beverages the total amount of vitamin B_1 favors the deposit of fat, the drinking interferes with adequate intake of protein and the action of some of the hormones is altered.

Certain persons are lean in spite of a high caloric diet; others are fat in spite of relatively low caloric diets, probably because of a constitutional predisposition. The naturally obese appear to be deficient in power of oxidation. It has been shown that if β-oxybutyric acid be injected into lean persons there is a slight elevation of temperature and complete combustion of the acid without the appearance of any of its products in the body. Conversely, when injected into obese individuals, there is no elevation of temperature, acetone appears in the urine and its odor may be detected in the breath. This indicates that in such persons there is reduced and slow oxidation insufficient to burn the fatty acid. This inefficiency of oxidation probably accounts for the accumulation of fat in the tissues.

Experimental observations have thrown some additional light on the subject. It is known that the liver of the depancreatized dog ultimately becomes the seat of marked fat infiltration, which is prevented by feeding pancreas. Best and his associates attribute this preventive effect to the presence of choline and perhaps other constituents of protein. Dragstedt and his coworkers are of the opinion that choline plays but a small part, if any, in this phenomenon. They have extracted a substance from the pancreas, called lipocaic, which they consider to be a hormone. It is not an external secretion because it is not found in pancreatic juice. This means that the pancreas provides two internal secretions, insulin and lipocaic.

Lipocaic is highly effective in preventing fatty liver in depancreatized dogs. When rats are given a high caloric fatty diet, there is well marked fat infiltration of the liver, that can be prevented by lipocaic and choline. Best agrees as to the effects of lipocaic but thinks that choline is also a factor and that both operate. Administration of extract of anterior pituitary favors this fat infiltration in the rat, but hypophysectomy does not interfere with it in dogs. Best's experiments with rats indicate that vitamin B_1 is essential for the production of fat infiltration, perhaps because it favors the synthesis of fat from carbohydrate, but contradictory evidence has been adduced. Many experimental studies of fatty changes in the liver are going on, but reports are somewhat confusing because there is little distinction made between simple fat deposit in the liver and destructive lesions with the appearance of fat. There is further discussion in the chapter on Liver and Pancreas.

The influence of ductless glands and hormones is observed in the increase of fat in pregnancy and lactation, following natural or artificial menopause, in eunuchs, and in patients with deficient action of the thyroid. The mode of operation is not clear, but in thyroid deficiency, the reduced metabolic rate plays a significant part, and the condition is relieved by administration of thyroid products. In all these instances the pituitary probably has an effect.

Obesity

Also physiologic is the obesity of those who consume more food than they oxidize. This adiposis simplex may be marked, but is corrected by diet and exercise. There are, however, certain forms of obesity that deserve to be called pathologic. In adiposis dolorosa, often called Dercum's disease, fat accumulates about the upper trunk, neck and axilla. It is usually tender to pressure and may be painful. Its cause is not known, but Wells draws attention to the association of the fatty growths with nerves.

Adiposis cerebralis, adiposogenital syndrome and Fröhlich's syndrome apply to the same condition. The body has a feminine conformation with a moderate deposit of fat, especially about the hips. In both sexes the external genitalia are small. In males, there is scanty growth of hair in the axilla, on the pubis, where it is usually of feminine distribution, and on the face. In females, the breasts are small. Growth and mental development are not disturbed. Although Fröhlich's original case had a tumor of the pituitary, he and others have found that this is not a common accompaniment and it is likely that the disorder is due to lesions of the hypothalamic region sometimes produced by pressure of supracellar tumors or other condition in the neighborhood (Kunstadter).

weeks in spite of restricted intake. Fat people who reduce weight by dry diets do not really decrease the actual amount of fat.

Lipodystrophy is not due to accumulation of fat, but rather the converse. It is not rare to see people who have a lean face with sunken cheeks, hence whose lower extremities and lower abdomen appear to be fat by contrast. It may be progressive and is sometimes given the name lipodystrophia progressiva. Since this begins to appear in child-

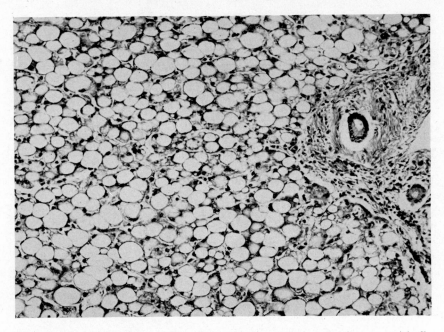

Fat infiltration of the liver. The large spaces in the parenchymal cells were originally fat globules which have been dissolved in preparation of the tissue.

Adenolipomatosis is rare and of unknown cause. Fat accumulation may be general or in the form of tumor-like masses in various parts of the body. Microscopically the fat contains many lymphocytes which may be in foci resembling tiny lymph nodes. This and other observations, according to Wells, indicate a relation between fat-organs and the lymphatic apparatus.

Steatopogy is a peculiar accumulation of fat about the buttocks of Bushmen and Hottentots, a sort of gluteal hump, evidently hereditary, but of unknown cause. There are other forms of obesity not readily classified.

In obesity of any form there is a disturbance of water balance. If such people drink large amounts of water, their weight increases and may remain up for several

hood, it is not due to congenital absence of fat-organs and it is not hereditary because it does not occur in families. Its cause is unknown. Much rarer is the loss of fat from the lower extremities. Insulin lipodystrophy is a localized loss of fat, not yet explained, which occurs in parts where insulin is repeatedly injected (Wirtschafter and Schultz).

Fatty Degeneration

Fatty degeneration differs from fat infiltration of neutral fat in that its effects are upon neutral fats and lipoids. It is fatty rather than simply fat. It is not merely an infiltration, but rather a true degeneration. It occurs principally in parenchymatous cells rather than connective tissue although it may affect the latter. Liver, kidney, myocardium, leukocytes and other cells may exhibit it. It is due to much the same causes as is cloudy swelling, operating more intensely or over a longer period of time. Thus infectious dis-

seat of fatty degeneration is somewhat variable dependent upon other associated conditions which may be present. In a fairly typical case the organ is soft, flabby, may be

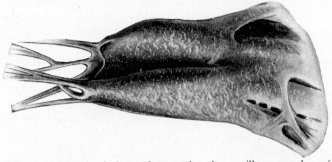

Gross appearance of fatty degeneration in papillary muscles of the heart.

eases are a frequent cause. High-grade anemias, notably pernicious anemia, often lead to fatty degeneration, especially in the heart. Yellow fever, acute diffuse necrosis of the liver and eclampsia are accompanied by fatty degeneration, particularly manifest in the liver. Diabetes may be accompanied by changes in metabolism of fat with resultant fat infiltration, fatty degeneration and lipemia. Local anemia, or ischemia, may lead after a lapse of sufficient time to fatty degeneration of the affected part. The margins of infarcts often show fatty degeneration, probably because the cells can bring about a liberation of fatty acids and glycerol, which diffuse out of the dead tissues, so that fat is formed.

Certain poisons, such as phosphorus, carbon tetrachloride, chloroform, phlorhizin, hydrazine hydrochloride, mercury and other metallic substances, etc., in addition to general effects, are noteworthy because of the production of fatty degeneration. Some of these, especially carbon tetrachloride, may be industrial hazards. Some are introduced accidentally, some are used for suicidal purposes and some are employed almost solely for experimental studies. Dietrich and Kleeberg quote various authors as indicating that fatty changes in cells are part of a response to various stimuli. Thus, as in cloudy swelling, fatty changes may well represent phases of physiologic excitation and depression of cells.

The gross appearance of an organ the

considerably reduced in size and in the case of an encapsulated organ shows a flaccid capsule. It cuts with normal or reduced resistance and the cross section is soft, bulging, moist and distinctly friable. The color of

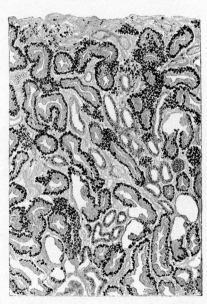

Fatty degeneration of the kidney, showing the osmicated fat globules lying near the basement margins of the cells.

both the outer and the cut surfaces is yellow. In the heart, the yellow may be distributed irregularly and when viewed through the endocardium, the patches of yellow may form small lines separated from each other so as to produce a "tabby cat" or "tigroid" appearance. In the liver, the central zones of the lobules are particularly the seat of this change. In the kidney, fatty degeneration appears rather in the cortex than in the pyramids.

Microscopically, the cell the seat of fatty degeneration is variable in size, sometimes slightly increased because of the accompanying cloudy swelling and sometimes reduced. Some form of degeneration other than the fatty change is always present. This is most commonly cloudy swelling, therefore the cytoplasm is usually granular. The fat is present usually in the form of small globules. The nucleus may exhibit no change whatever or may show a peripheral disposition of the chromatin similar to that seen in some cases of cloudy swelling. Occasionally the chromatin shows a failure to take the basic stain and therefore may be regarded as being in an early stage of solution. In contrast to fat infiltration, fatty degeneration affects particularly the parenchymatous cells. It therefore is likely to be confused with fat infiltration only in the liver. In addition to showing small globules, fatty degeneration in the liver usually affects the cells of the central zone more markedly than those of the peripheral zone, and the associated degenerative changes are of great importance in making the diagnosis. It is quite true that fat infiltration may also appear in the form of small globules, but this change is more marked in the peripheral zone, and unless complicated in some way is not associated with degenerative changes. It is extremely rare that fatty degeneration shows such a great accumulation of fat in the cells as to push the nucleus to one side, as is the case in fat infiltration. It is probable, according to Wells, that the fat globules accumulating in a normal cell, agglomerate by the pressure of the relatively firm cytoplasm to form a single large droplet, but in the degenerate cell the consistency of the cytoplasm is reduced and the small droplets of fat remain discrete. However, the old idea, namely that when the globules are smaller than the nucleus, fatty degeneration is present, does not meet acceptance in view of more modern studies. Fatty degeneration affects not only the heart, liver and kidney, but practically all the glandular organs of the body, the blood vessels, voluntary and involuntary muscles and nerve tissues.

The chief problems concerning the nature of fatty degeneration are as to whether the fat is produced in the cell, whether it is fat made visible by changes in the cell, or is fat transported to the cell from other situations. It is unlikely that fat can be made from protein and also unlikely that fat in the cell of fatty degeneration is due to changes in the cellular protein. Work with tissue cultures, however, suggests that there is a cellular endogenous mechanism that elaborates fat. There is no doubt that cells in cultures can ingest fat from the culture medium. Foot thought he could see direct transformation of cell granules into fat and Lewis maintained that cells growing in a medium devoid of fat can produce fat. Sims and Stillman have reported the presence in serum of a factor which can induce the formation of fat in cell cultures and in strips of adult tissues. Thus there is evidence to favor the view that cells can produce fat, but the application of this to degenerate cells is not yet clear.

The second of the propositions given above concerns the process called fat phanerosis: in fatty degeneration, fat may be rendered visible microscopically by intracellular changes. Thus an organ the seat of fatty degeneration may show no increase in weight but have an augmented amount of fat as demonstrated by quantitative chemical tests. If a tissue in which fat is not visible microscopically is digested with pepsin, fat globules can then be demonstrated. These facts gave rise to the theory of phanerosis, although it was not assumed that pepsin digestion is responsible for fatty degeneration. Dible, however, has studied the fat in heart, liver and kidneys and offers strong evidence that phanerosis is not responsible for fatty degeneration in these organs. Modern study gives no support for the theory of phanerosis in the sense of enzymatic processes. Somewhat different is the hypothesis of Fischer to the effect that intracellular fat of parenchymal cells is normally in extremely fine emulsion protected by proteins and electrolytes. As suggested in the discussion of cloudy swelling, cellular degeneration is accompanied by the production of hydrophilic acid-protein. The imbibition of water so alters the internal environment that the protective action of proteins and electrolytes is disturbed with a fusion of the emulsified fat globules to form microscopically visible droplets. This is supported by the fact that in fatty degeneration, the amount of water in the tissues is increased and the protein decreased.

The third proposition concerns transport of fat. Many years ago it was shown that if a dog be poisoned with phosphorus, which produces marked fatty degeneration of the liver, and then fed a fat that could be identified by melting point, iodine number, etc., the fat in the liver is largely the ingested fat. Variations of this experiment were all confirmatory. Furthermore, as a rule, organs the seat of fatty degeneration contain more fat, by quantitative chemical determination than is present normally. Various other facts, including the studies of Dible, quoted above, favor the view that fat is transported to and accumulates in the course of fatty degeneration. Thus it may be stated that the fat in fatty degeneration is largely transported fat and that perhaps intracellular processes of a nature not yet proven may lead to some local production of fat.

It was pointed out in the section on cloudy swelling that sometimes doubly refractile globules are present in the cells in this condition. This material is likely to be present in greater amounts in fatty degeneration than in cloudy swelling. Neutral fat is singly refractile and is spoken of as isotropic in contrast to these anisotropic droplets. Chemical analysis shows that these consist chiefly of cholesterol esters combined with variable amounts of phosphatids, fatty acids, soaps, and neutral fats. The constitution varies under different conditions and the change is to be regarded as a degenerative process affecting the various lipids of the cells. It is possible that the physical changes leading to liberation of fat also disturb the balance of fat, protein and lipoids so that the lipoid material accumulates in the form of microscopically visible droplets. Quantitative studies of the lipoid content of organs, the seat of cloudy swelling and of fatty degeneration, have not yet been made in sufficient number to determine positively whether the lipoids are actually increased in amount or not. Determinations on the basis of histologic studies do not sharply differentiate either fats or lipoids. Particularly is this true of lipoids, since the differential staining of these substances is subject to greater errors than is true of the fat stains.

Clinically, the manifestations of fatty degeneration may or may not be evident and often it is not possible to be certain whether they are due to the fatty degeneration or to other changes brought about by the causative condition. There is no doubt, however, that fatty degeneration may result in serious reduction of functional activity. This can be seen particularly well in the case of fatty degeneration of the heart, which is often associated not only with low blood pressure and pulse pressure but also with cardiac arrhythmia and in rare instances may be the only demonstrable cause of death. Similarly, fatty degeneration causes disturbance of renal function. In the more moderate cases of chronic glomerulonephritis, the changes in the interstitial substance and in the glomeruli may be relatively slight, and cloudy swelling and fatty degeneration of the epithelium are the most striking changes seen. Deficiencies of elimination are likely to be marked in this disease. In fatty degeneration of the liver there may be marked changes in protein metabolism, particularly in those cases where the lesion is severe. The disturbance of metabolism is seen particularly well in cases of accidental phosphorus poisoning and in acute yellow atrophy of the liver.

Recovery from fatty degeneration of an organ depends in large part upon the possibility of removing the cause. In young individuals where fatty degeneration is the result of infectious disease, recovery commonly occurs, but it may take months and years before all the functional defects are removed. As age advances, the possibility of recovery is decreased. With continued activity of the cause, fatty degeneration not infrequently is followed by death of the cell.

Diseases of Fatty Tissues

There are certain lesions that are peculiar to fatty tissues. Fat necrosis is one of these. Here the death of the fat is accompanied by splitting into fatty acid and glycerol, with a combination of the glycerol and calcium to form a soap. This is observed in the abdomen in cases of acute pancreatic necrosis and also occurs as a result of trauma to subcutaneous tissues. It is discussed in the chapter on Necrosis and Somatic Death.

Lipogranulomatosis is a condition in which a small, movable, poorly defined lump is felt in subcutaneous tissues. The patients do not complain of pain, but the lump is noticeable. Often there is a history of minor injury. Microscopically, there is a focus of dead fat surrounded by granulation tissue, rich in fibroblasts and usually with delicate capillaries. It should not be mistakenly diagnosed as sarcoma.

Sclerema neonatorum is observed in infants whose subcutaneous fat is firm and rigid, as if solidified. Wells states that it seems to be due to a deficiency of olein so that the fat is largely palmitic and stearic. This fat has a higher melting point than oleic fat and is thus relatively solid at body temperature. Injuries during labor readily induce necrosis of this fat. Such necrosis may be without known cause. The local lipodystrophy due to injections of insulin has been referred to earlier. Certain diseases of lipoid metabolism are discussed in the chapter on the Hematopoietic System.

Adipocere

Obese corpses buried in wet ground are sometimes partly converted into a soap-like mass which preserves the general conformation of the body. As a rule the face and the distal parts of the extremities are only poorly if at all preserved. This material is resistant to bacterial decomposition so that the corpse may retain its general form for many years. Early studies of the condition were interpreted to indicate that the muscle and other tissues are converted into fat and then into soap, but more recent studies indicate that the soap is formed entirely from the body fats. The fats are split by bacterial enzymes during decomposition and possibly also by the lipases of the body. The glycerol diffuses and the fatty acids combine with the ammonia of decomposition to form the soluble ammonium soaps, which flow into and replace the decomposed muscle. Subsequently, slow reaction with calcium and magnesium salts produces the firmer and less soluble soaps of these metals. The condition is seen in ground not only moist but rich in lime. The calcium may come from both the body and the ground or water.

THE HYALINS

Under pathologic conditions there may appear in tissues a clear, homogeneous, structureless material which is described by the term "hyalin." Grossly, the material is usually somewhat translucent or glassy and transmits the underlying color of the organ. The term is a broad descriptive one and includes in its scope a considerable number of substances which have these physical characters. By virtue of gross, microscopic and chemical reactions, it has been possible to separate and to differentiate certain particular forms which have a special character. These include mucin, colloid, glycogen, amyloid and several other clear structureless materials. The features which differentiate these special forms of hyalin will be described in connection with the discussion of the particular topics. In order to be specific in the application of terms, it is well to refer to that form of hyalin which is not to be differentiated by special characters as simple hyalin.

Hyaline Degeneration

The most common and the most widespread of the simple hyalins is that appearing in connective tissue. This may be found in dense tissue in old people, it may be seen in old scars and in situations where connective tissue is laid down as part of chronic inflammation. It is similar in all probability to the hyalin of cartilage and yellow elastic tissue. Grossly, this material is often seen in the thickened pleura of chronic pleurisy, in the thickened capsule of the spleen and in certain stages in the process of arteriosclerosis. To the naked eye it is a clear, homogeneous, structureless material and often has a faint blue tint. Microscopically the nuclei are seen scattered somewhat sparsely about the tissue and between these is the homogeneous material. This connective tissue hyalin is seen particularly well in chronic inflammation of lymph nodes in which it was first described by Von Recklinghausen in connection with chronic tuberculous lymphadenitis.

Epithelial cells are also capable of producing hyalin. This may be seen in the form of droplets within the cytoplasm of the cells and is especially well exemplified by the presence in tumor cells of the so-called Russell fuchsin bodies. At first supposed to be the causative organism of tumor formation, these

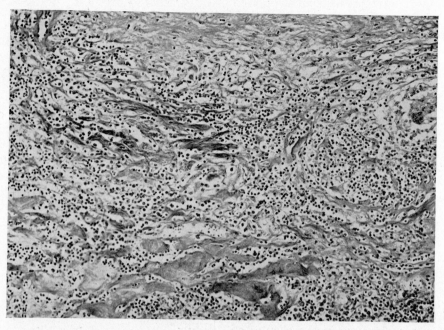

Connective-tissue hyalin in a tuberculous lymph node. Von Recklinghausen's hyalin.

sue. Epithelial hyaline droplets are found in various diseases of the liver and kidney. In

bodies were subsequently shown to be simple degeneration products of the cells. Similar bodies may be found in plasma cells and in the connective tissue cells of granulation tis-

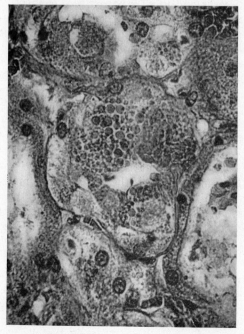

Hyaline droplets in renal epithelium.

the former, they can be reproduced experimentally by the injection of certain proteins and appear to be agglomerations of the protein (Weld et al.). That this is comparable to what occurs in man is not certain. In the kidney, the droplets in the tubular epithelium are protein which has passed through the glomerular tuft and has been resorbed in the epithelium. Experimentally the size of the droplets varies in proportion to the molecular size of the protein (Johnson and Smetana; Hein).

The urine in renal disease often shows tubular casts, some of which are hyaline. Although the origin of these casts is not known, it is generally believed that the hyaline droplets are extruded from the epithelial cells and agglomerated to form the hyaline casts. A peculiar tumor known as the cylindroma is characterized histologically by the presence of hyaline cylinders. These apparently are produced by the cells which surround the cylinders. It is not definitely known whether these cells are epithelial or endothelial in character but it seems likely that the hyaline substance is produced by the cells. The keratinization of squamous epithelium is also a form of hyaline change.

In connective tissue hyalin there is apparently a retrogressive physical change whereby the fibers of the connective tissue fuse to form the hyaline masses. Similarly, red blood corpuscles may conglutinate to

tion of these substances in quantity are devised, much of the future investigation depends largely on microchemical technic.

Zenker's Hyalin

Patients with typhoid fever, and sometimes those with influenza, pneumonia and

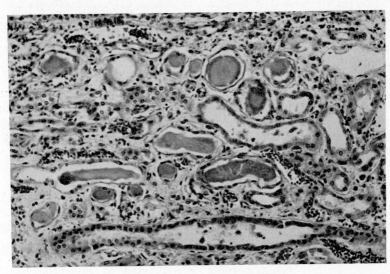

Hyaline casts in tubules of kidney.

form hyaline masses. Fibrin threads may fuse similarly. In certain types of necrosis (local death of tissues) small groups of cells of epithelial or other character may fuse to form hyaline areas. Blood clots may undergo similar change. In all these instances, it appears that the important alteration which occurs is physical rather than chemical, because the hyaline material retains essentially the same chemical constitution as the parent substance.

The important known characters of simple hyalin are physical rather than chemical. The fact that certain forms have been differentiated by chemical examination leads to the hope that further differentiation will be possible. Goodpasture draws attention to the fact that certain hyalins may be crystallized in the cells. The crystals behave toward solvents and other chemicals in the same way as does the noncrystallized material. This may mean that whereas the simple hyalins show variation of composition, yet probably each form has a fairly definite chemical structure. Unless methods of isola-

other infectious diseases, may suffer from rupture of the rectus abdominis or other

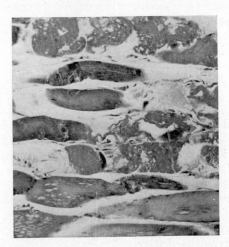

Zenker's hyalin of voluntary muscle. Army Medical Museum 45896.

muscles. This is due to what is variously called Zenker's degeneration, waxy degeneration, Zenker's hyalin or Zenker's hyaline necrosis. Grossly, the muscle is pale and translucent, somewhat like fish muscle; rupture and hemorrhage are not infrequent. Microscopically, the muscle fibers are found to be swollen, scattered, often fractured, and instead of the usual transverse striation, the muscle substance is clear, translucent, homogeneous and takes the acid stain. The softening of the muscle often gives the fiber a somewhat wavy appearance and between the fractured ends of the hyaline material the space is bridged by the muscle sheath. The muscle nuclei are usually completely absent. Thus the lesion is necrosis rather than degeneration. The Fishbacks found that if the destruction of the sarcolemma in the lesion produced experimentally be not too severe, regeneration may occur, but in man the result is usually scar formation. The lesion may also occur in the myocardium, as part of the acute myocarditis of infectious diseases, especially diphtheria.

Experimental studies have shown this lesion of muscle to be a nutritional myodegeneration or necrosis, a necrosis of coagulative type. In the discussion of vitamins in Chap. 1, it was referred to as accompanying deficiencies of vitamin C (as in scurvy) and of vitamin E or alpha tocopherol. Cod-liver oil in certain diets and overdosage of vitamin D may also produce it. Whether in infectious diseases it is due to reduced oxidation as suggested by Wells or to dietary deficiencies is not yet certain. (See Pappenheimer; Chor and Dolkart.)

Mucinous Degeneration

The gross characters of mucin are familiar in the structureless, clear, viscid material secreted from the nose and throat. Because of these gross characters the material is included among the hyalins. Microscopically, however, the character depends largely upon precipitation by the fixing agent. At times mucin appears under the microscope as a finely granular material and again as a clear structureless hyaline material. It can be differentiated from other forms of hyalin because it takes the basic dyes. It is soluble in weak solutions of alkali and is precipitated by weak acids, particularly acetic acid. Since it contains a sugar, it will reduce Fehling's solution after having been boiled with strong acid. The presence of a small amount of sulfuric acid is probably the reason for the fact that mucin takes basic dyes. In man and in other mammalia, mucin may be produced either by epithelium or by connective tissue cells. The normal prototype of that secreted by epithelial cells is seen in mucus from epithelial glands. The normal prototype of connective tissue mucin is seen in that of the umbilical cord. Following Cohnheim's suggestion the former is referred to as mucin and the latter as mucoid.

Wells describes mucin as a "compound protein consisting of a protein radical and a conjugated sulfuric acid which contains a nitrogenous sugar." Analysis shows slight differences in the composition of mucins from various origins and in a general way the mucins contain less sulfur than the mucoids. Levene found that certain of the connective tissue mucoids contain chondroitin-sulfuric acid and that others, including true mucins, contain mucoitin-sulfuric acid. The former group includes the mucoid of cartilage, tendons, aorta and sclera; the latter includes gastric mucin, Wharton's jelly, vitreous humor, cornea and ovarian cysts. The protein of the mucin or mucoid serves as an antigen in the immunologic sense, and the reactions indicate a close similarity of the protein of epithelial mucin and of connective-tissue mucoid.

The term mucinous degeneration refers to the formation of an excess of mucus with an associated degeneration of the epithelial cells. It is often difficult to be certain that cells are the seat of mucinous degeneration rather than simply the seat of an excess of mucin formation. For example, the cells of the large intestine and of the appendix often show typical goblet forms under normal circumstances. The diagnosis of mucinous degeneration in this situation depends upon the determination of an excess of mucin production in association with degenerative changes in the cells, more particularly cloudy swelling. In confined situations such as cysts, it is easily possible to determine an excessive production of mucin by the distension of the cyst. The condition is frequently seen in catarrhal inflammation of mucous membranes. It is also well exemplified in certain tumors of epithelial origin, formerly called colloid cancers but more properly designated as mucinous cancers. In these tumors the epithelial cells form acini and secrete considerable quantities of mucin. Secondary to the distension of the acini by the excess of mucin, the cells undergo cloudy swelling and atrophy.

Connective-tissue mucoid is present normally in the intercellular tissues. Pathologically, this may be increased by myxedema—a curious thickening and swelling of the skin seen in connection with deficiency of thyroid secretion. It is also found in myxoma and various combinations of myxoma with other tumors. Here it resembles the mucoid of the umbilical cord. The cells of

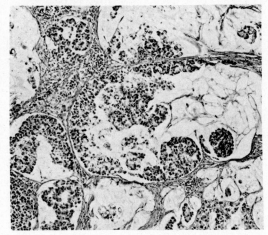

Mucinous adenocarcinoma. The spaces are partly filled by stringy mucus, a form of mucinous degeneration.

the tumor are of stellate and spindle shape with interlacing processes, between which the basic-stained mucoid lies. A somewhat similar histologic appearance is given by edema of certain fibrous tumors, particularly nasal polyps. The edematous material between the cells in these cases takes the acid stain faintly, whereas if mucoid be present the material takes the basic stain faintly. Not infrequently during the process of arteriosclerosis mucoid may be found lying between connective tissue cells and processes of the intima of the aorta and other large vessels.

Pseudomucin

Within the cysts of the simple multiple cystic ovary a pale yellow, clear, translucent, viscid, semi-solid or gelatinous material is sometimes found which is called pseudomucin. In the softer or fluid forms it resembles epithelial mucin very closely. Although on boiling with acids it will reduce Fehling's solution as does mucin, yet it is alkaline in reaction and is not precipitated by acetic acid. Microscopically it is clear, homogeneous and structureless, and in contrast to true mucin takes the acid stain. Similar material is found in some of the cysts of the congenital cystic kidney as well as occasionally in other cysts.

Colloid Degeneration

The term colloid was originally employed to indicate a clear, gelatinous, brown, hyaline material, similar in gross appearance to the colloid of the thyroid gland. With more careful study of the colloid of thyroid gland, it was found that this substance differs chemically from other hyaline materials which have essentially the same gross appearance. Considerable confusion in the employment of this term has resulted and it is considered advisable to restrict it to a material essentially the same as that secreted by the thyroid. The other substances of similar gross appearance may be called hyalin, or, if it be considered desirable to indicate the naked eye appearance, they may be referred to as pseudocolloid.

True colloid has its normal prototype in the thyroid gland. The material secreted by the thyroid epithelium is an albuminous fluid at first, but subsequently, either by inspissation or by the additional secretion of other substance, becomes a clear hyaline material. In the normal thyroid, this material appears perfectly hyalin under the microscope, takes the acid stain, occasionally shows a scalloping of the edges next to the cells and frequently, because of its density, shows a certain amount of marking by the section knife. In the condition known as colloid goiter, the amount of colloid is materially increased and the acini may attain large size. Sometimes the acinus may increase in size so that it becomes visible to the eye as a cyst. In cancers and other tumors of the thyroid, the colloid may be increased, and the metastases of thyroid cancers frequently show identical material. It was formerly supposed that the hyaline material seen in the anterior lobe of the hypophysis is similar to but not identical with the colloid of the thyroid gland, but Wells maintains that only when iodine is given therapeutically does it appear in the hypophyseal colloid. The particular material characteristic of colloid is iodine, which appears in the form of an iodine-containing protein or iodine-protein combination called thyro-iodine. Further refinement of examination shows this to be a thyreoglobulin. The activity of thyroid substance

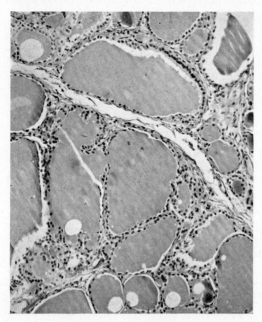

Colloid in colloid goiter.

depends upon the presence of iodine in some such combination.

Hyaline substances grossly resembling colloid may appear in a variety of circumstances. Usually, this pseudocolloid is formed by an inspissation or condensation of some other material. In the kidney, for example, it is not uncommon to find cystic dilatations of the tubules which contain a brown gelatinous material. Histologically, this takes the acid stain somewhat less deeply than do the simple hyaline casts. The same material may be found in the congenital cystic kidney which is a defect of development whereby the kidney is made up largely of numerous cysts containing either pseudocolloid, hyalin, or thin, serous fluid. The pseudomucin of the ovary may also become condensed after a long time and give the gross appearance of pseudocolloid. Numerous other conditions where cysts are formed may lead to the same appearance. This may be true regardless of whether the cysts contain old blood, old serum or old protein material of almost any nature. These substances then apparently represent a condensation of protein material not containing iodine and therefore differentiated sharply from true colloid. Histologically, practically all these materials take the acid stain and show an entirely structureless hyaline character.

Glycogen Infiltration

Glycogen appears in tissues as a hyaline substance with particular staining reactions and with a definite composition. It is the only one of the carbohydrates which can be demonstrated microscopically. It appears in the form of a labile or depot glycogen in the liver and in muscle. The amount in these situations varies with work performed and nutrition supplied. Whether glycogen appears in the cells in pure form only or whether it exists in combination with some other substance is an open question. The fact that, microscopically, the droplets of glycogen are often found in close approximation to, or in combination with, the cell granules leads to the supposition that perhaps there is combination between glycogen and protein. Even if this be true, it seems not to interfere with the lability of the substance or with its staining reactions. In contrast is the stabile form of glycogen which may appear in almost any tissue and is particularly evident in those tissues which are somewhat removed from direct contact with the blood stream, such as cartilage and the upper layers of cutaneous epithelium. Practically any cell in the body may contain glycogen although it may not be demonstrable microscopically.

Glycogen is likely to appear in many places which also show fat, and it is probable that essentially the same causes influence the appearance of both these substances. Glycogen is, however, much more labile than fat and disappears more readily. Studies of glycogen in skeletal muscle show a reduction after work and Richard's study indicates that the same is true of smooth muscle. The curve of disappearance of glycogen shows an abrupt fall after death of the cells or of the body, but in the course of eight or ten hours the decline is more gradual. Whether the enzyme concerned in glycogenesis and in glycolysis is the same or not is of little importance in the present connection, but certainly is of significance in general disturbances of carbohydrate metabolism. In order to demonstrate glycogen in tissue sections, it is necessary to use fixatives, such as alcohol, or watery fixatives saturated with dextrose, in which glycogen is not readily soluble. Embedded in paraffin or celloidin, it is stained brown with iodine. Its intracellular position distinguishes it from amyloid and even after fixation it is soluble in ptyalin or saliva. More useful is the Best carmine stain, which although not absolutely specific (Gierke) stains the homogeneous droplets in the cytoplasm, and sometimes in the nucleus also, a bright red color. Watery fixatives dissolve out the glycogen and leave only vacuoles in the cells. These are indistinguishable, except that when found in the loops of Henle in the kidney their presence is highly suggestive of glycogen infiltration.

In most instances, glycogen infiltration is secondary to other conditions. In inflammation around dead tissue, glycogen is deposited together with an accumulation of fat. Chronic inflammatory tissue of other sorts may contain glycogen. In acute exudative inflammation, the leukocytes in the circulating blood and those which infiltrate the inflamed region are likely to show iodophilic droplets of glycogen infiltration in the cytoplasm. Since embryonal cells are likely to be richer in glycogen than are adult cells, it has been thought that malignant tumors, the cells of which approach embryonal form, are more likely to contain glycogen than benign tumors with their more mature types of cells. This is often but not invariably true; it certainly is not a diagnostic feature. In these states the glycogen does not appear to injure the cells and glycogen infiltration is readily reversible except in glycogen disease.

Glycogen Disease. (von Gierke's disease, glycogen-storage disease and thesaurismosis glycogenica.) This is not simply a storage because the glycogen is fairly well fixed in the tissues and does not entirely dissolve out after prolonged immersion in such watery fixatives as formalin. It appears to be an inherent defect of glycogen metabolism, probably hereditary because of the instances of familial occurrence. There are irregular alterations of carbohydrate metabolism also. One type is manifested by enlargement of the liver, demonstrable clinically, and of the kidneys, a hepatorenal form. It is distinguished from congenital hepatic cirrhosis by the fact that the spleen is not enlarged. The other is characterized by enlargement of the heart, one of the forms of so-called congenital cardiac hypertrophy. These two forms are usually separate and do not occur together. Other organs may be rich in glycogen but are not enlarged. There is no regular involvement of the ductless glands and the cause remains unknown. The disease becomes evident in infancy or early childhood. Although usually fatal, there are cases of survival into adolescence with improvement. Van Creveld gives a full account of the disease.

Glycogen in Diabetes

In diabetes the glycogen is more or less exhausted from the ordinary depots such as the liver and muscles. Nevertheless, tissues which do not ordinarily contain much glycogen are likely to show it in considerable amounts. It may be found in heart muscle, in leukocytes, in capillaries of the brain and in the tissues of the eye. Of particular importance, however, is its presence in the kidney. This situation is fairly common in human diabetes and is also found in experimental diabetes caused by excision of the pancreas and by puncture of the floor of the fourth ventricle. It is seen particularly well in the cells of the loops of Henle, either in the form of numerous small globules or as larger masses which may exceed the size of the nucleus. The presence of large vacuoles in these particular cells, when special methods have not been employed, is almost diagnostic of glycogenic infiltration. With the special stain, the appearance is striking. Recent studies indicate that the epithelium of the convoluted tubules exhibits the glycogen more commonly than the loops of Henle.

Löschke showed that glycogen is synthesized in the epithelium of the capillary loops of the glomeruli, passes into the urine and is reabsorbed in the convoluted tubules. Perhaps subsequent reabsorption occurs in the cells of Henle's loops. Klestadt suggests that the excretion of large quantities of sugar in the urine, rather than the disease complex diabetes, determines the appearance of glycogen in the kidney. Klestadt's review of the literature would indicate that the loops of Henle are more frequently involved in human diabetes than are the convoluted tubules. The reason for the accumulation of glycogen in cells other than those of the glycogen depots and particularly in the cells of the kidney remains as yet unexplained. Von Gierke states in summary that the content of glycogen in the cells is dependent upon the type of cell, the state of nutrition and the nature of the injury.

Amyloid

The principal observable difference between amyloid and other hyalins is found in special staining reactions. In the gross specimen the application of iodine in watery solution (Lugol's solution) imparts a deep brown color to the glassy material. Subsequent treatment with dilute sulfuric acid deepens the color to reddish-brown, brownish-blue or blue-black. For microscopic sections, the metachromatic aniline dyes and Congo red are employed, as indicated below.

Classification. According to Reimann and associates, amyloid may be classified as (a) primary, (b) secondary, (c) tumor forming amyloid, and (d) that associated with myeloma. For the sake of clarity, secondary amyloidosis is discussed before the primary and tumor-forming types.

SECONDARY AMYLOIDOSIS. Most frequently, amyloid is secondary to other disease, particularly chronic suppuration. Usually this is the result of chronic tuberculosis of lungs, bones and joints, but chronic pyogenic osteomyelitis is often a cause. It may also be secondary to nonsuppurative tuberculosis, to syphilis, both congenital and acquired, to leprosy, to tumors, infected or not, to chronic nephritis, to hepatic cirrhosis, and rarely to other diseases. The distribution of secondary amyloidosis is one feature that distinguishes it from primary amyloidosis. It affects principally spleen, kidneys, liver and adrenals, but may also be present in other organs. The staining reactions given above are usually typical. As a rule, there are no reactions to its presence in the tissues.

Amyloidosis accompanies about 7 per cent of cases of MULTIPLE MYELOMA of bones and may be said to be secondary to that disease. It may occur in the usual secondary distribution, but 12 cases are on record in which it looked like the primary form (Tarr and Ferris).

PRIMARY AMYLOIDOSIS. Not infrequently small tumor-like nodules, so-called AMYLOID TUMORS, which contain a glassy substance, usually stainable by the special dyes but often atypically, occur in the larynx. Rarely, they may also be found in the base of the tongue, the nasal septum, trachea and bronchi. Local amyloid deposits have been reported in the bladder and in certain tumors of endothelial origin. Sometimes incorrectly interpreted as primary and local in amyloidosis of spleen or of lymph nodes in the drainage region of suppurative disease, these are probably only the first stages of what would prove to be widespread secondary amyloidosis.

Widespread primary amyloidosis is rare and is characterized by the deposition of amyloid, often massive, in mesodermal tissues, such as skeletal muscles, joints, bones, subcutaneous tissues, smooth muscle including the media of arteries, serous surfaces, etc. The organs characteristically affected in secondary amyloidosis usually escape. In Koletsky and Stecher's patient, one of the clinically conspicuous features was massive amyloid in the lips and tongue. The staining reactions of primary amyloid are much less regular than those of secondary amyloid. None of the causes of secondary amyloidosis is observed. Pearson, Rice and Dickens found that there may be reaction to the presence of primary amyloid in the form of lymphocytic infiltration and the production of foreign-body giant cells, together with the presence of amyloid rings about fat cells.

Grossly, amyloid is homogeneous and glassy in appearance and transmits the color of the organ in which it is found. Microscopically, it is a hyalin which takes the acid stain. It occurs principally in the small blood vessels, but it may be found in the aorta and endocardium, and in the primary form may be observed in almost any mesoblastic tissue (Reimann, et al.). In capillaries the amyloid is deposited immediately outside the endothelial lining (Ohmori). In slightly larger vessels it occurs in the connective tissues immediately outside the endothelium, whereas in arteries and veins it is found between the muscle cells of the media. It does not occur within cells, except rarely when it is broken down and taken up by phagocytes, often in the form of multinucleated giant cells. In order to identify it in tissue sections special

PLATE II

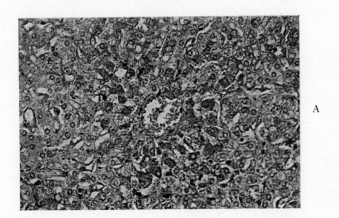

A

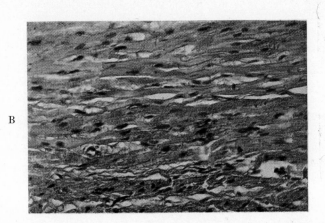

B

A. Heart in glycogen disease, Best carmine stain.
B. Liver in glycogen disease, Best carmine stain.

stains are often necessary. When microscopic sections are stained by such metachromatic

In the kidney, the change is seen first in the capillary loops of the glomerular tufts.

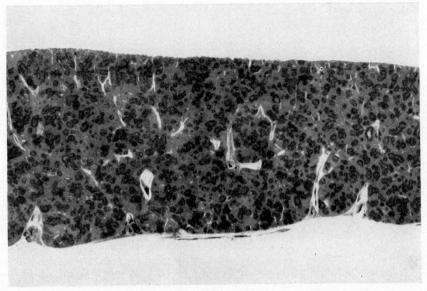

Cross section of a portion of the spleen, stained with Lugol's solution and dilute sulfuric acid to show amyloid—the so-called Sago spleen.

aniline dyes as methyl violet, aniline gentian violet, methyl green, etc., the amyloid is stained some shade of red and the tissues the color of the dye. Congo red has an affinity for amyloid, and its disappearance from the blood after intravenous injection is used as a clinical test (Lipstein).

The amyloid deposit is enabled to injure cells because it accumulates in amounts sufficient to produce pressure upon surrounding cells and thereby lead to atrophy of these cells, or the amount of amyloid may be so great as definitely to limit the internal caliber of the affected blood vessels, thereby leading to cloudy swelling and fatty degeneration and atrophy or necrosis, because of the limitation of nutrition. Cellular atrophy is best seen in the liver, whereas the nutritional changes, such as fatty degeneration and cloudy swelling, are best seen in the kidney.

In the spleen the amyloid is found first in the media of the central arteriole of the follicles. Subsequently, it appears in the follicles as a network made up of very coarse fibers which finally collect to form a solid mass of amyloid. Still later it extends out through the pulp of the spleen, usually along the walls of the splenic sinuses.

It is also likely to be found in the walls of the arteriæ rectæ of the pyramids and, to a

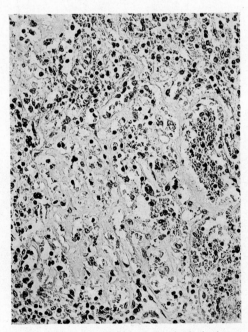

Slight deposit of amyloid in walls of splenic sinuses and a vein.

less extent, in the interlobular arterioles of the cortex. In advanced cases, amyloid may be found lying under the epithelial cells of the tubule, involving the basement membrane.

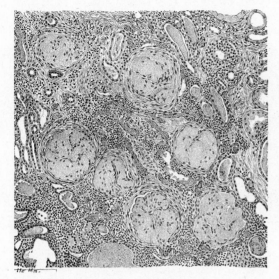

Amyloid in capillary tufts of renal glomeruli.

In the liver, amyloid in most cases affects primarily small arteries and veins of the capsule of Glisson. It is likely to be most extensive, however, in the sinusoids of the lobules. Here it appears immediately outside

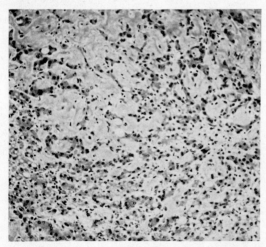

Amyloid of liver, situated between atrophic parenchymal cells.

the endothelium of the sinusoids, particularly in the middle part of the lobule. As it becomes more extensive the central and peripheral parts of the lobule also are affected. As the condition advances the pressure atrophy of the liver cells becomes more and more marked and amyloid from adjacent sinusoids may fuse to form a solid mass of considerable size.

Amyloid of the heart is most likely to be found in the subendothelial connective tissue of the endocardium of the right atrium. It may occasionally be found in the capillaries of the myocardium of the ventricular walls.

The intestines are affected particularly in the muscular coat, but occasionally amyloid may be found very sharply defined in the capillary loops of the villi.

In the adrenals it appears particularly in the capillaries of the cortex.

Grossly, organs the seat of amyloid disease are usually considerably enlarged, firm, show a tense capsule and a rounding of any sharp edges. Both on the outer surface and in the cross section the organ is pale, due principally to the limitation of blood supply brought about by the extent of the amyloid process. The organ cuts with slightly increased resistance and shows a cross section which neither bulges nor retracts unless other changes are present. This cross section is firm and nonfriable, showing a generalized glassy appearance in the more extensive cases. In certain instances, which will be mentioned, amyloid may appear as small points of glassy translucent material which transmit the color of the underlying organ. When the process is extensive, the organ resembles somewhat fresh hog fat and therefore the term "lardaceous" has been applied. In the cross section of the liver, the large, pale, firm organ may show irregularly distributed points of amyloid, which in association with hyperemia of the central zones may produce the appearance called "nutmeg amyloid liver."

The spleen in this disease is large and firm, but is not more pallid than is normally the case. To the naked eye the earlier stages of amyloid, affecting the follicles, show numerous small areas of glassy material transmitting the red color of the spleen. These small masses resemble boiled sago grains and the organ has been called the "sago spleen." In later stages the spleen may be diffusely involved and become the "lardaceous spleen." The kidney of amyloid is a large, pale, firm kidney which to ordinary inspection shows nothing characteristic of the amyloid. In any of these instances it is customary to apply gross staining in order to make the diagnosis of amyloid. Usually this is done by the application of Lugol's solution. If the organ be very bloody, it is well to wash with dilute acetic acid in order to remove most of the blood before applying Lugol's solution. The amyloid under these circumstances takes the iodine stain in the form of a deep reddish-brown color (mahogany brown). In the liver and spleen this can be seen very readily. In the kidney, however, it requires close inspection to make out the amyloid deposit in the glomeruli. In doubtful cases it is sometimes necessary to apply dilute sulfuric acid also, whereupon the changes mentioned above appear, namely, a brownish-red, deep blue, or brownish-black color. Occasionally, amyloid which gives neither of these reactions is found. In these instances it is usual to apply the methyl violet reaction to frozen sections, although the same reaction can be performed with the gross cross section. This can be stained intravitally by the use of Congo red or trypan blue.

The Nature of Amyloid. The exact chemical composition of amyloid is unknown. It responds positively to xanthoproteic tests and is of protein nature, but a purified protein has never been isolated. Hass and Schulz recovered two slightly different proteins from secondary amyloid and by physical methods found that there are three varieties of amyloid. Tentatively, it seems that amyloid is not a single substance and that there are variations in its composition. It is not starch-like as suggested by the name amyloid given by Virchow and there is no proof that it contains carbohydrates at all. The protein material is basic because it takes acid stains. It is said to be rich in amino-acids and in some respects to resemble gelatin, but the latter contains more monamino-acid nitrogen. Kuczynski found a rich content of tyrosin. For a long time it was thought that amyloid is a compound of protein and chondroitin-sulfuric acid, the latter derived from destroyed tissues, especially cartilage. When particles of amyloid were carefully picked out of organs, no chondroitin-sulfuric acid could be found even although it was present in the surrounding tissue. As a matter of fact, sulfur has not been identified in amyloid. Nevertheless the possible relationship of chondroitin-sulfuric acid and amyloid is still under study (Ehrström). Hass and Schulz concluded that amyloid has a matrix of protein, which may become complex by combination with other substances in the body fluids.

Numerous attempts have been made to produce amyloid experimentally in animals. Repeated failure has followed the use of chondroitin-sulfuric acid, either isolated and used pure or as a sodium salt, or in the form of cartilage and mucin. The feeding of flowers of sulfur was also ineffective. The same is true of nucleoprotein of pus, and of Witte's peptone. The production of long-continued suppuration by bacteria such as *Staphylococcus aureus*, or by the use of oil of turpentine has led to the formation of amyloid in experimental animals. Suppuration, however, is not essential, since the intravenous injection of bacteria not leading to pus formation, as well as the injection of bacterial toxins may be followed by the formation of amyloid. It is stated that injection of sterile pus and of certain ferments may lead to amyloid deposit. Although staphylococcal infections are important in man, the use of these organisms experimentally has led to conflicting reports. Bailey was successful with the use of *Bacillus coli communior*. Thomas has found a high incidence in rabbits experimentally infected with bovine tubercle bacilli, especially in the presence of advanced caseation. Amyloid is common in horses used for the production of immune sera.

Smetana suggests that the reticulo-endothelial system is active in the formation of amyloid, and Loeschcke believes that a reaction between leukocyte proteins and antibody occurs in relation to this system. Hass and Schulz, however, think that amyloid is not an antigen-antibody precipitate, because it is deposited slowly and other chemical substances may enter into intimate combination with it. Leupold had previously reported a positive Abderhalden reaction between amyloid as a substrate and the blood serum of patients with chronic suppurative disease. On this slender evidence he built up the theory that the presence of a specific protein stimulates the production of an enzyme which transforms the protein into amyloid.

In regard to the use of turpentine and other nonbacterial substances, there is the possibility that infection or destruction of tissue, or both, may have been an accompaniment, and any amyloid found may be due to these secondary factors rather than the agent employed. Nevertheless, when bacteria or toxins are administered intravenously, such tissue destruction is not likely to occur and yet amyloid may be formed.

Repeated injections of nutrose (sodium caseinate) into mice produce amyloid. A high carbohydrate diet appears to inhibit and a high protein diet to favor the incidence among the animals (Ku and Simon). This type as well as that in serum horses may be destroyed by organization, but it is not certain that this occurs in man. Leupold's statement that amyloid may be produced in vitro by the action of dilute sulfuric acid upon excised spleen requires confirmation. In summary it can be said that amyloid is a protein complex, differentiated chiefly by its staining properties.

Origin of Amyloid. It is now generally believed that amyloid is an infiltration rather than a degeneration. The origin and mode of deposit have been extensively studied without arrival at definite conclusions. Theories to the effect that it is derived from iodophilic granules of leukocytes or coalescence of erythrocytes are not adequately supported. The fact that amyloid does not contain chondroitin-sulfuric acid has led to abandonment of the idea that amyloid is the result of conjugation of this acid, derived from destroyed cartilage, with intercellular protein or cement substance. This applies also to the belief that suppuration or other destructive process leads to formation of a protein precursor of amyloid, circulating in the body fluids and precipitated as a gel by local accumulation of acid. There is probably some disturbance of protein metabolism, but its nature is not as yet known. The fact that animals, especially horses, used in the preparation of antisera, frequently show amyloidosis, has led to the belief that amyloid is the product of an antigen-antibody reaction. Letterer proposes the hypothesis that the antigen is a liquefied native protein, capable of stimulating specific antibody production and that the precipitate is in the form of amyloid. He claims that the antibody is present in the animals before the deposit of the amyloid and disappears as precipitation occurs. This does not explain the situation of the deposit, its occurrence without destructive disease, nor the primary forms. The deposit of amyloid in relation to endothelium, the difficulty of demonstrating reticulo-endothelial cells in the regions of deposit, the delay in appearance of amyloid after blockade of the reticulo-endothelial system, all suggest the importance of this group of cells, despite the variable results which accompany splenectomy. The situation of certain primary amyloid deposits, distant from capillaries, suggests that perverted fibroblastic activity may be significant (Warren). The exact mechanism of this cellular activity is unknown. The protein content of amyloid has, for a long time, suggested an abnormality of protein metabolism. Various observations have incriminated globulin. Certain of the diseases to which amyloidosis is secondary are accompanied by hyperglobulinemia. The production of antisera may be accompanied by increase in globulin of the blood. Prolonged repeated vaccination with bacterial antigens often produces hyperglobulinemia and in at least one case has been followed by amyloidosis. Eklund and Reimann have demonstrated persistent hyperglobulinemia in rabbits, in which amyloid was produced by injections of sodium caseinate. Similar results are reported by Dick and Leiter, following injections of certain strains of streptococci. Thus it would appear that cellular activity, especially of the reticulo-endothelial system, and increased protein content of the blood are established, and that these two factors operating together have much to do with the production of amyloid. The problem will probably be not entirely settled until the composition of amyloid is accurately determined.

REFERENCES

Bailey, C. H.: The Production of Amyloid Disease and Chronic Nephritis in Rabbits by Repeated Intravenous Injections of Living Colon Bacilli, Jour. Exper. Med., **23**: 773, 1916.

Bergmann, G. von: Das Enstehung der Fettsucht. Handbuch Biochem., **4 (2)**: 208, 1910.

Best, C. H.: The Role of the Liver in the Metabolism of Carbohydrate and Fat, Lancet, **1**: 1155, 1216, 1274, 1934; *see also* McHenry, E. W.: Vitamin B_1 and Fatty Livers, Jour. Physiol., **89**: 287, 1937.

——: The Significance of Choline as a Dietary Factor, Science, **94**: 524, 1941.

Bradley, H. C., H. Fletcher, M. Morse, and J. Taylor: Studies of Autolysis, Jour. Biol. Chem., **21**: 209, 1915; **22**: 113, 1915; **25**: 201; 261; 363, 1916; **29**: 281, 1917; **44**: 553, 1920.

Butt, E. M.: Experimental Subacute Amyloid Nephrosis in Rabbits, Arch. Path., 1: 859, 1930.

Chor, H., and R. E. Dolkart: Experimental Muscular Dystrophy of the Guinea Pig, Arch. Path., 27: 497, 1939.

Cutter, W. D., and W. J. Gies: The Composition of Tendon Mucoid, Amer. Jour. Physiol., 6: 155, 1901.

Davidman, A., and D. H. Dolley: Cloudy Swelling a Process of Stimulation, Jour. Med. Res., 42: 515, 1921-22.

Dible, J. H.: Is Fatty Degeneration of the Heart Muscle a Phanerosis? Jour. Path. and Bact., 39: 197, 1934.

Dible, J. H., and W. W. Gerrard: The Source of Fat in Experimentally Produced Fatty Degeneration of the Heart, ibid., 46: 77, 1938.

Dible, J. H., and J. D. Hay: The Nature of Fatty Change in the Kidneys, ibid., 51: 1, 1940.

Dick, G. F., and L. Leiter: Experimental Amyloidosis and Hyperglobulinemia, Trans. Asso. Amer. Phys., 52: 246, 1937.

Dietrich, A., and J. Kleeberg: Die Störungen des zellulären Fettstoffwechsels, Ergeb. Allg. Path. Anat., 202: 913, 1924.

Dragstedt, L. R.: The Present Status of Lipocaic, Jour. Amer. Med. Asso., 114: 29, 1940.

Duthie, E. S.: Mitochondrial Changes in Autoplastic Liver Transplants, Jour. Path. and Bact., 41: 311, 1935.

Ehrström, M. C.: Chondroitinschwefelsäuren, Heparin, Albuminurie, Amyloid und Serumproteine, Acta Med. Scandinav., 101: 551, 1939.

Eklund, C. M., and H. A. Reimann: The Etiology of Amyloid Disease, with a Note on Experimental Renal Amyloidosis, Arch. Path., 21: 1, 1936.

Fischer, M. H.: Fats and Fatty Degeneration, New York, Wiley, 1917.

Fishback, D. K., and H. R. Fishback: Studies of Experimental Muscle Degeneration, Amer. Jour. Path., 8: 193, 211, 1932.

Foot, N. C.: Ueber das Wachstum von Knochenmark in vitro, Beitr. Path. Anat. u. Allg. Path., 53: 446, 1912. The Growth of Chicken Bone Marrow in Vitro, etc., Jour. Exper. Med., 17: 43, 1913.

Fricke, O., H. Groll, and E. Meyer: Chemische Untersuchungen zur Frage der trüben Schwellung, Beitr. Path. Anat. u. Allg. Path., 83: 135, 1930.

v. Gierke, E.: Physiologische und pathologische Glykogenablagerung, Ergeb. Allg. Path. u. Path. Anat., 11²: 871, 1907.

————: Ueber ein Meckelsches Divertikel mit Magenschleimhaut. Zugleich über die mit Bestscher Glykogenfärbung sich rot färbenden Magenschleimepithelien, Zentralbl. Allg. Path. u. Path. Anat., 71: 81, 1939.

Goodpasture, E. W.: Crystalline Hyalin, Jour. Med. Res., 35: 259, 1916.

Hass, G., and R. Z. Schulz: Amyloid: I. Methods of Isolating Amyloid from Other Tissue Elements, Arch. Path., 30: 240, 1940.

Hein, A.: Ueber die Entstehung und Bedeutung der hyalinen Tropfen in den Hauptstücken der Niere auf Grund von Experimenten an Salamandra Maculosa, Virchow's Arch. Path. Anat., 301: 339, 1938.

Johnson, F., and H. Smetana: Experimental Colloid Droplets in Renal Epithelium (Abstract), Amer. Jour. Path., 17: 635, 1941.

Klestadt, W.: Ueber Glykogenablagerung. Ergeb. Allg. Path. u. Path. Anat., 15²: 349, 1911.

Koletsky, S., and R. M. Stecher: Primary Systemic Amyloidosis. Involvement of Cardiac Valves, Joints and Bones with Pathological Fracture of Femur, Arch. Path., 27: 267, 1939.

Ku, D. Y., and M. A. Simon: Influence of Various Diets upon Experimental Amyloidosis in Mice, Arch. Path., 18: 245, 1934.

Kuczynski, M. H.: Neue Beiträge zur Lehre vom Amyloid, Klin. Wochenschr., 2: 2193, 1923.

Kunstadter, R. H.: Adiposogenital Dystrophy, Jour. Amer. Med. Asso., 117: 1947, 1941.

Lauter, S.: Zur Genese der Fettsucht, Deutsch. Arch. Klin. Med., 150: 315, 1926.

Leathes, J. B.: The Fats, Monograph on Biochemistry, London, 1910.

————: The Functions of the Liver in Relation to the Metabolism of Fats. Harvey Lectures, Philadelphia, Lippincott, 1908-09.

Letterer, E.: Neue Untersuchungen über die Entstehung des Amyloids, Virchow's Arch. Path. Anat., 293: 34, 1934.

Leupold, E.: Amyloid und Hyalin, Ergebn. Allg. Path. u. Path. Anat., 21: 120, 1925-26.

Levene, P. A.: Hexosamines, Their Derivatives and Mucins and Mucoids. Monographs Rockefeller Inst. Med. Res., No. 18, 1922.

Lewis, P. A.: Hemorrhagic Hepatitis in Antitoxin Horses, Jour. Med. Res., 15: 449, 1906.

Lewis, W. H.: Degeneration Granules and Vacuoles in the Fibroblasts of Chick Embryos Cultivated in Vitro, Bull. Johns Hopkins Hosp., 30: 81, 1919.

Linoissier, G.: Les Lipoides dans l'Infection et dans l'Immunité, Paris, 1920.

Lipstein, S.: An Evaluation of the Congo-Red Test for Amyloidosis, Amer. Jour. Med. Sci., 195: 205, 1938.

Loeschcke, H.: Vorstellungen über das Wesen von Hyalin und Amyloid auf Grund von serologischen Versuchen, Beit. Path. Anat. u. Allg. Path., 77: 231, 1927.

Loevenhart, A. S.: On the Relation of Lipase to Fat Metabolism-lipogenesis, Amer. Jour. Physiol., 6: 331, 1902.

Lucké, B., and M. McCutcheon: Reversible and Irreversible Swelling of Living and Dead Cells, Arch. Path. and Lab. Med., 2: 846, 1926.

————: The Effect of Injury on Cellular Permeability to Water, Arch. Path., 10: 662, 1930.

Mallory, F. B.: Cirrhosis of the Liver. Five Different Types of Lesions from Which It May Arise, Bull. Johns Hopkins Hosp., 22: 69, 1911.

Münter, O. Ueber Hyalin im Magen und Darm sein Vorkommen, seine Bedeutung und Entstehung, Virchow's Arch. Path. Anat., 198: 105, 1909.

Ohmori, D.: Bedeutung der Membrana propria der Glomerulusschlingen in der Nierenpathologie Virchow's Arch. Path. Anat., 234: 53, 1921.

Pack, G. T., and A. H. Davis: Burns, Philadelphia and London, Lippincott, 1930.

Pappenheimer, A. M.: The Pathology of Nutritional Muscular Dystrophy in Young Rats, Amer. Jour. Path., 15: 179, 1939.

Pearson, B., M. M. Rice, and K. L. Dickens: Primary Systematic Amyloidosis: Report of Two Cases in Negroes, with Special Reference to Certain Histologic Criteria for Diagnosis, Arch. Path., 32: 1, 1941.

Pratt, J. H.: On the Causes of Cardiac Insufficiency, Johns Hopkins Hosp. Bull., 15: 301, 1904.

Richard, G.: Ueber den Einfluss der Funktion auf den Glykogengehalt der glatten Muskulatur, Beitr. Path. Anat. u. Allg. Path., 61: 514, 1916.

Schmidt, M. B.: Referat über Amyloid, Verhand. Deutsch. Path. Gesellsch., 7: 2, 1904.

Schmorl, G.: Pathologisch-histologischen Untersuchungsmethoden, Leipzig, 1914.

Simms, H. S., and N. P. Stillman: Production of Fat Granules and of Degeneration in Cultures of Adult Tissue by Agents from Blood Plasma, Arch. Path., 23: 316, 1937.

Smetana, H.: Relation of the Reticulo-endothelial System to the Formation of Amyloid, Jour. Exper. Med., 45: 619, 1927.

Tarr, L., and H. W. Ferris: Multiple Myeloma Associated with Nodular Deposits of Amyloid in the Muscles and Joints with Bence-Jones Proteinuria, Arch. Int. Med., 64: 820, 1939.

Thomas, R. M.: Occurrence of Amyloidosis in Rabbits Experimentally Infected with Tuberculosis, Amer. Jour. Path., 10: 419, 1934.

Van Vreveld, S.: Glycogen Disease, Medicine, 18: 1, 1939.

Warren, S.: Generalized Amyloidosis of the Muscular Systems, Amer. Jour. Path., 6: 161, 1930.

Weld, J. T., W. C. Von Glahn, and L. C. Mitchell: Production of Cytoplasmic Inclusions in Liver Cells of Rats Injected with Certain Proteins, Proc. Soc. Exper. Biol. and Med., 48: 229, 1941.

Wells, H. G.: Chemical Pathology, 5th ed., Philadelphia, Saunders, 1925.

——: Adipose Tissue, a Neglected Subject, Jour. Amer. Med. Asso., 114: 2177, 2284, 1940.

Wirtschafter, Z. T., and E. D. Schwartz: Note on Localized Lipoid Atrophy in Diabetes, Amer. Jour. Med. Sci., 202: 880, 1941.

4

Necrosis and Somatic Death

INTRODUCTION

Death signifies the complete cessation of functional and metabolic activities of the cell. In unicellular organisms death does not naturally occur because these bodies divide to form two, or sometimes more, new individuals from the original cell. Such reproduction does not leave as a product the dead body of any predecessor. As a group, such organisms may then be regarded as immortal. Accidents of various kinds may kill certain individuals or groups of individuals, but the main stem goes on uninterrupted. In addition, life may be preserved in the form of spores of bacteria, and fungi and seeds of plants, without any apparent metabolic activity. In multicellular organisms, reproduction depends upon the activity of a germ plasm. The germ plasm may be regarded as immortal in the same sense as are unicellular organisms. Each germ cell is the descendant of a previous germ cell and represents the ancestral strain, although during each generation its multipli-cation gives rise to the somatic cells of the individual. It is therefore essential in the consideration of death to differentiate between germ plasm and somatoplasm. The latter constitutes the body of the multicellular organism. Applying this principle to man it is seen that the family line is represented by the germ plasm and the individual members of the family represented by the somatoplasm.

In multicellular organisms, it is possible to differentiate between three forms of death. SOMATIC DEATH indicates death of the entire organism. NECROBIOSIS signifies death of certain groups of cells and replacement by new cells in the normal course of bodily activity. This is seen particularly in the skin of man where the desquamating superficial epithelium dies, is cast off and is replaced by new cells arising from the lower layers. It seems certain that essentially the same process goes on in connection with practically all the cells of the body with the exception of highly differentiated cells such as those of the central nervous system. The third form of death in the body is referred to as necrosis. NECROSIS indicates death of a group of cells or a localized part of an organ or tissue in connection with the living body.

SOMATIC DEATH

In normal life all the organs and tissues of the body co-operate in the preservation of life. Certain organs and tissues, however, are absolutely essential. These include the respiratory system, the cardiovascular system, and the central nervous system. Complete failure of function of any of these systems leads to death of the entire organism. Fundamentally, of course, the immediate cause of death is failure of circulation, because upon this function depend all the other activities of the body. Failure of the central nervous system not only leads to deficient co-ordination of various bodily functions, but results in death because of removal of those stimuli which lead to cardiac and respiratory activity. Failure of the respiratory system brings about cessation of the entire mechanism upon which depend oxidation and removal of carbon dioxide. With any of these functions removed, therefore, death must ensue. Certain other organs are essential to life, including the liver, kidneys and adrenals, but in case of their ablation death follows only after an interval of several days. Ligation of the ureters, or the removal of a kidney or adrenal when the other of the pair is hypoplastic or absent, are guarded against by careful surgeons. It has even been said that a human liver was removed because it was mistaken for a tumor.

Signs of Somatic Death

It is the duty of the physician to be certain that the patient is dead before he makes out the death certificate. Deep coma may simulate death and differentiation may require careful observation. Remarkable cases of restoration to life after what seemed to be death, if they ever do occur outside the boundaries of romantic writing, depend upon inadequate determination of the criteria of death.

Cessation of Circulation and Respiration. The criteria are primarily cessation of cardiac and respiratory activity. Within a short time, the cessation of functional and metabolic processes leads to the secondary changes which include algor mortis (cooling of the body), rigor mortis (postmortem rigidity of muscles), livor mortis (dependent lividity), clotting of blood, desiccation of the body and putrefaction. The textbooks of legal medicine give details of tests for death. It is reported that the San Francisco Board of Health has recommended certain observations as follows: I: cessation of respiration as determined by (a) stethoscope over larynx, (b) mirror held in front of nose to observe possible condensation of moisture and (c) movement of air currents against a wisp of cotton placed in the nares; II: cessation of heart beat determined by stethoscope on precordium; III: cessation of circulation as determined by (a) opacity of hands when held near a strong light, (b) failure of a bleb to appear on the skin after application of burning heat and (c) lividity

and dependent discoloration; IV: loss of body heat; V: rigor mortis; VI: desiccation as indicated in coarseness of cornea (not fully reliable, nor is the state of the pupil); VII: decomposition.

Sudden and unexpected death may be due to a variety of conditions affecting persons already ill or those who seem to be perfectly well, as well as those subjected to violent injury. In the last group, the cause of death may be quite evident, but in the former groups, a knowledge of the natural history of diseases and of their complications is necessary to arrive at any reasonable judgment as to cause of death; and no real conclusion can be reached without autopsy. There are often important relations to insurance and legal aspects. (See Moritz.)

Algor Mortis. Cooling of the body occurs as the result of the gradual equalization of its temperature with that of the surrounding medium. It has been shown that a dead human body in the nude state, under ordinary conditions cools at the rate of about 1° F. per hour. The temperature of the interior of the body, as indicated by rectal thermometer, equals that of the exterior in about 40 hours after death. Extremely cold outside temperatures may hasten, and warm temperatures retard cooling of the body; a thick layer of fat may retard cooling. Occasionally death is followed by a great increase in body temperature. This may occur following death from acute infectious disease, certain diseases of the nervous system, as well as death from certain other causes. Such an increase, however, is of short duration and probably depends upon active metabolism continuing after death without that element of radiation which depends upon circulation of the blood and body fluids.

Rigor mortis signifies the stiffening of muscles after death. It begins first in the involuntary muscles such as the heart. It usually affects the voluntary muscles within 12 hours after death, and usually passes off in three or four days. It is seen first in the muscles of the head, particularly the eyelids and the muscles of the jaw, and thence progresses to the muscles of the neck and downward over the body. Many times, however, the arms are involved last. As a rule, the flexors predominate over the extensors.

The appearance of rigor is hastened by

warm temperature and retarded by cold. Its disappearance is likely to be retarded by cold and hastened by heat. Metabolic activity at the time of death appears to play an important part in producing this condition. Accordingly, individuals who die from acute infectious fevers and those who are killed in the midst of great muscular activity are likely to show rigor mortis earlier than others. Heavily muscled individuals are likely to show early and pronounced rigor. Poisons such as strychnine and veratrum viride are likely to lead to marked rigor which may persist for a very long time. Ordinarily the rapid onset of rigor is followed by delayed disappearance.

When rigor disappears from a corpse or when it is broken by force it does not return again. Although it was formerly supposed that rigor represented a sort of tetanic contraction of muscles, not differing from the physiologic and probably dependent upon the removal of inhibition, at the present time there is no doubt that this condition represents a chemical change in the muscle. By vital staining it can be shown that in contraction of muscles during life there is no important histologic change, whereas in rigor mortis there is a definite precipitation of protein. Two substances can be extracted from muscle, myosinogen and paramyosinogen, both of which are changed into insoluble myosin at low temperature. This coagulation, however, is not identical with blood clotting. Proteins play a certain rôle but apparently the presence of acid is of the utmost importance. The normally amphoteric muscle becomes slightly acid when at work and the same is true when its circulation is occluded. This is due very largely to the formation of sarcolactic acid. The formation of myosin is probably a part of, or accompanied by, certain physical changes in the protein of the muscles. Wells states that the presence of the sarcolactic acid is sufficient to cause a swelling of the muscle colloid, which may be so great as to destroy the structure of the muscle cell and even be a cause of waxy degeneration of Zenker's hyalin. Collip finds that the point of maximum precipitation is between 6.3 and 6.6 index, which corresponds to the point at which muscle goes into rigor. Further acidification redissolves the precipitate. The swelling is due to the hydrophilic acid-protein and is reduced as the acidity is further increased, due to loss of hydrophilic property. Thus, as time goes on, the increasing acidity leads to loss of rigor. Neither postmortem decomposition nor autolysis is responsible primarily for loss of rigor.

Livor mortis is a red discoloration of dependent parts of the body due to settling of the blood into these parts. It is seen in the form of diffuse or localized reddening in the dependent superficial parts, and as hyperemia in dependent organs or parts within the body. On cutting into such areas the blood escapes from the vessels in fluid form, in contradistinction to hemorrhage into a part; in hemorrhage, the blood does not flow readily when the part is cut owing to the fact that it has clotted. Histologically, it is not difficult to distinguish between the simple hyperemia of livor mortis and the extravasation of blood in hemorrhage. If the position of the body be changed, the blood will slowly flow from the old into the newly dependent parts. After death, the blood corpuscles are dissolved with varying degrees of rapidity so that finally hemoglobin is found in solution in the blood serum. This material diffuses readily through, and visibly stains, the lighter colored tissues. This is particularly true of heart valves, and the lining of great vessels and of the larger serous cavities. Hemolysis and diffusion of hemoglobin are hastened particularly in death from infectious diseases, more especially when infection is due to hemolytic bacteria. The change is seen very strikingly in death from gas gangrene. There is, however, little reason for believing that such staining of tissues by hemoglobin occurs before death. For all practical purposes it is to be looked upon as a postmortem change.

Postmortem clotting of the blood appears very early. In cases of slow death, clotting may probably begin before death actually occurs; in these circumstances the clots are referred to as agonal. The postmortem clot is most commonly of the type called "cruor clot" or "currant jelly" clot, in which all the blood elements are coagulated in one mass; this type of clot has a characteristic bright red color and jelly-like consistence. In cases of slow death and in other circumstances where the clotting does not proceed very rapidly, the red blood cells sink to the lower part of the clot and the leukocytes, because of their lower specific gravity, accumulate in the upper part as a yellow, translucent mass. This is particularly well seen in the heart where the upper layer of clot, namely, that nearest the anterior chest wall, is likely to be fairly firm and of light yellow color. The consistency and color give it the name "chicken fat" clot. Some cases of rather slow death show a whipping out of fibrin by the chordæ tendineæ of the heart which produces a firm, somewhat friable, white, fibrin clot. Postmortem clotting and agonal clotting differ from antemortem clotting in a variety of ways, but the fact that the portmortem clot is not adherent to the vessel walls is particularly to be noticed. Sometimes the clot may, of course, be rather firmly formed about the chordæ tendineæ and papillary muscles of the heart. In these instances, it can readily be seen, however, that this is simply due to clot formation and not the result of adhesion to the heart wall. In the vessels the distinction is very readily made, but there may occasionally be confusion because of the difficulty in withdrawing long clots from smaller branches of blood vessels. The differentiation is more fully considered in the discussion of thrombosis.

Desiccation of certain parts of the body is very common after death. This is particularly true in the cornea of the eye and the fluid of the anterior chamber. The cornea becomes dry, glazed, and because of sinking of the fluid into the back of the eye, becomes wrinkled. Similar dryness of surfaces may be seen over wounds and abrasions or in other situations where the skin has disappeared or is extremely thin. Only rarely is drying of the tissues seen in the internal parts of the body. Occasionally, however, in marked emphysema of the lung, the lung itself may be dry and the dryness may be noticed in adjacent parts of the pericardium.

Putrefaction of the dead body is due to the entrance into the tissues of the rapidly multiplying saprophytic organisms of the intestinal canal. The growth of these organisms results in softening and putrefaction of tissues and the formation of numerous gases, particularly the offensive hydrogen sulfide. As has been pointed out in the chapter on pigmentation, these gases may alter body pigments so as to produce various color changes. The most prominent of these colors is the green discoloration which appears over the abdomen, due to interaction of hydrogen sulfide with the iron of blood and other tissue to form the greenish-blue iron sulfide. As has been said above, methemoglobin may be formed by the action of hydrogen sulfide; hematin may appear and other pigments are occasionally encountered. Putrefaction is retarded by cold and accelerated by warmth. It is also retarded by the use of chemicals such as formalin and arsenic. If obligate or facultative saprophytes gain access to the blood stream before death, decomposition is likely to proceed with great rapidity. This is seen particularly well in cases of gas gangrene. Gas formation in connection with decomposition of this sort is very rich and organs, particularly the liver, may become actually foamy because of the presence of bubbles of gas in the tissue. The presence of such foamy organs is practically diagnostic of the presence of the organisms of gas gangrene, and can be produced very readily by injecting a culture into a living animal, killing the animal and placing it for a few hours in an incubator.

Autolysis

Digestive glands secrete ferments which during life produce decomposition of food products and after death are likely to digest the organs themselves. This is especially well seen in the stomach where, if the body be examined a sufficiently long time after death, or if conditions of warmth be such that digestion may proceed actively, the lining mucosa of the stomach or even the entire wall shows softening and disintegration. The same may be true, but to a lesser extent, in the small intestine. The pancreas frequently shows marked digestion.

Autolysis is that process whereby tissues undergo digestion without the presence of bacteria or of ferments introduced from without. Two methods are employed to demonstrate autolysis: (1) the antiseptic method, (2) the aseptic method. The method of Salkowski, which is commonly employed, depends upon the employment of antiseptics. The organs are ground in a grinder and placed in a sterile vessel with some antiseptic such as toluene or chloroform. The tissue is allowed to stand for several days or weeks and subsequently examined. It is found that the coagulable nitrogen is considerably reduced, while the noncoagulable nitrogen in the form of albumose, peptone, ammonia, aminoacids, etc., is increased. In the aseptic method, the organs are removed under complete asepsis and preserved under aseptic conditions. Danger of infection is very great and the work of Wolbach, Saiki and Jackson shows that in the case of the dog it is practically impossible to secure aseptic organs, because bacteria are usually present in such organs before they are removed from the body.

The change in autolysis appears to be due to an enzyme or enzymes liberated upon the death of the cell and operating best in a slightly acid medium (see Bradley). Acid probably operates by alteration of the protein substrate upon which enzymes act. Nevertheless, a degree of acidity may be reached which is sufficient to inhibit the ferment action. Oka has confirmed the general principle that the more highly differentiated parenchymatous cells undergo autolysis more readily than the cells of the supporting tissues and the cellular derivatives of the latter. Glandular cells meeting death during active digestion undergo autolysis more readily than when at rest. Certain types of cell granules autolyze more rapidly than do those granules which have a special affinity for carmine.

Morphologic Changes in Death

Changes noticed in the exterior of the body following death have been indicated in the section given above. In a general way the same is true of the changes seen in the internal viscera following death. The most important changes in the viscera depend upon the processes of autolysis and putrefaction. If organs and tissues be examined immediately after death no change is noticed other than dependent hyperemia. If, however, degenerative changes have had time to occur, the organs show softening. Sometimes swelling may appear, the result of imbibition of water, probably due to changes of the tissue colloids by which they become hydrophilic. This swelling and softening of organs very closely resembles and is easily confused with cloudy swelling. The softening may go on to actual liquefaction.

Microscopic changes may occur very early after cell death, particularly in the re-action of cell granules to certain dyes. Subsequently, the normal granularity and even the outline of the cell may be lost, the cytoplasm may show a hyaline appearance and later coarse granules. Certain substances not ordinarily visible under the microscope may become so after autolytic and putrefactive changes, e.g., fats, myelin and other lipids. Neutral red and methylene blue do not stain the nuclei of living cells, but practically as soon as death has occurred the nuclei take these stains. This change appears before there are morphologic alterations in the nucleus. Later, however, the nucleus is likely to show paler staining and may finally undergo complete lysis. If a sufficient time elapse after death, mitotic figures which were in evidence at the time of death may go on to complete division and show the resting stage of the nucleus. Thus, the number of mitotic figures seen in a given preparation may not actually indicate the number present at the time of death. All these changes which have been described serve to emphasize the importance of examination of organs and tissues as soon after death as possible. Immediate fixation of tissues serves to preserve appearance more nearly like those in the living organism than is true if fixation be delayed.

NECROSIS

Necrosis indicates death of a group of cells, a part of tissue or an organ, in continuity with the living body. The most familiar example is death of an extremity or part of an extremity due to occlusion of an artery. Similarly, a part or even an entire viscus may die as the result of the occlusion of the main artery or of its smaller branches. Burns of the third degree produce necrosis of the tissue. Such burns differ from the ordinary reddening or blistering in that there is destruction of the underlying skin and even of deeper structures.

Etiology

Necrosis may be produced physically in a variety of ways.

Trauma. Of the utmost importance in this connection is trauma. Prolonged pressure on the tissues, or cutting by means of a sharp instrument causes necrosis, the former operating to produce large masses of necrosis and the latter producing necrosis in the track of the instrument. A characteristic form in which necrosis may appear as a result of prolonged pressure is known as decubitus. This signifies a chronic ulceration, which appears on the buttocks, over the sacrum, heels or other bony prominences. The ulcers arise usually after long confinement to bed and occur especially in debilitated patients and also in those suffering from certain lesions of the nervous system, where trophic disturbances are supposed to occur. Hence, factors other than pressure are operative, the most important of which are probably a general lowering of vitality and decreased nutrition. Injury to the cytoplasm of a cell does not necessarily lead to death but injury to the nucleus is probably never survived. This is apparently due to the importance of the part played by the nucleus in metabolic activity.

The thermal causes of necrosis include both heat and cold. The activity of these depends upon the degree of temperature and the duration of exposure. Temperatures of 45° C. applied locally may produce necrosis provided exposure is prolonged for five or ten minutes. Similarly, a temperature of 53° C. may produce necrosis following an exposure of three minutes. Local temperatures in the neighborhood of 100° C. may produce necrosis so slight as not easily to be demonstrable but indicated by the subsequent appearance of inflammation. Prolonged exposure to temperatures of about 100° C. produces deep necrosis of the tissues. Momentary exposure to higher temperatures may produce the same result. Less high degrees of temperature, when affecting the entire body, may lead to more serious changes, and it is stated that mammals succumb at temperatures of 47° C. The essential change appears to be the coagulation of cell proteins. Such coagulation may upset the colloidal equilibrium of the cells so as to lead to death. Most enzymes resist temperatures of 60° to 70° C. and are therefore probably of little significance in necrosis due to higher temperatures.

Local exposure to extreme cold may produce necrosis, for example in toes and fingers. It is probable that this can be due to vasoconstriction and the benefit of prompt use of the so-called vascular pumps supports this view. Crystallization of water in the parts would cause injury to cells and thrombosis in blood vessels, with consequent necrosis. Unicellular organisms and certain isolated cells of metazoa, such as blood cells, ciliated and surface epithelium, are highly resistant to cold, but if crystallization of intracellular water occurs, they do not survive.

Radiant Energy. Other physical causes of necrosis include electricity, light, the roentgen ray, and the rays of radium. The electric spark produces necrosis in the course of the spark. The passage of the electric current, if of sufficient amperage, may lead to cell death or death of the entire organism. Wells suggests that "the electric current causes a migration of ions toward one or the other pole of the cell, in this way separating the movable inorganic ions of the ion-protein compounds of the cell, from the immobile colloidal proteins with consequent serious alterations in the chemistry of the cell." This may serve to explain the vacuolization of cells dead as the result of the electric current. Light rays may produce death of unicellular organisms, as the result of the action of short wave-length rays. The longer wave lengths require oxygen and probably depend in part for their activity upon oxidation, but this does not appear to be true of the ultraviolet rays. In man, strong sunlight may produce slight necrosis and inflammation; in the presence of sensitizers such as the porphyrins it may produce more extensive necrosis and somatic death. Prolonged light exposure may injure enzymes and other similar bodies, but in the presence of sensitizers such as eosin, rose bengal, numerous metals and their salts, the activity of light may be much augmented. Sensitization may also intensify the destructive action of light upon organic substances and living cells. Roentgen rays produce necrosis provided the dose is sufficiently great. The effect appears to be directly upon the cells involved and causes deteriorative changes in the nuclei before the cytoplasm becomes affected. No cells are immune, but the effect is seen particularly in the lymphoid apparatus where necrosis of germinal centers is pronounced. Hall and Whipple have demonstrated that suitable doses given over the abdomen produce necrosis of the intestinal epithelium. Surface burns by roentgen rays show extensive necrosis which heals slowly. Radium rays have essentially the same effects.

The chemical causes of necrosis include particularly the corrosives such as strong acids, strong alkalis and phenol. The skin of different individuals shows variable degrees of susceptibility to necrosis by phenol, but this does not appear to be true of the corrosion produced in internal viscera such as the stomach. The direct effect of concentrated corrosives is coagulation of, and in some instances chemical combination with, the cell

poisoning by bichloride of mercury the mucosa of the lower ileum may become necrotic, probably because of excretion of the poison in this situation. The poison produced in the condition known as eclampsia and in acute yellow atrophy of the liver produces necrosis of liver cells. This is also true of phosphorus, chloroform, hydrazin, and other agents. Any marked alteration in the hydrogen ion concentration, either toward acid or alkaline reaction, may lead to the death of the cell.

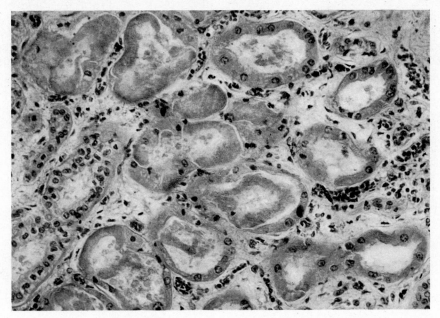

Necrosis of renal epithelium in mercuric chloride poisoning. Note that many cells have no visible nuclei, due to karyolysis. There is desquamation of necrotic cells in the lumina of the tubules.

proteins. Dilute phenol may cause necrosis by producing conglutination of red corpuscles with consequent obstruction of small vessels. Any chemical which coagulates the protoplasm or destroys the enzymes of a cell leads to its death.

Other causes in the same general category, often loosely called TOXIC, include certain chemical poisons and the poisons of parasitic or saprophytic organisms. In the former group are included such substances as bichloride of mercury, cantharidin, uranyl nitrate and other substances which, circulating in the blood appear to have a particular affinity for cells of the kidney, although other parenchymatous cells are affected to a less degree. In the later stages of

BACTERIA produce poisonous substances which lead to necrosis of the surrounding cells. This is particularly true of pyogenic bacteria. These are likely to lodge in small blood vessels, in interstices of the skin, in tonsillar crypts, or other situations, where they proliferate and form masses of organisms which become surrounded by a zone of necrotic tissue. Local necrosis may be produced on injection of diphtheria toxin and certain other toxins. The general effect of these toxins, however, even when leading to somatic death, does not necessarily lead to necrosis. It is possible so to concentrate the reacting substances in allergy as to produce necrosis.

Vascular Occlusion. Of particular

importance is necrosis due to occlusion of
the blood vessels. Unless there is collateral
circulation sufficient to maintain nutrition,
the abrupt occlusion of an artery leads to a
series of changes in the region supplied,
which ultimately go on to necrosis, the process being called infarction. The infarct is
likely to be irregularly conical in shape corresponding to the area of distribution of the
artery and its branches. Such occlusion of
arteries may be due to lodging of small foreign particles in the blood stream, spoken of
as emboli; it may be due to occlusion of vessels by intravascular clotting or thrombosis;
it may be due to occlusion by arteriosclerosis
of different forms; it may be due to prolonged constriction of the vessels, probably
of nervous origin; or may result from com-

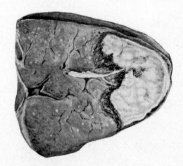

White or anemic infarct of
the spleen. The gross picture of
coagulation necrosis.

pression of the vessel, as for example, by
tumor growth. The necrosis of infarction is
due to removal of blood supply. Certain
types of cells, however, appear to resist this
lack of nutrition for longer periods than
others. Ganglion cells are especially susceptible. In a general way parenchymatous cells
are much more susceptible than connective
tissue cells and the surface epithelium of the
skin. The cause of necrosis in infarction is
probably a combination of factors, including
lack of oxygen and deficient nutrition. Cata-
bolic and anabolic changes are no longer bal-
anced, organic acids probably accumulate
and the proteolytic enzymes continue to
operate even after the death of the cells, especially in the acid medium produced.

Altered Nerve Supply. Necrosis is
also said to be due to alteration of the nerve
supply, so that the ordinary nutritional and

metabolic processes in the tissues are cut off.
Such a process of necrosis is seen in atrophic
necrosis or ulcer of the cornea. In association
with the loss of tissue which is seen in these
ulcers, there is an anesthesia of the cornea,
and it seems likely that the ulcer is due to
unsensed traumatism resulting from this anesthesia, rather than directly to the nerve
lesion. There is no doubt that muscle atrophy
of certain parts may be the result of a lesion
of the motor ganglia supplying that part, but
that this is due to trophic disturbance rather
than simple lack of use is a matter of great
doubt. In neural leprosy necrosis of fingers
and toes often occurs, but here again the
difficulty is probably due to trauma and
infection, rather than to interference with
nerve regulation. Similarly, in those curious
ulcers which develop on the feet, the so-called
perforating ulcers of the feet or "mal per-
forant du pied," there is an associated
anesthesia. Raynaud's disease shows symmetrical necrosis of peripheral parts, particularly the toes and fingers, and is associated with functional nerve lesions. The
disease is not trophic in the ordinary sense,
but depends almost certainly upon prolonged
constriction of arteries due to nerve stimulation. Certain diseases of the nervous system
associated with anesthesia, such as syringomyelia, may lead to traumatic necrosis because of loss of sensation.

Morphology of Necrosis

The gross morbid anatomy of necrosis
can best be described in the various forms
which are to be discussed, because these
forms are likely to show important differences in the naked eye appearance. Microscopically, however, the changes are fairly
uniform. Three important alterations are
found in the nucleus, namely, karyolysis,
karyorrhexis, and pyknosis. The term karyolysis signifies solution of the nucleus. There
may be, however, intermediate stages in the
lysis of the nuclei in which the nucleus stains
less deeply than normally. Nevertheless, it
must be assumed that the nucleus is dead
with the beginning of solution. Karyorrhexis
signifies fragmentation of the nucleus
whereby the nuclear substance is broken up
in small particles. These take the nuclear
stain deeply and sometimes are difficult to
distinguish from bacteria, but the fragments

are of irregular size and by reasonably careful study can easily be identified. Pyknosis indicates reduction in size and condensation of nuclear material, to form a solid, deeply basic-stained body. In addition to these more important changes, the nucleus may sometimes show vacuolization in the process of necrosis. This change, however, may be associated with other lesions and is not diagnostic

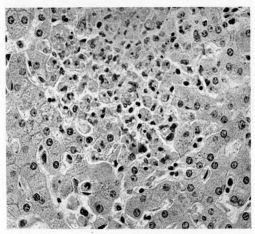

Necrosis of the liver. Note that some nuclei are poorly stained due to karyolysis. Some are shrunken—pyknosis; and many are fragmented—karyolysis.

of actual death of the cells. These alterations of the nucleus are not necessarily sequential and may be quite independent of each other, but karyolysis is the final stage and may affect the nuclei, either primarily or as the sequence of karyorrhexis, pyknosis or vacuolization.

The cytoplasm of the cells shows primarily those changes which have been described in cloudy swelling. Subsequently, however, cells may show either very coarse granules in the cytoplasm or hyaline transformation. Ultimately, the cell outline is completely lost and the altered cytoplasm of neighboring cells fuses. As autolysis proceeds the material disappears, very largely by absorption of the fluid products of autolysis. Fragments of cells and of nuclei may be taken up by phagocytic cells, transported to neighboring situations and ultimately destroyed. The presence of dead tissue in the body is irritant to the surrounding living structures, and gives rise to the sequence of changes described as inflammation. This re-

sults in the infiltration of migrating blood and tissue cells and finally to growth of new blood vessels and connective tissue. The new blood vessels and connective tissue collectively are called granulation tissue. These undergo a series of alterations with the final production of a scar. Uninfected dead tissues give rise to only slight acute reaction and the process is seen almost solely as fibrosis.

Types of Necrosis

Coagulation Necrosis. This form of necrosis is best exemplified by the so-called anemic or white infarct which is a region of local death of tissue, consequent upon the obstruction of its supplying blood vessel. In the early stages, the region is likely to be swollen, somewhat granular, pallid or clay colored, soft, relatively dry and friable. It is usually sharply defined, projects in the cross section and is likely to be surrounded by a small zone of redness due to early reactive inflammation. The changes indicated above are to be found microscopically. Such necrosis is given the name coagulation because of the fact that not infrequently fibrin, or so-called fibrinoid, formation may be demonstrated. As a rule, however, the fibrin is so small in amount as to be shown only by special staining. The necrotic material itself is not soluble in water, solutions of neutral salts or dilute acids and alkali, but a salt-solution extract of such foci may readily coagulate. If bacterial infection go hand in hand with necrosis, fibrin may be present in larger amounts. Fibrinoid is a substance which forms a network similar to that of fibrin, but does not react to stains in exactly the same fashion. Instead of taking the acid stain it is more likely to take the basic stain. As time goes on and the fluid is removed, the focus of necrosis loses its swollen appearance and shows decrease in size, increased firmness, and retraction. If it be not too large it ultimately becomes entirely substituted by scar tissue, but if its size be too great for this process it becomes surrounded by a zone of fibrous tissue and is said to be encapsulated. Gierke includes in this group of necrosis, focal necrosis due to infectious disease and Zenker's degeneration or necrosis of voluntary muscle. Zenker's hyalin has been described in connection with degenerations but it must be admitted freely that this change is a necrosis rather than a simple degeneration.

Cheesy or Caseous Necrosis. This form of necrosis is particularly well exemplified in the necrosis of the center of a tubercle. The gross appearance gives the condition its name. It is usually found in fairly well circumscribed foci and is characterized by its resemblance to cheese. This differs from other forms of necrosis, in that the degenerative and necrotic changes of the cells lead to the formation of fat and lipoid products which may readily be demonstrated by special staining. The percentages of fat, cholesterol and other lipids vary considerably in different specimens and in the hands of different investigators. Caseous necrosis is so complete that no remnant or outline of the original tissue remains. The direct cause of caseation is unknown. Whether it be due to the wax of the tubercle bacilli, some soluble product of the bacilli, enzymes from the surrounding lymphocytes or other agent has not been finally determined.

Microscopically, the cellular changes are found to be similar to those described above except for the fatty change. This means that with ordinary stains, the condition in itself is not characteristic. With the diagnosis, however, of tuberculosis of the area, it is very easy to assume that the necrotic change is caseous in character. Cheesy necrosis may be seen in conditions other than tuberculosis, particularly in cysts with necrosis of the contents, but for all practical purposes the change is confined to tuberculosis. The necrosis in the gumma of syphilis is much the same histologically but grossly more closely resembles a gummy or putty-like substance than cheese. In certain instances of caseous necrosis, fibrin can be demonstrated, and for this reason Gierke includes caseous necrosis as one of the varieties of coagulation necrosis.

Colliquation or Liquefaction Necrosis. This indicates an alteration of the dead tissue so as to produce fluid. In other words, the region softens considerably and finally liquefies. The change may follow any of the other forms of necrosis and is generally considered to be the result of activity of ferments or autolytic agents. Thus the infarct of kidney and spleen may finally show colliquation necrosis and the same is true of cheesy necrosis. This is particularly well exemplified in the softening of tuberculous foci of the lung so that the material is expectorated as a fluid or semifluid mass. The same general process operates in the softening of pneumonic exudate so that the material can either be absorbed or expectorated, and in the softening of abscesses so that the contents can be discharged. Infarcts of the central nervous system are not likely to show the early stage of coagulation necrosis but rapidly go on to liquefaction, producing cystic areas filled with fluid, which at first are surrounded by living nerve substance, and ultimately become encapsulated. The most common example of colliquation necrosis is seen in the liquefaction of pus in abscesses or other areas of suppuration.

Fat Necrosis. The particular type of death of fat included under this heading is that seen most commonly in man as a result of acute destructive disease of the pancreas. The fat of the neighboring omentum, of the pancreas itself, sometimes of the abdominal walls and even that of more remote situations such as the liver, shows the appearance of small, pale yellow or white nodules closely resembling soap. As a rule, somatic death results from the causative disease, so that subsequent changes are not observed. In experimental work, however, it is known that the lesion leads to reactive inflammation in the neighborhood, which finally results in the complete disappearance of the fat and healing of the region.

The death of the fat is due to liberation of pancreatic ferments resulting from the destruction of part of that organ. Wells has made extensive experimental studies of this condition, and finds that the injection of fresh pancreatic extract and even of commercial pancreatin can produce these lesions. Neal and Ellis have found that lipase of either animal or vegetable origin can produce fat necrosis and that there is no specificity as regards species. They have purified the material and consider that it fulfills the biologic and chemical criteria of a ferment or enzyme. The most serious lesion in man occurs in the pancreas and here it seems possible that both lipase and trypsin operate. It is conceivable that trypsinogen is activated by a kinase from leukocytes and other cells, the trypsin destroys tissue cells and subsequently the lipase splits the fat. As a result of fat splitting, fatty acids and glycerol are liberated, the latter to be absorbed and the former to crystallize or to combine with calcium to form soaps.

Microscopically, the fat cells, including cytoplasm and nuclei, show necrosis, which may produce large foci of complete destruction of tissue. The fat has disappeared, or is converted into a soap which,

The destruction may be a slow aseptic process due to the gradual action of lipases of tissue and blood, or it may be rapid. If the former, it is likely to excite little inflammation, but in time a heavy margin of fibroblasts with numerous capillaries may appear which may be mistaken for sarcoma (see Dunphy). In some cases, there is the same sort of granulation tissue plus foreign-body giant cells containing soapy material or fatty-

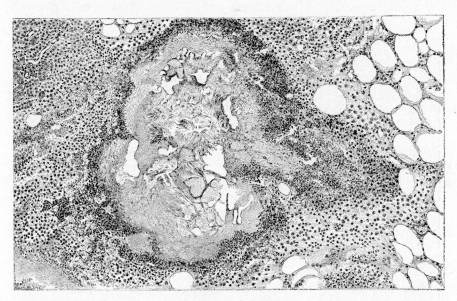

Experimental fat necrosis, showing disappearance of fat cells, granular mass of detritus, acicular spaces of fatty acid crystals and reactionary infiltration of polymorphonuclear leukocytes.

because of its calcium content, appears as a homogenous or finely granular mass taking the basic stain. Fatty acid crystals may be stained by Benda's copper-acetate method in fresh tissue and, if dissolved by fixation and staining, they leave acicular slits in the tissues. The necrotic foci are surrounded by inflammatory exudate of polymorphonuclear leukocytes, lymphocytes and large mononuclears. Hemorrhage is often observed because of destruction of blood vessels. Further reference to this subject is found in the chapter on Liver and Pancreas.

Fat necrosis may occur also in subcutaneous tissues, breast and other situations. There appear to be four groups of such cases, those due to injections of oils or various medicinal solutions, those due to trauma with or without penetration of the skin, those found in the neighborhood of inflammations, and those in which no cause can be found.

acid crystals and large mononuclear phagocytes which may take up fine droplets of lipid so that they resemble immature fat cells. This constitutes the LIPOGRANULOMA. Rarely lipogranulomas may be multiple and somewhat symmetrically situated, suggestive of a constitutional factor, the state of LIPO-GRANULOMATOSIS (Goldzieher). Fat necrosis may be observed in infants, usually from 8 to 20 days after birth, evidently due to birth injuries, and it may complicate scleroderma neonatorum. As concerns both infants and children, those who have a goodly supply of subcutaneous fat are the most susceptible to subcutaneous fat necrosis.

Liver Necroses. These represent an important chapter in both special and general pathology.

FOCAL NECROSIS of the liver is seen in connection with infectious diseases, most notably typhoid fever, although in diphtheria, scarlatina, measles, and other acute infections, necrosis, anatomically identical with that of typhoid fever, may occur. The foci of necrosis are so small that they are rarely, if ever, visible to the naked eye. Microscopically, they occupy a small part of the lobule of the liver; they appear as rounded areas of complete necrosis of the liver cells accompanied by infiltration of other cells, particularly large mononuclears mixed with a certain number of lymphocytes

minor significance and that more important probably is some cytolytic element conveyed by the cells. Jaffé, however, maintains that the proliferation of the Kupffer cells of the liver in focal areas leads to the lesion, and that if necrosis be actually present it is secondary to the focal proliferation of these cells.

CENTRAL NECROSIS of the liver is to a certain extent dependent upon passive hyperemia. It affects the cells near the central

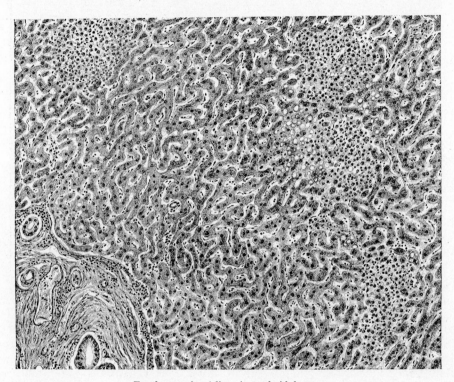

Focal necrosis of liver in typhoid fever.

and occasionally with polymorphonuclear leukocytes. Except for this infiltration there is likely to be no other reaction. According to Mallory, these foci of necrosis are due to blocking of the liver sinusoids by large endothelial cells from the spleen and other portions of the abdominal lymphatic apparatus. In typhoid fever these cells multiply in the lymphoid apparatus, and may become free so as to enter into the blood circulation and thus gain access to the liver. In a study of experimental necrosis of the liver due to injection of specific hemolytic immune serum, Karsner and Aub come to the conclusion that obstruction of the capillaries alone is of

veins and there is, in the acute cases, no indication of fixed tissue reaction. It has usually been assumed that damming back of blood into the central vein and neighboring capillaries, as the result of prolonged passive hyperemia, leads to such deterioration in the nutrition of the parenchymatous cells in that neighborhood that they finally undergo necrosis. Mallory, however, in a careful study of this condition comes to the conclusion that passive hyperemia alone will not produce central necrosis but that, in addition to the passive hyperemia, there must be present a circulating poison of some sort which so reduces the resistance of the cells that they cannot survive the nutritional reduction incident to passive hyperemia. The central cells show all the changes of necrosis, associated, as a rule, with some dilatation of the central ends of the liver sinusoids. The change is so minute as not to be observed by the naked eye.

The hepatic necrosis of yellow fever is often marked, but the gross changes are not marked. Microscopically, there is more or less extensive MID-ZONAL NECROSIS with peculiar cytologic changes. In the cytoplasm of the cells are acidophilic hyaline globules, the so-

particular affinity for liver cells. Chloroform is likely to produce well-marked necrosis affecting first the central zone of the lobule and subsequently the middle and even the peripheral zones. When produced experimentally in the guinea-pig, complete recovery ensues in about ten days. In the dog, the injury to the liver is increased when the animal is depleted of protein. When large amounts of protein, or of methionine or cystine are administered, the injury is reduced or absent. Other amino-acids have not been shown to be effective. Miller, Ross and Whipple sug-

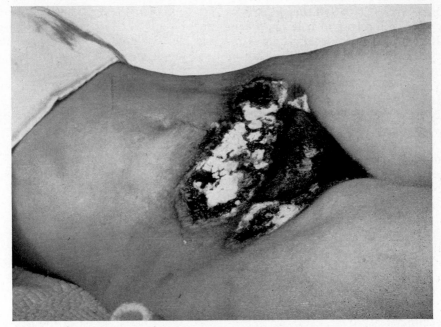

Progressive bacterial synergistic necrosis of the lower abdominal wall. Some of the white paste used in the treatment is present.

called Councilman bodies and there are also intranuclear inclusions (Klotz and Belt). In extensive surface burns with death, the liver shows identical changes (Belt). It is reported, however, that the use of tannic acid in the treatment of burns can produce necrosis, but this is central rather than mid-zonal (Wells, Humphrey and Coll).

Eclampsia may be accompanied by PERIPHERAL ZONAL NECROSIS of the liver. In acute diffuse necrosis of the liver, so-called acute yellow atrophy, the necrosis is primarily central but rapidly becomes diffuse. These changes are discussed further in the chapter on Liver and Pancreas.

Various poisons apparently have a

gest that a combination of chloroform and sulfhydryl groups inactivates the cellular enzyme systems and causes death of the cell unless there is an adequate reserve of methionine and cystine. Carbon tetrachloride produces central necrosis, with marked fatty change, often followed by extensive fibrosis or cirrhosis. Phosphorus produces necrosis of the liver affecting primarily the peripheral or middle zone and associated with extensive fatty changes. Hydrazine hydrochloride produces extensive necrosis throughout the entire lobule from which the liver may readily recover.

Progressive Bacterial Synergistic Necrosis. This is usually called gangrene, but since saprophytic bacteria are not concerned, necrosis is preferable. Meleney has shown it to be due to the synergistic action of a micro-aerophilic nonhemolytic streptococcus and an aerobic hemolytic *Staphylococcus aureus*, neither of which alone produces the disease. It is a progressively extending necrosis of the skin and subcutaneous tissues, occurring especially on abdomen and trunk, which follows wounds particularly such as are due to drainage of abscess. The region becomes tender, red and swollen. A purple zone appears in the center and enlarges; as it does so the red zone extends laterally. The central part breaks down and sloughs to produce an ulcer with a base of pale red granulation tissue, which slowly enlarges in diameter but only slightly in depth. The skin at the margin is gray and opaque, liquefies and becomes undermined. Microscopically, there is exudative inflammation with numerous polymorphonuclear leukocytes, surrounded by granulation tissue with only slight disposition to cicatrization. Resistant to ordinary modes of treatment, it usually responds to complete excision followed by application of zinc peroxide cream, but skin grafting may be necessary. (See Lichtenstein.)

Gangrene. Gangrene signifies necrosis to which is superadded invasion and multiplication of saprophytic organisms. The condition may affect any part of the body as the result of invasion of organisms through wounds or interruption of continuity of skin surface, or through the respiratory, intestinal, or genito-urinary tract. Clinically, a distinction is sometimes made between dry and wet gangrene. This applies especially to extremities and local areas in the skin.

THE SO-CALLED DRY GANGRENE is not true gangrene. It is bland infarction, due to embolic, thrombotic or arteriosclerotic occlusion of supplying artery or arteries. It may also be due, apparently, to prolonged spasmodic occlusion of arteries. The term ischemic necrosis, to replace dry gangrene, is gaining widespread use. Since there is reduction or absence of circulation and the part is exposed to air, variable degrees of desiccation occur. Because of deteriorative changes in the blood and blood pigments which remain in the part, discoloration appears. This is usually green, or yellow and finally dark brown or black. Drying of skin and other parts leads to a parchment-like skin with reduction in the size of the part, wrinkling of the skin and the general appearance spoken of as mummification. The presence of the dead tissue leads to inflammatory reaction in the neighboring tissue so as to form the so-called line of demarcation. This may be emphasized by liquefaction of that necrotic tissue situated near enough to the living tissue to imbibe fluids and their ferments.

WET GANGRENE, which is a true gangrene according to our definition, may appear in extremities or internal viscera. The invasion of saprophytic bacteria gives rise to rapid degenerative changes in the dead tissue, leading to liquefaction, gas formation and the development of foul odors. Discoloration appears but is very much modified by the moisture and gas formation. Owing to the irritant products of the bacteria, the surrounding tissues may react with considerably more violence than is seen in "dry gangrene." The absorption of the toxic products of these saprophytic bacteria leads to the general symptoms of sapremia and sometimes results fatally. Microscopically, the study of the tissues of ischemic necrosis shows the usual changes of necrosis, somewhat modified by desiccation. Many of the nuclei do not undergo complete solution, but pyknosis and karyorrhexis are likely to be common. The cell outline may not be lost. The failure of the usual microscopic changes of necrosis to make active progress is probably due to desiccation of the tissues, which inhibits the activity of autolytic ferments. In moist gangrene the solution of the tissues is likely to be so complete that no remnant of cells or nuclear structure is to be found.

Gas Gangrene. The importance of gas gangrene was emphasized by the experiences of World War I. Access for micro-organisms is provided by crushing wounds which destroy a considerable amount of tissue, permit introduction of the organisms into deep parts where there is little or no access of air, and thus provide favorable nutritional conditions for the saprophytic, anaërobic bacteria. The organism of most importance and of most common occurrence is the *Clostridium welchii*. Bull and Pritchett have demonstrated that the toxin of the *C. welchii* can, upon injection, produce necrosis of the tissue.

This being true, it seems likely that the disease extends because of neighboring necrosis due to absorption of the toxin, thus providing suitable conditions for further growth of the saprophytes.

Grossly, the part affected is swollen, discolored, has a foul odor and upon palpation is found to crepitate. Gas formation may

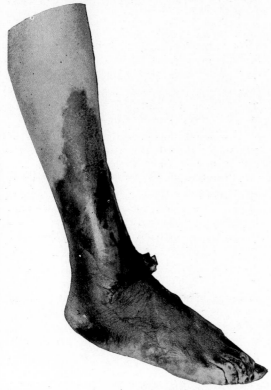

Ischemic necrosis of leg and foot due to arterial embolism.

be so extensive as to produce not only crepitation but visible bubbles and surface blisters. The discoloration which is due to secondary changes in blood and blood pigments is similar to that of the ordinary forms of gangrene. Muscle, the seat of this condition, first shows failure to contract on stimulation, followed by a peculiar, pale, glossy appearance resembling that of the muscle of fish. This is followed by extensive softening associated with gas formation and dark greenish-brown or black discoloration. Microscopically, the changes seen are similar to those seen in other forms of necrosis, except that even with ordinary stains the bacilli

may readily be demonstrated. This condition was found in soldiers because of contamination of wounds by infected earth, particularly those wounds associated with extensive destruction of tissue. The same is true of cases in civil life where certain wounds are similarly contaminated. This is not infrequently found in injuries to coal miners or other workers who come in contact with earth infected by animal carriers of the organisms.

Somewhat similar in gross appearance is a gaseous inflammation due to embedding in the tissues of splinters of metallic magnesium or other light metal, due to the liberation of hydrogen from the fluids of the body. Other gases may ultimately appear. Although called chemical gas gangrene, the lesion is a local inflammation. (See McCord, et al.)

REFERENCES

Belt, T. H.: Liver Necrosis Following Burns, Simulating the Lesions of Yellow Fever, Jour. Path. and Bact., 48: 493, 1939.

Bradley, H. C.: Studies of Autolysis: VIII. The Nature of Autolytic Enzymes, Jour. Biol. Chem., 52: 467, 1922.

Bull, C. G., and I. W. Pritchett: Identity of the Toxins of Different Strains of Bacillus Welchii and Factors Influencing Their Production in vitro, Jour. Exper. Med., 26: 867, 1917.

Child, C. M.: Senescence and Rejuvenescence, Chicago, 1915.

Collip, J. B.: Rigor Mortis, Jour. Biol. Chem., 50: xlv, 1922.

Corper, H. J.: Correlation of the Histological and Chemical Changes in the Spleen During Necrosis and Autolysis, Jour. Exper. Med., 15: 429, 1912.

Dunphy, J. E.: Surgical Importance of Mammary and Subcutaneous Fat Necrosis, Arch. Surg., 38: 1, 1939.

Fleisher, M. S., and L. Loeb: The Experimental Production of Necrosis of the Liver in the Guinea Pig, Jour. Exper. Med., 20: 169, 1914.

Flexner, S.: The Constituent of the Bile Causing Pancreatitis and the Effect of Colloids Upon Its Action, Jour. Exper. Med., 8: 167, 1906.

Goldzieher, M. A.: Lipogranulomatosis (Makai), Arch. Surg., 23: 690, 1931.

Hall, C. C., and G. H. Whipple: Roentgen-ray Intoxication: Disturbances in Metabolism Produced by Deep Massive Doses of the Hard Roentgen Rays, Amer. Jour. Med. Sci., 157: 453, 1919.

Jaffé, R. H.: Zur Histogenese der typhösen Leberveränderungen, Virchow's Arch. Path. Anat., 228: 366, 1920.

Karsner, H. T., and J. C. Aub: An Investigation of the Origin of Immune Serum Necrosis of the Liver, Jour. Med. Res., 28: 377, 1913.

Klotz, O., and T. H. Belt: The Pathology of the Liver in Yellow Fever, Amer. Jour. Path., **6**: 663, 1930.

Lichtenstein, M. E.: Progressive Bacterial Synergistic Gangrene: Involvement of the Abdominal Wall: Report of an Unusual Case, Arch. Surg., **42**: 719, 1941.

Mallory, F. B.: Necroses of the Liver, Jour. Med. Res., **6**: 264, 1901.

——: A Histological Study of Typhoid Fever, Jour. Exper. Med., **3**: 611, 1898.

McCord, C. P., J. J. Prendergast, S. F. Meek, and G. C. Harrold: Chemical Gas Gangrene from Metallic Magnesium, Industrial Medicine, **11**: 71, 1942.

Meleney, F. L.: Bacterial Synergism in Disease Processes, with a Confirmation of the Synergistic Bacterial Etiology of a Certain Type of Progressive Gangrene of the Abdominal Wall, Ann. Surg., **94**: 961, 1931.

Metchnikoff, E.: The Prolongation of Life, New York and London, 1910.

Miller, L. L., J. F. Ross, and G. H. Whipple: Methionine and Cystine, Specific Protein Factors Preventing Chloroform Liver Injury in Protein-depleted Dogs, Amer. Jour. Med. Sci., **200**: 739, 1940.

Minot, C. S.: The Problem of Age, Growth and Death, New York, 1908.

Moritz, A. R.: Sudden Death, New England Jour. Med., **223**: 798, 1940.

Neal, M. P., and M. M. Ellis: Experimental Fat Necrosis in Various Vertebrates, Amer. Jour. Clin. Path., **1**: 251, 1931.

Oka, D.: Zur Frage der postmortalen Autolyse der Zellgranula, Virchow's Arch. Path. Anat., **228**: 200, 1920.

Opie, E. L.: Diseases of the Pancreas, Philadelphia, 1903.

——: On the Relation of Combined Intoxication and Bacterial Infection to Necrosis of the Liver, Acute Yellow Atrophy and Cirrhosis, Jour. Exper. Med., **12**: 367, 1910.

——: Zonal Necrosis of the Liver, Jour. Med. Res., **12**: 147, 1904.

Pack, G. T.: The Pathology of Burns, Arch. Path. and Lab. Med., **1**: 767, 1926.

Pearce, R. M.: The Experimental Production of Liver Necroses by the Intravenous Injection of Hemagglutinins, Jour. Med. Res., **12**: 329, 1904.

Pearl, R.: The Biology of Death, Philadelphia, 1922.

Pütter, A.: Altern und Sterben, Virchow's Arch. Path. Anat., **261**: 393, 1926.

Rössle, R.: Wachstum und Altern, Ergebnisse Allg. Path. u. Path. Anat., **18**[2]: 677, 1917.

Wells, D. B., H. D. Humphrey, and J. J. Coll: The Relation of Tannic Acid to Liver Necrosis Occurring in Burns, New England Jour. Med., **226**: 629, 1942.

Wells, H. G.: The Relation of Autolysis to the Histological Changes Occurring in Necrotic Areas, Jour. Med. Res., **15**: 149, 1906.

——: Chemical Pathology, 5th ed., Philadelphia, 1925.

Whipple, G. H.: Insusceptibility of Pups to Chloroform Poisoning, During the First Three Weeks of Life, Jour. Exper. Med., **15**: 259, 1912.

Wolbach, S. B., T. Saiki, and H. C. Jackson: Anaërobic Bacterium and Autolysis of Liver, Jour. Med. Res., **21**: 267, 279, 281, 1909.

5

Mineral Infiltrates and Concrements

CALCIFICATION

Introduction

The deposit of calcium and other inorganic salts for the production of bone is under the influence of (1) endocrine glands, especially the parathyroids; (2) vitamins, especially C and D; (3) the supply of calcium and phosphorus as compared with the daily requirements; and (4) in certain species, the acid-base balance (Logan). Calcium and other salts are deposited in cartilage and osteoid tissue during the growth of the body and in osteoid tissue after endochondral growth of bone has ceased. Calcium is essential to clotting of blood and plays an important part in connection with irritability of nerve and muscle, as illustrated in parathyroid tetany considered in the discussion of diseases of that organ. Bones themselves are the seat of pathologic changes in deposition of calcium, covered in the chapter on Organs of Locomotion.

Pathologic Calcification

This differs from normal or pathologic ossification in that the calcium and salts are laid down without arrangement into trabeculae, canals and lacunae. Pathologic calcification is divided into dystrophic and metastatic forms.

Dystrophic calcification is that form in which the calcium is deposited in tissues and cells which are the seat of disease. Thus foci of dense fibrosis, especially if hyalinized, and necrotic masses may become infiltrated. The calcific mass is often referred to as a monument of tissue destruction. Calcium may be deposited around foreign bodies and may infiltrate dead parasites as for example *Trichinella spiralis* and the ova of schistosoma. Dystrophic calcification may attain sufficient size to be seen grossly, as for example in the wall of the aorta. The masses are firm, dense, coherent, usually pale gray, giving a metallic sound when struck with an instrument, usually fracturing easily and producing crepitus after fracture. In the early stages of calcification, microscopic examination may show simply the presence of a number of fine granules. Sometimes the calcium is found in the form of small globules called calcospherites, measuring 20 micra or more in diameter, with a dense center and sometimes distinctly laminated. As the process advances, the granules or calcospherites increase in number and fuse to form solid granular masses, in which the identity of the calcospherites is usually lost. Calcium takes the basic stain, and small masses with their neighboring granules sometimes resemble bacteria, but the lack of uniformity in size and outline of the calcium granules serves for ready differentiation. Usually the microscopic appearance is distinctive, but sometimes special stains such as the von Kossa are used. This silver method gives a characteristic picture but is not absolutely specific. The presence of calcific masses is not likely to excite those tissue reactions which usually occur about foreign bodies. Only occasionally is there a reactive zone of fibrosis, lymphocytic infiltration and foreign-body giant cells.

Dystrophic calcification is common in the late stages of intimal arteriosclerosis of the aorta. In this form of arteriosclerosis,

cium, so does hyalinized connective tissue. In senile arteriosclerosis, the media of peripheral arteries becomes fibrous and calcification takes place in the fibrous parts to constitute the so-called corduroy and pipe-stem arteries. Fibrosis in the pleura, pericardium, peritoneum and other serous membranes, especially when due to chronic inflammation rather than scarring, may be accompanied by calcification. In the pericardium it is sometimes extensive. Cardiac valves and their rings, es-

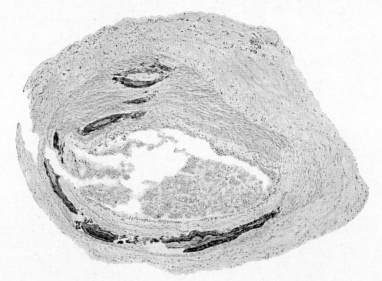

Calcification in media of small artery in senile arteriosclerosis.

fibrosis occurs first, followed by hyalinization and then by a form of necrosis called atheroma in which fats, fatty acids and lipoids are observed. Calcification occurs principally in this necrotic mass. Sometimes focal masses of necrosis and infarcts become slightly or markedly calcified. Calcium is not infrequently deposited in desquamated dead epithelial cells of the renal tubules, especially after mercuric chloride poisoning. Necrotic material in old cysts and in inspissated collections of pus often becomes calcified. Of especial importance is the calcification of the caseous necrotic material in tubercles, especially in the arrested stage of primary tuberculosis of the lungs and mediastinal lymph nodes, often visible by roentgen ray.

Calcification occurs also in tissues where there is marked fibrosis, but usually after the fibrosis becomes hyalinized. As hyaline cartilage favors deposition of cal-

pecially those of the left side, may be markedly calcified as a sequel of chronic inflammation. Calcium may be found in various calculi and concretions, as indicated subsequently. Calcification in scleroderma and dermatomyositis is probably dystrophic.

Metastatic calcification differs from the dystrophic form in that there is not any clearly identified tissue injury as a precursor and in that calcium is mobilized from its natural places of deposit. The term is used in a broad sense to cover any of the forms of calcification which are not known to be dystrophic. Important in man, although fortunately uncommon, is metastatic calcification due to disease of bone, such as osteomalacia, secondary tumors, that primary tumor of the marrow called multiple myeloma and rarely leukemia, myeloid and lymphoid, when bone is destroyed. The calcification occurs in the veins, capillaries and alveolar septa of the lungs, in the endocardium of the left side of the heart, in the tunica propria of the acid-secreting parts of the mucosa of the stomach, in tubules and connective tissue of the kidneys, as well as in other situations. Calcification is reported with similar distribution in chronic disease of the kidneys. Experimentally, widespread calcification can be produced by administration of large amounts of irradiated ergosterol, a hypervitaminosis

these situations injuries are common. Many of the patients have scleroderma. Furthermore patients may also exhibit vasoconstriction in the extremities of the nature of Raynaud's disease. Because of the possibility of injury, the presence of altered fats and of vasoconstriction, the absence of lesions of joints and a normal calcium metabolism, the calcification is probably dystrophic. Foreign body reaction may be seen microscopically.

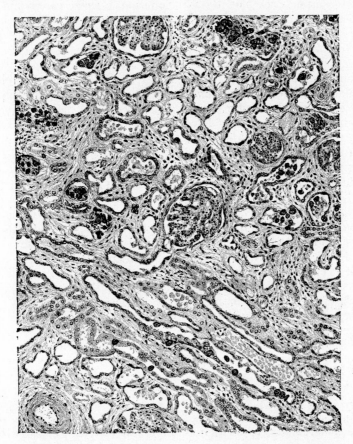

Calcification in renal tubules in a case of mercuric-chloride poisoning.

D (see Shohl, Goldblatt and Brown), and by hyperparathyroidism (Jaffe et al.). It follows intraperitoneal, subcutaneous and intravenous injections of calcium (Wells). It can be produced in mice by feeding an acid diet rich in calcium (Butler).

Calcinosis occurs in two forms, circumscribed and diffuse. The former affects adults as a deposit of calcium salts in the subcutaneous tissues of the fingers and toes and extensor surfaces of knees and shoulders; it is sometimes loosely called chalk gout. In

Diffuse calcinosis is rare and affects young children especially, but may appear in adults. Large portions of the subcutaneous tissues are converted into calcific plaques with fluctuant edematous masses, which may break through the skin and discharge gritty chalky material. Muscles, tendons and nerve sheaths are often involved. There is no evidence of previous inflammatory or other disease of the fat nor is it clear that calcium metabolism is altered. Microscopically the calcium is first deposited in fine granules at the periphery of fat cells and in later stages is found in fatty tissue and edematous connective tissue. The blood vessels often show endothelial proliferation and fibrosis of media, sometimes with fibrous obliteration. It cannot be said definitely whether the disease is metabolic or dystrophic. No cause has been ascertained (see Rosenberg; Lutz).

Mechanism of Pathologic Calcification. The chemical composition of pathologically calcified masses does not differ significantly from that of normal bone (Meeker and Kesten). Various theories are offered as to dystrophic calcification. In necrotic foci, oxidation is reduced and the amount of carbon dioxide present may be too small to maintain calcium in solution. This idea may not be valid because other acids are formed in necrotic tissue. A widely quoted theory is that of the "Kalkfänger," something which has a special affinity for calcium. This supposes that in the destruction of tissues rich in nucleoproteins, phosphoric acid is liberated to serve as the "Kalkfänger." The phosphate ions, electronegatively charged, combine with the positively charged calcium ions to form the calcified mass. Wells found, experimentally, that if comparable masses of dead tissues, rich and poor in nucleoproteins, be implanted, the deposit of calcium is the same in both. In tissues rich in fat, calcification may be due to an intermediate stage of soap formation. Hartsuch investigated the problem of how immiscible hydrolyzing fats and basic substances in aqueous systems can react. He found that there is an interchange of ions at the water-oil interphases to produce calcium soaps. Further molecular changes result in the formation of calcium salts. It is not established, however, that this is applicable to dystrophic calcification in tissues poor in fat. The calcification sometimes observed in masses of extravasated blood in tissues (hematoma) is in part due to the affinity of iron for calcium.

In metastatic calcification, the precipitation of calcium is due either to an increase of the amount of calcium in the blood and tissue fluids or to a decrease in its solubility. In that form due to diseases of bones in man, local alkalinization and decrease of CO_2 are evidently important. Thus there is probably a tissue alkalinization in the part of the stomach where acid is secreted. This may also be true in the kidney due to excretion of acid phosphates. After the blood passes through the pulmonary capillaries, there is a reduction in CO_2, so that with even a little hypercalcemia, the calcium is precipitated in the pulmonary veins and in the endocardium of the left side of the heart.

Nevertheless, calcification may occur elsewhere, where Wells' explanation of precipitation in elastica, a hyaline tissue, is not applicable. It may well be that in some of these situations there is injury of tissue due to the primary disease and that some of the calcification is dystrophic. The calcification which is occasionally observed in cases of chronic renal disease may be due to disturbance of colloidal balance. Hueper draws attention to the importance of albuminous substances and phosphates in keeping the calcium in solution and supposes that loss of albumins in the urine may disturb the balance so that calcium is precipitated. In all such cases, however, it is necessary to consider the possibility of retention of potassium and an accompanying overactivity of the parathyroids.

Hypercalcemia occurs in experimental hypervitaminosis D and hyperparathyroidism (produced by injections of parathormone), and the same is probably true of man. Precipitation may thus be due to local alkalinization and perhaps to local tissue injury, although there is still no final proof that in either condition a toxic factor operates. There is no satisfactory explanation of the phenomena in circumscribed or diffuse calcinosis. Excellent reviews of calcification are given by Barr and by Logan.

Pathologic Ossification

This differs from calcification in that a structure with lamellae, canaliculi, lacunae and sometimes bone marrow are formed. It may be observed in soft tissues (heteroplastic) and in bones.

In heteroplastic bone formation, the bone is found in abnormal situations and has been reported in pericardium, aorta, cardiac valves, kidneys, muscles, eyes, and, according to Harvey, in nearly every organ of the body. Grossly, ossification in soft tissues cannot be distinguished from calcification. Microscopically, the lamellae, canaliculi and lacunae are usually irregularly disposed.

When marrow is present it is likely to be fatty. Around the bone there is chronic inflammation but in man cartilage has not been observed. Experimental ligation of the ureter of the rabbit produces distention of the renal pelvis and atrophy of renal substance. After five or six weeks, calcification is marked and if circulation be adequate, ossification occurs. Harvey painted the adventitia of the aorta of rabbits with 2 per cent silver nitrate or 2 per cent cupric sulfate and found a sequence of necrosis, calcification and then ossification; occasionally there was an intermediate substance which resembled cartilage.

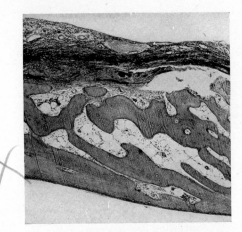

Heteroplastic bone formation in chronic inflammation of choroid coat of eye. Army Museum 46852.

The mechanism of pathologic ossification is not altogether clear, but it seems that calcification is a necessary precursor. Wells pictures it as like endochondral bone formation except that calcified masses take the place of cartilage. Inflammation precedes the ossification, granulation tissue erodes the calcareous mass, and the new connective-tissue cells of the granulation tissue undergo functional metaplasia and act as osteoblasts. It is unlikely that the cells are wandering osteoblasts derived from bone. The exact stimulus to this metaplasia is not known, other than that calcium salts are present. Ossification is favored by an appropriate blood supply; in the kidney of the rabbit, a poor blood supply delays ossification and if it be rich there is neither calcification nor ossification. Wells states that "in order to have ossification of calcific deposits, certain conditions of relationship between calcium salts, fibrous tissues and blood supply evidently must be exactly met."

Myositis ossificans occurs in two varieties, a local form and a progressive multiple ossifying myositis. The former is exemplified in "rider's bone." The latter occurs in growing children as a progressive calcification and ossification of muscles, tendons, ligaments, fascias and aponeuroses. Ossification takes place during the repair of fractures, may accompany inflammation of bone, may occur with certain primary and secondary tumors, and in certain obscure diseases of bone such as Paget's disease of bone and osteopetrosis (Albers-Schönberg). These are discussed in the chapter on Organs of Locomotion.

CRYSTALLINE DEPOSITS IN TISSUES

Urates

Minerals other than calcium may be deposited in tissues as crystals or as amorphous granules.

Gout is the most important disease of this order; it is due to faulty metabolism or excretion of uric acid. There is evidently an inherent predisposition which in some but not all instances appears to be hereditary. Overeating, large consumption of wines and malted beverages and lead poisoning may precipitate the acute attack in which there is deposit of sodium monourate around and in joints, especially of the great toe, with acute inflammation. With repeated attacks chronic gout ensues. Urates are deposited near joints to constitute the tophi of gout. Tophi may be found in other situations in dense connective tissue, as for example in the fibrous tissue of the renal pyramids, rarely in the valves in chronic endocarditis, and in cartilage such as that of the external ear. There is but little or no inflammatory reaction around the tophi.

Arthritis. Joints may be the seat of a chronic destructive arthritis. The urates are found in cartilage and dense connective tissue which may furnish physical conditions which favor deposit of urates much as the same states favor deposit of calcium.

Uric Acid Infarction. On postmortem examination, the kidneys of very young infants frequently show grossly in the pyramids radiating streaks of yellow, crystalline material. This is spoken of as uric acid infarction of the kidney. Microscopically, it is found to consist of deposits of crystals in small globules within the lumina of the collecting tubules. These are covered with a refractile colloidal substance. They are discharged into the pelvis of the kidney and excreted in the urine as a sandy material. Occasionally, they may serve as a centrum for the formation of calculi. The condition probably depends upon the altered metabolic condition incident to change from intra- to extra-uterine life. The material is usually uric acid and urates. The newborn excretes relatively larger amounts of uric acid than cholesteatoma. If deposited in sufficient amounts, the white or yellowish-white glistening material is easily visible to the naked eye. Microscopically, the crystals are found in the form of colorless rhomboid plates with broken or re-entrant corners. The ordinary methods of fixing and embedding tissues dissolve and remove the crystals, so that in preparations of this sort there occur only spaces representing the position formerly occupied by the cholesterol crystals. The formation of multinucleated giant cells, the so-called foreign-body giant cells, is common about the crystals.

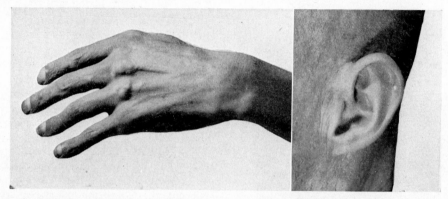

Gouty tophi near metacarpal-phalangeal joint. Tophus in pinna of ear of same patient.

the adult. This is probably due to the liberation of nucleoprotein and the consequent formation of uric acid, dependent upon transformation of the erythrocytes from nucleated to non-nucleated forms, and also to the active destruction of leukocytes said to occur immediately after birth.

Cholesterol

Cholesterol exists normally in the blood and in practically all body tissues. It is found in considerable amounts in the bile and in the adrenal cortex. Pathologically, it may be deposited in the tissues as a result of degeneration and of necrosis, particularly when these changes are associated with fatty metamorphosis of some kind. The crystals are found especially in the atheromatous plaques of arteriosclerosis as well as in certain chronic cysts. They are also found frequently in conditions where there is marked destruction of squamous epithelium, for example, in sebaceous cysts of the skin, dermoid cysts and in the tumor known as

CONCREMENTS

Introduction

Concrements or concretions are solid masses of material formed within hollow organs or passages in the body. They are of great clinical importance because they may obstruct passages such as the bile ducts and ureters, with violent colic. Retained in ducts, the output of secretion or excretion may be stopped and when this persists, the organ undergoes atrophy, for example, the kidney, pancreas and liver. Concrements may be composed of mineral or organic substances or mixtures of the two. When the mineral content is high and the mass solid, the name calculus or stone is applied. Most concrements have a centrum, nidus or nucleus. The nidus may be a small clump of desquamated cells, a mass of mucin, a clump of bacteria, a small mass of fibrin or of leukocytes, a small scybalous mass of feces or a foreign body of some sort. Upon such a centrum, salts from the surrounding medium may be precipitated to form an encrustation, which gradually increases in size and forms the concrement. Certain concrements, however, are not formed in this way, for example, the hair ball of the stomach which is made up of masses of swallowed hair. If these remain in the intestinal tract very long, they may become infiltrated with carbonate and phosphate to form relatively solid concrements. The principal calculi of man are those of the biliary and urinary tracts, but they are also found in other situations. The following discussion is amplified by sections in the chapters on systemic pathology.

Biliary Concrements

These are found most often in the gallbladder, are frequent in the extrahepatic ducts and occasionally occur in the intrahepatic ducts. In the gallbladder they may be single or multiple. The single stones usually attain large size and have been found as large as the gallbladder itself. When there are few stones they are spheroidal, but when there are many they are faceted and pyramidal or polyhedric in shape. The edges of the facets are rounded. Frequently, calculi are associated with inflammations of the gallbladder. In some cases the inflammation may be primary, and, by virtue of the exudate and influences upon the bile, leads to the formation of calculi. In other instances the inflammation is secondary to the presence of calculi, which operate as foreign bodies to produce irritation and inflammation. Lodgment of a calculus in the cystic duct may produce marked distention of the duct and alteration of the contents of the gallbladder. Lodgment in the common duct may produce jaundice, absence of bile pigments in the stools, and if long continued, may lead to obstructive biliary cirrhosis of the liver. Inflammation of the gallbladder or the extrahepatic ducts, either with or without obstruction by stones, may result in multiple abscess formation in the liver or, if the infectious agent be not particularly virulent, or the resistance of the individual great, the sequence may be a chronic intrahepatic cholangitis.

The chemical composition of gallstones is varied. Practically all the elements which go to make up bile may enter into the composition of the calculi. Occasionally, calculi are found made up almost entirely of cholesterol. They are likely to have an organic nidus of some sort and a certain amount of organic stroma holding the calculus together. They are not very clearly stratified but show a yellowish-white or creamy-white, glistening outer surface, and when incised the crystalline character of the cross section is easily seen. The commoner stones are made up very largely of bile pigment. Whether they are green or yellow depends upon the degree of oxidation of the pigment. These pigments are usually present not in pure form but as calcium combinations of the pigments.

Occasionally, calculi are found which are made up entirely of pigment. The main constituent is bilirubin but there is in addition the simply oxidized biliverdin, the more oxidized bilifuscin and the highly oxidized bilihumin. The more common gallbladder stones are usually distinctly laminated. In addition to the central nidus of organic material, concentric and more or less alternating laminae are found, made up of pigments and of cholesterol. As a rule, the pigmented layers predominate. Not infrequently when the gallbladder is the seat of inflammation, a previously formed calculus may serve as a nidus upon which occurs a deposit of calcium salts. It is only rarely, however, that a pure calcium concrement is found in the biliary tract. Aschoff and Bacmeister classify gallstones as pure cholesterol stones, stratified cholesterol calcium stones, cholesterol pigment calcium stones, composite stones composed of cholesterol and a superficial incrustation of a mixture of cholesterol and calcium, bilirubin calcium stones which are the form found within the bile passages of the liver, and, finally, calculi made of calcium carbonate.

Mechanism of Biliary Concretion. Aschoff and Bacmeister have laid down the general proposition that the first step in the formation of biliary concrements is precipitation of cholesterol. There are two possible causes of the precipitation, namely general and local. Elevations of cholesterol content of the blood, hypercholesterolemia, may cause an increase in the amount of cholesterol in the bile. Cholesterol is held in solution by certain constituents of the bile, but there is considerable dispute as to which of these is or are responsible. Nevertheless, supersaturation with cholesterol would lead to precipitation. Hypercholesterolemia has not been proved to cause gallstones in the human, because the two do not occur at the same time. As an example, biliary concrements occur in women who have previously been pregnant and hypercholesterolemia is common in pregnancy, but years may intervene before gallstones are observed. Nevertheless, women who have never been pregnant, as well as men, have gallstones, without any proof that they ever had hypercholesterolemia.

Local conditions in the gallbladder and ducts are definitely causative. Stagnation of the flow of bile is followed by concretion, although complete stoppage rarely has that sequel. Stasis may be due to disease of ducts or gallbladder and to delayed emptying of the gallbladder in sedentary life or to some interference with the stimulation of the gallbladder on taking food. This stagnation permits absorption of acids with consequent precipitation of cholesterol. Comparable absorption of acids may take place through an inflamed wall of the gallbladder or ducts. Inflammation may play a double part, because the exudate may alter constitution of the bile to cause precipitation and the stones may excite inflammation, a sort of vicious circle. The deposit of pigments is due to the same general disturbance of physicochemical relations. In inflammation associated with stones there may be sufficient alkalinization to cause encrustation of the stone by calcium salts, rendering the calculus opaque to the x-ray.

A nidus or centrum is found in nearly all biliary concrements, usually organic material such as necrotic cells or mucus. It was thought that bacteria such as typhoid bacilli, colon bacilli, streptococci and others might enter from the duodenum and provide the nidus. Aschoff and Bacmeister, however, showed that the concrements are permeable to bacteria and suggest that their presence in the calculi is secondary rather than primary.

In the light of present knowledge, it is reasonable to assume that a nidus is provided by disease of the gallbladder or ducts, by infection, by ulceration and possibly by bacteria, and that precipitation is determined by alterations of the physicochemical relations in the bile.

Urinary Concrements

These may be formed in the renal pelvis or in the urinary bladder. Those found in the ureter are calculi which have entered from the renal pelvis and some of those in the urinary bladder are passed into it through the ureters. They are composed of minerals derived from the urine. Precipitation may be due to supersaturation of sub-

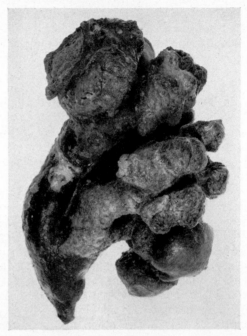

Uratic calculus from the renal pelvis, the so-called "stag horn" calculus. About natural size.

stances in the urine (for example uric acid and oxalic acid), or to alterations of composition of the urine so that certain components can no longer be held in solution. The nidus is more often a crystalline deposit than mucus or epithelial cells, but there is usually an organic matrix which binds the constituents together. Foreign bodies sometimes form the nidus of concrements in the urinary bladder.

Urinary concrements vary greatly as to size and shape. They may be multiple tiny sandy particles or so large as to fill the entire renal pelvis or the bladder. In the former they vary in shape from small irregular stones to a larger mass which fills several calyces, the "stag-horn" calculus, or a mass which may fill many of the calyces, the "mulberry stone." Calculi in the urinary bladder

PLATE III

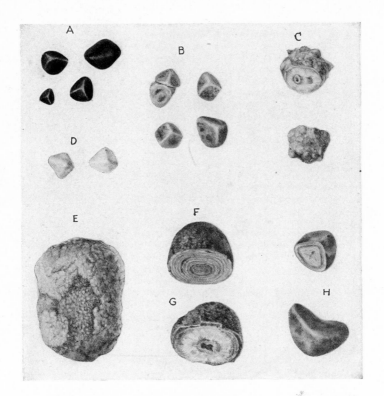

Various types of biliary calculi. A, Faceted pigment calculi. B, Faceted pigment calculi. C, Mulberry form of pigment calculi; upper figure shows cross section with nidus of pigment surrounded by layer of cholesterol and then a layer of pigment. D, Faceted pigment calculi covered with a layer of creamy white glistening cholesterol. E, Large solitary pigment calculus; encrusted with phosphates. F, Solitary pigment calculus showing in cross section multiple layers of pigment. G, Solitary calculus showing nidus of pigment, radiating crystals of cholesterol and covering layer of pigment. H, Large faceted calculi; upper figure shows pigment nidus and multiple layers of pigment.

are usually spheroidal. Urinary calculi may be composed of uric acid, urates, oxalates, phosphates and other materials. There may be mixtures but usually one component preponderates. The alterations of composition of the urine which determine precipitation are principally those of the salts and acids rather than of the colloids. Hyperparathyroidism is one of the conditions often associated with urinary concretion. In rats, deficiency of vitamin A frequently causes stone formation in the bladder and at times in the renal pelvis, in part because of the production of a nidus of desquamated cells of metaplastic epithelium and in part the alkaline reaction of the urine (see special article, Jour. Amer. Med. Asso., 105: 1983, 1935). Further discussion of urinary concretion is found in the chapter on the Urinary System.

Chemical Composition. CALCULI COMPOSED OF URIC ACID are fairly frequent. Uric acid is a relatively insoluble substance and is maintained in solution in the urine partly by virtue of the presence of sodium diphosphate and certain organic materials, particularly the urinary pigment. The margin between solubility and insolubility is so slight that not infrequently when the urine cools after excretion, sandy deposits of uric acid and urates may be thrown down. Uric acid is found in the urine combined chiefly with sodium, potassium and ammonium. Acidity of the urine, as is well known, is determined by the presence of acid phosphates. These possibly combine with the bases of the urate, thus liberating the uric acid which is precipitated because of its greater insolubility. Such precipitation is favored by concentration of uric acid in the blood and urine, a condition which may be caused by consuming food rich in nucleoproteins. Uric-acid calculi are usually of brownish-red or reddish-yellow color, very hard, irregular in outline, often showing sharp points which may be a source of irritation to the renal pelvis, the ureter or the bladder. The color is due to the presence of urochrome and urobilin. Calculi composed of urates are more frequent in infancy than in later life, and are probably formed about a nucleus of urates which enters the renal pelvis when the salts constituting the common uric-acid infarcts pass down the urinary tract. They are usually relatively soft and of a brilliant yellow color. When found in adults they are usually secondary to infection of the urinary passages which leads to alkalinity of urine. In either case the calculi are more likely to be composed of ammonium or sodium urate, but occasionally other salts may be found.

CONCREMENTS COMPOSED OF CALCIUM OXALATE are the most common calculi of the adult urinary tract. They are extremely hard, pale yellow, rough calculi which may not only irritate the mucous membrane but may also produce hemorrhage. Oxalic acid is a normal constituent of urine and is maintained in solution largely by reason of the presence of acid phosphates. Excessive ingestion of food containing oxalic acid such as rhubarb, spinach, grapes, may lead to supersaturation of this acid in the urine, which results in precipitation. Oxalic acid may be formed from uric acid in metabolism and may be produced in the urine by bacterial infection. The color depends upon the mixture of urinary pigment, but if hemorrhage has occurred, the calculi may assume a dark brown color due to hematogenous pigment.

CALCULI COMPOSED OF PHOSPHATES are usually secondary to the presence of other calculi which induce inflammation of the pelvis of the kidney or of the urinary bladder. Such inflammations are likely to be accompanied by decomposition, with the formation of ammonia from urea. This causes precipitation of several salts so that the calculi are composed largely of ammonium magnesium phosphate, with a certain amount of calcium phosphate, calcium oxalate and ammonium urate. In the renal pelvis they are practically always secondary to other calculi. In the bladder they may occasionally be primary, portions of desquamated epithelium from the bladder wall, mucus, pus cells, fibrin or other inflammatory products serving as a centrum. In fact, the deposit of phosphate in the urinary bladder may be so great as to form extensive encrustation of the bladder wall. The phosphatic calculi are usually grayish-white on the outer surface, although they too may be pigmented by urinary pigment or by blood pigment. The secondary calculi usually have a centrum composed of an oxalate or urate calculus. Phosphate calculi contain considerable organic material, which serves to bind the salts into a mass. These calculi are usually soft and friable.

OTHER TYPES of urinary concrements are rare, but reports have appeared of calculi made up of cystine, xanthine, indican, fatty substances, fibrin and cholesterol.

Miscellaneous Concrements

Pancreatic and Salivary Calculi. These are probably formed solely as the result of inflammatory disease of the ducts. Ligation of these ducts does not lead to the production of calculi. Such calculi consist very largely of calcium phosphate. In the case of the pancreas, numerous other substances may be present, owing to the digestive effect of pancreatic juice upon the organic material in the duct wall and in the secretion itself. Certain pancreatic calculi are made up largely of calcium carbonate. Usually, however, there is a mixture of substances other than the main salt comprising the calculus. As a rule, these calculi are of considerable size, are granular on the outer surface, pale yellow or grayish-white in color, soft and easily broken up. One stone came under our observation which occupied the entire length of the pancreatic duct, and showed projections corresponding to the smaller divisions of the main duct. Calculi in the salivary glands similarly are made up of calcium salts and present the same general appearance. They are likely, however, to show more organic material binding the salts together. Sometimes salivary calculi are found to have a centrum of some foreign body such as a fragment of tooth, a piece of filling, or other foreign material.

Intestinal Concrements. A variety of foreign bodies may serve as the centrum for calculus formation in the gastro-intestinal tract. These may be ingested foreign bodies such as pins, nails, fruit stones, pieces of bone, or foreign bodies which gain access in other ways, such as gall stones. Occasionally, hard masses of feces may remain in the intestine long enough to form the centrum of a calculus. As a rule, the intestinal calculi are made up very largely of ammonium magnesium phosphate, mixed sometimes with calcium salts, protein material and soaps. These calculi may occur in almost any part of the lower intestinal tract and may lead to partial or complete obstruction. Concrements of fecal material are not infrequently found in the appendix. They may have a nidus of some foreign body or may be composed entirely of feces. It is only rarely, however, that they are infiltrated to any considerable degree with mineral salts.

Other Forms of Concrements. Occasionally concrements are found under the prepuce in cases of phimosis and apparently are the result of deposition of urinary salts upon the accumulated smegma. Concrements are occasionally found in the prostate, originating in corpora amylacea upon which are deposited inorganic salts, particularly those of calcium, magnesium and phosphoric acid. Calculi are rarely found in the bronchi and sometimes may be expectorated. They are either deposits of lime salts and other materials upon a centrum of desquamated cells or exudate, or they represent calcified tuberculous masses which become extruded and lie in the bronchial tree. Foreign bodies in the nose sometimes lead to the deposit of calcium salts and the formation of the so-called rhinoliths. Such calculi may also form on a nidus of blood clot or nasal secretion. The necrotic material in the crypts of the tonsil may also occasionally serve as a nidus upon which salts of various kinds are deposited. Similar to these are the calcium deposits of sebaceous cysts of the skin, giving rise to the so-called cutaneous concretions.

Phleboliths or vein stones are usually more or less concentric deposits of lime upon and within thrombi in the veins. They occur in the spleen, but most of the calcific masses in that organ are calcified tubercles. Small veins in other situations may be affected, notably in the wall of the urinary bladder. Arterioliths, of the same nature, are occasionally encountered.

Corpora Amylacea. The most common situation is in the prostatic acini, the number increasing with age. Similar bodies occur in the lateral ventricles of the brain, as well as in sites of chronic inflammation or hemorrhage in the lung and other organs. They may be seen grossly as tiny pale yellow or brown nodules, but ordinarily they are visible only microscopically. In section, the corpus is a disk-like body, which takes the acid stain and is laminated. The center may be finely granular and the laminae radially striated. The outline may be faceted when several corpora occur in an acinus. Although they are stained by iodine, other staining reactions for amyloid are inconstant; they are not true amyloid. Chemical studies of those in the prostate show that they are composed largely of protein and nucleic acid, probably as a nucleoprotein. Lipids are present in small amounts, but double refraction with polarized light is due to crystalline purins. The corpora are formed from desquamated epithelial cells and prostatic secretion. Only rarely is a nidus discovered. Presumably interphasial phenomena between corpus and surrounding medium determine the deposit of the concentric laminae.

Prostatic concrements, which are granular bodies, usually dark brown in color and a few millimeters in diameter, occasionally considerably larger, have corpora amylacea as a basis. The corpora become infiltrated with calcium salts, probably because of their hyaline character, and often show a small amount of iron. Rarely urinary calculi gain access to prostatic ducts. (See Moore.)

Psammoma Bodies. These are small bodies of concentrically laminated calcareous deposit, usually microscopic in size, but sometimes with a diameter of 2 or 3 mm. Grossly, the psammoma bodies can best be described as sand-like particles. Microscopically, they are generally spherical bodies, which show concentric lamellation of finely granular basophilic calcareous material. They are composed of carbonate and phosphate of calcium mixed with organic material. They are found particularly in connection with chronic inflammation and tumor formation, and are said to be practically normal in the adult pineal gland in the form of the so-called "brain sand." The deposit of lime salts is usually upon a pre-existing hyaline matrix. They are not infrequent in chronic inflammations of the dura mater. They occur in both benign and malignant epithelial and connective tissue tumors, and such tumors are qualified as psammomatous. The true psammoma is a meningioma with numerous psammoma bodies.

REFERENCES

Aschoff, L., and A. Bacmeister: Die Cholelithiasis, Jena, 1909.

——: The Origin of Gall Stones, Lectures on Pathology, New York, 1924, p. 206.

Bacmeister, A.: Die Entstehung des Gallensteinleidens, Ergeb. Inn. Med., **11**: 1, 1913.

Barr, D. P.: Pathological Calcification, Physiol. Rev., **12**: 593, 1932.

Butler, M.: Experimental Calcification in Mice, Proc. N. Y. Path. Soc., **24**: 79, 1924.

Ham, A. W.: Mechanism of Calcification in the Heart and Aorta in Hypervitaminosis D, Arch. Path., **14**: 613, 1932.

Hart, D.: Ueber die Entstehung der Gallensteine, Med. Klin., **13**: 549, 1917.

Hartsuch, P. J.: The Chemical Reaction between Oleic Acid and Aqueous Solutions of Magnesium, Arch. Path., **25**: 17, 1938.

Harvey, W. H.: Experimental Bone-Formation in Arteries, Jour. Med. Res., **17**: 25, 1907-08.

Holt, L. E., Jr., V. K. LaMer, and H. B. Chown: Studies in Calcification, Jour. Biol. Chem., **64**: 509, **1925.**

Hueper, W.: Metastatic Calcifications in the Organs of the Dog after Injections of Parathyroid Extract, Arch. Path., **3**: 14, 1927.

Jaffe, H. L., A. Bodansky, and J. E. Blair: Fibrous Osteodystrophy (Osteitis Fibrosa) in Experimental Hyperparathyroidism of Guinea-Pigs, Arch. Path., **11**: 207, 1931.

Kahn, M.: Study of the Chemistry of Renal Calculi, Arch. Int. Med., **11**: 92, 1913.

Klotz, O: Studies upon Calcareous Degeneration, Jour. Exper. Med., **7**: 633, 1905; **8**: 322, 1906.

Kramer, B., and M. J. Shear: Composition of Bone. II. Pathological Calcification, Jour. Biol. Chem., **79**: 121, 1928.

Logan, M. A.: Recent Advances in the Chemistry of Calcification, Physiol. Rev., **20**: 522, 1940.

Lutz, J. F.: Calcinosis Universalis, Ann. Int. Med., **14**: 1270, 1941.

Mann, F. C.: The Effects of Complete and of Partial Removal of the Liver, Medicine, **6**: 419, 1927.

Meeker, D. R., and H. D. Kesten: Composition of Pathological Calcium Deposits, Jour. Biol. Chem., **113**: 289, 1936.

Moore, R. A.: Morphology of Prostatic Corpora Amylacea and Calculi, Arch. Path., **22**: 24, 1936.

——, and R. F. Hanzal: Chemical Composition of Prostatic Corpora Amylacea and Calculi, ibid., **22**: 41, 1936.

Roberg, O. T.: Sialolithiasis, Ann. Surg., **39**: 669, 1904.

Robison, J.: The Possible Significance of Hexose-Phosphoric Esters in Ossification, Biochem. Jour., **17**: 286, 1923.

Rosenberg, E. F.: Chalk Gout. A Report of Two Cases With a Brief Report of Some Previously Reported Studies on Calcinosis, Jour. Amer. Med. Asso., **115**: 1791, 1940.

Scheunert, A., and R. Bergholz: Zur Kenntnis der Pankreaskonkremente, Zeitschr. Physiol. Chem., **52**: 338, 1907.

Shohl, A. T., H. Goldblatt, and H. B. Brown: The Pathological Effects upon Rats of Excess Irradiated Ergosterol, Jour. Clin. Invest., **8**: 505, 1930.

Wells, H. G.: Metastatic Calcification, Arch. Int. Med., **15**: 574, 1915.

——: Chemical Pathology, 5th ed., Philadelphia, Saunders, 1925.

6

Atrophy

INTRODUCTION

Definition

Atrophy is an acquired reduction in size of an organ or cell that has reached mature size. It is not to be confused with agenesia, aplasia and hypoplasia. Agenesia implies complete absence of an organ, the result of faulty or absent anlage. Aplasia refers to a scanty and usually abnormal development, so that there is but little of the organ to be seen; indeed it may be represented only by a small mass of connective tissue. Hypoplasia is a failure of development of an organ up to its natural mature size although the essential structures of it are usually present. Hypoplastic organs, however, may become atrophic.

CLASSIFICATION

Atrophy was formerly classified as simple, when the reduction in size was supposed to be due solely to decrease in the size of the cells, and numerical, when due to decrease in the number of cells. It is true that individual cells may be the seat of atrophy, and it is possible that this may be sufficiently extensive to reduce the size of the organ, but for all practical purposes any organ, the seat of a noteworthy atrophy, can be regarded as having suffered a loss of many of its cells. Consequently, numerical atrophy is used synonymously with atrophy when that term is applied to an organ or tissue.

CAUSE

The cause of atrophy is inadequate nutrition. Atrophy is classified as primary and secondary. Primary atrophy is due to some fault within the cell whereby its utilization of nutrition is decreased or its growth energy is inadequate. Secondary atrophy is due to an excess of catabolism over anabolism, the result either of inadequate nutrition or of overwork. It is often impossible to distinguish between these two forms and it is probable that changes incident to primary atrophy are partly, if not largely, responsible for all forms of atrophy.

Theoretically an atrophic cell should be simply reduced in size but as a matter of fact there is usually also cloudy swelling and sometimes fatty degeneration. Indeed in some atrophic organs many cells disappear, for example in the heart (Karsner, Saphir and Todd). Bradley states that the changes in atrophy "are brought about by chemical liquefaction of the tissue proteins, catalyzed by enzymes present in the cells," and that the "same products are formed which appear as the end result of hydrolytic cleavage of protein by the digestive tract, namely, the peptides and amino-acids."

Atrophy of muscle and bone may produce functional disturbances and deformities. In internal viscera, atrophy may lead to no clinical disturbance unless it is marked. The atrophic heart may maintain circulation adequate for the ill-nourished, emaciated or chronically ill patient. Organs such as kidneys and liver have adequate reserve to compensate for atrophy of a good deal of substance. In certain instances, such as the atrophy of an immobilized group of muscles, removal of the cause is followed by full restoration to normal. Various manifestations of

88

atrophy are classified according to presumptive causes as indicated in the following paragraphs.

PHYSIOLOGIC ATROPHY

This includes the natural atrophy that occurs in certain organs at different times of life, as exemplified in the atrophy of the thymus gland in early life and the atrophy of ovaries and breasts at the menopause. These are physiologic but also appear to represent aging of those organs and thus are in another sense senile atrophies. After pregnancy the hypertrophic uterus returns to normal, but this is not a true atrophy because there is no reduction below the original adult size.

PATHOLOGIC ATROPHY

Atrophy of Inanition

The problems of inadequate nutrition have been studied with regard to the entire body and parts of it. General inanition may be partial when food is taken in insufficient quantities, or complete when food is withheld entirely. Well nourished adults can withstand abstinence from food for several weeks provided water is given. The individual studied by Benedict lost one pound per day for 31 days, but little else of great significance was observed. Dogs have survived complete starvation for periods of seven weeks. Complete lack of food results in utilization of stored glycogen and fat, and may ultimately produce disturbance of general metabolism of these substances. Fixed acid intoxication by ketones may occur, but affects the obese more seriously than the lean. Starvation affects different parts of the body variously and the losses may result in abnormality of form. The central nervous system and to a lesser degree the bones are more resistant than other parts. Muscles which are in active use suffer less than those at rest. Jackson points out that cells are reduced in size, show a modified nucleus-cytoplasm ratio and resemble the embryonal type, but mitosis is usually inhibited. Subsequently cloudy swelling, fatty metamorphosis and death may occur. In rats, Slonaker and Card found reduced growth, reduced reproductive capacity

and increased death rate. Jackson refers certain abnormalities of form to inanition and suggests that in addition to effects on somatoplasm, the germ plasm may perhaps be so affected as to be of importance in heredity and evolution.

Undernutrition, as distinguished from starvation, probably differs only quantitatively in effect. It may be due to deficiency of all the food factors or to deficiency of either carbohydrates, fats or proteins, or even to certain amino-acids. Usually there is also a deficiency of vitamins with the special features indicated in the chapter on General Phenomena of Disease. In addition to general atrophies of soft tissues, the bones may show extreme degrees of osteoporosis. Deficiency of proteins may so deplete the blood that nutritional edema occurs. Malnutrition either directly or through avitaminoses appears to reduce resistance to infectious diseases, but there are few exact studies of this.

Malnutrition and consequent atrophy may also be due to strictures of the alimentary tract, such as esophagus and pylorus, to disease of digestive glands or obstruction to their ducts. It may accompany destruction of the pituitary gland, as in cachexia hypophyseopriva or Simmonds' disease, and is a striking feature of anorexia nervosa, a profound loss of appetite probably of psychoneurotic origin.

Gradual reduction in the lumen of an artery leads to atrophy of the part supplied. Thus in a kidney whose arteries are sclerotic there are foci of atrophy of the parenchyma, accompanied by local fibrosis. The same is true in the heart. In the brain, atrophy due to arteriosclerosis leads to gliosis rather than fibrosis.

Pressure Atrophy

There are numerous examples of atrophy following prolonged pressure to a part, especially when continuous. It may occasionally follow interrupted pressure. This form of atrophy is probably entirely nutritional both by compression of cells in such a way as to interfere with their metabolism, and by pressure upon blood vessels. Arteries are more resistant than veins, so that a good deal of the interference with nutrition is due to passive hyperemia from pressure of veins. A frequent example is the bed sore or decubitus. Prolonged confinement to bed produces pressure over bony prominences, especially after fat is reduced by long illness. There is first atrophy of the skin and underlying tissues, followed by necrosis and ulceration. Tumors which grow by expansion may produce pressure atrophy in surrounding parts of the organ affected. The grooves that appear in the body surface of an infant due to the pressure of a displaced umbilical cord are due partly to atrophy and partly to hindrance to local growth. The ducts of glands may be occluded by pressure from without or by disease within the duct. The organ becomes atrophic and often distended; for example, occlusion of a ureter is followed by distention of the renal pelvis and atrophy of the kidney. Much of the atrophy is due to pressure of accumulated urine, but some of it may be due to cellular inactivity.

Toxic Atrophy

That this condition actually exists is open to doubt. Toxins and other deleterious products of infections produce degenerations and necrosis, rather than atrophy. In prolonged infections, as, for example, tuberculosis, various organs may become atrophic, but this is probably largely if not entirely nutritional. It may be that in continuous or frequently repeated fever, catabolism may exceed anabolism, with consequent atrophy, but this has not been proved. The wasting of flesh that occurs in patients with malignant tumors is due to malnutrition or to hemorrhage or both, and often to psychic loss of appetite, but there is no proof that the tumor produces poisonous effects except through the split protein products of necrosis. Roentgen rays and radium produce reduction in size of lymph nodes and genital glands, but this is due to destruction of cells rather than atrophy.

Atrophy from Inactivity: Neurotrophic Atrophy

These are considered together because they are not clearly distinguishable. Reference has been made to atrophy of glands due to occlusion of their ducts. Usually the accumulated secretion leads to a pressure atrophy, but even when distention does not occur, atrophy may supervene. An interesting example is atrophy of the acinar cells of the pancreas following occlusion of the ducts even when there is no distention of the ducts; the islets persist, probably because they are richly vascularized and are not concerned with external secretion.

Muscles may undergo atrophy while they are immobilized as in the treatment of fractures or as the result of ankylosis of joints. Experimentally this is found to be due to decreased size of the muscle fibers, without alteration of the ratio of water and solids and without effects on nerves or nerve endings. Full recovery follows removal of the cause. Quite different is the atrophy that follows disease or destruction of the motor neurons. Atrophy ensues much more quickly and there is disintegration of sarcoplasm and sarcostylic elements, soon followed by death of some of the fibers. Intramuscular nerves and nerve endings degenerate. The nuclei of the sarcolemma and muscle proliferate evidently because of stimulus in the direction of regeneration, but true regeneration does not occur. Chemically, however, the only regular change is an early decrease of total phosphorus. Interstitial fibrosis and deposit of fat may be a later sequel. If muscle of this sort is restored to activity, the function is assumed by the remaining undestroyed fibers. (See Chor et al.)

Atrophy from Overwork

Provided nutrition be adequate, increased work leads to development of parts and to hypertrophy. There are limits to which hypertrophy may progress, and if the increased work continue, atrophy may ensue. Examples are found in the atrophy in the arms of blacksmiths, and of the forearms in piano players, seamstresses, typists, etc. It is possible that exhaustion of peripheral motor neurons plays an important part in the process, and that it is due as much to neurotrophic influences as to alterations in the muscles themselves. In many of these cases the atrophy is preceded by a period during which effort is accompanied by spasm of the muscle, the so-called occupational neuroses, such as writers' cramp, telegraphers' cramp, etc. Whether there is a primary nerve disturbance which leads to both cramp and atrophy, or whether the atrophy is due to exhaustion from the cramp, is not known. Possibly the atrophy of thyroid gland cells following hyperplasia and hypertrophy may be due to overwork.

Senile Atrophy

The aged are likely to have atrophy of various organs. In part it may be due to inactivity and in part to reduced intake of food and ill-advised balance of diet. There is no doubt that much of it is a physiologic involutionary process perhaps due to diminution of growth stimulus. It has been remarked that the placenta is senile by the end of pregnancy. Involution of the thymus begins in early postnatal life. The gonads become atrophic in middle life in women and in later life in men, and in women give rise to the clinical phenomena of the menopause. Atrophy of brain, heart, elastica of lungs, liver, kidneys and other viscera appear at different times in the process of aging. Nevertheless, many of the atrophies that occur in old age are due to local malnutrition incident to arteriosclerosis. This is especially true in the brain, heart and kidneys, with their accompanying senile dementia, heart failure and renal insufficiency. The causes of arteriosclerosis, as indicated in the chapter on Cardiovascular System, are not clearly identified, but the condition is not to be looked upon as a simple involutionary change in the arteries. It has been shown that certain of the acute and chronic infectious diseases have deleterious effects on arterial walls and it is possible that these leave residual changes. Repeated infections of one kind or another may thus have a cumulative effect. Since much of the atrophy of the aged is due to arteriosclerosis, the atrophy is ultimately due to whatever incidents in a long life lead to the arterial disease, arteriosclerosis (Karsner).

The average duration of life has increased markedly in the last forty years and therefore population trends are in the direction of a greater proportion of older people than heretofore. This fact presents special problems in diagnosis and treatment. The effects of the so-called degenerative diseases of the heart, arteries, kidneys and other organs, as well as the incidence and manifestations of tumors become especially noteworthy. Older patients also are subject to diseases that occur in all age periods, but the symptoms, signs and course may be modified in the aged subject. Special attention has to be given to methods of surgical operations so that risks are reduced. Physicians, surgeons and others in the medical field, as well as insurance companies and statisticians, have intensified their study of the problems of aging, and are writing upon this subject of Geriatrics. The pathology of diseases of advanced life is covered in the chapters on Systemic Pathology, but certain references to the literature on the general topic of aging are given below.

THE MORPHOLOGY OF ATROPHY

In addition to reduction in size, organs the seat of atrophy show certain other changes. In a general way weight is reduced, but if the atrophy be moderate, and there be a considerable replacement of atrophic parenchymatous tissue by fibrous connective tissue, the weight may not be materially reduced and sometimes is found to be increased. The general shape of the organ is retained except in those instances where the atrophy is due to pressure. Superficial changes, however, are not infrequent. The brain, when it undergoes atrophy, is likely to show a reduction in the size of the gyri, accompanied by an increase in the width of the sulci. The liver is likely to show an increased sharpness of its edges. At times the atrophy may be so marked that the underlying structures may be easily apparent through the capsule. When replacement of atrophic parenchyma by connective tissue occurs, it is not uncommon for the connective tissue to undergo secondary contraction. This contraction may produce a nodular appearance of the outer surface, because of the contraction of masses of connective tissue between which the parenchymatous substance may bulge. The consistency of the organ is increased, for as the parenchymatous cells undergo atrophy, the connective tissue is relatively increased and, as has been indicated, is often absolutely increased. Because of the relative or absolute increase in connective tissue, the organ cuts with increased resistance. The cross section is likely to retract and may show changes due to the increase of connective tissue. As a rule, the blood content is about normal as is also the moisture of the cut surface. Occasionally, however, especially when fat undergoes atrophy, there may be some replacement by a serous fluid, the so-called edema of atrophy. This, of course, produces moisture in the cross section. Atrophy of voluntary muscles may be accompanied by partial replacement by fat. In these circumstances the muscles may not be reduced in size, but are of reduced consistence, greasy, and show the fat in cross section. The color of atrophic organs may not be altered from the normal. As has been pointed out, however, the atrophy of heart, liver and spleen may be accompanied by relatively or absolutely increased amounts of pigment, giving grossly a brown appearance to the organs.

Microscopically, pure atrophy of the cells shows simply reduction in their size. The shape is not altered except in cases of pressure atrophy where there is, in addition, condensation of the material within the cell membrane. For a time the nuclei may be relatively large, giving an increase of nucleo-cytoplasmic ratio, but ultimately they too are reduced in volume. Storage substances may remain in atrophic cells, especially in the pressure atrophy around tumor masses in the liver, and may persist in spite of their compression by surrounding nonatrophic cells. Pigments also remain, as in atrophic cardiac muscle. As said above, simple atrophy is not common; there is usually degeneration, both parenchymatous and fatty, and certain cells may disappear.

REFERENCES

Benedict, F. G.: Study of Prolonged Fasting, Carnegie Inst. Pub., No. 203, 1915.

Bradley, H. C.: Autolysis and Atrophy, Physiol. Rev., 18: 173, 1938.

——, and J. Taylor: Studies of Autolysis. III. The Effect of Reaction on Liver Autolysis, Jour. Biol. Chem., 25: 261, 1916.

Child, C. M.: Senescence and Rejuvescence, Chicago, 1915.

Chor, H., and R. E. Dolkart: A Study of "Simple Disuse Atrophy" in the Monkey, Amer. Jour. Physiol., 117: 626, 1936.

——, R. E. Dolkart, and H. A. Davenport: Chemical and Histological Changes in Denervated Skeletal Muscle of the Monkey and Cat, ibid., 118: 580, 1937.

Cowdry, E. V., Editor: Problems of Ageing. Biological and Medical Aspects, Baltimore, Williams and Wilkins, 1939.

Jackson, C. M.: Dystrophic Morphology and Its Significance, Science, 57: 537, 1923.

Karsner, H. T.: Involutionary Changes in the Cardiovascular System, University of Pennsylvania Bicentennial Conference, Philadelphia, 1940, p. 17.

——, O. Saphir, and T. W. Todd: The State of the Cardiac Muscle in Hypertrophy and Atrophy, Amer. Jour. Path., 1: 351, 1925.

Metchnikoff, E.: Prolongation of Life, New York, Putnam, 1908.

——: The Nature of Man, New York, Putnam, 1908.

Minot, C. S.: The Problem of Age, Growth and Death, New York, 1907.

Muhlmann, M.: Die Veränderungen im Griesenalter, Zentralbl. Allg. Path., 11: 204. 1900.

Slonaker, J. R., and T. A. Card: The Effect of Restricted Diet on Growth, Amer. Jour. Physiol., 63: 503, 1922-23; 64: 35, 167, 203, 297, 1923.

Warthin, A. S.: Old Age. The Major Involution, New York, Hoeber, 1929.

7

Disturbances of Circulation

INTRODUCTION

There are many conditions, of great practical importance, due to disease of heart and vascular tree, to alterations in composition of the blood and to nervous and endocrine disturbances. As indicated in the outline given above, they are divided, for the sake of discussion, into general and local disturbances. An understanding of these is valuable in the subsequent sections on general pathology and many are discussed in the material on Systemic Pathology, especially in the chapter on Cardiovascular System.

GENERAL CIRCULATORY DISTURBANCES

Disturbances Originating in the Heart

Normal circulation depends upon coordination of the functions of the myocardium, the valves of the heart, the elasticity and contractility of blood vessels, the nervous system, the conduction system, muscular activity and the movements of respiration. It is impossible to ascribe disturbances of circulation to any one of these factors. Nevertheless the disturbances may take origin in any of these, but the effects generally are observed in various other parts of the system. Those which have their origin in the heart may depend upon disturbances of the myocardium, the valves, the pericardium, the conduction system, and to a limited extent the nervous system.

Failure of Cardiac Muscle. As to the myocardium, various diseases may result in the reduction of its capacity as a pump. These include especially degenerations of the muscles and interference with coronary blood supply. In the course of infectious diseases, there may be accompanying disease of the cardiac muscle, manifested as cloudy swelling, fatty degeneration, necrosis, or acute inflammation of the myocardium. Despite the inefficiency of the myocardium, circulation may be maintained for a period because of the compensating action of other mechanisms of circulation.

The myocardium receives its supply of blood through the coronary arteries. Arteriosclerosis of these arteries may so reduce the lumens that there are focal or fairly widespread regions of atrophy, with corresponding reduction in bulk of functional muscle.

93

Local death of muscle, known as infarction, is due to abrupt occlusion of the artery, most often the result of thrombosis, infrequently of embolism, and rarely of arteriosclerosis. Anoxemia occurs in the part supplied by the affected artery and if the regions so deprived of oxygen are sufficiently extensive, the heart fails at once. Anoxemia of the myocardium may also be relative. For example, a heart the seat of extensive arteriosclerosis or one which has marked aortic stenosis may suddenly fail. This is presumed to be due to the fact that when there is marked increase in cardiac output and corresponding utilization of energy by the myocardium, the coronary flow, although considerably augmented as a part of the increased ventricular discharge, is still not sufficient to supply an adequate amount of oxygen to the muscle.

The most important causes of hypertrophy of the heart are persistent hypertension, including the essential form and that due to chronic renal disease, and disease of the cardiac valves. Although the vascular bed of the myocardium is progressively increased during the course of hypertrophy, there comes a time when the blood supply cannot support further hypertrophy. Failure of a hypertrophic heart may be due to any of the causes enumerated above, including the degenerative effects of infectious disease and disturbances in coronary circulation.

Diseases of the Valves. The valves of the heart may be the seat of acute or chronic inflammation and occasionally are ruptured. The mass of vegetations in acute vegetative valvulitis may be so great as to interfere seriously with the function of the valve. In the course of only six or eight weeks, hypertrophy may be evident in those chambers in which the valvular disturbances bring about diastolic stretching. The deformity due to chronic disease of the valves may give rise to insufficiency or stenosis, or both, with consequent effects upon the cardiac chambers. The resulting disturbances of circulation may be marked enough to be manifest clinically. Nevertheless, in such a disease as chronic mitral stenosis there is often a good deal of passive hyperemia in the lungs, even though the patient may not complain of any symptoms referable to it. As long as hypertrophy maintains circulation, these valvular defects may continue for years without serious disturbance. Nevertheless, because of intercurrent disease of the myocardium or advancement of the valvular deformity, the heart ultimately fails. Rupture of valves, more especially the aortic valve, leads to insufficiency with its chain of disturbances in circulation. Dilatation of valvular rings may also produce faulty circulation.

The pericardium may become filled with fluid because of transudation of edema fluid, acute inflammation with considerable volumes of serous exudate, or with blood due to rupture of the heart itself or the intrapericardial segments of great vessels. The gradual accumulation of fluid due to passive hyperemia of the pericardium or to acute inflammation permits of some stretching of the parietal pericardium. Nevertheless there is likely to be a certain amount of compression of the veins entering the heart, especially the pulmonary veins, so that inflow into the left atrium and correspondingly systolic discharge are much reduced. Pulsus paradoxus may occur. The sudden accumulation of a large quantity of blood in the pericardium due to rupture of the heart or of the proximal aorta leads also to a transfer of intraventricular or intra-aortic pressure to the pericardium so that diastolic expansion of the heart is reduced. The heart is said to be the seat of tamponade and the usual outcome is death within a very few minutes. Although it was formerly supposed that adhesions between the parietal and visceral pericardium can produce hypertrophy of the heart, this idea has been discarded because of observations on human material and because of experimental work. Nevertheless, adhesions may go on to obliteration of the sac and a mass of fibrous tissue grow to such an extent that the heart is surrounded by a dense rigid envelope. This so-called constrictive pericarditis or pericardial scar may lead to interference with diastolic expansion of the heart. The sequel is passive hyperemia in the body and accumulation of edematous fluid, especially in the peritoneal cavity. It is probable that nervous influences such as paroxysmal tachycardia may ultimately lead to hypertrophy of the heart with the possibility of consequent failure. Cardiac arrhythmias lead to comparatively little disturbance in circulation; ordinarily the fault in circulation is to be attributed to those conditions which of themselves bring about the arrythmia. The effect of congenital malformations upon circulation depends upon their situation and extent. Some are of little significance, for example patent foramen ovale, whereas others may lead to death upon birth or in early infancy. Still others are consistent with survival until early middle or later life.

Congestive Heart Failure. Patients in whom the heart fails are said to have congestive heart failure, manifested by shortness of breath or dyspnea, cyanosis or blueness of skin and mucous membranes, cough, edema of dependent parts and certain other phenomena. The principal factor in the muscular inadequacy is oxygen deficit because of the utilization of glycogen in production of energy. Since insulin is concerned in this mechanism, local deficiency of insulin or of glycogen could also be effective. Numerous studies have demonstrated reduction of amounts of creatinine, creatine, phosphorus and acid soluble phosphorus in the myocardium but whether this is the cause of the failure or the result is not yet certain (Herrmann and Decherd).

Disturbances Originating in the Vascular System

The hydrostatic pressure within the vascular tree is maintained by the activity of the heart and peripheral vascular resistance. The latter may be increased through various mechanisms to produce hypertension. As a rule, hypertension is not accompanied by any noteworthy disturbances of circulation until the heart fails or vessels in the brain rupture or the kidneys become insufficient. This matter is discussed further in the chapter on Cardiovascular System.

Low blood pressure which is of pathologic significance may be due to a variety of disturbances. For example, alterations of vasomotor activity, whether central or peripheral, are significant. The poisonous effects of acute infectious diseases, such as diphtheria, typhoid fever, pneumonia and the like, may lead to low blood pressure. Whether this is due solely to the effects upon the muscle of the heart and blood vessels or is contributed to in large part by poisonous effects on vasomotor mechanisms, is not altogether certain. The same may be said of the low blood pressure that frequently accompanies chronic wasting disease, such as tuberculosis and malignant tumors. The low blood pressure of Addison's disease is in part due to insufficiency of adrenal cortical influences and may perhaps be due in part to alterations in the composition of the blood. Ingested poisons such as alcohol, chloral hydrate and the cyanides may also cause low blood pressure but ordinarily, except for the cyanides, this has little or no significance. Hemorrhage, if sufficiently large in amount, may result in low blood pressure. Usually, however, following the loss of a moderate amount of blood, the volume is rapidly restored by withdrawal of fluid from the tissues. One of the most important causes of low blood pressure is shock, which is discussed in the next paragraph. Pathologic low blood pressure is of importance functionally because of the failure to supply nutrition and oxygen, and failure to provide for the natural circulation of fluids through the tissues. Even the heart itself suffers from the inadequate supply of nutrition and oxygen.

Shock. This term covers a group of signs and symptoms usually of abrupt onset, characterized by partial or complete loss of consciousness, apathy, depressed motor activity and reflexes, partial or complete loss of sensation, fall of temperature, rapid and shallow respiration, pallor and marked fall of blood pressure. The clinical manifestations of anaphylactic shock, anaphylactoid phenomena, pulmonary embolism, etc., are similar, but the mechanism is different. What is often called medical shock occurs in certain acute infectious diseases, especially influenza and pneumonia, in connection with certain violent poisons, as a sequel of severe burns, of intestinal obstruction, of acute perforation or rupture of a viscus. Traumatic shock is usually classified as primary or secondary; the former follows shortly after the injury or surgical operation and the latter is delayed for several hours.

Shock due to wounds of various kinds is ordinarily delayed and usually referred to as secondary. Traumatic accidents, injury to the central nervous system, crushing wounds of the extremities and of the testes, surgical operations, especially under a general anesthetic, may all be followed by shock. The fall of blood pressure is generally considered to be the key phenomenon and has been variously attributed to vasomotor depression, acidosis, acapnia, fat embolism, injurious products of tissue destruction, reduction of blood volume and hemorrhage. Vasomotor depression is probably of importance in certain forms of medical shock as in that which occurs in influenza and pneumonia, but it is not generally considered to be primary in most forms of shock. Acidosis is secondary rather than primary and can be explained by anoxemia of the tissues. Acapnia is somewhat similar clinically, but is not true shock. Fat embolism and other forms of pulmonary embolism are also similar clinically, but the physiologic and anatomic changes are quite different. Although still in dispute, the experimental evidence adduced by Moon and others strongly supports the view that products of disintegration of muscle produce shock, but some think this may not be the primary essential factor.

Massive hemorrhage gives rise to many of the phenomena of shock, which ultimately may progress to shock. Nevertheless, hemorrhage differs from shock in several important respects. In hemorrhage, the blood is diluted because of the withdrawal of fluid from the tissues. In shock, the blood is concentrated, a phenomenon called hemoconcentration. Moon points out that in the patient in shock, hyperemia and petechiae are often marked, whereas in profound hemorrhage there is anemia of the tissues. Furthermore, the administration of salt solution aids materially in the elevation of blood pressure following hemorrhage and is ineffective in shock. Transfusion of whole blood is effective in hemorrhage and considerably less so, if at all, in shock.

Hemoconcentration occurs because of loss of the fluid part of the blood. Moon is of the opinion that the fundamental change is an increased permeability of the capillaries. This would permit escape of water and of plasma proteins. Loss of the latter from the blood reduces its osmotic pressure so that water does not re-enter into the blood. The whole mechanism may thus become a vicious cycle. There is some question as to whether or not the increased permeability of the blood vessels is primary or secondary. Nevertheless it is certain that the administration of plasma and of its proteins, especially the albumin fraction, is beneficial in shock, whether it be due to trauma, burns or hemorrhage. This evidently increases the osmotic pressure of the blood and aids thus in restoration of its volume. Various other factors may be of considerable importance. For example, in the early stages of shock there appears to be peripheral vasoconstriction, although subsequently this is followed by dilatation of blood vessels in the viscera. Wiggers indicates that the peripheral vasoconstriction might so reduce the venous return to the heart that the systolic discharge would be depressed to a point where systemic blood pressure could not be maintained. Indeed it is possible, but not proved, that disturbance of cardiac muscle may be one of the early changes in shock. Scudder has found an increase of the potassium in the blood in both hemorrhage and shock but admits that this increase follows rather than precedes the drop in blood pressure. He offers the assumption that the increased amount of potassium may alter the heart in such a way as to reduce cardiac output.

Moon describes the autopsy on a patient dead of shock as disclosing collapse of superficial capillaries, distention of peritoneal capillaries, hyperemia and cyanosis of various viscera, a small contracted spleen, profound hyperemia and edema of the lungs together with some hemorrhage, and also the presence of bloody fluid in the serous cavities. Experimentally the hyperemia of the intestinal canal is most marked at the duodenal end and decreases in degree toward the ileocecal junction. The adrenal glands often show a fragmentation of the cortex due to necrosis of its deeper portions. It is not to be expected that every autopsy will show all the changes and furthermore some of the lesions may be observed in conditions other than shock.

Disturbances Originating in Mass and Constitution of Blood

It is ordinarily considered that the volume of the blood is one of the physiologic constants of the body but Barcroft states that it is "a physiological variable which is adjusted to the work required of it and to the size of the bed it occupies." If this be true, minor changes in volume are of no significance. Pathologically, however, there may be significant changes in volume in the direction of an increase or a decrease.

Plethora. The term plethora is applied to an increase in the total volume of the blood, including both the corpuscles and the plasma. This is especially well illustrated in polycythemia vera. In secondary plethora, although the total volume of blood is increased, this does not affect especially the corpuscular volume. In hydremic plethora the total number of corpuscles is not increased but the volume of fluid is. This increase in amount of fluid may depend upon failure of excretion of water or upon increased osmotic pressure of the blood. It may occur temporarily because of a large intake of fluid but such forms of plethora usually disappear rapidly. In certain instances where great intake of fluid persists for a long time, for example in the continued consumption of large quantities of beer, hydremic plethora may last as long as the habit is carried on.

In hydremia, as distinguished from hydremic plethora, there is an increase in the amount of fluid in the blood without an increase in the total amount of blood. Following hemorrhage there is a withdrawal of fluid from the tissues and the volume is restored to about normal, but the blood is watery and the seat of a true hydremia.

Anemia. A decrease in the volume of blood is referred to as anemia or oligemia. A decrease in total volume may be due to hemorrhage or to loss of fluids as exemplified in shock. In the former, the reduction in volume is only temporary because withdrawal of fluid from the tissues restores the volume. In the latter it lasts until the osmotic pressure of the blood is restored to satisfactory levels. Some of the phenomena of hemorrhage have been referred to in the discussion of shock and other features are discussed later. Reduction in the number of corpuscles may be due to a single hemorrhage, large in amount, to frequently repeated small hemorrhages or to disease of the hematopoietic system. The various forms of anemia in which there is reduction in the total number of circulating red blood cells are discussed in the chapter on Hematopoietic System.

Anhydremia. The term anhydremia refers to a reduction of the fluid part of the blood. It may be due to a variety of causes and gives rise to the clinical manifestations of dehydration. These include dryness of the skin and mucous membranes associated with loss in weight and with thirst. The blood itself exhibits increased concentration of the plasma proteins, of hemoglobin and of erythrocytes, together with increased viscosity. Although the crystalloids show little or no change, nonprotein nitrogen, including urea, is increased and sometimes reaches high figures, partly because of the fact that renal function is disturbed by the concentrated blood. Sugar may be increased in amount in the blood, there may be sugar in the urine, and there may be ketonuria. According to Marriott, there is a decrease of blood volume, an impaired circulation and a reduction in the oxygen carrying capacity of the blood, as well as vasoconstriction. The volume flow through the extremities is reduced and the capillaries usually contain a large number of red blood corpuscles. The reduction of blood volume reduces the effective pressure in the left atrium so that there is probably a decreased ventricular discharge, but for a considerable time this is compensated for by the increased viscosity of the blood and by vasoconstriction. Anhydremia results from restriction of intake of water as in psychic disturbances, from excessive output of water as in prolonged vomiting, watery diarrhea and Asiatic cholera, and, as indicated above, plays an important part in shock. There is little to show for anhydremia in the autopsy except that the weight of the body and the viscera may be reduced because of the relative dehydration of the tissues.

Edema

This term signifies the accumulation of fluid in excess in cells, tissues and various cavities of the body such as serous sacs and also in pulmonary alveoli. Ordinarily it applies to accumulations in tissues such as permit pitting on pressure and in body cavities to a point definitely in excess of that normally present. There are two main varieties of edematous fluid. One is a fluid called transudate and the other a fluid that is part of an inflammatory exudate. Unless otherwise specified, the term edema refers to transudates. Exudates rich in fluid are called serous exudates or inflammatory edema. The term effusion, as used in the clinic, usually refers to serous exudate, for example, "pericarditis with effusion" and "pleurisy with effusion." Because of lower concentrations of protein, transudates are of lower specific gravity than fluid exudate, richer in chloride and other electrolytes and usually poorer in cells. Wells states that the specific gravity of transudates is usually below 1.015 and that of exudates above 1.018. Exudates show a greater shift of hydrogen-ion concentration toward the acid side than do transudates. Inflammatory edema is discussed further in the next chapter.

Edema may be due to obstruction to lymphatics, increased venous pressure as in passive hyperemia, decreased osmotic pressure of the blood, increased osmotic pressure of the tissues, reduced physical pressure of tissues, and increased permeability of venules, arterioles, and especially of capillaries. Obstruction to lymphatics may be due to lesions in the draining lymph nodes or in the larger lymphatics. The conditions of significance in the lymph nodes are metastatic tumor and tuberculosis. Large trunks may be involved in the scars of surgical operations as in the removal of axillary lymph nodes in cases of carcinoma of the breast; the same effect may be due to scarring the result of roentgen-ray or radium therapy. Blocking of lymphatics by filaria may produce marked edema especially in the lower extremities and the scrotum, the so-called elephantiasis. Obstruction of the thoracic duct, most commonly due to tumor or tuberculosis, may lead to edema in peritoneal and pleural cavities, often rich in lipids, called chylous ascites or chylous hydrothorax. Rupture of the duct may also play a part. Pseudochylous fluids are due to fatty degeneration of cells in the fluid.

Edema due to increased venous pressure may be local or general. In both, the intravascular pressure becomes high enough to exceed the natural osmotic pressure of the blood. Local edema of this sort is the result of compression of veins by tumors, enlarged lymph nodes and other lesions, or to disease in the wall of the vein with partial or complete filling of the lumen. The ascites of hepatic cirrhosis is probably due to reduction of the vascular bed in the liver, resulting in increased pressure in the portal venous system. More widespread edema occurs in congestive failure of the heart, the causes of which have been outlined above and further

elaborated in the chapter on the Cardiovascular System.

If the colloid osmotic pressure of the blood be normal, the hydrostatic pressure in the venous end of the capillaries must be 20 mm. mercury in order for edema to occur. A tendency to formation of edema develops when the hydrostatic pressure in the same situation rises to within 2 mm. or less of the colloid osmotic pressure (Fahr and Ershler). Capillary dilatation increases filtration surface and this may favor production of edema, but anoxemia does not reach a degree sufficient to increase permeability. McLean thinks that in cardiac edema there is an increase of water content of the blood, which in dependent parts favors filtration. When the tissues are well filled with fluid, progress of the edema is slowed, probably due principally to the physical pressure in the tissues and perhaps in small part to an increase of osmotic pressure in the blood. Even early in this form of edema there is no proof of increased osmotic pressure in the tissues. There is no definite correlation between duration of edema and protein content of the fluid (Landis). It is interesting that increased pressure in the arteries, even in prolonged hypertension, does not cause edema. In hypertension there is no increase in osmotic pressure in the blood and no other satisfactory explanation for the absence of edema.

The principal forms of edema associated with reduced osmotic pressure of the blood are the edema of renal insufficiency and that of prolonged malnutrition. The decrease of osmotic pressure is attributed to decrease of plasma protein. Since the osmotic pressure of albumin is four times as great, gram for gram, as that of the globulin (Bruckman and Peters), the albumin must be the more important factor. It is unlikely that mere reversal of the albumin : globulin ratio is effective unless the quantity of albumin is significantly reduced. In human and experimental nephrosis, there is great loss of protein in the urine with reduction of plasma proteins, especially the albumin, and a resultant fall in osmotic pressure. The same is often true of edema accompanying glomerulonephritis, but this is by no means invariable. It occasionally occurs in cardiac edema, but if so is probably due to passage of protein through the kidneys rendered permeable because of passive hyperemia. The lipids of the blood also play a part in maintenance of osmotic pressure. Usually a fall of proteins in the blood is accompanied by a rise in cholesterol. Fishberg has found that if lipemic blood be reduced in volume and diluted by hemorrhage, the osmotic pressure per gram of protein is greater than if blood be diluted to the same concentration of pro-

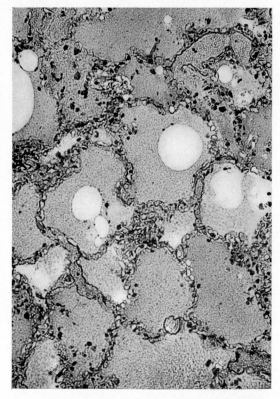

Edema of the lung. The protein of the fluid has been precipitated in preparation of the specimen, in the form of finely granular material in the air spaces.

tein. Murphy reports that in nephritis with edema the blood cholesterol is increased but that if edema be not present the cholesterol is not increased. Other factors also appear to operate. Van Slyke and his collaborators are of the opinion that in renal edema the plasma protein deficit is the controlling factor but it may be modified by the action of salts and perhaps capillary permeability. It is easily possible, but not finally proved, that the general metabolic disturbances of renal disease may produce injury to capillary endothelium.

In general the same mechanisms ap-

pear to operate in nutritional edema, a phenomenon common in the victims of famine. Because of inadequate intake of protein, there is reduction of osmotic pressure of the blood incident to decrease of plasma proteins but without noteworthy alteration of the albumin : globulin ratio.

The part played by increase of colloid osmotic pressure in the tissues is still not finally agreed upon. Schade and Claussen could demonstrate none, but McClure and Aldrich, and Andrews and others state that early in the course of edema there is an increased affinity of the tissues for water. Fahr and Erchler maintain that the edema fluid of various origins contains about the same amount of protein, but this is not sufficient to explain the edema. Much attention has been paid to the part electrolytes, especially salt, may play. Diffusibility is so great that it is hard to understand how there could be a significant difference in concentration in the blood and tissues. Nevertheless, Kerkhof has found that salt retention in the tissues appears to be essential to the development of edema in the dog. This problem continues to be studied in man and in experimental animals.

Edema following reduced resistance to capillary pressure may occur in the neighborhood of atrophy of the brain and in the substance of atrophic fatty tissue. Cupping produces marked reduction in extravascular pressure and leads to a readily reversible edema.

Injury to the endothelium appears to be responsible for the edema of inflammation and of paraphenylendiamine poisoning. It also is significant in the edema of the lungs due to inhalation of irritant gases, especially the war gases. Urticarial edema and that of various diagnostic skin tests is inflammatory and due to allergic reactions or to bacterial products.

The influence of the nervous system upon inflammatory edema will be discussed subsequently. There has been much study of pulmonary edema in the acute paroxysmal or neuropathic form. Luisada maintains that it is due to neurogenic vasodilatation and indicates that this is true of pulmonary edema in mitral stenosis and conditions in which the left heart fails. Nevertheless when the vasodilatation is present, dynamic factors of passive hyperemia augment the edema. It cannot be said that this matter is finally settled. (See Luisada.)

Morphologically, tissues, the seat of edema, are swollen, boggy, of doughy consistency, and when pressed leave the imprint of the finger. The area is pallid, except where associated passive hyperemia gives a dusky red or purple color. Incision releases the fluid and these characters are thereafter less marked. The cross section is pale, semitransparent or gelatinous, and from it can be expressed a thin, limpid, colorless or blood-tinged, salmon-colored fluid. In the serous cavities such as the pleura, pericardium and peritoneum, fluid is normally present, and edema is said to be present when the amount of fluid found is materially in excess of the normal. Histologic examination of edematous tissues shows the essential tissue elements separated from one another by the fluid accumulation. In stained specimens the spaces thus formed are occupied by fine, acidophilic granules due to precipitation of the protein content of the fluid. Accordingly, the number and size of granules vary with the protein content. Overheating of specimens in their preparation may produce similar separation of fixed tissue elements, but the acidophilic precipitate is absent.

LOCAL CIRCULATORY DISTURBANCES

These may result in either an increase or decrease of blood in a part. An increased volume is often called congestion, but since that term has various applications, the specific term hyperemia is preferable. Active hyperemia is due to increased supply from arteries. In passive hyperemia there is stagnation of blood in the venous side of the circulation.

Active or Arterial Hyperemia

This is a natural physiologic process in secreting glands, functioning skeletal muscle, is seen in pregnancy in the enlarged uterus and occurs in the skin in warm environments. It is probable that vasomotor reflexes and local physicochemical changes are involved. Pathologically, the most important form of active hyperemia is that which occurs in the first stages of inflammation, discussed fully in the next chapter. Nervous influences and diseases may result in active hyperemia. This is sometimes seen in neuralgia, is exemplified in emotional flushing (blushing) and probably accounts for dilatation of the vessels in the interior of the body following the vasoconstriction in the surface due to chilling. Neuroparalytic hyperemia, the result of interruption of stimuli through the vasoconstrictors, is well exemplified in Horner's syndrome, in which destruction of the cervical sympathetics by wounds, disease of the vertebrae, invading tumors, or inflammation, leads to active hyperemia of the corresponding side of the face and neck, sometimes with profuse sweating, dilatation of the pupil and drooping of the eyelid.

Morphology of Active Hyperemia. An organ or part the seat of arterial or active hyperemia is of bright red color, but slight pressure will force the blood out so that the part becomes pallid. By close examination of the living part, provided the covering membranes are not too thick, it is possible to see the smaller vessels distended and pulsating. If the hyperemia be sufficiently severe the organ may be tense. There is usually some swelling and, both objectively and subjectively, an increase in temperature when hyperemia is on or near the surface of the body. Microscopic observations are best made in living objects, because after death the blood sinks rapidly out of the part and the hyperemia may not be visible. Exception to this is found in acute inflammation where certain secondary changes preserve the caliber of the vessels as in life. Active hyperemia may be apparent in life as in some of the cutaneous rashes, but after death these rapidly disappear and histologic examination may show little or no vascular change. Edema, wandering out of blood cells and other phenomena occurring in passive hyperemia, such as will be described subsequently, are not to be found in simple active hyperemia. When disease of the smaller vessels or a deterioration of the vessels, such as is seen in old age, complicates the hyperemia, small hemorrhages may occur. Diagnosis of active hyperemia at autopsy is usually postulated only in those cases where infection or inflammation is known to be present. Without some such condition it is practically impossible to differentiate active from passive hyperemia after death.

Passive or Venous Hyperemia

This is one of the most frequent conditions found at autopsy and one of the most important sequels of chronic disease of heart, lung and liver. It varies from slight or moderate stagnation of blood in the veins and capillaries to complete cessation of flow or stasis. It may be of short duration or may become chronic. It is called passive because it is due to various conditions which interfere with venous drainage. Since vis-a-tergo plays but a small part in production of venous pressure, low arterial pressure is of little or no significance except in as far as it is due to myocardial insufficiency. Here the fault of propulsion is due to dilatation of cardiac chambers, with consequent venous stagnation.

Cardiac disease is the most frequent cause of widespread passive hyperemia, usually the outstanding phenomenon in congestive heart failure. Disease of pericardium, myocardium and valvular endocardium is significant, as indicated in the section above on disturbances of circulation originating in the heart and in the chapter on Cardiovascular System. Chronic fibrous disease of the lungs, emphysema, fibrous obliteration of the pleural sac, fluid or tumors in the sac and deformities of the thoracic spine, may result in decrease of negative pressure in the thorax, but are not likely to cause any marked degrees of passive hyperemia. In as far as any of these increases pulmonary arterial pressure with hypertrophy of the heart, especially of the right ventricle, and subsequent failure, it may ultimately cause marked passive hyperemia. Emphysema with its reduction of vascular bed in the lungs and chronic disease of the smaller arteries and arterioles are important in this connection. Reduction of vascular bed in the liver in hepatic cirrhosis causes passive hyperemia in the tissues and organs drained by the portal system. Lack of muscular activity may be significant in the accumulation of blood in the venous system of the lower extremities and be a factor in the production of varicose veins. Constipation, with its straining at stool, plays a part in development of anal hemorrhoids. The physiology of passive hyperemia is well discussed by Harrison.

In addition to these more general causes, there are numerous causes for local passive hyperemia referable to narrowing of the lumen of veins. This reduction in lumen may result from disease within the vein such as thrombosis or thrombophlebitis, disease in the vein wall such as phlebosclerosis, or from pressure upon the vein from without. Passive hyperemia due to local causes, where the circulation is dammed back in only a limited region, may be somewhat ameliorated by the establishment of collateral circulation. The passive hyperemia of a lower extremity, resulting from thrombosis of a femoral vein, may not lead to long standing or extensive hyperemia because of collateral circulation established in the deeper veins. In cirrhosis of the liver, veins of the abdominal wall may be conspicuously enlarged, because of a collateral circulation established through connections of the lower abdominal veins. The increased pressure in the portal venous system is gradually communicated to these veins, which become enlarged and provide for collateral venous drainage from the abdomen.

Morphology of Passive Hyperemia. The most conspicuous feature in the living patient is cyanosis of skin, lips, finger ends and mucous membranes. The same blue or reddish-blue discoloration is seen on gross examination of internal organs, the seat of passive hyperemia. These organs are likely to be somewhat increased in size and if encapsulated the capsule is tense. The weight and consistency are increased. Upon death or removal from the body, the blood may drain out of the organ in considerable amounts, so that the weight may be reduced below that which existed in life. Hyperemic organs removed by surgical operation may lose one-third of the weight or more by bleeding, as soon as the organ is cut open. Even after this loss of weight the dark red or purple color persists. The cross section bleeds freely. In the liver, the bleeding from the central zones of the lobules results in retraction of those portions so that they are on a lower level in the cross section than the peripheral zones. Microscopically the veins, venules and venous capillaries are found engorged with blood.

A simple, uncomplicated picture of passive hyperemia is rarely seen because secondary changes, including cellular degenerations, hemorrhage, pigmentation, edema and fibrosis, soon occur. The more severe or the more prolonged the passive hyperemia, the more pronounced are these degenerative disturbances. They lead to important functional

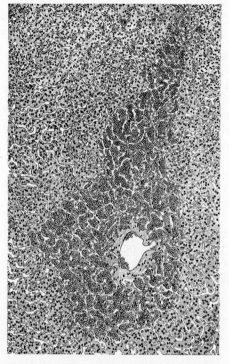

Passive hyperemia of the liver, showing the accumulation of blood in the central sinusoids and distention of central vein.

disturbances in certain areas. For example, the degeneration in the gastro-intestinal glands may lead to severe digestive disturbance. The deterioration of tissues may involve the walls of the venules and capillaries to such a degree that hemorrhage occurs. In passive hyperemia of the lung it is not at all uncommon for patients to expectorate blood-stained sputum. The deterioration affects not only the tissue cells but also the blood corpuscles themselves, especially those that have become extravasated, so that in cases of prolonged hyperemia, hematogenous pigmentation of the tissues is likely to be marked. In the liver the pigment is found in the parenchymatous cells near the center of the lobules. In other viscera the pigment is likely to be

found in macrophages in the neighborhood of the hyperemic vessels. This is likely to be easily demonstrable in the spleen, and is also seen in the lung, where the macrophages filled with blood pigment appear both within the alveoli, in the infundibula, within the lymphatic spaces and other structures. In the kidney the pigment may be found in the epithelial cells of the tubules but this is not commonly observed. Pigment may also be found in extracellular positions.

Edema frequently accompanies prolonged passive hyperemia. This is especially true in congestive heart failure where it is observed in dependent parts of the body, especially in skin and subcutaneous tissues, occurs as hydrothorax, hydropericardium, ascites and pulmonary edema. It may also be found as an interstitial or even intracellular edema of various viscera. This form of edema has been discussed previously, the fluid being a transudate.

Chronic passive hyperemia is characterized especially by the formation of fibrous tissue. Several factors contribute to cause the fibrosis. In the chapter on Atrophy, it was pointed out that fibrosis occurs incident to cellular atrophy, and this is true of the cellular atrophy which accompanies prolonged passive hyperemia. As cells are injured and destroyed, the products of disintegration stimulate a low-grade inflammation that results in fibrosis. Furthermore, continued presence of edema incites fibrosis. Grossly, organs the seat of chronic passive hyperemia are firm, cut with increased resistance and have a somewhat retracted, bloody cross section. Atrophy of the parenchyma and retraction of the fibrous tissue ultimately bring about reduction in size.

Microscopically the fibrosis is found particularly near the hyperemic vessels. In the kidney it is likely to be found in glomeruli and around the smaller vessels of the cortex and medulla. In the liver it is seen around the central veins. In the lungs it appears about the smaller vascular trunks and the capillaries of the alveolar walls. The fact that in the spleen the fibrosis is diffuse, leads to the belief that irritation of accumulated toxic products, incident to passive hyperemia, may result in the fibrosis, because in the spleen there is no true parenchymatous tissue and until passive hyperemia is very marked there is likely to be no atrophy. Passive hyperemia when affecting veins not well supported within organs causes dilatation, as seen in the lower part of the esophagus, the hemorrhoidal plexus and veins of the lower extremities. These may become thickened, elongated and tortuous, probably because the increased venous pressure operates on veins which are inherently less resistant than normal. Tributary lymphatics may become distended and thickened.

Local Anemia or Ischemia

When, for any reason, the blood vessels of a part are constricted, there naturally follows a diminution of the blood content of the part, a local anemia or ischemia. Associated with this there is local blanching or pallor and, in certain areas, disturbances of sensation. Local anemia is commonly of nervous origin and is usually spasmodic in character. An example is seen in Raynaud's disease, in which there is symmetrical blanching

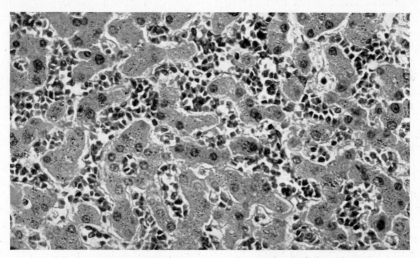

Passive hyperemia of the liver. Distention of the sinusoids by blood.

ACTUAL STASIS OF BLOOD in the vessels, which means complete cessation of current, may be the result of complete occlusion of the vessel. It appears in the margins of ulcers and old wounds, apparently as the result of evaporation of fluid in the superficial vessels. This increases the viscosity of blood and favors stasis. Cooling to –7° C. or heating to over 50° C. also leads to complete stasis. In the latter instance it is probable that evaporation also plays a contributing part, and in the former the crystallization of the water is of importance. Numerous chemical irritants may produce stasis: the corrosive alkalies and acids, hypertonic salt solutions, sugar, glycerol, croton oil and other substances. This may be due to chemical clotting of the blood or to precipitation of the blood proteins, or to the inflammation produced. Provided stasis be not too prolonged, circulation may be restored, but, if the process continue, thrombosis occurs and circulation is completely obstructed.

of fingers or toes on both sides of the body, associated with tingling or pain and fall in local temperature. Somewhat similar, although apparently not of nervous origin, is the disease known as thrombo-angiitis obliterans. Ergotism also exhibits areas of local anemia. The local application of cold, of adrenalin, or of certain other drugs may also lead to local anemia. Reflex anemia of the skin surfaces may be produced by psychic disturbances such as anger and fear. Local or general anemia of the brain may be the direct cause of fainting, as the result of pain, fright, or other emotion. Reflex disturbances of this sort are likely to be only temporary and do not lead to serious secondary effects. Provided the constriction be of sufficient duration, the coincident reduction of nutrition may lead to a series of secondary changes such as cloudy swelling, fatty degeneration, atrophy, necrosis, or gangrene. Local interference with circulation may also be produced by obstruction to an artery. This may result from pressure from without, from disease of the arterial wall, from thrombosis or embolism. Thrombosis signifies the formation of a clot in a living vessel. Embolism signifies the lodging in a vessel of some material foreign to normal circulation, including particles of thrombi, bacterial clumps, air, oil, and other foreign substances. For the sake of clarity, disturbances incident to obstruction of an artery will be discussed under the heading of infarction.

Infarction. The process of infarction is the series of events which follows the sudden and continued occlusion of an artery. The region supplied by the artery shows a sequence of hyperemia, hemorrhage, degeneration, necrosis, inflammation and either encapsulation by connective tissue or conversion into a fibrous scar. Necrosis is the essential feature in identification of an infarct. Rarely, infarction may be due to gradual occlusion of an artery as in marked arteriosclerosis. Infarction due to occlusion of veins is also infrequent. Infarcts are classified as either bland or infected and as either hemorrhagic or white. Infarcts may be infected because of infection in the causative condition or because of infection already existent in the tissue of the infarct. The ultimate result is a hematogenous abscess. The description of infarcts follows the discussion of mechanism of infarction.

The process has been extensively studied experimentally in spleen, kidney, heart, lung and brain. Observation of infarcts in man shows states of infarction, comparable to those of the experimental animal so that the results of the latter can be used in interpretation of infarction in man. The earliest stage is hyperemia in the region affected. This statement has been the subject of considerable discussion, but the series of papers by Karsner and associates are convincing. Although the cause of the hyperemia has not been proved, it is probably a vasomotor phenomenon. The occlusion stops the flow of blood and it remains in the dilated vessels where it is solidified by thrombosis. The accumulation of blood is slightly less if all collaterals are tied off and slightly greater if draining veins are ligated. In the lungs, however, occlusion of a branch of the pulmonary artery leads only to hyperemia, which lasts for a week or two. This is a form of temporary postoperative pulmonary complication. Only when pulmonary circulation is disturbed by conditions other than the arterial occlusion does stasis, thrombosis and infarction occur. Passive hyperemia of the lungs due to cardiac incompetency, pleural effusions, multiple emboli, occlusion of a main trunk of the pulmonary artery and perhaps other conditions may lead to this disturbance in circulation. Without it, blood continues to flow in the hyperemic focus because of the rich capillary bed in the lungs. Thus the older idea that infarcts may be anemic is not structurally valid, even though the region is anoxemic. Nor is it true that differences between white and hemorrhagic infarcts are due to occlusion of an end-artery in the former and communicating arteries in the latter. This assumption is contradicted by the observation of hemorrhagic and white infarcts in the same spleen. The degree of hyperemia, however, is greater in richly vascularized organs such as lung and spleen than in compact organs such as myocardium and kidney.

The essential factor in the development of the infarct is the local anoxemia and because of this the subsequent changes take place. Within two hours after the obstruction of the vessel, the blood corpuscles in the affected part begin to fuse together and form conglutinated masses. The part becomes swollen as the result of hyperemia and of edema but the edema soon disappears. Cloudy swelling appears usually in about two hours and retrogressive changes progress until, at the end of 48 hours, necrosis is present in the center of the infarct. The necrosis affects particularly the parenchymatous cells in the earlier stages but ultimately affects also the connective-tissue elements. Hemorrhage is constant but varies in amount dependent upon the vascular supply of the organ. For example, hemorrhage in the spleen and the lung is much more marked than that in the kidney or in the heart. In these latter organs it may not be demonstrable grossly, but is always present upon microscopic examination.

When necrosis appears, the margin of living tissue around the area shows a so-called reactive or collateral hyperemia, due in all probability to the irritant effect of the necrotic tissue. The necrotic mass becomes anemic, or pallid, or white, because of decoloriza-tion following degeneration of the blood. The removal of the pigment is probably by plas-matic diffusion. The pigment is probably removed as hemoglobin because, with the ex-ception of the spleen and the brain, pig-mentation by granular or crystalline blood pigment is not common. The decolorization appears first in the center of the infarct and then progresses peripherally. Blood injected into the lungs experimentally is removed by large mononuclear phagocytes and carried to the regional lymph nodes; and there is little doubt that this process serves to remove cells and granular pigment from the margins of the infarcts. The mononuclear phagocytes do not penetrate deeply into the infarct. The most important sequence of infarction is organiza-tion. This is a process whereby, as the result of a very low grade inflammation, connective tissue and capillaries grow to form a capsule around larger infarcts or to replace small in-farcts completely. By gradual alteration of this tissue into adult type connective tissue, the infarct becomes either encapsulated or cicatrized. The details of this growth of con-nective tissue will be considered in the discus-sion of inflammation. When any mass of tis-sue is destroyed there is, in some degree, regeneration of the destroyed tissues, depend-ing upon the type of tissue affected. Regen-eration is discussed in the chapter on in-flammation.

HEMORRHAGIC INFARCTS. Infarcts in general show early hemorrhage. The hemor-rhage may not be visible grossly. It is custom-ary to describe as hemorrhagic infarcts those in which the naked eye examination dis-closes a rich blood content. Such infarcts are seen in tissues where the blood supply is rich and the arrangement of the tissues rather loose. Consequently, the lung and the spleen show hemorrhagic infarcts to the best advan-tage. The infarct is generally conical in form, and occurs near the periphery of the organ with the apex toward the point of occlusion. The conical form may, however, be altered by the conformation of the outer surface of the organ. Affecting a margin of the spleen, the infarct may resemble a double cone or spin-dle. Affecting an oblique surface of the lung the form may be that of a truncated cone. Superficially the area involved is found to be swollen, solid, red, and firm. Not infrequently

in the case of the lung, the pleural surface may be covered by a thin film of fibrinous exudate. The color is dark red and any zone of reactionary hyperemia in the margin can be differentiated by its brighter red color. The cross section of such an infarct is gener-ally triangular in outline, sharply defined, shows the same color as the outer surface, bulges above the surrounding tissue and, be-cause of clotting of the blood with fibrin for-mation, usually is less moist than the sur-rounding tissue. The cross section bleeds very little because of the fact that the blood is coagulated.

Microscopically, the infarct is usually well defined, and shows beneath the capsule or surface of the organ a narrow zone of tissue, uninvolved save for the marginal hy-peremia. In the early stage, hemorrhage is the most notable feature; the parenchymatous cells show cloudy swelling or even fatty de-

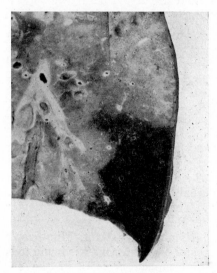

Hemorrhagic infarct of lung.

generation. Later the parenchymatous and less resistant parts of the tissues show com-plete necrosis, whereas the connective-tissue frame-work may be fairly well preserved. Ultimately, however, all tissues including the blood undergo necrosis. The necrotic areas show necrosis in the form of granularity or hyalinization of the cytoplasm, loss of cell outline, karyorrhexis, pyknosis or complete solution of the nuclei. In the earlier stages, the margins show the reactionary hyperemia in the form of distention of the blood vessels and, in addition, the exudation of a few poly-morphonuclear leukocytes and infiltration of lymphocytes and large mononuclear phago-cytes. Phagocytosis of cell fragments by the large mononuclear phagocytes is present but not striking. Accompanying these changes the marginal cells may show fat infiltration or fatty degeneration. Subsequently, this mild inflammatory reaction is followed by the growth of new blood vessels and connective tissue, constituting the process of organiza-tion spoken of above. Still later there is a dense margin of connective tissue around the infarct which may partially or completely replace the infarct.

WHITE INFARCTS. Since the white, or "anemic" infarcts are pallid because of de-colorization of the blood in the original re-gion of infarction, it follows that the less the hemorrhage the earlier does the infarct be-come pale. Hence those organs which do not have an extremely rich blood supply are more likely to show white infarcts than are others. Thus, of those organs where infarc-tion is most frequent, white infarcts are com-moner in the kidney and heart. Such infarcts, however, are not uncommon in the spleen and are occasionally seen in the lung. In the earlier stages of the process white infarcts are swollen, but in the later stages, they show, as a rule, a certain amount of retraction of the outer surface. They are of the same shape as hemorrhagic infarcts; they are solid, are well defined and paler than the rest of the organ. The usual color of the pale infarcts is a light yellow. The cross section is dry, granular and friable. Reactionary hyperemia about the margin is almost constant. Microscopically, the greater part of the mass is found to be the seat of complete necrosis. If the original hemorrhage has been slight, all traces of blood corpuscles have disappeared. If the hemorrhage has been marked, there may re-main, especially near the margins, the out-lines of erythrocytes without hemoglobin, the so-called shadow cells. Toward the margin, red cells may be fairly well preserved and, in general, necrosis is less marked at the mar-gin than centrally. Reactive hyperemia is more apparent and organization further ad-vanced than in the red infarcts. An infarct may progress to the white stage and may still show microscopically an outline of the connective-tissue structure, but even though

the outline remains, the connective tissue itself is usually completely necrotic. The ne-crotic cellular material of the organ substance is made up almost entirely of coarse granules, which take the acid stain. Infarcts of the spleen usually show blood pigment in the

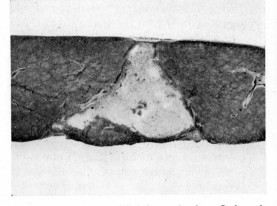

White or "anemic" infarct of spleen. It has al-ready undergone retraction. Note the living tissue be-tween the infarct and the capsule of the organ.

form of hematoidin, deposited in fine needle-like crystals collected together in sheaf-like bundles, the so-called "burrs." Hemosiderin is not commonly found in old infarcts except those of the brain, where it is collected in phagocytes at the margin.

Usually over the base of the infarcts there is a small line of living tissue which fails to become necrotic because of a more or less independent circulation, in and under-neath the organ surfaces. In the case of the kidney and spleen this is provided by the cap-sular circulation. In the lung the pleural vessels course parallel to the surface of the pleura, and are not involved by the obstruc-tion which produces the infarct. In the case of the heart the base of the infarct is toward the endocardium, where both endocardium and underlying cardiac tissue obtain their nutrition from the blood in the chambers of the heart and the thebesian vessels. With the exception of the brain, infarcts of which will be described in the section on neuropathology, other organs than those mentioned above are very rarely the seat of infarction. Such lesions are described in the liver, in the adrenal, in the pancreas, and are of particular impor-tance in the intestinal canal. In the intestine, however, white infarcts do not occur, because with the onset of necrosis the penetration of bacteria from the lumen leads to gangrene, which causes widespread peritonitis and death either by direct extension of infection to the peritoneum or by rupture of the gut.

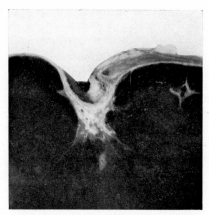

Cross section of cicatrized infarct of spleen.

If diagnosed in time, the surgeon removes the gangrenous segment.

FUNCTIONAL DISTURBANCES following infarction depend upon the size, number and region involved. In the brain, areas important for motor or sensory function or even struc-

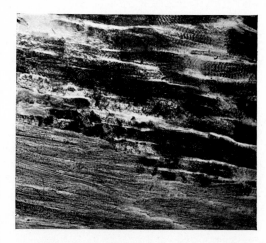

Photomicrograph of experimental infarction of dog's heart, showing hyalin and granular necrosis of muscle.

tures necessary for life may be involved. In the lungs, the infarcts are usually relatively small and of little functional significance, although at times the pleurisy over the surface may give pain and the sputum may be bloody. In the heart, small infarcts can be survived with little difficulty, but if the in-

farcts be sufficiently large the wall may be weakened and local dilatation ensue. Subsequently, this may rupture because of the intracardiac pressure. Sudden death may follow embolic occlusion of a sufficiently large part of the coronary circulation. The amount of circulation which must be obliterated to produce death depends, to a certain degree, upon the condition of the heart muscle. Large infarcts of the spleen may produce pain for a short time but otherwise are of no functional significance. Infarcts of the kidney may produce pain and rarely lead to hematuria, but in the absence of other disease of the kidney, infarcts must be multiple and large to produce any clinical manifestation. If the tissue destruction be sufficiently extensive, there may be fever, due presumably to the absorption of protein split products.

The retrogressive changes in the dead cells depend upon autolysis, a process that has been discussed in connection with the

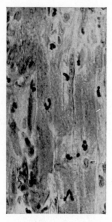

Photomicrograph of experimental infarction of dog's heart, showing migration of a few leukocytes into the necrotic muscle.

subject of necrosis. The fact that, in infarcts of the spleen and of certain other organs, the connective-tissue nuclei and the nuclei of the lymphocytes fail to disappear until relatively late has led to the suspicion that there may be an enzyme which operates especially upon cytoplasm.

The removal of the necrotic material depends in part upon the activity of the phagocytic cells, but anatomic study of infarction shows a relatively small participation on the part of these cells. Corper found that during the earlier stage of infarction when the nuclei show relatively little change, there is practically no solution of protein or protein products. Even when nuclei can no longer be found, from 30 to 50 per cent of the protein material is still in the insoluble form. This is in harmony with the customary slow reduction in the size of infarcts. In our own experimental observation the infarcts were only slightly reduced in size at the end of six weeks. In human cases there may be completely healed lesions of cardiac valves, from which emboli were probably discharged during the acute stage, but the resultant infarcts may be only slightly shrunken even though they must be very old. Wells points out that the inhibition of autolysis is probably due to

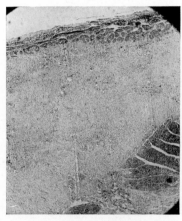

Low-power photomicrograph of experimental infarction of dog's heart in stage of complete cicatrization. Note pyramidal outline and the preservation of muscle under the endocardium.

the seeping of the alkaline tissue fluid through the infarct. Our own studies would indicate that phagocytosis plays only a small part in the removal of the necrotic material and that the materials which are rendered soluble by the lytic processes are removed by plasmatic diffusion. Large mononuclear and perhaps other cells at the margins of infarcts not uncommonly contain fat. It is not limited to infarcts, however, and may be seen about any mass of necrosis. The destruction of tissue is accompanied by breaking of fat into glycerol and fatty acids. These diffuse to the margin of the infarct where remaining cell lipase synthesizes the fat.

Postmortem Blood Clots. Of great importance at autopsy is the determination of whether solid masses of blood constituents found in heart and blood vessels are clots formed in the death agony and after death, or are thrombi formed in life. Upon this distinction may rest the establishment of the cause of death, a matter of broad scientific interest and also often practically significant in legal medicine and insurance claims. The diagnosis is made on the basis of gross and microscopic study. Usually the blood in the vessels clots rather suddenly after death, and in the clots are enmeshed all the elements of the blood, producing a red clot similar to that seen outside the body. This is called the "currant jelly" clot. Infrequently, however, where death occurs rather slowly, the elements of the blood may separate out to a considerable degree by virtue of differences in specific gravity, so that portions of the clot which lie in a superior position in the body may be of rather brilliant yellow color, and are called "chicken fat" clots. Sometimes, also, in the neighborhood of the chordæ tendineæ of the atrioventricular valves, the whipping action of these cords may separate the fibrin to produce a white fibrin clot, enmeshing very few cells. The "currant jelly" clot, therefore, contains all the cellular blood elements; the "chicken fat" clot contains principally white blood corpuscles, and the white fibrin clot has little or no corpuscular content.

The presence of fibrin is that which differentiates clots from simple clumping together of corpuscles. The fibrin serves to bind together the elements of the clot and give it a certain degree of firmness. If present in large quantities it gives a gray color to the clot and in cross section a dry appearance. Microscopically fibrin appears in the form of fine, refractile, acid-staining fibrils varying somewhat in size, branching and anastomosing to form an irregular mesh, which may resemble somewhat the fibrils of connective tissue. The fibrin mesh represents a precipitate from the fluid of the blood, and at the lines of junction there is an increase in amount of material which produces the so-called fibrin nodes. Not infrequently, certain small centers of platelets or leukocytes appear from which the lines of fibrin radiate to form the so-called fibrin asters or stars.

Under certain conditions blood in small vessels may, by virtue of stasis, undergo conglutination or congelation, in which the corpuscles fuse together in a relatively solid mass without any fibrin formation. Numerous substances, including specific agglutinating sera, as well as a wide variety of colloids, may produce agglutination in the circulating blood and these agglutinated masses may lodge in small vessels to occlude them.

Thrombosis

The term "thrombosis" indicates the formation in living vessels of more or less solid masses of constituents of the blood (or lymph). It may occur in any part of the vascular system. In one form or another, it is observed in from 14 to 22 per cent of autopsies (Bela; Dietrich). It may occlude the vessels and may also be the source of embolism.

Conditions which favor thrombosis include injury to the vessel wall, slowing of the stream and eddies in the current, and alterations of the constitution of the blood. The smooth lining of vessel walls is disturbed in arteriosclerosis and aneurysm, in infectious processes producing endothelial degeneration or actual inflammation, and in injury to the wall. With these disturbances of lining, slowing of the current favors thrombosis but is not an essential factor. It probably plays little if any part in the thrombosis which is often observed upon the roughened areas due to ulceration of arteriosclerotic plaques in the aorta, except that the current may be retarded by failing circulation. The influence of slowing of the current is seen in the fact that thrombosis is distinctly more common in veins than in arteries, and especially in those veins where under certain circumstances the current is likely to be especially slow. Similarly, the fact that thrombosis occurs in aneurysm and in dilatations of the veins is probably due in large part to the slowing of, or production of eddies in, the current.

General passive hyperemia also produces a tendency toward thrombosis, probably because of increased viscosity due to accumulation of carbon dioxide. When the stagnation of the current goes on to cessa-

tion, as is seen following ligation of a vessel, thrombosis in some degree almost invariably appears. Although careful ligation of vessels may produce thrombosis simply at the site of ligation, yet, as a general rule, thrombosis appears in the entire column of blood which is interrupted. Therefore, it extends to the next branch above and the next branch below. In addition to the slowing of the current and alterations of the vessel walls, any of the fac-

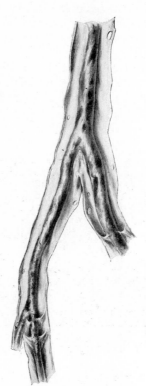

Extensive thrombosis of a vein and its tributaries. The vein has been laid open and shows the valves.

tors described above as favoring clotting also operate to favor thrombosis. The term "hyperinosis" is sometimes used to indicate an altered state of the blood favoring clotting, whereas "hypinosis" indicates a condition which inhibits clotting. These alterations are probably of physicochemical and chemical nature, which affect surface conditions, as for example in the agglutination of platelets to form white thrombi; probably similar is the activity of those products of tissues which have been shown to favor coagulation. (See Silberberg.)

Relation of Bacterial Infection to Thrombosis. Bacterial infection is of the utmost importance in thrombus formation, and may operate through any of the three methods outlined above. Bacteria may produce roughening of vascular walls, they may produce slowing of the current or they may produce alteration in the constitution of the blood. To lead to any or all of these alterations, bacteria may be present in foci in the body or may actually invade the blood stream. In the first instance, damage is due to products of the bacteria which are absorbed. In the second instance, the damage is due to both the bacterial bodies and to their products. The presence of bacteria in the body may lead to local inflammatory reac-

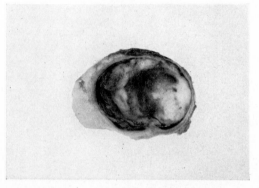

Gross photograph of cross section of a thrombus in inferior vena cava to show mottled character.

tion, which in the case of the pyogenic bacteria and certain other organisms, results in the formation of abscesses or other types of suppuration. As the bacteria proliferate and the inflammatory process extends, the latter comes in contact with blood vessels. In thin walled vessels thrombosis may ensue without direct involvement of the vessels by the lesions. This is believed to be due to diffusion of bacterial products, which so injure the endothelial lining of these vessels as to produce roughening and thrombosis. When the inflammatory processes involve the vessel walls the same phenomenon occurs, and when by extension they penetrate through the wall, thrombosis is the natural reaction. Bacteria in the blood stream may lead to thrombosis either by breaking off fragments of an infectious primary thrombus, with subsequent lodgment in other vessels, or by the actual deposit of bacteria or clumps of bac-

teria in vessels. In either case, inflammation is set up and thrombosis occurs.

Bacterial infection in the body may alter the constitution of the blood in two ways. In intense infection, it is not uncommon to find clotting retarded so that multiple hemorrhages may occur, particularly under the skin and serous surfaces. On the other hand, bacterial infection may so alter the blood constitution as to favor thrombosis. These changes are probably due to products of the bacteria rather than the bacterial bodies themselves, but exactly what constituent of the blood is affected is not precisely known. As has been pointed out in discussing degenerations, bacterial products may produce parenchymatous degeneration of heart muscle and of vascular muscle, which reduce blood pressure and lead to slowing of the current, favoring thrombosis. In a study of thrombosis in man, Lubarsch was able to exclude an infectious agent in only 13 per cent of the cases.

In the two preceding sections, attention has been drawn to thrombi without bacterial invasion, i.e., bland thrombi, and to infected thrombi. In the former, reaction in the wall of the vessel is moderate or slight and not exudative. In the latter there is acute exudative inflammation in the vessel wall. This is of practical importance, for example, in the great veins of the lower extremities where it is essential, both therapeutically and prognostically, to distinguish between phlebothrombosis (bland) and thrombophlebitis (infected). (See Ochsner and DeBakey.)

Construction of Thrombi. Depending upon construction, it is possible to differentiate mixed thrombi, red thrombi and hyaline thrombi. The most common and most important are the mixed thrombi. Grossly, these are found adherent to the vessel walls, and in this way can be distinguished from postmortem clots. The thrombus is firm and on cross section shows a mottled mixture of gray, yellow and red. Microscopically, it has a rather complicated architecture which shows an irregular network of fibrin, masses of blood platelets more or less fused together, masses of leukocytes, masses of red blood corpuscles and places in which these cells are mixed together. Aschoff's demonstration that the primary change is a deposit of platelets

PLATE IV

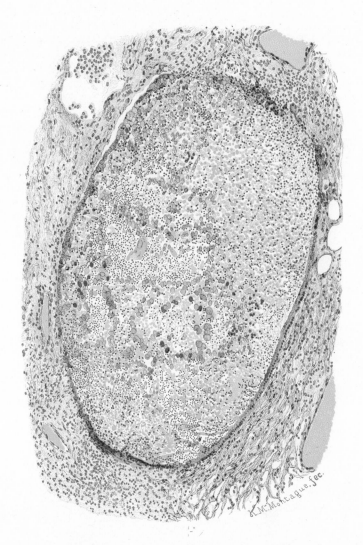

Early thrombosis of a vein, showing red and white corpuscles, agglutinated platelets and a small amount of fibrin.

has been confirmed anew by Apitz who finds that there is no fibrin in the early deposits. The agglutination of platelets and their adherence to the vessel walls is associated with degeneration of the endothelium but is in larger part determined by changes in the plasma. Secondarily, there is a deposit of fibrin and further accumulation of platelets which form a tree-like or coral-form support, or scaffolding, for the deposit of the other cells. As the primary thrombus is laid down, this leads to alteration and whorling of the circulating blood in the neighborhood, so

be present in the same vessel, but if so they are usually well delimited one from the other and readily distinguishable.

RED THROMBI are those which are made up of the blood constituents in about normal proportions. When a vessel is ligated the sudden stoppage of blood in that vessel leads to the formation of a red thrombus. At first this is not adherent to the vessel wall, but soon becomes so owing to degenerative changes in the vessel wall and to the process of organization which will be discussed later. The same thing occurs when a vessel be-

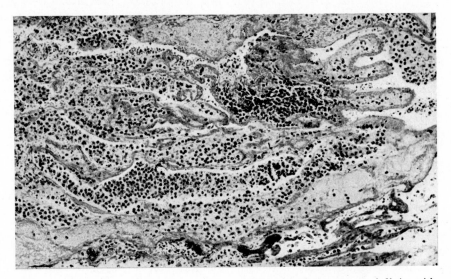

Thrombus of a vein, to show the so-called coral structure of the masses of fibrin, with enmeshed leukocytes and erythrocytes.

that under different conditions the deposit of cells may be white blood corpuscles, or red blood corpuscles or mixtures of the two.

It is of importance to differentiate between the gross appearance of postmortem clots and antemortem thrombi. The postmortem clots are usually of the type called "currant jelly." They are of jelly-like consistence, elastic, moist and of homogeneous character, not attached to the vessel wall, easily removed and may upon removal appear as a branching cast of the vascular tree. The antemortem thrombi are usually firm, friable, dry, laminated or mottled in character, sometimes with a softened center; they are more or less firmly attached to the vessel wall and when removed may leave a somewhat roughened vessel wall. Both postmortem clots and antemortem thrombi may

comes completely occluded by thrombosis, or is blocked by means of an embolus or tumor growth. If the blood current be extremely slow, due to other disease, the presence of a small white or mottled thrombus in the vessel wall may lead to the development of an occluding red thrombus, probably because of a disturbance of relation of blood constituents in that particular place. If, however, the circulation be fairly rapid, this type of thrombus is not likely to occur secondary to anything other than complete occlusion. Microscopically, such a thrombus is found to be made up of a loose network of fibrin enmeshing many red blood corpuscles, a few leukocytes and a moderate number of platelets.

WHITE THROMBI are made up almost entirely of platelets, and are deposited as a rule because of a lesion of a vessel wall, apparently regardless of whether the circulation be slowed or normal. They can be produced experimentally by injuring the vessel wall with a corrosive such as silver-nitrate solution, which when painted on the outside of a vein leads to the development of thrombi within. In man, such thrombi may be seen on the roughened aortic wall of arteriosclerosis. As a rule, however, there is a small admixture of fibrin and leukocytes. It is supposed that the normal smoothness of vessel walls permits the free passage of such sticky cells as the leukocytes and the platelets, but when the continuity of the lining is interrupted, these no longer flow with normal freedom, adhere to the roughened surface and produce thrombi. These thrombi are not infrequently the primary change in that disease of the heart called acute endocarditis, where they develop quite independently of slowing of the circulation. In those instances where the leukocytes predominate, the thrombus has a pale yellow appearance and is referred to as a "leukocyte thrombus."

The "fibrin thrombi" mentioned in connection with postmortem clotting of blood rarely appear during life, but apparently are thrown down rather in the agonal period. "Hyaline thrombi" occur particularly in smaller vessels such as the capillary loops of the renal glomerulus, the capillaries of the lungs, the sinusoids of the liver. They are not visible grossly, but microscopically are found to be made up of masses occluding these vessels and exhibiting simply a hyaline acidophilic character. It is probable that they may originate in small masses of fibrin which occlude the vessels, or small agglomerations of red blood corpuscles which plug the capillaries. In either case subsequent changes lead to the formation of hyaline substance. Hyaline thrombi occur in infectious diseases such as diphtheria, scarlatina, pneumonia and peritonitis. They may also be produced by poisoning such as that of snake venom, poisonous fungi, certain enzymes, extensive burns, eclampsia, and may be produced experimentally by the injection of certain poisons such as uranyl nitrate. They may be produced experimentally also by the injection of an agglutinating serum, which leads to the lodgment of small clumps of cells in vessels and subsequent hyaline transformation. Hyaline thrombi may occur in blood

transfusion in man as the result of the injection of incompatible blood which produces agglutination of the donor's corpuscles.

Types of Thrombi. Certain terms are applied to thrombi depending upon their form and situation. The so-called autochthonous thrombi are those which are laid down upon the wall of a vessel as a sequence of alteration in the lining of the vessel. These may be either simple mural thrombi, or they may have a point of attachment with a pedicle thus constituting valve-like thrombi. Occluding or obstructive thrombi are those which obliterate the lumen of the vessel. From these may develop secondary thrombi which extend in a progressive manner either up or down the vessel. This type of progressive thrombus must be differentiated from the obscure disease known as progressive thrombosis, in which thrombi appear, either as the result of injury or spontaneously in the veins of an extremity, subsequently involve the veins of other extremities, and may become fairly widely generalized. A thrombus originating a short distance below a branch in a vessel may extend up that vessel to the branching point, and then down the other branch to form a Y-shaped clot, the so-called "saddle thrombus." In the heart, thrombi may be situated upon the walls of the ventricle to form mural thrombi, upon the valves to form vegetations, or may lie in the cavities to produce globoid thrombi; if these be attached to the heart wall by a pedicle, they constitute the so-called "ball-valve thrombi." The marantic thrombus is one which occurs where the circulation is slowed and is seen most commonly in the auricular appendages. The association of slowed circulation and the irregularities of the internal surface produced by the pectinate muscles favor the deposition of mottled thrombi.

Sequels of Thrombosis. Aside from interrupted or altered circulation produced by thrombosis, there are certain changes which occur in the thrombus itself. The clotting of blood, whether within the vessels or outside the vessels, signifies the death of that fluid tissue. Leukocytes are embedded in practically all thrombi and when death occurs are likely to liberate proteolytic enzymes. These lead to softening of the clot. The softened mass is usually grayish-red in color and of semifluid or granular character. Lysis may extend to the surface of the clot and liberate fragments into the blood stream. This bland or aseptic softening is to be distinguished from septic softening due to the presence of, or invasion by, bacteria. Bacteria may be present at the time of the thrombosis, they may invade from surrounding

thrombus itself is a focus of suppuration, which may invade and extend through the vessel wall to produce hemorrhage or infect surrounding tissues.

ORGANIZATION AND CANALIZATION. A thrombus in a vessel is made up of dead blood and, as is the case with dead tissue elsewhere, serves as a foreign body to excite a

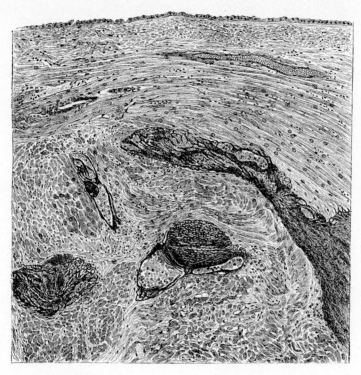

Thrombosis in an auricular appendage, the so-called marantic thrombus. The irregular spaces of the appendage appear as lakes in the heart muscle and are filled with a clot rich in fibrin.

suppurative lesions, or may be conveyed to the thrombus by the blood stream. The softening of a bland thrombus leads in most cases simply to the presence of small infarcts in other tissues, or if the emboli lodge at vital points, serious symptoms or death may follow. The softening of an infected thrombus discharges infected emboli, which lodge in small vessels and lead to the development of multiple abscesses in various parts of the body, a condition called pyemia. Not only may infected thrombi produce pyemia, but they may serve as a point of bacterial growth from which poisonous substances enter the blood to produce toxemia, or bacteria may be discharged into the blood stream to produce septicemia. The infected

low grade of inflammation. As the fluid part of the clot is removed by absorption, the contraction of the clot brings to bear a certain amount of tension on the vessel wall. These factors operate as a stimulus to connective-tissue growth, which proceeds from the vessel wall into the thrombus and, in order to provide nourishment, small capillaries accompany the connective-tissue growth. This leads ultimately to practically complete substitution of the thrombus by a connective tissue and capillary mass. The connective tissue subsequently becomes of adult type, the small blood vessels disappear and the thrombus is said to have become organized. While this is going on the end surfaces of the thrombi become covered with endothelial cells, which grow from the endothelial lining of the vessel.

As a part of the organization, canalization sometimes occurs. The canals in the thrombus probably develop from the small lumen of the vessel. If this occur on the end upon which the impact of circulation is felt; the pressure of the circulation may dilate these vessels and establish irregular lines of communication through the clot. By further

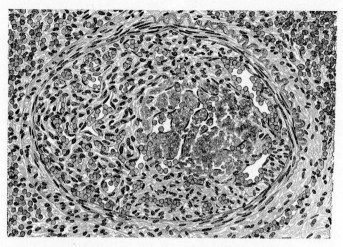

Almost complete organization of a thrombus in a small branch of the pulmonary artery. The new connective-tissue cells are accompanied by minute capillaries.

capillaries which accompany the connective-tissue growth. These capillaries constitute an

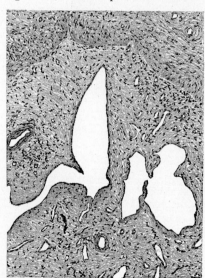

Canalization of a thrombus. A section of an old thrombus of the jugular vein. The connective tissue is dense and poor in nuclei. The canals are variable in size and outline.

intricate network throughout the thrombus. As they appear near the end surfaces of the thrombi, they may break through to the dilatation of the communicating vessels, circulation may be to all practical intents completely restored. In large vessels a certain amount of the canalization may be participated in by the vasa vasorum. In certain situations, notably the spleen, thrombi may undergo calcification to form the so-called phleboliths.

Other Forms of Thrombosis. In addition to the forms of thrombi mentioned above, attention may be called to certain other forms which occur. Not only do the acute infections lead to thrombosis but the more chronic infections may do likewise. Tuberculosis in its development may directly invade vessel walls and induce thrombus formation, or in cases where the bacilli float in the blood stream they may lodge and produce tubercles of the intima. Syphilis may lead to thrombosis because of syphilitic inflammation of the vessel walls, or its special lesion, the gumma, may extend directly into a vessel wall and induce thrombosis. Of great importance is the invasion of blood vessels by malignant tumors. The malignant connective-tissue tumors or sarcomas are the common offenders, but the malignant epithelial tumors or carcinomas may also act in this way. This invasion leads to tumor formation in the vessel, spoken of as tumor thrombus. Such a thrombus may grow along the walls of vessels and become very extensive. When the tumor growth does not occlude the vessel, secondary red or mottled blood thrombi are likely to appear and produce obstruction. Numerous instances of widespread extension of sarcoma are on record, but the commonest instance is the spread of carcinoma of the kidney through the renal vein into the cava. Such extensions of carcinomas are not so common.

Thrombi in the lymphatic vessels are commonly made up of tumor masses. Neighboring acute inflammation may bring into the lymphatics sufficient plasma and leukocytes to produce lymphatic thrombi.

Embolism

Embolism is defined by Welch as "the impaction in some part of the vascular system, of any undissolved material brought there by the blood current. The transported material is an embolus. Embolism may likewise occur in lymphatic vessels." Emboli may be solid, liquid or gaseous.

Solid Emboli. The term embolus usually indicates that the material is a fragment of a thrombus. As has been indicated above, thrombi readily undergo softening, and may easily be broken down so as to liberate fragments in the blood stream. Common sources of emboli include thrombosis upon heart valves in acute endocarditis and thrombosis of veins. Other sorts of solid emboli include fragments of tissues such as small pieces of heart valves, tumor cells, parenchymatous cells, vegetable parasites, particularly bacteria, animal parasites such as the cysticercus of tenia echinococcus, small masses of calcified material, pigment granules and foreign bodies. From the point of origin, the emboli are carried by the blood current until they reach a projecting point in a vessel or more usually until they reach a vessel whose lumen is too small to permit passage of the material. Thus an embolus which originates in a tributary of the inferior vena cava may be carried to the right heart and thence to the lungs. Similarly an embolus originating in an acute endocarditis, may be carried to practically any part of the arterial circulation. Welch states that the order of frequency of lodgment

of emboli is approximately as follows: pulmonary, renal, splenic, cerebral, iliac and lower extremities, axillary and upper extremities, celiac axis with its hepatic and gastric branches, central artery of the retina, superior mesenteric, inferior mesenteric, abdominal aorta, coronary arteries of the heart. He points out, however, that judgment is somewhat difficult owing to the fact that minute emboli may lodge in small vessels of the extremities, or in the hepatic artery or other situations, with no apparent damage and no reason for suspecting their presence. Very rarely emboli may be so large as to obstruct the orifices of the heart. It is noteworthy that embolism is much more often multiple than single. Petitpierre believes that fixation at the point of lodgment is favored by vascular spasm due to the impact of the embolus.

PARADOXIC OR CROSSED EMBOLISM. There are unusual and aberrant forms of embolism such as paradoxic and retrograde embolism, that form in which an embolus originating in the venous system lodges in systemic arteries. It is paradoxic in that it is too large to have passed through the pulmonary capillaries. In such cases the foramen ovale is patent and cases are reported in which an embolus actually lodged in the foramen. This presupposes an alteration of pressure, so that it is higher in the right than in the left atrium (Gross; Thompson and Evans). Although the pulmonary capillaries are larger than the systemic and dilate readily, solid masses of sufficient size to produce infarction elsewhere do not ordinarily pass through. Tumor cells sometimes pass this barrier and produce secondary nodules, but ordinarily they lodge in the lungs, produce growths there and cells from these may enter the pulmonary veins to be distributed by the systemic arteries.

RETROGRADE EMBOLISM is that form in which an embolus originating in a thrombus of a vein lodges farther away from the heart than the thrombus itself. Some suppose that this is due to back pressure in the vein the result of positive pressure in the thorax incident to coughing or forced respiration. Others think that with markedly slowed circulation in the vein, the embolus may drop backward by gravity. Neither of these suppositions has been proved. Rare cases of retrograde arterial embolism have been recorded (Ciechanowski).

THE SADDLE OR RIDING EMBOLUS is one which lodges at a bifurcation of a vessel and remains there astride the bifurcation with segments extending down the branches.

CELLS may be dislodged from their normal situation and become emboli. Cord cells of the liver may lodge in pulmonary capillaries as a result of hepatic necrosis. Cells of the bone marrow may lodge in the pulmonary capillaries because of disease of the marrow, fractures of bones and for some unexplained reason following surface burns, chorionic cells may be found in hepatic sinusoids and in pulmonary capillaries. Even the squames from the fetal skin may gain access to the maternal lungs. Usually cellular emboli are of little importance, except that tumor cells may grow to produce a new secondary tumor.

SEQUELS OF SOLID EMBOLI. Infarction as a result of bland and infected emboli has been discussed previously. Pulmonary embolism, with its likelihood of sudden death, is described in the chapter on Respiratory System. If tissue cells, pigment granules, masses of calcareous material, foreign bodies be of sufficient size they may cause infarction, but this is rare. Foreign bodies may be transported in the blood as emboli. We recently found a carpet tack embedded in the myocardium; it could only have got there by transport through blood vessels. Bullets, shell fragments, needles are reported in places remote from the site of entry or lodgment and the only explanation is by transport as emboli. The lodgment of clumps of tumor cells may lead to metastatic tumor, but this development depends to a considerable degree on environmental factors, as discussed in the chapter on Tumors.

When emboli lodge they produce conditions favorable to the formation of thrombi, so that secondary thrombosis is practically always present. If the embolus completely occlude the vessel, the thrombus is usually a red thrombus, extending to the next branch of this vessel. If it simply lodge in the side of a vessel owing to a projection from the wall, it may lead to the formation of a mural thrombus, which increases in size until occlusion results. If the vessel be examined shortly after the lodging of the embolus, it is easily possible to distinguish between the embolus and the secondary thrombus, but if considerable time has elapsed, this distinction may not be possible. The identification of the embolus rests on its similarity to the thrombus or tissue from which it originated. As has been pointed out in the discussion of infarction, if collateral circulation be sufficient, the only interference in circulation, beyond the lodgment of the embolus, is a dilatation of vessels and hyperemia. If, on the other hand, collateral circulation be not sufficient to maintain nutrition, infarction occurs. If pathogenic bacteria be present in an embolus, the secondary changes include those incident to the presence of bacteria, ordinarily suppuration. If the embolus be such a body as the scolex of the tenia echinococcus, it may increase in size to produce an echinococcus cyst. Tissue cells and fragments produce effects not differing from those produced by the ordinary type of embolus, and the same is true of the lodgment of pigment granules, masses of calcareous material and of foreign bodies. In World War I, the transport of fragments of projectiles sometimes occurred and even in civil life the transport of foreign bodies, such as a fragment of needle introduced through the skin, sometimes occurs. The lodging of tumor cells leads usually to the development of secondary tumors or metastases.

EMBOLISM IN THE LYMPHATIC CIRCULATION is difficult to demonstrate except in the case of embolism of tumor cells. In these circumstances, the tumor grows and invades the lymphatic vessel, and certain small cells or groups of cells are broken off and carried in the lymphatic current. These usually find lodgment in the neighboring lymph nodes. After growth of the tumor in the lymph nodes, the latter may become so obstructed as to establish a retrograde lymphatic flow, as a result of which retrograde transport of tumor cells may occur. This is discussed more fully in the chapter on Tumors. Other conditions may also obliterate the lymphatic flow in lymph nodes, and establish retrograde flow, such as tuberculosis. Thus bacteria may be carried from the site of infection to the lymph nodes, excite disease there and then be carried in other directions by retrograde flow. This applies not only to tuberculosis but to the more acute infections such as those produced by the pyogenic bacteria.

Fat Embolism. There are two important forms of liquid embolism, due to entry into the blood of substances not miscible with blood. The most common is fat embolism, but important also is embolism of amniotic fluid. Vance gives as true etiologic factors of fat embolism (a) trauma to adipose tissue,

(Gauss). The fat is transported to the lungs where it lodges in small arteries and capillaries. It may pass through in considerable quantities to lodge elsewhere. There are two clinical forms of disturbance, pulmonary and cerebral. In the pulmonary form, symptoms usually appear after 12, 24, 36 or more hours and include rapid respiration, fall in blood pressure, pulmonary edema and small rapid

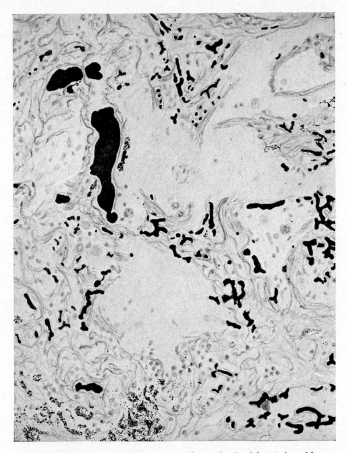

Fat embolism of pulmonary vessels; stained with osmic acid.

including injuries to the osseous system, fractures, jarring of skeleton and operations on bones, (b) injury to subcutaneous fat (surgical operations, especially on obese persons), interosseous fat and fatty viscera. A possible factor is therapeutic intravenous injection of oils, but only one case is reported in which the large volume of 50 cc. oil was injected. He considers dubious such factors as burns, poisons and postmortem processes. It is doubtful that in lipemia, the lipids are agglomerated to form emboli, and it has not been shown that osteomyelitis is a cause

pulse. In the cerebral form symptoms may be even further delayed up to seven days, and include vomiting, convulsions and coma (Winkelman). Death may follow either form.

Gross examination at autopsy reveals dilatation of right heart, hyperemia and edema of lungs and often petechiae in various organs. Upon cutting the lungs, visible droplets of fat may be seen on the knife. Bacon and LeCount found that if blood be withdrawn from the main pulmonary arteries into a glass tube and the contents allowed to settle, a layer of fat rises to the top. Microscopically, fat stains on frozen sections of lungs show a fairly uniform distribution of fat in the small arteries and capillaries as globules, short or long cylinders and as stellate figures at branchings of vessels. Globules may be found in alveoli and are said to be demonstrable in sputum. There are hyperemia and edema sometimes with exudation in the alveoli and fibrinous thrombi in the vessels. Fat may be found in any part of the central nervous system accompanied by ring-like hemorrhages and infarction. The heart may show streaky hemorrhages grossly, which are seen also microscopically, sometimes associated with small foci of necrosis of the muscle. In the kidneys, the fat is in the capillaries of the glomerular tufts and sometimes elsewhere. In the liver it is in the sinusoids and may be taken up by Kupffer cells. If lodging in cutaneous capillaries, petechiae occur. It may be discovered in spleen, adrenals, pancreas and thyroid.

Provided the amount of fat is large enough to be significant, physiologic studies show a rise in pulmonary arterial and right intraventricular pressure, associated with fall in systemic arterial pressure and rise in systemic venous pressure. This chain of phenomena is due to the resistance to pulmonary circulation caused by the fat in the smaller vessels. (See Simonds; Wiggers.)

The reaction to fat embolism is quantitative. Simonds found that it requires about 2 cc. of oil per kilogram of body weight to produce death in the dog and somewhat similar amounts are necessary to kill a rabbit. In cases of fracture, in subjects dead of other causes, it is not rare to find a few fat droplets but without any indication that the small fat embolism was of any importance; how much it takes to be fatal for man is not known. Fat may also be found in the lungs due to postmortem putrefaction and in lipemia of diabetes, but in both the amount is small. In case of recovery, the fat is probably removed by phagocytes before or after saponification.

EMBOLISM FROM AMNIOTIC FLUID. Certain cases of death, about seven to 10 hours after labor (especially when this was difficult) have been found to be due to embolism in the pulmonary arteries and capillaries of materials from amniotic fluid. Mucin, derived from meconium, appears in the same situations as described for fat. There are also amorphous masses containing fat, the latter derived from sebaceous glands of the fetus. In addition, squames, desquamated from the skin, are found. The manifestations are much the same as those of fat embolism and constitute a form of so-called obstetrical shock (Steiner and Lushbaugh).

Air and Gas Embolism. Air embolism is due to entry of air into the venous system, but the quantity must be fairly large and the time during which it enters fairly short. It occurs in man as a complication of surgical operations and wounds about the neck, shoulder and thorax, where the negative pressure may suck air into the large veins. It may also occur by way of the uterine veins in cases of placenta previa, induced abortion and diagnostic injections into the uterus, and has been demonstrated after washing of maxillary antra.

The utmost importance attaches to its proper demonstration at autopsy. Two meth-

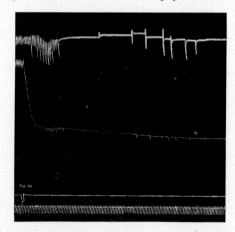

Tracing of air embolism in 5 kilo dog. Upper line shows respiration, middle line blood pressure in femoral artery. The lower lines are signal and time in 2 seconds. Before the final injection of 70 cc. air into the femoral vein the animal had received 150 cc. in fractions of 10, 30 and 50 cc. Heart stops before respiration; the latter increases in depth and becomes gasping. The deep respirations record on the blood-pressure tracing.

ods are available. In one, the thorax is filled with water and the right ventricle punctured to determine whether or not air escapes. In the second, which is preferable, all the great vessels are ligated, including the inferior vena cava, the lungs and heart removed together and immersed in a basin of water and the right ventricle incised. No case of air embolism is proved unless one of these two methods is followed. The manipulations incident to the usual autopsy are such that it is not uncommon to draw bubbles of air into vessels, and this artefact must not be mistaken for air embolism. Death occasionally follows diagnostic and therapeutic punctures of the thorax, but there is dispute as to the cause of death. Some think it is due to a pleural cardio-inhibitory reflex (Capps; Mersheimer and Colmer) but others believe it to be due to entry of air into the pulmonary veins with consequent embolism in the arterial supply, especially that of the brain (Jones and Lockhart). It seems possible that either of these mechanisms may be effective in different cases. Certainly the amount of air that can be harmful is less when injected so as to enter the arteries than is true of entry into the veins. In the cases of air embolism in the lungs, the organs usually exhibit hyperemia and edema and the right heart is dilated; microscopic examination adds little further except for petechiae in both these organs and myocardial degeneration.

Physiologically, the phenomena are much the same as in fat embolism, dependent upon increased resistance in the pulmonary circuit to the passage of foamy blood. Experiments have shown that with constant pressure, the passage of foamy blood through a capillary requires about 50 per cent more time than for normal blood. The presence of foamy blood in the right ventricle may also be a factor because the compressible foam can be expelled less readily than the relatively noncompressible blood, so that there is probably a considerable residue after systole. The amount of air required to kill a dog depends in part on the speed of injection. The rapid injection of about 25 cc. of air into the femoral or jugular vein of a dog produces a temporary fall of mean systemic arterial and pulse pressure, with a rise of venous pressure. In a dog of 10 kilograms we produced death by injection of 450 cc. of air in amounts of 20, 30, 50 and 70 cc. in the course of 25 minutes. Nevertheless, twice as much may be injected if the time be extended to about 90 minutes. Oxygen is more readily absorbed than air, but as much as a liter of oxygen may be injected into man in the course of an hour without the effects of air embolism (Ziegler). Although aspiration into the great veins of the thorax is said to be important in man, a glass cannula may be introduced into the superior cava of the dog without significant entry of air. When injected into the dog's vein, a bubbling sound can be heard by stethoscope as the air enters the heart and the same is said to be true of man.

The distribution of such air as may pass through the pulmonary capillaries is not well known. Certain observations indicate that it may enter the brain. Rukstinat lays much stress on the experimental demonstration of air in the coronary arteries as a cause of death from myocardial anoxia, but this has not been found in man.

It is said that gas-forming bacteria may produce enough to cause gas embolism, but the proof of this is open to question. This is a different proposition from the occurrence of foamy organs in death following infection by anaerobic gas bacilli such as *C. welchii*. These are saprophytes which, after death, may produce gas bubbles in various organs of the body, the so-called foamy organs. These organs are swollen, tense, soft, cut with decreased resistance, crepitate and show fine and large bubbles throughout. An interesting confirmatory experiment is to inject the organisms intravenously in the rabbit, kill the animal and place it in an incubator for 6 to 12 hours. The autopsy demonstrates the foamy organs.

CAISSON DISEASE. Too sudden release of pressure in work under compressed air, as with divers and caisson workers, causes a variety of symptoms and signs. The laws of physics govern the solution of gases under pressure. When the body is in compressed air, the tissues and body fluids contain increased amounts of nitrogen, oxygen and carbon dioxide in proportion to the pressure. The latter two can be absorbed but the nitrogen is inert. Furthermore nitrogen is five times more soluble in fat than in other tissues. Sudden release of pressure produces bubbles in tissues and fluids, and the bubbles contain principally if not solely nitrogen. Bubbles in the blood may act as emboli but this is less significant than the presence of bubbles in the tissues, especially the nervous system. Nevertheless, emboli may lodge in the brain, pulmonary vessels and perhaps coronary arteries. Since the myelin of the nervous system absorbs great quantities of nitrogen, the bubbles formed there as a result of the released pressure may be numerous. The consequence, in cases where recompression and slow decompression are not done or are much delayed, is necrosis of nerve tissues. The emboli or gas bubbles may often be accompanied by small hemorrhages in various viscera and skin.

The symptoms usually occur in the first hour after decompression, but may be delayed for 12 hours. Permanence of the lesions of central nervous system may lead to death subsequently because of the complications of paralysis. Pain of "the bends" may be due to lesions of nerves or joints, and in

vomiting forces air into the lymphatics and there is a sort of air embolism into the lymphatics with transport to somewhat distant sites. This is discussed further in the chapter on the Alimentary Canal.

Hemorrhage. Hemorrhage means the passage of blood from the blood vessels into any extravascular position. The hemorrhage, depending upon its origin, may be arterial, venous or capillary. When the blood passes outside the body, the condition is spoken of as external hemorrhage, whereas the entrance of the blood into the tissues or cavities of the body is called internal hemorrhage. Petechiae or ecchymoses are hemorrhages in the tissues

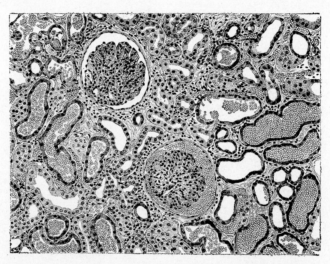

Hemorrhage into a subcapsular glomerular space and into numerous tubules of the kidney.

abdominal bends is probably due to emboli in abdominal vessels. The vertigo of "the staggers" is due to cerebral lesion or bubbles in the internal ear. The air hunger of "the chokes" is probably due to pulmonary embolism. Bubbles in the skin or cutaneous vessels lead to "the itch." (See Thorne.)

The rapid reduction of barometric pressure, such as occurs when aviators are compelled by military needs to ascend quickly to great heights, may have much the same effects (Fulton).

Further discussion is to be found in the chapter on Nervous System.

GAS CYSTS OF THE INTESTINE, or intestinal emphysema, are gas-filled cysts of the lymphatics of the intestinal wall. They are probably due to entry of gas through ulcers, especially those of the stomach. Increased pressure in the stomach due to distention or

from 1 to 3 or 4 mm. in diameter. These are not infrequently referred to as purpuric spots. Sometimes the blood collects in the tissues in a fairly large, tumor-like mass, called hematoma. According to the origin of the hemorrhage various terms may be applied. Epistaxis signifies hemorrhage from the nose; hematemesis signifies vomiting of blood; melena signifies the discharge through the rectum of blood, which originates from intestinal hemorrhage; hemoptysis signifies the coughing up of blood from hemorrhage in the lungs or respiratory tract; hematuria signifies blood in the urine; menorrhagia signifies profuse bleeding during the menstrual period, and metrorrhagia signifies bleeding from the uterus between periods; hematocolpos is a retention of blood or menses in the vagina. Hemorrhage into the various serous cavities may be referred to as hemothorax, when in the pleura; hemopericardium, when in the pericardium; hematocele, when in the tunica vaginalis testis.

According to the mechanism of extravasation, hemorrhage is distinguished as per rhexis and per diapedesis. Hemorrhage per rhexis is that form which results from rupture of the vessel wall. The rupture is usually traumatic as by wounds of various kinds, but may also result from erosion as by extension of ulcers. Disease of blood vessels may so alter their resistance to pressure that increases of pressure may lead to rupture, but it is hardly likely that any pressure can be present in the body sufficient to produce rupture of normal vessels, other than capillaries and vessels of almost capillary size. Such bleeding is seen in conjunctival hemorrhage resulting from vigorous coughing or violent vomiting. Diapedesis means the passage of relatively few red blood corpuscles through the vessel walls. In hemorrhage per rhexis all the blood elements and the plasma appear, but in diapedesis practically only red blood corpuscles are found. It has been thought that in diapedesis the red blood cells pass out through the lines of junction between the endothelial cells, but it seems likely that this is not altogether true, and that in certain if not all cases the red blood corpuscles pass directly through the endothelial cells as one colloid may pass through another. The common example is the passage of a small globule of mercury through a column of soft gelatin without leaving a tract in the gelatin. Diapedesis is a very common accompaniment of passive hyperemia, occurring in the lungs, liver, and other organs.

The destruction of the extravasated cells is responsible very largely for the pigmentation that accompanies prolonged passive hyperemia. Minute hemorrhages are also likely to follow the lodgment of emboli whether they be solid, liquid or gaseous, and the hemorrhage that is seen in infarction results from diapedesis in the earlier stages and probably from rhexis in the later stages. It must be said, however, that many investigators consider that diapedesis rarely, if ever, occurs and believe that the small amounts of blood supposed to be the results of diapedesis are really from small points of rupture.

The hemorrhagic diatheses will be considered more fully in diseases of the blood, but it may be mentioned here that several diseases exist in which hemorrhage plays a constant part. The hemorrhage is usually in the form of ecchymoses but may be more massive. These diseases include purpura hemorrhagica, and infectious and obstructive icterus, scurvy, hemophilia and others. Leukemias and pernicious anemia, as well as profound secondary anemias, may also be accompanied by hemorrhage. Whether the hemorrhage in these instances is due to alteration in the blood or alteration in endothelial lining of the vessels is problematic, but it seems likely that the latter is of importance in hemorrhagic anemias of various kinds, because of the lack of nutrition of these cells.

Bacterial infection is not uncommonly a cause of hemorrhagic tendencies, as exhibited in cases of streptococcal and staphylococcal septicemia, as well as in such specific infectious diseases as anthrax, plague, etc. It is now known that infectious icterus is due to a spirochete, the *Leptospira icterohemorrhagiae*, and therefore this disease cannot be regarded as bacterial.

Certain poisons such as phosphorus, some of the snake venoms, and poisonous fungi, may also in their action on the body be accompanied by hemorrhages, and this is now believed to be due to a direct specific action upon the capillary endothelium which permits the extravasation of blood. Phosphorus and chloroform poisoning are accompanied by a reduction in fibrinogen, and this alteration in the blood reduces its clotting capacity to favor continuance of hemorrhage. As has been indicated, passive hyperemia is an important condition in the production of certain forms of hemorrhage, and it is possible also that depression of vasomotor activity may lead to circulatory disturbances, which in their turn accentuate a tendency to hemorrhage. Hemorrhage appears frequently in the inflammatory reaction, and is discussed further in that connection. The relation of deficiency of vitamin K and reduction of prothrombin to hemorrhagic disease of the newborn and the bleeding tendency of hepatic disease have been discussed in the earlier chapters.

The general effects of hemorrhage depend upon the amount of blood lost and the suddenness of the loss. The symptoms of large hemorrhage taking place fairly quickly, i.e., in about 20 to 30 minutes, include weakness, which may go on to collapse, nausea, blurred vision, pallor, sweating and fall of blood pressure. Slower bleeding would not have such effects. Just how far blood pressure may fall without fatality is not known, but in dogs recovery is uncertain if the mean pressure reaches 20 to 30 mm. mercury. Robertson and Bock found in wounded soldiers that the total volume may fall to 60 per cent of normal and recovery ensue, but this is probably the limit. Reduction in the percentage of hemoglobin may be marked, provided the volume is maintained and may go as low as five-sixths the normal. Nevertheless death may occur when the hemoglobin is not reduced to that point. The restoration of volume begins at once by withdrawal of protein-poor fluid from the tissues, and is complete in about 72 hours. With this early dilution, the percentage of proteins is decreased but is then gradually increased and the proportion of proteins is not disturbed at any time (Ebert, Stead and Gibson). The restoration of volume does not go to a point where it would dilute the hemoglobin percentage to low figures. Usually, decrease of plasma proteins is accompanied by increase of lipids, especially cholesterol, and as indicated above, this favors maintenance of osmotic pressure. Naturally the number of erythrocytes per cmm. is reduced, but the number of leukocytes is often moderately increased. Reticulocytes and large erythrocytes are usually found. Whipple has shown that restoration of erythrocytes takes place in about 10 days, but this is retarded by starvation and accelerated by certain foods, especially liver and muscle. Restoration of fluid may be retarded by previous dehydration, lack of intake of water, shock and extremely low levels of hemoglobin. Repeated small hemorrhages, such as those which occur in eroding tumors, varices, etc., may cumulatively result in secondary anemia, as discussed in the chapter on Hematopoietic System.

The effects of internal hemorrhage depend upon the amount and the situation. Thus hemorrhage into the brain may produce paralysis and, in larger amounts, death. Hemorrhage into the pericardial sac, together with transmission of intraventricular or intra-aortic pressure may produce fatal cardiac tamponade. Hemorrhage into pleura or abdomen may be sufficient in amount to be fatal. Hemorrhage into the respiratory passages and lungs may lead to suffocation; the patient "drowns in his own blood." Large hemorrhage into the upper intestinal tract, most often due to bleeding peptic ulcer, is followed by absorption of products of destruction of erythrocytes and leads to increased nitrogen content of the circulating blood, the so-called alimentary azotemia (Chunn et al.). Following hemorrhage into the tissues the corpuscles disintegrate and pigments are produced, hemosiderin in the margins where oxygen is available, sometimes hematoidin in the center and often bilirubin by action of endothelial cells. The clotted blood acts in much the same way as a foreign body and excites a variable degree of inflammation. The leukocytes and large mononuclear cells of the reaction penetrate only a limited distance into the margin of the hemorrhage, phagocytose the hemosiderin and remove it to the surrounding living tissue. A moderate amount of transport may occur to the neighboring lymph nodes. The fact that the blood acts as a foreign body leads to a fixed tissue reaction in the neighborhood, so that fibroblasts and capillaries appear with the ultimate formation of adult connective tissue. If the hemorrhage be small, this adult connective tissue may entirely replace it, but if it be fairly large the connective tissue forms a capsule and the softened blood appears as a cyst. Blood pigment usually gives to the contents of this cyst only a light yellow color, because most of the pigment is removed by the diffusion and by the action of phagocytes. Bile pigment may also be formed. The margins of such regions, however, are likely to be deeply pigmented because of the presence of the hemosiderin contained in the phagocytes.

REFERENCES

Andrews, E.: Water Metabolism, Arch. Int. Med., **37**: 82, 1926.

Apitz, K.: Ueber den Bau jüngster Blutplättchenthromben und den Einfluss des Novirudins auf ihre Entstehung, Zentralbl. f. Allg. Path. u. Path. Anat., **50**: 9, 1930-31.

Aschoff, L.: Thrombosis, Lectures on Pathology, New York, 1924, p. 253.

Bacon, L. H., and E. R. LeCount: Automobile Injuries. A Study from Records of Postmortem Examinations, Arch. Surg., **18**: 769, 1929.

Bela, H.: 20 Jahre Thrombosenstatistik, Virchow's Arch. Path. Anat., **292**: 629, 1934.

Bruckman, F. S., and J. P. Peters: The Plasma Proteins in Relation to Blood Hydration. V. Serum

Proteins and Malnutritional or Cachectic Edema, Jour. Clin. Invest., **8**: 591, 1929-30.

Capps, J. A.: Air Embolism versus Pleural Reflex as the Cause of Pleural Shock, Jour. Amer. Med. Asso., **109**: 852, 1937.

Chunn, C. F., H. N. Harkins, and R. T. Boals: Alimentary Azotemia and the Bleeding Peptic Ulcer Syndrome, Arch. Surg., **43**: 773, 1941.

Ciechanowski, S.: Ueber retrograde arterielle Embolie, Virchow's Arch. Path. Anat., **302**: 784, 1938.

Corper, H. J.: Correlation of the Histological and Chemical Changes in the Spleen During Necrosis and Autolysis, Jour. Exper. Med., **15**: 429, 1912.

Dietrich, A.: Thrombose. Ihre Grundlagen und ihre Bedeutung, Berlin, Springer, 1932.

Ebert, R. V., E. A. Stead, Jr., and J. G. Gibson, 2d: Response of Normal Subjects to Acute Blood Loss, with Special Reference to Mechanism of Restoration of Blood Volume, Arch. Int. Med., **68**: 578, 1941.

Fahr, G., and I. Ershler: Studies of the Factors Concerned in Edema Formation. II. The Hydrostatic Pressure in the Capillaries during Edema Formation in Right Heart Failure, Ann. Int. Med., **15**: 798, 1941.

Fishberg, E. H.: The Relations of the Serum Proteins and Lipids to the Osmotic Pressure, Jour. Biol. Chem., **81**: 205, 1929.

Fulton, J. F.: Physiology and High Altitude Flying: With Particular Reference to Air Embolism and the Effects of Acceleration, Science, **95**: 207, 1942.

Gauss, H.: The Pathology of Fat Embolism, Arch. Surg., **9**: 593, 1924.

Gross, P.: The Patency of the So-called "Anatomically Open but Functionally Closed" Foramen Ovale, Amer. Heart Jour., **10**: 101, 1934.

Harrison, T. R.: Arterial and Venous Pressure Factors in Circulatory Failure, Physiol. Rev., **18**: 86, 1938.

Herrmann, G., and G. M. Decherd, Jr.: The Chemical Nature of Heart Failure, Ann. Int. Med., **12**: 1233, 1939.

Jones, T. R., and J. A. Lockhart: Air Embolism in Artificial Pneumothorax, Jour. Amer. Med. Asso., **117**: 2064, 1941.

Karsner, H. T., J. H. Austin, J. E. Ash, J. E. Dwyer, and A. A. Ghoreyeb: Studies in Infarction. I. Kidney and Spleen, Jour. Amer. Med. Asso., **57**: 951, 1911; II. Lungs, Jour. Med. Res., **27**: 205, 1912; III. Heart, ibid., **34**: 21, 1916; IV. Pulmonary Embolism, Jour. Exper. Med., **18**: 507, 1913.

Kerkhof, A. C.: Plasmapheresis Experiments upon the Influence of Colloid Osmotic Pressure, Water and Salt in Edema Formation, Ann. Int. Med., **11**: 1407, 1938.

Krogh, A.: The Anatomy and Physiology of the Capillaries, New Haven, 1929.

Landis, E. M.: The Passage of Fluid through the Capillary Wall, Harvey Lectures, Williams & Wilkins, **32**: 70, 1936-37.

Lubarsch, O.: Thrombose und Infektion, Berliner Klin. Wochenschr., **55**: 225, 1918.

Luisada, A.: The Pathogenesis of Paroxysmal Pulmonary Edema, Medicine, **19**: 475, 1940.

Marriott, W. McK.: Anhydremia, Physiol. Rev., **3**: 275, 1923.

McClure, W. B., and C. A. Aldrich: Time Required for Disappearance of Intradermally Injected Salt Solution, Jour. Amer. Med. Asso., **81**: 293, 1923.

——: The Intradermal Salt Solution Test, ibid., **82**: 1425, 1924. *See also* C. A. Aldrich: A Study of the

Clinical Course of Generalized Edema, Jour. Amer. Med. Asso., **84**: 481, 1925.

McLean, F. C.: Edema as a Problem in Physiological Regulation, Physiol. Rev., **5**: 618, 1925.

Mersheimer, W. L., and M. L. Colmer: Pleural Shock—A Reflex, Jour. Lab. and Clin. Med., **27**: 148, 1941.

Moon, V. H.: Shock and Related Capillary Phenomena, New York, Toronto and London, Oxford Press, 1938.

——: Shock, Its Dynamics, Occurrence and Management, Philadelphia, Lea and Febiger, 1942.

Ochsner, A., and M. DeBakey: Thrombophlebitis and Phlebothrombosis, South. Surg., **8**: 269, 1939.

Peters, J. P.: Body Water: The Exchange of Fluids in Man, Chicago, Thomas, 1935.

Rukstinat, G.: Experimental Air Embolism on the Coronary Arteries, Jour. Amer. Med. Asso., **96**: 26, 1931.

Schade, H.: Colloid Chemistry and Internal Medicine, in Colloid Chemistry by H. Alexander, New York, 1928, vol. 2, p. 629.

——, and F. Claussen: Der onkotische Druck des Blutplasmas und die Entstehung der renalbedingten Oedem, Zeitschr. Klin. Med., **100**: 363, 1924.

Scudder, J.: Shock. Blood Studies as a Guide to Therapy, Philadelphia, Lippincott, 1940.

Silberberg, M.: The Causes and Mechanism of Thrombosis, Physiol. Rev., **18**: 197, 1938.

Simonds, J. P.: A Study of the Low Blood Pressures Associated with Anaphylactic and Peptone Shock and Experimental Fat Embolism, with Special Reference to Surgical Shock, Jour. Exper. Med., **27**: 539, 1918.

Steiner, P. E., and C. C. Lushbaugh: Maternal Pulmonary Embolism by Amniotic Fluid as a Cause of Obstetric Shock and Unexpected Deaths in Obstetrics, Jour. Amer. Med. Asso., **117**: 1245, 1941.

Thompson, T., and W. Evans: Paradoxical Embolism, Quart. Jour. Med., **23**: 135, 1930.

Thorne, I. J.: Caisson Disease. A Study Based on Three Hundred Cases Observed at the Queens-Midtown Tunnel Project, 1938, Jour. Amer. Med. Asso., **117**: 585, 1941.

Vance, B. M.: The Significance of Fat Embolism, Arch. Surg., **23**: 426, 1931.

VanSlyke, D. D., E. Stillman, et al.: Observations on the Courses of Different Types of Bright's Disease, and on the Resultant Changes in Renal Anatomy, Medicine, **9**: 257, 1930.

Welch, W. H.: Hemorrhagic Infarction, Tr. A. Am. Physicians, **2**: 121, 1887.

——: Embolism, Albutt's Syst. of Med., London, 1899, vol. 7, p. 228; *also* Welch, Papers and Addresses, Baltimore, 1920, vol. 1, p. 193.

Whipple, G. H.: Hemoglobin Construction within the Body as Influenced by Diet Factors, Amer. Jour. Med. Sci., **175**: 721, 1928.

Wiggers, C. J.: Physiology in Health and Disease, Philadelphia, Lea and Febiger, 3d ed., 1939.

——: The Present Status of the Shock Problem, Physiol. Reviews, **22**: 74, 1942.

Winkleman, N. W.: Cerebral Fat Embolism: A Clinicopathologic Study of Two Cases, Arch. Neurol. & Psychiat., **47**: 57, 1942.

Wolf, L. P.: Experimentelle Studien über Luftembolie, Virchow's Arch. Path. Anat., **174**: 454, 1903.

Ziegler, E. E.: The Intravenous Administration of Oxygen, Jour. Lab. and Clin. Med., **27**: 223, 1941.

8

Inflammation

INTRODUCTION

There are many features in the normal structure and physiology of the body which serve to protect against injury. The continuity of skin and mucous surfaces protects to a considerable extent against minor in-

juries. Bones are so constructed that they are susceptible to major injury only. The conformation of the skull, thoracic cage and pelvis is such that they and the organs within them are not easily injured. Normal or increased secretion such as of the eyes, nose, urinary tract; movements, such as of the eyelids, or cilia of the tracheal mucosa; chemical constitution such as that of the gastric juice are other examples of reaction to injury or bacterial invasion. Other effective mechanisms are reflexes, such as sneezing, coughing, dodging, etc. Within the body fluids there are certain substances called immune bodies, some of which may be increased in amount following recovery from infectious diseases and by artificial immunization. They play an important part in the various reactions to infection.

The very existence of life represents a series of physiologic responses to stimuli of various kinds. Inflammation is a physiologic response to injury, but that kind of stimulus is in a sense abnormal or pathologic. The mechanisms concerned in the reaction are basically like those which occur in response to the stimuli of normal life, but they differ in quality and quantity. Therefore, although the reaction is physiologic, the term inflammation connotes also a pathologic process. In most people, inflammation follows a fairly regular course with but minor variations. In some, however, it is altered because of deviation from the usual, a state called allergy. Since this state is abnormal it has also been named pathergy; it can be in the form of hyperergy and hypoergy. Allergy or pathergy may be specific, as in response to a protein or other agent to which the body is unusually sensitive, or it may be nonspecific. As commonly employed, the term allergy refers to hyperergy, in which the reaction is more marked than is natural to the species and may exhibit special departures in various phases of the process.

124

DEFINITION

The inflammatory reaction takes place in blood vessels and in fixed tissues. The changes in the blood vessels begin a few seconds after injury and those in the fixed tissues begin only a short time thereafter, probably a matter of a half hour. The vascular alterations lead to exudation. Cells of the exudate and some of those of the fixed tissues remove debris and bacteria; they "cleanse" the region. Proliferation of vascular endothelium and of connective tissue develops ultimately into the scar; other cells may provide for regeneration of destroyed cells and tissues. The processes go on at the same time; they are interrelated and overlapping. The details are given in subsequent paragraphs. Inflammation is complex in manifestations and implications, and many say that inflammation cannot be exactly defined. This is probably true, but some statement of what is covered by the term is essential for discussion. The inflammations which lead to the formation of pus are of great concern clinically, but whether there be a large amount of pus or only a red spot on the skin, the process is basically the same. Also the character of the exudate may change. For example, in meningitis the exudate at first may be serous and a day or so later clearly purulent, but in both stages there is inflammation.

The principal difference of opinion among pathologists and biologists has centered about the questions: (a) whether or not the primary injury can be considered a part of the process, (b) the limitation of the definition to the vascular reactions and consequent exudation, and (c) the inclusion in the process of fixed tissue proliferation, repair, regeneration and cicatrization. The injury which stimulates the reaction is not part of the reaction itself. The reaction, however, is the physiologic response to the stimulus and in this case includes the vascular changes and tissue proliferation. The scar is the ultimate result of proliferation of vascular endothelium and fibroblasts. Thus, right up to the end, the process is one of reaction. In the same sense, regeneration is a response to death of cells and is properly to be considered a reaction. A further point of discussion concerns the inclusion of certain lesions of parenchymatous viscera, in which the degeneration of the parenchymatous cells dominates the picture. An organ may be the seat of degeneration without any signs of inflammation, but if there be exudation or tissue proliferation as a part of the local process the name inflammation or, as Marchand suggests, inflammatory disease, is justified. Inflammation is often spoken of as a defense reaction and likened to a battle between invader and host. This teleologic conception lends no aid to understanding the process, and is not in harmony with the fact that inflammation may produce serious and even fatal functional disturbances.

It is, therefore, possible to accept under the heading of inflammation either a definition limited by agreement, or to include various stages or all stages of the reactive and reparative mechanism. We modify the definition of Marchand to include in inflammation all the phenomena observed from the time of injury to the time of complete repair, thus including a series of reactive processes in the vessels and tissues, which follow upon injuries of physical, chemical or infectious nature, run a more or less regular course, and, in favorable cases, result in the destruction and removal of the injurious substances and lead to repair and healing.

CARDINAL SIGNS AND SYMPTOMS

The gross manifestations of inflammation have been clearly known since the time of Celsus, who pointed out four cardinal signs of the condition, redness, swelling, heat and pain (rubor, tumor, calor, dolor). As a result of later studies, a fifth cardinal sign, disturbance of function (functio laesa), was added. The redness is due to the hyperemia. The swelling is due to the exudate and tissue proliferation. The heat is due to transfer of internal heat to the surface because of the increased content of blood. The pain is probably due to involvement of sensory nerves by exudate and swelling. The disturbance of function may be due to pain, to interference with nerve supply and to destruction of functioning components of the tissue. Reference must be made to the work of those who have contributed to the investigation of the problem as a whole and its constituent parts.

Cohnheim studied the actual progress of inflammation in the web of the frog's foot. He saw the alterations of vessels and blood flow, the passage of fluid and cells through the vessel walls and explained many of the features of the process. Metchnikoff studied phagocytosis and pointed to its importance in inflammation. Other names that should not be overlooked are Leber, Councilman, Adami, Beitzke, Ricker, Klemensiewicz, Marchand and Aschoff. This by no means exhausts the list.

CLASSIFICATION

Inflammation shows variations depending upon the nature of the injury, the presence of diffusible substances, the violence and duration of reaction, the capacity for reaction and repair, and upon certain other factors. It is possible to classify the process in a variety of ways. Simplest perhaps is the division into acute and chronic inflammation depending particularly upon the duration of the process. Finer shadings of meaning are indicated by the terms subacute, of longer duration than acute, and subchronic, of shorter duration than chronic. Inflammation is also classified as exudative and as alterative or parenchymatous. The former is subclassified according to the preponderance of various constituents of the exudate into serous, fibrinous, purulent or suppurative, hemorrhagic and catarrhal forms. If two of the elements are conspicuous, combined terms are used, such as serofibrinous, fibrinopurulent, etc., the suffix indicating the major constituent. Alterative or degenerative inflammation occurs in the viscera and is a form in which degeneration of the parenchymal cells is the major part of the picture, associated with only slight exudation. It is sometimes divided into parenchymatous and nonsuppurative interstitial forms; in the latter the exudate is more marked than in the former. In some instances of alterative inflammation, as in certain forms of nephritis, cellular multiplication may be the principal indication of reaction. The term productive or proliferative inflammation indicates that multiplication of fixed tissue cells is notable; it is seen especially in chronic inflammation.

CAUSES OF INFLAMMATION

There have been many studies of the factors directly responsible for the various phases of the inflammatory reaction. These are discussed in the paragraphs on each of the phenomena, especially the primary vascular reactions and the response of the fixed tissues. Practically, however, the causes of inflammation are those which produce cellular changes varying from minor degenerations to actual death of cells. Certain agents injure cells without killing them. These include especially circulating poisonous substances such as may occur in infectious diseases; the consequent deterioration of cells may excite alterative or degenerative inflammatory disease. The common forms of inflammation, in which exudation is a major feature, are due to agents which lead to death of a few or many cells, and therefore the causes of necrosis are important causes of inflammation. They may be physical, such as mechanical injury; lesions due to electricity and light; thermal; the chemical corrosive poisons; the poisonous substances produced by bacteria; products of abnormal metabolism and certain poisons introduced from without; circulatory disturbances, particularly occlusion of a supplying artery; such neurotrophic disturbances as may lead to death of the tissues; and "allergic" or anaphylactic manifestations.

In as far as acute inflammation is concerned, the most important of all causes is bacterial infection. Pyogenic organisms, the pus producers, are among the most frequent causes of acute inflammation. In addition, a wide variety of bacteria may excite inflammation: the pneumococcus and members of that group, the diphtheria bacillus, the *Pseudomonas pyocyanea*, etc. The colon bacillus is one of those organisms which, occupying certain positions, for example the intestinal canal, does no damage, but when implanted in other situations, such as bladder or peritoneum, may serve to produce severe inflammation. Bacteria may gain access to the body through any of its surfaces including the skin, and the mucous membranes of the respiratory, alimentary and genito-urinary tracts. Protection is afforded against entrance by the continuity of these surfaces, by secretions, movements of secretion, constitution of secretion, and other protective mechanisms. Organisms vary considerably in virulence and may lodge in situations only to be discharged in various ways. If virulence be sufficient, the lodging of organisms in the body may readily lead to inflammation. A common example is the lodging of bacteria in the hair follicles of the skin, where their growth and multiplication not infrequently gives rise to minute or even very large abscesses. Lodgment in tissues about the teeth or in the crypts of the tonsils, or in other situations where removal is difficult, gives rise to similar manifestations. If the inflammation be not sufficiently pronounced to prevent further dissemination of the bacteria, they may be transmitted to other parts by the lymphatic current or by the blood stream. They may thus lodge in lymph nodes or in finer divisions of the blood vascular tree and set up secondary foci of inflammation. Bacteria in their growth produce certain poisonous substances which because of their diffusibility may result in necrosis of the surrounding tissue. In order that saprophytes may grow, they must be introduced into dead tissues, but the production of soluble poisons and toxins may kill surrounding tissues and provide a larger field for growth. Animal parasites and ova may injure and destroy immediately neighboring tissue.

When bacteria enter the blood stream they may be destroyed by two mechanisms, the action of bactericidal substances in the plasma and of phagocytic cells. If the bacteria survive, they may be injurious in two ways. They may lodge in capillaries and small arteries with resultant tiny infarcts, or they may multiply in comparable sites to produce products which kill the adjoining tissues. They then may multiply further and excite abscess formation. Those in the circulation or those which lodge, or both, may produce soluble poisons and toxins, which are a common cause of alterative inflammation. Furthermore, bacteria may grow on a surface and produce poisons which are absorbed. An example is diphtheria with its local lesion in the throat and with general illness due to absorption of the toxin. These matters are discussed in the chapter on Infectious Diseases.

It is not to be supposed that entry of bacteria into the blood invariably produces disease because some may not be pathogenic. As shown by studies of autolysis, this is common in normal experimental animals, in which bacteria are often observed in the liver, having been brought there by the blood. Adami expressed the view that, in man, bacteria may often enter the blood from alimentary and respiratory tracts, to be destroyed in a short time. He called this condition "subinfection." It is often difficult, however, to draw a sharp line of distinction between subinfection with no clinical manifestations and mild infection with very slight manifestations.

Mechanical injuries of various kinds may lead to inflammation. In fact, the production of a wound under strictly aseptic conditions results in minor degrees of inflammation (see Carscadden). Mechanical injury serves often as a ready means of access for bacteria. Thermal injury may result in burns varying in degree from a slight reddening of the skin to severe burns with actual destruction of deep tissues; in response to all these there are different degrees of inflammation. The death of parts as the result of exposure to cold leads to an inflammatory reaction in the surrounding living tissues. Burns by the electric current also produce injury with inflammatory reaction. The influence of light is manifested in sunburn. It has been pointed out that the tissues may be sensitized so that the reactions to light may be more severe. If the dose be sufficiently large, the use of radium and of roentgen rays produces injury and necrosis of tissues which, in the form of the so-called burn by these agents, shows the inflammatory reaction. Chemical corrosive poisons kill tissues and lead to inflammation, unless immediate death of the subject does not permit time for reaction. Of the toxic substances which may produce inflammation, the bacterial poisons are of the utmost importance. Metabolic poisons probably are active in such diseases as gout, chronic rheumatism and the like. Exogenous poisons include lead, arsenic, mercury and other substances. Some of these may produce actual parenchymal necrosis, for example mercuric chloride, but the injury may be of minor degree and may result in alterative inflammation only after prolonged administration. Circulatory disturbances uncomplicated by infection, as in bland infarction, produce only slight inflammation. Chronic passive hyperemia leads to variable degrees of connective-tissue proliferation. Inflammation of neurotrophic origin is probably due to loss of sensation, trauma and infection.

"Allergic" inflammation is exemplified by the Arthus phenomenon, in which the injection of a substance into an animal previously treated with the same substance, results in severe local reaction. From the many experiments dealing with its nature, hypotheses have been advanced that it is due to local antibody-antigen reactions, to local concentration of foreign protein, or to a general alteration of the mesenchyme, a "hyperergy" which increases local reaction to the degree of inflammation (see Opie, Nordmann). The theory of allergy has been applied to several diseases of man, including syphilis, tuberculosis, rheumatic fever, periarteritis nodosa, etc., to be discussed in subsequent chapters. Acute inflammation of this sort is seen in cutaneous wheals, diagnostic skin reactions, coryza, bronchitis, enteritis and other conditions which develop in those who are hypersensitive to specific substances, especially proteins. The reaction is like that of other forms of inflammation except that the exudate is often rich in eosinophiles. It should be remembered that eosinophiles occur in other forms of inflammation and that while allergic inflammation shows many eosinophiles in the exudate, the presence of these cells does not prove that an inflammation is allergic.

VASCULAR CHANGES

Changes in Caliber. The problems of importance deal with alterations in the caliber of the vessels, alterations in blood flow and the increase of permeability of the walls which plays a part in exudation. The first change in the blood vessels is a matter of controversy, but it is generally accepted that there is a primary and evanescent constriction of the vessels. This is rapidly followed, however, by a more lasting dilatation of the vessel. As a result of this dilatation, the arterial pressure is more directly communicated to the small vessels than is true when their caliber is normal. Hence, the rate of flow in the small vessels is accelerated. Klemensiewicz found an increase in arterial pressure in the early stage of inflammation in the leg of a dog from 174 to 190 mm. mercury, which could increase the rate of flow in the inflamed capillaries above that of a normal physiologic active hyperemia. The pressure is probably communicated through the capillaries to the veins, for the capillary and the venous pressure is also increased. The increased rate of flow persists, however, for

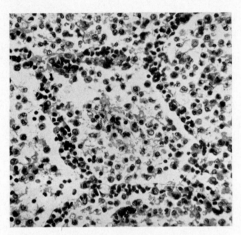

Capillary hyperemia in early pneumonia. Alveolar outlines made clear by the hyperemia. Within the air spaces are precipitate of edema, a few delicate fibrils of fibrin, mononuclear cells both large and small, and a few polymorphonuclear leukocytes.

only a short time and is replaced by a slowing of the current, which may progress to complete stagnation. If stagnation persist, clotting occurs. The dilatation appears first in the small arteries and arterioles and subsequently in the small veins, venules and capillaries. The chief problems to be dealt with are the mechanism of the vascular dilatation and the manner of slowing of the blood current.

Although the vascular dilatation is essentially an active hyperemia, yet there are important differences between inflammatory and simple active hyperemia. Adami would emphasize the difference by using the term capillary hyperemia for that occurring in inflammation. Samuel pointed out many years ago that if hyperemia of the rabbit's ear be produced by constriction at its base, puncture of the ear between the larger visible vessels leads to no hemorrhage, but if the ear be inflamed, puncture in the same situation leads to profuse bleeding. An important difference was also pointed out by Meltzer and

Meltzer, who found that the injection of adrenalin into a rabbit's ear, the seat of inflammation, produces no effect, whereas similar injection into an ear the seat of simple active hyperemia produces immediate pallor. Another difference of importance is that in ordinary active hyperemia the blood flow is continuously accelerated, whilst in inflammatory hyperemia the blood flow is only temporarily accelerated and for the most part slowed. Inflammatory hyperemia is likely to be of much greater duration than is ordinary active hyperemia. These differences may have an important bearing upon the fact that inflammatory hyperemia results in exudation, whereas ordinary active hyperemia does not.

Of importance is an understanding of the anatomy of the small vessels. Hooker points out that the arterioles are provided with a distinct muscular wall, and that the musculature continues for a certain distance along the arterial segments of the capillaries which are then devoid of musculature until they enter into the venules. These possess a musculature relatively less in amount than the corresponding arterioles. Nerve terminals, almost certainly of motor type, are found in connection with this smooth muscle. Nerves are found in the tissues in which the capillaries are embedded, but there is no clear and final indication that these communicate with the capillary endothelium. Hooker concludes that the evanescent vasoconstriction is probably due to the influence of nerves and the more lasting vasodilatation is due to chemical factors.

Nervous influences control the caliber of arterioles and venules. Furthermore it is now accepted that capillaries possess tonus and contractility, as shown by Krogh, but just what control the nervous system has is not certain. The question of the regulation of the inflammatory reaction by the nervous system has been the subject of many investigations. Samuel cut the sympathetic nerve supplying one ear of the rabbit and the auricular nerve of the other ear. Division of the sympathetic led to vasodilatation, and of the auricular to vasoconstriction. Both ears were then placed in water at 50° C. The ear in which capillary dilatation was present went on to severe inflammation, whereas that in which vasoconstriction was present responded much more slowly. Meltzer and Meltzer also

found that an ear from which the sympathetic control had been removed, responded somewhat more violently than a normal ear. It is therefore possible to influence inflammation by manipulation of the nervous control. Herpes zoster, an inflammatory lesion of skin over the course of nerves, is accompanied by lesions of spinal-root ganglia and the inflammation is attributed to the central disturbances. So-called sympathetic inflammation wherein irritation of one nerve may lead to inflammation in areas supplied by associated nerves has not been sufficiently studied to justify clear inferences. The same is true of reports of the influence of hypnosis and hysteria upon inflammation. Although questioned by some, it is probable that nervous influences operate in considerable part through axone reflexes as originally proposed by Bruce.

For completeness of discussion of the nervous influences, reference must be made to the hypothesis of Ricker, even though it is not widely accepted. He maintains that the inflammatory process depends upon nervous control and explains most of the phenomena upon this basis. Under normal conditions there may be a local hyperemia due to dilator action with still irritable constrictors and increased rate of blood flow because of wide patency of the arterioles. Ischemia may also be observed normally, due to action of vasoconstrictors, with decreased blood flow as the result of narrowing of the arterioles. Slightly in excess, abnormal stimuli produce pathic hyperemia. This may be succeeded by pathic ischemia, but the latter is especially likely to occur directly as the result of stronger stimuli. These processes then are only pathologic in that they exceed in degree what may be normally observed. In both instances the nerves are irritable. Still stronger stimuli lead to temporary paralysis, first of the constrictors and then of the dilators, with increased blood flow, but the stimulus may act upon arteriolar segments nearer the heart to reduce inflow of blood to capillaries and venules. Thus there occurs what Ricker calls prestatic slowing of the current (prestasis). Paralysis of the nerves supplying the proximal arterial segment may be followed by constriction of the next segment above, and as time elapses the slowing goes on to stasis, called red stasis or rubrostasis. This is a stage of extreme slowing with disorderly arrangement of the cells. Complete constriction of the arterioles may result in standstill of the current. The condition of stasis passes on to poststasis or postrubrostasis. As the arteriolar constriction is reduced by the action of dilators, which regain their irritability before the constrictors, the flow of blood is resumed gradually and in steps, and may return to normal. Under the proper conditions, the margination of leukocytes, which may appear in the stage of prestatic slowing of the current, is replaced in the poststasis period by a stage in which the small vessels are filled with leukocytes, white stasis or leukostasis. If this stage occur it is not certain that circulation is again restored in the affected vessels. Leukostasis never occurs without a preceding rubrostasis. In the stage of prestatic slowing of the current, escape of fluid is said to occur through the thinned intercellular substance of the dilated capillary wall, and erythrocytes are said to pass out through intercellular openings which open and close. Leukocytes pass out of the venules in small numbers in prestasis, but in large amounts only in leukostasis.

Many of the premises upon which this hypothesis has been built have been established by Ricker and his associates, but some have not been clearly demonstrated. Several of the studies quoted above controvert the Ricker hypothesis and Shimura brings evidence against its validity. Ricker, however, maintains that Shimura's experiments are technically inadequate. Direct observations of circulation in the rabbit's ear in the Clark window preparation shows, according to Sandison, that the arterioles regulate the blood flow in capillaries, which harmonizes with Ricker's studies. It is to be emphasized that the prolonged dilatation is in large part a paralytic phenomenon, which as yet cannot be attributed solely to exhaustion. Thus, it is possible to assume that the vascular changes when viewed in association with the series of exudative and fixed tissue changes of inflammation may be ascribed at least in part to physicochemical influences of the various incitants of inflammation.

The dilatation is probably in large part due to chemical and physicochemical factors. Certain studies indicate that there is a decrease of oxygen or an increase of carbon dioxide or both. Cohnheim and later Groll thought that vasodilatation is due to decreased oxygen concentration. Support was given by Amberg, Loevenhart and McClure, who found that injection of o-iodoso- and o-iodoxy-benzoic acid, which increases the availability of oxygen in the tissues, inhibits inflammation. Krogh showed that increase of carbon dioxide favors capillary dilatation. This he thinks is a part of the general phenomenon of dilatation by acids because carbon dioxide forms a weak acid with water. That there is acidity is illustrated by the work of Gilding who found that small foci of necrosis are on the acid side of neutrality, and that of Rous and Drury who showed that vasoconstriction may result in a shift toward acidity in the affected region.

The products of tissue injury have also been extensively studied, especially with a view to isolation of a single agent producing vasodilatation. Roessle found that many of the products of protein disintegration can cause various phenomena of inflammation. Histamine is an important product of tissue destruction and acts as a capillary poison to produce dilatation (Dale and Laidlaw). The H-substance of Lewis, found in cutaneous inflammation, produces much the same effects as does histamine and may well be identical. In certain types of inflammation the content of histamine is increased, perhaps because of accumulation of platelets which release histamine, whereas in other forms of reaction, the histamine content of the tissue is reduced (see Zon et al.).

We agree with Rous and Gilding that probably no single substance can be held accountable for the vasodilatation, because there are many that appear in the inflamed region. Because the primary vascular changes occur within a few seconds after the injury, it is unlikely that they are induced immediately by chemical factors. In summary, it is likely that the primary vasoconstriction and perhaps early vasodilatation are due to nervous influences and that the prolonged dilatation, presumably paralytic, is due either to decrease of oxygen, increase of carbon dioxide, local production of substances poisonous to the small vessels, or a combination of these factors.

Slowing of the Current

The slowing of the blood current has been attributed to various influences including alteration of the viscosity of the blood, swelling of the vascular endothelium, or an obscure increase in stickiness or diminution in smoothness of the vessel lining. There can be no doubt that if the proper physical conditions to establish increased rate of flow be present at the beginning, the subsequent decrease of rate must be due to local changes. Wooley, after a careful study of the literature, comes to the conclusion that the decrease in the rapidity of the blood stream is the result of two factors: an increase in the volume of the cells of the blood and of the endothelial cells lining the blood vessels, and increased viscosity of the blood as a whole. The evidence to support these conclusions is abundant and important. It must be obvious that the local activities in inflammation produce increased rate and volume of metabolism. Therefore, it is to be presumed that the products of metabolism are present in increased concentration. Studies of the red blood corpuscles indicate that an increase in the carbon-dioxide content increases the size of the corpuscles. This fact has been pointed out by numerous physiologists, and probably depends upon the increased hydrophilic character of the protein of the red blood corpuscles, incident to the increase in carbon-dioxide content. The same general principle applies to the increase in size of endothelial cells, whose intimate relation to the surrounding tissue affords a ready access not only to carbon dioxide but also to fixed acids such as lactic acid, the combination of which with the protein of the cells increases the hydrophilic properties and therefore leads to swelling. It is indeed possible to observe this swelling of endothelial cells during the period of increased rapidity of blood flow, followed in a short time by a slowing of the blood current and continued increase in the size of the lining cells. It is well known that the addition of acids to protein causes a swelling in the protein due to imbibition of water. The proteins of the blood fluid are no exception to this rule, and it may be readily assumed that as the plasma becomes increasingly hydrophilic, there is a resultant increase in viscosity. Landis states that injury of vascular endothelium is accompanied by increased stickiness. This may well be a factor in slowing of the current. After exudation has occurred, compression of the venous portions of the capillaries contributes further to the slowing of the current, as explained in the discussion of Klemensiewicz's views on exudation in the next section. Thus, it appears that the slowing of the current is due to various factors, including vasodilatation, increase in volume of red cells, increased viscosity of the blood and swelling and stickiness of the endothelium.

As the current is slowed, the distinction between axial (cellular) and peripheral (plasmatic) zones, especially in the venules, is disturbed. If stagnation occur, the cells are intermingled irregularly. Slowing of the current causes a significant accumulation of leukocytes in the peripheral zone (Nordmann and Rüther). It is generally believed that vortical or centripetal force maintains the zonal arrangement and that as circulation is slowed this force is reduced. It may be that the lighter specific gravity of the leukocytes is a factor in their margination, but Fåhraeus, as a result of his studies of blood sedimentation, considers that the red cells are more vigorously pulled into axial position because they become agglomerated to form masses greater in bulk than the individual leukocytes. This explanation is based on the conception that vortical force is more a matter of size of particles than of their specific gravity. Chemotaxis, discussed in connection with migration of leukocytes, may also be a factor in their margination. The leukocytes move slowly in the marginal zone and become attached to the endothelium, perhaps because of reduction of surface tension, exhibited first in the endothelium and then in the leukocytes. This is supposedly due to diffusion of products elaborated in the diseased tissues. Evidently the flow of blood produces some elongation of the attached leukocytes and ultimately many of them migrate through the capillary walls.

EXUDATION

This term means the passage through the walls of the vessels of water and dissolved solids, as well as of blood corpuscles. The product in the tissues is the exudate. The mechanisms of exudation have been extensively studied and in order to understand them it is necessary to consider the constituents of the exudate, the mode of their passage, the factors which favor passage and the functions of the various components.

Fluid of the Exudate

The mechanism of exudation of fluid is somewhat like that of the production of

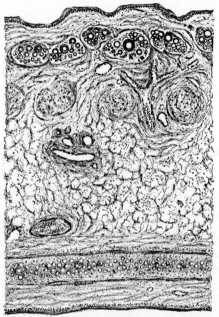

Inflammatory edema of rabbit's ear, due to painting of one surface with croton oil. The marked swelling of the painted side is contrasted with the slight swelling on the opposite side of the cartilage. Note the capillary dilatation, the marked separation of tissue fibrils by edema and the relatively slight cellular exudate.

lymph but there are significant differences. For example, the amount of fluid, rate of flow and the pressure in the lymphatics during the course of inflammation are vastly increased over the normal (Drinker et al.). The fluid of inflammation, or inflammatory edema fluid, is of high specific gravity (over 1.018), considerably greater than that of lymph or of the transudate of the edema incident to passive hyperemia. This increase of specific gravity is due principally to the content of plasma proteins. The fluid of the exudate contains practically all the solid constituents of the blood plasma, but their concentration

shows certain differences. In addition, the fluid of the exudate contains materials contributed from the inflammatory tissues. Thus, the inflammatory fluid contains salt in very much the same concentration as the plasma, extractives of various kinds including urea, fibrin forming elements, soaps, mucin, ferments and immune bodies. Oxidases, lipase, and trypsin are found. Anti-enzyme is also present, as in the plasma, but frequently the proteolytic enzyme contributed by the cells of the exudate not only neutralizes the anti-enzyme but may be present in excess. All types of immune bodies may be found including cytolysins, hemolysins, bacteriolysins, agglutinins and opsonins, as well as complement-fixing bodies. Complement is also present but in extremely variable amounts; it is particularly likely to be low in amount if the exudate be rich in leukocytes (pus). As a rule, the enzymes and immune substances are distinctly higher in inflammatory edema than in edema from other causes.

In the discussion of edema in the chapter on Disturbances of Circulation, attention was given to disturbances of osmotic pressure and capillary permeability. Probably the main factor in the problem of inflammatory edema is increased permeability. This is supported by the fact that the fluid is rich in solids, as indicated above, and that fibrin is precipitated from it. Landis reports that if capillaries are injured to a degree that stasis occurs, the walls permit the passage outward of proteins, colloidal dyes and colloidal starch. The loss of protein reduces the colloidal osmotic pressure of the blood and this furthers the development of edema. In fact the fluid may exude seven times as fast as in the formation of lymph, at a time when internal hydrostatic pressure within the capillary would otherwise permit of flow of fluid from the tissues into it. In inflammatory edema, then, capillary pressure and colloidal osmotic pressure of the blood are significant factors, but the most important feature is increased permeability. The participation of the inflamed extravascular tissues is not firmly established, even though there is a shift of pH toward the acid side, with the possibility of production of hydrophilic-acid proteins, as well as relative anoxemia and increase of carbon dioxide. The dilatation of the capillaries increases the filtration surface

PLATE V

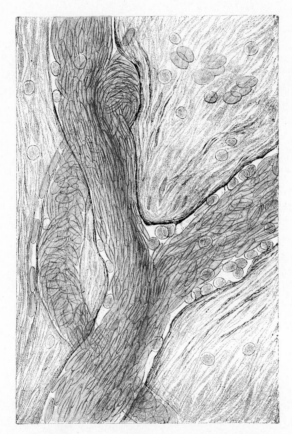

Margination of leukocytes in dilated capillary of frog mesentery. The leukocytes are rounded uncolored cells in the peripheral zone of the current.

but even more important is the development of pores in the endothelium and separation of the cells so that spaces develop which are estimated to have a diameter of 5 to 200 millimicra.

The cause, or causes of the increased permeability have been extensively studied. Histamine or H-substance can do it, but they are not solely responsible. Menkin reports the isolation and crystallization, from exudates, of an intermediate product of pro-

stances can bring about the increase of permeability, without there being as yet a positive identification of which is most significant.

Rous has shown that in certain capillaries there is normally a gradient of permeability that increases toward the venous ends, thus tending to equalize the passage outward of fluid as the internal physical pressure decreases. The hypothesis of Klemensiewicz, modified to meet the observations of Rous,

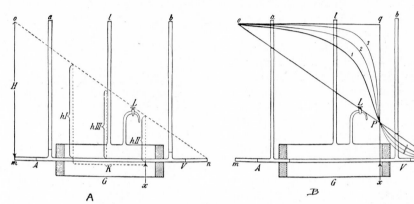

Diagrams from Klemensiewicz' *Die Entzündung*, to illustrate causes of slowing of current and fluid exudation. *A* shows normal capillary circulation. The glass cylinder *K* is plugged at each end with rubber stoppers. The tube *m-n* is of glass except within the vessel *K* where it represents a capillary and consists of a piece of rabbit intestine. The uprights *a, l, b,* are glass water manometers, and *L* is an outlet from *K*. A flow of water is established through *m-n* so that at *m* the pressure is up to the point *o*. The fall in pressure follows a diagonal represented by the line *o-n*. Fluid accumulates in the vessel *K* by transudation through the capillary and represents normal tissue pressure when the pressure indicated by *hI, hIII, hII* are attained, and may be maintained by dripping out of *L*, which represents lymphatic drainage.

B shows the changed pressure relations in inflammation, where owing to excessive outflows of fluid from the capillary and inadequate drainage, the fall of pressure, instead of following the line *o-n*, is represented by the curves *1, 2* and *3*. This is due to the fact that the increased pressure in *K* compresses the gut part of tube *m-h* at its point of least intravascular pressure, namely at *x*. Thus, pressure is increased in the part toward *m*. As pressure is increased near *m*, there is increased outpouring of fluid, due to the increased intravascular pressure, and this results in increased pressure in *K* which operates more strongly to compress at *x*. Pressure progressively increases in the tube toward *m*, and decreases between *x* and *n*. Thus, circulation is slowed in rate and fluid exudation increases until circulation is stopped by complete compression at *x*.

tein disintegration, probably a polypeptide, which he calls leukotaxine. This produces vasodilatation, but he states that it is not histamine. This differs from the saline extract of normal tissues prepared by Rigdon, which also increases permeability. Duthie and Chain prepared polypeptides from normal blood proteins and found them to increase permeability. They were unable to confirm Menkin's claims of crystallization. They thought that histamine is responsible for the permeability factor of leukotaxine, a view shared by Bier. Evidently various sub-

draws attention to the fact that the flow of blood through capillaries depends upon the progressive fall of pressure as the venous ends of the capillaries are approached. If capillary poisons increase the permeability of the walls, the outward passage of fluids is augmented. Failure of adequate drainage determines the occurrence of edema. As the fluid in the tissues accumulates it exerts pressure upon the capillaries, which is effective in the segments of low pressure near the venous ends, thus increasing pressure in the arterial segments and in the arterioles. This increased pressure, together with increased permeability, accelerates the passage of fluid from the arterial segments, which in turn further compresses the venous segments. The vicious circle so established may result in complete stagnation and clotting with cessation of further exudation. Ricker's assumption that the fluid passes out through stretched intercellular spaces requires confirmation.

Important functions are served by the fluid of the exudate. It dilutes soluble poisons and irritants, and thereby reduces their direct effect. Its flow into the lymphatics and venules, although inadequate for the large amount of fluid formed, is in excess of normal, as shown by Samuel, and aids in carrying off the noxious soluble materials. It also provides avenues of escape for the metabolites which are probably formed in excess. Its flow tends toward maintenance of the normal hydrogen-ion concentration. Its content of enzymes may operate to neutralize toxic bacterial products. The proteolytic enzymes serve to complete the solution of tissues which have been injured or killed, and thus aid in their removal. It is known that the fluid drained from the inflamed part contains digested products of protein, particularly peptone, and the fluid is of increased hydrogen-ion concentration. The enzymes and immune bodies serve in part to complete the destruction of tissues, and aid in destroying bacteria. The soluble materials so removed pass ultimately into the blood stream, undergo destructive changes in the body, and are excreted through normal routes. It is true, however, that the flow of fluid into the lymphatics and ultimately into the blood stream is not always an unmixed good, for living bacteria may be carried to lymph nodes, to remote parts of the body by the blood stream, and be generally distributed. If the amount of injurious material absorbed be sufficient, it may irritate the parenchymatous and other organs of the body and lead to alterative or degenerative inflammations. The work of Opie and others indicates that certain antibodies may be concentrated in the inflamed area, but this is not shown to be common to all antibodies. It is possible that the exchange of large volumes of fluid may bring to the part increased quantities of immune substances, but not necessarily an increased concentration. Can-

non and Pacheco suggest that agglutinating and opsonizing antibodies aid in preventing the dissemination of bacteria. Conversely various substances, including bacteria, may be concentrated in the injured area because of increased permeability of the vessels.

Fibrin Formation

The elements concerned in the formation of fibrin, normally present in the plasma, are also found in the fluid of the exudate. This fluid, however, is in an abnormal extravascular position which favors clotting. The death of cells of tissues and exudate liberates fibrin ferment. Fibrin is likely to be found in

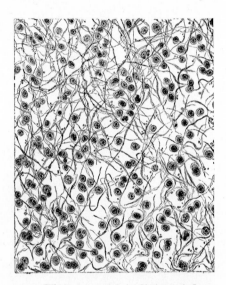

Fibrin formation in fibrinous inflammation of pleura; nodal points are evident. The cells are principally large lymphocytes, since the patient was a victim of lymphoid leukemia.

the early stage of almost any acute exudate. It is particularly prominent, however, in exudates upon serous surfaces. It may occur as the result of inflammation produced by practically any cause, but is especially likely to be found in inflammation induced by the diphtheria bacillus, by the pneumococcus and related organisms. On the serous surfaces and in pneumonia and diphtheria, the fibrin is likely to persist in the exudate for a considerable time, but in most cases ultimately disappears. Its disappearance, according to Opie, is probably due to proteolytic enzymes which originate in the blood and are contained in the fibrin precipitate. If large num-

PLATE VI

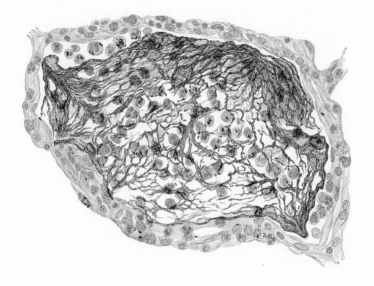

Special stain of fibrin in a pulmonary alveolus in lobar pneumonia. The fibrin fibrils are stained greenish-blue and are attached
at the pores of Cohn. The leukocytes enmeshed in the fibrin and cells
of the alveolar walls are stained pink.

bers of leukocytes be present in the exudate and suppuration ensue, or if other destructive elements appear in the exudate, the fibrin is likely to disappear, owing particularly to solution by the proteolytic enzymes of the leukocytes and of the fibrin. It may be deposited as a fine network, in heavy bands, or in large hyaline masses. When fibrinous exudates appear upon serous or mucous surfaces, the fibrin is deposited in large part outside the line of the surface cells, but frequently is found to be intimately connected with a fibrin deposit within the superficial tissues. Destruction of the surface cells is not an essential feature in the formation of the fibrin but frequently accompanies it. Further description is to be found in the section on fibrinous inflammation.

If bacteria, other particulate matter, or proteins be injected intravenously at appropriate times they are concentrated in foci of inflammation probably because of increased vascular permeability. If injected into inflamed foci, they may stay there. Menkin found that colloidal dyes and also staphylococci do not disperse into the lymphatics and attributed this to the formation of fibrin in draining lymphatics to constitute a filter. Cannon and Hartley injected streptococci into inflamed foci and saw no hindrance to dissemination of these bacteria. Kenton found the same to be true of staphylococcus toxin. Both Rigdon and Landis think that retention of particulate matter in inflamed foci is due to physicochemical factors in the cells and exudate rather than to a filter of fibrin. Other evidence points to the same conclusion. Fibrin may produce adhesions, as in the peritoneum, and prevent the extension of inflammation. It serves as a scaffolding for the growth of fibroblasts but does not contribute in itself to granulation or cicatrization.

Mucin Formation

Mucin may be found in minute quantities in almost any fluid exudate. It does not appear, however, as the product of exudation but is formed by fixed tissue cells, usually epithelial cells of mucous or other glands, or the glands and surface epithelium of mucous membranes. It is well known that connective tissue may, under certain conditions, form mucoid and the endothelial cells may do the same. Mucin is present in larger quantities in acute inflammations of mucous surfaces, the so-called catarrhal inflammation. There is, in such catarrhal exudates, a certain amount of exudation from blood vessels, but the main body of the exudate is the mucin provided by hypersecretion on the part of stimulated epithelial cells, principally glandular.

Cells of the Exudate

The Polymorphonuclear Leukocyte. Pathologists commonly use the term leukocyte to mean the polymorphonuclear

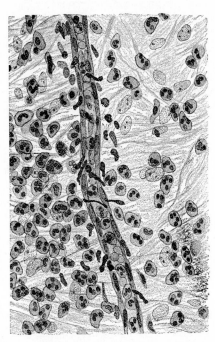

Emigration of leukocytes through the walls of a minute capillary, and further migration into tissues.

neutrophil. When other cells of the same general order are referred to, they are given their special names. This discussion takes up the migration through the vessel walls, passage through the tissues and functions of the leukocyte in the exudate. As the blood current slows, the marginal zone contains numerous leukocytes, which adhere to the lining of the vessel, pass through this lining and then wander along lines of least resistance, such as tissue and fascial spaces, toward the point of irritation. They may accumulate in very large numbers to form a limiting zone about the focus of injury. The predominant leukocyte is the neutrophil but the eosinophil may take part, and if the patient be the victim of a leukemia the cells of the exudate may include all those which appear in the leukemic blood. In the exudate of lobar pneumonia there are many polymorphonuclear leukocytes, but if, as shown by Winternitz and Hirschfelder, the blood be deprived of most of its granular cells by benzol poisoning, the exudate contains almost no leukocytes. Thus, the cellular content of the exudate is determined to a certain degree by the cellular content of the blood. The leukocyte migrates by virtue of its ameboid movement, a capacity shared by the eosinophil, the myeloblast, and the myelocyte. Maximow demonstrated the ameboid movement of lymphocytes, and the same property is possessed by the plasma cell, the endothelial cell and the fibroblast. The phenomenon of ameboid movement is now generally conceded to be due to alterations of surface tension, although other physical properties of the cell and medium are not without considerable importance. The phenomenon is explained very clearly by Wells as follows:

Imagine a drop of fluid suspended in water—let it be a drop of protoplasm, or oil, or mercury; the drop owes its tendency to assume a spherical shape to the surface tension, which is pulling the free surface toward the center and acting with the same force on all sides. The result is that the drop is surrounded by what amounts to an elastic, well-stretched membrane, similar to the condition of a thin rubber bag distended with fluid. If at any point in the surface the tension is lessened, while elsewhere it remains the same, of necessity the wall will bulge at this point, the contents will flow into the new space so offered and the rest of the wall will contract; hence the drop moves toward the point of lowered surface tension. Conversely, if the tension is increased in one place, the wall at this point will contract with greater force than elsewhere, driving the contents toward the less resistant part of the surface, and the drop will move away from the point of increased tension.

The ameboid movement of leukocytes is due to chemical stimulation. This is called chemotaxis or chemotropism. It may be positive or negative according to whether it attracts or repels cells. The chemotactic substance must be diffusible in order to reach the cells. Experimentally, a variety of substances are positively chemotactic, for example aleuronat, inulin, turpentine, and salts. These, however, are probably of no importance in naturally occurring inflammation. Here products of bacterial metabolism and of destruction of tissues operate. It is generally agreed that histamine is not chemotactic. It is also probable that the hydrogen-ion concentration plays no important part, although salt concentrations may (Karsner and Merrill). Nevertheless, as the exudate becomes more and more acid, the leukocytes are less in number and the large mononuclears more numerous (Menkin and Warner). Certain unidentified products of bacteria are positively chemotactic, but some are inert and a few are negatively chemotactic. The extracts of exudates and of normal tissues, referred to in the discussion of vascular permeability, are usually positively chemotactic. Chemotropism determines the direction in which the cells move, but does not increase their rate of motion (Dixon and McCutcheon). In addition to chemotactic attraction, other factors may be of importance. Thus, that leukocytes move toward solid materials, as a piece of glass or other foreign element, upon which they can get a hold, is attributed to physical rather than chemical attraction (Wright and Colebrook). Nevertheless, chemotaxis explains best the mass and direction of leukocytic migration.

Apparently the leukocytes serve two important functions in inflammation. They ingest and remove bacteria, solid particles of cell and tissue debris; they also provide proteolytic enzymes, pepsin, cathepsin and trypsin (Weiss and Czarnetsky) which liquefy the injured cells, thus favoring their removal. The fluid is readily absorbed and the cell fragments removed by phagocytes. Thus, the leukocyte aids in removal of debris and preparation for repair.

Phagocytosis. This term means ingestion of foreign particles by a cell; the cell is called a phagocyte. The process involves first the approximation of the cell and the foreign substance and second the ingestion by the cell. A third step, the solution of the particle by enzymes of the cytoplasm, does not always take place, because the body may be insoluble or, in the case of bacteria, they may resist solution or even kill the cell. Chemotaxis is the principal cause of approach of the cell to the material to be ingested. Pseudopodia extend out, surround the particle and by fusion ingest it. Thus both the approach and the ingestion depend upon the motility of the cell. Other factors are also important, such as the internal structure of the cell, the nature of the foreign particle and properties of the medium, including temperature and isotonicity. The process appears to depend on free energy at the interfaces of cell and particle. After ingestion, the particle becomes enclosed in a vacuole filled with fluid containing enzymes which act best in an acid medium. If the particle is not soluble by these enzymes, it may remain in the cytoplasm during the life of the cell or be extruded. Many of the activities of the ameba can be imitated by inert bodies such as a drop of oil or metallic mercury when placed in suitable media. The phagocytes in the body differ from free living amebae in several respects. They depend upon the body fluids for nutrition and live outside the body only for a short time. They do not move freely in a liquid medium but progress over solid surfaces. Their type of movement and irritability are different.

The chief phagocytes active in inflammation are the polymorphonuclear leukocyte and the large wandering mononuclear cell, the microphage and the macrophage of Metchnikoff. Other cells such as the eosinophil, the myelocyte, the myeloblast and the lymphocyte may be phagocytic but in considerably smaller degree. Usually the leukocytes ingest and destroy bacteria, while the large mononuclear cells ingest and dissolve debris of cells and tissues. In vitro, however, both act about equally well on bacteria and debris (Lucké et al.). Bacteria are usually taken up more readily if they are dead than if they are alive. If ingested alive they may be killed and dissolved or they may multiply within the cell and may destroy it. Migration and transportation of phagocytes which contain living bacteria may result in carriage of the bacteria to neighboring tissues and to the blood, when widespread dissemination may occur.

According to Wolf, phagocytosis may be favored by dead or living bacterial cultures, pathogenic or nonpathogenic, the products of protein disintegration such as peptone, amino-acids and amines, as well as by carbon dioxide and many crystalloids. Nevertheless other crystalloids may be negatively chemotactic and inhibit phagocytosis.

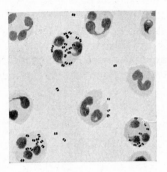

Drawing showing phagocytosis of gonococci by leukocytes in urethral exudate.

The amino-acids and amines are positively chemotactic and favor phagocytosis.

Normally the fluids of the body contain a substance, the opsonin of Wright, or the bacteriotropin of Neufeld, which renders the material to be taken up more favorable for ingestion. Opsonins act on bacteria, animal cells, fragments of cells and perhaps upon inorganic particles although this last has not been conclusively proved. Opsonins may be increased in amount by disease or by artificial immunization. Complement favors the action of normal and immune opsonins, but it is not essential to the operation of either. Indeed, normal opsonins reside in certain components of complement (Ecker et al.). In a general way it can be said that the more virulent the bacteria, the more resistant they are to phagocytosis and to opsonization, and this resistance is still effective after death of the organisms. Whether there are definite alterations of the bacterial membrane or whether the bacteria produce antiopsonic and antiphagocytic substances is not known. An excellent review of phagocytosis is furnished by Mudd, McCutcheon and Lucké.

This brief discussion of phagocytosis is not complete without reference to the possibility that bacteria may penetrate into cells by some mechanism other than phagocytosis. The immature form of the parasite of malaria invades erythrocytes, a situation in which phagocytosis is almost certainly not a factor, and it develops in the cell. In typhoid fever, bacteria enter large mononuclear cells in the lymphoid apparatus of the intestine and multiply. It is by no means certain that phagocytosis operates in this instance and there seems to be a sort of symbiosis between cell and infective organisms.

Cells Other than Leukocytes. Lymphocytes appear in the exudate but are not likely to be numerous in the more acute

is not well known. Some think they give rise to the large mononuclear cell, but that has not been finally proved. Opie's work indicates that they may be a source of a proteolytic enzyme which operates best in a weakly acid medium. This reaction of medium occurs in necrosis and inflammation; it would favor the action of this enzyme and inhibit anti-enzymes. Jobling and Petersen found that lymphocytes also contain a lipase, leading to the suggestion that the lymphocytes in the tubercle, liberating this enzyme, may serve to break down the wax of the tubercle bacilli.

Erythrocytes may be present in exudates in such small numbers as to be seen only microscopically or in such large numbers

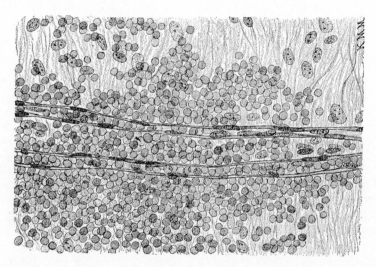

Hemorrhage in acute inflammation of mesentery.

inflammations. As inflammation becomes subacute and then chronic, lymphocytes may be found in larger numbers. Lymphocytes are capable of ameboid movement, but are only rarely phagocytic. Dixon and McCutcheon have shown that under experimental conditions they have no chemotropic properties, even though they are present in exudates and at times in great numbers. There is discussion as to whether they are derived from the blood or from the tissues, i.e., whether they are hemal or histogenous. The evidence in favor of the former is stronger than for the latter, but probably both play a part. The function of the lymphocytes in inflammation

as to render the exudate grossly hemorrhagic. They pass through the vessel walls by diapedesis, or vessel walls are ruptured and they are said to enter the exudate per rhexis. The latter is principally in the form of numerous ruptures of small vessels due to destructive effects of the process on the walls. Since erythrocytes are not motile, the process of diapedesis must be passive as far as these cells are concerned. How they pass through the walls is not known. Nevertheless, in the discussion of increased permeability, mention was made of the fact that with this change and dilatation, holes appear in the walls with an estimated diameter of 5 to 200 millimicra and it may be that these can be stretched to permit of diapedesis at a time when pressure is greater within than outside the vessels. A second theory is that the reduced permeability allows the erythrocytes to pass through the endothelium as one colloid of greater density passes through another of lesser density. The example offered is that in which a droplet of mercury is placed on top of a column of gelatin; it sinks through the gelatin and leaves no trace of its passage. This is offered because of the uncertain assumption that the endothelial cells do not separate at their junctions. The function of erythrocytes in the exudate is not known. They may carry oxygen, but probably in no greater amount than can be provided by diffusion.

Platelets are found in small numbers in the inflammatory exudate and may be seen to constitute the centrum of the fibrin asters. They are rarely seen as free bodies, probably because of the rapid clotting of the fluids and the consequent agglutination of the platelets. They probably pass through the vessel walls in much the same way as the erythrocytes. Aside from the influence in fibrin deposition, little is known of their functions. They appear to have a property called thigmotropism, by virtue of which certain bacteria may be clumped around masses of platelets. This is favored by opsonins and is probably determined by interfacial relations. Clumping and immobilization of bacteria favors phagocytosis. Platelets are deposited quickly on injured endothelium and may perhaps plug small injuries to the vessel walls. As indicated above they may liberate histamine.

The Large Mononuclear Cell. Microscopic study of exudates reveals large mononuclear cells, which become more numerous as time passes. Some of these are phagocytic and some are not. The latter are principally fibroblasts in an early stage of development. The number of large mononuclears varies considerably and they are especially conspicuous in the reactions to tubercle bacilli, lepra bacilli, typhoid bacilli and foreign bodies. They phagocytose tissue debris, dead cells, inert granules such as pigment, and erythrocytes. In the tissues they are not so active toward bacteria as are the polymorphonuclears. They act in a sense as scavengers to remove these various substances and prepare the field for repair. They vary considerably in form in various exudates, but look a good deal like the monocytes of the circulating blood. Monocytes may participate in exudation, but probably to only a small degree, and exercise phagocytic activity. The origin of the other large mononuclears has been extensively studied by comparative cytology and tissue culture, without final conclusion. All these cells have the same phagocytic function but have been given various names. Thus, such names as primitive wandering cell, resting wandering cell, clasmatocyte, polyblast, adventitial cell, pyrrhol cell, carmin cell, histiocyte, macrophage, endothelial leukocyte, splenocyte, monocyte, and transitional cell have been applied. The studies of Maximow indicate that practically all the cells of the exudate, furnished either from the circulating blood or from the tissues involved, originate from essentially the same primary cells of the mesoderm. How they are subsequently differentiated is a matter of no great moment in this discussion. Inasmuch as these various names for cells appear in the literature, it is well to consider a few of these forms.

THE PRIMITIVE WANDERING CELL is, according to Maximow, the small, mononuclear cell of the embryo, which arises from the mesoderm and subsequently by differentiation gives rise to either hematogenous or histogenous wandering cells of the body.

THE CLASMATOCYTE of Ranvier is a cell which in its actively motile state is found to have a large nucleus, and a somewhat granular cytoplasm which divides into numerous processes, and as it passes through the tissue spaces is likely to leave behind small particles of cytoplasm.

THE POLYBLAST of Maximow is a cell which varies considerably in form but is essentially a large mononuclear with a deeply stained nucleus, sometimes of irregular form, and an abundant cytoplasm which shows no granules. These he considered might originate from migrating lymphocytes, or from pre-existing wandering cells of the tissues which might be directly transformed into polyblasts, or become transformed by passing through a stage in which they resemble clasmatocytes.

THE ADVENTITIAL CELL described by Marchand is a small round cell found in the tissue especially in the region of the blood vessels, and in our opinion is probably identical with the small cells described by Councilman as lymphocytes, which appear in the perilymphatic, and probably also perivascular, structures.

THE PYRRHOL CELL AND THE CARMIN CELL are cells which are especially susceptible to vital staining, that is, to staining following injection of dyes into the circulating fluids of the body.

THE HISTIOCYTE is described by Aschoff as a large mononuclear cell, including those which take the vital stain and probably others, and is derived either from the monocytes or from comparable cells in the tissues such as reticulo-endothelial cells.

THE TERM MACROPHAGE was employed by Metchnikoff to designate phagocytic cells which originate in the tissues.

ENDOTHELIAL LEUKOCYTE is the term Mallory employs to designate the large wandering cell, both of the circulating blood and the tissues, which has notable phagocytic properties. He believes that all these cells originate from vascular endothelium, that they appear in the blood stream following multiplication of the endothelial lining and desquamation of cells, that they migrate in the course of inflammation through the vascular walls and may subsequently multiply in the tissues.

Pappenheim uses the term SPLENO-CYTE to indicate the macrophage of histogenous origin which migrates to the spleen and continues to exist there, possibly, according to him, as the local producer of hemolysin. The MONOCYTE is a similar cell appearing in the circulating blood. Both of these he believes to be descendants of those cells which take vital stains. The TRANSITIONAL CELL, originally described by Ehrlich as the transition form between the large mononuclear and the polymorphonuclear cells of the blood, is regarded by F. A. Evans as a cell probably originating from the bone marrow and to be grouped, because of its positive oxidase reaction, with the granulocyte series. It is a phagocytic cell which occasionally appears in the tissues in the course of inflammation, but is far outnumbered by the vitally staining histogenous cells which contain no oxidase.

In the numerous studies of this group of cells, various origins have been ascribed. It is generally admitted that they have the same embryologic origin, but their more immediate derivation is differently interpreted. We may quote F. A. Evans as follows:

> From the literature, then, although it is manifestly unfair to interpret the opinions of the more prominent students of the subject along such narrow lines and without further exposition, one may formulate in general the following different hypotheses: that the different types of mononuclear cells of the blood and tissues are (1) lymphoid (Maximow), (2) endothelial (Mallory), (3) histogenous (Tschaschin), (4) in part histogenous and in part hematogenous (Marchand, Aschoff, Pappenheim, Kiyone).

The investigations of Evans, Downey, McJunkin, Foot and others based upon morphologic and functional studies of blood and tissues indicate that these cells are identical functionally and probably all originate from endothelium of blood vessels or lymphatics. McJunkin supports Mallory's view that they originate from vascular endothelium and migrate from the blood stream. Foot concludes that they are derived in part from the proliferating vascular endothelium in the immediate neighborhood of the injury rather than from vascular endothelium in general, and that they do not originate in the omentum or connective-tissue cells or from lymphocytes. Sabin describes distinguishing morphologic features between monocytes of the blood and clasmatocytes of the tissues, but the Lewises and others believe them to be identical. Their functional importance in inflammation is apparently the same whether they be determined ultimately to originate either from circulating cells in the blood originally derived from vascular endothelium, or in large part are the direct descendants of proliferating vascular endothelium in the inflamed area. Their motility depends upon the same conditions that determine this property of the leukocyte. Their phagocytic activity toward bacteria and cell débris is influenced undoubtedly by the action of the opsonins.

This was shown clearly by Hektoen and others and confirmed by Karsner, Amiral and Bock. It is of especial importance to note that the discussion as to nature and mode of origin of the mononuclear cells revolves about special methods of preparation, reactions and staining. Routine tissue sections do not exhibit the features upon which many of the finer distinctions are based. There is no generally accepted terminology, but we usually refer to them as large mononuclear cells or mononuclear phagocytes.

The Plasma Cell. Since the discovery of this cell, descriptions have varied somewhat but that of v. Marschalkó is now accepted as representing the typical plasma cell. This cell is round or oval, slightly larger than the lymphocyte. The cytoplasm is basophilic, usually homogeneous or finely granular but without specific granular character, and with a perinuclear zone which takes the stain faintly or not at all. The nucleus is eccentrically situated. The chromatin is principally near the nuclear margin in the form of angulated masses with the base outward, radially arranged so as to produce the appearance of the "cart wheel" nucleus. Although these cells may be found in acute exudates, they are observed principally in subacute and chronic forms of inflammation. They are common in chronic gonococcal inflammations of tubes and ovaries. Their origin is still controversial. Michels' summary points out four theories: (1) a histogenous derivation from connective tissue cells such as tissue lymphocytes, fibroblasts, clasmatocytes, etc., (2) a hematogenic derivation from emigrated lymphocytes, (3) mixed origin from emigrated lymphocytes or tissue lymphocytes, and (4) an origin from immature blood cells. It is difficult to say that any of these hypotheses is adequately supported. Miller believes that the precursor is a primitive cell of the connective tissues and that the plasma cell is an entity. Nevertheless they may be grown in tissue culture from explants of lymphoid tissue. Degenerations occur and the cytoplasm may contain acidophilic hyaline granules, Russell bodies. The function of these cells in inflammation is not well known, except that they may be slightly phagocytic toward inert particles and bacteria. It seems unlikely that they give rise to other cells.

The Mast Cell. The mast cell is normally present in the blood stream in very small percentage and is also said to occur within normal tissues. It plays a very small part in the inflammatory reaction and probably is derived very largely from the blood stream, since in inflammation in leukemic patients mast cells may be found in considerable numbers. These are the basophilic leukocytes of the blood, and show a slightly indented or polymorphonuclear nucleus. The cytoplasm is fairly rich and contains granules variable in size and form, which take the basic stain deeply. Such cells are found more commonly in mild subacute and subchronic inflammations than in the acute forms. They are especially prone to degenerative changes so that the nucleus may be very faintly stained, or the cell may be fragmented and its granules distributed about the region. These granules may be mistaken for bacteria and sometimes for minute animal parasites. Certain authorities regard the cells as a degenerative form of the plasma cell or of the endothelial cell. It has slight ameboid movement but apparently plays little part in phagocytosis and has no other known function in inflammation.

Eosinophils may be conspicuous in acute inflammation of allergic nature, in response to certain parasites and in chronic inflammation. In allergic forms of asthma, in skin reactions, natural or diagnostic, and in occasional other inflammations of the same order, there may be many eosinophils in the exudate. In the early stages of reaction to the larvae of *Trichinella spiralis*, eosinophils take part. During the attack of asthma and in well-marked cases of trichinosis, there may be an increase of eosinophils in the circulating blood. Eosinophils are often found in the inflammation near carcinoma of the uterine cervix and in inflammations of the intestine, especially of the appendix. As indicated above, the presence of eosinophils in the exudate is common in allergic inflammation but is not pathognomonic because it occurs in other conditions. Eosinophilic leukocytes are capable of ameboid movement and migrate into the exudate, but the additional question of their origin in tissues is not settled. Liebreich maintains that other cells may become eosinophils as in foci of hemorrhage, due to the presumptive influence of some substance formed during clotting. In the movement of these cells, the pseudopodia do not contain the granules. There is no doubt that eosinophils can be phagocytic, but not in great degree. Other functions in the exudate are not known.

TYPES OF INFLAMMATION

As has been indicated, certain elements of the exudate are likely to predominate in any given inflammation, and the process is designated as serous, fibrinous, purulent, etc. In all the acute exudates, practically all the elements described above play a part, and although an exudate may be described as serous, this does not exclude the participation of leukocytes, fibrin and other elements. Sometimes it is difficult to determine the predominance of one particular element. If two elements appear to predominate, it is customary to employ combined terms such as serofibrinous, seropurulent, fibrinopurulent, etc., the second part of the term indicating the relative preponderance of the one element over the other. The personal equation often decides the designation of the inflammation in questionable instances. Of further importance is the fact that the character of an inflammatory process may change from day to day or even from hour to hour, so that any such designations as indicated here refer to the condition at the moment of observation. Thus a fibrinous pleurisy may in a few hours become a fibrinoserous pleurisy and may subsequently become a purulent pleurisy. A serous meningitis may rapidly become a purulent meningitis and similar changes may be noted in practically any type of inflammation.

Serous Inflammation

One of the most common examples of serous exudation is the formation of blisters of the skin following a burn or the action of corrosive chemicals. The blisters contain principally serum, only little fibrin and a few exuded cells. If infected, the blisters may become purulent. Serous inflammation may occur in almost any situation but is especially frequent in serous membranes and the serous cavities. The amount of fluid accumulated in the peritoneum may exceed several liters and in the pleura may be a liter or more.

Even in the pericardium a liter of fluid is occasionally found. Invariably, however, a certain amount of fibrin is deposited on the surface, and in the microscopic examination of such a membrane, the inflammation may be designated as fibrinous if no knowledge be possessed of the general condition of the cavity. Such fluids are of high specific gravity, contain considerable quantities of protein, and upon microscopic examination show desquamated endothelium and many leukocytes. When removed, such fluids are likely to clot in the containers. If clotting has occurred *in situ*, further clotting is not likely to occur upon removal. Experimentally serous exudation is observed in the rabbit's ear by painting it with croton oil or immersing it in hot water.

Fibrinous Inflammation

Fibrinous inflammation is well exemplified in the local reaction to diphtheria. The implantation of the diphtheria bacilli in

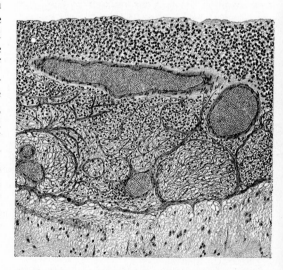

Acute fibrinopurulent inflammation of the meninges. Note the dilated vessels.

the tonsil leads first to redness, swelling and tenderness or pain in the tonsil and rapidly to the formation of the fibrinous exudate. This appears upon the surface as a white or pale yellow, smooth mass, sharply defined and of semisolid consistency. Subsequently, it shows roughening of the surface due to solution of the fibrin, and may become yellow in color due to an increased number of leukocytes. When examined microscopically, it is found to be made up of a network of fibrin strands, arranged very irregularly in the form of small hyaline bands or masses and a fine network of intercommunicating fibrils. The fibrin is found also in the surface epithelium and sometimes beneath the basement membrane in the substance of the tonsil. The same general principle is applied to fibrinous diphtheritic exudate anywhere. Fibrin formation is also well exemplified in lobar pneumonia. Fibrin may be formed in numerous other parts of the body and various names have been used. The term "diphtheritic inflammation" is now restricted to that form produced by the diphtheria bacillus. Exudates similar in gross and microscopic character appear also in the intestinal canal, particularly in the small intestine in various forms of enteritis and in the large intestine in dysentery. Although the term "diphtheritic" was formerly applied to these inflammations, it has now been abandoned, and although some apply the term "diphtheroid" it seems preferable to refer to these simply as fibrinous exudates or fibrinous inflammations of the gut. The term "croupous" inflammation was designed to apply to fibrinous inflammation of the respiratory tract below the level of and including the larynx. This is preserved in the term "croupous" pneumonia which is now used synonymously with lobar pneumonia. Inflammations of the serous surfaces are almost constantly accompanied by the formation of a considerable amount of fibrin. In the early stages the fibrin is deposited in the form of a soft, pale yellow or white substance, which adheres to the serous surface very much as butter adheres to bread, when two pieces are buttered and subsequently pulled apart. The old term "bread and butter" pericardium or pleura or peritoneum is still sometimes applied to these early fibrinous inflammations of serous surfaces, with their dull, light yellow, slightly roughened surface. As the fibrin continues to be formed, however, the movement of these membranes may whip the fibrin into more or less heavy bands. Thus, in the pericardium, the whipping action of the heart may form heavy, stringy masses of fibrin which gives the designation "shaggy" or villous heart.

The microscopic diagnosis of fibrin is important. Fibrin takes the acid stain in the tissue section and although it appears as hyaline bands or masses, the more delicate fibrils may be confused with connective-tissue fibrils. The distinction is usually not difficult if it be remembered that at the junction of the fibrils "nodal points" are found, which is not true of overlapping fibrils of connective tissue. The nodal points are tiny points produced by fusion at the junctions of fibrils as fibrin is precipitated, a fluid crystallization. Fibrin asters or stars are sometimes found and are helpful in identification of fibrin. These have a centrum of platelets or leukocytes from which the wavy fibrils of fibrin radiate. Intermingled with the fibrin there is usually a finely granular acidophilic precipitate from edematous fluid and variable numbers of exudative cells are often enmeshed.

Hemorrhagic Inflammation

The hemorrhagic character appears to depend variously upon virulence of infecting organism, upon character of infecting organism, upon disease of the vessels, upon alterations of circulation, and upon the state of the blood, the so-called blood dyscrasias. Organisms which ordinarily produce suppurative or other types of inflammation sometimes are so highly virulent as to injure vascular walls, with resultant rupture. Their absorbed products may reduce the clotting time of the blood. The local lesions of certain diseases may be hemorrhagic as in "black" smallpox, measles and diphtheria. The products of the hemolytic streptococcus, of the diphtheria bacillus and of the anthrax bacillus may cause hemorrhage in the inflamed regions and elsewhere. Some bacteria acting in special situations may produce hemorrhagic inflammation, for example tuberculous pericarditis. In infancy, blood vessels are more fragile than in later life and inflammation may become hemorrhagic. In adult life, disease of arteries and veins may do the same. When malignant tumors excite inflammation, especially in pleura, pericardium and peritoneum, the hemorrhagic character of the exudate is probably due to actual invasion of blood vessels or weakening of their walls. Inflammation in regions the seat of passive hyperemia are sometimes hemorrhagic. The blood dyscrasias of importance include leukemias, profound anemias and the forms of purpura. When inflammation occurs in patients with these diseases it may be hemorrhagic. These conditions are discussed further in the chapter on Hematopoietic System.

Suppurative Inflammation

The mere presence of large numbers of leukocytes in the exudate is not necessarily an indication of suppuration. An inflammation is truly suppurative only when pus is formed. In the stage of gray hepatization of lobar pneumonia, the exudate in the alveoli of the lung is principally leukocytic, but pus

proceeded. In man, suppurative inflammation is almost invariably caused by bacteria but, as in smallpox, a virus may produce the condition.

Microscopically the field of suppuration usually shows a great predominance of leukocytes, sometimes a moderate amount of serum, but only in the early stages is fibrin present. In the later stages the exudate is made up almost entirely of leukocytes with a few lymphocytes and endothelial cells. The pus cell is the leukocyte in which certain sec-

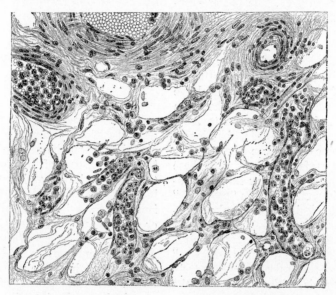

Masses of leukocytes within the capillaries and tissues of the vermiform appendix in early suppurative inflammation.

in the true sense of the word is not formed. In the instances where leukocytes predominate but pus is not formed, it is preferable to designate the inflammation as leukocytic. With very few exceptions, however, the presence of large numbers of leukocytes is sufficient for the diagnosis of suppuration.

Pus is a semifluid yellow or greenish-yellow material, opaque, creamy, and more or less granular. The color is sometimes determined by the organism which produces the inflammation. Thus, the ordinary pyogenic bacteria produce light yellow pus. The *Ps. pyocyanea*, on the other hand, produces green pus. The odor, as a rule, is only mildly foul but if gas-forming organisms be associated, as for example colon bacillus, the odor may be offensive. The consistency of the pus depends upon how far autolysis has

ondary changes have occurred. Cloudy swelling is not uncommon; the cells are usually rich in glycogen; not infrequently fat is present in considerable amounts. Necrosis of the neighboring tissues is usually conspicuous.

It is possible to distinguish three main forms of suppurative inflammation, namely that upon surfaces, the abscess, and the phlegmon. Inflammation of the skin and mucous surfaces may become suppurative in character. In the common cold, the earlier stages show a serous inflammation, then a thick, sticky, mucinous exudate, and in a later stage a thick, yellow, mucopurulent exudate, the color of which is due to a rich infiltration of leukocytes; if the condition progress further, discharge of actual pus from the nose may occur. The abscess is a localized collection of pus. The phlegmon is a collection of pus spread through tissue spaces usually parallel with a body surface. An example of

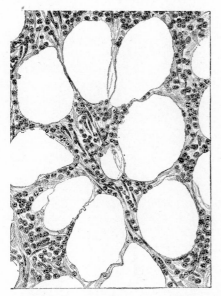

Leukocytes in tissues in early suppurative inflammation of animal omentum.

the phlegmon is seen in suppurative inflammation of the floor of the mouth, which sometimes starts as a small abscess and then extends to involve the entire floor of the mouth, the so-called Ludwig's angina. "Cellulitis" of subcutaneous and intermuscular tissues may be a serous inflammation or may be a phlegmon. As an example, a suppurative inflammation may be established in part of the thigh; extending deeply it may progress along the lines of the great fascias of the thigh to produce an extensive flat area of suppuration.

THE ABSCESS is probably the most common manifestation of suppuration. The typical picture of the acute abscess grossly is that of a swollen region, with all the cardinal signs of inflammation, which on palpation gives a sense of fluid material underneath, called fluctuation. If the abscess has extended near the surface, a yellow or greenish-yellow area in the center indicates the presence of pus. The typical picture of the abscess microscopically is that of a generally circular area, in the center of which are bacteria, surrounded by necrotic material, and this in turn surrounded by a wall of leukocytes, centrally degenerate and peripherally healthy. Lymphocytes and large mononu-

clears are found intermingled with the leukocytes. Around this is found the usual vascular dilatation and prominence of capillaries, and still further out the beginning of the process of repair and the forming of new capillaries and fibroblasts. As has been mentioned above, the abscess or any other form of suppuration in man is likely to be of bacterial origin. Small abscesses are very common on the skin surface as the result of implantation of bacteria, usually in the hair follicles, or as the result of small abrasions. These small abscesses are referred to as boils or furuncles; the condition may be multiple and give rise to furunculosis.

Carbuncles occur in certain places, such as the back of the neck, where the skin is thick and there are large columns of subcutaneous fat connecting the skin with more deeply placed fat. The carbuncle is an extensive zone of suppuration, usually of rather long duration, affecting the subcutaneous fat and communicating with the surface through fat columns which run at right angles to the skin surface. Thus, the carbuncle may have several points of discharge. Microscopically, the carbuncle differs from the abscess in that there are more lymphocytes and endothelial cells, indicative of its longer course. Necrosis and pus formation are present. Careful examination will show the extension toward the surface along the fat columns.

In addition to these superficial foci, abscesses may also be found in practically any situation in the body including brain, bone and all the viscera.

An abscess of any considerable size is to be regarded as a serious manifestation of inflammation. It may be accompanied by secondary inflammation of great importance. Thus, abscess of the hand may lead to an inflammation of the lymphatics which drain this area, and this in turn may lead to inflammation of the lymph nodes. Such inflammation of the lymphatics may subsequently become suppurative in character. The veins draining the part may also become the seat of inflammation, which may subsequently become suppurative leading to the establishment of a suppurative thrombophlebitis. Either as the result of this thrombophlebitis or by more direct entrance into the blood stream, bacteria may be carried to remote parts. General resistance may be so great that

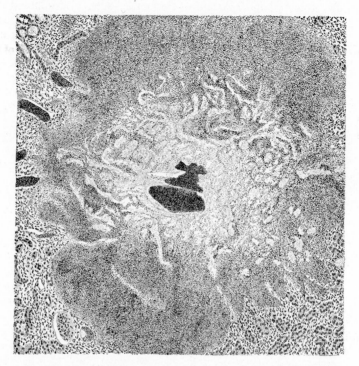

Experimental embolic staphylococcus abscess in kidney of rabbit. Note the mass of bacteria in the center surrounded by completely necrotic tissue, and this in turn by a mass of exuded cells.

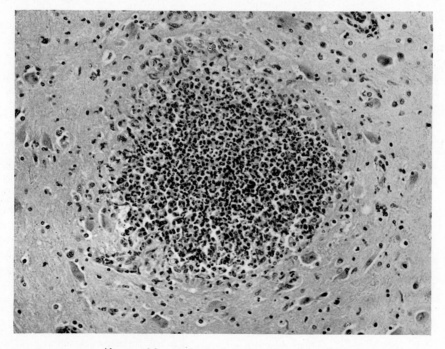

Abscess of human brain, a focal collection of pus.

bacteria are quickly destroyed in the blood stream and tissues, or resistance may be so low that the bacteria continue to exist in the circulating blood, a condition known as septicemia. As a result of septicemia, the organisms may set up inflammation in numerous situations. Thrombi may develop on the heart valves as the result of lodgment of bacteria, producing acute endocarditis. The bacteria may continue to proliferate in the thrombus and the lesion thus be a reservoir for a further supply of organisms to the blood stream. The lodging of fragments of thrombi from heart valves, or from a suppurative thrombophlebitis, or even the lodgment of small clumps of bacteria, may lead to secondary abscesses in numerous organs of the body, such as the lung, heart, kidney and other situations. The whole chain of events may be represented somewhat as follows: The presence of the abscess may lead to a condition in which simple absorption of toxic products, a toxemia, is primary. If bacteria gain entrance to the blood stream, their presence associated with the toxemia constitutes a septicemia. If to this be added the formation of multiple abscesses, the condition becomes a pyemia. Such a sequence of events may follow any suppurative infection from a minute furuncle to the most severely infected wound.

The progress of the abscess locally is variable. If the infection be rapidly suppressed, the dissolved material is removed by absorption and the solid debris is removed by leukocytes and large mononuclear cells. Granulation tissue fills the defect and the area is cicatrized. If the infection persist, the abscess may extend and enlarge. Its extension is along the lines of least resistance and if confined by heavy fascias, a phlegmon may develop, as exemplified in the palmar abscess, or cellulitis of various parts. "Pointing" of the abscess means approximation to a surface. Subsequently, the abscess may rupture on to the surface. Abscesses may point on the skin, mucous or serous surfaces, depending upon their location. The pus is discharged through the opening and carries off numerous bacteria and soluble irritants. What is essentially an ulcer is formed. This fills with granulation tissue and finally cicatrizes. If the abscess be deep-seated, the route to the surface is called a sinus.

Parenchymatous or Alterative Inflammation

Parenchymatous inflammation is essentially synonymous with alterative inflammation as used by some schools, or with degenerative inflammation as used by others. Marchand prefers to call it "inflammatory disease" and defines it as composed, on the one hand, of the degenerative sequences of an injurious etiologic agent, the acute and chronic reactive processes in the vessels and tissues, the proliferative and reparative tissue changes, and, on the other hand, of secondary functional and morphologic disturbances. Thus, cloudy swelling, fatty degeneration, hyaline necrosis or other degenerative process may be present. In establishing the identity of the process as an inflammation, it is necessary to have associated with the degenerative changes either exudation or cellular proliferation. Such types of acute inflammation may occur in the heart, liver, brain, spinal cord, and particularly in the kidney. They are caused by circulating poisons of exogenous or endogenous origin, particularly those of infectious diseases, or may be the result of lodgment *in situ* of bacteria, particularly those of relatively low virulence. As concerns the kidney, there is evidence that sensitization of the organ to bacterial products plays an important part in alterative inflammation. Nevertheless, it seems true that most inflammations of degenerative or parenchymatous type occur as the result of circulating injurious substances. Those introduced from without include such drugs as cantharides, mercuric chloride, arsenic, phosphorus, lead and other poisons. Those produced within the body include particularly the poisonous substances of bacterial infection, as well also as certain poisons probably produced in the body by faulty metabolism. It is important to keep in mind the exact interpretation of the term degeneration, as discussed in the chapter on that subject. There has been great discussion as to what type of degenerative changes, associated with other tissue changes, should properly be classified as inflammation and what should be looked upon as purely degenerative processes. This controversy arises particularly in reference to acute and chronic diseases of the kidney. Simple cloudy swelling of the kidney may lead to much the same clinical phenomena as does mild acute nephritis, but in the former the changes are likely to be of less severity and of shorter duration than in the latter. This, however, is not a satisfactory mode of pathologic differentiation. So much doubt exists as to the truly inflammatory character of the parenchymatous inflammations of the kidney, that the term nephropathy has been suggested and is frequently employed in literature. If, however, a distinction between simple degeneration and degenerative inflammation be based upon microscopic indications of exudation or proliferation, it is possible to differentiate the vast majority of cases, although a few instances arise in which the differentiation is difficult and depends upon the personal equation. All forms of acute nephritis show degeneration of the parenchyma, but in addition there are changes which vary from slight proliferation of endothelium of the capillary tufts, to the most marked exudation and proliferation.

In the heart, degeneration of the muscle may appear without any associated change in other parts of the tissue, or may be accompanied by infiltration of lymphocytes, large mononuclears, and plasma cells. In the more severe cases actual invasion of leukocytes is noted. The muscle may show cloudy swelling and fatty degeneration, hyaline necrosis or other severe degenerative manifestations. Similar inflammations of the liver occur but are by no means common. In infectious diseases, the brain and spinal cord may show degeneration of the ganglion cells, nerve fibers and of the myelin sheaths, accompanied by severe neurologic manifestations, but show little exudation or proliferation pathologically. In order to designate this as an inflammatory process, however, it is necessary to find either exudation or proliferation. Proliferation is commonly observed in multiplication of glia cells and fibers. Catarrhal inflammation may also be regarded as essentially degenerative in type, for it shows degeneration of the parenchymatous cells, that is, the epithelial cells, usually mucinous in type, associated in many instances with only moderate infiltration of leukocytes and lymphocytes. Inasmuch, however, as the hypersecretion of the cells and the outpouring of fluid from the vessels are prominent, it seems justifiable to place catarrhal inflammation in a category subordinate to the general group of alterative inflammations.

In contrast to the parenchymatous inflammations, the same organs may show interstitial inflammatory disease of much the same nature, except that the interstitial changes predominate. They may be more specifically referred to as nonexudative interstitial inflammations. Cells appear in interstitial tissues and the process academically may be regarded as an interstitial inflammation, but both acute and chronic diseases of parenchymatous viscera may occur in which exudation plays little part; the tissues may show infiltration of lymphocytes, plasma cells and large mononuclear cells which do not appear to be exudative in origin, or the interstitial connective tissue may be notably hyperplastic. The accompanying degenerative changes may be slight. Thus, the inflammatory disease of the viscus, although diffuse, may affect more particularly either the special parenchymatous cells or the interstitial tissues, and the condition is designated as parenchymatous or interstitial depending upon the predominance of the one change over the other.

Catarrhal Inflammation

This type may appear upon any mucous surface. The exudate is contributed by the mucous cells and by the blood vessels. It varies from a thin, watery secretion with very little mucin to a secretion which may be so rich in mucin as to be semisolid. The material may be colorless or slightly gray, or if there be a mixture of leukocytes, pale or deep yellow, depending upon their number and condition. Microscopically, such exudates show mucin, a small amount of protein, as well as leukocytes, lymphocytes and desquamated epithelial cells in variable numbers. Examination of a mucous membrane, the seat of this condition, shows it to be red, swollen, irritable and tender, and with increased temperature. Disturbance of function is exhibited in the hypersecretion. Microscopically, the surface epithelium is the seat of cloudy swelling, sometimes associated with mucinous degeneration of the cells. Desquamation of the cells, either singly or in groups, is common. The deeper cells, particularly those of the glands, are likely to show advanced mucinous degeneration. The tunica propria and submucosa show hyperemia and prominent capillaries. There is usually an infiltration of cells from the tissues and blood, composed in the milder cases principally of lymphocytes and large mononuclears with a small number of leukocytes. These cells appear not only in the position mentioned but may also be found infiltrating between the epithelial cells. In the severe cases, or later in the course of the reaction, leukocytes are found in greater numbers and the exudate may finally become purulent in type. There are various causes of catarrhal inflammation. The most frequent example of the disease is the common cold, caused by a virus. Catarrhs may be caused by irritant gases and dusts. Among the latter are the various plant and animal proteins to which patients may be hypersensitive or allergic. In the genito-urinary tract, the gonococcus is an important cause of acute and chronic catarrhs, which in the florid stage are purulent. Catarrhs of the intestinal tract may be caused by many types of bacteria, both saprophytic and parasitic, aërobic and anaërobic; irritation from spoiled foods, irritant or caustic liquids, solid foreign bodies may excite intestinal catarrh.

REPAIR

Almost as soon as the inflammatory reaction becomes evident, the processes leading toward repair begin. Although described in series in this discussion of inflammation, it is of the utmost importance to consider all the processes as going on hand in hand. In inflammations with little injury to the tissues, repair may be complete, so-called *restitutio ad integrum*. If there be any notable degree of destruction of tissues, the condition may completely heal with production of a scar but without full restitution of some of the destroyed tissue.

Granulation, Organization, Cicatrization

For the sake of simplicity, repair may be said to take place in three stages which are more or less intermingled, namely, granulation, organization, and cicatrization. Regeneration of other structures in the destroyed regions is also found during connective-tissue repair, but is a variable phenomenon, sometimes of importance, sometimes entirely in abeyance.

The first real evidence of repair is that

proliferation of fibroblasts and capillary endothelium (angioblasts) called granulation

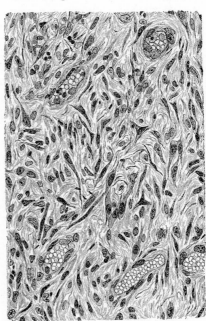

Young connective tissue (fibroblasts) in early experimental granulation in tongue.

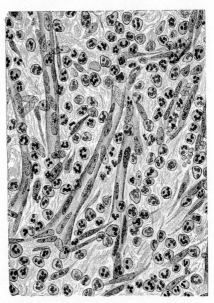

Newly formed capillaries in infected wound.

tissue. The proliferation is due to mitotic cell division. The mesenchyme appears to be disturbed and activated early in the course of inflammation. It is thought that this results in the formation of young cells with the potencies of embryonal cells. Werthemann believes these capable of differentiation into fibrous tissue, smooth muscle and elastica as well as large mononuclear phagocytes. It is possible that large mononuclear wandering cells in the tissues may be mistaken for young fibroblasts because these show short spindle and rounded forms with large round vesicular nuclei. Various theories have been expressed as to conversion of monocytes into large wandering mononuclears and thence into fibroblasts. The work of Hall and Furth gives no evidence that such conversion takes place.

It is probable that various stimuli operate to incite multiplication of fibroblasts.

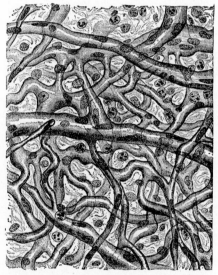

Reconstruction drawing of newly formed capillary loops in granulation tissue.

Carrel has demonstrated a product of leukocytes which excites fibroblastic proliferation. Thiocresol and similar products stimulate wound healing perhaps by the influence of sulphydryl (Reimann). Sperti and his associates draw attention to a substance produced by injury of tissues, capable of stimulating proliferation, which they believe to be a hormone. According to Fischer the most favorable hydrogen-ion concentration is about that of the animal body and departures toward either acidity or alkalinity depress the rate of growth. In tissue culture he finds that the rate of growth of new cells filling in a wound in a colony is about the same as that of the colony and that it is generally inversely pro-

portional to the age of the colony. Harvey and Howes report that an increase of protein in the diet favors the growth of fibroblasts. It is probable that vitamin C is also of importance (Lund and Crandon; Hartzell, et al.). The growth energy varies with different types of fibroblasts, so that those derived from periosteum, for example, have a greater growth energy than those from epichondrium, or skeletal muscle or myocardium. Respiration and glycolysis, although different in various animals, is in general like that of young or embryonal cells (Neuhaus). Howes, Sooy and Harvey find that "the tensile strength of a healing wound is a function of the fibroblastic process." For the first four or five days the tensile strength of the wound is negligible, but thereafter a rapid rise in strength occurs which becomes slower and reaches its maximum in from ten to fourteen days.

The formation of new capillaries occurs almost as soon as does proliferation of fibroblasts. Clark has shown, by direct observation, that the new capillaries are formed from pre-existing capillaries and venules by means of multiplication of endothelial cells. These grow out into the surounding tissues as pointed buds into the base of which the lumen projects. The bud grows until it meets another bud or capillary and circulation is established. Buds may retract or undergo dissolution so that not all survive. Some may ultimately be transformed into veins and arteries, the adventitia, muscle and elastica by differentiation of cells of the interstitium, which according to Werthemann are multipotential. Lymphatics multiply in much the same way, but usually follow the lines of the blood vascular spaces; their growth is sporadic and irregular. The mass of fibroblasts and new capillaries is called granulation tissue, because when seen grossly at the base of an ulcer, or in an evacuated abscess cavity, the surface is roughened by the projection of soft red granules, 1 or 2 mm. in diameter. These granules contain fibroblasts and new capillaries. In the unopened abscess, microscopic examination shows the granulation tissue outside the wall of leukocytes. In more diffuse inflammations, the granulation is more irregularly distributed. Inflammations of serous surfaces show the granulation beginning in the subserous tissues and growing into the exudate. In experimental inflammations, granulation may be found within an hour or so after injury. Clinical observation indicates that granulating surfaces are not likely to become secondarily infected and this has been found to be true in animal experiments by Halley, Chesney and Dresel. The mechanism of this resistance is not clear.

The granulations may grow into and fill up foci of necrosis or may extend into surface exudates to replace tissues or exudate.

but exactly how these cells operate in the development of collagen is not yet known. It appears, however, that fluids of granulation tissue favor increased deposit of collagen and also may favor its absorption.

When the defect is filled, or the exudate replaced, by granulation tissue, those processes which ultimately result in scar formation occur. The capillaries decrease in size and for the most part undergo gradual atrophy until they disappear. At the same

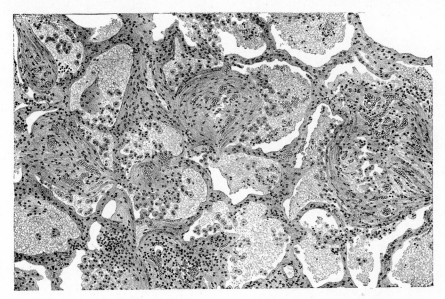

Organizing pneumonia, showing the growth of new connective tissue following the lines of fibrin.

This process is referred to as "organization." The latter term is often employed to include both the granulation and the filling of defects or substitution for exudates. In the case of fibrinous exudates, the line of growing fibroblasts and capillaries may follow the meshes of the fibrin net. This is well seen in organization of fibrinous exudates on serous surfaces, and is particularly well exemplified in the organization of the alveolar exudate of pneumonia in those cases where solution of the exudate does not occur.

It is during the stage of organization that formation of the collagenous fibrils of the connective tissue becomes notable. Hass defines collagen as a homogeneous or fibrillary protein which serves as the organic matrix of white fibrous connective tissue, bone and cartilage. Its formation seems to depend upon the viability of the fibroblasts,

time, the connective tissue shows shrinkage and condensation of the nuclei and the cytoplasm becomes more and more fibrillar, until the whole mass assumes the character of adult connective tissue with its numerous fibrils and sparsely scattered, dense, spindle form nuclei. This transformation is cicatrization and the product is the cicatrix or scar. Regarding the organizing mass as a growing tissue of capillaries and fibroblasts, the capillaries are seen to be reduced in size and number as the growth energy of the fibroblasts is diminished. Although the disappearance of the capillaries may be due to maturation of fibroblasts, fibril formation, condensation and contraction, it may also be a manifestation of the limitation of growth by tissue tension or growth balance. Failure of such limitation upon surfaces may lead to excessive granulation or "proud flesh." Epithelialization of surface wounds is due first to ameboid movement of surrounding epithelial cells, followed by rearrangement and multiplication to produce an epithelial membrane (Hartwell). DuNoüy's exponential formula

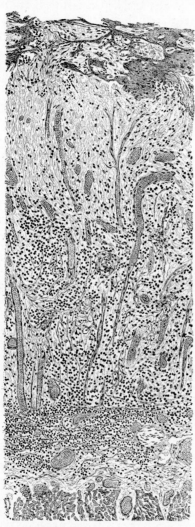

Organization of acute fibrinous pericarditis. The new granulation has grown from the myocardial margin of the picture so as partly to replace the exudate, some of which in the form of fibrin and leukocytes remains distal to the myocardium.

serves to predict the rate of surface healing and he finds that it is accelerated by epithelialization.

The gross appearance of a scar is familiar. In its earlier stages it is red, soft and almost coextensive with the original inflamed area. It gradually becomes paler until it is

pearly white, at the same time decreasing in size, and contracting until it is likely to be

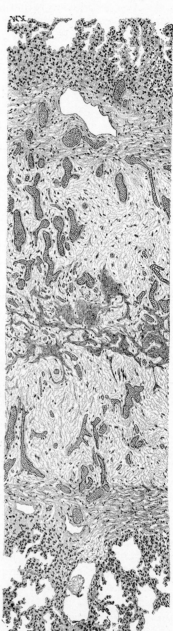

Formation of adhesion in interlobar pleura. Organization has proceeded from both pleural surfaces and meets in the middle, where a small amount of fibrinous exudate is still present.

smaller than the original injured region. With the shrinkage comes increased density. If situated in a place where a distending force is applied, the scar may subsequently stretch. Thus, abdominal scars, if the incisions be not repaired to provide adequate muscle support, may stretch and permit a hernial projection of abdominal contents. Scars in tissues over joints, cicatricial adhesions between joint surfaces, adhesive bands in pericardial, peritoneal or pleural cavities may stretch so as to provide no impediment to function.

Adhesions constitute an important manifestation of scar formation. Fibrous adhesions occur as the result of inflammation of serous surfaces. In the pleura and pericardium, an inflammation of visceral sheets is communicated to the parietal membrane and vice versa; thus inflammations involve the entire sac. In the peritoneum, inflammations may be localized to small areas but by contact involve apposing surfaces, such as those of a few coils of gut or coils of gut and parietal peritoneum. The cause may be bacterial or chemical, or as is frequently the case in the peritoneum or omentum, the result of surgical trauma. Regardless of the general type of the exudate, the surfaces show fibrin deposit, and if the fluid exudate be removed or absorbed, the fibrin of the apposing surfaces comes into contact and a loose fibrinous adhesion is formed. Granulation proceeding from the two surfaces meets and a somewhat firmer adhesion is formed. As organization goes on to cicatrization, the scar tissue unites the two surfaces by a firm, fibrous union, the fibrous adhesion. The ultimate condition may vary from a few areas, often stretched into fibrous bands by the movements of the viscera, or may be seen as an extensive adhesion which in the case of the pleura or pericardium may completely obliterate the sac. Such obliteration of the pericardium may result in serious functional disturbance of the heart; in the peritoneum it may lead to limitation of intestinal motility; in joints it may restrict or completely inhibit motion.

Reaction to Foreign Bodies

Foreign bodies may be introduced into the body purposely, as in the case of sutures and ligatures in surgical operations or as metallic substances in orthopedic operations, etc. They may get in accidentally as in industrial accidents, war casualties and the like. They may be formed in the body as in the case of crystals, such as those of cholesterol and fatty acids; blood clots and necrotic masses are foreign bodies. If the foreign body is infected, suppurative inflammation ensues and the foreign body is extruded with the pus or may ultimately be encapsulated in the healed scar. Even when sterile, the foreign body excites a certain amount of inflammation. Examination of early lesions produced experimentally, shows traumatic hemorrhage and a moderate amount of vascular dilatation,

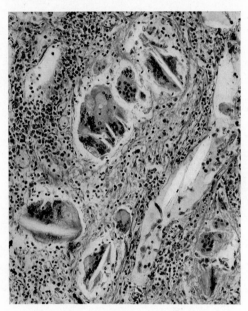

Foreign-body giant cells formed about cholesterol crystals which have been dissolved in preparation and are represented as slits.

and an exudate of leukocytes, serum and fibrin. This is followed by the reaction of the fixed tissues. Lymphocytes, macrophages, sometimes plasma cells and others of similar nature put in their appearance. These cells outnumber the leukocytes except when infection is present simultaneously. The cells migrate toward the foreign body, and at about the same time the earlier signs of granulation appear with the multiplication of fibroblasts and the formation of new capillaries. Small fragments of the foreign material may be taken up by mononuclear phagocytes and carried away, but the bulk of the foreign substance remains *in situ*. In many cases foreign-body giant cells occur. It is now established that the foreign body giant cell is formed by cytoplasmic fusion of large mononuclear wandering cells (Haythorn). The foreign-body giant cell shows multiple nuclei, usually of vesicular character and resembling rather closely those of the large mononuclear cells. As the giant cell matures, the nuclei tend to condense, and may show little remnant of the vesicular character. The cytoplasm is closely apposed to the foreign body, and if the latter be small enough, it may be completely surrounded by cytoplasm. Thus, the foreign-body giant cell has essentially the same phagocytic properties as the large mono-

ments of necrotic material. These cells may remain *in situ* for a considerable time, but in the usual experimental lesions the ingrowth of granulation tissue soon replaces them. Granulation progresses into very close apposition to the foreign body and in the case of sutures, such as those of silk, penetrates between the fibrils of the suture material. Following this infiltration of granulation tissue, cicatrization occurs. Thus, the foreign body becomes encapsulated by cicatricial tissue. If

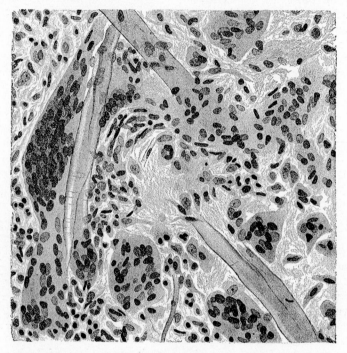

Foreign-body giant cells formed in response to the presence of insoluble suture material.

nuclear cells from which it originates. Cells of the same sort may occur in any area of granulation, provided sufficient foreign or dead material be present to stimulate their formation, but as a rule they are most commonly found in those reactions which occur as the result of foreign body implantation. Not only do they form about foreign bodies introduced from without, but in instances where crystals are formed in the body, the secondary formation of giant cells enclosing the crystals is not uncommon. Destruction of tissues leaving a considerable amount of necrotic material, which is not liquefied and absorbed, may also be followed by foreign-body giant cell formation about the frag-

the foreign body be of absorbable material such as catgut, the early reaction occurs in practically the same way, but as the enzymes destroy the gut, this is dissolved and absorbed. Nevertheless, the process of replacement by granulation tissue goes on in the same manner, and a small scar appears in the situation originally occupied by the ligature. The same general principle applies to noninfected foci of necrosis, as described in connection with infarction. The reaction is essentially the same as that to a foreign body except that giant cells are not commonly encountered in infarcts. The growth of granulation tissue progresses to form a band around the necrotic mass, which upon subsequent cicatrization constitutes a fibrous capsule. If the necrotic mass be small in extent, the granulation tissue may entirely replace the necrotic focus and the final result be a complete cicatrization.

Healing of Wounds

If a wound be inflicted aseptically and no infection occur subsequently, the process of healing is very closely similar to that about appear and granulation tissue is rapidly formed. The granulation starting from each side of the wound soon meets, so that in the wounded area there is a fused mass of granulation tissue. The enzymes, large mononuclears and leukocytes dissolve the exudate and remove the necrotic tissue, so that in the course of 24 or 48 hours little remains but the mass of granulation tissue with only a few leukocytes and large mononuclears. This

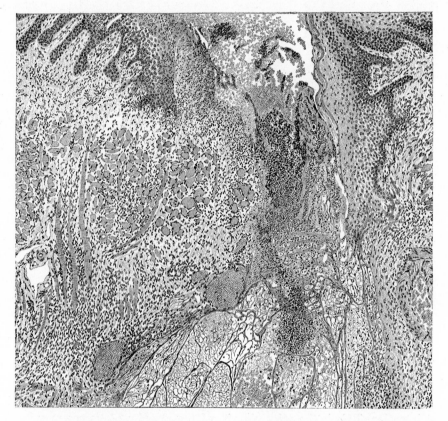

Tongue of rabbit on third day after incision with knife. Line of incision shows remnants of hemorrhage, deep necrosis, fibrin formation. Reaction is noted about margins of wound. Epithelial proliferation and downgrowth are apparent.

a foreign body. The wound causes a certain amount of hemorrhage, and necrosis of tissue through which the instrument has passed. After the edges of the wound are brought together, the reaction of inflammation appears in the margins. Thus, in even the cleanest wounds a small zone of reddening is found shortly afterwards. Microscopic examination shows the early signs of inflammation in the form of vascular dilatation and exudation of a few leukocytes, and serum, and fibrin formation. Large mononuclear cells granulation is soon replaced by cicatrization and the wound is healed. The clean healing of wounds is referred to in the surgical clinic as healing by first intention. Wounds, however, may break down because of bacterial infection, in which case the bacteria grow most readily in the loose tissues and blood of the wounded area and suppuration occurs. Although essentially like an abscess, the area is primarily open, and from it pus is discharged upon the surface. As the infection subsides, granulation tissue grows into the open area, gradually fills it up, becomes cicatrized and the wound is closed as the result of healing by second intention. In certain cases it is advisable to reopen wounds that have become infected secondarily, to clean the surfaces and bring them freshly into apposition. Sometimes this results in healing by what is essen-

similar to, that which has been destroyed. Physiologic regeneration occurs to replace cells which have been destroyed in the normal wear and tear of bodily activity. This goes on actively throughout life and results in complete restoration of the destroyed cells. In old age, however, it is possible that part

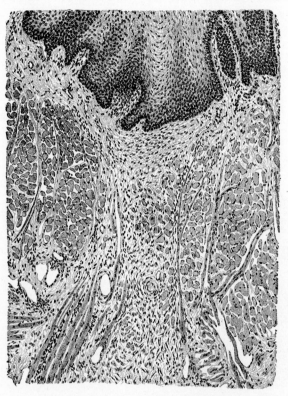

Healed wound of rabbit's tongue. Surface epithelium is completely regenerated but shows deep position. Cicatrix occupies space of tissues destroyed in wound.

tially first intention. This is the principle of the operation, called "debridement," used successfully in the treatment of wounds infected before having adequate surgical treatment. Infected wounds may be kept open until the bacterial content is reduced. Then the edges are brought together by suture and the wound heals after what is called delayed primary suture. Healing under a crust or scab is referred to in the discussion of ulcer. Healing of the skin surface is discussed under regeneration. (See Arey.)

Regeneration

By this term is understood a reproduction of tissue identical with, or closely

of the atrophy of tissues may be the result of faulty or incomplete replacement. The so-called pathologic regeneration represents the process carried on in repair of diseased processes or defects. Regeneration in this instance goes on according to the regenerative capacity of the type of tissue destroyed, and this capacity varies greatly with different tissues, is better in the young than in the old, and in a general way is in inverse ratio to the amount of tissue destroyed. If tissues be destroyed which have a great capacity for regeneration, the defect may show ultimately a complete regeneration of original structure. As a rule, however, many tissues are involved in lesions of any considerable size, so that regeneration is often incomplete. There is a general rule, with many exceptions, to the effect that the higher the degree of specialization of a cell, the less the capacity for regeneration following pathologic processes.

Surface Epithelium. The regeneration of surface epithelium is usually active and complete. In case of wounds involving only the surface epithelium, it is found that very shortly after infliction of the wound, the epithelium of the deeper layers, namely the malpighian layers, moves slightly over the uncovered connective tissue surface. Mitotic cell division results in the formation of intermediate cells, and finally of keratinized squamous cells. In the case of mucous membranes essentially the same process of regeneration follows. If the underlying tissues be involved, the regeneration of surface epithelium may be delayed until the defect is fairly well organized. At the margins, the epithelium may proliferate downward to be intermingled with the organizing tissue and is sometimes mistaken for carcinoma. As a matter of fact it may actually become carcinomatous.

As the defect is filled by granulation tissue, the epithelium grows over the surface until it meets with that of the opposite side. During this period, in the case of skin, the intermediate layers are also formed and keratinization proceeds from the margins. After the defect is entirely replaced, the epithelium covering it cannot be differentiated from other stratified squamous epithelium, except that the line between epithelium and underlying corium is not thrown into ridges or papillae as is the case with normal skin, and the area is devoid of hair follicles, sweat glands and sebaceous glands, since these do not regenerate. Surface epithelium in other situations follows the same general rule. The surface of the endometrium undergoes complete regeneration after menstruation, pregnancy or curettage. In the bladder, the stratified structure is easily restored. In the case of the intestine and similar structures, the surface epithelium is likewise restored. If glands be involved in the wound, they are not likely to be regenerated from the surface epithelium, and if they be completely destroyed, they have little capacity for regeneration themselves. In those mucous membranes where the glands represent merely crypts, new cryptlike structures may be formed by the growth of the surface epithelium. When skin surfaces are restored through the application of Thiersch skin grafts, the graft carries to the new area remnants of glandular structures and these may continue to grow to form oil glands, sweat glands and hair follicles.

Glandular epithelium, considered as a whole, does not regenerate readily. On the other hand, provided the ducts remain, they may take on what is essentially an embryonal function of growth so that the ducts extend, enlarge at the end and reproduce glandular structures similar to, and sometimes identical with, those that have been destroyed. This is well exemplified in the liver where destruction of parenchyma, provided it involve connective-tissue supporting framework, is not followed by regeneration of the essential liver cells, but a proliferation of bile ducts occurs, which sometimes forms not only club-shaped extremities made up of cells resembling liver cells, but may reproduce lobules somewhat similar to those of the normal liver. In the case of salivary and lachrymal glands, and even in the breast, regeneration of glandular structure from pre-existing ducts may be functionally adequate and almost complete morphologically.

Endothelium. In the term "endothelium" we include the lining cells of blood vessels, lymphatic vessels and the larger serous cavities of the body. From the consideration of the formation of granulation tissue, it will be seen that vascular endothelium has great capacity for proliferation and regeneration. Lesions involving larger blood vessels, such as thrombosis, may become completely covered by endothelium. Defects of serous membranes, produced by trauma or by inflammation, are rapidly lined by newly formed endothelium. The first change seen is a spreading out of the remaining endothelium to cover the margins of the thrombus or inflammatory exudate, rapidly followed by cell multiplication so that the areas are soon covered. The cells at first are cuboidal in character and only subsequently undergo flattening to resemble the normal type of surface endothelium.

Fibrous Connective Tissue. As can readily be understood from the discussion of organization, the fibrous connective tissue of the body regenerates readily. The stimulus to closing in defects determines a growth of connective tissue slightly in excess of that originally present. When scars are formed, the scar tissue is often quite indistinguishable from pre-existing connective tissue. In the case of skin, the only differentiation between scar tissue and pre-existing connective tissue lies in the fact that the scar tissue contains none of the skin glands and is covered by epithelium without papillae. Elastic tissue represents a differentiation of connective tissue. Nevertheless, in healed areas elastic tissue may appear to have regenerated. This is the result of differentiation of newly formed connective tissue.

Fat. The regeneration of fat may originate in some pre-existing fat cells which remain, or may perhaps be a transformation of regenerating connective-tissue cells which assume the special function of fat formation. Regeneration proceeds from the remnant of fat cells, including those without fat content but with intact nuclei. The fat is deposited first in minute globules which subsequently fuse to form the single large globule of the adult fat cell. In this early stage, the fat cells with their numerous small globules are morphologically identical with embryonal fat cells. The regeneration of fat tissues may, however, be much restricted by the mechanical limitation of dense cicatricial tissue.

Cartilage. The regeneration of cartilage occurs by activity of the cells of the perichondrium. Their multiplication gives rise to forms morphologically similar to the fibroblasts. Cell processes increase in size and multiply to form a fairly solid mass of these cells. As these increase in number, the cytoplasm of adjacent cells fuses to form a solid, hyaline mass or matrix. The nuclei are surrounded by a thin rim of cytoplasm, enclosed in small lacunae. In regenerating areas, transition stages between the fibrillar form of these cells and true cartilage cells in matrix are observed. Cartilage may similarly be formed by cells of the periosteum and of the endosteum, as well perhaps as from connective tissue which apparently originally had no connection with cartilage.

Bone formation in newly formed cartilage follows the general rule seen in ossification of cartilage in early life, namely, the ingrowth of osteoid tissue, which replaces the cartilage and finally becomes calcified with true bone formation. New bone is formed by the activity of cells of the periosteum and to a certain extent of the endosteum. These cells grow in the form of morphologically undifferentiated cells, similar to those in regenerating perichondrium. They proliferate and form numerous fibrils, which intermingle with one another to constitute a loose network. In the formation of spongy bone, the cells finally lodge in spaces between the fibrils. Subsequently, the fibrillar material becomes homogeneous and calcified to form spongy bone. As the calcareous material is deposited, the differentiation into haversian systems occurs; subsequently osteoclasts may appear and rarify the new bone to proper proportions. The formation of compact bone follows essentially the same program, originating in the periosteum, as a rule, by the laying down of parallel rows of cells which produce fibrils, become calcified and form compact bone layer after layer. The marrow may also regenerate from pre-existing marrow cells and blood vessels. This follows the general process whereby marrow is formed in embryonal bone.

The capacity of cartilage and bone for regeneration is great. In each case, there is little anatomic or functional differentiation of the generating cells. It is true that they form very definitely outlined masses, but the final differentiation depends either upon homogenization (hyalinization) of fibrils or upon calcification. When bones are fractured, hemorrhage occurs about the fractured ends. Growth of granulation tissue replaces the hemorrhage and disposes itself about the fractured ends. The granulation becomes firmer by calcification and irregular ossification to form a dense mass called callus. Callus appears about the periosteum (periosteal or ring callus) between the ends of the fracture (intermediary callus) and for a short distance up and down the marrow cavity (internal callus). The excess of callus, the provisional callus, is reduced in amount as the granulation tissue cicatrizes, and the definitive callus, between the bone ends, is converted into true bone. Types of fractures and their repair are discussed further in the chapter on Organs of Locomotion.

Muscle. SMOOTH MUSCLE shows little or no capacity for regeneration. Healing is almost entirely by cicatrization.

STRIATED MUSCLE. The study of the regeneration of striated muscle includes the myocardium and skeletal muscle. Our own experimental studies of signs of regeneration of cardiac muscle, following such an injury as infarction, led to the conclusion (in conformity with that of the majority of workers on this subject) that there is no evidence that cardiac muscle undergoes actual regeneration following traumatic or other injury. Very rarely mitotic figures may be found in the muscle nuclei, and occasionally the ends of

of sarcoplasm branch out. These may be club-shaped or pointed and usually contain numbers of nuclei. In favorable cases where the defect is not too large, the muscle sprouts or buds coming from adjacent ends may meet and lead to the formation of well-differentiated and functional muscle fibers. The nuclei in part disappear and in part move toward the sarcolemma. Longitudinal striation appears first and is followed by transverse striation. Whether the sarcolemma is formed by the muscle or by the adjacent con-

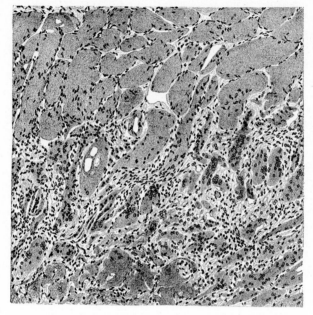

Regeneration of skeletal muscle following Zenker's necrosis. Muscle giant cells are numerous and in left lower part of field muscle buds can be seen.

injured muscle show the presence of a number of nuclei resembling somewhat the formation of multinucleated cells. In no instance, however, was actual regeneration observed. Skeletal muscle may show very much more active nuclear proliferation (Millar). Following injury, there is a certain amount of retraction and swelling of the living end of the muscle fiber. An increase in the number of nuclei rapidly appears as the result of multiplication of the nuclei underlying the sarcolemma. This apparently is usually the result of direct division of the nuclei, but occasionally mitotic figures are found. From the margin of the muscle fiber, usually a short distance from the seat of injury, small processes

nective tissue is in doubt, but majority opinion is that it is contributed by connective tissue.

Occasionally, where large masses of muscle are destroyed, a different type of regeneration is observed. Isolated cells resembling the embryonic myoblast appear, become elongated, fuse with adjacent similar cells, and ultimately by further differentiation are formed into muscle fibers. Generally speaking, however, when the amount of muscle is fairly large, repair is not due to regeneration, but rather to the formation of scar tissue. This forms a band which seals the two ends of the muscle together so that function is practically restored.

Nerve Tissue. Regeneration of nerve tissues will be discussed as it affects the supporting tissue of nerve substance or the neuroglia, the ganglion cells and the nerve fibers. Studies of regeneration in injuries of the brain in animals show that the neuroglia regenerates with little difficulty. In fact, it may fill up a defect in very much the same way that mesoblastic connective tissue does in other organs. Where a brain injury involves the white matter, there may be regeneration of the nerve fibers distal to the point of injury. This regeneration follows much the same rule as that of peripheral nerves to be described subsequently. Injury to ganglion cells is not followed by any regeneration whatever in higher animal life. While regeneration may occur to a moderate degree in lower forms, such as reptiles and amphibia, the phenomenon has never been conclusively proved in higher vertebrates. Regeneration of peripheral nerves has been carefully studied both in man and in experimental animals. Regeneration of this sort depends upon preservation of integrity of the ganglion cells contributing the nerve fibers. When injury to the nerve occurs, degeneration follows. This extends along the central end to the next node of Ranvier, but occasionally may extend through several more segments. The degeneration extends distally to the termination of the nerves. It affects both the axis cylinder and the sheath of Schwann. This wallerian degeneration is described more fully in the chapter on the Nervous System. Two views exist as to the regeneration of the axis cylinder. The generally accepted view is that regeneration proceeds entirely from the central end of the neuron. The axis cylinder elongates and passes through the injured area to the old distal tract. It is accompanied by new medullary sheath, provided in all probability by cells of the original sheath, which seem to be stimulated to proliferation by the degenerate axon (Ingebrigsten). Meeting the degenerate distal nerve, the axis cylinder follows this line to, and including, the terminals. New medullary sheath is formed and regeneration is complete. The beautiful studies, by R. G. Harrison, of the growth in vitro of embryonic nerve tissue, strongly support this conception of regeneration. He regards the growth of axis cylinders as a form of protoplasmic movement, or ameboid outgrowth

of the cytoplasm. The sheath cells proliferate and, as the axis cylinders grow, become arranged in tubular fashion. Apparently, the reproduction of new myelin is the result of combined action of axis cylinder and sheath cells, since no myelin is formed until the axis is present. Spielmeyer believes that regeneration of axis cylinders is due to the activity of neuroblasts derived from sheath cells, but Harrison, restudying the matter, maintains that sheath cells play no part in formation of the axon. Ssamarin finds that in the spinal cord, axon regeneration is slow and of no functional significance.

In case of amputation, it is common for the degeneration of the central end to extend as far as the ganglion cell and sometimes involve the latter in degeneration or atrophy. In certain cases, however, growth of nerve fibers continues in the stump and gives rise to intricate masses of nerve fibers, called the amputation neuroma. These structures are explained much more satisfactorily by the theory of centrifugal growth of fibers than by the Bethe-Spielmeyer hypothesis. Regeneration may be hastened by approximation of the severed ends of nerves, but it is found that the greater the space to be bridged by regeneration, the slower the process and the less likelihood of complete restoration.

Blood Vessels. The essentials of the regeneration of blood vessels have been described in connection with granulation. Injuries to vascular regions show replacement of blood supply by the multiplication of capillaries. These are easily provided with adventitia by the accompanying multiplication of connective-tissue cells. It is claimed that muscular regeneration may also appear, but this is not proved. Injury of larger vessels is not followed by regeneration of the vessels themselves. Circulation may be re-established by collateral communication extending through capillaries and slightly larger vessels. In the case of obstruction to circulation by thrombosis, the process of canalization may occur as described in the chapter on Disturbances of Circulation. Capillary lymphatics may regenerate in a manner similar to that of the regeneration of blood capillaries. The new formation of larger lymphatics from older lymphatics of the same type does not occur.

Blood, looked upon as a circulating tissue, can be destroyed by hemorrhage or by the action of poisonous substances of various kinds. Following hemorrhage, the blood cells may be restored to normal within the course of a few days, up to ten days or two weeks. When hemorrhage is marked and there is an accompanying depression of blood formation, complete regeneration may be delayed for a longer period. Destruction of blood by poisons such as carbon monoxide, nitrobenzol or the toxic products of infectious disease, may be more or less rapidly restored. The blood as it circulates in the vessels is an adult tissue. The cells normally found in the circulating blood are no longer capable of multiplication so that restoration of the cellular element depends upon the bone marrow and lymph nodes. Poisons which may destroy blood in circulation may also depress or destroy bone marrow. If the latter occur, regeneration is slow. If the bone marrow be not markedly damaged, or if following injury to the circulating blood, it remain normal, multiplication of the various hematogenous cells goes on and results in delivery into the blood of adult cells. If multiplication in the bone marrow be rapid, immature forms of cells may be discharged in the circulating blood, so that following certain injuries we may find myelocytes of various types, nucleated red blood corpuscles and large lymphocytes (see Sabin).

Summary. In a general way it may be seen from the foregoing that regeneration occurs with varying degrees of readiness in connection with different types of tissue. Aside from the inherent capacity of a tissue to regenerate, there are numerous other factors which play a part in regeneration following injury of inflammatory or other origin. It is easily understood that the larger the injury, the less likelihood is there of adequate regeneration. In these instances, cicatrization fills the defect. Nutrition, in the broadest sense, including proteins, fats, carbohydrates, electrolytes and certain vitamins, plays an important part in the regeneration, so that in individuals who are improperly nourished, either as the result of actual starvation or because of diseases which interfere with assimilation and metabolism, regeneration may be very much decreased. As Morgan points out, growth may be regulated by many factors other than oxygen and food supply. The regeneration of animal tissue depends to a considerable degree upon the age of the individual. In early life regeneration is undoubtedly carried out with much greater effectiveness than in late life. As age advances, the capacity for regeneration is much reduced. In the lower forms of animal life, cellular differentiation is not carried out to the same degree as in higher forms, so that in the lower animals regeneration may be active and complete. The same is true in regard to the lower vegetable forms. In the higher vegetable forms, regeneration follows much the same rule as in the higher animals: after tree branches have reached adult size their destruction is not followed by regeneration; new shoots from the trunk may form new branches but this is not a regeneration of the original branch.

CHRONIC INFLAMMATION

This is characterized by proliferation of connective tissues, especially the white fibrous connective tissue and also, to a limited degree, of the capillaries and even larger vessels. Exudation occurs and varies from the appearance of a few lymphocytes, plasma cells and large mononuclears, as in chronic endocarditis, to a suppurative exudate such as occurs in chronic osteomyelitis. Chronic inflammation is the principal form of productive inflammation. Whereas acute inflammation is limited as to duration and usually ends in recovery, chronic inflammation is progressive and, although it may heal, more frequently continues indefinitely. It differs in this respect from cicatrization; the scar is an end stage, is fixed, permanent and entirely quiescent. It is often difficult to distinguish grossly between a scar and a chronic inflammation, but microscopically the latter shows some of the manifestations of exudation, even if it be only a number of lymphocytes. As indicated above, acute inflammation in process of organization is not chronic inflammation.

Chronic inflammation may affect structures made up largely of connective tissue, especially the serous membranes such as endocardium, pericardium, pleura, synovia and meninges, and various parenchymatous viscera, notably the kidneys and liver. In certain of the infectious diseases, some or many of the lesions may be chronic, for example, in tuberculosis, leprosy and syphilis.

Chronic inflammation may be the outcome of one or several attacks of acute inflammation and it is believed that in some instances it is chronic from the beginning. The causes include bacteria, higher vegetable forms, animal parasites, injurious materials ingested or produced in the body, certain vaguely defined allergic phenomena, local irritations, and nutritional disturbances including some of the vitamin deficiencies. If the cause be infectious, there must be a peculiar host-parasite relationship, determined by virulence of the organism and resistance or chronic inflammations. Ingested poisons, such as lead and arsenic, may produce chronic inflammations of parenchymatous viscera. Deleterious substances produced in the body are possibly responsible for gout and some of the forms of chronic rheumatism. Allergic phenomena are held to be responsible for the chronic lesions of rheumatic fever, syphilis, tuberculosis and certain other diseases. There are various examples of the effects of prolonged irritation, good examples being chronic ulcers of tongue and oral mucosa from carious teeth and ill-fitting dentures. Illustrations of nutritional disturbances are to be found in cirrhosis of the liver, a form of

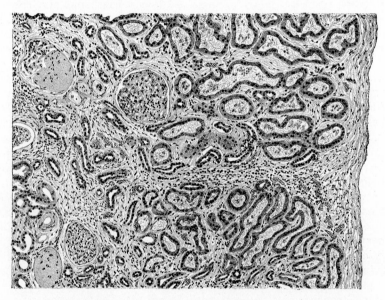

Chronic nephritis. Note the marked increase of connective tissue between the tubules, infiltration of mononuclears and the late stage of cloudy swelling of the tubular epithelium.

of the host. Staphylococci usually produce acute inflammation, but are also the cause of chronic osteomyelitis, chronic furunculosis and carbuncles. This may be due in part to differences in virulence, but seems to be due largely to factors of resistance. Local manifestations of resistance also are effective. For example, the tubercle bacillus may produce chronic inflammation in the lung but usually leads to acute inflammation when entering the meninges. The higher vegetable organisms more often lead to chronic than acute inflammations, but this is by no means invariable. Animal parasites such as *Trichinella spiralis* and *Schistosoma* may produce acute chronic inflammation, and certain forms of chronic gastritis.

In serous membranes, the gross features of chronic inflammation are fibrous thickening, opacity, fibrous adhesions and variable degrees of vascularization. These are well exemplified in chronic adhesive pericarditis and pleurisy. The adhesions may be so extensive as to obliterate the sac. In chronic inflammation of cardiac valves, thickening, rigidity, retraction and commissural adhesions occur. Vascularization occurs in all these situations. Microscopically, dense fibrosis with few nuclei and much collagen is usually seen, but various stages may be found

from immature fibroblasts to mature fibro-
cytes. Cellular infiltration is principally of
lymphocytes, but large mononuclears are not
infrequent and plasma cells may be found.

The gross changes in parenchymatous
viscera depend upon the fact that there are
associated lesions of parenchymatous cells
and that the connective tissue often retracts.
The organ usually has a nodular outer surface, a thick opaque capsule (when it is an
encapsulated organ), is firm, cuts with increased resistance and shows a firm, retracted
cross section. The vascularity and blood content vary considerably. Microscopically, there
is interstitial fibrosis, variable in degree even
in the same organ. Infiltration of lymphocytes and other mononuclear cells may be
slight or marked. The parenchymal cells may
show a variety of retrogressive changes such
as cloudy swelling, fatty degeneration, atrophy and necrosis. These alterations are described more specifically in the chapters on
systemic pathology.

Clinically, the signs and symptoms
vary from the unnoticeable to the most profound disturbances. A joint may be slightly
limited in motion, or a patient may be profoundly and fatally ill from such diseases as
chronic endocarditis and chronic nephritis.
The common severity of anatomic change and
functional disturbance justify Marchand's
term, "chronic inflammatory disease."
Chronic disease in one organ is usually reflected in disturbances of others. Chronic inflammations, as exhibited in chronic ulcers
and in cirrhosis of the liver, etc., may be the
forerunners of malignant tumors, especially
carcinoma.

Subacute Inflammation

There must certainly be stages in the
process of inflammation in which a transition
period between acute and chronic inflammation is to be found. The demarcation of this
period is difficult because the transition from
exudative to proliferative types of inflammation is by no means sharply defined. In a
sense, the term subacute inflammation may
frequently depend entirely upon the personal
equation of the observer. Similarly, the finer
division into subchronic inflammation as differentiated from subacute is extremely difficult. Nevertheless, if exudative inflammation
be still present, and proliferative changes

have occurred to a point indicating chronicity
of the process, the term "subacute" is usually
employed. If, on the other hand, the chronic
changes be well advanced with only a slight
remnant of exudative change, the term "subchronic" is frequently employed. Thus, in
those instances in which there is a considerable connective-tissue growth associated with
the presence of numbers of lymphocytes,
large mononuclears, and plasma cells, the condition is usually considered as subacute or
subchronic, depending upon the amount of
connective-tissue growth. Many pathologists,
however, prefer to make no such differentiation and would call a process of the sort just
indicated chronic rather than subacute or
subchronic. Inasmuch as a pathologic diagnosis must indicate the essential nature of the
process, this differentiation seems to us quite
justified. It is possible to indicate as subacute
or subchronic, inflammations in which a few
polymorphonuclear leukocytes may still be
present. This cell is distinctly more characteristic of exudation than the other cells
noted and its presence leads to the supposition that the acute stage of the inflammatory
process is still in evidence. These types of
inflammation must be considered as progressive in the same sense as are the chronic inflammatory processes. In the subacute forms
the probability of self-limitation of the process is greater than in the chronic.

INFLAMMATION IN AVASCULAR TISSUES

Inflammation may affect such avas-
cular tissues as the cornea and lens of the eye,
parts of cartilage and the free edges of heart
valves. Experimental inflammation of the
cornea has been studied by Grawitz, Leber,
Councilman and others, and their results may
be applied to other avascular tissues. Traumatic or bacterial injury affecting only the
epithelial cells of the cornea is followed by
regeneration, which may for a short time be
slightly in excess of actual replacement
and result in multiplication of layers. Aseptic
injury of the corneal tissue may result in
multiplication of corneal corpuscles to fill
the defect. More serious injury, such as may
be produced by injection of pyogenic bacteria, leads first to necrosis in the immediate
area, multiplication of bacteria which pene-

trate into the tissue spaces, subsequent swelling, degeneration and death of neighboring cells and fibers. Only after several hours have elapsed is neighboring vascular reaction observed. The marginal vein and small vessels become dilated and grossly visible as a zone of hyperemia at the margin of the cornea. This delay in vascular reaction is due, presumably, to the time necessary for passage of the bacterial poisons into the peripheral tissues. Microscopic examination shows typical vasodilatation, margination and emigration of leukocytes. As an evidence of chemotaxis, the leukocytes migrate directly and rapidly to the point of injury, and may take part in the formation of an abscess. If the injury be eccentrically placed, the part of the margin nearest it shows the most marked hyperemia. In unfavorable cases, the inflammation may extend widely in the eye, especially in those cases where the local lesion perforates the cornea and infection extends into the chambers. In favorable cases, repair occurs by multiplication of corneal corpuscles and of surface epithelium. In the more severe cases, granulation proceeds from the margin by proliferation of capillaries and fibroblasts, which grow in toward the injury. In either case there remains an area of opacity and, after cicatrization is complete, some of the new vessels may remain permanently in the cornea.

ULCER

The ulcer may be defined as an interruption of surface continuity with an inflammatory base. Certain authorities believe that in order properly to be qualified as an ulcer, the inflammation must be suppurative, but the broader conception is not limited in this way. Ulcers may be found on any surface of the body and may be due to traumatic destruction of the surface, or result from degeneration, necrosis or inflammation in the neighborhood, which leads to the sloughing of the injured superficial tissue from the underlying parts. Ulcers of the skin and mucous membranes are common. On the skin surface they may result from direct physical injury of various kinds. Ulcers may occur in the oral mucosa because of cuts, sharp foreign bodies, the edges of carious teeth, trauma of poorly fitted dentures, etc. In the intestinal canal they are most commonly the result of inflammation of the gut wall, with subsequent necrosis and sloughing of the epithelial and sometimes of the submucous lining of the gut. In certain other mucous surfaces, for example, the gallbladder and the genito-urinary tract, ulcers may result from abrasion by calculi. In any surface accessible to the exterior of the body, ulcers may be caused by direct trauma. Ulcerations also appear in the arteries as the result of breaking down and sloughing off of degenerate and necrotic portions of the arteriosclerotic intima and deeper parts. The necrosis is accompanied by surrounding inflammation so that ulcers in this situation meet the broader definition. The course of ulceration, that is, whether it heals rapidly or slowly, depends upon the nutrition and reactive capacity of the tissue. One of the commonest chronic ulcers is that type seen on the leg in older people. These may persist for months or years, and the failure to heal is probably due to damming back of the circulation incident to posture, or to general failure of the circulation. This may bring about delay in the growth of granulation tissue and organization, together with poor epithelialization.

In the ordinary forms of ulcer, the inflammation at the base depends upon the number and character of infective organisms. If kept fairly clean, the base may show little actual suppuration. There is always a moderate amount of serous exudation which may dry on the surface to produce a crust or scab. If the infection underlying the crust be slight, the crust formation may aid materially in healing. In the more prolonged types of ulcer, the base is likely to show, in addition to the serous exudation, considerable infiltration by the cells seen late in the course of inflammation, namely, lymphocytes, large mononuclears, and plasma cells. Somewhat deeper, granulation is found proceeding with different degrees of activity. Gross inspection shows the small knobs of projecting capillaries and connective tissue which gives the name granulation tissue. Ordinarily, in a favorable case, the granulation proceeds until it fills the defect, is covered by epithelium and gradually cicatrizes. In other instances, granulation may be excessive in amount and form a projecting mass above the general level of the surface, the so-called exuberant granulation, or "proud flesh." The surface epithelium grows over such superfluous granulation with greater difficulty than if the granulation merely fill the defect. This may delay healing, but if the excess be removed, healing proceeds and the final results are improved. Trauma may produce bleeding from the delicate new vessels and the edges may show phagocytes containing blood pigment. Epithelial proliferation sometimes proceeds to the production of carcinoma.

REFERENCES

Adami, J. G.: Inflammation, London, 1909.

Amberg, S., A. S. Loevenhart, and W. B. McClure: The Influence of Oxygen upon Inflammatory Reactions, Jour. Pharm. and Exper. Ther., 10: 209, 1917.

Arey, L. B.: Wound Healing, Physiol. Rev., 16: 327, 1936.

Aschoff, L.: Zur Begriffsbestimmung der Entzündung, Beiträge Path. Anat. u. Allg. Path., 68: 1, 1921; Lectures on Pathology, New York, 1924.

Beitzke, H.: Ueber den Entzündungsbegriff, Ergeb. Allg. Path. u. Path. Anat. 20²: 344, 1923.

Bier, O., and M. Rocha e Silva: Untersuchungen über Entzündung. I. Mechanismus der Erhöhung der Capillarpermeabilität bei der Entzündung, mit besonderer Berücksichtigung der Rolle des Histamins, Virchow's Arch. Path. Anat., 303: 325, 1939.

Bruce, A. N.: Vaso-dilator Axon-reflexes, Quart. Jour. Exper. Physiol., 6: 339, 1913.

Cannon, P. R., and G. A. Pacheco: Studies in Tissue-Immunity—Cellular Reactions of the Skin of the Guinea Pig as Influenced by Local Active Immunization, Amer. Jour. Path., 6: 749, 1930.

——, and G. Hartley, Jr.: The Failure of Allergic Inflammation to Protect Rabbits against Infection with Virulent Pneumococci, Amer. Jour. Path., 14: 87, 1938.

Carrel, A.: Tissue Culture and Cell Physiology, Physiol. Rev., 4: 1, 1924.

Carscadden, W. G.: Early Inflammatory Reactions in Tissues Following Simple Injury, Arch. Path. and Lab. Med., 4: 329, 1927.

Clark, E. R.: Growth and Development of Function in Blood Vessels and Lymphatics, Ann. Int. Med., 9: 1043, 1936.

Cohnheim, J.: Vorlesungen über allgemeinen Pathologie, Berlin, 1882; English Trans., London, 1899.

Councilman, W. T.: An Anatomical and Bacteriological Study of Acute Diffuse Nephritis, Amer. Jour. Med. Sci., 114: 23, 1897.

——: The Character of the Cellular Exudation in Acute Keratitis of the Rabbit, Jour. Boston Soc. Med. Sci., 3: 99, 1898-99.

Dale, H. H., and P. P. Laidlaw: Histamine Shock, Jour. Physiol., 52: 355, 1919.

Dixon, H. M., and M. McCutcheon: Absence of Chemotropism in Lymphocytes, Arch. Path., 19: 679, 1935.

——: Chemotropism of Leucocytes in Relation to Their Rate of Locomotion, Proc. Soc. Exper. Biol. and Med., 34: 173, 1936.

Downey, H.: Histiocytes and Macrophages and Their Relations to the Cells of Normal Blood in Animals Stained Intra Vitam with Acid Colloidal Dyes, Anat. Rec., 11: 350, 1916-17.

Drinker, C. K., and M. E. Field: Lymphatic, Lymph and Tissue Fluid, Baltimore, Williams and Wilkins, 1933.

DuNoüy, P. L.: Cicatrization of Wounds. X. A General Equation for the Law of Cicatrization of Surface Wounds, Jour. Exper. Med., 29: 329, 1919.

Duthie, E. S., and E. Chain: A Polypeptide Responsible for Some of the Phenomena of Acute Inflammation, Brit. Jour. Exper. Path., 20: 417, 1939.

Ecker, E. E., A. S. Weisberger, and L. Pillemer: The Opsonins of Normal and Immune Sera. I. Methods: A Comparison of the Effects of Normal and Immune Opsonins on Staphylococcus aureus, Jour. Immunol., 43: 227, 1942.

——, L. Pillemer, and A. O. Kuehn: III. The Opsonins of Different Species, the Role of Complement in Opsonic Activity, etc., ibid., 43: 245, 1942.

Ernst, T.: Ueber die ersten Stunden der Entzündung, Beit. z. Path. Anat. u. Allg. Path., 75: 229, 1926.

Evans, F. A.: Experimental Study of Mononuclear Cells of the Blood and Tissues with Special Reference to the So-called Transitional Cell, Arch. Int. Med., 18: 692, 1916.

Fåhraeus, R.: The Suspension Stability of the Blood, Physiol. Rev., 9: 241, 1929.

Fenn, W. O.: The Adhesiveness of Leucocytes to Solid Surfaces, Jour. Gen. Physiol., 5: 143, 1922.

——: Effect of Hydrogen Ion Concentration on the Phagocytosis and Adhesiveness of Leucocytes, ibid., 5: 169, 1923.

Field, M. E., C. K. Drinker, and J. C. White: Lymph Pressures in Sterile Inflammation, Jour. Exper. Med., 56: 363, 1932.

Fischer, A.: Regeneration. Versuche an Gewebekulturen in vitro, Virchow's Arch. Path. Anat., 279: 94, 1930.

Foot, N. C.: Studies on Endothelial Reactions, Jour. Med. Res., 40: 353, 1919; Jour. Exper. Med., 32: 513, 1920; 32: 533, 1920; 33: 271, 1921.

——: The Endothelial Phagocyte, A Critical Review, Anat. Rec., 30: 15, 1925.

Gilding, H. P.: The Relative Reaction within Living Mammalian Tissues. XIII. The Reaction Prevailing During the Autolysis in Vivo of Small Tissue Masses, Jour. Exper. Med., 52: 953, 1930.

Groll, H.: Experimentelle Untersuchungen zur Lehre von der Entzündung, Krankheitsforsch., 2: 195, 1926; see also G. Borger, and H. Groll, ibid., 3: 443, 1926.

Hall, J. W., and J. Furth: Cultural Studies on the Relationship of Lymphocytes to Monocytes and Fibroblasts, Arch. Path., 25: 46, 1938.

Halley, C. R. L., A. M. Chesney, and I. Dresel: On the Behavior of Granulating Wounds of the Rabbit to Various Types of Infection, Bull. Johns Hopkins Hosp., 41: 191, 1927.

Harrison, R. G.: The Outgrowth of the Nerve Fiber as a Mode of Protoplastic Movement, Jour. Exper. Zool., 9: 787, 1910.

——: Neuroblast versus Sheath Cell in the Development of Peripheral Nerves, Jour. Comp. Neurol., 37: 123, 1924.

Hartwell, S. W.: Surgical Wounds in Human

Beings—A Histologic Study of Healing, etc., Arch. Surg., **19:** 835, 1929.

Hartzell, J. B., J. M. Winfield, and J. L. Irvin: Plasma Vitamin C and Serum Protein Levels in Wound Disruption, Jour. Amer. Med. Asso., **116:** 669, 1941.

Harvey, S. C., and E. L. Howes: Effect of High Protein Diet on Velocity of Growth of Fibroblasts in the Healing Wound, Ann. Surg., **91:** 641, 1930.

Hass, G., and F. McDonald: Studies of Collagen. I. The Production of Collagen in Vitro under Experimental Conditions, Amer. Jour. Path., **16:** 525, 1940.

——: Studies of Collagen. II. Methods and Results of Implantation of Collagen-Forming Cultures in Granulation Tissue, ibid., **16:** 549, 1940.

Haythorn, S. R.: Multinucleated Giant Cells with Particular Reference to the Foreign Body Giant Cell, Arch. Path., **7:** 651, 1929.

Hektoen, L.: Opsonins Distinct from Other Antibodies, Jour. Infect. Dis., **6:** 78, 1909.

Hooker, D. R.: Evidence of Functional Activity on the Part of the Capillaries and Venules, Physiol. Rev., **1:** 112, 1921.

Howes, E. L., J. W. Sooy, and S. C. Harvey: The Healing of Wounds as Determined by Their Tensile Strength, Jour. Amer. Med. Asso., **92:** 42, 1929.

Hueck, W.: Ueber das Mesenchym. Die Bedeutung seiner Entwicklung und seines Baues für die Pathologie, Beiträge z. Path. Anat. u. Allg. Path., **66:** 330, 1920.

Ingebrigtsen, R.: A Contribution to the Biology of Peripheral Nerves in Transplantation, Jour. Exper. Med. **23:** 251, 1916.

Jobling, J. W., and W. A. Petersen: A Study of the Ferments and Ferment Inhibiting Substances in Tuberculous Caseous Material, Jour. Exper. Med., **19:** 383, 1914.

Kaiser, P.: See Year Book of Pathology and Immunology, Chicago, Year Book Publishers, 1940, p. 28.

Karsner, H. T., H. H. Amiral, and A. V. Bock: The Influence of Splenectomy and of Certain Organs and Organ Extracts on the Hemopsonins of the Blood Serum, Jour. Med. Res., **30:** 383, 1914.

——, and J. E. Dwyer: Experimental Bland Infarction of the Myocardium, Myocardial Regeneration and Cicatrization, Jour. Med. Res., **39:** 21, 1916.

——, and A. T. Merrill: Migration of Leucocytes in Blood Clots, Arch. Path., **7:** 101, 1929.

Kenton, H. B.: The Influence of Inflammation on the Skin Necrotizing Action of Staphylococcus Toxin, Amer. Jour. Path., **15:** 185, 1939.

Klemensiewicz, R.: Die Entzündung, Jena, 1908.

Krogh, A.: Nervous and Hormonal Control of Capillary Contractility, Harvey Lectures, Philadelphia, Lippincott, 1922-23, p. 232.

——: Anatomy and Physiology of the Capillaries, 2d ed., New Haven, Yale Univ. Press, 1929.

Landis, E. M.: The Passage of Fluid Through the Capillary Wall, Harvey Lectures, Baltimore, Williams and Wilkins, **32:** 70, 1937.

——: Capillary Pressure and Capillary Permeability, Physiol. Rev., **14:** 404, 1934.

Leber, T.: Die Enstehung der Entzündung, Leipzig, 1891.

Lewis, T.: The Blood Vessels of the Human Skin and Their Responses, Shaw, London, 1927.

Lewis, W. H.: The Transformation of Mononuclear Blood Cells into Macrophages, Epithelioid Cells, and Giant Cells, Harvey Lectures, Philadelphia, Lippincott, Series 21, p. 77, Baltimore, 1927.

Lucké, B., M. Strumia, S. Mudd, M. McCutcheon, and E. B. H. Mudd: On the Comparative Phagocytic Activity of Macrophages and Polynuclear Leucocytes, Jour. Immunol., **24:** 455, 1933.

Lund, C. C., and J. H. Crandon: Human Experimental Scurvy and the Relation of Vitamin C Deficiency to Postoperative Pneumonia and to Wound Healing, Jour. Amer. Med. Asso., **116:** 663, 1941.

Marchand, F.: Ueber den Entzündungsbegriff, Virchow's Arch. Path. Anat., **234:** 245, 1921.

——: Lehre von der Entzündung, Krehl and Marchand, Handbuch der Allg. Path., Leipzig, 1924, vol. iv, p. 78.

Maximow, A. A.: Relation of the Blood Cells to Connective Tissues and Endothelium, Physiol. Rev., **4:** 533, 1924.

McJunkin, F. A.: Origin of the Perivascular Phagocytes of Granulation Tissue, Amer. Jour. Path., **6:** 39, 1930.

Meltzer, S. J., and C. Meltzer: On a Difference in the Influence upon Inflammation Between the Section of the Sympathetic Nerve and the Removal of the Sympathetic Ganglion, Jour. Med. Res., **10:** 135, 1903-04.

Menkin, V.: Dynamics of Inflammation, an Inquiry into the Mechanism of Infectious Processes, New York, Macmillan, 1940.

——, and C. R. Warner: Studies on Inflammation. XIII. Carbohydrate Metabolism, Local Acidosis, and the Cytological Picture in Inflammation, Amer. Jour. Path., **13:** 25, 1937.

Metchnikoff, E.: La Pathologie Comparée de l'Inflammation, Paris, 1892. The Comparative Pathology of Inflammation, London, 1893.

Michels, N. A.: The Plasma Cell: A Critical Review of Its Morphogenesis, Function and Developmental Capacity under Normal and under Abnormal Conditions, Arch. Path., **11:** 775, 1931.

Millar, W. G.: Regeneration of Skeletal Muscle in Young Rabbits, Jour. Path. and Bact., **38:** 145, 1934.

Miller, F. R.: The Induced Development and Histogenesis of Plasma Cells, Jour. Exper. Med., **54:** 333, 1931.

Moon, V. H.: Mechanism of Acute Inflammation, Arch. Path, **20:** 561, 1935.

Morgan, T. H.: The Physiology of Regeneration, Jour. Exper. Zool., **3:** 457, 1903.

Mudd, S., M. McCutcheon, and B. Lucké: Phagocytosis, Physiol. Rev., **14:** 210, 1934.

Neuhaus, C.: Ueber den Stoffwechsel des Granulationsgewebes (Atmung und Glykolyse), Beitr. Path. Anat. u. Allg. Path., **83:** 383, 1929.

Nordmann, M.: Local Reactions in Sensitized Animals. Arthus Phenomenon. "Hyperergic Inflammation," Physiol. Rev., **11:** 41, 1931.

——, and A. Rüther: Ueber die Bedingungen der Leukodiapedese, Virchow's Arch. Path. Anat., **279:** 45, 1930.

Opie, E. L.: Inflammation. Harvey Lectures, Philadelphia, Lippincott, 1910, p. 192; Arch. Int. Med., **5:** 541, 1910.

Opie, E. L.: Inflammation and Immunity, Jour. Immunol., **17**: 329, 1929.

Reimann, S. P.: Use and Reasons for the Use of Thiocresol to Stimulate Wound Healing, Jour. Amer. Med. Asso., **94**: 1369, 1930.

Ricker, G.: Pathologie als Naturwissenschaft—Relationspathologie, Berlin, 1924.

——: Angriffsort und Wirkungsweise der Reize an der Strombahn, Krankheitsforschung, **1**: 457, 1925.

Rigdon, R. H.: Relation of Capillary Permeability to Inflammation, Southern Med. Jour., **34**: 292, 1941.

——: Observations on Capillary Permeability in Areas of Inflammation Produced by Staphylococci, Surgery, **9**: 436, 1941.

——: Capillary Permeability and Inflammation in Rabbits with Staphylococcic Septicemia: An Experimental Study, Arch. Surg., **44**: 129, 1942.

Rössle, R.: Referat über Entzündung, Verhandl. Deutsch. Path. Gesellsch., **19**: 18, 1923.

Rous, P., and D. R. Drury: Outlying Acidosis due to Functional Ischemia, Jour. Exper. Med., **49**: 435, 1929.

——, and H. P. Gilding: Is the Local Vasodilatation after Different Tissue Injuries Referable to a Single Cause? Jour. Exper. Med., **51**: 27, 1930.

——, ——, and F. Smith: The Gradient of Vascular Permeability, Jour. Exper. Med., **51**: 807, 1930.

Sabin, F. R. et al.: Studies on the Maturation of Myeloblasts and on Amitotic Cell Division, etc., Jour. Exper. Med., **40**: 845, 1924.

Sabin, F. R.: Bone Marrow, Physiol. Rev., **8**: 191, 1928.

——, and C. A. Doan: The Relation of Monocytes and Clasmatocytes to Early Infection in Rabbits with Bovine Tubercle Bacilli, Jour. Exper. Med., **46**: 627, 1927.

Samuel, S.: Ueber anämische, hyperämische und neurotische Entzündungen, Virchow's Arch., **121**: 396,

1890; Entzündung, Ergeb. d. Allg. Path. u. Path. Anat., **2**: 64, 1895.

Shimura, K.: Der Einfluss des zentralen und peripheren Nervensystems auf der Entzündung, Virchow's Arch. Path. Anat., **251**: 160, 1924.

Silverman, D.: A Chemotropic Substance Derived from Normal Tissues, Arch. Path., **25**: 40, 1938.

Sperti, G. S., J. R. Loofbourow, and M. M. Lane: Effects on Tissue Cultures of Inter-cellular Hormones from Injured Cells, Science, **86**: 611, 1937.

Spielmeyer, W.: Zur Frage der Nervennaht, Münch. Med. Wochenschr., **62**: 58, 99, 1915; *see also* G. Hohmann and W. Spielmeyer: Zur Kritik des Edinger'schen und des Bethes'chen Verfahrens der Ueberbrückung grosserer Nervenlücken, ibid., **64**: 97, 1917.

Ssamarin, N.: Zur Frage über die Regeneration des Rückenmarknervengewebes nach aseptischen Verletzungen, Virchow's Arch. Path. Anat., **260**: 369, 1926.

Weiss, C., and E. J. Czarnetsky: Proteolytic Enzymes of Monocytic and Polymorphonuclear Pleural Exudates, Arch. Path., **20**: 233, 1935.

Werthemann, A.: Ueber den Aufbau der Blutgefässwand in entzündlichen Neubildungen, etc., Virchow's Arch. Path. Anat., **270**: 605, 1929.

Winternitz, M. C., and A. D. Hirschfelder: Studies upon Experimental Pneumonia in Rabbits, Jour. Exper. Med., **17**: 666, 1913.

Wolf, E. P.: Experimental Studies on Inflammation, Jour. Exper. Med., **34**: 375, 1921; **37**: 511, 1923.

Woolley, P. G.: Factors Governing Vascular Dilatation and Slowing of the Blood-Stream in Inflammation, Jour. Amer. Med. Asso., **63**: 2279, 1914.

Wright, A. E., and L. Colebrook: Technique of the Teat and Capillary Glass Tube. London, 1921.

Zon, L., E. T. Ceder, and C. Crigler: Presence of Histamine in Inflammatory Lesions, Arch. Path., **33**: 452, 1942.

9

Principles of Infectious Disease

INTRODUCTION

Infectious diseases include those diseases which are transmissible from one individual to others, either by direct contact, in which instance we deal with contagious disease; or by the mediation of inanimate carriers of infections, such as water, food, clothing; or of animate carriers. The inanimate carriers may serve as culture media upon which the organisms multiply or simply act as inert carriers as in the case of clothing, utensils or other fomites. The animate carriers may carry from host to host, or con-

taminate foods and waters, or they may serve as intermediate hosts in which a definite cycle of the parasite takes place. Human carriers may convey disease on hands or clothing, or they may harbor (in the gallbladder, throat or elsewhere) organisms to which they are temporarily or permanently immune, but which upon discharge are virulent for others.

Infectious diseases may be caused by bacteria, higher vegetable organisms, protozoa, metazoa, rickettsia and viruses. They may be conditioned by alterations in the reaction of the body, i.e., some form of allergy. Metazoan parasites, such as worms and insects, are as a rule infestations of surfaces, intestinal, skin, etc., rather than infections entering into the body, although they may produce absorbable injurious substances as in the case of infestation by *Diphyllobothrium latum*, the fish tapeworm.

Primary: Secondary: Terminal. Primary infections are those which occur without any decrease of resistance due to another infection. Secondary infections occur in individuals already suffering from infections of another nature. The latter is well exemplified in the secondary infection of a tuberculous cavity of the lung by staphylococcus. Terminal infections are those which occur near the fatal termination of some other disease, whether that other disease be of bacterial nature or of some other origin. Infections of this type are seen in the terminal bronchopneumonias and septicemias which occur in the course of certain chronic diseases.

Mixed: Multiple: Complex. Infection by more than one organism may occur. This is spoken of as mixed, multiple, or complex infection. It is also possible to find an infective organism and one which is not pathogenic in the same case. For example, Kanof and Kramer studied 320 cases of septicemia. In 8 per cent of these there was an additional organism but in only 3 per cent were both the organisms definitely pathogenic. In about half the latter group the second organism appeared some time after the original infection. It is often difficult to decide which of the infections is the more significant for the patient. In order to determine that one infectious agent only is responsible for the disease, all the features of the disease should be accounted for as being due to that one organism (Shope). Furthermore there can be no doubt that one infection influences another existing at the same time and usually in a manner deleterious to the patient. Measles or lobar pneumonia may excite latent tuberculosis into activity. Latent syphilis may become active as the result of an attack of typhoid fever, and latent gonorrhea from an attack of tonsillitis. The removal of one chronic infection may favorably influence another, as is seen in the relief of certain cases of pyorrhea alveolaris by the removal of infected tonsils, and in numerous other instances of multiple, chronic infections. This is not necessarily due to action of a focal infection, the theory of which will be discussed in connection with streptococcal infections.

The purpose of this chapter is to present a discussion of some of the general effects of infectious diseases; that is, it is a discussion of principles rather than a detailed catalogue of all the disorders in this category. Nevertheless, a few examples are selected to illustrate different types of infectious diseases. The next chapter gives an account of those diseases which are called "infectious granulomata" and in the chapters on systemic pathology, certain others are discussed. A more exhaustive consideration of infection and resistance is to be found in the special textbooks on these subjects.

INFECTIOUS DISEASE

Disease of any kind represents the effects of a cause or several causes. Infectious disease, however, represents the interaction of two living bodies, namely the infecting organism and the host in which the disease is observed. It is therefore a host-parasite interrelationship. The relationship is reciprocal, for not only does the infecting agent bring about certain effects and reactions in the host but it is possible also that the host may cause certain changes in the infecting organism and its products. Indeed, these may be sufficient to kill the agent. Some of the effects in the host are represented by the destruction of tissues and cells by organisms and their products, whereas others are responses by the reactive capacities of the host to stimuli produced by the organism. It has been pointed out that inflammation is a local reaction to injury and in many instances a local reaction to infective agents. Infectious disease is something more, in that it is a reaction on the part of the whole body. It is a general reaction and shows various general manifestations. These disturbances may vary from minor malaise to profound exhaustion. There may be widespread disturbances of circulation, of respiration, of the nerves, of metabolism, of secretion, of excretion, etc. Chills and sweats are not uncommon but the most striking phenomenon of all is fever.

Varieties of Dissemination

These general effects are due to dissemination, throughout the body, of the infecting organisms themselves, of certain of their injurious products and also of more or less well-defined toxins. The dissemination may be manifested as sapremia, toxemia, bacteremia, septicemia and pyemia.

Sapremia is due to the production of injurious substances by saprophytic organisms. These multiply in dead tissues and the products are absorbed to produce special signs and symptoms.

Toxemia differs in that it represents the absorption of the products of parasitic organisms. The term is broadly used to include the absorption of true toxins, as in diphtheria, or of other products which may be injurious but do not have all the characters of toxins.

Bacteremia means simply the presence of bacteria in the blood. It is usually evanescent and may be due to transient entry of either pathogenic or nonpathogenic organisms.

Septicemia is much more important from both clinical and pathologic aspects. The term connotes not only the presence of bacteria in the blood but also of their poisonous products. Whether they actually multiply in the blood, or enter it repeatedly or continuously from a focus in organs and tissues, is not positively known, but the latter explanation is probably correct.

Pyemia. Although literally "pyemia" means pus in the blood, this is not the real significance of the term. Simply stated, pyemia is septicemia plus the production of abscesses in various parts of the body. For example, abscesses may develop in the kidney because of infection of the urinary tract, but from these abscesses organisms may gain access to the blood, circulate with it and be deposited in various locations, such as the lungs, brain, myocardium or elsewhere, with the production of secondary or metastatic abscesses. Basically, pyemia can only be diagnosed as such when metastatic abscesses are demonstrated.

CLASSIFICATION OF INFECTIONS

Acute, Chronic, Subacute. Infectious diseases may be classified as acute or chronic. Sometimes the term "subacute" is employed. These terms carry with them the idea of duration. No definite time limit can be assigned but in a general way those that have a duration of a few days or a few weeks are called acute; those which have a duration of a few months are called subacute; and those that last for several months to a year or more are called chronic. For example, diphtheria, pneumonia, typhoid fever and diseases of this kind are acute infectious diseases. In the ordinary course of events, tuberculosis and syphilis are likely to be chronic in course. Intermediate between these may be such a disease as subacute bacterial endocarditis. Furthermore, infectious diseases may be continuous, intermittent or remittent; these terms are self-explanatory. In addition, infectious diseases are often given further names to indicate type and course.

Entrance of the Invader

In order to enter the body, the organisms or their products must penetrate through one of the body surfaces, such as the skin, conjunctiva or the mucous membranes of the respiratory, alimentary and genito-urinary tracts. As a rule invasion through the skin requires interruption of continuity such as occurs in traumatic injury, in growth of the organism in the crypts of the skin (par-ticularly hair follicles and sweat glands), and after the bite of blood-sucking insects. Similar interruption of surface continuity of the various mucous membranes is of importance, but it is known that bacteria may penetrate the surface of the respiratory tract and of the alimentary canal without definite lesion of the mucous surface (see Moody and Irons). Certain organisms appear to enter almost exclusively through special surfaces; for example, the pneumococcus by way of the respiratory tract, the typhoid bacillus in the intestinal canal, and the gonococcus in the genito-urinary tract.

The mere fact of invasion does not of itself mean infection; the organisms must become established in the body, multiply and elaborate their injurious products. They may form exotoxins and endotoxins. The proteins of the organisms may be injurious and the destruction of bacteria and the tissues of the host may liberate the injurious split protein products. Virulence varies with different organisms and with different strains of the same organism, but may be modified by various mechanisms in the host so as to increase or inhibit virulence.

Factors Favoring the Invader

Bacteria and other minute forms of life are widely present in nature. Organisms which produce disease constitute only a small proportion of these many varieties. They are limited further by the fact that most are obligate parasites. Certain organisms are transmitted by insects or other carriers, either passively, as is the typhoid bacilli by the fly; or they pass a part of their life cycle in intermediate hosts, as the malaria parasites in the mosquito. Lice and ticks ingest and nourish rickettsiae, until these are transmitted by bites. The small size of infective agents makes their detection difficult and hence favors their transportation in water and foods, and their persistence in the air in droplets of moisture and the nuclei of these droplets after the moisture has evaporated. Rapid multiplication, the formation of resistant spores and cysts, adaptability to differing environmental conditions, capacity to utilize various forms of nutriment, all favor the infective agents in maintenance of their life, survival under variable conditions and penetration into the body.

Factors Favoring the Host

The host is favored by the normal continuity of body surfaces. There are, perhaps, special intrinsic factors in the skin injurious to invading organisms. By their movement, various secretions may wash away infecting organisms; and in certain instances, by their chemical composition, operate against the organism. Factors, such as hairs in the anterior nares and ciliated epithelium in various parts of the respiratory tract, aid in filtering out organisms or in transporting them so that they can be expelled. The intelligence of the higher forms of animal life aids in the avoidance and elimination of infecting organisms. Intelligence leads to purposive voluntary movements; in addition the more or less involuntary movements of reflex character, such as sneezing, coughing, diarrhea, increased flow of tears, etc., may aid the host. Of utmost importance are cellular activities in the interior of the body, such as phagocytosis and the process of inflammation. In addition there are the important humoral mechanisms of the body. These include antitoxins which neutralize toxins, agglutinins which operate to favor deposition of organisms in places where they may be readily phagocytosed, precipitins which may throw poisonous protein substances out of solution, cytolysins which may kill and dissolve bacteria or other invading organisms, and opsonins which prepare bacteria and other particles for ingestion and destruction by phagocytes. These humoral factors are treated in detail in texts on immunology.

Factors Unfavorable to the Host

The structure and activities of man may well counterbalance the favorable features just enumerated. The surfaces of the body, both external and internal, are relatively large; this fact and the intricacy of structures such as crypts, ducts, and folds, offer opportunities for lodgment and multiplication of infective agents. Ingestion of food and water may bring pathogenic organisms into the body. The ready availability of the superficial orifices such as the nose, ears, mouth, anus, and genital orifices may favor the invader rather than the host. The body temperature, and the darkness and moisture of the body interior, offer favorable conditions for the multiplication of organisms. Particularly, there are certain structures in the body which are relatively inactive such as the appendix vermiformis and crypts of the tonsils, where organisms find moisture, warmth, and darkness suitable for their development. The circulation of lymph and blood may favor widespread dissemination of organisms. Phagocytes may carry bacteria to other parts of the body; they may offer favorable and even necessary conditions for intracellular growth of certain pathogenic bacteria (Goodpasture and Anderson).

Another contributing factor is man's migratory tendency, in part brought about by his modern means of transportation. He travels into regions of endemic infection, such as those where typhus fever occurs. He carries infection in his body from one place to another, in a variety of diseases which range from smallpox to the common cold. His ships may carry plague-ridden rats. His airplanes may transport infected mosquitoes. He has increased his hazard of infection and has had to build up a system of public-health regulations.

The Course of Infectious Disease

The exact moment of invasion of an infectious agent is difficult to determine, but, in many cases of infectious disease, the time of exposure to infection can be determined within the limits of a few hours.

Moment of Infection. Incubation. Following the moment of infection there is a period of incubation during which the host exhibits no symptom of disease. This period of incubation in some diseases is extremely variable, whereas in others it is relatively fixed. In diphtheria, incubation may apparently vary from 24 hours up to nine or ten days, and certain other diseases show similar variation. In scarlet fever, on the other hand, the incubation period is usually five days, and other diseases show a comparative fixity of incubation time. When bacteria are planted in artificial culture media more or less distinct physical and chemical changes occur before growth becomes active. It is possible that the incubation period in the living animal represents somewhat similar changes preparatory to active multiplication. The lag, or latent period, in the growth of bacteria when implanted on culture media does not correspond in point of time to the incubation period in infectious disease; thus, other factors must be involved.

Prodromal Symptoms: Invasion or Effervescence: Fastigium or Acme. Following the period of incubation, the less violent infectious diseases show a short period of prodromal symptoms in which headache, malaise, and other minor manifestations may appear. The next period, that of onset of disease or so-called invasion or effervescence, may be frank or insidious. Lobar pneumonia may develop within a period of a few hours and exemplifies frank onset. In contrast, typhoid fever is likely to occupy a week or ten days between the period of prodromal symptoms and the full development of disease, thus illustrating insidious onset. That period during which the disease is at its height is called the fastigium or acme. Following the fastigium comes the period of decline or defervescence. This may be by crisis or lysis. Crisis is seen in approximately half the cases of lobar pneumonia, in which the decline occurs in a period of a few hours. Defervescence by lysis is seen in a large number of infectious diseases and is particularly well exemplified by typhoid fever in which several days, a week or more, may be consumed.

Convalescence is that period during which the symptoms of disease have practically disappeared and the patient gradually recovers and is restored to normal. Most of the acute infectious diseases are more or less self-limited in their course. Thus, lobar pneumonia runs a course of seven to eleven days, typhoid of about three weeks, scarlet fever and diphtheria a few days. This means that with an individual of average resistance and an organism of average virulence, the various reactive mechanisms of the body are adequate to destroy the invading organisms and the process ends in recovery. Disproportion, in the form of too great virulence or too low resistance, may delay recovery or cause death. Chronic infectious diseases exhibit no such regularity of development and course. In contrast to the acute infections, these are not likely to be self-limited, but progress until they have reached a point of such great severity, or of such complete exhaustion of the host, that death ensues.

Two of the most important general phenomena of infectious disease are fever and hyperleukocytosis.

General Manifestations

Fever. This term, in its narrow sense, signifies elevation of body temperature. In its broader interpretation it is a syndrome, comprising not only hyperthermia but also other conditions which vary with the degree of temperature elevation, and include dryness of skin and mouth, herpes, decreased output of urine, respiratory disturbances, increased heart rate and nervous symptoms varying from minor muscle twitchings to active delirium. In addition, there are important but not marked alterations of metabolism.

Mammals are homothermic, or warm-blooded, as contrasted with the poikilothermic, or cold-blooded, animals. Warm-blooded animals maintain a temperature that is constant with a possible normal variation not exceeding 5 or 6 per cent. In man the normal variation may range between 36.3° and 37.5° C., with a diurnal rhythm from the minimum in the early morning to the maximum in the later afternoon (Benedict). In other mammals the temperatures are usually higher and in birds may reach 43° C. Body heat is regulated by the mechanism of thermotaxis, which properly balances the production and the dissipation of heat. Heat is produced by absorption of food, especially proteins, by the general chemical changes of metabolism and especially by muscular work. It is dissipated by radiation, conduction and water evaporation. Circulation in the skin is therefore of the utmost importance in heat dissipation, since the blood flow to the skin aids in assuring proper heat elimination both by radiation and conduction, and by sweating and evaporation. The thermotaxic center in the midbrain is apparently influenced by the temperature of the blood and by afferent sensory impulses, particularly from the skin. The involuntary regulation is principally in the direction of dissipation. Increased heat production occurs as the result of shivering or perhaps less noticeable activity of the muscles, by eating and by voluntary exercise.

Body temperature may be increased by high external temperatures, by violent exercise and by certain drugs and chemicals such as strychnine, caffeine, xanthine. Injections of sodium-chloride solution may produce hyperthermia, but it does not ensue if calcium and potassium salts, as in Ringer's solution, be added. The hyperthermia of salt solutions made with old distilled water is probably due to the presence of minute traces of organic matter, according to Hort and Penfold. These various forms of hyperthermia are not necessarily to be regarded as fever, according to the conception offered above.

THE EXACT MODE OF OPERATION OF THE CAUSES OF FEVER is unknown, and correspondingly the identity of the various causes ascribed is not clear. The poisonous products of bacteria produce fever. Products of protein disintegration, whether the split-proteins of Vaughan or other products, induce fever. Foreign proteins, when introduced parenterally, often lead to fever, probably as the result of subsequent disintegration in the body. Water and hypotonic or hypertonic salt solutions induce hyperthermia. Allergic and anaphylactic phenomena are often accompanied by fever. Acute anaphylactic shock in animals, however, usually produces a fall in temperature because there is more profound intoxication than is present in the usual human cases. Lesions of the brain including cerebral hemorrhage, especially when it involves the ventricles, and traumatic lesions of the head, sometimes are accompanied by fever. There is also a so-called hysterical fever, not well established, supposed to occur in the psychoneurotic type of individual due to excitement. A reflex fever is said to occur as the result of painful excitation, as exemplified by biliary colic, but it is possible that infection plays a part. The studies of Cramer indicate that disturbances of sympathetics and adrenal-thyroid relations may produce a distinct hyperthermia similar to that of heat stroke.

The toxic fevers do not occur experimentally if the spinal cord be sectioned in the cervical region or the midbrain be removed; therefore they are probably due to influences upon the centripetal part of the mechanism of thermotaxis. Lesions of head and brain probably operate directly upon thermotaxic centers.

ARTIFICIAL FEVER. Only since the introduction of the so-called fever treatment by means of the different forms of cabinets for this purpose has it been possible to study fever in man without the influence of infections or foreign proteins. Most of the effects of artificial fever are due to sweating and hyperventilation. Both of these are responsible for loss of water from the blood and consequent hemoconcentration. This is not identical with the hemoconcentration of shock because there is no corresponding loss of plasma proteins. With a dry environment in the fever cabinet, dehydration may go as high as 15 to 20 per cent, but if the air is almost completely humidified the degree of dehydration and hemoconcentration is much less. Sweating also causes loss of blood electrolytes; the most significant of these is chloride, because cramps and exhaustion are relieved by administration of sodium chloride. The hyperpnea causes loss of carbon dioxide with a resultant tendency toward alkalosis. Indeed it is said that the greatest degrees of alkalosis are observed in marked artificial hyperthermia. Metabolism is increased, glycogen reduced and lactic acid elevated. Increase in nonprotein nitrogen in the blood is probably due in part to increased metabolism and in part to hemoconcentration. The number of erythrocytes and leukocytes is increased; that this is not altogether due to dehydration is indicated by the fact that immature forms of both are encountered evidently because of stimulation of the bone marrow. Lymphopenia is common, due apparently to destruction of lymphocytes in the lymph nodes (Doan).

CHANGES IN ORGANS AND TISSUES have been studied in man and animals. In animals hyperemia of viscera and periphery, cloudy swelling, fatty degeneration, glycogen depletion, focal hemorrhages especially in the gastro-intestinal tract, epithelial hyperplasia in parenchymatous viscera and stimulation of bone marrow occur (Jacobson and Hosoi). Few fatal cases in man have been studied, but the changes are much the same as in animals except that hyperemia, edema and small hemorrhages are conspicuous in various organs including brain. Vascular lesions include necrosis of small arteries, and thrombosis in small veins and capillaries. Thus foci of necrosis and true infarcts may occur. The hyperemia, edema and alveolar hemorrhage in the lungs may be responsible for bronchopneumonia in those who survive these more marked changes (Lichtenstein). Doan draws attention to the destruction of the lympho-cytes in lymph nodes and stimulation of large wandering mononuclear cells of the tissues, especially in the spleen, lymph nodes and the liver.

In the naturally occurring fevers of man, elevations of temperature rarely equal those obtained by the fever cabinet. The ob-servations which follow apply principally to the infectious diseases, where the fever is not simply a hyperthermia but is complicated by various metabolic disturbances incident to the disease. Heat production is increased, but not markedly. For example, DuBois found that heat production was increased 23 to 44 per cent in typhoid fever. In six different febrile diseases he observed an average heat-production increase of 13 per cent for each degree of temperature above normal. In con-trast, muscular exercise may increase heat production 300 or 400 per cent without any elevation of temperature. As a matter of fact, some patients with fever have no in-crease in heat production and even decreases are reported. With these slight alterations of heat production, heat dissipation is not ma-terially altered. According to Hewlett, the in-crease of body temperature in fever is not due primarily "to an increase of heat produc-tion or an absolute deficiency of heat dissi-pation but to a lack of adjustment between the two." The heat center is either "set" for a higher level of temperature or is in a state of altered excitability.

The respiratory rate remains about normal as does carbohydrate metabolism, but fat metabolism is increased in much the same manner as in starvation. Protein me-tabolism is increased together with consider-able destruction of body proteins, again prob-ably due to the relative starvation. With this go increases in output of uric acid, purin bases and creatinine. Although alkalosis may occur in the acute stages, in prolonged fevers acidosis may be observed probably because of a disturbance of ketogenic balance, the result of consumption of carbohydrates. In addition, there may be excessive and altered destruction of fat with consequent produc-tion of betahydroxybutyric acid, acetoacetic acid and acetone. The increased metabolism is an incident in fever, but there is no cer-tain evidence that it causes fever.

Although water and chloride are lost by sweating in high artificial fever, this is usually not the case in febrile diseases. In-deed, retention of salt is common. In this connection, pneumonia is a striking example, for during the course of the disease salt out-put is reduced and upon recovery distinctly increased. It has been shown that the reduced output is due to retention in the tissues. In contrast to the hemoconcentration of arti-ficial hyperthermia, the blood in infectious fever may be dilute. This hydremia might be expected to increase heat dissipation, but this is not necessarily true. Balcar, Sansum and Woodyat support the hypothesis that water in the body is in the form of "bound" water and "free" water. The bound water is supposed to be in combination with colloids and salts so that it is not available for ex-cretion by skin, lungs and kidneys. Thus, even though the blood may be hydremic, much of the water is bound and not avail-able for heat dissipation. It is thought that this applies to "thirst" fevers, inanition fevers of infants and the salt, lactose and glucose fevers. Nevertheless, Barr, Cecil and DuBois, as the result of study of fever due to injection of proteoses and foreign proteins, comparable in many respects to infectious diseases, state that there is "no evidence that the body is unable to mobilize water for heat elimi-nation."

The chill, which often precedes the development of fever, may be due to en-vironmental cold or to internal causes, espe-cially infection. There are minor differences in these two forms, but in general the effects are much the same. The surface temperature may be reduced, but the rectal temperature, normal at first, soon begins to rise. In ex-posure to cold the heart rate may be slowed, but in any case rises as the chill progresses. Respiration is variable, but may be shallow, jerky and even show periods of apnea. The changes in blood count are principally a drop in number of leukocytes with the ap-pearance of a few immature forms. Other-wise the blood and also the urine show no constant changes. The muscles show rhyth-mic contractions and increased tonus. There is an increased production of heat, but the rate of dissipation is variable. It is suggested that a center for chilling is situated in the posterior hypothalamic region, but this is not proved. (See Perara.)

Leukocytosis. Leukocytosis is a transient increase in the number of white blood corpuscles in the circulating blood, in contrast to the long-standing increase observed in the leukemias. The normal number of leukocytes varies within rather large limits; usually 5,000 to 10,000 per cu. mm. of blood is considered normal but not infrequently larger numbers are encountered. The number varies with age, diet, posture, altitude and numerous other conditions. In early infancy the number may be as high as 20,000 per cu. mm. or even more, diminishing during later infancy and reaching the adult figures at about the fifteenth year. Cummer suggests as standards for the proportion of the different types of leukocytes: polymorphonuclear neutrophils, 62-64 per cent; lymphocytes, 22-28 per cent; monocytes, 7.5-10 per cent; polymorphonuclear eosinophils, 1-3 per cent; and polymorphonuclear basophils (mast cells), 0.2-0.6 per cent. These estimates are only approximate and much wider ranges of the normal may be expected. During the period of high counts in infancy and childhood, the lymphocyte proportion is higher and the polymorphonuclear neutrophils lower than in adult life. With or without increases in the total number of leukocytes, various pathologic conditions may induce marked alterations in the proportion of the constituent cells. With a total increase, these may be referred to according to the type cell showing most marked increase, for example polymorphonuclear leukocytosis or eosinophilic leukocytosis. Without total increase, increases of constituent types are referred to as relative lymphocytosis, relative eosinophilia, etc.

PATHOLOGIC LEUKOCYTOSIS. Leukocytosis may be physiologic or pathologic. The physiologic form includes that incident to digestion, to pregnancy, and to muscular exercise. Pathologic leukocytosis is classified as posthemorrhagic, toxic and inflammatory. Leukocytosis also appears in association with some cases of malignant tumor and other exhausting diseases, but it is likely that this form belongs in one of the other groups.

Posthemorrhagic leukocytosis appears within 10 minutes after severe hemorrhage and may persist for several days or more. It is probable that the immediate increase in number of leukocytes is due to washing out from capillaries as fluid enters the blood from the tissues. The more lasting increase is probably due to the stimulation of the bone marrow incident to the hemorrhage.

The toxic leukocytoses include those due to drugs and those due to bacterial products. Certain chemicals such as the coal-tar drugs, chlorates and carbon monoxide may produce leukocytosis by the destruction of erythrocytes or by a relative asphyxia with resultant stimulation of bone marrow. The action of narcosis may be asphyxial. Leukocytosis due to the local application of such irritants as mustard oil, croton oil, and cantharidin may be attributed to products of the local inflammatory reaction. Various products of bacteria, including toxins, tuberculin, vaccines, and protein extracts may produce leukocytosis, and this probably bears directly upon the problem of leukocytosis in infectious disease. Its mechanism is discussed under the inflammatory leukocytoses. Peptone, pus, and various tissue and organ extracts produce leukocytosis probably in the same way. Bacon, Novy and Eppler take the view that the activating substances are essentially the intermediate products of protein cleavage such as proteoses, peptones and polypeptides.

Inflammatory or infectious leukocytosis depends upon the severity of the infection and the response of the body. Thus, fulminant infections may produce such immediate depression of the entire body as to lead to no leukocytosis. Other conditions may also produce decrease or absence of reaction. Within limits, the more severe the infection the greater the leukocytosis. Leukocytosis represents part of the general reaction, but it is difficult to say that any local inflammation associated with leukocytosis is necessarily to be regarded as an infectious disease in the narrower sense of the term. As a general rule, infectious leukocytosis shows primarily a marked proportional increase in the polymorphonuclear neutrophils, then a relative increase of lymphocytes and later of eosinophils, but these latter increases do not blot out altogether the proportional increase of polymorphonuclear neutrophils. Such leukocytoses show counts of about 15,000, 20,000 per cu. mm. or more, of which 80 to 90 per cent or more are polymorphonuclear neutrophils.

Nearly all the infectious diseases are

accompanied by leukocytosis, the notable exceptions being typhoid fever (often showing a decrease in leukocytes and later a slight relative increase of lymphocytes), tuberculosis (except when secondary infection is present), measles, mumps, influenza, glanders and acute poliomyelitis. Malaria may show a leukocytosis at the time of the chill but otherwise either a normal or decreased leukocyte count.

In Malignancy. Malignant tumors, of themselves, do not produce leukocytosis. Leukocytosis may result, however, from secondary changes in tumors such as infection or marked necrosis. Metastatic invasion of bone marrow may also stimulate a leukocytosis. The so-called cachectic leukocytosis of malignant tumors is probably to be explained by any of the secondary changes just mentioned, invasion of bone marrow or terminal infections such as pneumonia. Many patients, seriously ill as the result of malignant tumors, show little or no leukocytosis.

Agonal leukocytosis is that which often appears just before death. This may be due to slowing of the circulation of blood so that the leukocytes accumulate in upper parts of the body or it may be due to terminal infections. It has also been supposed that the approach of death releases those forces which normally hold the immature blood cells in the bone marrow, thus permitting their entrance into the circulating blood; there is as yet no definite support for this hypothesis.

ORIGIN OF LEUKOCYTOSIS. Both mature leukocytes and immature forms appear in leukocytosis. The mature forms are incapable of dividing and only with great rarity is mitosis seen in very young forms. Thus leukocytosis is not due to cell multiplication in the circulating blood. The cause must be something which both stimulates production of white cells and accounts for their release into the blood from the cell-forming organs, especially from the bone marrow and lymph nodes. This might be the action of chemotactic agents. Thus, positive chemotaxis could cause leukocytosis and negative chemotaxis cause leukopenia. In typhoid fever there is hyperplasia of the lymphatic apparatus and the leukopenia might be due to negative chemotaxis. On the other hand, leukocytosis does not occur in uncomplicated tuberculosis, but Wartman has demonstrated that protein

of the bacilli is positively chemotactic. Menkin has extracted a substance from inflammatory exudates which induces leukocytosis; it is probably a globulin or closely associated protein; it is different from the positively chemotactic leukotaxine mentioned in the discussion of inflammation. The influence of chemotaxis in exciting leukocytosis is not yet determined. There is a vague suggestion that leukocytosis is part of the general immune responses of the body to infection, but there is no reason to state that they contribute to the formation of immune bodies or of complement. It may be that leukocytosis is related to other factors incident to alterations of water balance in the body, to fever, and to protein cleavage products.

Metchnikoff indicated a certain degree of specificity of function of phagocytic cells when he differentiated micro- and macrophages. That there is, however, a qualitative difference in the type of cell in leukocytosis as the result of special stimuli is open to question. Infestations by animal parasites, particularly the *Trichinella spiralis*, may lead to an increase in the number of circulating eosinophils, as is true also of certain inflammatory skin diseases, of which dermatitis herpetiformis is a striking example. The function of this eosinophilia is unknown. In infectious diseases of early childhood the leukocytosis may be predominantly lymphocytic, but what seems to be the same type of infection in other children and in adults is accompanied by a polymorphonuclear leukocytosis.

Pathologic Effects of Infectious Disease. Infectious diseases have certain special effects and also lesions that are common to nearly all. The cutaneous lesions of the exanthemata are usually characteristic. Pneumonia, typhoid fever, acute anterior poliomyelitis, epidemic meningitis and many other infectious diseases exhibit phenomena that are more or less peculiar to each disease. The conditions that are common to most of the infectious diseases include various degrees of hyperplasia of the lymphadenoid structures and of anemia. Of especial importance, however, are the effects of injurious products of the disease or the organism, or both, upon the parenchymatous viscera. Cloudy swelling occurs and, in more severe or long-standing infections, fatty degeneration; still greater severity may lead to local necroses or to parenchymatous inflammations. Thus, cloudy swelling or more serious lesions of the myocardium may lead to low blood pressure and cardiac arrhythmias. Acute inflammations of the endocardium, particularly its valvular portions, may lead to death directly or give origin to crippling, chronic valve lesions. Pyemias may show abscesses in the myocardium. Fatty degeneration of the intima of the aorta is extremely common and more serious disease of arteries sometimes occurs, in rare instances leading to such important lesions as mycotic aneurysms of small vessels. Veins are not uncommonly the seat of thrombophlebitis, especially as a sequel of typhoid fever. Serous membranes, more especially pericardium and pleura, often show acute inflammations which in case of recovery result in chronic fibrous adhesions. In the pericardium such adhesions may lead to serious disturbances of the heart. Voluntary muscles may apparently suffer from cloudy swelling and fatty degeneration. In typhoid fever, influenza and other infections, Zenker's hyaline necrosis may occur. Degenerative lesions of the liver, pancreas and glands of the alimentary tract lead to digestive and nutritional disturbances. Cloudy swelling of kidneys may cause albuminuria and the appearance of hyaline casts. The process may become more severe and an acute nephritis develop. The nervous system may be affected by degenerative changes, but this is not common save in connection with diphtheria and those diseases where the nervous system is primarily involved.

The acute degenerative conditions are not only of import in the course of the disease but may be persistent for a long time after the disease has disappeared. Such sequels are more common with greater severity of the infection, and young individuals recover more readily than older ones. If acute parenchymatous inflammations develop, particularly in the kidney, they may become chronic and result in serious disability and ultimately in death. Acute infectious diseases are directly responsible for most of the chronic diseases of man, and represent the most common and most important group of conditions to be considered in any general study of etiology. This fact will become more and more apparent as the sections in special pathology are studied.

SPECIAL TYPES OF INFECTION

Pyogenic Infections

The foregoing is merely a brief outline of the general principles of infectious disease. Further discussion of numerous infectious diseases will be found in the chapters on Systemic Pathology. In this chapter, consideration is given to a few of the infectious diseases only which serve as examples. Various organisms are pus producers, but there are variations with a single organism and with organisms operating in various situations. The pyogenic cocci regularly lead to production of pus and consideration will be given to staphylococcal and streptococcal infections.

Staphylococcal Infections. Those due to *Staphylococcus aureus* are the most important. There are two type-specific forms of the organism, identifiable by precipitins. Type B is essentially nonpathogenic. Type A, the pathogenic form, has a type-specific carbohydrate, sometimes is encapsulated, and produces toxins of different orders including hemolytic, dermatonecrotic, gastrointestinal (food poisoning), leukocidal and a lethal toxin which kills animals rapidly upon intravenous injection. Type B produces a coagulase acting upon blood plasma and perhaps a fibrinolysin. Types A and B, as well as other staphylococci, may produce local suppuration in the form of abscess, phlegmon or cellulitis. Toxins may be absorbed from these especially if due to type A, but usually only in small quantity and with only slight toxemia. More important is the entry of the bacteria into the blood stream. The portals of entry, including skin, respiratory, alimentary and genito-urinary tracts, can usually be identified because of localized suppuration. Unless the local focus goes on to healing, dissemination occurs either by way of the lymphatics or directly into the blood stream.

The entry of organisms into lymphatics takes place by the usual routes of drainage. Furthermore, phagocytes may ingest bacteria and travel along the lymphatics. If the bacteria are not killed, they may be released by death of the phagocyte and multiply. Commonly a lymphangitis is produced and in cases where the infection is in or near the skin, this lymphangitis is evident as a red, tender and sometimes painful streak. The regional lymph nodes may become the seat of acute hyperplasia or may actually suppurate.

If the organisms are not stopped in the lymph nodes they may then be transported into the venous system. It is also possible that as an abscess extends, it may erode small blood vessels so that bacteria enter the blood stream directly. Here again migration of phagocytes may play a part. Since these organisms are pathogenic and toxin-producers, the condition is not simply a bacteremia but an actual septicemia. Bacteria may lodge in various organs, perhaps in part as the result of phagocytic activity by cells lining the blood vessels, or because small clumps become stopped in tortuous capillaries or at the point of division of vessels. In these situations they may give rise to abscesses similar to those at the portal of entry. When these secondary abscesses develop, the condition is pyemia. The gross and microscopic characters of these abscesses are not materially different from those of the original focus, except that septic infarcts occur when small arteries are occluded by bacterial emboli. Such secondary or metastatic abscesses are found in the kidneys, spleen, myocardium, lungs, brain and other viscera but are uncommon in the liver. Acute bacterial endocarditis may also develop. Hepatic abscesses are found particularly when there is a focus of infection in the portal drainage area, or in the gallbladder or the ducts of the liver. The toxins indicated above may have their special and general effects so that cloudy swelling frequently occurs and if the disease be intense or of long duration, may be succeeded by fatty degeneration and even focal points of necrosis together with acute parenchymatous inflammation. The hemolytic toxin may be responsible for a marked degree of anemia. In 122 cases of staphylococcal infection, studied by Skinner and Keefer, the gross mortality rate was about 82 per cent. Of those who recovered, the majority were less than 30 years of age. When recovery took place it usually followed a protracted course.

Streptococcal Infections. The course of these varies somewhat according to the type of streptococcus responsible, as to whether it is the hemolytic form, the viridans form or the nonhemolytic form. Infections by *Streptococcus viridans* (alpha streptococcus) are likely to run a somewhat protracted course. Infections with the hemolytic streptococcus (beta streptococcus) and with the nonhemolytic streptococcus (gamma streptococcus) are likely to be more acute.

The principles of entry, the production of localized suppuration and further extension of the disease are much the same as is true in connection with staphylococci, except that with hemolytic streptococci the lesions are likely to spread more rapidly and give rise to early toxemia. Acute streptococcal septicemia is prevalent in the extremes of life and is secondary especially to infections of the throat and ear in early life and to cellulitis and erysipelas in later life. About 30 per cent of the cases of septicemia become pyemic and of the septicemic cases there is approximately a 70 per cent mortality (Keefer et al.). The relationship of streptococcal infection to rheumatic fever will be taken up subsequently. Nevertheless, streptococcal septicemias are especially likely to be accompanied by acute alterative inflammations, especially in the heart and kidney. In the heart there is cloudy swelling and even necrosis of the muscle-fiber cells together with foci of lymphocytes and plasma cells in the interstitial tissue. Sometimes polymorphonuclear leukocytes and eosinophils are present. The same general manifestations may occur in the kidney, as well as in the liver, pancreas and other organs. These lesions may precede or be quite independent of the metastatic abscesses of streptococcal pyemia. (Mallory and Keefer.)

Much prominence has been given the studies of E. C. Rosenow on the elective localization of streptococci. The principle briefly stated is that streptococci, freshly isolated, tend to produce lesions in experimental animals similar to those of the patient. Thus, streptococci from endocarditis produce endocarditis in the rabbit, those from infected gallbladders produce gallbladder inflammation, and so on with streptococci from a wide variety of sources. It has also been maintained that hidden and more or less latent foci of streptococci, more especially the green-producing form (*viridans*), at tooth apices, in tonsils and other places are responsible for a wide variety of vague symptoms, particularly muscle pains, and for serious lesions such as endocarditis, nephritis, anemia, etc. The hypothesis is attractive, but confirmation is not convincing and contradiction has been offered by many well qualified workers. (Reimann.)

Suppuration may be produced by organisms other than the staphylococcus and streptococcus and follow the same general course. Colon bacilli, innocuous in the intestinal canal, may be extremely virulent in other situations, especially the peritoneum. Pneumococci, diphtheria bacilli, Friedlander's bacilli, and a host of others, under special conditions and situations, may be pyogenic.

Diphtheria (Toxemia)

This disease, due to the Klebs-Loeffler bacillus or *Corynebacterium diphtheriae*, produces local and general symptoms. The local symptoms arise at the point of invasion of the organism and the general symptoms are due to its toxin. In so far as general manifestations are concerned, they are to be regarded as those of toxemia. The primary invasion is usually in the upper respiratory tract, particularly in the tonsils and fauces. Primary or secondary local invasion may occur in other situations such as skin, conjunctiva, etc. The lesions in the latter situations are likely to be limited and rarely produce serious toxemia. When the tonsils and fauces are involved, functional disturbance is evident, especially in swallowing; this is probably due to pain. Extension into the nose may occur, or the disease may be primary in the nose, in which case nasal breathing becomes difficult or impossible. Extension may also occur to the larynx, and obstruction to breathing is often serious or disastrous.

The inflammation set up by the diphtheria bacillus is characteristically a fibrinous or fibrino-purulent inflammation. Destruction of the superficial epithelium is rapidly followed by fluid exudation and fibrin formation. The fibrin is deposited through a relatively small amount of the superficial part of the tissue, and is most massive as the so-called membrane or pseudomembrane on the surface. The fibrin mesh of the pseudomembrane and that of the tissues inter-

communicate. Included in the exudate are desquamated epithelial cells, more or less degenerate or necrotic, a number of leukocytes, lymphocytes, diphtheria bacilli, and other

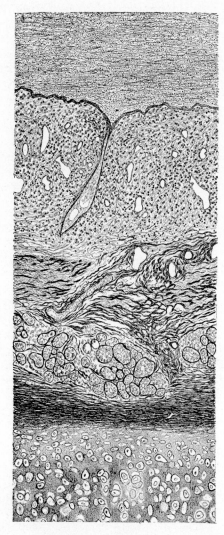

Laryngeal diphtheria. Note the fibrinous exudate on the surface, the large capillary spaces, edema and leukocyte infiltration of the underlying connective tissue.

bacteria. In the early stages, this pseudomembrane appears as a smooth, well-defined, creamy white or pale yellow material which, when detached, leaves a somewhat raw, slightly bleeding surface. As the disease progresses, the color may become distinctly yellow due to the increasing infiltration of leukocytes. The exudate may become more or less necrotic thus producing a shaggy or ragged surface, owing to dropping out of necrotic material. The underlying tissues are hyperemic and show less dense but similar exudation. Extension along the bronchi may lead to bronchopneumonia which is usually distinctly fibrinous in character. Bronchopneumonia may also be produced by aspiration of small masses of exudate and bacteria. It appears probable that when the lung is involved, further extension may occur because of transmission along lymphatic tracts by a fibrinous lymphangitis.

Formerly the term "diphtheritic inflammation" was applied to any type of inflammation which formed a pseudo-membrane on a mucous surface. Thus, a similar membrane may be formed upon the surface of the intestine in bacillary dysentery. It seems wiser to apply to these other forms the term "fibrinous inflammation," and to reserve the term "diphtheritic inflammation" solely for that due to the diphtheria bacillus. The term "croupous inflammation" has been applied to fibrinous inflammation involving the respiratory tract from and including the trachea, downward. This term should be abandoned. The term "croup" is a clinical term indicating difficulty of respiration due to lesions within the larynx. This has no direct bearing on the pathology of the condition, and as a rule diphtheritic croup and spasmodic croup can be distinguished clinically.

GRAVIS DIPHTHERIA. It has been found, however, that there is an especially malignant form of diphtheria, with relatively little exudate in the throat but with local destruction of tissue and marked inflammatory edema of the neck, and with profound toxic effects upon viscera and nerves. (See MacLeod et al.). This is due to *C. diphtheriae gravis*. The *mitis* form may occasionally act similarly, but most often it shows considerable exudate, which is usually superficial but may extend laterally, and produces only a relatively mild toxemia. Between the two is the *intermedius* form. Immunization with toxoid sometimes fails to prevent gravis diphtheria, and treatment with antitoxin, even in massive doses, may be disappointing. O'Meara reports that in addition to the usual toxin, diphtheria bacilli produce another antigenic substance which can be extracted in salt solution from the bacterial bodies. These he calls A and B respectively. The *mitis* form,

used in the production of antitoxin, produces mainly the A substance and only little B. The *gravis* form produces relatively little A, but large quantities of B. The B substance is highly toxic, with marked local effects in animals. These facts appear to explain the differences in manifestations, prevention and treatment of diphtheria.

The pathologic effects in viscera and nerves are different in degree, depending upon amounts of unneutralized toxin. Thus, the heart and vascular muscle, the liver, kidneys

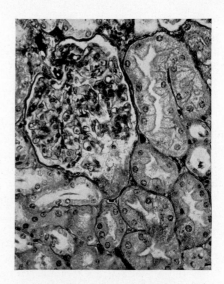

Cloudy swelling of the tubular epithelium of the kidney in diphtheria. Army Medical Museum 44904.

and other parenchymatous organs show varying degrees of parenchymatous degeneration, from simple cloudy swelling to severe fatty degeneration and even necrosis. Circulatory deficiency is very common in man and in experimental animals. It has been thought that the circulatory failure is primarily vasomotor, but the lesions of the heart and the studies of Edmunds and Cooper indicate that the myocardium is principally at fault. There is little good reason to believe that the transmission bundles of the heart are diseased. In addition to degenerations of the muscle, the myocardium may show acute interstitial inflammation. Occasionally acute endocarditis and pericarditis occur. Digestive disturbances are common and are believed to be due to parenchymatous degeneration of the glands. The liver, particularly, is likely to show severe cloudy swelling and even fatty degeneration. Focal necrosis of the liver is occasionally observed. The spleen and lymph nodes generally, including the Peyer's patches of the intestine, are likely to show varying degrees of acute hyperplasia. The kidneys are frequently involved by cloudy swelling, which may be evident clinically by the presence of albuminuria and hyaline casts. It is not uncommon, however, for this change in the kidney to proceed further to an acute nephritis. In addition to cloudy swelling, the tubular epithelium may show fatty degeneration, hyaline droplet formation, and even necrosis; the interstitial tissues may be infiltrated by leukocytes, plasma cells and lymphoid cells. The glomerular capsules occasionally show proliferation of their epithelium, but more common is involvement of the glomerular tufts. In this situation, there may be swelling and proliferation of capillary endothelium and frequently the formation of hyaline masses, or hyaline thrombi, within the capillaries. The lesions in peripheral nerves are due to the toxin (Feiner). They are principally degenerative and affect the axis cylinders and myelin sheaths. Occasionally there is also a slight infiltration of lymphocytes and plasma cells, but this inflammatory component is not marked. Recovery or cicatrization may follow. As a result, paralyses occur in palatal muscles and in other skeletal muscle; lesion of the vagus may lead to death from its influence on the heart. Skeletal muscle occasionally shows fatty degeneration and sometimes Zenker's hyaline necrosis. In experimental animals, hyperemia and hemorrhage of the adrenals occur; such lesions are common but not constant in man.

It will thus be seen that diphtheria in its more serious manifestations is principally a toxemia. Nevertheless, death may be due to local effects particularly in the case of laryngeal diphtheria.

Typhoid and Paratyphoid Fevers (Septicemia)

Typhoid Fever. This is due to the typhoid bacillus, often called the bacillus of Eberth and properly designated as *Eberthella typhosa*. The organisms multiply in the lymph nodules of the intestine and soon enter the blood so that septicemia develops early. Blood cultures become positive at about the time of onset and remain so for about a week. Although the bacilli disappear from the blood they may remain in organs, such as lymph nodes and spleen, and have been recovered from bone marrow up to 3 weeks after onset (Sacks and Hachtel). The organisms, which are derived from the feces or, rarely, the urine, of a patient or carrier of the disease, are ingested with food or drink and enter the body through the intestine, presumably by way of the lymphoid structures. Goodpasture presents evidence that young plasma cells of the lymph nodes are essential cellular hosts in the process of infection. Rare cases are reported which are septicemic throughout and evidence no local lesions; in some of these the bacteria probably enter through some portal other than the intestine. The intoxication which accompanies the septicemia is probably due in large part to endotoxin liberated by the death of organisms, but since it has been shown that the bacillus of paratyphoid fever *B* elaborates an exotoxin, it is possible that an exotoxin can be produced by *Eberthella typhosa*, which plays a part in typhoid fever. The general symptoms include particularly: varying degrees of prostration, fever which reaches its maximum in the second or third week of the disease and gradually declines by lysis, and a very pale red macular eruption on the abdomen, in the axillae and sometimes in other parts of the body. Diarrhea is a common manifestation of the disease, but this is not always the case. The "pea soup" stools of the older writers probably depended more upon the diet given the patient than upon the disease itself.

LESIONS. The principal local lesions of typhoid fever are observed in the lymphoid apparatus of the abdominal cavity, including the Peyer's patches and solitary follicles of the intestinal canal, mesenteric and retroperitoneal lymph nodes and the spleen. The course of events in these lymphoid aggregates is hyperemia, hyperplasia and necrosis. The hyperplasia of the spleen is observed at first as an enlargement which may reach a weight of 300 to 400 grams or more; it is a large, firm, red spleen, with a tense smooth transparent capsule. The organ cuts with decreased resistance and shows a slightly bulging, pink, fairly firm, moist cut surface. The Peyer's patches of the intestine enlarge in all diameters. They are sharply defined, somewhat pink, considerably elevated above the intestinal surface and superficially give a somewhat convoluted appearance suggesting the cortical surface of the brain of a small animal. The solitary follicles may show the same appearance except that they are not likely to be convoluted on the surface. Microscopically, the enlargement of all these organs is found to be due partly to hyperemia, infiltration of plasma cells and occasional leukocytes and lymphoid hyperplasia, and partly to hy-

visible grossly, except that these organs become distinctly softened. Microscopically, however, minute foci of necrosis may be demonstrated.

The same process occurs in the Peyer's patches, but inasmuch as these are upon a body surface, namely the surface of the intestinal canal, necrotic material is likely to slough out of the Peyer's patch leaving an ulcer. At first the ulceration appears as multiple small ulcers in the surface of the Peyer's

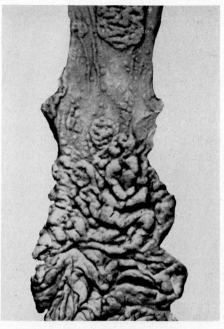

Hyperplasia of Peyer's patches and of solitary follicles in typhoid fever. The lower portion is just above the ileocecal junction and shows the convoluted surface.

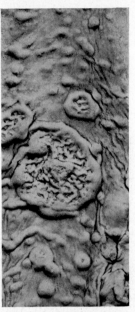

Early ulceration of Peyer's patches in typhoid fever, also in some of the hyperplastic solitary follicles.

perplasia and multiplication of the endothelium of the lymphatic sinuses and of the pulp. The endothelial cells frequently show phagocytosis of nuclear fragments, of entire lymphocytes, of red cells, and of tissue detritus. Special staining will demonstrate typhoid bacilli, which are likely to be present in considerable numbers in the large mononuclear cells.

Necrosis appears following the stage of acute hyperplasia. The necrosis is probably due to interference with the free flow of nutritive fluid, due to the general hyperplasia and possibly in part due to substances elaborated by the organism. In the spleen and lymph nodes the necrosis is not usually

patch; the ulcers subsequently fuse together to be coextensive with the patch. The edges are likely to be somewhat undermined and the base rough and often stained by the intestinal contents. In the uncomplicated cases the necrotic areas of the spleen and lymph nodes are removed in the usual way. The Peyer's patch becomes covered with surface epithelium under which is cicatricial tissue due to organization. In young individuals there is undoubtedly some regeneration of the lymphoid structures, but the glandular epithelium does not regenerate. No attempt is made in this discussion to correlate the anatomic changes with the stages of the disease in terms of weeks. No such correlation is accurately possible. In the same case, for example, one frequently sees simple hyperplasia in the upper part of the ileum, whereas necrosis may be well advanced in the lower ileum. The lymphoid nodules in the bone marrow may also show the same sort of hyperplasia and this disturbance may be responsible for the leukopenia of typhoid fever.

infection is likely to extend more deeply into the intestinal wall. It may progress as far as the peritoneal coat. As the ulceration extends, the margin shows a definite inflammatory reaction, and, as the peritoneal coat becomes involved, inflammation appears on the peritoneal surface, particularly in the form of a fibrin deposit. The further extensions of the

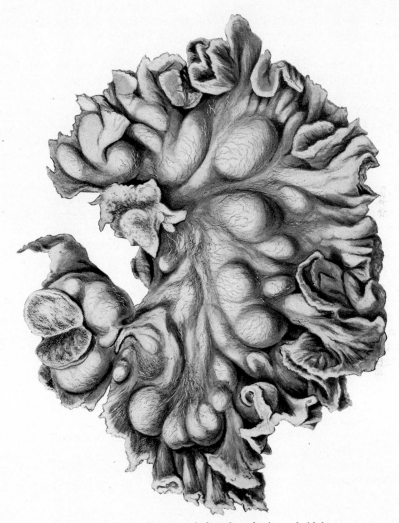

Acute hyperplasia of mesenteric lymph nodes in typhoid fever.

Complications. The local lesions in the intestinal tract may show serious complicating features. When necrosis occurs in the Peyer's patches and material drops into the intestinal canal, a raw surface is exposed which is susceptible to secondary infection from the intestinal contents. Thus, the ulcer in its later stages represents not simply a necrotic ulcer, but because of the secondary

ulcer may cause perforation of the intestinal wall allowing the escape of the intestinal contents and bacteria into the peritoneal cavity. If the perforation has progressed slowly, the preceding deposits on the peritoneal surface may bring about adhesion with neighboring coils of gut or to the abdominal wall, so that when the perforation occurs, it may open into a small cavity entirely surrounded by fibrin and fibrinous adhesions. Often, however, this protective fibrinous adhesion does not occur or is torn by distention and movement of the gut, and widespread peritonitis ensues. In the ordinary course of events, when an ulcer occurs in any situation, the inflammatory reaction in the margin includes a reactive thrombosis of any blood vessels which happen to be in the path of extension. If, however, the ulceration be extremely rapid, this thrombosis may not be sufficient to protect against the pressure in the blood vessels, the thrombi may be expelled and hemorrhage occurs. In the intestinal wall a further danger comes from intestinal movement and particularly from distention by gas which may be sufficient to dislodge thrombi and thereby lead to hemorrhage into the lumen of the gut. The two important complications of typhoid fever referable to the intestines are perforation and hemorrhage. The hemorrhage may lead to severe secondary anemia or even to death.

PATHOLOGIC ANATOMY. As in all serious infectious diseases, typhoid fever also is likely to be accompanied by cloudy swelling of parenchymatous organs and in the more severe cases, fatty degeneration. Various organs may be involved in the course of typhoid fever with lesions more or less characteristic of the disease.

In the alimentary canal as a whole, the mouth and pharynx may be the seat of mild inflammation which occasionally goes on to ulceration and sometimes membrane formation. The esophagus is sometimes ulcerated immediately posterior to the larynx. The stomach may show a mild catarrh, and in extremely rare cases the lymphoid follicles of the stomach are involved as are those of the intestine and may go on to ulceration. A general catarrhal inflammation of the ileum sometimes occurs, particularly if there be severe secondary infection of the ulcers. This may be accompanied by pseudomembrane formation and sometimes gangrene of the gut.

In the respiratory system, enlargement and even ulceration of the tonsils may be encountered. A low grade inflammation of the larynx is not rare and occasionally may show pseudomembrane formation with serious disturbance of respiration. Ulceration may also appear in this situation. A common accompaniment of typhoid fever is passive hyperemia of the dependent parts of the lungs. A low-grade catarrhal bronchitis is fairly frequent and this, in association with the passive hyperemia and edema, may finally result in a bronchopneumonia. The association of lobar pneumonia with typhoid fever is not rare. Pleurisy may occur and occasionally empyema is observed.

The circulatory system shows important disturbances; general blood pressure is low and the pulse is almost constantly dicrotic. The cardiac muscle usually shows cloudy swelling, may show fatty degeneration and occasionally shows hyaline necrosis. Inflammations of the pericardium and endocardium may occur. Not uncommon is thrombophlebitis, particularly in the iliac and femoral veins.

In the genito-urinary system, aside from cloudy swelling of the kidney, occasional cases of acute nephritis are encountered. The bladder may be the seat of catarrhal or pseudomembranous inflammation. Orchitis and epididymitis occur rarely. In the nervous system degenerative changes are encountered in the ganglion cells and thrombosis of venous sinuses may occur. Typhoid meningitis has been reported in several instances. In the bone, low-grade periostitis sometimes occurs and in rare instances actual suppurative periostitis. In the muscles, particularly in the recti abdominis, a common change is Zenker's hyaline necrosis.

Focal necrosis of the liver is more common in typhoid fever than in any other disease. Grossly, the necrosis is only rarely visible. Microscopically, the foci of necrosis are irregularly distributed and occupy only a small part of the lobule. In the section they are generally circular, with complete disappearance of cord cells, and in their place is a mass of endothelial cells with which there may be a few lymphoid cells and an occasional polymorphonuclear leukocyte. The origin of these lesions has been discussed in the chapter on Necrosis and Somatic Death.

Survival from an attack of typhoid fever usually, but not invariably, confers a lasting immunity. The immunity to paratyphoid fever conferred by an attack of typhoid fever is probably not so great as with the homologous disease. Agglutinins appear in the blood toward the end of the first week, usually reach a maximum in the third week, but persist in lower titer for years. Vaccina-

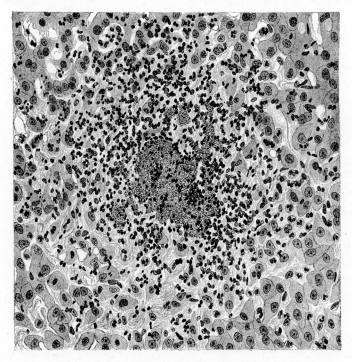

Early focal necrosis of the liver in typhoid fever, showing infiltration of large mononuclear cells and an unusual number of leukocytes.

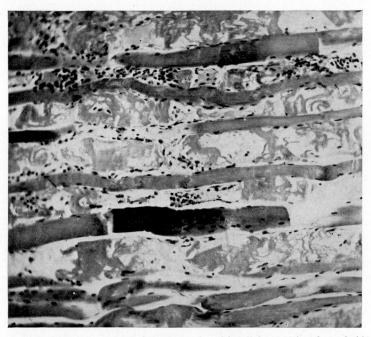

Zenker's hyaline necrosis of skeletal muscle, with cellular reaction, in typhoid fever. Army Medical Museum 46831.

tion also induces agglutinin formation, lasting for years. The agglutinins are of two forms, the O agglutinin against the somatic portion of the bacilli and the H agglutinin against the flagellar portion. In the course of the disease the O agglutinins usually but not invariably reach higher titers than the H form, whereas the agglutinin due to vaccination is principally the H form. Precipitins, opsonins and complement fixing antibodies develop, and skin reactions can be produced with typhoid antigen. The titer of the various immune bodies is not a safe guide to the degree of immunity to the disease. Some consider the mouse protection test an index of resistance to infection (Siler).

Paratyphoid Fevers. In principle these fevers follow the same general rules as those laid down for typhoid fever. Whereas the course of typhoid fever runs over a period of three or four weeks before convalescence sets in, in the case of paratyphoid A (*Salmonella paratyphi*) the course may be shorter, and in the case of paratyphoid B (*S. schottmülleri*) considerably longer. Moreover, these types are usually not so severe as is typhoid fever. The pathologic lesions and the immunologic reactions are much the same. Certain forms of the typhoid bacillus not included in these three categories have been described and are generally grouped under the comprehensive heading of paratyphoid C (*S. hirschfeldii*).

SPIROCHETAL DISEASES

Syphilis and yaws are discussed in the chapter on Infectious Granulomata. Spirochetes presumably are symbionts with fusiform bacilli in causing Vincent's angina. Of the acute infectious diseases which are due to spirochetes, the most important are Weil's disease and rat-bite fever.

Leptospirosis

Weil's disease, spirochetal jaundice or infectious jaundice, occurs in most parts of the world. Since it may be subclinical and varies from mild to severe in its manifestations, the term "leptospirosis" has been adopted. It is generally milder in the United States than in other parts of the world. The disease is usually due to *Leptospira icterohaemorrhagiae*, transmitted by the wild gray rat. Occasional cases are caused by the *Leptospira canicola* of the dog. The excreta of more than 10 per cent of the common wild gray rat contain the leptospira of Weil's disease. These are found also in the field mouse, cat, pig, fox and horse. In a sense the disease is an occupational hazard because it occurs in those who work in moist places which may be contaminated by the urine or feces of the wild rat. Thus it occurs in miners in wet places, sewer diggers, cutters and cleaners of fish, tunnel workers and those working about poultry yards. It is also reported to have followed swimming in contaminated places (Havens, et al.). Only with great rarity does it follow the bite of the wild rat and it is not identical with rat-bite fever. About 90 per cent of the cases occur in males. Although rare in children, it can occur at any time of life and is most frequent in the age period between 10 and 40 years.

The clinical picture is divided into three stages.

In the first stage, following a sudden onset, there are headache, vomiting, fever, pains in muscles of the body, more particularly the calf muscles, and prostration. Leukocytosis may be marked. This is a septicemic stage; the organisms can be found in the circulating blood but during this time they are not present in the urine. Although the organisms can be identified fairly satisfactorily by darkfield illumination of blood films, the use of either blood cultures or intraperitoneal inoculation into young guinea pigs is more satisfactory. Agglutinating and lytic antibodies develop from about the eighth to the tenth day and are most important in diagnosis.

Second Stage. After about a week the patient enters the second, or toxic stage. Here the general manifestations are well marked and, in the more severe cases, jaundice appears. Organisms have disappeared from the blood but they occur in the urine at about the same time that antibodies appear. In the fatal cases the jaundice increases, the output of urine decreases and there is retention of nitrogenous products in the blood due to the development of renal disease. Purpura appears on the skin and mucous membranes, there is a fall of blood pressure and death ensues.

IN THE THIRD OR CONVALESCENT STAGE of the favorable cases, the antibodies in the blood are of high titer and organisms continue to be excreted in the urine. In this convalescent stage attacks of secondary fever sometimes ensue.

The anatomic lesions include degenerations of the parenchymatous viscera and hemorrhages due to deterioration of the walls of small blood vessels. This is one of the infectious diseases in which spleen and lymph nodes are not likely to show hyperplasia, although the lymph nodes may be hemorrhagic. The kidney is the organ most markedly involved. It is slightly enlarged, soft, generally pallid but with tiny hemorrhages and is sometimes icteric. Microscopically, the tubular epithelium shows cloudy swelling, necrosis and desquamation. There may be a slight proliferation of endothelium in the capillary tufts but this is not conspicuous. Organisms are found in the lumina of the tubules, and to a limited degree in the interstitial tissues.

The liver is slightly enlarged and bile stained. Occasionally there is a mild acute cholangitis affecting the smaller bile passages but in general it cannot be said that the icterus is due to this disorder. The cells of the cords show marked cloudy swelling, sometimes with considerable dissociation. Irregularly distributed foci of necrosis are also found. Fatty change is not marked. Stagnation of bile may be found in the central zones. Organisms are sometimes found in the lymphatic spaces around the sinusoids.

The heart may show marked cloudy swelling or even a slight acute alterative or interstitial myocarditis. The lungs are hyperemic and hemorrhages are often observed. The process may go on to a hemorrhagic type of bronchopneumonia. The skeletal muscles are usually normal to gross inspection except for a few punctae of hemorrhage. Microscopically, however, the muscles of the calf and also the pectoral muscles show a change comparable to that seen in Zenker's hyaline necrosis. The principal difference is that in typhoid fever the rectus muscles of the abdomen are affected, whereas in Weil's disease the lesions are in the calf and the pectoral muscles. Inflammations of serous membranes occur and an occasional case of meningitis is reported.

The deterioration of capillaries results in minute hemorrhages throughout the body. These are most commonly observed in the peritoneum, the pleura, the stomach and intestines, the kidneys, the mucosa of the nose, and the skin and are not infrequently massive in the adrenals. The brain and meninges may also show these hemorrhages. The hemorrhages may be severe enough to induce epistaxis, hemoptysis, hematemesis, hematuria or melena. For the first few days, the spirochetes are entirely in extracellular positions. They then enter various parenchymatous cells where they may remain for a considerable period of time, but they persist longer in the kidney than elsewhere. (Ashe, et al.; Havens, et al.; Rathbun and Waghelstein.)

The form of the disease due to the *Leptospira canicola* of the dog is much the same except that the tendency to icterus is less and the likelihood of hemorrhage greater (Raven).

Rat-Bite Fever

This disease, also called Sodoku, is caused by the *Spirochaeta morsus muris*. It is usually induced by the bite of an infected wild rat; other rodents may carry the infection, however, and it has been reported in the cat. Children are more often affected than older people because of rat bites during sleep. The bite itself usually heals promptly but after an incubation period varying from a few days to a month or even more, there is an abrupt onset of fever, together with swelling, redness and tenderness of the site of the original bite. Together with this, a local lymphangitis and acute hyperplasia of the regional nodes often occur, followed by general lymph node hyperplasia. The spleen is affected in the same way. There is an erythematous rash over the trunk and extremities. Leukocytosis appears with an increase in eosinophils and a reduction in the relative number of lymphocytes. After a few days there is a remission of the disease but relapses may occur several times. The course of the disease ranges over a few weeks and may last for months. Death is uncommon.

The anatomic manifestations are not especially striking. There is acute hyperplasia of spleen and lymph nodes, together with cloudy swelling of myocardium, liver and kidneys. Sometimes there is acute inflammation of serous cavities, mainly pericardium and pleura. Disease of the small blood vessels is not common but when it occurs there are minute hemorrhages in various situations. In the lungs this may develop into a hemorrhagic pneumonia.

Haverhill Fever. Not to be confused with rat-bite fever is Haverhill fever, contracted by bites of rats and from contaminated milk. This is also given the descriptive name "erythema arthriticum epidemicum." The onset is abrupt and the manifestations include chills, fever, vomiting and headache, a macular eruption chiefly on the extremities and inflamed, painful and tender joints. The causative organism, grown from blood and fluid of joints is *Haverhillia multiformis* of Parker and Hudson. Its exact classification is not final, but it probably is one of the order actinomycetales, family mycobacteriaceae. (See Farrell, et al.)

RICKETTSIAL DISEASES

The rickettsiae are defined by Wolbach as micro-organisms adapted to arthropods (insects) and pathogenic for vertebrates. They are characterized by small size (1 to 2 micra), pleomorphism, slight affinity for aniline dyes and the fact that they are intracellular in the insect host. They are gram-negative and grow only in media in which there is fresh tissue. There are many forms, but only three or perhaps four are pathogenic for man. *Rickettsia prowazeki* causes typhus fever; *Dermacentroxenus rickettsii* causes Rocky Mountain spotted fever, and *Rickettsia nipponica* causes Japanese river sickness or tsutsugamuchi disease. It is probable that trench fever is due to *Rickettsia quintana*. Typhus fever and Rocky Mountain spotted fever are the diseases that occur in the United States. Typhus in mild forms in Mexico is called tabardillo and in the eastern United States, Brill's disease. Body lice and head lice harbor and, by biting, transmit the organism of typhus, which is ultimately fatal for the louse itself. The wood tick is the vector of Rocky Mountain spotted fever and may transmit it from generation to generation of tick to furnish a continuous reservoir of the disease. Rabbit ticks are occasional vectors. An eastern form of the disease is transmitted by the dog tick. Bites usually transfer the organisms but in some instances merely crushing the ticks in the hand is sufficient.

Rocky Mountain Spotted Fever

This is selected as an example of rickettsial diseases because it is the principal form in the United States. The anatomic lesions are like those of typhus. The western and eastern varieties are much the same save for the greater severity of the former. The western form occurs largely in adults as an occupational hazard; the eastern form occurs in children because of playing with dogs. The disease runs a course of about three weeks; when fatal, death occurs from about 11 to 17 days after onset. The mortality of the western form is variable in different regions, ranging from 4 per cent in Idaho to as much as 90 per cent in the Bitterroot Valley of Montana. The eastern form has a low mortality rate. The incubation period lasts from a few days to about two weeks. The onset is usually sudden, with chill, high fever, headache, vomiting, and pains in the muscles, bones and joints, especially the back and the legs. An eruption of pale red macules, about 2 to 5 mm. in diameter, begins on the first day or up to five days after onset, first on the distal parts of the extremities and then extending to trunk and face. In severe cases it becomes hemorrhagic and marked purpura may develop. Jaundice may supervene. Hemorrhage may occur via mouth or rectum. Delirium, the "typhoid state," rigidity, coma and cyanosis usually precede death.

The principal lesion is found in the smaller blood vessels in various parts of the body. Swelling and proliferation of endothelium, sometimes occlusive and often accompanied by thrombosis, occur. The arterioles may show necrosis of their walls and a surrounding leukocytic exudate. There are also perivascular accumulation of lymphocytes, plasma cells and large mononuclear cells, some of which are phagocytic. These lesions account for petechiae in various organs. The perivascular infiltrations are found in many organs and in the serous membranes including the meninges. The corium of the skin shows the perivascular lesions as well as necrotizing arteriolitis and thrombosis. In the later stages, foci of hemorrhage and occasionally necrosis and ulceration of the epidermis occur; these are especially marked in the scrotum, but also occur about fingers and toes and elsewhere. The heart is of about normal size but the muscle is soft. Microscopically there is cloudy swelling, not infrequently with acute myocarditis.

The lungs are hyperemic, edematous, with hemorrhagic spots and often bronchopneumonia. The liver is swollen and soft and often icteric. Microscopically passive hyperemia, cloudy swelling, fatty degeneration, focal necrosis and, in the portal spaces, the cellular infiltrations of acute hepatitis are found. The Kupffer cells are often phagocytic for red cells and nuclear fragments.

The kidneys show slight swelling and hyperemia grossly; microscopically the tubules show cloudy swelling, hyperemia, occasionally foci of hemorrhage, vascular lesions and perivascular cellular infiltration. The spleen is moderately enlarged, the pulp firm or soft and the follicles not visible. Microscopically the follicles are small, the pulp markedly hyperemic, the large mononuclear cells actively phagocytic. The lymph nodes are hyperplastic and sometimes hemorrhagic. Bone marrow is active and may show vascular and perivascular lesions. The adrenals are usually not much affected, but vascular lesions may occur together with small hemorrhages. The brain and meninges show vascular and perivascular lesions; the brain may show foci of necrosis and tiny infarcts as the result of the vascular disease. Hassin found a nonsuppurative meningo-encephalitis in one case. Rickettsiae are found in vascular endothelium and in large mononuclear phagocytes as well as in muscle of the vessels. They have been reported in skin, brain, heart, pancreas, kidneys and elsewhere, especially in the testis. (See Wolbach; Cowdry; Blumer; Lillie.)

DISEASES DUE TO PROTOZOA

These are in part diseases which represent infections of one or another surface of the body and in part those due to entry of the protozoa into the viscera. In the latter, man is usually only one host in the life cycle of the parasite. The other host is often an insect but may be some other animal. Amebiasis is transmitted from man to man by way of water and food. In most instances the infection is confined to the mucosa of the colon, the so-called amebic dysentery, but sometimes the *Endamoeba histolytica* produces hepatic abscess. Other protozoa affect blood and viscera. In addition to amebiasis, the diseases of this group of importance to man are malaria, kala-azar, granuloma inguinale, oriental boil and other comparable diseases due to Leishman-Donovan bodies, trypanosomiasis which is especially exemplified in African sleeping sickness, and toxoplasmosis. The diseases selected to represent this category of infection are malaria and toxoplasmosis. Reference to others is found in the chapters on Systemic Pathology.

Malaria

In this disease the sexual cycle of the parasite takes place in the mosquito and the asexual cycle in man. The disease is transmitted by the bite of the anopholene mosquito. The clinical manifestations of the disease, with chills, fever and often prostration, occur in three principal forms: Tertian malaria in which the chill appears every other day is due to the *Plasmodium vivax*. The quartan form in which the chill occurs every third day is due to *Plasmodium malariae*. The estivo-autumnal form in which the chills appear at irregular periods is due to the *Plasmodium falciparum*. The organisms enter the red blood corpuscles and continue their asexual cycle in those cells. The regularity of growth, rupture of the red blood corpuscle and discharge of the segments into the blood is such as to determine the periodicity of the chills. In the case of estivo-autumnal fever, this cycle is less regular. The consequence of rupture of the red blood corpuscles is anemia. Malaria may occur in a pernicious form in which the destruction of blood is great and hemoglobin appears in the urine, the so-called black-water fever. As recovery from the attack ensues, there is a tendency for selective localization of the parasites in the spleen, liver and bone marrow. In the liver the parasites and their pigment are taken up by the Kupffer cells. In the spleen and bone marrow they are taken up by reticulo-endothelial cells in the spleen and reticular cells in the bone marrow.

The pathologic disturbances other than those of the blood, are found principally in liver, spleen and bone marrow. The liver is somewhat enlarged and shows cloudy swelling, sometimes fatty degeneration and even focal necrosis. Segments of parasites and more especially pigment granules are found in the Kupffer cells. In cured or chronic cases, the only manifestation is pigment in the Kupffer cells, but this may be sufficient in quantity to give the liver a brown color grossly. The spleen is enlarged, firm and has a tense capsule. Microscopically, hyperplasia of cell elements, especially the reticulo-endothelial cells, and sometimes focal necrosis and small infarcts are found. Parasites and especially pigment granules are found in the reticulo-endothelial cells. In chronic cases there is likely to be great enlargement of the spleen due to hyperplasia of connective tissue. It has a thick capsule, is firm and the cross section is brown.

The bone marrow is usually not remarkable grossly but microscopically shows pigmentation and hyperplasia, particularly of the reticular cells. This form of hyperplasia may well account for the absence of leukocytosis or the presence of leukopenia in malaria. The hyperplasia of lymphoid cells and of the large mononuclears may determine a relative lymphocytosis and a relative monocytosis. Localization in other organs is not common and is due principally to the accumulation of large numbers of parasites in the capillaries, sometimes referred to as embolic occlusions. This occurs in the brain and may lead to hemorrhage in ring form and to destruction of cells and tissues of the brain. The same sort of phenomenon may occur in the heart and in the gastro-intestinal tract, as well as occasionally in other organs of the body, including kidneys, pancreas, thyroid, lungs and adrenals. (See Cannon.)

Toxoplasmosis

Although not certainly identified, the evidence points strongly to the view that toxoplasma is a protozoan parasite. The identity of toxoplasmosis of animals and man has been established by Sabin. Thus, there exists in the rabbit, dog, guinea-pig, rat, probably cat and other animals a reservoir of infection, but exactly how it is transmitted is unknown. In infants and children the disease is usually manifested by an encephalomyelitis.

Pathology. Pathologically there are foci of destruction of cells and fibers in the central nervous system with complete necrosis in these regions, which may go on to the formation of cysts. The inflammatory reaction is not marked except that the neighboring leptomeninges may show edema, hyperemia, infiltration of lymphocytes and plasma cells, mononuclear cells and eosinophils. In the lesion and in the reacting zones there are large mononuclear phagocytes which contain the parasite; these generally measure 4 to 6 micra long and 2 to 3 micra wide. They may be in the form of single bodies, oval or rounded in shape, or as clusters. Each parasite has a fairly deeply staining margin and in the middle or near the margin a darkly staining compact mass. Rarely, the nodules may become abscesses (Reid, et al.). In adults much the same form of disease may be encountered, but clinically, according to Pinkerton and Henderson, it may also resemble Rocky Mountain spotted fever with its great depression and widely disseminated cutaneous eruption. In these instances the parasites are found widespread in the body, including heart, lungs (where there is often a focal type of pneumonia) and other viscera. In the lungs the pneumonia shows comparatively few leukocytes and but little fibrin and the inflammatory response is especially in the form of mononuclear cells similar to the viral pneumonias. Wolf, Cowen and Paige suggest that some of the cases in infants are due to congenital transmission but this has not yet been proved.

DISEASES DUE TO FUNGI

Higher forms of vegetable parasites are responsible for many surface infections. Thus there are varieties of mycosis of the skin, such as the tineas, etc., discussed in books on dermatology. Fungi may affect the mouth, as in thrush and other forms of stomatitis. They occur in tonsils and in respiratory tract, in urethra and vagina. Internal viscera may be affected in blastomycosis, coccidioidal granuloma, torula infections, sporotrichosis and aspergillosis, which are discussed in the next chapter. Disease due to the higher bacteria are also included in that chapter. Much has been written of disease due to fungi, but in certain instances the postulates of Koch have not yet been fulfilled. In many, the clinical manifestations are more striking than the pathologic features. (See Castellani.) Of the acute diseases involving viscera and caused by fungi, there is one which claims increasing interest in North America, namely histoplasmosis.

Histoplasmosis

This disease is sometimes called reticulo-endothelial cytomycosis. The organism, *Histoplasma capsulatum,* was first described by Darling in the Panama Canal Zone. The organism is round or oval, 3 to 5 micra in diameter and gram-positive. It consists of a round or crescent-form central mass, sometimes vesicular, surrounded by a clear zone and a refractile capsule. It can be transferred to monkeys, young dogs, young mice,

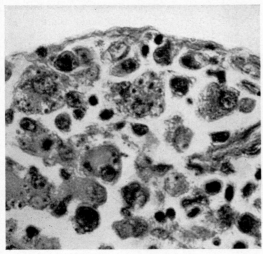

Histoplasmosis. Parasites, surrounded by areolae in reticulo-endothelial cells at base of ulcer in intestine.

guinea-pigs and rabbits and has been reported to occur naturally in a dog. The mode of transmission is not known, but insect bites are suspected. It occurs both in infancy and childhood and is usually fatal. The patients show enlarged liver and spleen, local or widespread enlargement of lymph nodes, profound anemia and leukopenia with relative lymphocytosis, often superficial abscesses and chronic inflammation of the lungs. Clinically, the organisms may be demonstrated in the blood, in punctures of bone marrow, spleen, liver or lymph node and by animal inoculation. Van Pernis and associates have described a skin test with supernatant fluid from a growth in dextrose broth, which appears to give promise as a diagnostic aid.

The lesions grossly are nodules of necrosis a few millimeters in diameter or much larger. Their presence in the skin leads to abscess formation, in the intestine to ulceration and in serous surfaces such as the pleura to fibrinopurulent pleurisy. They may be found in almost any organ of the body either widely scattered or confined to a few organs. In a few cases they have been observed in the adrenals alone. Microscopically there is central necrosis around which are fibroblasts, new capillaries, many lymphocytes and variable numbers of large mononuclear phagocytes. These phagocytes may contain only a few organisms but are often crowded with them. Similar phagocytes may be found in various parts of the reticulo-endothelial system without nodule formation. In culture, chlamydospores may occur and mycelial forms develop, but mycelia are rare in tissues. (See Meleney; Wright and Hachtel; Anderson, et al.; Shaw and Reid.)

Viral Diseases ⟵ ——— Caps?

The exact nature of viruses is not finally settled. Indeed there is no assurance that they are all of the same nature. They have in common the facts that they are very small and that they propagate solely within cells. Their composition appears to vary but they all contain nucleoprotein. Each virus is fairly uniform as to shape but there are differing forms, from slender rods to spherules. Their size varies from that of a protein molecule to that of the smallest bacteria. They are measured in terms of millimicra rather than micra and by various methods of determination have been found to vary from 8 to 12 millimicra for the virus of foot and mouth disease to 125 to 175 millimicra for the virus of vaccinia and lymphogranuloma venereum. Many have been propagated in culture media but only when live cells are present. Some also have multiplied in the chorio-allantoic membrane of the chick and in the chick embryo (see Saunders). If they be living organisms, they are obligate parasites. Some of the viruses of plant diseases have been crystallized, suggesting but not proving that they are inanimate agents. It is also suggested that they are nonliving autocatalytic agents in the cell; and some propose to place them as transitional forms between the living and the inanimate. Not only do they exist within cells but they have a high degree of specificity as to the cells in which they propagate. They are cytotropic and for the most part specifically so. In some viral diseases, the virus is recoverable from blood and body fluids, but this is not true of all. The necessity for propagation in cells means that there is an interdependent relationship and that they are not phagocytosed.

All the known viruses are pathogenic and their effects are known only by the way they act in their respective hosts. Immune reactions have been studied in relation to the elementary bodies of several of the viruses, which have been obtained in quantity, washed and put in suspension. The most important antibody is a protective substance in the serum, demonstrably capable of protecting against infection by the virus. Many, but not all, of the viral diseases of man confer lasting immunity. Nevertheless the cell-virus relationship may protect the virus against circulating antibody.

The viral diseases can be placed in three groups (Goodpasture). In the first are diseases that affect only epithelial cells such as cutaneous warts and molluscum contagiosum. The virus is epitheliotropic, presumably obligate, and does not enter the blood. The second group includes such diseases as smallpox, chickenpox, and probably measles. Here the virus enters the blood, probably through the upper respiratory tract, and then localizes in the skin where it affects epithelium, fibroblasts, vascular endothelium and sometimes other cells. In the third group are viral diseases of the nervous system. The viruses of poliomyelitis and rabies appear to be obligate neurotropic, enter the peripheral nerves and require neurons for multiplication and spread. The viruses of St. Louis encephalomyelitis and equine encephalitis affect other cells as well. They probably enter the blood and are then localized. The viruses which affect more than one type of cell are called pantropic or preferably polytropic.

The pathology of viral diseases varies considerably. One of the features most extensively studied is the development of intracellular inclusion bodies. These have not been demonstrated in all the viral diseases but have been found in many. Most of them are well-defined, globular masses included in the cytoplasm and often surrounded by an areola. With ordinary stains they appear to be homogeneous but many have been found to have a net-like structure. In some instances, for example molluscum contagiosum, there is a matrix in which are enmeshed innumerable infective elementary bodies. That this structure is common to all inclusion bodies is not yet certain. In addition to these intracytoplasmic inclusions, intranuclear inclusions are sometimes observed. The effects upon cells are largely degenerative and in some of the diseases, as in poliomyelitis, the anterior horn cells may be completely dissolved. Reaction to the destruction of cells is also variable. In some diseases there is none. In others there may be a preliminary exudation of polymorphonuclear leukocytes rapidly succeeded by lymphocytes and large mononuclear phagocytes. In some instances the entire reaction is on the part of lymphocytes and large mononuclears. Exudation of fluid may produce vesicles, as in smallpox. In this and certain other diseases vesiculation is followed by actual suppuration. Generally speaking, however, inflammatory response in viral diseases is minor. (See Goodpasture; Rivers; K. M. Smith.)

The viral diseases in man include various minor illnesses and some that are severe and fatal. A partial list includes the common cold, herpes simplex or fever blisters, influenza, certain forms of pneumonia, measles (probably), trachoma, chickenpox, molluscum contagiosum, psittacosis, lymphogranuloma venereum, yellow fever, smallpox, vaccinia, rabies, poliomyelitis and various forms of encephalitis. Also of importance to man are the bacteriophages. Although viruses are known to produce tumors in animals, there has been no proof that they do so in man except for the common wart of the skin and the papilloma of the larynx. Certain of these diseases are discussed in the chapters on Systemic Pathology. It is impossible in the scope of this book to present the features of all, hence smallpox is selected in order to provide an example.

Smallpox

Technically called variola, this disease is due to a virus, resistant to drying, carried in the air and also on fomites (clothing, towels, etc.), which probably enters the body by the respiratory tract. The virus is carried by the blood and localized most conspicuously but not exclusively in the skin. The incubation period, from 12 to 14 days, is followed by rather sudden onset with fever, headache, severe backache and vomiting. A macular rash sometimes precedes the eruption. The papular eruption, the firm or "shot like" nodules being 2-3 mm. in diameter, appears on about the third day, particularly on hands and forehead but spreading widely over the body. After another 2 or 3 days these become vesicles, often umbilicated. In 2 or 3 days more the vesicles become pustules and then crust over. If these lesions extend into the corium, scarred pock marks result. In endemic form, the disease is usually mild and the eruption not extensive. In epidemics it may be severe, the pustules may become confluent, the mouth and respiratory tract are similarly involved and the mortality rate is high. Strains of the virus vary considerably in virulence and this may determine the severity of the disease. In nonfatal cases, recovery ensues in two or three weeks. The virus of vaccinia is a smallpox virus modified by passage through animals, especially the calf and rabbit. Following Jenner's publication in 1798, vaccination gradually became more and more widely practiced and has almost eliminated the disease in civilized countries.

The specific lesion begins in the epidermis, with swelling of groups of cells in the intermediate layers, preceded by swelling and degeneration of their nuclei. The cell borders become condensed to form a sort of reticulum. Fluid exudate enters from below and the increasingly swollen cells rupture, with the formation of a loculated vesicle. Only when necrosis is evident is there exudation of polymorphonuclear leukocytes together with the appearance of large mononuclear phagocytes. Suppuration, when it occurs, is probably not due solely to the virus but to secondary pyogenic infection. If the lesions enlarge sufficiently they extend into the corium. If this occur, healing involves scar formation, but if only the epidermis be involved, the epithelium can regenerate completely.

Intracellular inclusion bodies (Guarnieri bodies) are found in the epithelial cells beginning with the earliest lesions. For the most part these are globules 1 to 3 or 4 micra in diameter, surrounded by a vacuole. Within the larger forms are smaller, more deeply stained granules and the body may have a reticulated ("mulberry") appearance. Similar but smaller inclusions may be found

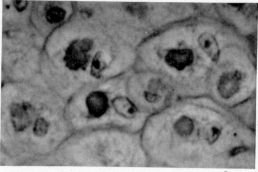

Cytoplasmic inclusion bodies in fowl pox. These can be distinguished from nuclei in this photomicrograph because of the vesicular character of the nuclei and the presence of nucleoli.

in the nuclei. They represent agglomerations of elementary bodies, which in this disease are among the largest known.

The lesions in the mucous membranes are much the same except as they are modified by the structure of the mucosa and moisture. This is the picture of uncomplicated variola vera, but it is modified in abortive cases. Hemorrhage may occur at any stage, but more especially when the pustule has formed. Rarely the lesion is purpuric.

More or less peculiar to the disease are foci of necrosis, which may perhaps be due to localization of the virus. These are practically constant in the outer portion of the testis, but occur also in kidney, liver, adrenal and bone marrow. The lymph nodes are usually hyperplastic. The hyperplasia of the bone marrow and spleen gives rise to many cells of the order of monocytes and large mononuclear phagocytes. The proliferation of monocytes is responsible for the relative monocytosis of the blood; leukocytosis is not marked. The cloudy swelling of the parenchymatous viscera which may be exceptionally severe in the liver is presumably due to the secondary pyogenic infection rather than to the virus. The studies of the pathologic anatomy of smallpox by Councilman,

Magrath and Brinckerhoff have not been surpassed even though they were mistaken about the etiology.

Psittacosis

Parrots, parakeets and related birds suffer from a gastro-enteritis due to one of the larger viruses. This is readily transmitted to man by unknown routes. After an incubation period of a few days, it produces high fever, severe headache, cough and delirium, and is often fatal. The virus is polytropic and induces the formation of intracytoplasmic inclusion bodies in which elementary bodies can sometimes be seen. The autopsy on a fatal case shows the degenerations in parenchymal viscera common to acute infections, but with little or no hyperplasia of spleen and lymph nodes. It is evidently septicemic, but the outstanding lesion is pneumonia. There is likely to be extensive consolidation, with moderate hyperemia and marked edema. Edema and variable amounts of fibrin are found microscopically. There are numerous large mononuclear cells, many of which contain inclusions. Desquamation of the lining cells of the bronchi and the alveoli may be marked. Capillaries and small blood vessels may be the seat of thrombosis, together with necrosis of alveolar walls. The brain and cord show hyperemia and edema with vascular disease and ring-shaped hemor·rhages.

DISEASE PERHAPS OF ALLERGIC NATURE

Rheumatic Fever

This was formerly called acute articular rheumatism, but it is now known to be systemic and can occur without arthritis. The geographic distribution of the disease is not known, but it certainly occurs in many parts of the world. There is no positive indication of racial distribution. It is more common in cold than in warm climates, and is more frequent in late winter and spring than in summer and early autumn. It affects those of poor and moderate economic status more often than the well-to-do. It may be that this has to do with reported low content of vitamin C in the blood, but this may well be due to utilization of that vitamin in the course

of the disease. There is probably a hereditary susceptibility and this may perhaps account for the fact that it sometimes affects several members of a family. Although the first attack may occur in adolescence or early adult life, it most commonly starts in childhood, at about six to eight years of age, a little later in boys than in girls. The sex incidence is somewhat higher in girls than in boys, but may be equal in certain regions. It may be preceded by an attack of upper respiratory infection, but this is true of only about half the cases. It is characterized by fever, sweating, malaise, moderate leukocytosis, moderate anemia, increased sedimentation rate, often migratory polyarthritis of larger joints—especially ankles, knees and wrists—cutaneous manifestations such as erythema marginatum and multiforme in a few patients, and rarely purpura; subcutaneous nodules also occur. It is essentially a cyclic disease, but many patients have only one cycle. It is probable that not less than 90 per cent of affected children develop rheumatic cardiac disease. Rheumatic endocarditis is the usual precursor of endocarditis lenta (subacute bacterial endocarditis).

Etiology. The predisposing factors have just been enumerated, but the exciting cause is unknown. The most important current theories are that it is due to bacteria, or to a virus, or that it is allergic in nature. Various bacteria have been recovered from the blood, joints and throat, but none is constantly found. The most frequent is the hemolytic streptococcus. Coburn and his associates are proponents of the view that rheumatic fever is a streptococcal infection. They have noted that the sore throat which sometimes precedes the attack shows hemolytic streptococci and that antibodies to streptococci are found in the course of the disease. There is said to be a seasonal and geographic relation between streptococcal infections and rheumatic fever. Corroboration has not been sufficiently frequent to justify acceptance and Wilson points to facts that appear to be contradictory. Moon and Stewart suggest that the bacteria are of low virulence and Oettel suggests that they are attenuated because of autovaccination. Again, confirmation is wanting. Jones believes that there may be some association between streptococci and rheumatic fever, but that these bacteria are not the only important factor. Elementary bodies, agglutinable by the serum of these patients, have been recovered from rheumatic exudates, suggesting that a virus is the cause, but injections of these bodies into monkeys have failed to reproduce the disease (Eagles et al.).

tion in joints of both exudative and productive mononuclear-cell type. Lesions of similar form, closely resembling those of rheumatic fever were found in blood vessels, endocardium and muscle. These, he states, are practically identical with conditions which he observed in autopsies on patients dead of the

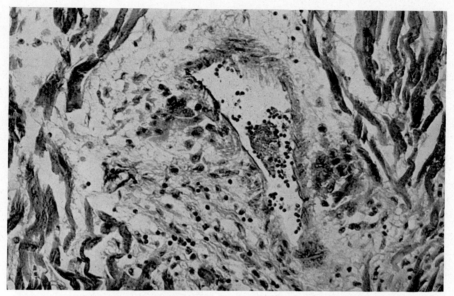

Aschoff nodule in myocardium. Note two clusters in perivascular position.

THE THEORY OF ALLERGY is attractive and has numerous supporters. On the basis of clinical, anatomic, bacteriologic and immunologic observations, Swift has proposed that

the pathogenesis of rheumatic fever can be explained by the existence in certain individuals of a condition of hypersensitiveness (allergy or hyperergy) to streptococci resulting from repeated low grade infection or the persistence of foci of infection in the body. When under suitable circumstances streptococci or products of streptococci are disseminated in the tissues, these tissues overreact and the characteristic picture of the disease results.

Experimental support to this theory is furnished by Klinge, but without special reference to streptococci of any variety. By regulating the sensitizing and intoxicating doses of horse serum in experimental animals he has produced acute and subacute inflamma-

disease. The exudative reaction and the later infiltration, diffuse or focal, are probably all

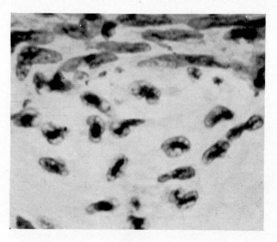

Character of nuclei in cells of Aschoff nodule. Above are smooth-muscle nuclei of vascular wall. Cytoplasm only faintly stained.

part of the same general response. Swift found that animals can be sensitized somewhat similarly to streptococci, but that repeated injections finally lead to immunity. Neither he nor Klinge has proved that the condition is specific. Coburn, however, introduces another theory which involves specificity. He thinks that because of hereditary and environmental conditions there are persons who do not respond in the usual way to infections with hemolytic streptococci. In them the cells of the reticulo-endothelial system become sensitized, so that subsequent infections produce contact between antigen and antibody within these cells, which then react to produce the rheumatic type of inflammation. No one has as yet reproduced in animals the exact counterpart of the

swelling is probably due to changes in the mucoprotein ground substance (Coburn). At the center of a fresh Aschoff nodule there is usually a small focus of necrosis. Around this are a few lymphocytes intermingled with peculiar cells called Anitschkow myocytes, or more often Aschoff cells. This cell has abundant cytoplasm but is characterized by the nucleus, which is vesicular with chromatin arranged in a central mass from which delicate fibrils radiate to or near the nuclear membrane. Such cells may be present normally in the connective tissues of the heart and valves, but they proliferate especially in rheumatic inflammation. The cell itself is not diagnostic (Clawson). In the Aschoff nodule,

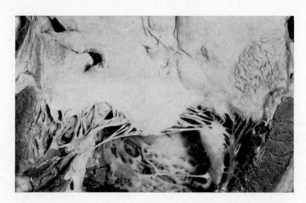

Chronic rheumatic endocarditis of the mitral valve and left atrium.

Aschoff nodule. It is not to be assumed that the theory of allergy is uniformly accepted. Nevertheless, pending the discovery of some other exciting cause of the disease, allergy or some stage resembling it appears to be the most acceptable theory yet offered.

Pathologic Anatomy. Fundamentally, rheumatic fever is a disease of the heart and blood vessels. The lesions found in joints, lungs, pleura, aorta and elsewhere are primarily due to vascular disease. Many of the inflammatory effects are fairly characteristic because of their common occurrence in rheumatic fever, but the specific lesion is the Aschoff nodule, found in the myocardium and occasionally elsewhere. Whatever the result, whether exudative, subacute or chronic inflammation or the production of the Aschoff nodule, the primary changes are necrosis, often only slight, swelling of the collagenous tissues and edema (Klinge). This primary

these cells often fuse to produce multinucleated forms. Somewhat similar nodules are seen in which there are many lymphocytes and a few polymorphonuclear leukocytes, the Bracht-Waechter bodies, thought to be the earliest stage of the Aschoff nodule. In the myocardium the Aschoff nodules are characteristically in a perivascular position. They may even extend for a considerable distance along vessels and sometimes appear to compress thin-walled veins.

The myocardium in the florid cases often shows a diffuse acute myocarditis in addition to the Aschoff nodules. In adults, the myocardium contains masses of mature connective tissue which in the progressive cases is probably a chronic myocarditis, but in the healed cases represents cicatrization; in either event Aschoff nodules are infrequent or absent. Myocardial hypertrophy occurs when valves are deformed.

RHEUMATIC ENDOCARDITIS begins in the subendocardial connective tissue, with edema, swelling of collagen, an infiltration of lymphocytes, proliferation of cells of the Aschoff type and, rarely, Aschoff nodules (Coombs). Presumably the surface endothelial cells deteriorate and are injured by the trauma of closure of valves so that verrucae, made up principally of fibrin, are formed. This may heal with little cicatrization or may become a chronic inflammation with thickening, stiffening, adhesion and retraction of cusps or leaflets and vascularization. The consequent deformity leads to stenosis or insufficiency of the valve or both. The mural endocardium may be similarly affected, especially in the posterior wall of the left atrium. The pericardium is often the seat of acute fibrinous or fibroserous inflammation and may contain Aschoff nodules. The organization and cicatrization may be followed only by adhesions in the atrioventricular sulci, or the adhesions may be more widespread and even lead to complete obliteration of the sac. The effects on the heart are discussed further in the chapter on the Cardiovascular System.

Various members of the arterial tree may be affected. Pappenheimer and Von Glahn found exudative and proliferative lesions in the adventitia of the aorta, with extension into the media and in one case involvement of the intima in the form of translucent, pale-brown plaques (Klinge describes the intimal plaques as "sausage-like"). They observed that the lesions are diffuse rather than nodular, but Aschoff cells are present. Similar lesions occur in other arteries including renal, superior mesenteric and celiac axis. Karsner and Bayless found lesions in the coronaries in all of 56 hearts examined. Kugel and Epstein found comparable changes in the pulmonary arteries together with Aschoff nodules. Similar disease occurs in the renal arteries and Fahr placed rheumatic fever among the possible causes of nephrosclerosis. Formation of verrucae in arteries is rare. Thrombophlebitis may occur but usually without destruction of the walls of the veins.

RHEUMATIC PNEUMONIA. Although ordinary bronchopneumonia may occur in rheumatic fever, there are occasional cases in which the pneumonia appears to be of rheumatic origin. In this the pulmonary arteries, especially smaller divisions, exhibit infiltration of lymphoid cells and disruption of elastica; and the cells lining the alveoli are desquamated. Paul describes cell clusters in the interlobular septa similar to Aschoff nodules. Gouley has noted focal cellular accumulations in alveolar walls. Acute fibrinous or fibrinoserous pleurisy, with or without pneumonia, occurs in rheumatic fever, sometimes with cellular foci resembling Aschoff nodules in the underlying connective tissue.

THE AFFECTED JOINTS are red, swollen, tender and painful. In the florid stage, the joint cavity is distended by a fluid exudate which contains fibrin and leukocytes. The synovial membrane is edematous, hyperemic and may show petechiae. The periarticular structures are the seat of edema and hyperemia, together with rheumatic lesions of the blood vessels. Aschoff cells and even Aschoff nodules may be found in the periarticular tissue and in the capsule of the joint. These persist after the acute inflammation subsides.

SUBCUTANEOUS NODULES occur especially in children. They are moderately firm, sometimes tender, round masses which push up the skin; they measure from a few millimeters to a centimeter or more in diameter. In early lesions, the cross section is gray and translucent, sometimes with minute yellow foci of necrosis. Microscopically, these are made up of edematous connective tissue, fibroblasts, large mononuclear cells, lymphocytes, leukocytes and eosinophils without regular arrangement. Aschoff cells have been described but Clawson denies their occurrence in these nodules. The nodules usually disappear but may persist for a long time during which they are converted into firm masses of dense collagenous connective tissue. Secondary changes, including hyalinization, fatty degeneration, calcification and even bone formation, may take place. Many other forms of subcutaneous nodule may be confused with those of rheumatic fever (Keil).

CHOREA (Sydenham's chorea) is now accepted as a form of rheumatic fever. This is so rarely fatal that but few autopsy reports are recorded. There are various forms of rheumatic vascular disease in the brain and meninges, widely disseminated and associated with secondary necrosis of the brain and inflammation in both brain and meninges. The changes may be slight or marked and constitute a meningo-encephalitis.

SEPTICEMIA. In rare cases various lesions of rheumatic fever, especially those in the blood vessels (the heart sometimes escapes) are associated with severe and fatal streptococcal septicemia. This has been called rheumatoid sepsis (Oettel) and although the evidence favors the view that it is essentially a form of rheumatic fever, this is not finally established.

The reader is referred to Sacks and to de la Chapelle for excellent reviews of the pathologic anatomy of rheumatic fever and to Wilson for a comprehensive survey and analysis of the disease.

Disseminated Lupus Erythematosus

There are certain other diseases such as erythema nodosum and periarteritis nodosa (see chapter on Diseases of the Cardiovascular System) which appear to be allergic in nature, although their infectious character is not positively proved. In the same category is disseminated lupus erythematosus. This only remotely resembles other forms of lupus and is not tuberculous. It is perhaps different also from discoid lupus erythematosus. It is a systemic disease characterized by fever, a maculopapular eruption on exposed parts and sometimes generalized, inflammation (usually sterile) of serous membranes including pleura, pericardium, peritoneum and joints (migratory and evanescent in smaller joints), anemia, leukopenia and thrombopenia as expressions of depression of the bone marrow, and renal disturbances in the form of albuminuria, casts and erythrocytes in the urine but usually without renal insufficiency. Cardiac murmurs are common and occasionally there are enlarged lymph nodes. It is a disease of the white race and is much more frequent in females than in males. It has been reported in age periods for 10 to 50 years. The duration varies widely, from 4 weeks to 9 years.

The important pathologic changes are found in the skin, serous membranes, blood vessels, heart and kidneys. The cutaneous lesions, microscopically, are not characteristic. Lymphocytes, plasma cells and a few polymorphonuclear leukocytes, form an infiltration into the corium which is only vaguely perivascular in situation. Fibrino-serous inflammation may be encountered in the serous cavities and there may be chronic inflammation and fibrous adhesions. Vascular lesions include dilatation of capillaries with extravasation of blood, proliferation of vascular endothelium, necrotizing inflammation of smaller arteries and sometimes thrombosis. Acute chronic and healed endocarditis of the cardiac valves occurs, the acute form corresponding to the indeterminate endocarditis of Libman. The kidneys show changes which vary considerably. Marked degeneration of tubular epithelium, sometimes nonsuppurative interstitial nephritis may occur and in the glomeruli there may be foci of necrosis, subacute glomerulitis and a peculiar thickening of the capillary walls in the form of the "wire loop" lesions. (See Bunim; Stickney and Keith.)

See Klemperer et al Arch Path 32 56

REFERENCES

Anderson, W. A. D., I. D. Michelson, and T. M. Dunn: Histoplasmosis in Infancy. Report of a Case, Amer. Jour. Clin. Path., **11**: 344, 1941.

Andrews, F. W., W. Bullock, et al.: Diphtheria: Its Bacteriology, Pathology and Immunology, London, 1923.

Ashe, W. F., H. R. Pratt-Thomas, and C. W. Kumpe: Weil's Disease. A Complete Review of American Literature and an Abstract of the World Literature. Seven Case Reports, Medicine, **20**: 145, 1941.

Bacon, D. K., F. O. Novy, and H. H. Eppler: Factors in Leucocytosis, Arch. Int. Med., **30**: 229, 1922.

Balcar, J. O., W. D. Sansum, and R. T. Woodyatt: Fever and the Water Reserve of the Body, Arch. Int. Med., **24**: 116, 1919.

Barbour, H. G.: The Heat-Regulating Mechanism of the Body, Physiol. Rev., **1**: 295, 1921.

——, E. Tolstoi, E. Lozinski, and W. Bourne: Heat Regulation and Water Exchange, Amer. Jour. Physiol., **67**: 366, 378, 388, 399, 1924.

Barr, D. P., R. L. Cecil, and E. F. DuBois: Clinical Calorimetry, XXXII. Temperature Regulation after the Intravenous Injection of Proteose and Typhoid Vaccine, Arch. Int. Med., **29**: 608, 1922.

Blaisdell, J. L.: The Renal Lesions of Rheumatic Fever, Amer. Jour. Path., **10**: 287, 1934.

Blumer, G.: Rickettsial Diseases, with Special Reference to Those of Importance Along the Atlantic Seaboard, Bull. New York Acad. Med., **17**: 280, 1941.

Bunim, J. J.: Lupus Erythematosus Disseminaatus, Ann. Int. Med., **13**: 1399, 1940.

Cannon, P. R.: Some Pathological Aspects of Human Malaria, Publication 15, Amer. Asso. Advanc. Sci., p. 214.

Castellani, A.: Fungi and Fungous Diseases, Chicago, Amer. Med. Asso., 1928.

de la Chapelle, C. E.: The Pathological Aspects of Rheumatic Fever, Bull. New York Acad. Med., **16**: 659, 1940.

Clawson, B. J.: Experimental Streptococcic Inflammation in Normal, Immune and Hypersensitive Animals, Arch. Path., **9**: 1141, 1930.

———: The Relation of Experimental Rheumatoid Inflammation to Allergy, Ann. Int. Med., **4**: 433, 1930-31.

———: Relation of the "Anitschkow Myocyte" to Rheumatic Inflammation, Arch. Path., **32**: 760, 1941.

Coburn, A. F.: The Factor of Infection in the Rheumatic State, Baltimore, Williams and Wilkins, 1931; Faulty Disposal of Streptococcus Hemolyticus in Relation to Development of Rheumatic Lesion, Trans. and Stud. Coll. Phy. Philadelphia, **8**: 91, 1940.

Coombs, C. F.: Rheumatic Heart Disease, New York, 1924.

Councilman, W. T., G. B. Magrath, and W. R. Brinckerhoff: The Pathological Anatomy and Histology of Variola, Jour. Med. Res., **11**: 12, 1904.

Cowdry, E. V.: Rickettsiae and Disease, Arch. Path. and Lab. Med., **2**: 59, 1926.

Cramer, W.: On Sympathetic Fever and Hyperpyrexial Heat-stroke, Brit. Jour. Exper. Path., **1**: 31, 1920-21.

Cummer, C. L.: Manual of Clinical Laboratory Methods, 2d ed., Philadelphia, 1926.

Doan, C. A.: Peripheral Blood Phenomena and Differential Response of Bone Marrow and Lymph Nodes to Hyperpyrexia, Radiology, **30**: 382, 1938.

DuBois, E. F.: Metabolism in Fever and in Certain Infections, Endocrinology and Metabolism, edited by L. F. Barker, New York and London; v. 4, p. 95.

Eagles, G. H., P. R. Evans, J. D. Keith, and A. G. T. Fisher: Infection Experiments with Virus-like Bodies from Rheumatism, Jour. Path. & Bact., **46**: 481, 1938.

Edmunds, C. W., and R. G. Cooper: Action of Cardiac Stimulants in Circulatory Failure Due to Diphtheria, Jour. Amer. Med. Asso., **85**: 1798, 1925.

Fahr, T.: Kurze Beiträge zur Frage der Nephrosklerose, Deutsches Arch. Klin. Med., **134**: 366, 1920.

———: Beiträge zur Frage der Herz-und Gelenkveränderungen bei Gelenkrheumatismus und Scharlach, Virchow's Arch. Path. Anat., **232**: 134, 1921.

Farrell, E., G. H. Lordi, and J. Vogel: Haverhill Fever. Report of a Case with Review of the Literature, Arch. Int. Med., **64**: 1, 1939.

Feiner, R. R.: Experimental Diphtheric Paralysis, Jour. Immunol., **42**: 273, 1941.

Goodpasture, E. W.: Etiological Problems in the Study of Filterable Virus Diseases, Harvey Lectures, Baltimore, Williams and Wilkins, **25**: 77, 1931.

———: Immunity to Virus Diseases. Some Theoretical and Practical Considerations, New England Jour. Med., **222**: 901, 1940.

———: The Pathology of Virus Disease, Jour. Pediatr., **18**: 440, 1941.

———: Concerning the Pathogenesis of Typhoid Fever, Amer. Jour. Path., **13**: 175, 1937. *See also* Adams, J. W., Jr., Intracellular Bacilli in Intestinal and Mesenteric Lesions of Typhoid Fever, Amer. Jour. Path., **15**: 561, 1939.

———, and K. Anderson: The Problem of Infection as Presented by Bacterial Invasion of the Chorio-Allantoic Membrane of Chick Embryos, Amer. Jour. Path., **13**: 149, 1937.

Goulev, B. A.: The Evolution of the Parenchymal Lung Lesions in Rheumatic Fever and Their Relationship to Mitral Stenosis and Passive Congestion, Amer. Jour. Med. Sci., **196**: 1, 1938.

Gross, L., L. Loewe, and B. Eliasoph: Attempts to Reproduce Rheumatic Fever in Animals, Jour. Exper. Med., **50**: 41, 1929.

Hassin, G. B.: Cerebral Changes in Rocky Mountain Spotted Fever, Arch. Neurol. and Psychiatr., **44**: 1290, 1940.

Havens, W. P., C. J. Bucher, and H. A. Reimann: Leptospirosis: A Public Health Hazard. Report of a Small Outbreak of Weil's Disease in Bathers, Jour. Amer. Med. Asso., **116**: 289, 1941.

Hewlett, A. W.: Pathological Physiology of Internal Diseases, New York and London, 1919.

Hort, E. C., and W. J. Penfold: A Critical Study of Experimental Fever, Proc. Royal Soc., London, **85** (series B): 174, 1912.

Jacobsen, V. C., and K. Hosoi: The Morphologic Changes in Animal Tissues Due to Heating by an Ultrahigh Frequency Oscillator, Arch. Path., **11**: 744, 1931.

Jones, T. D.: The Etiology of Rheumatic Fever, A Discussion, Jour. Pediatr., **15**: 772, 1939.

Kanof, A., and B. Kramer: Multiple Invasion of the Blood Stream, Jour. Lab. and Clin. Med., **27**: 173, 1941.

Karsner, H. T., and F. Bayless: Coronary Arteries in Rheumatic Fever, Amer. Heart Jour., **9**: 557, 1934.

Keefer, C. S., F. J. Ingelfinger, and W. W. Spink: Significance of Hemolytic Streptococcic Bacteremia: A Study of Two Hundred and Forty-six Patients, Arch. Int. Med., **60**: 1084, 1937.

Keil, H.: The Rheumatic Subcutaneous Nodules and Simulating Lesions, Medicine, **17**: 261, 1938.

Klinge, F.: Der Rheumatismus. Pathologisch-anatomische und experimentell-pathologischen Tatsachen und ihre Auswertung für das ärztliche Rheumaproblem, Ergebn. Allg. Path. u. Path. Anat., **27**: 1, 1933.

Kugel, M. A., and E. Z. Epstein: Lesions in the Pulmonary Artery and Valve Associated with Rheumatic Cardiac Disease, Arch. Path., **6**: 247, 1928.

Lichtenstein, L.: Pathological Changes Following Therapeutic Hyperthermia. Report of a Case, Amer. Jour. Path., **15**: 363, 1939.

Lillie, R. D.: Pathology of Rocky Mountain Spotted Fever, Nat. Inst. Health Bull. 177, Washington, D. C., 1941.

Maclachlan, W. W. G., and de W. G. Richey: The Histopathology of the Tonsil in Acute Rheumatic Fever and Chorea, Ann. Int. Med., **1**: 506, 1927-28.

Mallory, F. B.: Pathology of Diphtheria, Nuttall and Graham-Smith's Bacteriology of Diphtheria, Cambridge, 1913, p. 82.

Mallory, G. K., and C. S. Keefer: Tissue Reactions in Fatal Cases of Streptococcus Haemolyticus Infection, Arch. Path., **32**: 334, 1941.

McLeod, J. W., J. W. Orr, and H. E. deC. Woodcock: The Morbid Anatomy of Gravis, Intermedius and Mitis Diphtheria: Observations on a Series of 51 Post-mortem Examinations, Jour. Path. and Bact., **48**: 99, 1939.

Meleney, H. E.: Histoplasmosis (Reticulo-Endothelial Cytomycosis): A Review with Mention of Thirteen Unpublished Cases, Amer. Jour. Trop. Med., **20**: 603, 1940.

Menkin, V.: Mechanism of Leukocytosis with Inflammation. The Nature of the Leukocytosis-Promoting Factor in Exudates, Arch. Path., **30**: 363, 1940.

Moody, W. B., and E. E. Irons: Invasion of Body by Bacteria from Intestinal Tract, Jour. Infect. Dis., **32**: 226, 1923.

Moon, V. H., and H. L. Stewart: Experimental Rheumatic Lesions in Dogs and Rabbits, Arch. Path., **11**: 190, 1931.

Oettel, H.: Rheumatoide Sepsis, Deutsch. Arch. Klin. Med., **138**: 773, 1940.

O'Meara, R. A. Q.: *C. Diphtheriae* and the Composition of its Toxin in Relation to the Severity of Diphtheria, Jour. Path. and Bact., **51**: 317, 1940.

Ott, I.: Fever, Its Thermotaxis and Metabolism, New York, Hoeber, 1914.

Pappenheimer, A. M., and W. C. VonGlahn: A Case of Rheumatic Aortitis with Early Lesions in the Media, Am. Jour. Path., **2**: 15, 1926; Studies in the Pathology of Rheumatic Fever, Two Cases Presenting Unusual Cardiovascular Lesions, ibid., **3**: 583, 1927.

Paul, J. R.: Pleural and Pulmonary Lesions in Rheumatic Fever, Medicine, **7**: 383, 1928.

Perera, G. A.: Clinical and Physiologic Characteristics of Chill, Arch. Int. Med., **68**: 241, 1941.

Petersen, W. F.: Serum Changes Following Protein "Shock" Therapy, Arch. Int. Med., **20**: 716, 1917.

Pinkerton, H., and R. G. Henderson: Adult Toxoplasmosis. A Previously Unrecognized Disease Entity Simulating the Typhus-Spotted Fever Group, Jour. Amer. Med. Asso., **116**: 807, 1941; *see also* Pinkerton, H., and D. Weinman: Toxoplasma Infection in Man, Arch. Path., **30**: 374, 1940.

Pribram, E.: Distribution of Water and Salts in the Human Organs during Fever, Arch. Path. & Lab. Med., **2**: 1, 1926.

Rathbun, H. K., and J. M. Waghelstein: Weil's Disease: Report of Six Cases, Ann. Int. Med., **15**: 395, 1941.

Raven, C.: Canine Leptospirosis in Pennsylvania, Jour. Infect. Dis., **69**: 131, 1941.

——: Clinical and Laboratory Diagnosis of Leptospirosis, Ohio State Med. Jour., **38**: 29, 1942.

Reimann, H. A., and W. P. Havens: Focal Infection and Systemic Disease: A Critical Appraisal. The Case Against Indiscriminate Removal of Teeth and Tonsils, Jour. Amer. Med. Asso., **114**: 1, 1940.

Rivers, T. M.: Filterable Viruses, Baltimore, Williams and Wilkins, 1928.

——: The Nature of the Viruses, Physiol. Rev., **12**: 423, 1932.

——: Viruses and Virus Diseases, Lane Medical Lectures, Stanford Univ. Press, 1939.

Sabin, A. B.: Biological and Immunological Identity of Toxoplasma of Animal and Human Origin, Proc. Soc. Exper. Biol. and Med., **41**: 75, 1939.

Sacks, B.: The Pathology of Rheumatic Fever. A Critical Review, Amer. Heart Jour., **1**: 750, 1925-26.

——, and F. W. Hachtel: A Note on the Bacteriologic Culture of Bone Marrow in Typhoid Fever, Jour. Lab. and Clin. Med., **26**: 1024, 1941.

Saunders, M.: Cultivation of the Viruses. A Critical Review, Arch. Path., **28**: 541, 1939.

Sharp, W. B., and M. B. John: Climate and the Streptococcus-Rheumatism Relationship, Jour. Infect. Dis., **60**: 15, 1937.

Shaw, F. W., and J. D. Reid: Fungi and Fungous Diseases, Jour. Lab. and Clin. Med., **26**: 256, 1940.

Shope, R. E.: Complex Infections, Arch. Path., **27**: 913, 1939.

Siler, J. F., and Associates: Immunization to Typhoid Fever, Baltimore, The Johns Hopkins Press, 1941.

Skinner, D., and C. S. Keefer: Significance of Bacteremia Caused by Staphylococcus Aureus: A Study of One Hundred and Twenty-two Cases and a Review of the Literature Concerned with Experimental Infection in Animals, Arch. Int. Med., **68**: 851, 1941.

Smith, K. M.: The Virus. Life's Enemy, Cambridge University Press, 1941.

Stickney, J. M., and N. M. Keith: Renal Involvement in Disseminated Lupus Erythematosus, Arch. Int. Med., **66**: 643, 1940.

Swift, H. F.: Rheumatic Fever, Jour. Amer. Med. Asso., **92**: 2071, 1929.

Van Pernis, R. A., M. E. Benson, and P. H. Holinger: Specific Cutaneous Reactions with Histoplasmosis. Preliminary Report of Another Case, Jour. Amer. Med. Asso., **117**: 436, 1941.

Wartman, W. B.: Attraction of Human Polymorphonuclear Leukocytes by Tubercle Protein, Am. Jour. Path., **13**: 612, 1937.

Wilson, M. G.: Rheumatic Fever. Studies of the Epidemiology, Manifestations, Diagnosis, and Treatment of the Disease During the First Three Decades, New York Commonwealth Fund, 1940.

Wolbach, S. B.: The Rickettsiae and Their Relation to Disease, Jour. Amer. Med. Asso., **84**: 723, 1925.

Wolf, A., D. Cowen, and B. H. Paige: Toxoplasmic Encephalomyelitis, Amer. Jour. Path., **15**: 657, 1939.

Wright, R. B., and F. W. Hachtel: Histoplasmosis of Darling; Report of a Case, Ann. Int. Med., **15**: 309, 1941.

10

The Infectious Granulomata

INTRODUCTION

In this category of infectious granulomata is included a group of diseases, which at some time during their course exhibit more or less characteristic nodules that in most instances are inflammatory. In some, the infectious character is fully established; in others this is only suspected. In some, the causative organism is proved, in others the associated organism is probably but not certainly the cause, and in still others no organisms have yet been found. In the outline given above, some of the diseases listed under the various causes are probably but not certainly due to them. Some have pronounced systemic manifestations and others appear to be local inflammations. The common feature of nodules or granules is the principal reason for grouping them together. The nodules may be the most noteworthy or indeed the only lesion, or they may occur infrequently in the course of the disease. Thus the tubercle is common in tuberculosis, but the gumma is much less frequent in syphilis. The suffix "oma" suggests tumor, but it refers really to local swelling. The term "granuloma" is accepted by common usage, not because the nodule is necessarily like granulation tissue either grossly or microscopically, but rather because of the occurrence of a nodule or granule. The gumma of syphilis contains capillaries as does granulation tissue, but the tubercle is devoid of them; some of the granulomas are principally foci of suppuration, for example, actinomycosis. Thus the microscopic picture of the granuloma in the different diseases is by no means constant. Furthermore, some of the organisms which cause the formation of a granuloma may also, under various conditions of virulence, dosage, resistance, or allergic alteration of reactive capacity, produce inflammatory responses with little or no resemblance to granuloma. For example, the tubercle bacillus although commonly inducing the tubercle may also produce acute exudative inflammation.

DUE TO BACTERIA

Tuberculosis

Introduction. Tuberculosis is one of several mycobacterial diseases, including leprosy, Johne's disease (paratuberculosis of cattle), so-called rat leprosy and certain other diseases of animals. Long points out that they have in common their causation by mycobacteria, characterized by acid-fastness, and a host reaction in which mononuclear phagocytes and epithelioid cells play a prominent part. Variables occur in the organisms and in the host, but the chemical constitution of the bacteria is relatively constant.

The lesions produced by *Mycobacterium tuberculosis* differ, apparently depending upon strain, number and virulence of the organism, portal of entry, situation in the

201

body, the susceptibility or resistance of the host and perhaps local immune phenomena. The most characteristic lesion is the tubercle, but the reaction may also be in the form of acute exudative inflammation, which may or may not exhibit distinguishing morphologic features.

The human variety is responsible for most of the tuberculosis of man at all periods of life. The bovine form is more often encountered in childhood than in adult life, especially in tuberculosis of the cervical lymph nodes, bones and joints (Griffith). From 6 to 10 per cent of deaths in infancy have been attributed to the bovine bacillus, but the number is probably decreasing. It may occasionally affect adults (Cobbett). Infection of man by the avian bacillus is exceedingly rare; this form has been reported as causing tuberculosis of the skin and of the kidney and as appearing in septicemic form. There is no satisfactory proof that it is the cause of Hodgkin's disease. (See Feldman.) Very rare, also, are the mixed infections with human and bovine forms (Griffith).

Modes of Entry of the Tubercle Bacillus. The tubercle bacillus can gain access to the body through any of the surfaces which are connected with the exterior, but the most important is through the respiratory tract, with a small number of cases of entry through the intestine (Reichle). It is doubtful that tubercle bacilli ever gain access to the body through the genito-urinary canal, except in those rare instances where open lesions of the external genitalia permit transmission by sexual contact. Implantations occur in the skin through accidental infection, such as pricks with infected syringe needles or cuts with infected instruments.

A discussion of infection with the tubercle bacillus must consider modes of dissemination, primary infection, reinfection, superinfection, and transport within the body. It was formerly thought that by the time adult life is reached, about 90 per cent of the population have acquired tuberculosis. Modern methods of study by tuberculin testing and roentgenogram indicate that the figure is much lower, probably in the order of 50 per cent for the white race and somewhat higher for Negroes. This means that although the first infection by tuberculosis is likely to occur in childhood, it may

and does take place in adolescence and early adult life. Various hypotheses are advanced concerning modes of dissemination of the organisms, and there is little doubt that all may have a basis in fact. The most frequent origin is undoubtedly infected human sputum, but infected cow's milk is also an important source. Dust containing dried sputum may be aspirated; droplets forcibly exhaled in coughing, sneezing, etc., may be aspirated in the moist or dry state; these presumably lead to tuberculosis of the lungs or mediastinal lymph nodes. Tuberculous cow's milk may upon ingestion lead to intestinal or mesenteric lymph-node tuberculosis and by transfer from the abdomen give rise to pulmonary tuberculosis. The infection is indoor rather than outdoor. Without minimizing the importance of the modes of infection just listed, Krause considers that the most common mode of infection in infancy and childhood is by more or less fresh sputum on floors, furniture, etc., which contaminates the child's hands, is conveyed to the mouth and thence to respiratory or alimentary tract. Experimental epidemiology demonstrates both air borne and enteric infections in animals, shows that crowding increases the incidence of the infection, and that if enteric infection be eliminated the incidence is decreased (Lurie).

There are two great clinical and pathologic types of tuberculous infection, primary and secondary. The former is common in childhood but may occur later. In certain instances, it has been possible to establish an incubation period of from 3 to 9 weeks. The secondary form is usually called the adult type. In order for infection to develop, the bacteria must pass through the epithelial covering of the various portals of entry. It is said that this may take place both in lung and intestine without evidence of the disease at the portal of entry. If this be true, it is exceedingly rare. The most frequent portal of entry is the lung. The work of Ghon, Opie and others provides convincing evidence that in practically all instances the lesion is primary in the lung and secondary in the tracheobronchial or bronchopulmonary lymph nodes. When the bacilli enter the lung or the skin, the lesion occurs in the interstitial tissues, but in the intestine is found in the lymph nodules.

PLATE VII

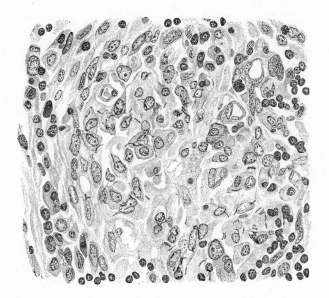

Microscopic drawing of tubercle bacilli (carbolfuchsin) in an early tubercle. Bacilli are found in and between epithelioid cells. Lymphoid cells and plasma cells are found in the margins.

IN INFANCY AND CHILDHOOD the primary pulmonic lesion rapidly becomes a focalized caseous pneumonic lesion a few millimeters in diameter, located in well ventilated parts of the lung; it usually occurs under the pleura of the periphery or near the hilum. This lesion may become fibrotic and even calcified, or it may be the source for a widespread dissemination of the disease, especially in colored children. The local disease is called the primary focus. This plus the comparable disease in the lymph nodes at the apex in the adult form. This is due to superimposed infection. In many cases this is a new infection introduced into the body, called superinfection. In others it is a reactivation in some part of the primary complex; this is called reinfection, or endogenous reinfection (Reichle and Gallavan; Long). It is generally believed that the difference in character of the adult type of tuberculosis is a result of a change of reactivity due to the pre-existing disease, but Long is of the opinion that the decisive factors are dosage of

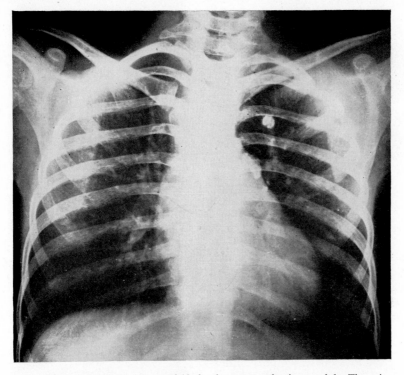

Roentgenograph to show calcified primary complex in an adult. The primary focus is in the left upper lobe and the lymph node is just behind the left upper border of the cardiac shadow.

the hilum which drain the affected region constitute the primary complex. The same course of events may follow primary infection in later life, but frequently here the disease is progressive and may be rapidly fatal (Israel and Long).

THE ADULT TYPE OF TUBERCULOSIS differs in that it is more destructive locally and tends to become chronically progressive; it also shows other features. Whereas the primary lesion in the lung in childhood is likely to be in the middle parts of the lung near the periphery or the hilum, it is most common in bacteria and constitution, including heredity and also environment in the sense of nutrition and general hygiene.

The Ranke hypothesis indicates that the primary complex may become cicatrized, or may give rise to a generalized miliary tuberculosis which may in turn either heal or produce organ tuberculosis. He assumes three stages, namely (1) the primary focus, (2) generalization of the virus, and (3) isolated organ tuberculosis. He believes the generalization to be due to sensitization and the localization to subsequently developed resistance. (See Reisner.) Since hypersensitiveness and resistance may be present simultaneously, the sharp distinction made by Ranke is not justified. The operation of these factors is not

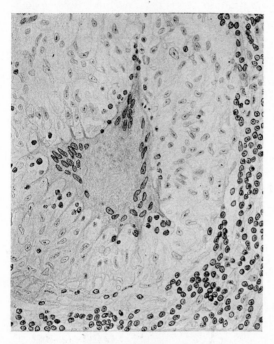

Giant cell in center of miliary tubercle, showing cytoplasmic processes.

clear, but the morphological distinctions appear to be valid.

Types of Lesion. The early reaction to tuberculous infection may be exudative or, as is more commonly the case, tubercles may be formed.

THE TUBERCLE is essentially interstitial in situation, whereas acute tuberculous inflammation affects surfaces such as pulmonary alveolar surfaces, and serous membranes such as pleura, meninges and joints. This does not, however, exclude the possibility of tubercle formation upon such surfaces. The tubercle is a lesion which histologically is extremely characteristic and grossly is, as a rule, easily distinguishable. The simple discrete tubercle is composed of a central mass of large oval or elongated cells with fairly large vesicular nuclei. These are called the endothelioid or epithelioid cells. (Their nature is referred to later in the discussion of the histogenesis of the tubercle.) Surrounding these is a mass of lym-

phocytes. As this lesion develops, the tissues occupied are destroyed, so that within the lesion no remnant of original tissue is likely to be found. Secondary changes occur very early in the course of the process. Endothelial cells often fuse together to form the so-called giant cells of Langhans. When fully developed these are large multinucleated cells with a finely granular cytoplasm. The outline is frequently irregular because of the projection of small cytoplasmic processes, which may extend as minute fibrils out into the surrounding tubercle. The nuclei are somewhat more deeply chromatic than in the original epithelioid cell. The nuclei are oval and frequently arranged in a circle around the margin of the cell with their long axes in a radial position. Sometimes the cell is elongated in character and shows nuclei only at the poles. If the line of section of the cell include only the pole, then the nuclei may appear to be centrally disposed in the cell. Special staining frequently demonstrates tubercle bacilli within the cytoplasm of the giant cell. Not infrequently the center of the cell is the seat of caseous necrosis.

Caseous necrosis of the center of the tubercle appears early in the course and involves the endothelial cells and giant cells particularly. Microscopically, the caseation

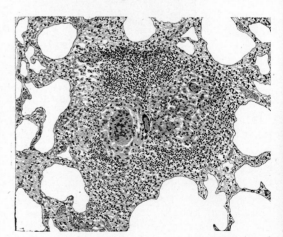

Miliary tubercles of lung with several giant cells.

shows simply a granular necrotic mass. As the process continues and the tubercle enlarges the central caseation also increases in amount. Of great importance is the fact that in the construction of the tubercle, blood vessels do not play a part; the lesion is avascular. The central necrosis in the tubercle is the result in part of the lack of vascularization, and in part perhaps of cellular enzymes, although these have not been satisfactorily demonstrated (Reed). The caseous material and the wall of the tubercle are, as has been shown by Caldwell and others, richer in alcohol-ether soluble substance than is normal tissue. This soluble material consists largely of cholesterol, phospholipins and unsaturated fatty acids and their soaps. The protein content is chiefly in the form of coagulated pro-

ance. The antitryptic effect of the soaps of fatty acids is insufficient to prevent action by the proteolytic enzymes and liquefaction of the mass takes place. When this occurs the microscopic picture is considerably altered and may show nothing characteristic of tuberculosis. Regardless of secondary changes the essential cells of the characteristic tubercle are the epithelioid cell and lymphocyte.

The tubercle may increase in size either by growth of the original tubercle or by the formation of satellite or daughter tubercles. It is believed that the migration of phagocytic mononuclear cells containing live

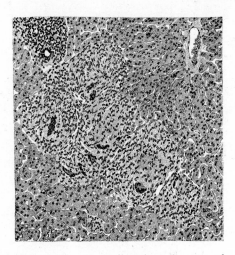

Miliary tubercles of liver in early stage of coalescence.

Miliary tubercles in pia-arachnoid of the cerebrum.

tein which undergoes little or no digestion (see Wells, De Witt and Long). Caseous foci tend to remain caseous or to become even more solid. Ordinarily, they show no disposition toward softening or liquefaction and this is believed by Jobling and Petersen to be due to the presence of soaps of fatty acids, which have a marked antitryptic effect and therefore inhibit the action of autolytic enzymes. There is no doubt that many of the earliest reactions to tuberculous infection show polymorphonuclear leukocytes, especially in previously tuberculous animals, but they disappear as the characteristic tubercle develops. If secondary pyogenic infection occur, leukocytes again make their appear-

bacilli, or the transmission of bacilli in the flow of tissue juices serves to implant a few organisms in the immediate neighborhood. These lead to the production of secondary tubercles. As these enlarge they join with the original mass to produce a more rapid enlargement. This process of secondary tubercle formation and successive enlargement of the original mass may go on to the production of large solitary tubercles, such as are found in the brain or in the liver where diameters of 1, 2 or 3 cm. are not uncommon. At any stage during the progress of the tuberculous lesion, resistance may become sufficient to prevent further spread. When this occurs, fibroblasts take part in the reaction and a zone of proliferating connective tissue is found around and sometimes within the zone of lymphocytes and epithelioid cells. This may be of granulation tissue type and be fairly well vascularized. In the majority of instances, however, the growth of connective tissue is slow and little vascular participation is observed. The entire mass may be completely encapsulated by the growth of this connective tissue. After encapsulation has occurred, the lesion may remain quiescent throughout life or may exhibit renewed activity as indicated by the development of fresh active tubercles in the margin.

Histogenesis of the Tubercle

The primary lodgment of the tubercle bacilli, notably in the liver of experimental ing clasmatocytes of the tissues or to fibroblasts. Long believes that they may originate in some more or less distant situation and are transported to the site of tubercle formation. Good reasons are given for all these views but it seems most likely that they are derived ultimately from reticulo-endothelial cells.

In support of the view that cells of the reticulo-endothelial system are affected is the demonstration by Rosenthal that tuberculosis induces a generalized swelling and proliferation of the reticulo-endothelial system. Certain other investigators interpret this as a hetero-allergic reaction and suggest that the

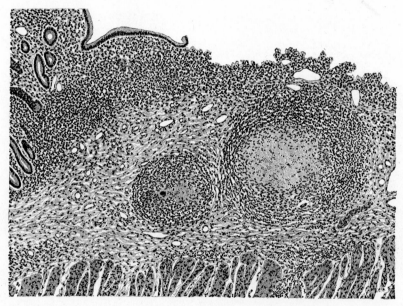

Miliary tubercles in an intestinal ulcer. Note incomplete regeneration of surface epithelium.

animals, may be followed immediately by an accumulation of leukocytes and the formation of a small amount of fibrin. This may sometimes be observed in early tubercles in man, but the polymorphonuclears do not remain permanently in the lesion. The type cell of the usual tubercle as seen in tissue sections is a large mononuclear cell, variously called "endothelial," "endothelioid" and "epithelioid." The origin of these cells has been studied extensively. Some investigators believe they originate locally from endothelium of the blood and lymphatic vessels. Others attribute their origin to the monocytes of the circulating blood, to the wandering focal accumulation of the cells in the tubercle is a manifestation of local allergy (Dienes and Mallory). Another presumptive indication of this sort of change is found in the increase of monocytes in the circulating blood (Cunningham and Tompkins; Finner). Advantage has been taken of the chemical partition of tubercle bacilli by Anderson and his associates, to determine how the fractions operate in the living animal. Sabin reports that the phosphatide of the bacteria, principally because of the content of saturated fatty acid, can produce the tubercle; that the unsaponifiable wax attracts monocytes; that the protein attracts plasma cells;

and that the polysaccharide attracts polymorphonuclear neutrophils. In animals which are already tuberculous, Holley finds that the protein induces degenerative changes, but that the phosphatide has no effect upon the tuberculous which it does not have upon nontuberculous animals. Experiments with the chemical fractions in vitro are not complete, but Wartman has found the protein to be chemotropic for leukocytes.

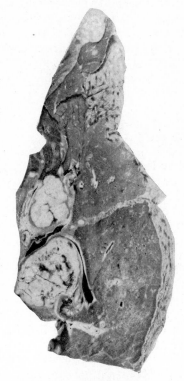

Conglomerate caseous tuberculosis of bronchiopulmonary lymph nodes.

Although the Langhans' giant cell has special morphologic features, as pointed out above, it is fundamentally of foreign-body type for it usually appears only after necrosis has begun. It is formed largely by fusion of epithelioid cells, but perhaps in part by nuclear division without cell division. Supravital staining shows the rosettes of the monocyte in these cells. Lymphocytes also appear and in the older lesions may be present in large numbers, but no convincing explanation has been offered for their occurrence or mode of origin.

LESIONS OTHER THAN THE TUBERCLE. Infection by tubercle bacilli does not invariably lead to the development of the tubercle. Acute inflammatory reactions may appear especially when the bacilli are implanted upon serous membranes such as the meninges, the pleura, pericardium and peritoneum. Rich primary implantation in the lung may lead to the development of a tuberculous pneumonia. Experimentally, such is the case in rabbits. That these exudative types of inflammation in man are entirely the result of rich implantations is open to doubt, however. In the serous membranes, implantation of the organisms must be secondary to a primary focus. This being true, it is conceivable that the primary focus has so influenced the body that new implantations result in more violent reactions. The tuberculin reaction is almost certainly an allergic manifestation; it persists in the body after the establishment of a primary lesion; the acute inflammatory types of tuberculosis are to be grouped in the same general category, but are not to be regarded as purely allergic.

In the serous membranes, the acute reactions show an outpouring of leukocytes, lymphocytes and a fair amount of fibrin formation. In most instances the number of leukocytes is less than that of the lymphocytes and endothelial cells. Tuberculous pneumonia is characterized by considerable edema, moderate fibrin formation and infiltration of leukocytes, lymphocytes and endothelial cells in the alveoli. Necrosis of the exudate and of the tissues involved is common in these diffuse types of tuberculous inflammation. In the meninges, it is not uncommon to find small, generally spherical foci of necrosis of the exudate, which may extend and involve the superficial parts of the brain or cord. In tuberculous pneumonia, necrosis may be much more extensive and involve not only the exudate but also the pulmonary tissue. In these acute inflammations the number of organisms may be extremely great. According to Jobling and Petersen, the necrosis is probably due to the activity of material liberated by the tubercle bacilli. The caseous character of the necrosis is determined by the same factors that determine caseous necrosis in the center of a tubercle, namely, the inhibition of autolytic ferments by the presence of large quantities of soaps of unsaturated fatty acids. Pagel has presented evidence that allergic phenomena are of fundamental importance in the production of the necrosis.

GROSS LESIONS OF TUBERCULOSIS. It is improbable that the earliest form of tubercle is grossly visible except in such a transparent tissue as the eye. Primary discrete tubercles, however, can be seen as minute bodies measuring less than a millimeter in diameter, projecting into a cross section or upon a serous surface, firm, rounded, sharply demarcated and of gray color. As the lesions become larger, however, the color is changed by the central caseous necrosis and the mass becomes yellow. Both these forms of lesions are spoken of as miliary tubercle—the earlier, as the gray miliary tubercle; the later, as the yellow miliary tubercle. These are called miliary because they approximate the size of a millet seed.

Conglomerate tubercles are formed by the fusion of neighboring miliary tubercles or by growth of, and fusion with, secondary or daughter tubercles as already described. The conglomerate tubercle is larger than the miliary and may attain considerable size. It shows the central caseous mass characterized by a relatively dry, finely granular, yellow, often somewhat soapy cross section, surrounded by a thin rim of gray material made up of the reacting cells. The color varies from a very pale grayish-yellow to a deep yellow, and the consistency from a firm, slightly friable mass to a distinctly softer and sometimes almost semifluid mass. Secondary infection determines more distinct softening and pus formation. The outline of the smaller conglomerate tubercle may be distinctly irregular or lobulated when the lesion is due to fusion of several miliary tubercles. When the size is greater, attaining a diameter of 0.5 to 1.0 cm., the term conglomerate tubercle is usually employed, but the lesion is sometimes referred to as diffuse tuberculous tissue. The mass may attain a diameter of several centimeters. This lesion is frequently called the solitary tubercle, or, if the size be impressive, it may be referred to as a tuberculoma.

Secondary changes in the tubercle are of considerable importance. As the tuberculous mass enlarges or extends, it may grow into and penetrate a surface communicating with the exterior. Thus, a conglomerate tubercle in the lung may involve a bronchus, or bone lesions may communicate with the skin surface either directly or by way of muscle sheaths; tuberculosis of the epididymis may rupture directly through the scrotum; tubercles of the intestinal lining usually rupture into the lumen. Communication with these surfaces exposes the lesion to additional infection by pyogenic organisms and leukocytes infiltrate. They bring enzymes which overbalance the anti-enzymatic activity of the soaps of the unsaturated fatty acids, and softening and liquefaction occur. Thereafter, open cavities form in the lungs, sinuses develop from lesions of the bones, and ulceration occurs in the intestines. The suppuration incident to the secondary infection may result in rapid extension of the lesion. On the other hand, this infection may stimulate more sturdy granulation than does the tubercle bacillus, and the resulting fibrosis may lead to sharp delimitation of the tuberculous process. As Opie has demonstrated in the pleura of the dog, the presence of large numbers of leukocytes may aid materially in limiting the tuberculous process. It is generally stated that the chills, fever and night sweats of advanced pulmonary tuberculosis are due to the secondary pyogenic infection. However, the capacity of the tubercle bacillus to excite acute inflammation makes it at least possible that these clinical signs are due to the tubercle bacillus alone in some instances.

When the tubercle grows in the neighborhood of vessels thrombosis occurs as the vessel walls are involved. If secondary infection has occurred, this thrombosis is likely to be well pronounced. As the thrombus becomes organized the vessel is converted into a fibrous mass. Involvement externally of bronchi, particularly smaller branches, leads to fibrosis of the walls and finally conversion into a fibrous mass. These are more resistant to the destructive action either of the tuberculous process or of the secondary infection, and in cavities of the lung it is common to find trabeculae made up of those fibrous blood vessels and bronchi.

Tuberculosis may be disseminated in various organs of the body in the condition called disseminated or generalized miliary tuberculosis. The mode of dissemination will be discussed subsequently. Such dissemination usually occurs as the result of pulmonary tuberculosis but may originate in secondary situations such as bone or epididymis. The lesions are usually of uniform size, distributed through the substance of the organs. In addition to the lungs, the liver, the spleen and the kidneys commonly show the miliary

and endothelial cells, fewer polymorphonuclear leukocytes, and a distinct disposition to undergo caseation necrosis. Giant cells and more or less well-defined tubercles are usually found. Where resistance to tuberculous infection is manifest varying degrees of cicatrization occur. This may progress through

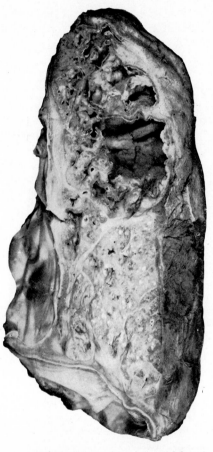

Tuberculous cavity of upper lobe of lung. Note trabeculation of cavity, thickened pleura, caseous tuberculous pneumonia of lower lobe.

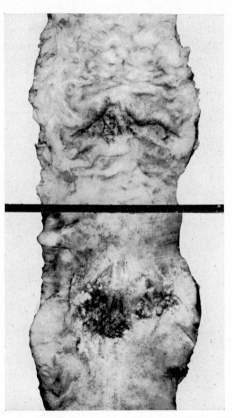

Tuberculous ulcer of small intestine, the mucosal aspect above, the peritoneal below.

tubercles. No organ is immune to invasion in this disease, but the pancreas is only rarely affected, the uterus is usually free and although the pericardium may be tuberculous the myocardium usually escapes.

LATER LESIONS OF TUBERCULOSIS. A tuberculous granulation tissue is seen around open lesions of tuberculosis, that is lesions communicating with surfaces. It resembles nontuberculous granulation tissue, but is likely to show a richer content of lymphoid

the intermediation of granulation tissue or may surround nonulcerated tubercles. Small primary or even secondary lesions may become so densely encapsulated as to arrest the progress of the lesion. Under certain vaguely defined conditions the lesion may permit dissemination of the remaining living organisms, with local extension of the tuberculous process. On the other hand, the surrounding fibrosis may be incomplete or inadequate to arrest the process and the disease becomes chronic.

Chronic fibrous tuberculosis shows tubercle formation in places but is characterized by progressive growth of dense fibrous connective tissue. Fibrous adhesions are common on surfaces such as the pleura. Chronic tuberculosis of the serous membranes often shows extensive hyalinization of the inflammatory fibrous tissue. Calcification is common in the older lesions of tuberculosis. Small lesions may be almost completely calcified after caseous necrosis and encapsulation, yet the bacilli remain alive for many years. It is probable that the soapy materials in the caseous necrosis favor, in a physicochemical manner, the infiltration and deposition of calcium salts (see Maver and Wells). Increased calcium content of the blood appears to favor calcification of tuberculous foci (Spies).

bercle but are not altogether satisfactory in determining whether the lesion is due to the bacterial body or to its products. It is probable that both play a part. It cannot be said that the tubercle bacillus produces a toxin in the strict sense of the word and we agree with Krause that "it is the general opinion that no true toxin of the micro-organism has ever been demonstrated."

Thus it cannot be said that the tuberculin reaction is due to a toxin. Although various constituents of the organisms have been held responsible, it is now known that it is produced by water soluble tuberculoprotein, which can be recovered from the organisms and also from certain media in

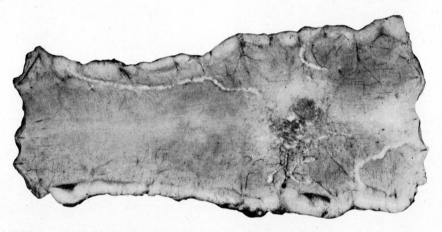

Miliary tubercles in peritoneal lymphatics, extending from tuberculous involvement of peritoneum by tuberculous ulcer of ileum.

Immunity in Tuberculosis. The tubercle bacillus produces its effects partly as the result of the presence of the bacterial bodies and partly as the result of more or less soluble products of its growth. It has long been known that the injection of killed tubercle bacilli and of the lipids of tubercle bacilli and other acid-fast bacteria, as well as defatted tubercle bacilli, may induce the formation of tubercles. As indicated previously, Anderson has fractionated tubercle bacilli chemically, and Sabin and others have worked with these fractions. Thus the phosphatide of the bacteria, principally because of the content of saturated fatty acid, can produce the tubercle. The unsaponifiable wax attracts monocytes. The proteins attract plasma cells, and the polysaccharide attracts polymorphonuclear leukocytes. These facts explain the cellular constituents of the tu-

which they are grown. The protein in the medium is probably the result of liberation upon death of the bacteria. The reaction is an acute exudative inflammation, with hyperemia, exudation of leukocytes and infiltration of large mononuclear cells, together with formation of a certain amount of fibrin. There is usually a central focus of necrosis. It is agreed that lysins which act upon the bacillus and the soluble protein are developed in the animal or man. The product of this action excites the inflammation. (See Long; Seibert.)

Agglutinins and precipitins have been demonstrated in experimental animals, but they are rare in man. Complement-fixing antibodies have been found in experimental animals and in the human disease; they appear to be greatest in the active stages and tend to disappear in quiescent stages. These are of interest but have not been shown to be a measure of resistance or immunity.

TUBERCULIN REACTION. The various types of tuberculin reaction are of great importance clinically, and the results have been widely utilized in epidemiology and in hypotheses concerning the immunology of the disease. The tuberculin may be applied intradermally, subcutaneously (for general reactions), in the conjunctival sac or percutaneously as in a salve. Positive local reactions are of inflammatory character; positive general reactions are febrile. The test becomes positive soon after infection and persists indefinitely, although decreases may be observed when the disease is in an active stage. Reactors may become negative also during the course of acute infections. It is a highly specific test when due consideration is given to the dosage employed; thus the most careful interpretation is required. Sensitivity of the test is variable, but cases in which animal inoculation was the only way to prove the existence of the disease have been diagnosed on this basis. That subcutaneous injections of tuberculin can excite a latent lesion to activity is unquestioned, but it is doubtful if this occurs often. There has been dispute as to whether the reaction is one of immunity or of sensitization, but general opinion favors the latter.

Tuberculosis is generally thought of as a disease of civilization; this is not necessarily true because it does occur in primitive races. Nevertheless the environmental conditions of civilization which produce intimate contacts favor transfer of infection from one person to another. In isolated communities where tuberculosis is ordinarily infrequent the disease, when it does affect individuals, is likely to run a progressively severe course. When people of these groups are transplanted to civilized communities they show much the same disposition to severe disease. It has been thought that the milder course of disease in civilized communities is due to the fact that those who are susceptible have been killed off. However, as will be mentioned later, the severity or mildness may be determined by heredity and constitution. Just why tuberculosis in primitive peoples is likely to be severe and that in civilized communities likely to be mild is not yet definitely settled. This has a bearing on the problem concerning

race. Long states that there is no question of there being a greater mortality from tuberculosis in Negroes than in whites, but the negro mortality rate is no higher today than the white mortality rate 35 years ago. Thus there is little to support the view that there is an innate racial susceptibility. He says further that "it seems much more likely that the difference in mortality rate in negroes is in large part a difference in environment, and it has been proved that both races have responded to improving environment with a continuously dropping death rate."

Age and sex appear to play a certain part in the disease. It is well known that children become the victims of tuberculosis in its primary stage more often than do adults. Nevertheless, in the age period from 4 to 14 years, children rarely acquire tuberculosis in spite of exposure. Sex is of some importance because adolescent girls, in spite of relatively less exposure to infection, succumb to tuberculosis more frequently than boys in comparable age groups.

In addition there is the problem of why the adult type of tuberculosis usually runs a course different from that of the primary infection. Whether the induction of chronicity in the adult type of disease is related to immunity cannot definitely be said. If immunity be involved, it probably depends upon local cellular resistance. Certainly the establishment of reinfection and superinfection is now well known, and this is hardly in line with the idea that there is a general immunity. Although not proved by laboratory experiments, it is reasonably evident that malnutrition, such as occurs in famine; the existence of acute diseases, such as measles and influenza; and the existence of chronic exhausting diseases of various kinds all favor renewed activity in patients with minor tuberculous disease. However, the exact mechanism of this disturbance of resistance is not yet known.

The tubercle is surrounded by a wall of lymphocytes. Jobling and Petersen have demonstrated a lipase in lymphocytes and suggest that this may attack the bacilli by dissolving the waxy shell, but Reed was unable to find such a ferment. Pavlow, however, found that lymphocyte extracts destroy tubercle bacilli. Reticulo-endothelial cells, particularly those of the liver and spleen, have a high phagocytic power for tubercle bacilli, as is true also of the giant cells. Anatomic studies indicate that cellular reactions constitute a most important mechanism in tuberculosis and play a large part in its arrest.

Dissemination of Tuberculosis. The dissemination of tuberculosis may occur through the blood stream, the lymphatic stream, over surfaces, by direct extension or, as Permar points out, by the migration of epithelioid cells which contain bacilli. The

berculosis usually shows lesions of about the same size and presumably of about the same age in various organs. It is therefore assumed that dissemination results from rupture of a lesion through the vessel wall, thus discharging into the blood stream a large number of organisms, a "shower" of tubercle bacilli, at one time. Nevertheless, smaller discharges into the blood stream must occur. On this basis are explained tuberculous lesions of bones and joints as well as those of the genito-urinary tract, of the meninges and of

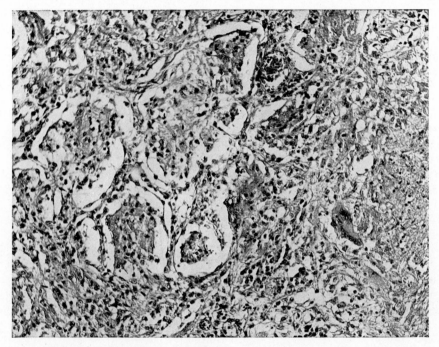

Tuberculous pneumonia. To the lower right is a tubercle. The alveoli show mononuclear cells and fibrin, and the exudate is in process of organization.

growth of tubercles may involve blood-vessel walls, either veins or arteries. If reactive thrombosis does not occur, the tubercles may project into the lumen of the vessel and tubercle bacilli thus gain access to the blood stream. In more rapidly extending lesions, preëxisting tubercles may rupture directly into the blood stream. In the case of rupture into a pulmonary artery, the dissemination through the blood stream may be limited to the part of the lung supplied by that artery. In most cases, however, rupture into the blood stream determines widely disseminated tuberculosis throughout the body.

This so-called disseminated miliary tu-

other situations in which transmission from the primary focus of infection must be by the blood. According to Krause, the secondary tubercles arise in the immediately neighboring tissues not within the blood vessels; the bacteria must penetrate the tissues before they produce lesions.

Dissemination through lymphatic tracts is much more common, but does not result in such widespread lesions as dissemination through the blood channels, except where a tuberculous thoracic duct supplies organisms to the blood stream. Tubercle bacilli may be carried in the lymphatic stream either free or within phagocytic cells.

Lesions are most commonly established in lymph nodes which drain the affected regions. Nevertheless, tubercles may also appear in the walls of lymphatic vessels. This is particularly well seen in the lymphatics of the intestine about an area of ulceration of the mucosa. In certain situations, particularly the lung, the involvement of draining lymph nodes may block them so that no further drainage is possible. The result is retrograde flow to other nodes or to other situations. Involvement of the nodes of the hilum of the lung may cause retrograde flow of lymph through the lung toward the pleura, and consequent dissemination of tuberculosis along the perivascular and peribronchial lymphatics. This results in the formation of numerous tubercles about the vessels and smaller bronchi, the so-called peribronchial and perivascular tuberculosis. Dissemination over surfaces is observed sometimes in the lung, where aspiration of tuberculous material along the bronchial tree may result in secondary tuberculous foci in the branches. There is little doubt that a few foci in the peritoneum may spread over that surface by direct dissemination and the same is undoubtedly true in relation to pleura, meninges, and pericardium. Patients with a long standing tuberculous cavity of the lung frequently have an associated ulcerative tuberculosis of the intestine. This may be due to swallowing organisms with the sputum. It might be expected that the gastric secretion would destroy the bacilli, but such work as that of Kopeloff leaves no doubt that with reduced acidity, bacteria survive exposure to gastric juice. Calmette is of the opinion that intestinal involvement is more frequently due to dissemination through the blood stream than to swallowing. It might also be due to transfer by migrating phagocytic mononuclear cells. Dissemination by direct extension is seen in those instances where enlargement of a focus in a lung involves the pleura. Similarly, tuberculosis of the spinal vertebrae may extend directly and involve kidneys or other neighboring organs. Tuberculosis of the ends of bones may extend directly into joint cavities. Meningeal infections are sometimes observed as the result of direct extension from tuberculosis of the vertebrae and, more rarely, of the cranium.

Heredity and Tuberculosis. Heredity is the transmission of characters through the germ plasm. It is impossible, however, for infectious disease actually to be transmitted by heredity, for the germ cell could not multiply and probably would be destroyed. Thus, heredity of tuberculosis can be dismissed. Two things in this connection need consideration; hereditary constitutional predisposition and congenital infection. It was formerly thought that a certain type of body form indicated a susceptibility to tuberculosis, but modern studies indicate that this is not strictly true. Evidently brunettes are infected quite as often as the patients who are thin skinned, blond, gazelle-eyed, with long narrow flat chests. The fact that the disease appears in various members of the same family is due in large part to exposure to infection. Nevertheless, there is probably a certain degree of constitutional predisposition or resistance upon a hereditary basis. Experimentally, Lurie has found that in the rabbit, resistance to naturally or artificially acquired tuberculosis depends upon genetic constitution. Even this, however, is related in some measure to the dosage of the organisms because with massive dosage the resistance can be overcome.

CONGENITAL INFECTION occasionally occurs, but most of the cases of tuberculosis in early childhood are acquired and do not occur until the patient is four to six months of age. Including infection of placenta or fetus or both, Whitman and Greene collected 113 cases of prenatal infection and add seven additional cases including one of their own. It is possible that some cases have escaped detection or have not been reported, but the whole number is small as compared with the enormous number of children of tuberculous mothers free from the disease at birth. Tuberculosis in the fetus may be widely disseminated by the infected placental blood, or there may be widespread tuberculous pneumonia due to aspiration of amniotic fluid containing bacilli. It is said that there are records of tuberculous stillborn fetuses from mothers whose clinical examination showed no tuberculosis, whereas the fathers were obviously tuberculous; had the mother died and been examined postmortem this story might have been different. It is to be emphasized that tuberculosis in infants is usually a disease acquired from the mother or other member of the family, by infection from sputum. If the infants be removed from this environment immediately after birth, they are likely to escape infection. Although it is conceivable that an infant may be infected from the mother's milk, this is unlikely because the obviously tuberculous mother will not or cannot nurse the infant.

Leprosy

Introduction. Leprosy is a chronic infectious disease, whose effects are observed especially in the skin and nervous system. The *Mycobacterium leprae*, discovered by Hansen in 1871, is believed by many to be the cause of the disease. The disease seems to have originated in some part of the Orient, probably India, and, transmitted in epidemics and by infected individuals, has appeared in practically every part of the world. Nevertheless, it appears to be more frequent and more firmly established in endemic form in tropical and subtropical than in colder regions.

Numerous types of bacteria have been isolated from leprous lesions, varying considerably in morphology, staining properties and conditions of cultivation. Neither by minced material from the lesion nor from cultures has it been possible to reproduce in animals a disease that even closely resembles leprosy. The only postulate of Koch that has been nearly met is the fact that the acid-fast Hansen bacillus is constantly present in some, but not all, of the lesions. There is no final proof that *Mycobacterium leprae* has been cultivated in vitro. (See McKinley.)

Clinical Manifestations. The infection usually occurs in childhood, but the disease may not become manifest for many years. The portal of entry has not been determined but is probably through the skin, although some suspect that it is through the mucosa of the nose. Usually an exposure prolonged over many months precedes development of the disease, but a few cases have given a history that indicates only brief exposure. Individual susceptibility appears to be more important than length of contact. The incubation period is unknown, but it is probably several months and in some instances may be years. Patients do not necessarily have the same type of disease as those from whom they seem to have contracted it.

The onset is usually gradual except that in children it may start fairly quickly with fever, moderately widespread erythema or a mottled swollen skin. Although leprosy tends to become a generalized disease, local manifestations may be conspicuous. Clinically there are two main forms, lepromatous and neural. A third form, tuberculoid leprosy,

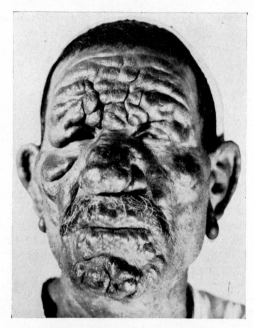

Lepromatous leprosy showing leonine face and loss of hair of eyebrows.

is described, but it is probably a subgroup of the neural form.

THE LEPROMATOUS FORM is manifested especially in the skin either by diffuse involvement in which the skin becomes erythematous, swollen and often smooth and glistening; firm, usually painless, projecting nodules may develop, either discrete or fusing to form large conglomerate masses. When the latter involve forehead and face, together with loss of eyebrows and eyelashes, the face is described as leonine. Involvement of conjunctiva leads to blindness; hearing, smell and taste are sometimes lost. This form of disease progresses fairly rapidly as compared with the neural form. Death, however, is usually due to intercurrent disease such as tuberculosis.

IN NEURAL LEPROSY, formerly called the maculo-anesthetic form, the peripheral

PLATE VIII

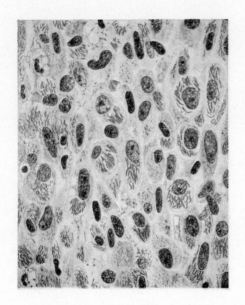

Lepra bacilli in cells of nodule.

nerves are affected. A few or many nerves may be involved. Sometimes beginning with tingling in the region supplied, the first manifestation is usually anesthesia to temperature, followed by loss of pain and tactile sense. The skin shows areas of pallor, which are smooth, finely scaly and inelastic. The cutaneous lesion is usually macular. Atrophy, stiffness and weakness of the muscles occur and contractures, especially of the hands, are common. The nerves become thick, cordlike or nodular, tender, and the nodules occasionally suppurate. The bones of the phalanges may show absorption, which sometimes is especially notable near the joints. Ulcers may develop on the hands, the feet and over the bony prominences.

IN TUBERCULOID LEPROSY, the skin shows elevated plaques, often flat, slightly

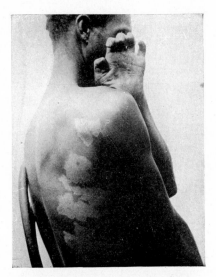

Photograph of neural leprosy, showing depigmented macules on back and claw-hand. Courtesy Guthrie McConnell, M.D.

firmer and often darker in color than the surrounding skin. Some of the lesions are anesthetic. The lesions progress and recede, and some entirely disappear while new ones develop. Periodically the lesions may be greatly accentuated, in what is called the reactive stage, and the same is sometimes true of lepromatous leprosy. It is not to be supposed that one form of the disease occurs without others. Mixtures, with one form predominating, are the rule.

Pathologic Anatomy. The nodules of the lepromatous form vary in size from the microscopic miliary lepromata, which occur in viscera such as the liver, to those 1 or 2 cm. or more in diameter in the skin. These larger nodules are well defined, have a tense overlying epiderm, are firm, cut with resistance and show a slightly bulging, pale-yellow or light-gray cross section. Situated in the

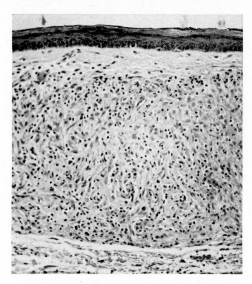

Lepromatous leprosy in corium. Note epithelioid and other types of cells and intervening corium between lesion and flat atrophic epidermis.

corium, they may extend deeply. Microscopically, the nodule is made up principally of large mononuclear cells with an irregular intermingling of lymphocytes, plasma cells and multinucleated giant cells of Langhans type. The large mononuclears and giant cells are often foamy and contain the acid-fast bacteria, identical morphologically with tubercle bacilli. These foam cells may also contain fat. The bacteria may also be found in vascular endothelium, in occasional polymorphonuclear leukocytes and even in epithelium. They are present as small clusters of organisms, the so-called cigar packs, and as large masses called globi. Extracellular organisms are also found and may be in the form of globi, but these globi are originally intracellular (Cowdry). MacCallum describes the lesion as somewhat like a granulation tissue, fairly rich in blood vessels and lymphatics. Fibrous tissue may develop near or in the lesion, and progress so that the lesion is entirely replaced by scar tissue.

The macules in the earlier stages may show a slightly elevated erythematous border. Microscopically the epidermis is usually thin and atrophic and the corium atrophic. Perivascular infiltrations of large mononuclear and lymphoid cells often occur in the corium. In the quiescent lesions this infiltration may be scanty and composed entirely of lymphocytes. In the tuberculoid lesions, microscopic study may disclose merely tiny groups of lymphocytes or there may be larger clusters in which epithelioid cells and even Langhans giant cells are present. Such foci also occur in lepromatous leprosy. The microscopic appearance of tuberculoid leprosy may closely simulate that of Boeck's sarcoid.

Gross examination of the nerve trunks will show either diffuse or nodular enlargement. Microscopically, the epineurium and endoneurium are infiltrated with cells similar to those found in the lepromatous form. Large round cells are distributed irregularly through the connective tissue and are sometimes accompanied by fibroblasts. There is degeneration of both myelin sheath and axis cylinder.

The distribution of bacilli is of importance both anatomically and clinically because in the living patient they may be demonstrated in scrapings from skin and mucous membranes in lepromatous leprosy. They may occasionally be demonstrated in puncture material obtained from the nerves in neural leprosy. It is exceedingly uncommon to find them in tuberculoid leprosy except in the reactive stage. Anatomically, the bacilli are found in the lepromatous lesions in considerable numbers, both as intracellular forms, as globi and as smaller clusters of organisms. They are not so numerous in the nerve lesions and as a rule are not to be found in tissue sections of tuberculoid lesions.

After leprosy has continued for a long time the patient may show a generalized fibrosis of many of the internal viscera. Independent of the development of tuberculosis, amyloid is common.

Immunity. The fact that *Mycobacterium leprae* has never been grown in culture makes it difficult to make statements concerning immune bodies. Nevertheless, with some of the organisms that have been cultivated it has been possible to demonstrate agglutinins and complement-fixing antibodies. The periodic occurrence of crops of leprous lesions indicates a cyclic process. This, together with the fact that reactive stages occur, strongly suggests that there is an alternation of bacterial activity and host resistance, allergic in nature. (See Wade; Cowdry.)

Tularemia

Caused by *Pasteurella tularensis* (McCoy and Chapin, 1912) and described fully by Francis, this disease occurs in rabbits, ground squirrels, wild rats and field mice. Man is highly susceptible to infection but more resistant to the disease than the animals mentioned, the human mortality rate being about 4 per cent, or higher among those seriously ill. Man is most frequently infected by dressing diseased rabbits, but infection is also transmitted by the horse fly and wood

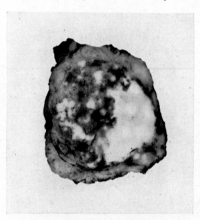

Cross section of lymph node in tularemia. Note the small pole nodules characteristic of the disease. The large mass is an abscess.

tick. Incubation in man is from one to 10 days, most often three days. The disease is always febrile, often with moderate leukocytosis. Agglutinins and opsonins appear in the second week and have persisted as long as 24 years after the attack. The organism is not found in smears or tissues from man and is usually isolated by inoculation of guinea pigs. The gross lesions are diagnostic in inoculated rabbits and guinea pigs. The lesions are miscropic in white mice, in which the cord cells and Kupffer cells of the liver contain large numbers of organisms.

The **clinical manifestations** include chills, fever, and varying degrees of prostration. The course may be acute with recovery, or fulminating and fatal, or it may become subacute with recovery. The disease has different forms. The ulceroglandular form shows a primary lesion in the skin, usually accompanied by enlargement of the neighboring lymph nodes. In the oculoglandular form the primary lesion is a conjunctivitis. A glandular form involving lymph nodes occurs without primary lesion, and occasionally there is a typhoidal form without either primary lesion or lymph-node enlargement. Diagnosis is aided by demonstration of agglutinins and by skin tests with bacterial antigens. Treatment by antibacterial immune serum has reduced morbidity and mortality (Foshay); chemotherapy with sulfonamides has also been helpful.

Pathologic Anatomy. The primary lesion in the skin may arise in a wound or apparently without a wound. It starts as a red, tender papule, sometimes painful, which soon breaks down to form a punched-out sloughing ulcer, usually with a crust over it. In a few instances a secondary cutaneous lesion is described, with small papules on the hands or arms. In the ocular form the conjunctiva is hyperemic, inflamed and may show small pale foci and occasionally considerable fibrinopurulent exudate. The lymph nodes are large and soft in the earlier stages but become firm later on. Small necrotic foci, 1 or 2 mm. in diameter, are seen in cross section and occasionally abscesses form. In the fatal cases, similar small necrotic foci are likely to be found not only in the lymph nodes, but in the spleen, liver, lungs and sometimes on the surfaces of the peritoneum and pleura. Generally speaking, the microscopic observation of these lesions shows basically the same condition. Around foci of necrosis there is a more or less marked infiltration of polymorphonuclear leukocytes and large mononuclear cells, sometimes with other cells of the exudate. In the healing stages, there is an increase in the large mononuclear cells which take on the appearance of elongated epithelioid cells, and Langhans giant cells may be formed. Fibrosis progresses and may encapsulate or completely replace the lesion.

The primary cutaneous lesion shows essentially the same features except for the superficial ulceration beneath which there is desiccated necrotic material with a considerable number of polymorphonuclear leukocytes. Nevertheless, beneath that there is the

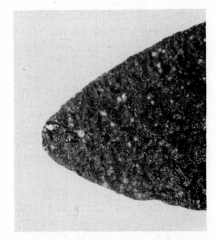

Segment of cross section of spleen, to show tularemic nodules.

focus of necrosis with surrounding cellular infiltration. The secondary cutaneous papules are likely to show necrosis in the corium surrounded by leukocytes and mononuclears,

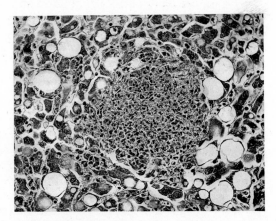

Tularemic nodule in liver, late stage.

and sometimes vesiculation of the epidermis resembling that of smallpox. Foci of necrosis may also be found in the inflamed conjunctiva. The peritoneum may contain a good deal of fluid exudate in which the organisms can be identified together with the formation of the small pale foci on the peritoneal surface. The pleura may show a considerable degree of fibrinoserous pleurisy. In the lungs, in addition to the necrotic foci, there may be a fairly widespread bronchopneumonia, which microscopically is characterized by the fact that the exudate is made up principally of large mononuclear cells with moderate edema and a few other cells. Fibrin is not conspicuous. Where the pneumonia approximates the foci of necrosis there may be necrosis of the alveolar walls. (See Francis; Lillie.)

Glanders

Introduction. Glanders is a specific infectious disease, which, more particularly in the prolonged and chronic cases, exhibits lesions which microscopically are definitely granulomatous. Although principally a disease of the horse and ass, it affects other animals and occasionally is observed in man, particularly those in contact with horses. It has also been observed in man as a laboratory infection. The disease has been known since the middle ages and is one of the first in which definite infectious character was demonstrated, this having been proven in the latter part of the eighteenth century. The causative organism is the *Pasteurella mallei*, a gram-negative, somewhat beaded, nonmotile, curved or straight rod.

Clinical Features. Both in horse and in man the disease may appear in either acute or chronic form. In man the acute form has an incubation period of four to eight days and is usually fatal within three to four weeks. Infection is usually by implantation of material from infected horses into the nose, or in abrasions or cuts in the skin. At the site of inoculation a red, swollen papule develops which rapidly becomes pustular and then breaks down leaving an ulcer with granular base and undermined edges. The disease is febrile and may be introduced with chills or other violent symptoms. Enlargement of the regional lymph nodes is common, and cases are likely to show a more or less diffuse erythematous or erythematopapular eruption. Beginning in the nose, the first symptoms may be the discharge of bloody mucopus, following which the local and general symptoms progress as described. Extension from the nose may involve the pharynx, the soft palate and the larynx. The spleen and liver are likely to be enlarged and not uncommonly rheumatic pains are observed in the joints. Secondary subcutaneous nodules which soften

and ulcerate may occur. In the chronic form, the incubation time is probably longer and the development of the individual lesion is slower. The local and general symptoms are not so severe. The superficial lesions are sometimes taken for syphilis, and metastasis in the deeper tissues of the body may resemble tuberculosis. Although practically all acute cases are fatal, according to Kolle and Hetsch about half the chronic cases recover spontaneously.

The acute disease in the horse is very much like that in man, prostration is extremely marked and the outcome is usually fatal. The chronic disease in horses may last over years, with discharge from the nose, and after the course of time, considerable destruction of the nasal septum. In addition, the lymph nodes are enlarged and not uncommonly break down. These are the "farcy nodules," particularly likely to be seen along the tendons of the extremities, either as deep-seated putty-like nodules or as somewhat deep eroding ulcers.

Pathologic Anatomy. The superficial lesions are described above; on section it is

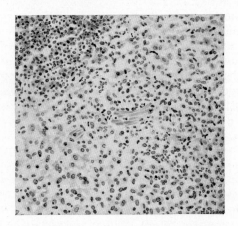

Histology of glanders. Note the variety of cells present and in the upper part of the field the pleomorphic character of chromatin masses.

found that, as a rule, there is some reactive fibrosis in the surrounding tissue. Of the internal viscera, the lung is most likely to show specific lesions. Here the lesion appears somewhat like small conglomerate and large conglomerate tubercles, although in some instances there is a resemblance to bronchopneumonia. The spleen is the seat of an acute hyperplastic enlargement. The liver, kidneys and heart are likely to show cloudy swelling or fatty degeneration. Microscopically, the lesion differs with the duration of the disease. The study of the disease in man and animals, as well as by experimental methods, indicates that the lesions probably vary depending upon the virulence of the organism. The lesion may be destructive, accompanied by acute inflammation, or it may be granulomatous. Duval and White point out that in experimental animals, lesions of different types are produced, depending upon virulence. The more virulent organisms produce an early destruction of tissues, followed rapidly by an infiltration of leukocytes and formation of fibrin. Less virulent organisms produce little or no immediate destruction of the tissues, but their injection is followed rapidly by an inflammatory infiltration. Organisms of low virulence produce primary tissue proliferation with epithelioid cells in large numbers, and giant-cell formation.

As ordinarily seen in man the lesions show various foci, with central necrosis of the tissues and of the exudate. Karyorrhexis of tissue nuclei and of the nuclei of invading leukocytes, as well as pyknosis, lead to the formation of irregular and bizarre masses of chromatin. In the neighborhood are found masses of polymorphonuclear leukocytes with a few lymphocytes. Fibrin may be present in the form of small fibrils. In addition, irregular masses of epithelioid cells are observed, either outside a layer of leukocytes or immediately adjacent to a necrotic mass. Giant cells are not common in the human lesion but may be found in the form of typical Langhans giant cells or more nearly like the foreign body type of giant cell. Granulation tissue is often abundant. Hemorrhage is not uncommon. The bacilli may be demonstrated in the large mononuclear cells or in the giant cells. Duval calls attention to lesions of the smaller blood vessels, in which there is fatty degeneration of the musculature underlying the intima, preceded by, or associated with, proliferation of the intimal endothelium. Lesions examined microscopically early in the disease show principally necrosis and suppuration, whereas those examined later show a greater prominence of epithelioid cells. Provided the lesion be old enough, a considerable amount of reactive fibrosis appears in the marginal areas. In the neighborhood of the glanders nodule, pulmonary lesions show a reactive bronchopneumonia which may exhibit organization.

Immunity. Natural infection with the disease leads to the production of precipitins, agglutinins and complement-fixing antibodies. Furthermore, hypersusceptibility occurs. Agglutinins are at their height at the 5th and 11th day of the disease, and complement-fixing bodies appear at about the same time or slightly later. Hypersusceptibility is demonstrated by the use of mallein, prepared from cultures of the organism. Within a few hours, subcutaneous injection leads to a fairly large local reaction with tenderness, swelling and redness, together with fever which may last for several days. Instillation of mallein into the conjunctival sac is followed rapidly by inflammaation and even suppuration of the conjunctiva. These tests are used largely in animals but because of their profound reaction are not commonly employed in man. The diagnostic test in man is the Strauss reaction. This is performed by intraperitoneal injection of suspected material or culture into the male guinea-pig. Within two or three days the spermatic cord becomes swollen and this is followed rapidly by enlargement of the testes. The latter lesion may break down and lead to superficial discharge of pus in which organisms are readily demonstrated. The animal usually dies in one or two weeks. In addition to the lesions of the testes and spermatic cord there may be a more or less marked acute peritonitis.

A moderate degree of immunity can be obtained in animals by vaccination but this is by no means absolute.

Melioidosis. This disease occurs in Indo-China, Ceylon and the Malay states. It has been observed in guinea pigs, rabbits, rats, cats, dogs and the horse. It may affect man and appears to be highly fatal. The lesions are somewhat like those of glanders and the organism isolated is called *B. whitmori*, which is closely related to *Pasteurella mallei* (Flescher).

Rhinoscleroma

Introduction. Rhinoscleroma is a chronic granulomatous infection, which begins in the anterior part of the nasal fossa and often extends to the soft palate, pharynx and even larynx, and to the anterior nares and upper lip and may perforate the hard palate. It occurs rarely in larynx and bronchi. Since it is not confined to the nose, the name scleroma has been suggested but not widely adopted. The disease is endemic in various parts of the world and is most prevalent in southeastern Europe, "the shores of the Danube." It is almost certainly caused by *Klebsiella rhinoscleromatis*, the bacillus of Frisch, an organism much like Friedländer's bacillus, but clearly identified by Morris and Julianelle. It grows readily in culture, but the

nodule comprises a mass of plasma and lymphoid cells, the latter predominating near the surface. Large mononuclears and an occasional polymorphonuclear may be found. The lesion is well vascularized in the second stage, but this decreases as the connective tissue increases in the later stages. Globular hyaline masses may replace the cytoplasm of large mononuclears and appear also in lymph spaces and blood vessels. The specific cells are the Mikulicz cells, which are either irregularly distributed through the lesion or are clumped in masses of a dozen or more. These

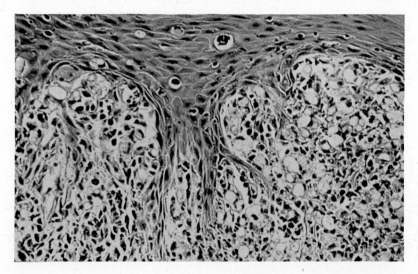

Rhinoscleroma. The large vacuolated cells with shrunken eccentrically placed nuclei are Mikulicz cells.

disease has not yet been reproduced in experimental animals and thus all the postulates of Koch have not been met.

Pathologic Anatomy. The lesion, which originates in the nose, progresses through three stages. The first is a chronic nasal catarrh, the second shows granulomatous nodules and the third a long period of cicatricial contraction. Only the granuloma of the second stage is morphologically characteristic. Small, firm, pale-brown nodules arise in the deeper mucosa and fuse later to form larger masses which may attain a diameter of 1.5 to 2.0 cm. or more. Manipulation may produce bleeding, but ulceration is uncommon. The nodules cut with resistance and show a red or reddish gray, bleeding, slightly retracted cross section.

Microscopically, the granulomatous

are large oval or round cells, four to five times the diameter of the plasma cell. The cytoplasm contains large vacuoles known to be neither fat nor glycogen. They contain the bacilli either sparsely around the margin of the cell or crowding the entire cytoplasmic mass. Fine technic may demonstrate capsules. The nuclei are relatively small, frequently pyknotic and so shrunken as to present a serrated outline. Although thought to be derived from plasma cells, the Mikulicz cells are probably large mononuclear phagocytes of reticulo-endothelial origin. The vacuoles probably are the result of the presence in the cells of the bacteria, although other hypotheses have been offered.

Immune Reactions. Bailey found that the serum of a patient fixed complement in the presence of both homologous and heterologous strains, in higher dilutions than Friedländer's bacillus. Precipitin and agglutination reactions were not specific. Anderson found that vaccines were not permanently beneficial to one case so treated.

The introduction of radium therapy has proved highly beneficial, whereas formerly the disease was usually fatal (see Figi and Thompson). Stelwagon reports a case in which malignant change occurred.

DUE TO SPIROCHETAL ORGANISMS

Syphilis

Introduction. Syphilis is often called lues and, in olden days, great pox. Known for centuries, but confused with other venereal diseases, it was not until the early part of the nineteenth century that it was clearly distinguished from gonorrhea. There has been lengthy dispute as to whether it was introduced into Europe as a result of the voyages led by Columbus or whether it had previously existed there. Whatever the truth of that matter, the disease now occurs in all parts of the world. For the most part it is acquired in early adult life, the number of congenital cases being relatively small. The incidence varies widely in different countries and in different social groups. In the United States, serologic tests are positive in from 5 to 20 per cent of dispensary patients. In our dispensary, about 15 per cent of the Negroes and about 2 per cent of the whites are positive. In the general population, the incidence is much lower and in a group of 10,000 voluntary donors of blood for plasma, the incidence of positive tests was 0.24 per cent. In men between the ages of 20 and 39, it is estimated that about 1.6 per cent are infected. In general, men are more often infected than women, but according to Turner, whereas the disease is almost twice as frequent in white males as in white females, it is more common in Negro females than in Negro males.

Marital transmission is so frequent that the wife of a syphilitic husband acquires the disease in nearly half the marriages. The more remote the acquisition of the disease and the more thorough the treatment, the less likely is marital infection. Congenital transmission is less common.

Causative Organism. That the disease is infectious has long been recognized, but it was not until 1903 that transmission to animals was accomplished, when Metchnikoff and Roux produced lesions in the chimpanzee by inoculation of material from early human disease. In 1906, Bertarelli reported the inoculation of rabbits and, in 1907, Parodi introduced a method of injection of syphilitic material into the rabbit testis, a procedure widely used for study of the disease. Since then lesions have been produced in the guinea-pig and transiently in the dog, sheep and horse. Brown and Pearce, in classical studies, showed that the rabbit may exhibit primary, secondary and probably tertiary lesions.

In the meantime (1905) Schaudinn and Hoffmann announced their demonstration of the presence in the disease of *Treponema pallidum*, commonly but incorrectly called *Spirochaeta pallida*. This is a slender coiled organism, 3 to 15 micra in length and about 0.5 micron in diameter. The coils are regular and closely spaced; the ends are pointed and continue into a flagella-like strand. It exhibits active movement, both rotary and progressive. It can be demonstrated in the moisture of the primary lesion and in other conditions by darkfield illumination. It can be seen when India ink is used to produce a black background and may be stained by the Giemsa and the Fontana methods. In tissues it is best demonstrated by the Levaditi technic or some modification of it. The organisms are readily killed by heat, by drying and by soap solutions, but they may remain active on moist towels for as much as 11 or 12 hours (Zinsser and Hopkins) and in the refrigerator for as much as seven days (Rosahn). In the laboratory it and other organisms may survive a temperature of $-78°$ C. for as much as three years (Turner). Many attempts have been made to cultivate the *Treponema*, but although they remain alive for several days, there is no proof that they multiply. The organism is practically constant in the lesions of man and the rabbit, but otherwise the postulates of Koch have not been met. The supposed occurrence of different morphologic strains is due to environmental conditions (Pearce). The idea that there are neurotropic and dermatropic strains has not been given conclusive support. For a time doubt was thrown on the experimental disease in rabbits because they are subject to a natural disease caused by *Spirochaeta cuniculi*, but Warthin and his associates, as well as others, found that the two diseases are distinguishable and that the experimental work with syphilis can be accepted.

In the secondary stage several recrudescences may appear, separated by periods of latency. The lesions of the later recrudescences tend to be more destructive and somewhat more deep seated, and it is often difficult to determine whether these lesions (e.g., the

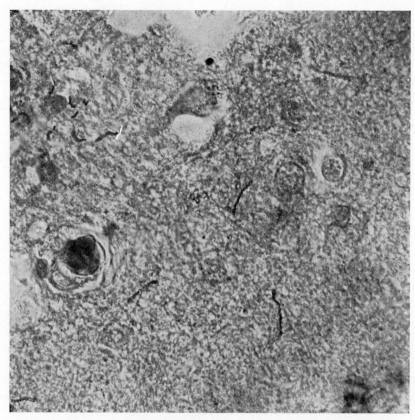

Spirochetes in brain of paresis. From Noguchi and Moore, Jour. Exper. Med.

Lesions in Man. It is customary to divide the manifestations of syphilis in man into a primary stage, a secondary stage, and a tertiary stage. Formerly a parasyphilitic or metasyphilitic stage was described, in which sclerotic lesions, particularly of the central nervous and vascular systems, appear. It is now known that these lesions are directly attributable to the treponema and are therefore truly syphilitic rather than parasyphilitic. The division into stages is convenient but not always practicable.

The primary stage is usually distinctive, but sharp separation between the secondary and tertiary stages is sometimes impossible. It is essential to regard syphilis as a disease which shows recurring cycles of manifestations.

serpiginous skin ulcers and the syphilitic rupia) should be classed as secondary or tertiary. This stage may also show cycles of recurrence, or may be evidenced simply by the functional deficiency of organs the seat of advanced syphilitic fibrosis.

INFECTION is usually by sexual contact and the primary lesion, the chancre, is found upon the glans penis or prepuce, upon the labia, vaginal wall or uterine cervix. Chancres of the lip, tongue, tonsil, nipple, finger or other extragenital situations are the result of accidental contamination by towels, drinking and eating utensils, pipes, clothing, etc., kissing, sexual perversions, or may represent accidental infections, as on the hands of physicians and nurses or the breasts of wet-nurses; rarely it may be transmitted from

PLATE IX

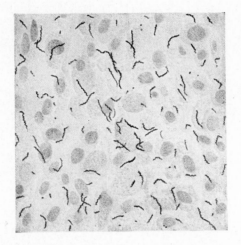

Spirochetes in a chancre of the penis, stained
by the Levaditi technic.

sputum in tattooing and in ritual circumcision. The lesions that are most likely to be a source of infection for others are the chancre, mucous patches of mucous membranes, moist papules and open lesions of the skin in late secondary and early tertiary syphilis. There are so few treponemata in late tertiary lesions that they are not highly infectious. The period of incubaton is from two to five weeks, usually about three weeks. The chancre appears at the site of inoculation. Chancres, however, may be concealed, for example in the anterior urethra of males and in the vagina and uterine cervix of females. In syphilis due to transfusion, chancre

Before the development of the primary lesion there is, as has been stated, a period of incubation in which symptoms are absent. After the subsidence of the chancre there is a period of latency, variable in duration, before secondary lesions occur. After the secondary stage a period of latency is observed which may be short or may last over many years. Tertiary lesions may occur and subside, particularly when treated, only to recur at some later time. The fibrosis and sclerosis of late syphilis progress in spite of clinical and even immunologic evidence indicating quiescence of the disease. Furthermore, patients apparently cured may suffer relapses.

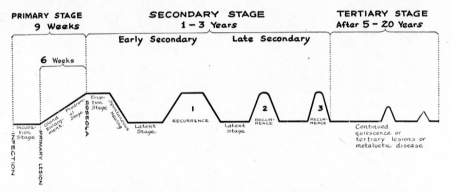

Diagram to show cyclic development of symptoms and signs in syphilis; the peaks indicate clinical manifestations in general, not necessarily fever. Modified from Kolle and Hetsch, Die Experimentelle Bakteriologie und die Infektionskrankheiten, Berlin, 1919.

is not observed; there is an incubaton period of about 10 weeks (Klauder and Butterworth). After entrance through the usual portals, the organisms are rapidly disseminated. In animals they appear in the blood and the regional lymph nodes in less than 5 minutes, and in animals and man are recoverable from the blood for long periods of time (Raiziss and Severac). Dissemination takes place through lymphatics and after the regional nodes are affected others follow suit. Dissemination through the blood stream results in deposit of the organisms throughout, but apparently they may remain latent for years as far as the production of local lesions is concerned. Clinically the excision of the chancre does not prevent full development of the disease, and the same is true of excision of the primary testicular lesion in animals. Warthin's work indicates that once the disease is established, the organisms are probably never entirely removed from the body.

THE PRIMARY LESION is the hard chancre or hunterian chancre or true chancre and is to be differentiated from the soft chancre or chancroid, ascribed to an entirely different organism. The typical hunterian chancre begins as either an acuminate or flat papule, firm, slightly reddened and painless. The induration may extend beyond the margin and upon palpation feel like a subcutaneous "button." Owing to a superficial necrosis, ulceration appears comparatively early but may be preceded by the formation of a vesicle. As usually observed, the chancre is a single ulcer varying in diameter from a few millimeters to more than a centimeter, with a red moist base sometimes covered with a crust of dried exudate, and surrounded by an elevated dense margin, the remnant of the original papule. As the lesion becomes older the marginal density or induration may extend several millimeters beyond the edge of the ulcer. Shortly after the appearance of the chancre, the regional lymph nodes become enlarged and firm, painless and rarely tender.

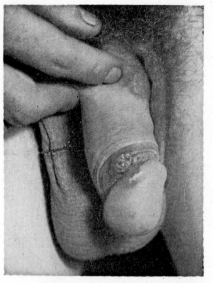

Photograph of chancre of reflected layer of prepuce. From White and Martin's Genito-Urinary Surgery.

Microscopically, the fully developed chancre is a generally spherical mass of various kinds of mononuclear cells, provided

with a variable number of new capillaries. It is situated in the corium but may extend more deeply; involvement of the epiderm

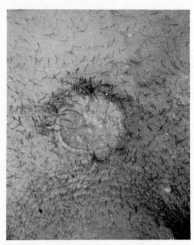

Chancre on mons veneris.

occurs principally during the formation of the ulcer. In the stage of ulceration, superficial necrosis is observed with slight acute inflammation at the base. Secondary infection of the ulcer, with pronounced acute inflammation, may obscure the picture microscopically, grossly and clinically. The cells of the

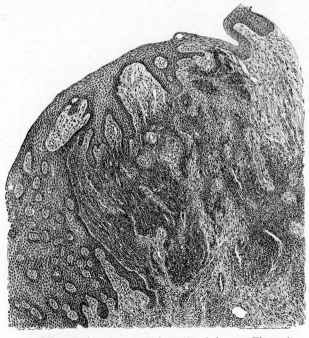

Microscopic appearance of margin of chancre. The corium is diffusely infiltrated with mononuclear cells. The lesion has existed for some time as indicated by the well marked epithelial proliferation at the margin of the ulcer.

chancre are principally lymphoid cells with a number of large mononuclears. Multinuclear giant cells with vesicular, centrally disposed nuclei are occasionally encountered. The investigations of Fordyce and of Brown indicate an early lesion of the smaller blood vessels and capillaries. Brown finds that as soon as the organisms proliferate they are grouped about the capillaries, probably in association vessels within the lesion or near its margin show moderate or marked fibrotic thickening of their walls. Special staining demonstrates numerous organisms both within the cells and between them. The fibroblasts rarely produce significant amounts of connective tissue, and hence the chancre heals with very slight scar formation save for that due to the secondarily infected ulcerated surface.

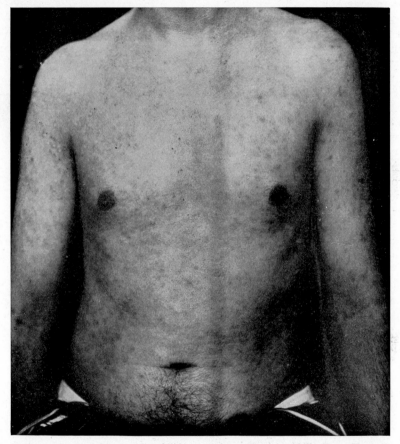

Photograph of erythematous syphilide, secondary stage of syphilis. From Hartzell, Diseases of the Skin.

with injury of the endothelium (personal communication). There is a slight exudation of leukocytes accompanied by local necrosis, rapidly followed by infiltration of lymphoid cells in mantle form about the pre-existing and new vessels; this soon spreads into the surrounding tissues to form a solid mass of cells. The vascular endothelium swells and probably proliferates.

As the condition progresses, fibroblasts may be found intermingled with the other cells, and, in the later stages of the lesion, it is not uncommon to find that the smaller

THE SECONDARY STAGE of syphilis is characterized by lesions of the skin and mucous membranes and widespread enlargement of lymph nodes. The skin lesions may be macular erythematous, maculopapular, papular and even pustular. Microscopically, the macular eruptions show only a dilatation of the small vessels of the papillary bodies and adjacent corium, sometimes with slight perivascular infiltration of lymphocytes and plasma cells. In the papular varieties the lesion is a circumscribed mass of lymphocytes, plasma cells and large mononuclears with a varying number of fibroblasts. According to Fordyce, the pustular forms are due to secondary pyogenic infection and consequently show acute suppurative inflammation. Mucous patches appear in the mucous membranes of the mouth, vagina and anal margin. These are at first flat papules but rapidly ulcerate to form shallow flat ulcers, well defined, reddened at the base and with slightly elevated margins.

Microscopically, the lesion of the corium is like that of the papular skin lesions, although not so sharply circumscribed, and in the depths there is a well-marked perivascular distribution of the cells. The epithelium is swollen at first, then becomes necrotic and exfoliates. The exposed surface is essentially granulation tissue and is resistant to secondary infection. The lymph nodes are moderately enlarged, easily palpable, firm and usually neither painful nor tender.

Microscopically, there is subacute or chronic hyperplasia. The secondary nodules may be enlarged and active, the sinuses show a moderate endothelial hyperplasia and fibrosis is usually pronounced. Pain or tenderness in the periosteum of the long bones, especially of the tibia, is common and is due to a mild subacute periostitis. Areas of baldness, or alopecia, may result from mild cutaneous lesions of the scalp.

THE THIRD STAGE of syphilis, as now understood, includes the entire period of the disease following the secondary stage. There may be a period of clinical latency following the subsidence of secondary lesions, but that there are no anatomic lesions in the body during this stage is doubtful. Although diffuse fibrosis in various organs occurs in the tertiary stage, the characteristic lesion is the gumma.

The Gumma. The primary and secondary lesions of syphilis are not granulomatous in character but the gumma is typically so. It may appear in any tissue in the body. The classical gumma is a solitary, fairly large nodule without secondary or daughter lesions. It may attain a diameter of several centimeters but usually averages about 1 to 1.5 cm. Nevertheless, small gummata of microscopic or miliary size may occur and these are usually multiple. The solitary gumma is a relatively firm, elastic structure

surrounded by a granulomatous cell mass and fibrous connective tissue.

Upon cross section the center of the lesion is a slightly gelatinous, elastic, somewhat hyalinized necrotic mass. The consist-

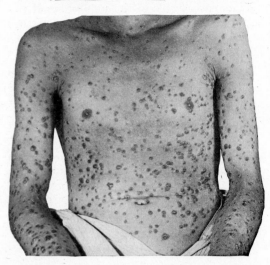

Pustular syphiloderm of secondary stage of syphilis.

ency is that of fairly firm rubber and from this is derived the name, "gumma." The necrosis is essentially a coagulation necrosis, likened by some to infarction. Microscopically it is granular rather than hyaline. It is more likely to show tissue and cell shadows than is tuberculous caseation and special stains demonstrate a denser arrangement of reticulum (Coronini). Around the necrotic focus is a rim of cells, principally epithelioid cells and lymphocytes. As a rule, the lymphocytes far outnumber the epithelioid cells. Giant cells similar to those of the tubercle are sometimes present; as a rule, however, they are not numerous and usually are entirely absent. Intermingled with the layer of lymphocytes is found a proliferation of fibroblasts or of adult connective tissue which contains numerous capillaries. The vascularization of the gumma often extends well down toward the necrotic area, and in this respect the gumma differs markedly from the tubercle. In the later stages of the lesion, cicatrization or encapsulation is likely to be marked and the fibrosis may extend widely into the surrounding tissue. Not infrequently the blood vessels of the neighborhood show distinct fibrous thickening of their walls. Special stains may show the treponemata in small numbers, but usually they escape detection.

Gummata in the skin or mucous membrane may show deep ulceration. Hemorrhage from the ulcerated lesion may lead to serious anemia and even death. Sometimes marginal thrombosis of vessels occurs so that the lesions extend progressively to form large ulcers, which are likely to be chronic and progressive so as to produce the so-called ser-

clusion of the meningeal vessels. In the nervous tissue there may be focal areas of gliosis or perivascular infiltrates of lymphocytes and plasma cells. More extensive gliosis occurs in cases of paresis, associated with cortical atrophy; the foci are irregularly distributed in cerebrospinal syphilis and affect the posterior columns in tabes dorsalis or locomotor

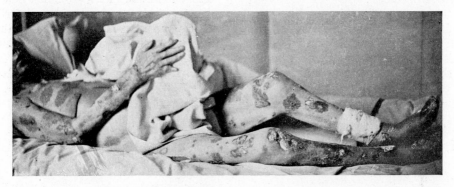

Photograph of tertiary syphilide of skin. Patient subsequently completely relieved by specific treatment. Patient of Dr. H. N. Cole.

piginous ulcers. Miliary gummata may appear in considerable numbers in the skin and are not infrequent in the media of the aorta.

Systemic Lesions. The structure of the gumma is usually so characteristic that upon identification a diagnosis of tertiary syphilis can be made. Nevertheless, it is uncommon in autopsy material. Much more frequent is fibrosis of various viscera, often associated with infiltration of lymphocytes and plasma cells, especially near blood vessels and lymphatics and accompanied by atrophy of parenchyma. These lesions are so common in late syphilis that they must be part of the effects of the disease, but their structure, gross or microscopic, is not diagnostic except in a few situations. These changes require years for their development and are due to the presence of treponemata in the tissues. Grossly, the more advanced lesions are recognizable as small areas, but the fibrosis usually is of only microscopic size. The nervous system, heart, aorta, pancreas, adrenals, and testis are likely to be affected, and morphologically similar lesions are found in the kidney and other organs.

In the central nervous system the pia-arachnoid may show diffuse or localized thickening, the latter being associated with fibrosis of the walls or complete fibrotic oc-

ataxia, with associated destruction of cells and neuraxons. It is possible that these more

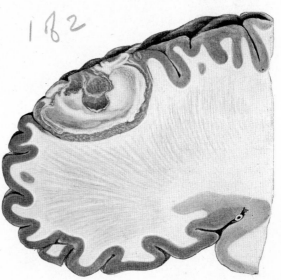

Gumma of the cerebrum.

serious lesions represent progression from the minor lesions.

The heart may or may not show fibrosis grossly. Microscopically there are perivascular infiltrates in the myocardium, especially near the endocardium. This fibrosis is usually patchy but may be diffuse. The local lesion may consist of small accumulations of lymphocytes and plasma cells, with slight fibrosis between the muscle fibers, or larger accumulations about larger vessels, and may approach miliary gummata in size. They do not show the necrosis, the vascularization, nor the giant cells of gumma. The muscle may show hypertrophy, atrophy, fatty degeneration or even necrosis.

The endocardium is not likely to be affected except for the aortic valves, which are often involved by extension from syphilitic disease of the aorta so that widening of the commissures or retraction of leaflets or

common. The pulmonary artery may be similarly involved. The peripheral arteries may show medial disease, but more often only infiltration of lymphocytes in the adventitia. Sometimes, especially in the cerebral arteries, there is a subacute granulomatous inflammation.

The characteristic lesion of the liver is "hepar lobatum." More common is a diffuse fibrosis of the liver like that described in other organs, but it is thought that this may progress to an alteration of the architecture like that seen in Laennec cirrhosis. The lobated liver is produced by the contraction

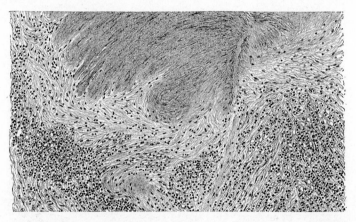

Section of gumma. Note necrosis above. In margin of necrotic area are a few epithelioid cells. There is a rich infiltrate of lymphoid cells in a well vascularized mass of granulation.

both may cause aortic insufficiency. Syphilis may cause simple intimal sclerosis of the aorta, but the specific lesion is syphilitic mesaortitis. This occurs at the root of the aorta and often extends to the arch but only rarely further in the aorta. The intima shows numerous depressed lines which produce an irregular or stellate wrinkling. Intimal plaques of thickening, which tend to become hyalinized, are often associated. Tiny foci of scar tissue in the media under the wrinkled intima may be visible to the naked eye.

Microscopically there are perivascular infiltrates of lymphocytes and plasma cells around the vasa vasorum of the adventitia and media. In the media these are associated with destruction of muscle and elastica. From these foci, strands of fibrous tissue radiate and their retraction causes the depressions in the intima. Dilatation of the aorta and development of aneurysms are

of masses of fibrous tissue which leads to lines of depression in the surface and the formation of pseudolobes. The bands of connective tissue often radiate from gummata in the liver, but occasionally no gumma is found. The pancreas frequently shows irregularly disposed interstitial fibrosis and an associated atrophy of the parenchyma.

The testis is almost constantly the seat either of cellular infiltrates or of fibrosis of the interstitial substance, which may be general or focalized and associated with fibrosis of the basement membrane and decreased spermatogenesis.

The kidneys may also show fibrosis. It is said that acute glomerulonephritis may be due to pyogenic infection of syphilitic lesions. Nephrosis occurs and is supposed to be a syphilitic manifestation because it clears up with antisyphilitic therapy; this theoretical assumption is applied to other lesions arising during the course of syphilis, with equal lack of conviction. Rich describes an occasional lesion of the kidneys which he believes to be syphilitic, but without final proof. In the interstitial tissues there is an infiltration of lymphocytes, large mononuclear phagocytes, plasma cells and an occasional eosinophil. This encroaches on tubules

quent stages until dense cicatricial tissue develops, when they are no longer demonstrable. They have been found in the aorta in syphilitic aortitis and in the brain in paresis. Claims have been made that they have been demonstrated in many organs of the body, but it is probable that spirals thought to be treponemata are artefacts.

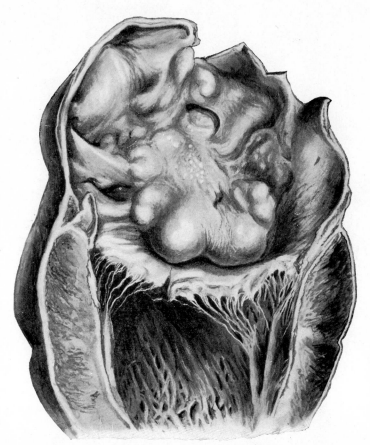

Multiple gummata of the atrium of the heart.

and may penetrate into them. Cholesterol crystals, sometimes within foreign-body giant cells, may be found in the tubules. Cicatrization may be extensive. There are no clear-cut clinical manifestations.

Some of the visceral and other lesions of syphilis are about equally distributed between the sexes, but Turner's study of 10,000 cases of syphilis showed that males are more often affected by syphilis of the central nervous system, the cardiovascular system and the bones than are females.

Warthin has found treponemata in the earlier cellular infiltrates and in the subse-

CONGENITAL SYPHILIS. Syphilis is not hereditary; the infection is acquired by the fetus in the uterus and is thus congenital. Treponemata are found in the placentas of syphilitic mothers and directly infect the embryo or fetus. The organisms may be found in the semen of syphilitics, but it is unlikely that an ovum invaded by the organisms could multiply because it is known that the disturbance of a single blastomere in the lower vertebrates leads to arrest of development or production of malformations; if this be true of lower vertebrates with their high power of regeneration, the effect would probably be much more severe in the higher mammals and man. Infection of the embryo probably only occurs by infection of the mother at or preceding the time of conception. Hata

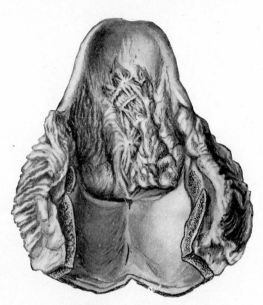

Syphilitic scars in epiglottis.

many of the surviving children are defective or die young, owing to syphilis. Congenital syphilitics may live to adult life with few or no signs or symptoms of the disease. Their children may show obvious syphilis. There are records of syphilis transmitted through three generations.

Analysis of the cause of stillbirths shows that syphilis is only one cause and not an especially frequent one. Bell found only 3.38 per cent of stillborn babies to be syphilitic. Of infants who died before the end of the first year, syphilis was present in but 2.63 per cent and it was even less frequent thereafter.

Among the skin lesions of stillborn congenital syphilitics, the more important are bullae of the palms of the hands and soles of the feet, and general maceration of the skin. The internal viscera may or may not be enlarged but show faulty development microscopically. The kidney, liver, pancreas, and the lung are dense, relatively fibrous organs. On microscopic examination, however, it is found that this density is not due to an increase in fibrous connective tissue, but rather to a failure of development on the part of ingrowing epithelium or other structure which fails to displace the original mesoblastic tissue. Thus, the alveoli of the lungs are not fully developed and are separated from one

Gross section of multiple gummata of liver, with heavy bands of fibrous connective tissue radiating through the organ.

found that of syphilitic women married for at least three years only 60 per cent were impregnated. As a result of the pregnancies there were 28 per cent abortions, 42 per cent living infants which died within two years of birth and 30 per cent of living children which survived for two years or more. He states that

another by masses of tissue made up particularly of small round cells resembling very closely those of the mesoblast ("white pneumonia"), but comparable pictures are found in nonsyphilitic infants (Ammich).

The liver is likely to show large, thick, perilobular spaces filled with connective tissue and the same types of cells as are seen in the lung. This may be true not only of the perilobular connective tissue but the cells

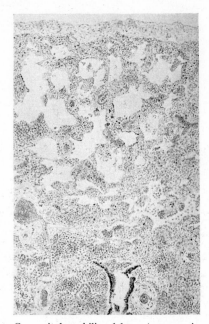

Congenital syphilis of lung (pneumonia alba) showing thick alveolar walls.

may be present in fairly large numbers between the liver cords. The development of the pancreas is similarly delayed so that between small and imperfectly developed acini the mesoblastic tissues or its descendants remain undifferentiated. The same mesoblastic remnants are found in the kidney. Bone formation is also delayed so that the development of the diaphysis is particularly affected. The gross examination of the ends of long bones shows a thick, yellow, irregular line between the diaphysis and the epiphysis. This is in contrast to the sharp, narrow white line that appears normally. Microscopically, the development of the trabeculæ in the primary spongiosa, instead of proceeding regularly with the formation of parallel columns of tissue, proceeds irregularly so that there is an alteration of the normal parallelism. The vis-

cera are likely to be crowded with treponemata.

Infants born alive are likely to be undersized, wizened and to have widely open fontanelles. The angles of the mouth show radiating linear scars, the syphilitic rhagades. There may be a syphilitic rhinitis or "snuffles." Sometimes infants are born apparently healthy and at about the second month exhibit snuffles, rhagades, not infrequently discharge from the ears and deafness. Ulcerations of the nose with necrosis of the septal bones may lead to perforation of the septum and to dropping of the bridge of nose, the so-called saddle nose. Cutaneous lesions and mucous patches similar to those of acquired syphilis may occur. The bone ends, liver and spleen are usually enlarged. These patients frequently die and show visceral lesions similar to but of less marked degree than those of the stillborn. Treponemata are not numerous in these lesions. Primary dentition is often delayed and secondary dentition accompanied by deformity of incisors and molars, the Hutchinson and Fournier teeth, discussed further in the chapter on Alimentary Canal. There is no satisfactory evidence that this is due to local invasion by spirochetes. The disease may become quiescent after the early outbreak, to appear again at puberty or later. Iritis and chronic interstitial keratitis may appear in early infancy but the keratitis is more common at puberty or later. Hutchinson's triad of congenital syphilis includes malformation of the teeth, keratitis and deafness. Gumma formation is not common in congenital syphilis but is sometimes seen in the stillborn and less often in the living infants and children. In those who survive longer, the condition is often called "lues tarda."

Immunity in Syphilis. Because of the failure to cultivate virulent *Treponema pallidum*, studies of immunity in syphilis must be approached in the living animal or patient. No method of vaccination has been devised. The disease itself appears to confer immunity but how often and for how long is uncertain. Chesney and his associates found that early treatment of the experimental disease in rabbits apparently results in a cure so that reinfection can occur; this is not readily effected if treatment be delayed. The second infections may occur without primary lesions and the resistance established appears to be in certain measure strain specific. In both animals and man it is likely that the disease must have been present for a considerable period for lasting immunity to develop. As Chesney has shown the disease may be cured in rabbits, but in man it is difficult to be certain of cure because, as Warthin has shown, the body may harbor spirochetes after the Wassermann test has become negative.

a syphilitic mother are immune to the acquired disease is no longer tenable: such children as do not exhibit syphilis are resistant because they are victims of the disease, even though it be latent.

The general reaction of the body to *Treponema pallidum* is more nearly like that to protozoa than to bacteria. The primary reactions of the body have some influence on the subsequent disease, since Brown and

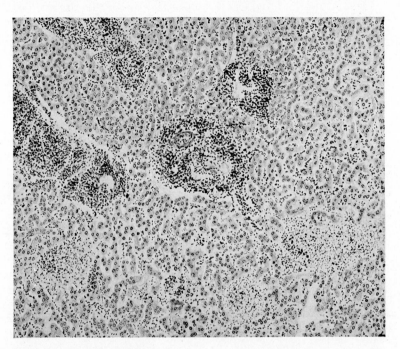

Congenital syphilis of liver, showing cellular infiltrate in perilobular connective tissue and foci of necrosis in parenchyma.

By observation of rigid criteria as to the incontestible evidence of first infection and reinfection, Stokes, Schoch and Ireland conclude that no fully proved human case has been reported. If the standards be only moderately rigid, 116 cases can be accepted, but even with average standards only 120 cases can be included. Further study, with attention to exclusion of local relapses, is necessary before the matter can finally be settled. Colles' or Colles-Baumes' law to the effect that mothers who give birth to syphilitic children and who give no evidence of syphilis are immune to the disease has been abandoned. It has been shown that in the vast majority of instances such mothers react positively to the Wassermann test and are the victims of latent syphilis. Profeta's law that children of

Pearce have shown that removal of the primary lesion in the rabbit or depression of the primary reaction by drugs favors more rapid development of subsequent generalized manifestations of disease. The presence of syphilis in the body leads to an alteration of the tissues and fluids which apparently represents an unstable balance between resistance and hypersusceptibility, but a high degree of immunity does not seem to occur. By good technic and proper dosage, it is possible to inoculate organisms locally at almost any stage of the disease, but the incubation is short, the lesions are less pronounced and regress more rapidly. The lesions resemble those of the stage of the disease during which inoculation takes place. Thus, in the primary stage a chancre-like lesion is produced, in the secondary stage a papular skin lesion, in the tertiary stage a destructive lesion resembling the gumma.

The cycles of syphilis show periods of active lesions alternating with periods of latency. The explanation of these cycles is at this time largely hypothetical, since it is evidently difficult to work with concrete manifestations of immune bodies or of susceptibility. In the primary stage there is probably a rapid increase in resistance of the body, since reinoculation is difficult and multiple chancres rare. The subsequent period of latency shows little resistance and may represent even depressed resistance or a "negative phase." This is probably a true incubation period of the disease, but not of generalization of the organisms since they spread rapidly from the primary lesion.

Only after the development of the secondaries does a true resistance develop, as represented in the next period of latency. In the primary and early secondary lesions the organisms are numerous, progressively decreasing in number with subsequent lesions. The later lesions, however, with smaller numbers of organisms, are progressively more and more destructive. This is assumed to be due to an alteration of tissue reactivity, a state of allergy or a true hypersensitiveness. Even with hypersensitiveness, the activity of the disease is presumably sufficient to lead again to resistance, with latency followed by new hypersensitiveness as the resistance gradually disappears. In the stage of gumma formation, only a few organisms are associated with the marked tissue destruction and severe local reaction. It is possible, however, that the number of organisms may be so small that the gumma is not formed; the reaction then is solely in the form of the low-grade inflammation and fibrosis described above. That these cycles are due to alterations of virulence of the treponemata is unlikely, since they are equally infective at all stages of the disease.

Studies of agglutinins and opsonins in vitro have been carried out with various spirochetes grown in culture, but since these are not *Treponema pallidum* the results throw no real light on immunity in syphilis. The same can be said of treponemocidal bodies and of skin tests. Complement-fixation tests have been done with cultivated spirochetes and are closely correlated with absence or presence of the disease, but this does not necessarily mean specificity in the strict immunologic sense of the word. Humoral bodies, so-called protective antibodies, have been demonstrated in the serum of syphilitic rabbits and syphilitic humans. When the serum is mixed with infective tissue before injection, a great majority of the experimental animals do not acquire the disease (Turner et al.).

The Wassermann Test. This is not considered as an immune reaction in a strict sense. The antigens ordinarily employed are not antigens in the strict biologic sense, but rather finely suspended colloidal emulsions of lipoids, particularly lecithin and lipoids of the diaminophosphatide group, as well as fatty acids and certain proteins or protein fractions usually extracted from beef heart. The "fixing body" or "amboceptor" of the luetic serum is a substance apparently closely related to the globulins, especially the euglobulins; the globulins are known to be increased in syphilitic blood and spinal fluid. According to Wells "a favorite interpretation of the Wassermann reaction, which seems to harmonize with the facts, is that there is a precipitation of serum globulin by the lipoidal colloids of the antigen and adsorption of the complement by this precipitate."

The Wassermann test is positive in a large proportion of all syphilitics. Craig found 85.9 per cent positive in 5,600 cases diagnosed clinically as syphilis, and it must be remembered that there is at least a small factor of error in the clinical diagnosis. It is therefore apparent that the presence of a syphilitic infection leads to some change in the body, by which a substance is elaborated capable of fixing complement in the presence of the antigen. That this substance is an immune body is not as yet proved. The test shows a greater percentage of positive results in secondary syphilis, i.e., during the most active stages of the disease; therefore, it is not indicative of resistance nor is the "fixing body" indicative of immunity. The Wassermann test cannot be regarded as an indication of immunity or lack of it. It is the result of changes which occur in the body as the result of infection, referable rather to alterations in the body fluids than to production of immune bodies.

Craig found the Wassermann test positive in 89.8 per cent of primary syphilis, 96.1 per cent of secondary syphilis, 87.4 of tertiary syphilis and 82.2 of congenital syphilis. Various modifications of the test give results as good or better, but the adjustment of sensitivity and accuracy (so-called specificity) is difficult in all. In the course of some of the acute infectious diseases, in malaria, leprosy, trypanosomiasis, there may be false positives, but in some of these cases adequate investigation has shown them not to be false but due to syphilis clinically unrecognized at the time.

Criticism has been directed against the test because of the fact that results do not always agree with clinical findings, and because of differences in results upon the same serum in different laboratories. It must be admitted that the factors of error in the test are numerous. Discrepancies in reports from different laboratories may, in part, be due to inherent faults in the test, to faults in technic, to faults in selection of materials and to insufficient training of the worker. With modern methods and skillful performance, the test is reliable, not as an absolutely specific diagnostic measure but as supplementary to the clinical observations.

OTHER TESTS. Certain flocculation and precipitation tests have been introduced. Utilizing only antigen and serum, these are simpler, more expeditious and economical than the Wassermann. They are also useful because they can be readily varied in sensitivity. Thus it is possible to increase sensitivity so that a negative result can safely be interpreted as excluding syphilis. Otherwise they can be interpreted and applied in the clinic in the same manner as the Wassermann test or its modifications. Although in many laboratories, the tests have supplanted the Wassermann, the best practice is to use them in parallel with the Wassermann. As a result of national and international surveys, it can be safely said that tests such as the Kline and the Kahn tests are as accurate as the Wassermann or more so. (See Venereal Disease Information, U. S. Treas., 1935, 1937.)

Yaws or Frambesia Tropica

Introduction. This disease is confined almost entirely to tropical and subtropical countries. Although it resembles syphilis in some of its clinical manifestations, it is almost entirely a disease of the skin and rarely of the mucous membranes, is not likely to be transmitted by sexual contact, and has a fairly strict geographic distribution. The presence of the one disease does not confer immunity against the other. The *Treponema pertenue* is regarded as the cause by those who accept the separate identity of yaws. This resembles the treponema of syphilis, but the coils of *pertenue* are not so close and regular, the body is somewhat thicker and the ends likely to be hooked or coiled.

The Lesion. The incubation period is variable but is approximately two to four weeks. The disease is somewhat cyclic in course and is said to have three stages. The primary lesion is usually on some exposed part such as leg, ankle, foot, forearm or hand, and it is probable that trauma provides the portal of entry. A slowly growing papule appears in the skin, which shows a moist yellow secretion, tends to become encrusted and shows an ulcer with granulomatous base under the crust. This may extend to produce a large, moderately erosive ulcer several centimeters in diameter, and heals either before or after the secondary lesions appear.

The secondary stage appears in from one to three months after the primary and shows an eruption of papules over a large part of the body surface, which sometimes ulcerate and coalesce to form large lesions. These clear up and recur after variable intervals, the recurrences being less widespread. In the late secondaries the palms and soles may show a psoriasis-like lesion resembling that of syphilis, and on the soles there may be deep-seated nodules with circumvallate ulceration (clavus). The nodule may be extruded leaving a deep ulcer. Lymph-node enlargement is common and persistent. In the third stage, gummatous lesions appear, which may ulcerate deeply and produce great deformity. Bones may be involved but deep visceral lesions are practically never found. The primary and secondary lesions do not differ materially and are well described by Moss and Bigelow:

In the frambesic papules the surface epithelium is greatly thickened and numerous elongated downgrowths are seen. In patches the epithelial cells are swollen, vacuolated and degenerating. Circumscribed areas contain polymorphonuclear leukocytes. The layers near the corium are almost normal, but the corium itself is edematous. There is a diffuse, cellular infiltration consisting of polymorphonuclear leukocytes, large and small mononuclears, eosinophils, plasma cells, mast cells, connective tissue cells and some extravasated erythrocytes.

The organisms are found principally in small nests in the epiderm, but may also be found in the perivascular connective tissue of the corium. The study of the histopathology of the disease furnishes no satisfactory criteria for distinguishing it from syphilis (Ferris and Turner). The arsenicals used in syphilis are also effective in yaws. An excellent description is given by Wilson and Mathis.

Experimentally yaws can be transmitted to apes and to the testis of the rabbit, and the organism can be recovered from the lesions. The organism has been grown in pure culture and upon inoculation produces lesions in the rabbit's testis. There is, therefore, little doubt as to its causative relation. The work of Nichols and of Craig and Nichols shows that the serum of syphilitic patients gives crossed reactions with antigens made of pure cultures of *Treponema pertenue*, but the reaction is not so strongly nor so frequently positive as with syphilitic antigens. Syphilis of the rabbit does not protect against yaws and vice versa. The Wassermann test is positive in a large percentage of victims of yaws and probably depends more on the crossed reaction than on the coincident presence of syphilis. (See Schobl.)

DUE TO HIGHER BACTERIA

Actinomycosis

Introduction. Actinomycosis is a subacute or chronic inflammatory process, leading to suppuration and the formation of granulation tissue, from which pus may be collected containing characteristic, small, white or brownish-white masses, the "sulfur granules" or actinomyces "drusen." It occurs most commonly in cattle and swine as "lumpy jaw," "big jaw" or "wooden tongue."

The causative organism is the *Actinomyces bovis* Harz, a member of the order of higher bacteria, actinomycetiales, which show long filamentous forms and true branching. In man, the *Actinomyces israeli* and certain other related organisms may cause the disease (see Franklin). The branching filaments occur in cultures and only rarely in tissues. If a sulfur granule be pressed between two glass slides, there is a central tangle of threads with radiating threads at the margins. In stained preparations and granules in the tissues the ends of these radiating threads are in the form of clubbed termini. For cultivation, the granules should be well washed and inoculated in large quantity upon a variety of media, both aerobically and anaerobically. Secondary infection is so common that contamination is frequent.

The Disease in Animals. In addition to cattle and man, the disease has been reported in swine, horse, sheep, ass, deer, elephant, dog and cat. The primary lesion is in the alimentary canal, jaw, cheek, pharynx, tongue, and intestinal canal, particularly the ileocecal junction. It may also affect the skin. From the primary site, other structures may be affected, as liver, lung, brain or other viscus. Lymph nodes may be enlarged as the result of an inflammatory hyperplasia but rarely by the disease itself. Dissemination appears to follow invasion of blood vessels large enough to carry the organism rather than by the small lymphatic vessels.

Transmission of the Disease. The disease may be produced experimentally, but does not show the progressive character of the nonexperimental disease. The organisms must be implanted in order to lead to disease, and it is probable that in man and animals it gains entrance through abrasions. Such abrasions may be induced by carious teeth or by accidental trauma. It is possible that minor abrasions may be produced by uncooked grains and cereals or by straws. The organisms may be found in teeth, tartar, carious tooth cavities and tonsil crypts (Colebrook) and upon kernels of grain. Grain kernels are found in the abscess in some cases. Whether the grains carry in the infection or are incidentally present is not certain. The organism flourishes on moist grains, but is extremely resistant to drying. The disease prevails in rainy years, wet seasons, and the damp regions of Austria, Germany, Switzerland, Russia, the upper

Mississippi valley and northwestern States (Sanford) where cereal cultivation and cattle raising are the chief occupations. It may also occur elsewhere.

Actinomycosis in Man. The disease occurs in adult life and is four times more frequent in males than females. A history of chewing wheat, oat or barley spears is very common. Infection usually takes place through an abrasion and in the focus there may sometimes be found particles of grain. Entry may be through the surface of the skin, the respiratory tract or the alimentary canal. It is uncommon to find lesions in the skin except over the cheek, and here a clinical form known as the cervicomaxillary type develops. Entering through the respiratory tract, the clinical picture may somewhat resemble that of tuberculosis. When swallowed the organisms are likely to lodge in the cecum or in the flexures of the large intestine. Here the clinical manifestations may resemble those of appendicitis. From this situation the lesion may extend retroperitoneally to produce draining sinuses of flanks or groins, or may be the source of acute and chronic abscesses of the liver. Although essentially a local inflammatory process, it may spread extensively and metastasize; by virtue of secondary infection it may be febrile and may result in a bacterial septicemia or pyemia.

GROSSLY, the lesion may be either a moderately or greatly swollen, red, tender mass, dense on the outer surface, often with a soft or semifluctuant center. Sometimes, however, there is little redness and the mass resembles a tumor. Single or multiple sinuses appear, from which is discharged a creamy yellow or brownish-yellow pus containing the characteristic granules, usually somewhat less than a millimeter in diameter.

MICROSCOPIC EXAMINATION of tissues has shown that the lesion begins as an accumulation of polymorphonuclear leukocytes about the organism, followed by a massing of large mononuclears and then a layer of granulation tissue and fibrosis. Giant cells are occasionally encountered. The lesion enlarges by progressive extension of the process accompanied by destruction of the invaded tissue, and necrosis of the central parts with abscess formation. As the disease advances, the abscesses rupture on surfaces and chronic sinuses result; the lesion is highly invasive

and appears to break down bone as readily as soft tissues. Blood vessels become the seat of thrombosis and may be invaded so that organisms can be transmitted to neighboring organs. As in the pus, so in the tissue sections, fat and lipoids can be demonstrated in a few of the leukocytes and in many of the large mononuclears. The diagnostic feature is the presence of the organism in the typical granules. In tissue sections, with the ordinary stains, the central mass of organisms takes the basic stain and may be distinctly granular as the result of degeneration. Around this is a band of radiating threads terminating in clublike extremities. The core of each club is a thread of organism and takes the basic stain; the club, however, is a transformation product probably degenerate in character, and takes the acid stain. Only fine technic demonstrates the thread in the center of the club. The termini may, however, be bare.

An organism, which grows as a bacillus, the actinobacillus, may produce lesions resembling actinomycosis. Actinobacillosis is rare in man, but cases of meningitis and bacillemia have been reported (Beaver and Thompson).

Staphylococcic actinophytosis (Botryomycosis) is referred to here because the abscesses are of nodular type and within them are masses of bacteria in an acidophilic matrix of dead tissue, with radial clubs at the margin covered with doubly refractile cuticula. The abscesses originate at a point of injury in the skin or mucous membranes such as intestine and progress slowly, evidently because of a balance of resistance and virulence. The center of the abscess is often widely necrotic and the margin is likely to show granulation and fibrosis. Secondary abscess may occur in the viscera. Although *Staphylococcus aureus* is the chief cause, other bacteria may produce the same lesion. (See Fink; Kimmelstiel and Easley.)

Madura Foot or Mycetoma

This disease, first described and prevalent in India, also occurs elsewhere. It usually is seen in the foot as firm, relatively painless nodules from a millimeter to a centimeter or more in diameter. These break down with the discharge of minute granules which in different cases may be white, black, red or of an intermediate shade. Suppura-

PLATE X

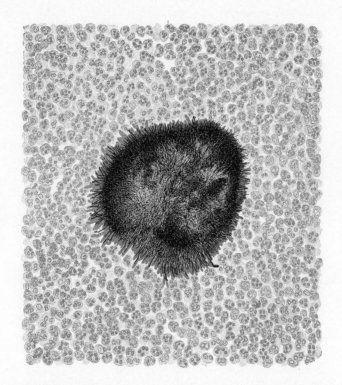

Actinomyces granule surrounded by leukocytes. Note the basophilic central mass of mycelium and the radiating marginal acidophilic clubs.

tion may occur with the discharge of viscid pus which may contain granules. Rarely there is extensive destruction of tissue with exposure of tendons. The color of the granules may be due partly to blood pigment but is mainly contributed by the causative organism, which does not of necessity produce the same color in all cases with which it is associated.

Microscopically the lesion shows a tangle of nonsegmented mycetial filaments, which usually is surrounded by radiating threads with club-shaped extremities. Around this are a variable but usually small number of leukocytes, many large mononuclears, sometimes multinucleated foreign-body giant cells and a dense fibrous tissue which may exhibit Russell fuchsin bodies. The pigment appears as fine granules, some of which may be hemosiderin. It is generally agreed that there are two types of the disease, maduromycotic and actinomycotic. In maduromycotic mycetoma, the mycelium of the granules is well defined and has chlamydospores or other spores. From it 17 species of fungi of different genera and classes have been isolated. In actinomycotic mycetoma the mycelium of the granules is poorly defined, spores are not found, and 13 species of actinomyces have been described. (See Jones and Alden.)

Other actinomycetes producing abscesses include the *Actinomyces thibiergi* which produces the so-called cutaneous discomycosis; the *Actinomyces asteroides*, isolated from a brain abscess; and certain others of less importance.

Streptothricosis

Cases of disease of the lungs have been reported, apparently caused by a branching filamentous organism which cannot be definitely classified as *Actinomyces bovis* or *Actinomyces maduræ*. The organisms of streptothricosis probably represent a group rather than a single organism, since in different cases they vary as to staining properties and when cultivated (with difficulty) are sometimes aerobic and sometimes anaerobic. Claypole would include in the group of streptothrices acid-fast bacteria, such as tubercle bacillus and lepra bacillus diphtheria bacillus, the mycelium forming organisms and the higher sporulating fungi.

The disease clinically may resemble tuberculosis, as in Flexner's case, gangrene as in Ophül's cases or pneumonia as in Lenhartz' case. The gross morbid anatomy may be that of tuberculosis, and the condition may be combined with tuberculosis. The lungs, however, are likely to show extensive consolidation with necrosis and multiple cavity formation. There may be either acute fibrinous pleurisy, empyema or chronic fibrous pleurisy. Microscopically, the lungs show a rich infiltration of leukocytes both in the alveoli and tissues of the lung, necrosis, and in some areas an infiltration of large mononuclear cells. In the more chronic cases, there may be extensive formation of granulation tissue, associated with small giant cells. Isolated lesions may resemble tubercles very closely. They show central necrosis, epithelioid cells and giant cells, but in the layer of epithelioid cells and surrounding lymphoid cells there is a definite formation of fibroblasts and new blood vessels. The organisms may be demonstrated in the tissues. The lesions are commonest in the lungs but may appear in lymph nodes, omentum and other viscera. The sputum may sometimes show granules like those of actinomycosis. They are usually gram positive and stain with carbolfuchsin; they may or may not be acid-fast. They can also be demonstrated in the pus of open lesions. (See Singer and Ballon).

DUE TO HIGHER VEGETABLE PARASITES (FUNGI)

Blastomycosis or Oïdiomycosis

Introduction. Blastomycosis, or as it is usually called, American blastomycosis, is a specific granulomatous process which occurs in two forms, (a) cutaneous and (b) systemic. It is more common in males than females. The causative organism is *Blastomyces* or *Blastomycoides dermatidis*, an oïdium which multiplies in the tissues by budding but in cultures shows features of growth like fungi. In the tissues the organisms appear as gram-negative bodies, with a homogeneous doubly contoured capsule and a granular or slightly vacuolated central protoplasmic mass. The mode of transmission is not known, but such organisms occur free in nature and accidental trauma may permit entry into the skin.

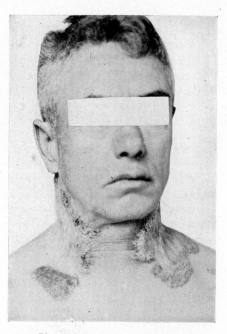

Photograph of late lesion in blasto-mycosis. Note central healing and marginal active lesions. Patient of Dr. H. N. Cole.

Morbid Anatomy. The disease is far more common in males than in females, occurs most frequently in middle life but is seen at other periods. The skin lesion often follows a minor injury and appears first as a papule which becomes pustular, ulcerates, discharges tenacious pus and gradually extends. The surface of the larger ulcer is studded with soft nodules, and is surrounded by a red areola in which can be found many minute intracutaneous abscesses. As the lesion advances, healing is likely to occur in the older central part, and in the prolonged cases cicatricial contraction may be marked. The hands, forearms, and head are most often attacked, although the disease occurs in other parts. The disease progresses slowly, usually over many months.

Microscopically, the ulcerated area shows absence of epithelium. Other parts show a thickened horny layer, and also extensive downgrowth of irregular processes of the interpapillary epithelium; the prickle cells are enlarged and show prominence of the cell bridges. The epiderm commonly

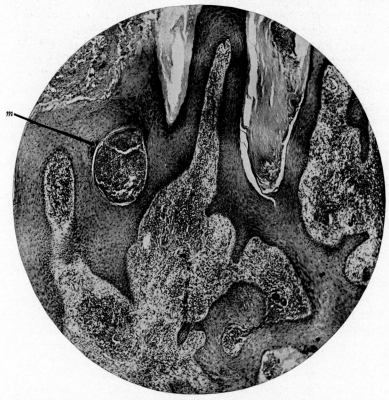

Blastomycosis cutis, showing interpapillary prolongations of the rete mucosum and at *m* a miliary abscess. From Hartzell, Diseases of the Skin.

shows a diffuse but scanty infiltration of polymorphonuclear leukocytes and lymphoid cells. Miliary abscesses are common in the epiderm at the margins of the lesion; these are made up principally of leukocytes, but other inflammatory cells appear and sometimes a few threads of fibrin are present. The corium, particularly in the upper layers, is infiltrated with leukocytes, lymphoid cells, large mononuclears, plasma cells, granular mast cells and giant cells. In the older cases, granulation tissue is likely to be found, partly or completely converted into scar tissue. Giant cells are found in epiderm and corium, are of the foreign-body type with large cytoplasm and irregularly distributed large vesicular nuclei. They usually contain one or more blastomyces. Ricketts was of the opinion that the giant cells originate from epi-

duce marked lesions in the mediastinal nodes. Essentially the same lesions are found in the other viscera attacked. (See D'Aunoy and Beven.)

Immunity. Hektoen was able to produce agglutinins by successive inoculations of the organism. Davis found that the vaccinated guinea-pig walls off infection more readily than the normal animal, and that immune serum reduces the growth activity of the organisms in vitro. Agglutinins were absent and low-titer precipitins variable in the guinea-pig immune sera. Lytic and complement-fixing bodies were not demonstrable, nor were cutaneous and ophthalmic reactions obtainable. Anaphylactic manifestations were not definitely demonstrated. Phagocytosis by peritoneal cells is fairly active, but opsonins appear to have no great influence on the

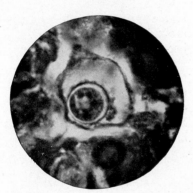 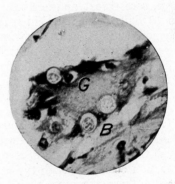

High power photomicrographs showing parasite in lesion, and a giant cell.
From Hartzell, Diseases of the Skin.

thelial cells, but it is possible that those in the corium are of reticulo-endothelial origin.

Systemic blastomycosis may involve any of the deep tissues of the body. Entrance is through the skin or the respiratory tract, rarely through the intestinal canal. Entering through the respiratory tract, the organisms lodge in the smaller bronchi or bronchioles and a bronchopneumonic patch is established, followed by growth of the organisms. The lesions resemble tubercles grossly, but microscopically may be either a collection of blastomyces with a small surrounding area of necrosis; a tubercle-like lesion with central necrosis, epithelioid and giant cells; or an abscess rich in polymorphonuclear leukocytes. In any of these, the lesion is identified by the presence of the organism. The disease extends through the lymphatics and may pro-

process. Intracutaneous tests are valuable in diagnosis in man but not absolutely dependable. Other immune reactions in man are not demonstrable. It may be said that natural and artificial infection with blastomyces lead to little or no immune reaction.

Experimental animals are susceptible to inoculation, but as a rule natural healing results; only occasionally are widespread or fatal experimental lesions encountered except following intravenous inoculation.

The human cutaneous disease runs a chronic course with remissions and exacerbations. Under proper treatment cures are effected. The systemic disease is fatal after a less prolonged course. (See Smith; Martin and Smith.)

Chromoblastomycosis is due to *Hormodendron pedrosoi*, an organism of the same general order as the blastomyces. It occurs principally in tropical and subtropical regions. The lesions are usually on the foot or leg, with pink or violaceous color and verrucous or papillomatous lesions of the skin; it is commonly of long duration (Emmons et al.). Similar is chlamydoblastomycosis due to *Phialophora verrucosa* (Shaw and Reid).

Coccidioidal Granuloma: Coccidioidomycosis

Introduction. Although this disease resembles systemic blastomycosis there is no question as to its separate identity. It occurs in two forms, which have been called coccidioidomycosis and coccidioidal granuloma. Coccidioidomycosis, sometimes called valley fever or desert fever, is observed particularly in children. It begins with sudden onset of fever, dry cough, sore throat and headache. From three to 18 days later the skin may show erythema nodosum. Pulmonary symptoms and signs predominate and pneumonia may develop. In contrast, the coccidioidal granuloma runs a progressively chronic course and is fatal in more than half the cases.

Clinically the condition behaves somewhat like tuberculosis and the pulmonary changes are much the same. In both forms of the disease, infection occurs through the respiratory tract but there are occasional instances of cutaneous infection. The causative organism is the *Coccidioidis immitis* or *Blastomycoides immitis,* which evidently has two cycles. It occurs in the tissues as a yeast-like form; there are spherical bodies from 4 to 25 micra in diameter, with a double contour, which contain small globules evidently indicative of endosporulation. The other cycle is found in cultures as a fungous type of growth. Although the highest incidence of the disease is in the San Joaquin Valley of California, cases have been reported from other states and in Europe. It is not certain that the acute stage of coccidioidomycosis is a precursor of the chronic stage, but what appear to be primary foci have been observed in the lungs of those cases in which the granulomatous appearance occurs. It has been observed in cattle, sheep and dogs. It affects all ages of man and is distinctly more frequent in males than females.

After infection occurs in the lung, dissemination takes place either through the blood or lymphatic stream. Practically any organ in the body may be affected but it is most commonly seen in the lungs, bones, lymph nodes and meninges. The lesions grossly resemble small tubercles but microscopically the difference is striking. There is a collection of lymphocytes and polymorphonuclear leukocytes together with a few large mononuclears. The organisms are observed in the center of this mass. As the disease progresses the central part may become necrotic. A few cases have been observed in which the disease in the lungs and mediastinal lymph nodes appears to have been arrested because calcified nodules were found in these sites in patients dead of other diseases. The center of these nodules was necrotic and contained the organism. A considerable growth of fibrous tissue occurred around this necrotic focus. The disease has been transmitted to guinea-pigs and to rats. Precipitins have been demonstrated and skin tests devised with filtrates of cultures; skin tests with this material, coccidioidin, aid in diagnosis but are not absolutely specific. (See Farness; Dickson; Cox and Smith; Cronkhite and Lack; Stewart and Kimura.)

Torula Infections

Distinct from blastomycosis and coccidioidal granuloma, but apparently somewhat confused with these, are cases due to infection with the *Torula* or *Blastomycoides histolytica* of Stoddard and Cutler. There is an occasional association with Hodgkin's disease (Warvi and Rawson). The infection may appear in the brain and meninges, lungs, liver, spleen and kidneys but does not affect skin or bones. The lesions grossly resemble tuberculosis and in the meninges may suggest syphilis. Microscopically, there is destruction of tissue, which may be visible grossly as a gelatinous mass. In connection with the necrotic focus is an infiltrate of lymphoid, large mononuclear and plasma cells, often associated with some fibrin formation and practically always with multinuclear giant cells; polymorphonuclear leukocytes may appear but not in large numbers. The organisms appear free or within giant cells and epithelioid cells. They are small spherules, 1 to 13 micra in diameter, which stain well with ordinary basic dyes and in the larger forms show a refractile capsule. Proliferation in tissues is by budding. Upon inoculation the organism is highly pathogenic for mice and rats, slightly so for guinea-pigs, rabbits and dogs, and has an especial affinity for the central nervous system. Culturally, it proliferates by budding and never produces mycelium. (See Holt.)

Sporotrichosis

This is caused by one of the pathogenic fungi, *Sporotrichium schenckii*. Because it is common on plants of various kinds, it is an occupational hazard for farmers, gardeners, nurserymen, florists, etc. The primary lesion is usually on the finger or hand and may be ascribed by the patient to the prick of a thorn, such as barberry, but this is by no means always true. This lesion begins, after an incubation period of from 10 days to several weeks, as a small painless subcutaneous papule several millimeters in diameter, slightly reddened and sometimes slightly tender. Secondary nodules appear along the course of the draining lymphatic vessels. These may remain as of somewhat gummy consistency without ulceration, but usually break down and discharge a viscid, white, yellow or brown pus. The usual forms are localized with neighboring lymphangitis and lymphadenitis. Disseminated gummatous sporotrichosis with multiple subcutaneous nodules, distributed throughout the body without ulceration; disseminated ulcerative sporotrichosis with multiple ulcers over the body, resembling the ulcerative lesions of tuberculosis, syphilis or furunculosis; and extracutaneous sporotrichosis appearing in mucous membranes, muscles, bones, joints, eye, synovia, kidney and lungs, also occur. Warfield's case is one of a few of widely disseminated sporotrichosis reported in this country, but cases with less extensive lesions are not uncommon. In the more usual forms of the disease, the primary lesion breaks down and discharges pus, and this is followed after variable periods by secondary lesions along the lymphatics, which also break down. The ulcers show a red suppurating base and firm elevated margins. Microscopically, the lesion may appear as an abscess with surrounding organization or, in the more prolonged forms, as a focal accu-

mulation of polymorphonuclear leukocytes, large mononuclears, and in the margins, fibroblasts, newly formed blood vessels and plasma cells. Although the organism may be found in the pus, the microscopic tissue section rarely shows it, except that occasionally fragments of more or less degenerate mycelium may be found within large mononuclear or giant cells. The diagnosis depends upon recovering the organism, which can frequently be obtained in pure culture. Local lesions may be produced experimentally in animals but upon intraperitoneal injection into rats lesions are produced in the testicle and cord from which pure cultures may be obtained and which show the organisms in microscopic section. Using spore suspension as antigen the patient's serum may agglutinate in dilutions of from 1:80 up to 1:1000. Using either spores or culture material as antigen, complement-fixation tests with patients' sera are positive. Both intracutaneous and subcutaneous reactions with killed spores usually give definite positive reactions.

The same disease occurs in the horse, dog, rat and certain other animals. In the horse it closely resembles epizoötic lymphangitis but is distinguishable by cultural methods. Certain cases in man are due to infection from contamination by diseased animals. (See Gastineau et al.)

Aspergillosis

Fungi of the genus *Aspergillus* may be pathogenic for man, and no less than 11 species have been recognized in lesions of varying situation and severity. The commonest in nature and the commonest found in man is *Aspergillus fumigatus* Fresenius. It produces a dark green or brown growth in culture and shows branching mycelia 2 to 3 micra in diameter and produces conidia. It occurs in various cereals, unmilled grain, hay and stock feeds. Birds, such as ducks, pigeons and chickens may be infected. Evidently prolonged exposure, or ill health, is required for infection in man, which is in a sense occupational. The disease occurs among the feeders of geese in producing the fat liver, in sponge cleaners and wig-makers. The disease has been produced experimentally in monkeys, guinea-pigs and rabbits. A true endotoxin has been found in the sap of the mycelium (Henrici).

The disease may be superficial, involving eye, ear, nose, urethra and skin, and may complicate wounds and ulcers. It may be superficial also as concerns bronchi, with a bronchitis which may ulcerate. Much more serious is involvement of the lungs to produce *Pseudotuberculosis aspergillini* or *Pneumomycosis aspergillini*. The clinical course is like that of chronic pulmonary tuberculosis. The lesions grossly resemble tuberculosis in miliary and conglomerate forms; they may be pneumonic in type and may also exhibit cavitation (see Schneider). Coarse granules may be found in the lesion, made up of organisms; if *A. fumigatus*, dark brown or green, if *A. niger*, black in color. Microscopically, the earlier lesions show an infiltration of leukocytes, followed later by the presence of epithelioid and a few giant cells. The latter are of the foreign-body type and may contain parts of the organism. Central necrosis begins early, but does not progress far because of the early fibrosis and marginal vascularization. The surrounding lung may show reactive pneumonia and extensive diffuse fibrosis. Cavitation occurs as the result of secondary infection. The early lesions may show mycelia and spores, but they are sparse and difficult to find in the later stages. The cultures develop toxic bodies which produce tetanic convulsions and paralysis in animals.

Aspergillosis of the lungs is likely to be associated with similar lesions in liver, kidney and other organs. Apparently organisms may enter through the intestine and infect the mesenteric lymph nodes. Lesions may be produced in superficial parts such as the eye, ear, nose, urethra, skin, and may infect wounds and ulcers. Secondary lesions may develop in liver, kidney, meninges and other organs, presumably because of transport of organisms in the blood stream (Linck).

DUE TO OTHER AGENTS

Granuloma Inguinale

This disease, characterized by nodular lesions and chronic serpiginous ulceration, affects the perineum and inguinal region, and also external genitalia, lower abdomen, inner surface of thigh, anus and vagina. It is endemic in tropical and subtropical countries and has been called granuloma venereum and granuloma pudendi ulcerativum. Cases occur in other regions, most commonly in large general hospitals and almhouses. Although the lesion is principally around the genital organs there is no absolute proof that it is a venereal disease. Syphilis may be associated but not in a causative relation. Various bacteria may be found in the lesion as secondary invaders. The spirochetes that are observed are probably those from the surfaces of the genitalia. The organism constantly found is

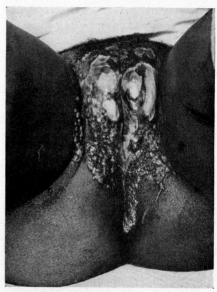

Extensive ulceration of the perineum in granuloma inguinale.

the Leishman-Donovan body. The disease has been transmitted experimentally to man but not to any other animal. The Donovan bodies, however, have not been grown in culture. They appear to be specifically cytotropic and multiply only within large mononuclear and plasma cells. The bodies are small, rounded, or rod-like forms, deeply basophilic and surrounded by an areola that suggests capsule formation. Both in smears taken from the surface of the ulcer and in tissue sections, the characteristic mononuclear cells with Donovan bodies in the cytoplasm are found and because of rupture of the cells, some are free in the tissue.

The incubation period is not definitely known but ranges from perhaps 25 to 50 days. The first lesion is nodular but this is soon followed by a serpiginous type of ulceration which tends to extend. Adjacent smaller lesions may occur but whether they are due to auto-inoculation or to transfer through the lymphatics is not certain. Nevertheless, the inguinal nodes may become swollen and firm. The ulcer is well defined, with an irregular, slightly elevated base and a sluggish red granular surface on which there is a thin serous fluid which sometimes condenses to form a crust. Microscopically, the earlier stages show exudate in the upper corium, often associated with hyperplasia of the epidermis and prolonged downward sprouts of interpapillary epithelium. As the condition continues, however, the epidermis becomes thin and finally ulceration takes place. At this stage there is extensive granulation tissue with fibroblasts and new capillaries. The most numerous cells are plasma cells but there are some polymorphonuclear leukocytes and occasionally eosinophils. Lymphocytes are not abundant. Conspicuous are the large mononuclear cells containing parasites.

Secondary infection may cause deep erosion of the lesions which, when they heal, leave marked mutilation of the region. (See D'Aunoy and von Haam; Pund and Greenblatt; Greenblatt et al.)

Treatment by intravenous injections of tartar emetic has been highly successful, although Lynch is of the opinion that if syphilis be associated, the antimony treatment should be supplemented with antiluetic therapy.

Lymphogranuloma venereum

Various names have been given this condition but the term "lymphogranuloma venereum" is the one most widely adopted. The disease is transmitted by sexual contact and after a short incubation period a primary lesion may be observed on penis or vulva, or may be extragenital. The disease is practically worldwide but is prevalent especially in tropical, subtropical and temperate climates. It occurs in the lower social classes and is more frequent in Negroes than in whites and is about twice as common in males as in females. As with other venereal diseases, the age incidence is in the group between 20 and 40 years. The primary lesion may be either a small herpes-like vesiculation or a somewhat larger ulcerative lesion somewhat resembling a small chancre. Soon the regional lymph nodes become enlarged, soft, tender, and may break down with discharge of pus. In the male the inguinal nodes are likely to be affected and in the female those in the pelvis.

Microscopically, the vesicular primary lesion shows hyperplasia of the epidermis with edema and infiltration into the deeper parts of the epidermis of small and large mononuclear cells and leukocytes. The chancre-like lesion is like that of chancroid, with necrosis of the epithelium and underlying corium, some infiltration of inflammatory cells and hyperplasia of the surrounding epithelium. The lymph nodes grossly are large, firm, red and, because of surrounding fibrosis, adherent to one another. The cross section is soft and bulging and contains tiny pale or white nodules about a millimeter or so in diameter, which at first are discrete and may later fuse. Abscesses may be found in the more advanced cases. Microscopically, there is acute or chronic hyperplasia of the node and the pale foci seen grossly show a necrotic center surrounded by epithelioid cells, often with their long axes radially disposed toward the mass. Leukocytes may participate and are conspicuous when abscess develops.

The disease is caused by a virus which is one of those of large size, measuring 75 to 125 millimicra. It has been grown in tissue culture and produces disease in experimental animals. In these animals, although the inoculation is usually intracerebral, with production of an acute meningo-encephalitis, the virus can be recovered from other organs. In man the virus is disseminated by lymphatics and perhaps also by the blood. Demonstration of immune bodies in the animal is not as yet convincing. In man, however, there is a lasting state of sensitivity indicated by the Frei test. This is a skin test with filtrates from pus of the human lesion, filtrates from the cerebral lesions in mice and other animals or virus cultivated in the chick embryo. It may be demonstrated many years after the acute disease and is positive in at least 95 per cent of all cases.

Low rectal strictures, especially in women, are most frequently due to lymphogranuloma venereum and represent extension of the disease from the pelvic lymph nodes. It is probable that a few of the cases of chronic colitis are also caused by this disease. The chronic ulcerative lesion of the vulva called esthiomenè is now known to be due to lymphogranuloma venereum. The chronic lesions of the rectum may develop into carcinoma. It has become realized that the disease is systemic as well as local. Fever may occur in the acute stage and the blood film may show relative monocytosis or eosinophilia. The infection often is accompanied by marked increase of plasma proteins, especially the globulins and an associated increase in sedimentation rate. There are also reports of involvement of kidneys, bones and joints, but these are not yet positively proved to be a part of the disease. The Frei test also indicates the systemic character of the disease. (See D'Aunoy and von Haam; Gutman; Sanders.)

Tropical ulcer or ulcus tropicum is a different condition attacking the legs and feet and due in large part to trauma. According to Wolbach and Todd the lesion is not to be regarded as a granuloma and is due in all probability to the *Spirochaeta schaudinni* (see also Corpus).

WITHOUT PROVED CAUSE

Hodgkin's Disease

Introduction. Hodgkin's disease exhibits a progressive enlargement of the lymph nodes, occurring in chains or groups rather than in individual nodes, extending over a period of months or years, accompanied by anemia and cachexia. The clinical features were described by Hodgkin in 1832. The disease was subsequently described in greater detail and differentiated as a clinical entity by Wilks in 1856, who gave it the name which it now bears. Numerous other terms have been applied including pseudoleukemia, lymphogranulomatosis and lymphogranuloma malignum. Some investigators have thought the disease to be a variety of malignant tumor, but most regard it as granulomatous. Nevertheless there are occasional instances in which the lesions become so invasive as to justify the conclusion that it may become sarcomatous. In 1898, Sternberg published the first of a series of papers indicating that the disease is probably of tuberculous nature. This was followed in

1902 by the work of Reed which indicated beyond question that the disease is a clinical and pathologic entity and, on both pathologic and experimental grounds, not caused by the tubercle bacillus. This was further confirmed by Longcope in 1904, who described the histologic picture in great detail. The histologic differences between diffuse tuberculosis of the lymph nodes and Hodgkin's disease were pointed out by Karsner in 1910. The lesions

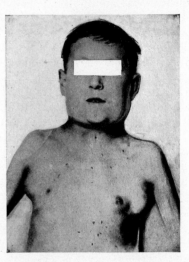

Photograph of patient, the victim of Hodgkin's disease involving cervical and axillary lymph nodes.

are usually well confined by the capsule of the involved nodes or spleen and practically never appear in situations where there is not pre-existing lymphoid tissue. Invasion, therefore, is slight, if present at all, and there is little indication that metastasis occurs.

Despite innumerable investigations, the cause of Hodgkin's disease remains unknown. Various claims have been made for causation by nonacid-fast bacilli resembling those of tuberculosis, by spirochetes and by diphtheroid bacteria, but these views have been abandoned because definitive proof is lacking. L'Esperance suggested that the disease is due to an attenuated strain of avian tubercle bacilli but there has not been adequate confirmation and tuberculin tests give no indication that Hodgkin's disease is due to any variety of tubercle bacillus (Parker, et al.). The view that it is due to a virus has been contradicted by several investigators (Edward). *Brucella melitensis* and *suis* have been isolated from the disease and although no claim has been definitely made that they cause it, yet the suggestion is made that this infection may significantly influence the course (see Wise and Postow; Forbus and Gunter). Definite confirmation has not been made.

Clinical Manifestations. The disease may occur at almost any time of life, but the greatest incidence is in the third decade. In general it is about twice as common in males situation in which lymphoid tissue is found. It is likely to progess slowly with augmentation and recession of local signs. Fever may be continuous for long periods or may be the intermittent type called Pel-Ebstein fever. Loss of flesh and strength are usually slight or moderate until the disease is advanced. Secondary anemia of moderate degree may occur. Leukocytosis is not frequent, but some cases show a relative increase in eosinophils and some a relative increase of monocytes

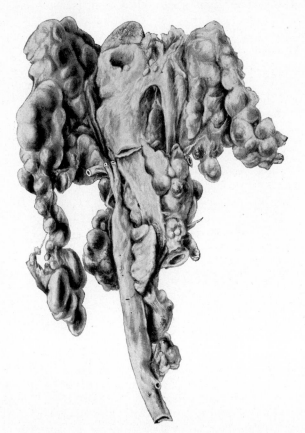

Hodgkin's disease involving cervical and upper mediastinal lymph nodes.

as females, but in childhood the proportion of males is much higher. Usually the first manifestation is a painless, slowly progressing enlargement of lymph nodes, but occasionally pruritus, cough, or dyspnea may be the first sign. As a rule, chains of superficial lymph nodes are the first to become enlarged, especially those of the neck, but it may occur first in the spleen, gastro-intestinal canal, mediastinal or retroperitoneal lymph nodes, in the spinal canal, or any other and decrease of lymphocytes. Platelets are sometimes increased in number and occasionally megakaryocytes appear in the blood. There is, however, no characteristic blood picture. Cutaneous lesions, in the form of a macular, often itchy, eruption, due to infiltration in the skin, are not uncommon. Various other clinical manifestations may be due to the situation of the lesions. For example, blood vessels may be compressed, lesions in the spinal canal or in the brain may cause paralysis. Gastro-intestinal disturbances, cough, dyspnea, vomiting, etc., may be due to special localizations. The course may last for a few months to several years, the average being somewhat less than four years. (See Goldman; Wallhauser; Winkelman and Moore.)

Of interest is the Gordon test, performed by the intracranial injection of filtrates of lymph nodes into rabbits (or guinea pigs). This is followed in a few days by paralysis; sections of the cerebellum show loss of Purkinje cells. The test is positive in about 75 per cent of cases and only rarely gives false positives (Steiner). It is not spe-

according to the stage. The earliest changes noted are proliferation and hyperplasia of the lymphoid cells with partial or complete obliteration of the architecture. Hyperplasia of germinal centers can be found in the germinal centers of remaining follicles and in situations which can safely be estimated as the original position of follicles. The sinuses show extensive endothelial hyperplasia. It cannot definitely be stated whether this hyperplasia is from the lining endothelium or is also participated in by the cells of the reticulum.

As time goes on, the architecture of the node is definitely obliterated and the cell

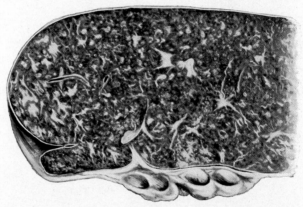

Cross section of spleen in Hodgkin's disease, showing extensive fibrosis and small areas of necrosis.

cific and can be caused by material from normal bone marrow and spleen. Biopsy is the most successful method of diagnosis, but the Gordon test may be of aid in doubtful cases.

Morbid Anatomy. The lymph nodes are found to be enlarged in chains or groups. They are pale in color and of increasingly dense consistency as the disease is of greater duration. There is usually a chronic inflammatory change in the tissues surrounding the individual nodes, so that they are adherent to one another. Cross section of the nodes shows that they are discrete and there is little tendency for invasion of the capsule or fusion of the lymphadenoid tissue. The cross section is moist, pale, bulges in the earlier stages and in the later stages does not. It is firm in the later stages, and in any stage may show small foci of yellow or yellowish-gray necrosis. Microscopically, the picture differs

picture is characteristic: hyperplasia of the lymphoid cells and an associated increase in large mononuclear cells, numerous plasma cells, an occasional mast cell and varying numbers of large mononuclear and multinuclear giant cells. The giant cells are several times the diameter of the endothelial cells and show a generally homogeneous cytoplasm. The nuclei are large and distinctly vesicular and in the multinuclear forms override one another. These are often called Sternberg cells or Dorothy Reed cells. Their exact nature is not established, but, on the basis of their behavior in tissue cultures, Lewis believes them to be myeloid rather than lymphoid or monocytic in origin. Eosinophils are frequent in many cases but absent in a considerable number of others. An important feature of the histology is the proliferation of the connective tissue. In the earlier stages this is slight but as the disease progresses, fibrosis may form a very prominent part of the picture. Longcope divided the disease into three stages on the basis of the degree of fibrosis, but it can readily be seen that such a division is purely arbitrary. Nevertheless, it is possible to distinguish early and late cases on this basis. Necrosis appears in the form of small foci with loss of cell outline, pyknosis, karyolysis and

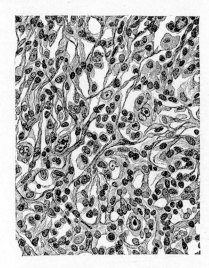

Histology of lymph node of Hodgkin's disease, showing extensive fibrosis and several types of cells.

karyorrhexis; it affects the cellular rather than the fibrous parts. Granules of golden-brown pigment are often present but their nature is not definitely known.

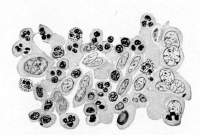

Cell detail in Hodgkin's disease. Note the various forms of giant cells, endothelial cells, a plasma cell, polymorphonuclear leukocyte, and several granular eosinophils.

Of the other organs of the body, the spleen is frequently and in fact almost constantly involved. This organ is large, firm, dense, shows a thick slaty capsule and in cross section is firm, red, and may show foci of necrosis. Connective tissue is obviously increased but the follicles may or may not be visible. The histology of the spleen is essentially the same as that of the lymph node, although in this situation pigmentation may be more prominent. The liver is usually somewhat enlarged, but shows no particular gross characters. Microscopically, however, cell masses similar to those in the lymph nodes are sometimes found in the perilobular connective tissue. These, however, are not encapsulated and may appear to invade the liver tissue.

Bones may be involved by enlargement of marrow foci of the disease or by direct extension from neighboring lymph nodes. Both osteoplastic and osteolytic changes may occur. The bones especially affected are the vertebrae and pelvis, with less frequent involvement of other spongy and long bones (Craver and Copeland).

Mycosis Fungoides

Mycosis fungoides is a chronic disease, of unknown cause, with special manifestations in the skin. It is most common between 40 and 60 years of age, and affects the sexes about equally. Clinically there are four stages. The first stage of dermatitis, including erythema, eczematoid, urticarial or mixed forms of eruption, lasts for months or years. The second stage of infiltration of the skin with papule formation is of shorter duration. In the third stage, tumor-like nodules appear and the patient becomes systemically ill. In the fourth stage, the nodules break down and fungating ulcers appear. Anemia is common and the blood films may show a relative eosinophilia, and cells of the order of monocytes may be frequent. Formerly thought to be a cutaneous disease, it is now known that involvement of internal viscera is frequent.

Microscopically, in the lesions of the early, the premycotic, stage, there occurs a thickening of the epidermis, prolongation of the interpapillary portion, and an infiltration into the corium (especially the papillae) of lymphoid cells with a few plasma and new connective tissue cells. The nodules are made up of lymphocytes, plasma cells, large mononuclears, leukocytes, eosinophils, mast cells, multinucleated giant cells and connective tissue cells irregularly intermingled. Karyorrhexis is common and mitotic figures in cells closely in relation to the small areas of necrosis are not infrequent. The giant cells show vesicular over-riding nuclei; the nuclei are somewhat more numerous than is usual in the similar cells of Hodgkin's disease. The connective tissue may not increase until late in the disease. The blood vessels are dilated and in late stages may show hyaline degeneration of the walls and thrombosis, the latter leading to edema of the tissues. Various bacteria are commonly present as the result of secondary infection.

The nature of the disease is not clear, except that it is not a mycosis caused by fungi or other vegetable parasites. It is not a local neoplasm in the ordinary sense. Modern studies suggest that the disease belongs in the large group of lymphoblastomas, a systemic disease of the reticulo-endothelial cells of various parts of the body. It would thus be related in some vague way to, but not identical with, leukemia, especially the monocytic form, Hodgkin's disease and lymphosarcoma. (See Berman; Symmers.)

Sarcoidosis

Lupus pernio of Besnier, lymphogranulomatosis benigna of Schaumann and sarcoidosis of Boeck are probably slightly different manifestations of the same disease. It affects young adults and sometimes those of later life. In Europe the disease occurs in whites, but in this country, although the same is true, it is more common in the Negro and has been reported in an American Indian. It begins insidiously and progresses slowly. It is not often fatal and recoveries or prolonged remissions are frequent. The patients exhibit enlarged superficial lymph nodes, cutaneous lesions, pulmonary infiltrations which may be sufficiently marked to reduce vital capacity, enlarged mediastinal lymph nodes, foci of bone destruction in the distal parts of the extremities, iridocyclitis and the manifestation known as uveoparotid fever. It is rare to see all these phenomena in each case; one or more may predominate.

The blood may show anemia, increased sedimentation rate and occasionally eosinophilia or monocytosis. The lesions may be found in lymph nodes, subcutaneous tissues, lungs, the parotid gland, various viscera including the heart (rarely) and skeletal muscle. Grossly, they are firm, gray, noncaseating nodules, varying in size from the barely visible up to a centimeter or more.

Microscopically, there are tubercle-like granulomas, usually multiple in the single gross lesion. These are composed of epithelioid cells and giant cells, usually of foreign-body type, sometimes containing one or two vacuoles. A few lymphocytes may be found in the periphery, but the granuloma is

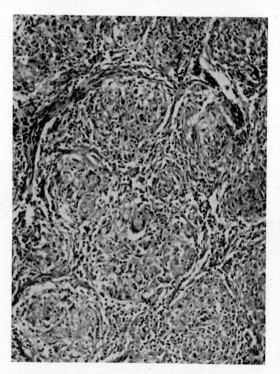

Boeck's sarcoid. Lesion in lymph node.

well circumscribed. Fibrosis occurs in this lesion and often for a very short distance around it. Central necrosis or caseation is absent except for a rare tiny focus. Bacterial stains are negative.

The cause is quite unknown. The lesions have a certain resemblance microscopically to those of tuberculosis, syphilis and leprosy, but careful investigations have failed to show that any of these causes Boeck's sarcoid. Allergy, nonspecific in type, has been suspected but not proved. (See Longcope; Harrell; Tice and Sweaney; Kissmeyer.)

REFERENCES

Tuberculosis

Anderson, R. J.: The Chemistry of the Lipoids of Tubercle Bacilli, Physiol. Rev., **12**: 166, 1932.

Baldwin, E. R., S. A. Petroff, and L. U. Gardner: Tuberculosis: Bacteriology, Pathology and Laboratory Diagnosis, etc., Philadelphia, Lea and Febiger, 1927.

Caldwell, G. T.: Chemical Changes in Tuberculous Tissues, Jour. Infect. Dis., **24**: 81, 1919.

Calmette, A.: L'Infection Bacillaire et la Tuberculose chez L'Homme et chez les Animaux, Paris, 1928.

Cobbett, L.: The Rôle of the Three Types of Tubercle Bacilli in Human and Animal Tuberculosis, Lancet, **1**: 979, 1922.

Cornet, G.: Acute General Miliary Tuberculosis, New York, 1914.

Cunningham, R. S., and E. H. Tomkins: The Epithelioid Cell, Amer. Rev. Tuberc., **23**: 71, 1931.

Dienes, L., and T. B. Mallory: Influence of Allergy on Development of Early Tuberculous Lesions, Proc. Soc. Exper. Biol. and Med., **34**: 59, 1936.

Feldman, W. H.: Avian Tuberculous Infection, Baltimore, Williams and Wilkins, 1939.

Finner, L. I.: The Clinical Value of the Monocyte Count in Pulmonary Tuberculosis, Amer. Rev. Tuberc., **21**: 764, 1930.

Gardner, L. U.: The Cellular Reactions to Primary Infection and Reinfection with the Tubercle Bacillus, etc., Amer. Rev. Tuberc., **22**: 379, 1930.

Ghon, A.: The Primary Lung Focus of Tuberculosis of Children, New York and London, 1916.

Griffith, A. S.: The Types of Tubercle Bacilli in Human Bone and Joint Tuberculosis, Jour. Path. and Bact., **31**: 875, 1928.

———: Mixed Infections with Human and Bovine Tubercle Bacilli in the Human Subject, Tubercle, **18**: 193, 1937.

von Hayek, H.: Immunobiologie, Dispositions und Konstitutions-Forschung, Berlin, 1921.

Hoefert, B.: Ueber Bakterienbefunde in Duodenalsaft von Gesunden und Kranken, Zeitschr. f. Klin. Med., **92**: 221, 1921.

Holley, S. W.: Corneal Reactions of Normal and of Tuberculous Guinea Pigs to Tuberculo-protein and Tuberculo-phosphatide, Amer. Jour. Path., **11**: 937, 1935.

Israel, H. L., and E. R. Long: Primary Tuberculosis in Adolescents and Young Adults, Amer. Rev. Tuberc., **43**: 42, 1941.

Jobling, J. W., and W. A. Petersen: A Study of the Ferments and Ferment Inhibiting Substances in Tuberculous Caseous Material, Jour. Exper. Med., **19**: 383, 1914.

Kageyama, S.: Ueber die frühzeitigen Reaktionen des retikulo-endothelialen Systems bei phthisishtuberkulöser Infektion, etc., Beit. Path. Anat. u. Allg. Path., **74**: 356, 1925.

Kopeloff, N.: The Bacterial Content of the Stomach as Influenced by Saliva, Proc. Soc. Exper. Biol. and Med., **19**: 110, 1921.

Krause, A. K.: Tuberculosis: Infection, Pathology, Etiology, and Bacteriology, Nelson Loose Leaf Manual, Vol. I, p. 309, 1921.

———: The Spread of Tuberculous Infection in the Body, Amer. Rev. Tuberc., **9**: 83, 1924.

Letulle, M.: La Tuberculose Pleuro-pulmonaire, Paris, 1918.

Long, E. R.: Tuberculin and the Tuberculin Reaction, in Jordan and Falk's The Newer Knowledge of Bacteriology and Immunology, Chicago, Univ. of Chicago Press, 1928, p. 1066.

———: A Chemical View of the Pathogenesis of Tuberculosis, Harvey Lectures, Baltimore, Williams and Wilkins, **25**: 144, 1929-30.

———: The Inflammatory Reaction in Tuberculosis, Amer. Jour. Med. Sci., **185**: 749, 1933.

———: Tuberculosis, Leprosy and Allied Mycobacterial Diseases, Science, **87**: 23, 1938.

———: Pathogenesis of Primary and Reinfection Tuberculosis, New England Jour. Med., **223**: 656, 1940.

———: Constitution and Related Factors in Resistance to Tuberculosis, Arch. Path., **32**: 122, 286, 1941.

Lurie, M. B.: Experimental Epidemiology of Tuberculosis, Jour. Exper. Med., **51**: 729, 743, 753, 769, 1930.

———: Heredity, Constitution and Tuberculosis. An Experimental Study, Amer. Rev. Tuberc., Suppl. **44**: 1, 1941.

———: Studies on the Mechanism of Immunity in Tuberculosis. The Fate of Tubercle Bacilli Ingested by Mononuclear Phagocytes Derived from Normal and Immunized Animals, Jour. Exper. Med., **75**: 247, 1942.

Maver, M. E., and H. G. Wells: The Alimentary Absorption of Calcium and Its Deposition in the Tissues in Experimental Tuberculosis, Amer. Rev. Tuberc., **7**: 1, 1923.

Maximow, A.: Tuberculose des Tissus de Mammiferes en Culture, Ann. d'Anat. Path., **3**: 1, 1926.

Opie, E. L.: The Pathogenesis and Transmission of Tuberculosis, Harvey Lectures, **24**: 197, 1928-29; Amer. Jour. Med. Sci., **179**: 104, 1930.

———: Cellular Reactions of Tuberculosis and Their Relation to Immunity and Sensitization, Arch. Path., **14**: 706, 1932.

———, and H. Anderson: First Infection with Tuberculosis by Way of the Lungs, Amer. Rev. Tuberc., **4**: 629, 1920.

Pagel, W.: The Rôle of the Bacillus and of "Hetero-allergy" in Tuberculous Liquefaction, Jour. Path. and Bact., **42**: 417, 1936.

Pawlow, M.: Einwirkung von Lymphocyten auf Tuberkelbazillen in Vitro, Zeitschr. f. Immunitätsf., **38**: 181, 1923.

Permar, H. H.: The Function of the Endothelial Cell in Pathological Conditions, Especially in Tuberculosis, Amer. Rev. Tuberc., **9**: 507, 1924.

Prudaen, T. M., and E. Hodenpyl: Studies on the Action of Dead Bacteria in the Living Body, New York Med. Jour., **53**: 637, 697, 1891.

Ranke, K. E.: Primäraffekt, sekundäre und tertiäre Stadien der Lungentuberkulose, Deutsches Arch. f. Klin. Med., **129**: 224, 1919.

Ravenel, M. P.: The Passage of Tubercle Bacilli Through the Normal Intestinal Wall, Jour. Med. Res., **10**: 460, 1903.

Reed, C. C.: Studies of the Biochemistry and Chemotherapy of Tuberculosis XXVI, Fat-Splitting Ferments in Lymphocytes, Amer. Rev. Tuberc., **7**: 105, 1923.

Reichle, H. R.: Primary Tuberculous Infection of the Intestine, Arch. Path., **21**: 79, 1936.

———, and M. Gallavan: Reactivation of a

Primary Tuberculous Complex as a Source of Tuberculous Reinfection, Arch. Path., 24: 201, 1937.

Reisner, D.: The Relations between Extrapulmonary and Pulmonary Tuberculosis, Amer. Rev. Tuberc., 30: 375, 1934.

Rosenthal, S. R.: General Tissue and Humoral Response to an Avirulent Tubercle Bacillus (BCG), Trans. Nat. Tuberc. Asso., 33: 146, 1937.

Sabin, F. R., K. C. Smithburn, and R. M. Thomas: Cellular Reactions to Wax-like Materials from Acid-fast Bacteria. The Unsaponifiable Fraction from the Tubercle Bacillus, Strain H-37, Jour. Exper. Med., 62: 751, 1935.

Seibert, F. B.: The Chemical Composition of the Active Principle of Tuberculin, etc., Jour. Biol. Chem., 78: 345, 1928; see also Amer. Rev. Tuberc., 17: 402, 1928; Jour. Infect. Dis., 51: 383, 1932.

Spies, T. D.: The Calcification of Tubercles by Means of Irradiated Ergosterol in Experimental Chronic Tuberculosis, Amer. Rev. Tuberc., 23: 169, 1931.

Thompson, W. P., and M. Frobisher, Jr.: The Filterability of the Tubercle Bacillus, Amer. Rev. Tuberc., 18: 823, 1928.

Wartman, W. B.: Attraction of Human Polymorphonuclear Leukocytes by Tubercle Protein, Amer. Jour. Path., 13: 612, 1937.

Wells, H. G., L. M. De Witt, and E. R. Long: The Chemistry of Tuberculosis, Baltimore, 1923.

Whitman, R. C., and L. W. Greene: A Case of Disseminated Miliary Tuberculosis in a Still-born Fetus, Arch. Int. Med., 29: 261, 1922.

Wolbach, S. B., and H. C. Ernst: Observations on the Morphology of Bacillus Tuberculosis from Human and Bovine Sources, Jour. Med. Res., 10: 313, 1903.

Syphilis and Yaws

Ammich, O.: Über die nichtsyphilitische interstitielle Pneumonie des ersten Kindesalters, Virchow's Arch. Path. Anat., 302: 539, 1938.

Bell, E. T.: Frequency with Which Syphilitic Lesions Are Encountered in Postmortem Examinations, Arch. Path., 26: 839, 1938.

Bertarelli, E.: Ueber die Transmission der Syphilis auf das Kaninchen, Centralbl. f. Bakteriol., 1 te Abt. Orig., 41: 320, 1906; 43: 238, 1907.

Bronfenbrenner, J., and H. Noguchi: On the Resistance of Various Spirochaetes in Cultures to the Action of Chemical and Physical Agents, Jour. Pharm. and Exper. Ther., 4: 333, 1912-13.

Brown, W. H., and L. Pearce: Experimental Syphilis in the Rabbit, Jour. Exper. Med., 31: 475, 709, 729, 749, 1920; 32: 445, 473, 1920; 33: 495, 515, 525, 1921; 34: 167, 1921; Proc. Soc. Exper. Biol. and Med., 17: 164, 167, 1920.

———: Superinfection in Experimental Syphilis Following the Administration of Subcurative Doses of Arsphenamine or Neoarsphenamine, Jour. Exper. Med., 33: 553, 1921.

Chesney, A. M.: Acquired Immunity in Syphilis, Harvey Lectures, 25: 103, 1929-30.

———, T. B. Turner, and F. H. Grauer: Studies in Experimental Syphilis. X. Observations on Cross-inoculations with Heterologous Strains of Syphilitic Virus, Bull. Johns Hopkins Hosp., 52: 145, 1933.

Cole, H. N.: Report of a Series of Sixty-one Extragenital Chancres, Jour. Amer. Med. Asso., 67: 1805, 1916.

Coronini, C.: Ueber mikroscopische Unterscheidungsmöglichkeiten zwischen tuberkulöser und luischer Nekrose, Virchow's Arch. f. Path. Anat., 274: 560, 1929-30.

Craig, C. F., and H. J. Nichols: A Study of Complement Fixation in Syphilis with Spirochaeta Culture Antigens, Jour. Exper. Med., 16: 336, 1912.

Currie, D. H., M. T. Clegg, and H. T. Hollmann: Studies upon Leprosy, XIV. The Artificial Cultivation of the Bacillus of Leprosy, XV. Attempts at Specific Therapy in Leprosy, Public Health Bulletin, No. 47, Sept. 1911.

Ferris, H. W., and T. B. Turner: Comparative Histology of Yaws and Syphilis in Jamaica, Arch. Path., 24: 703, 1937.

Hata, S.: On the Ravages of Congenital Syphilis and Its Prevention, Inter. Jour. Public Health, 2: 354, 1921.

Kahn, R. I.: The Kahn Test, a Practical Guide, Baltimore, Williams and Wilkins, 1928.

Klauder, J. V., and T. Butterworth: Accidental Transmission of Syphilis by Blood Transfusion, Amer. Jour. Syph. Gonor. and Ven. Dis., 21: 652, 1937.

Kline, B. S.: Microscopic Slide Precipitation Tests for the Diagnosis and Exclusion of Syphilis, Baltimore, Williams and Wilkins, 1932.

Kolle, W., and H. Hetsch: Die experimentelle Bakteriologie und die Infektionskrankheiten, Berlin, Urban, 1922.

Levaditi, C., and A. Marie: Plurality of Syphilis Virus, Presse Medicale, 28: 646, 1920.

Moss, W. L., and G. H. Bigelow: Yaws, an Analysis of 1046 Cases in the Dominican Republic, Bull. Johns Hopkins Hosp., 33: 43, 1922.

Nichols, H. J.: Observations on a Strain of Spirochaeta Pallida Isolated from the Nervous System, Jour. Exper. Med., 19: 362, 1914.

———: Further Observations on Certain Features of Experimental Syphilis and Yaws in the Rabbit, Jour. Exper. Med., 14: 196, 1911.

Noguchi, H.: The Spirochetes, Jordan and Falk's. The Newer Knowledge of Bacteriology and Immunology, Chicago, 1928.

Parodi, U.: Ueber die Uebertragung der Syphilis auf den Hoden des Kaninchens, Centralbl. f. Bakteriol, 1 te Abt., Orig., 44: 428, 1907.

Pearce, L.: Specificity of Spirochetes in Diseases of the Eye, Ear, Nose, and Throat, Arch. Otolaryngol., 1: 680, 1925.

Raiziss, G. W., and M. Severac: Rapidity with Which Spirochaeta Pallida Invades the Blood Stream, Arch. Derm. and Syphilol., 35: 1101, 1937.

Reasoner, M. A.: The Effect of Soap on Treponema Pallidum, Jour. Amer. Med. Asso., 68: 973, 1917.

Rosahn, P. D.: The Infectivity of Treponema Pallidum in Excised Syphilitic Tissue, Amer. Jour. Hyg., 22: 283, 1935.

Schaudinn, F., and E. Hoffmann: Ueber Spirochaetenbefunde im Lymphdrüsensaft Syphilitischer Deutsch. Med. Wochenschr., 31: 711, 1905.

———: Ueber Spirochete Pallida bei Syphilis und die Unterschiede dieser Form gegenüber anderen Arten dieser Gattung, Berlin, Klin. Wochenschr., 42: 673, 675, 1905.

Schobl, O.: Immunity in Yaws, Jour. Philippine Islands Med. Asso., 8: 6, 1928.

Stitt, E. R.: Practical Bacteriology, Blood Work and Animal Parasitology, Ea. 8, Philadelphia, 1927.

Stokes, J. H., A. G. Schoch, and F. A. Ireland: The Clinical Concept of Reinfection in Syphilis: A Critique Based on Five Cases, the Reported Literature and a Study of Early Relapse, Arch. Derm. and Syphilol., 23: 829, 1931.

Turner, T. B.: The Race and Sex Distribution of Lesions of Syphilis in 10,000 Cases, Bull. Johns Hopkins Hosp., 46: 159, 1930.

——: Protective Antibodies in the Serum of Syphilitic Rabbits, Jour. Exper. Med., 69: 867, 1939.

——, and W. L. Fleming: Prolonged Maintenance of Spirochetes and Filtrable Viruses in the Frozen State, ibid., 70: 629, 1939.

——, ——, and N. L. Brayton: Protective Antibodies in the Serum of Human Syphilitics, Jour. Clin. Invest., 18: 471, 1936.

Warthin, A. S.: The New Pathology of Syphilis, Harvey Lectures, 1917-19, p. 67, Lippincott, Philadelphia.

——: Sex Differences in the Pathologic Picture of Syphilis, Amer. Jour. Syph., 12: 301, 1928.

——, E. Buffington, and R. C. Wanstrom: A Study of Rabbit Spirochetosis, Jour. Infect. Dis., 32: 315, 1923.

Wile, U. J.: Experimental Syphilis in the Rabbit Produced by the Brain Substance of the Living Paretic, J. Exper. Med., 23: 199, 1916.

Wilson, P. W., and M. S. Mathis: Epidemiology and Pathology of Yaws: A Report Based on a Study of One Thousand Four Hundred and Twenty-Three Consecutive Cases in Haiti, Jour. Amer. Med. Asso., 94: 1289, 1930.

Zinsser, H., and J. G. Hopkins: The Viability of the Spirochaeta Pallida in Diffuse Daylight at Room Temperature, Jour. Amer. Med. Asso., 62: 1802, 1914.

Other Granulomata

Bailey, C. H.: Serologic Reactions in a Case of Rhinoscleroma, Jour. Cutan. Dis., 37: 447, 1919.

Beaver, D. C., and L. Thompson: Actinobacillosis of Man. Report of a Fatal Case, Amer. Jour. Path., 9: 603, 1933.

Bennett, R. A.: Hodgkin's Disease, Bristol, 1923.

Benzancon, F.: Precis de Microbiologie Clinique, Paris, 1920.

de Beurmann, L., and H. Gougerot: Les Nouvelles Mycoses, Paris, 1912.

Berman, L.: Pathologic Nature of Mycosis Fungoides, Arch. Path., 29: 530, 1940.

Blair, J., and N. C. Yarian: Two Cases of Sporotrichosis Infection Due to Barberry, Jour. Amer. Med. Asso., 91: 96, 1928.

Bridge, N.: Streptothricosis (Actinomycosis) of the Lungs, Jour. Amer. Med. Asso., 57: 1501, 1911.

Brown, P. K., and W. T. Cummins: A Differential Study of Coccidioidal Granuloma and Blastomycosis, Arch. Int. Med., 15: 608, 1915.

Busse, O.: Die Hefen als Krankheitserreger, Berlin, 1897.

Campbell, M. F.: Etiology of Granuloma Inguinale: With Report of Eighteen Cases, Amer. Jour. Med. Sci., 174: 670, 1927.

Castellani, A., and A. J. Chalmers: Manual of Tropical Diseases, New York, 1919.

Claypole, E. J.: Human Streptothrichosis and Its Differentiation from Tuberculosis, Arch. Int. Med., 14: 104, 1914.

Claypole, E. J.: On the Classification of the Streptothrices. Particularly in Their Relation to Bacteria, Jour. Exper. Med., 17: 99, 1913.

Colebrook, L., and others: Discussion on Actinomycosis Common to Man and Animals, Proc. Roy. Soc. Med. (Sect. Compar. Med. and Surg.) 23: 61, 1930 (p. 861 of entire volume).

Coleman, W., and J. Ewing: A Case of Septicemic Glanders in the Human Subject, Jour. Med. Res., 9: 223, 1903.

Corpus, T.: A Survey of Ulcus Tropicum, Jour. Amer. Med. Asso., 82: 1192, 1924.

Cowdry, E. V.: Cytology of Leprosy, Puerto Rico Jour. Publ. Health and Trop. Med., 14: 95, 1938.

——: Cytological Studies on Globi in Leprosy, Amer. Jour. Path., 16: 103, 1940.

Cox, A. J., and C. E. Smith: Arrested Pulmonary Coccidioidal Granuloma, Arch. Path., 27: 717, 1939.

Craver, L. F., and M. M. Copeland: Changes in the Bone in Hodgkin's Granuloma, Arch. Surg., 28: 1062, 1934.

Cronkhite, A. E., and A. R. Lack: Primary Pulmonary Coccidioidomycosis. Experimental Infection with Coccidioides Immitis, Jour. Exper. Med., 72: 167, 1940.

D'Aunoy, R., and J. L. Beven: Systemic Blastomycosis, Jour. Lab. and Clin. Med., 16: 124, 1930-31.

——, and E. von Haam: The Pathology of Granuloma Venereum, Amer. Jour. Path., 14: 39, 1938.

——: Venereal Lymphogranuloma, Arch. Path., 27: 1032, 1939.

Davis, B. F.: The Immunological Reactions of Oidiomycosis (Blastomycosis) in the Guinea Pig, Jour. Infect. Dis., 8: 190, 1911.

Dickson, E. C.: Coccidioidomycosis: The Preliminary Acute Infection with Fungus Coccidioides, Jour. Amer. Med. Asso., 111: 1362, 1938.

Duval, C. W., and P. G. White: The Histological Lesions of Experimental Glanders, Jour. Exper. Med., 9: 352, 1907.

Edward, D. G. ff.: Observations on the Nature of Gordon's Encephalitogenic Agent, Jour. Path. and Bact., 47: 481, 1938.

Emmons, C. W., H. Hailey, and H. Hailey: Chromoblastomycosis. Report of the 6th Case from Continental United States, Jour. Amer. Med. Asso., 116: 25, 1941.

Farness, O. J.: Coccidioidomycosis, ibid., 116: 1749, 1941.

Ferris, H. W., and T. B. Turner: Comparison of Cutaneous Lesions Produced in Rabbits by Intracutaneous Inoculation of Spirochetes from Yaws and Syphilis, Arch. Path., 26: 491, 1938.

Figi, F. A., and L. Thompson: Rhinoscleroma, Jour. Amer. Med. Asso., 91: 637, 1928.

Fink, A. A.: Staphylococcic Actinophytotic (Botryomycotic) Abscess of the Liver with Pulmonary Involvement, Arch. Path., 31: 103, 1941.

Fischer, O.: Erfolgreicke Behandlung eines Falls von chronischem Nasenrotz mittels Autovakzine, Deutsch. Med. Wochenschr., 46: 73, 1920.

Fletcher, W.: Melioidosis, in A System of Bacteriology in Relation to Medicine, Medical Research Council, London, 1930; v. 5, p. 56.

Flexner, S.: Pseudo-Tuberculosis Hominis Streptothricha, Jour. Exper. Med., **3**: 435, 1898.

Foerster, H. R.: Sporotrichosis, an Occupational Dermatosis, Jour. Amer. Med. Asso., **87**: 1605, 1926.

Forbus, W. D., and J. U. Gunter: Pathogenicity of Strains of Brucella Obtained from Cases of Hodgkin's Disease, South. Med. Jour., **34**: 376, 1941.

Fordyce, J. A.: Some Problems in the Pathology of Syphilis, Harvey Lectures, Philadelphia, Lippincott, **10**: 221, 1915.

Foshay, L.: Tularemia: A Summary of Certain Aspects of the Disease Including Methods of Early Diagnosis and the Results of Serum Treatment in 600 Patients, Medicine, **19**: 1, 1940.

Fox, H.: Granuloma Inguinale; Its Occurrence in the United States, Jour. Amer. Med. Asso., **87**: 1785, 1926.

Francis, E.: A Summary of Present Knowledge of Tularaemia, Medicine, **7**: 411, 1928.

Franklin, G. C. H.: Actinomycosis: A New Species, Pathogenic for Man, Ann. Int. Med., **13**: 1205, 1940.

Frothingham, L.: The Diagnosis of Glanders by the Strauss Method, Jour. Med. Res., **6**: 331, 1901.

Fulmer, S. C., and M. J. Kilbury: Tularemic Peritonitis, Jour. Amer. Med. Asso., **89**: 1661, 1927.

Gastineau, F. M., F. M. Spolyar, L. W. Spolyar, and E. Haynes: Sporotrichosis. Report of Six Cases Among Florists, Jour. Amer. Med. Asso., **117**: 1074, 1941.

Gilchrist, T. C., and W. R. Stokes: A Case of Pseudo-lupus Vulgaris Caused by a Blastomyces, Jour. Exper. Med., **3**: 53, 1898.

Goldman, L. B.: Hodgkin's Disease. An Analysis of 212 Cases, Jour. Amer. Med. Asso., **114**: 1611, 1940.

Greenblatt, R. B., R. B. Dienst, E. R. Pund, and R. Torpin: Experimental and Clinical Granuloma Inguinale, ibid., **113**: 1109, 1939.

Gutman, A. B.: Systemic Manifestations of Lymphogranuloma Venereum, New York State Jour. Med., **39**: 1420, 1939.

Hamburger, W. W.: Sporotrichosis in Man, Jour. Amer. Med. Asso., **59**: 1590, 1912.

Harrell, G. T.: Generalized Sarcoidosis of Boeck: A Clinical Review of Eleven Cases, with Studies of the Blood and the Etiologic Factors, Arch. Int. Med., **65**: 1003, 1940.

Hektoen, L.: The Organism in a Case of Blastomycetic Dermatitis, Jour. Exper. Med., **4**: 261, 1899.

Henrici, A. T.: An Endotoxin from Aspergillus Fumigatus, Jour. Immunol., **36**: 319, 1939.

Holt, R.: The Identification of Blastomycoides histolytica in Three Infections of the Central Nervous System, Jour. Lab. and Clin. Med., **27**: 58, 1941.

Hooper, P.: The Symptomatology and Treatment of Leprosy, Jour. Trop. Med. and Hyg., **24**: 137, 1921.

Jones, J. W., and H. S. Alden: Maduromycotic Mycetoma (Madura Foot): Report of a Case Occurring in an American Negro, Jour. Amer. Med. Asso., **96**: 256, 1931.

Karsner, H. T.: A Study of Cases of Hodgkin's Disease and Certain Allied Conditions, Arch. Int. Med., **6**: 175, 1910.

Kimmelstiel, P., and C. A. Easley, Jr.: Experimental Botryomycosis, Amer. Jour. Path., **16**: 95, 1940.

Kissmeyer, A.: La Maladie de Boeck, Copenhagen, Levin and Munksgaard, 1932.

Lenhartz, H.: Ueber Lungenstreptotrichose, Deutsch. Arch. Klin. Med., **136**: 129, 1921.

L'Esperance, E. S.: Experimental Inoculation of Chickens with Hodgkin's Nodes, Jour. Immunol., **16**: 37, 1929.

——: Study of a Case of Hodgkin's Disease in a Child, ibid., **18**: 127, 1930.

Lewis, M. R.: The Behavior of Dorothy Reed Cells in Tissue Cultures, Amer. Jour. Med. Sci., **201**: 467, 1941.

Lillie, R. D.: The Pathology of Tularemia, Nat. Inst. Health Bull., No. 167, Washington, D. C., 1937.

Linck, K.: Tödliche Meningitis aspergillina beim Menschen, Virchow's Arch. Path. Anat., **304**: 408, 1939.

Longcope, W. T.: On the Pathological Histology of Hodgkin's Disease, etc., Bull. Ayer Clin. Lab. Penna. Hosp. No. 1, p. 4, 1903.

——: Hodgkin's Disease, Osler and McCrae's Modern Medicine, Philadelphia and New York, 1915, vol. IV, p. 755.

——: Sarcoidosis or Besnier-Boeck-Schaumann Disease, Frank Billings Lecture, Jour. Amer. Med. Asso., **117**: 1321, 1941.

MacCallum, W. G.: A Text-Book of Pathology, Philadelphia and London, 5th ed., 1932.

MacNeal, W. J., and R. M. Taylor: Coccidioides Immitis and Coccidioidal Granuloma, Jour. Med. Res., **30**: 261, 1914.

Martin, D. S., and D. T. Smith: Blastomycosis, Amer. Rev. Tuberc., **39**: 488, 1939.

McKinley, E. B.: The Etiology of Leprosy, Medicine, **13**: 377, 1934.

Metchnikoff, E., and E. Roux: Études expérimentales sur la Syphilis, Ann. l'Inst. Pasteur, **17**: 809, 1903.

Moore, J. J., and D. J. Davis: Sporotrichosis Following Mouse Bite, with Certain Immunologic Data, Jour. Infect. Dis., **23**: 252, 1918.

Morris, M. C., and L. A. Julianelle: A Biological Classification of the Bacillus of Rhinoscleroma, Jour. Infect. Dis., **55**: 150, 1934.

Naussac, G., and others: Symposium on Actinomycosis, Internatl. Clinics, Lippincott, Philadelphia, series 31, vol. 3, 1921.

Netherton, E. W.: Tularemia with Reference to Its Cutaneous Manifestations, Arch. Derm. and Syph., **16**: 170, 1927.

Oliver, J.: The Origin of the Lepra Cell, Jour. Exper. Med., **43**: 233, 1926.

Ophüls, W.: Acid-proof Bacilli in Five Cases of Pulmonary Gangrene, Jour. Med. Res., **8**: 242, 1902.

Page, C. G., L. Frothingham, and J. B. Paige: Sporothrix and Epizoötic Lymphangitis, Jour. Med. Res., **23**: 137, 1910.

Parker, F., Jr., and N. P. Hudson: The Etiology of Haverhill Fever (Erythema Arthriticum Epidemicum), Amer. Jour. Path., **2**: 357, 1926.

——, H. Jackson, Jr., G. Fitz Hugh, and T. D. Spies: Studies of Diseases of the Lymphoid and Myeloid Tissues, IV. Skin Reactions to Human and Avian Tuberculin, Jour. Immunol., **22**: 277, 1932.

Pund, E. R., and R. B. Greenblatt: Specific Histology of Granuloma Inguinale, Arch. Path., **23**: 224, 1937.

Reed, D. M.: On the Pathological Changes in Hodgkin's Disease with Especial Reference to Its Relation to Tuberculosis, Johns Hopkins Hosp. Rep., 10: 133, 1902.

Rich, A. R.: The Pathology of Nineteen Cases of a Peculiar and Specific Form of Nephritis Associated with Acquired Syphilis, Bull. Johns Hopkins Hosp., 50: 357, 1932.

Ricketts, H. T.: Oidiomycosis (Blastomycosis) of the Skin and Its Fungi, Jour. Med. Res., 6: 374, 1901.

Rothwell, T. A.: Experimental Aspergillosis, Jour. Path. and Bact., 7: 34, 1901.

Sanders, M.: Studies on the Cultivation of the Virus of Lymphogranuloma Venereum, Jour. Exper. Med., 71: 113, 1940.

Sanford, A. H.: Distribution of Actinomycosis in the United States, Jour. Amer. Med. Asso., 81: 655, 1923; see also L. J. Halpern, and A. Levinson: Pulmonary Actinomycosis, etc., ibid., 91: 13, 1928.

Schneider, L. V.: Primary Aspergillosis of the Lungs, Amer. Rev. Tuberc., 22: 267, 1930.

Shaw, F. W., and J. D. Reid: Fungi and Fungous Diseases, Jour. Lab. and Clin. Med., 26: 256, 1940-41.

Simpson, W. M.: Tularemia, History, Pathology, Diagnosis and Treatment, New York, 1929.

Singer, J. J., and H. C. Ballon: Streptothricosis, Amer. Rev. Tuberc., 22: 233, 1930.

Smith, L. M.: Blastomycosis and the Blastomycosis-like Infections, Jour. Amer. Med. Asso., 116: 200, 1941.

Steiner, P. E.: Reliability and Significance of the Gordon Test in Hodgkin's Disease, Arch. Path., 31: 1, 1941.

Stelwagon, H. N.: Rhinoscleroma Undergoing Malignant Change, Jour. Cutan. Dis., 36: 185, 1918.

Stewart, R. A., and F. Kimura: Studies in the Skin Test for Coccidioidal Infection. I. The Preparation and Standardization of Coccidioidin, Jour. Infect. Dis., 66: 212, 1940.

Stoddart, J. L., and E. C. Cutler: Torula Infection in Man. Monographs of Rock. Inst. for Med. Res., No. 6, New York, 1916.

Sutton, R. L.: Sporotrichosis in America, Jour. Amer. Med. Asso., 55: 2213, 1910.

Symmers, D.: Mycosis Fungoides as a Clinical and Pathologic Nonexistent, Arch. Derm. and Syph., 25: 1, 1932.

Tanner, F. W.: Bacteriology and Mycology of Foods, New York and London, 1919.

Thom, C.: The Aspergilli; A Typical Group of Molds, Jordan and Falk's The Newer Knowledge of Bacteriology and Immunology, Chicago, 1928.

Tice, F., and H. C. Sweaney: A Fatal Case of Besnier-Boeck-Schaumann's Disease with Autopsy Findings, Ann. Int. Med., 15: 597, 1941.

Wade, H. W., and G. S. Bel: A Critical Consideration of Systemic Blastomycosis With Notes on Certain Special Features and Report of 5 Cases, Arch. Int. Med., 18: 103, 1916.

Wade, H. W.: Reports on the International Congress of Leprosy Held in Cairo, March, 1938, Internatl. Jour. Leprosy, 6: 389, 1938.

Wallhauser, A.: Hodgkin's Disease, Arch. Path., 16: 522, 672, 1933.

Warfield, L. M.: Report of a Case of Disseminated Gummatous Sporotrichosis with Lung Metastasis, Trans. Asso. Amer. Phys., 36: 5, 1921.

Warvi, W. N., and R. W. Rawson: Torula Meningitis, Arch. Int. Med., 69: 90, 1942.

Winkelman, N. W., and M. T. Moore: Lymphogranulomatosis (Hodgkin's Disease) of the Nervous System, Arch. Neurol. and Psychiatr., 45: 304, 1941

Winslow, C. E. A., and Committee: The Families and Genera of the Bacteria, Jour. Bact., 5: 191, 1920.

Wise, N. B., and M. A. Poston: The Coexistence of Brucella Infection and Hodgkin's Disease. A Clinical, Bacteriologic and Immunologic Study, Jour. Amer. Med. Asso., 115: 1976, 1940.

Wolbach, S. B.: The Life Cycle of the Organism of "Dermatitis Coccidioides," Jour. Med. Res., 13: 53, 1904-05.

——, and J. L. Todd: A Study of Chronic Ulcers, Ulcus Tropicum, from the Gambia, Jour. Med. Res., 27: 27, 1912.

Wright, J. H.: A Case of Mycetoma (Madura Foot), Jour. Exper. Med., 3: 421, 1898.

Yates, J. L., and C. H. Bunting: The Rational Treatment of Hodgkin's Disease, Jour. Amer. Med. Asso., 64: 1953, 1915.

11

Progressive Tissue Changes

INTRODUCTION

The first six chapters of this section on General Pathology deal with processes that are clearly retrogressive. In the chapter on Inflammation, attention is drawn to retrogressive changes which initiate the reaction, but it is pointed out that in the fixed tissue reaction proliferation is the most important feature. Thus the inflammatory reaction is in considerable part progressive and continues on to organization and cicatrization. In repair, regeneration plays a variable part and this in itself implies a progressive rather than a retrogressive process. The progressive changes discussed in this chapter include multiplication of cells, increase in their size and certain alterations in architectural arrangement. The multiplication of cells in the growth of tumors is considered in the next chapter.

The Cell

Multiplication of cells depends upon cell division. In mammalian organisms, this is due in largest part to mitotic division. Perhaps amitotic division occurs but it probably is not frequent. What appears to be amitotic division in diseased tissues is largely the result of pathologic alterations of nuclei and of mitoses. The stimulus to cell division may arise within the cell or it may be ex-

trinsic. For example, the fertilization of the ovum provides an intracellular stimulus to multiplication. Nevertheless, the studies of artificial parthenogenesis show that changes in osmotic pressure of the surrounding medium excite cell division. Multiplication of cells is influenced by various factors, such as temperature which may be inhibitory, optimal or stimulating. In infectious diseases, products of the infective organisms, or substances elaborated in the host, often induce cellular multiplication, especially in the lymph nodes and spleen. Anemia stimulates bone marrow. Deficiencies of food, vitamins and minerals usually lead to retrogressive changes but may in certain instances induce cell multiplication. In the growth of tissues, there appears to be a balance between the cellular constituents, and it is at least possible that removal of restraint by one component may stimulate multiplication of another. This hypothesis enters into the discussion of tumors, but cell multiplication is only one of the features of tumor growth; there is unlimited and autonomous multiplication which characterizes tumors. In normal growth and development, hormones play an important part. The integration of hormonal activities may be disturbed so that alterations in one or several glands may induce hyperplasia in others.

The factors which control size of a cell are much the same, but operate on the cells in such a way that growth of the individual cell is especially influenced. Various stimuli may induce increase in size, for example the stretching of a hollow muscular organ to excite hypertrophy of the muscular elements, and deficiency of iodine in leading to enlargement of cells of the thyroid acini. In the higher forms of life, blood and lymph supply, nervous influences, functional stimuli, and other forces and conditions play a part in the multiplication and increase in size of

254

cells. The "organizers" of Spemann refer to tissues rather than cells, but in the further study of the matter, it becomes evident that the views of the older school of embryologists to the effect that cells can only differentiate along strictly specific lines is not invariably true, especially as concerns pathologic processes.

In the following paragraphs, metaplasia, hyperplasia and hypertrophy are discussed. In essence, these processes differ, but sharp distinctions are often impossible; overlapping and combinations are not infrequent.

METAPLASIA

In normal embryonal development, cells undergo alterations in size, form and

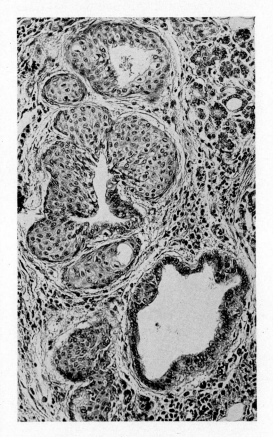

Metaplasia of cells lining ducts of pancreas.

function, the processes of differentiation and development. The term "metaplasia" refers to a change in the form of adult cells. It is a substitution of one form of cell for another and in a certain sense is atypical regeneration. In most instances, any accompanying functional alterations are retrogressive, but in some there may be an increase in functional capacity. A few examples are given before the discussion of causes and mechanisms.

Epithelial metaplasia is seen in places where the surfaces are exposed to unusual conditions. The columnar epithelium of the gallbladder may become stratified squamous in type as the result of concrements in the bladder or of chronic catarrhal inflammation. Chronic catarrhs may induce the same change in that part of the larynx normally covered by cylindrical epithelium. Prolapse of the uterus, in which the organ drops into the vagina and eventually may protrude through the vulva, leads to eversion of the organ so that the epithelium of the cervix and even of the fundus is exposed. If the condition persist for a sufficient time, the columnar epithelium becomes stratified squamous. In congenital exstrophy of the urinary bladder the reverse process occurs, namely, a transformation of transitional into columnar epithelium, sometimes with goblet-cell and crypt formation. Less common are similar changes in other situations, such as metaplasia of bronchial epithelium into stratified squamous epithelium due to chronic inflammation, and of duct epithelium of the pancreas into stratified squamous due to obstruction, chronic inflammation, or calculi.

Connective-tissue metaplasia is strikingly illustrated in heteroplastic bone formation which was discussed in the chapter on Calcification. This may be a direct transformation or occur through the intermediation of cartilage. It may follow a preceding calcification or appear as primary ossification, but in either case it is usually associated with some type of inflammation.

The regeneration of certain structures may be accompanied by metaplasia. Thus it is reported that excision of part of the lining of the rabbit stomach is followed not only by regeneration but also by metaplasia of the epithelium to the stratified squamous form (Fütterer). Somewhat different is the picture in the remaining parts of the salivary glands following partial extirpation, the cuboidal acinar cells becoming cylindrical (Carraro). What part inflammation following operation plays in such changes is not certain. A somewhat similar change may take place in tumors. For example the adenocarcinoma of the uterus, made up largely of columnar epithelium, may show places in which there has been a transformation into stratified squamous epithelium.

Retrogressive and Prosoplastic Metaplasia

In these various illustrations of metaplasia it is evident that changes take place in the direction of lower orders of differentiation and also in the direction of higher differentiation. The former is called regressive metaplasia, or sometimes anaplastic metaplasia. The term "anaplasia," however, as will be explained in the chapter on Tumors, has a broader meaning and is not desirable in this connection. When the transformation is toward higher degrees of differentiation, it is called prosoplastic metaplasia, or prosoplasia.

Most of the examples of metaplasia given above show its connection with inflammation, particularly when chronic, and thus in many instances, the cause is inflammation. There are some forms, however, in which inflammation plays little or no part, but these occur in processes of regeneration or of tumor growth. Here, the rapid proliferation may determine some intrinsic fault in processes of differentiation. The influence of vitamin deficiencies is well illustrated in deficiency of vitamin A, in which there is a "substitution of stratified keratinizing epithelium for normal epithelium in various parts of the respiratory tract, alimentary tract, eyes, paraocular glands and the genito-urinary tract." (Wolbach and Howe; Goldblatt and Benischek.) Thus some of the metaplasias, supposedly due to inflammation or irritation, may be caused in whole or in part by vitamin deficiencies.

Mechanism of Metaplasia

The theories of the mechanism of metaplasia include those of direct change, indirect change, environmental factors and embryonal inclusions. The original proposal of Virchow was that cells of one form may be directly transformed into another, but although this may possibly occur, the view is not widely held now. The theory of indirect metaplasia is widely adopted. This supposes that in the course of inflammation, regeneration or tumor growth, new formation of cells is from primitive forms, a reversion toward embryonal types of cells. As new cells are formed, some do not differentiate as they would under normal conditions, but produce forms that are abnormal to the part. The reasons for this are not clear, but it may have to do with tissue balance, or, more likely, is due to the presumptive fact that in a tissue one type of cellular component may act as a sort of organizer for other cellular components, in the Spemann sense. Thus altered connective tissue may not exercise its natural influence in the organization of newly formed epithelium. The theory that embryonal inclusions of cells of a somewhat different order from those normally present may be stimulated to growth by destruction of normal cells could account for but few of the metaplasias. Indeed, it is likely that some of the supposed illustrations are really the result of altered environmental conditions that disturb tissue organization. (See Foulds.) In certain epithelial tumors, factors of pressure and arrangement of cells may lead to the production of spindle-form epithelial cells, and in connective-tissue tumors or the connective tissues of chronic inflammations, there are cells which resemble epithelial or endothelial cells; this is spoken of as false metaplasia.

HYPERPLASIA

Hyperplasia is an increase in the number of cells of a part, usually due to stimulation by various forms of irritation or by inflammation. The cells are often of mature form, but there may also be many cells which are in developmental stages. Generally, such reversionary cells as may be present do not show the immaturity of tumor cells and hyperplasia can readily be distinguished from neoplasia. Hyperplasia is usually accompanied by enlargement of the organ, but it is to be distinguished from that variety of hypertrophy in which there is multiplication of cells, because in hypertrophy there is increased functional capacity.

Examples of hyperplasia are numerous and frequent. In most of the acute infectious diseases, hyperplasia of lymph nodes and spleen occur, with multiplication of lymphocytes, reticulo-endothelial cells and endothelial cells of the sinuses. An example is typhoid fever with enlargement of abdominal lymph nodes, of lymphoid follicles of the intestine and of the spleen. In some of the chronic infectious diseases, the hyperplasia involves these same cells to lesser degree, with an associated hyperplasia of connective tissue; a good illustration is syphilis. Chronic inflammations of mucous membranes may lead to hyperplasia of epithelium and also of connective tissue, as in the nasal polyps associated with chronic sinusitis. Prolonged irritation of epidermal structures may lead to hyperplasia of the epithelium, for example,

be offered, some of them discussed fully in the section on Systemic Pathology.

Causes of Hyperplasia

The causes of hyperplasia are varied. The hyperplasia of the lymph nodes and the spleen in infectious diseases is probably due to irritative soluble products elaborated in the course of the disease. Local irritation is certainly a cause, but perhaps low-grade inflammation plays a part. Chemical factors are of importance, as deficiency of iodine in thyroid hyperplasia. Hormonal factors operate. The hyperplasia in mammary ducts can be

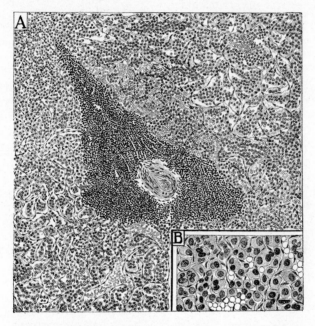

Endothelial hyperplasia in spleen. A. Low power. B. High power of cells of pulp.

the hyperplasia and hyperkeratosis of the lip due to smoking. Hyperplasia also occurs in glandular organs, as in thyroid and mammary gland. This may result in a heaping up of epithelial cells in acini and ducts, sometimes with enlargement or multiplication of acini. The line of distinction between such adenomatous hyperplasia and adenoma is not sharp, but the adenoma grossly is a well-outlined circumscribed nodular lesion. Mixed hyperplasias occur in benign enlargement of the prostate where epithelium, connective tissue and even smooth muscle may be hyperplastic. Many other examples of hyperplasia might

produced in animals by use of estrogenic substances. The hyperplasia of the prostate probably depends on irregularity of action or other abnormality of androgenic substances.

Aplasia, agenesia and hypoplasia are explained in the chapter on atrophy.

HYPERTROPHY

This term is commonly interpreted to mean the enlargement of an organ due to enlargement or multiplication of its constituent cells. The term should, however, carry with it the conception of an increase in functional capacity. In the examples of hypertrophy given below, it will be seen that this correlation of size and increased functional capacity applies to all.

Kinds of Hypertrophy

Simple and Numerical Hypertrophy. When hypertrophy is due to the enlargement of the constituent cells it is usually called simple, but when it results from an increase in the number of cells it is called numerical hypertrophy. It is not always possible to draw a sharp line of distinction between a hypertrophy that is a natural physiologic process and one that carries

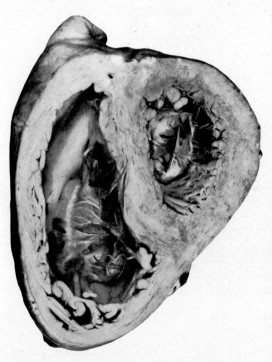

Cross section of ventricles of heart to show great thickening of the right ventricular wall due to hypertrophy, cor pulmonale.

with it a connotation of disease. The favorite example of simple hypertrophy is the blacksmith's arm. There is no increase in number of muscle elements but they are certainly increased as to size. A common example of numerical hypertrophy is to be found in the pregnant uterus where the individual muscle cells are not only enlarged but they are also increased in number. In both these instances the implication of increased functional capac-

ity is unquestioned. The forms of hypertrophy that are associated with pathologic changes of one kind or another or with disturbances of the internal environment of the body are classified as adaptive, compensatory and chemical.

Adaptive Hypertrophy. An illustration of adaptive hypertrophy is to be found in the heart. Fundamentally this is due to diastolic stretching of the muscle. It may be brought about by defects in the valves, by hypertension, by local disturbances in the myocardium which bring about diastolic stretching, such as infarction, and perhaps by nervous and hormonal influences. Normally the number of cardiac muscle-fiber cells increases until early adult life. In hypertrophy of the adult heart, however, there is no increase in number of fibers. A distribution curve shows that the fibers of larger sizes increase in number to constitute a majority (Karsner, et al.). Intestinal obstruction when due to prolonged lesions such as stricture or tumor, is accompanied by a hypertrophy of the intestinal muscle above the point of reduction in size of lumen. Hypertrophy of the urinary bladder may be the sequel of stricture of the urethra or of enlargement of the prostate. In all of these instances the hypertrophy is accompanied by increase in functional capacity. In the heart, however, that increase is accompanied by a relative loss of reserve power.

The term "compensatory" as applied to hypertrophy should not be interpreted to mean that this is a purposive reaction on the part of the body. It is undoubtedly due to stimuli that operate through a variety of mechanisms. One of the best examples is to be seen in paired organs. Thus, if a kidney be congenitally aplastic, the opposite kidney grows so that it is equal in weight to both kidneys. If one kidney be removed surgically the other undergoes hypertrophy, a hypertrophy which is functional as well as morphologic. The removal of the spleen is followed by enlargement of lymph nodes in various parts of the body, but that this is truly a hypertrophy cannot be said because of ignorance concerning the function of these structures. Destructive lesions of one adrenal may be accompanied by hypertrophy of the opposite adrenal.

Chemical stimulation to hypertrophy may be exogenous or endogenous. The former is rare, but experimentally it has been found that minute doses of phosphorus may increase the growth of bone and that minute doses of arsenic and phosphorus may produce enlargement of liver and kidneys. Again it is not certain that this is a true hypertrophy. The best example of endogenous stimuli is found in the hormones. The close interrelation of the endocrine glands means that there illustration is found in the hypophysoadrenal relationship, as in the so-called Cushing syndrome, in which lesions of the pituitary are accompanied by enlargement, presumably with increased function, of the adrenal glands. Morphologically this is a hyperplasia or a numerical hypertrophy rather than simply an enlargement in the constituent cells. Somewhat similar seems to be the adrenogenital relationship because it has been shown experimentally that extirpation

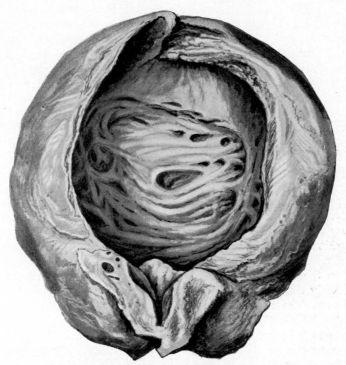

Hypertrophy of wall of bladder as result of obstruction by enlarged prostate. Note the heavy muscular trabeculæ.

is a constant action of stimulation and depression, one upon another. Cramer has divided these activities into antagonistic and synergistic. For example, the increased activity of one endocrine gland may bring about increased function on the part of its antagonist and decreased function on the part of its synergist. A depression of function of one endocrine may lead to depression in its synergist and increase in function in its antagonist.

Stimuli to increased function probably take place periodically or regularly in ordinary life, but if continued over a long period may lead to actual morphologic change. An of the ovaries is commonly followed by increase in size of the adrenal. The effects of activity of endocrines is not always confined to the endocrine system itself. Thus in pregnancy the breast undergoes hypertrophy, evidently due to the stimulation of estrogen. In males with tumors of the testis there may be the peculiar condition known as gynecomastia, in which the breasts become hypertrophic, again due to stimulation by estrogenic hormone. Hypertrophy of the heart may accompany hyperthyroidism, but just why this occurs is not certainly known. It may be that nervous stimuli may excite the heart to greater activity or it may be that deterioration of the cardiac muscle leads to diastolic stretching.

Etymologically, hypertrophy means overnutrition but it must not be thought that overnutrition can cause true hypertrophy. Nor is it necessary to assume that in order for hypertrophy to take place overnutrition is required. As a matter of fact, there are certain indications that hypertrophy may occur even in the presence of reduced nutrition, for instance in a heart the seat of arteriosclerosis. Furthermore, hypertrophy may take place even when a cardiac muscle is degenerated, as in acute infectious disease.

Pseudohypertrophy is best illustrated by pseudohypertrophic muscular atrophy. Grossly, the muscles seem to be enlarged, but upon microscopic examination it is found that the muscle fibers are the seat of atrophy, and between them is so rich an infiltration of fat as to increase the gross size of the muscle.

FUNCTIONAL ADAPTATION

This term means certain alterations in structure and arrangement of tissues due to pressure, tension and perhaps other influences. It is a reaction to stimuli of various kinds and does not require interpretation as a purposive action on the part of the body to fulfil a need. Probably the most striking examples are in bones. The arrangement of bony trabeculæ, especially in the ends of long bones, and in the spongy bones, is such as to provide maximum strength. Acquired deformities, such as ankylosis, scoliosis, union of fractures in poor position, lead to differences in mechanical stresses upon the bone, which are ultimately met by a rearrangement of the internal trabeculæ better to meet the new conditions. The transplantation of bone segments results in new bone, adapted in form to meet the mechanical strains and stresses of the part. Transplanted tendons show alterations in form and proportions of elastic and connective tissue fibers adapted to the new position. Occasionally, the endocardium in the ventricles immediately below insufficient semilunar valves is thrown into valve-like folds as the result of mechanical stresses during the development of a fibrosis (Saphir). Following removal of the gallbladder, there is often a notable enlargement of the common

duct, but although this permits and probably is due to accumulation of bile, there is no indication that gallbladder function is replaced. It will be seen that in all these phenomena, altered mechanical and physical factors play a large part and that the changes called functional adaptation or, by Jores, "metallaxy" are in the nature of a readjustment of the tissues concerned.

TRANSPLANTATION

Marchand defines transplantation as the healing of a living part within or upon a different individual or another part of the same individual. This excludes the IMPLANTATION of dead and inert materials, such as metals, ivory, celluloid, etc., sometimes used to aid the surgical repair of defects of various kinds. The success of transplantation depends upon a variety of factors many of which are unknown. Autoplastic transplantation, the grafting of one tissue into the same individual, is more likely to be successful than isoplastic or homeoplastic transplantation, the grafting of tissue of one individual into another of the same species. Heteroplastic transplantation, the grafting of tissue into another species, rarely meets with success. In plastic surgery, a segment of skin is partially removed and placed over a defect, leaving a portion of the segment still attached in the original site. This is sometimes called attached or pedunculated transplantation, a form of autotransplantation. It is not strictly included in the definition of transplantation, however, because it is merely a shift in position of a tissue with part of its original blood supply intact. The index of success of transplantation is the permanency of life in the transplant, for many grafts live for a few weeks only to die and disappear.

Factors Governing Transplantation

Numerous factors governing transplantation have been studied: genetic relationship of donor and recipient or host, age, chemical factors of various kinds, blood supply, nerve supply, functional need of the transplant and others. As has been indicated, autografts are most likely to be successful, homeografts less so and heterografts rarely. Successful transplanting of skin, blood, bone and ductless glands is of the utmost practical importance and may be extended to include the transplantation of organs and limbs. Autografting is necessarily restricted in scope, and is practically limited to the transplantation of skin and bone, and, to a lesser extent, of ductless glands, most notably the ovary. Homeografting may be understood to include also the transplanting or transfusion of blood. Heterografting, if it could be placed upon a satisfactory basis, would throw open a large field for transplantation of various tissues and organs which cannot be removed from human donors without great sacrifice or until death has occurred. Experimentally, transplantation is somewhat more widely applicable than in human medicine, as for example the results obtained by Carrel in the transplantation of kidneys and limbs in animals, which depends upon careful maintenance of circulation by accurate suture of blood vessels.

The age and phylogenetic development of the subjects is of importance. In protozoan and lower animal forms, success is greater than in the more highly differentiated species. Transplantations in embryo and fetus are likely to be more successful than in adults. The studies of Marine and others indicate that youth is more favorable than later life. In vegetable life, transplantation is highly successful under proper conditions.

The tissue to be transplanted must be viable and the conditions to which it is exposed in the period between its transport from the donor to the recipient must not be injurious. Carrel has found that tissue may be transplantable after several hours and that ice chest temperature is suitable for preservation. Skin is still transplantable after an hour or more in gauze moistened with saline, at room temperature. Preservation in chemicals has not been satisfactory save in the case of blood corpuscles, in which instance formolized cells are still useful after several weeks. That such blood cells operate in all ways as living cells has not been determined, but there is no doubt that they serve for interchange of gases. Transfusion, however, does not represent permanently successful transplantation, since the cells are incapable of multiplication. Nevertheless, Ashby has shown that they may survive for more than thirty days, and Wearn, Warren and Ames

found that such cells survive for an average of 83 days.

The fact that chemical conditions must be nicely adjusted is indicated by the failure of heterografts and the relatively higher degree of success of autografts over homeografts. The fact that blood transfusion is successful only with properly adjusted blood groups is due in large part to the action of isohemagglutinins and isohemolysins. Although Ingebrigtsen found, as the result of animal experiments, that interagglutination has no influence on transplantation of arteries, it has been indicated by Masson and conclusively demonstrated by Shawan that skin grafting is successful according to the same rules as hold for blood transfusion. That the failure of skin grafts from antagonistic donors is due to isocytolysins has not been conclusively proved although it is highly probable; that other chemical adjustment plays a part must also be considered. The chemical factors probably reside both in the transplant and the host.

Success may depend upon conditions of internal environment, especially those that stimulate the transplants to functional activity. Thus, Halstead and others found that transplants of thyroid do better in animals from which the thyroid had previously been removed and reported that the same principal applies to parathyroids. Loeb and Hesselberg, however, did not find this to be true of thyroid transplants. Manley and Marine reported that splenectomy favors transplantation of the spleen and that thyroid grafts do better in iodized animals than in others. These are but a few examples of improved chances of success when conditions are such as to stimulate the grafts to functional activity.

There is little doubt that the better the supply of blood to the transplanted part the greater the chance of success. An index of this is the success of Joannovics in transplanting parathyroids into blood vessels, and the importance of the vascular supply is demonstrated in innumerable other experiments. Carrel's success with transplantation of entire organs is dependent upon maintenance of circulation. That nerve supply is of importance is indicated by the fact that innervated muscle appears to do well, but that it is essential is certainly not proved.

The behavior of transplants varies with different tissue but as a rule there is a certain amount of necrosis of parts of the transplant. Some of the cells, however, retain sufficient bioplastic energy to survive and proliferate. The transplants set up reactive processes in the host just as do foreign bodies, so that new vessels and connective tissue penetrate to support and nourish. Unsuccessful transplants undergo necrosis, and are either encapsulated or disappear, to be replaced by organization and cicatrization.

urine. Transplanted nerves, muscle, periosteum, bone, pancreas, and other tissues may continue to function. Discussion of the transplantation of individual tissues and organs is too extensive to be included here, but is to be found in reviews such as that of Goldzieher and Makai, and the article by Goodman.

Parabiosis

The term "parabiosis" indicates the anatomic and physiologic union of two animals of either the same or different species.

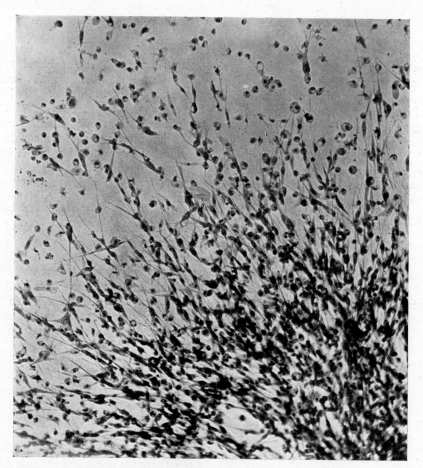

Photomicrograph of connective-tissue culture. (From Carrel and Burrows, Jour. Exper. Med.)

There is no doubt that transplanted tissue may continue to function. The maintenance of thyroid and parathyroid function has already been mentioned. Ovarian function may be maintained in every way, as pointed out by Guthrie and Lee and others. Carrel's transplanted kidneys secreted normal

Double monsters demonstrate the condition as it occurs naturally. Experimentally, it has been found practicable in animals of the same (Rous) or closely related species such as mouse and rat (Lambert), but in different species the death of one or the other individual soon supervenes. As a method of experimental work the condition has been utilized to study immunity, function of kidneys and pancreas, and other problems, all of which are considered in detail by Goldzieher and Makai.

TISSUE CULTURE. EXPLANTATION

The fact that tissues may survive outside the body has long been known and utilized in the study of function. That cells may grow and multiply in vitro, an entirely different proposition, has developed in the present century. In 1897 Leo Loeb was able to cul-

fields. Thus, there is definite information that calcium and potassium ions, maltose, dextrose and certain protein decomposition products favor multiplication and growth, and that the presence of a solid supporting framework, such as a network of fibrin, is of importance although not absolutely essential. It is known that certain cells may be kept growing outside the body for long periods, as for example the Carrel connective-tissue culture which has passed through more than 1800 generations in more than 18 years (Ebeling) and is still growing. Burrows showed that embryo heart muscle can grow and multiply in vitro, and

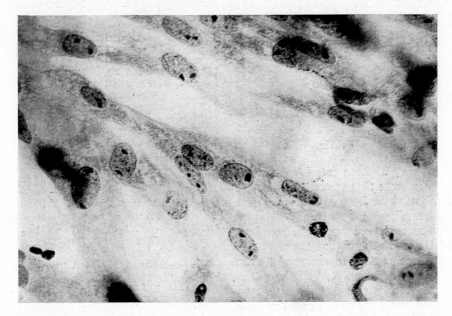

High-power photomicrograph of connective tissue culture. From Carrel and Burrows, Jour. Exper. Med.

tivate and observe the multiplication of epithelium upon culture media and thus is the pioneer in this field, but his method is apparently not widely applicable. It remained for Harrison, in 1907, to adapt, as he says, the tissue isolation method of the embryologist and the hanging drop method of the bacteriologist, in order to study the growth of nerve fibers. The method was soon elaborated and extended by the work of Carrel, Lambert, L. Loeb, the Lewises, Strangeways and others. At first applied to the general biologic problems of cell multiplication and growth, it was soon extended to include physiologic, pathologic and immunologic

that the primary and descendant cells retain an intrinsic capacity for rhythmic contraction over several weeks. Cells may grow in plasma of widely different species, and certain features of their metabolism have been studied. It has been found that most cells in culture exhibit ameboid movement, and there is reason to believe that surface tension phenomena are of great importance in cytoplasmic division. Culture of white cells of the blood has yielded a pure strain of monocytes and it is claimed that these may give rise to fibroblasts.

Lambert found that foreign-body giant cells are produced by fusion of large mononuclear cells. His work also indicates that fat globules in culture cells are derived from fat in the medium. Lewis maintains that fat is formed in cells growing in fat-free media. Nasu is doubtful that the material in the cells is fat and found that cells living, or perhaps vegetating, in salt solution show no such globules. Nevertheless, the work in general indicates that some cellular endogenous

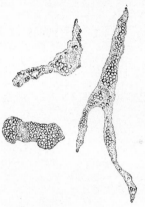

Isolated culture cells containing fat globules.

mechanism can elaborate fat. Lambert was able to demonstrate that sarcomal cells show atypical mitosis in culture as compared with normal mitosis in nontumorous cells, that sarcoma cells are more readily affected by heat, and Drew has found that the stroma of tumors behaves more like embryonal than like adult cells. Lambert studied the movement of tumor cells and estimated that by this process alone, tumor cells could migrate from the breast to the axillary lymph nodes in six to eight weeks. It has been shown that plasma from sarcoma-immune animals does not inhibit growth, thus indicating that tumor immunity does not reside in the plasma. Carrel and Ingebrigtsen have demonstrated that cells in vitro are capable of producing specific hemolysins and Fischer has demonstrated increased resistance on the part of cells against injurious antigens. Lambert has shown that isohemagglutinins have no influence upon human cell cultures.

At first the work was limited to the use of cells from lower animals, embryo and adult, but was extended by Lambert to include human cells. Media capable of forming permanent fibrin nets were considered essential but later fluid and solid media were em-

ployed. Carleton draws attention to the relationship in cultures between connective tissue and other cells. The connective tissue seems to be an important factor in restraining unlimited cell multiplication and upholding differentiation. The field of work is now broadened by studies, notably those of A. Fischer who has succeeded in growing intestinal segment with multiplication of all elements and the secretion of mucus by the epithelium. The extent and possibilities of this mode of investigation cannot be predicted, but it seems likely that much light will be thrown upon the natural history of cell growth in health and disease. (See Silberberg.)

REFERENCES

Ashby, W.: The Determination of the Length of Life of Transfused Blood Corpuscles in Man, Jour. Exper. Med., **29:** 267, 1919.

Borst, M.: Das pathologische Wachstum, Aschoff's Pathologische Anatomie, 5th ed., Jena, 1921, vol. 1, p. 615.

Burrows, M. T.: The Tissue Culture as a Physiological Method, Trans. Cong. Amer. Phys. and Surg., **9:** 77, 1913.

Carleton, H. M.: Tissue Culture: a Critical Summary, Brit. Jour. Exper. Biology, **1:** 131, 1923-24.

Carraro, A.: Ueber Regeneration in den Speicheldrüsen, Frankfurt. Zeitschr. Path., **3:** 26, 1909.

Carrel, A.: Growth-promoting Function of Leucocytes, Jour. Exper. Med., **36:** 385, 1922.

——: Transplantation in Mass of the Kidneys, ibid., **10:** 98, 1908.

——: Latent Life of Arteries, ibid., **12:** 460, 1910.

——: The Ultimate Result of a Double Nephrectomy and the Replantation of One Kidney, ibid., **14:** 124, 1911.

——: Ultimate Results of Aortic Transplantation, ibid., **15:** 389, 1912.

——, and M. T. Burrows: Cultivation of Tissues in Vitro and Its Technique, ibid., **13:** 387, 1911.

——, and A. H. Ebeling: Heat and Growth-inhibiting Action of Serum, ibid., **35:** 647, 1922.

——, and R. Ingebrigtsen: The Production of Antibodies by Tissues Living Outside of the Organism, ibid., **15:** 287, 1912.

Cramer, W.: The Sex Hormones and the Endocrine Balance, Bull. New York Acad. Med., **17:** 3, 1941.

Drew, A. H.: A Comparative Study of Normal and Malignant Tissues Grown in Artificial Culture, Brit. Jour. Exper. Path., **3:** 20, 1922.

Ebeling, A. H.: A Ten Year Old Strain of Fibroblasts, Jour. Exper. Med., **35:** 755, 1922.

Fischer, A.: Cultures of Organized Tissues, ibid., **36:** 393, 1922.

——: Action of Antigen on Fibroblasts in Vitro, ibid., **36:** 535, 1922.

——: Tissue Culture, London, 1925.

Fleisher, M. S.: Immunity and Tissue Transplantation, Jour. Med. Res., **37**: 483, 1917-18.

Foot, N. C.: The Growth of Chicken Bone Marrow in Vitro, and Its Bearing on Hematogenesis in Adult Life, Jour. Exper. Med., **17**: 43, 1913.

Foulds, L.: The Histological Analysis of Tumours. A Critical Review, Amer. Jour. Cancer, **39**: 1, 1940.

Fütterer, G.: Ueber Epithelmetaplasie, Ergeb. Allg. Path. u. Path. Anat., 9^2: 706, 1903.

Goldblatt, H., and M. Benischek: Vitamin A Deficiency and Metaplasia, Jour. Exper. Med., **46**: 699, 1927.

Goldzieher, M., and E. Makai: Regeneration, Transplantation und Parabiose, Ergeb. Allg. Path. u. Path. Anat., 16^2: 344, 1912.

Goodman, C.: Thyroid Transplantation, Internatl. Clinics. **32**(3): 54, 1922.

Guthrie, C. C., and M. E. Lee: Ovarian Transplantation, Jour. Amer. Med. Asso., **64**: 1823, 1915.

Halsted, W. S.: Auto- and Isotransplantation in Dogs of the Parathyroid Glandules, Jour. Exper. Med., **11**: 175, 1909.

Harrison, R. G.: The Life of Tissues Outside the Organism from the Embryological Standpoint, Trans. Cong. Amer. Phys. and Surg., **9**: 63, 1913.

Ingebrigtsen, R.: The Influence of Isoagglutinins on the Final Result of Homoplastic Transplantations of Arteries, Jour. Exper. Med., **16**: 169, 1912.

Joannovics, G.: Beitrag zur intravaskulären Transplantation, Wien. Klin. Wochenschr., **24**: 698, 1911.

Jores, L.: Metallaxie, Virchow's Arch. Path. Anat., **221**: 14, 1916.

Karsner, H. T., O. Saphir, and T. W. Todd: The State of the Cardiac Muscle in Hypertrophy and Atrophy, Amer. Jour. Path., **1**: 351, 1925.

Konschegg, T.: Zur Epithelmetaplasie, Virchow's Arch. Path. Anat., **259**: 89, 1926.

Lambert, R. A.: The Influence of Mouse-Rat Parabiosis on the Growth in Rats of a Transplantable Mouse Sarcoma, Jour. Exper. Med., **13**: 257, 1911.

——: The Life of Tissues Outside the Organism from the Pathological Standpoint, Trans. Cong. Amer. Phys. and Surg., **9**: 91, 1913.

——: Technique of Cultivating Human Tissues in Vitro, Jour. Exper. Med., **24**: 367, 1916.

Lane-Claypon, J. E., and E. H. Starling: An Experimental Enquiry into the Factors which Determine the Growth and Activity of the Mammary Glands, Proc. Roy. Soc., B., **77**: 505, 1905.

Lewis, M. R.: The Importance of Dextrose in the Medium of Tissue Cultures, Jour. Exper. Med., **35**: 317, 1922.

Lewis, W. H.: Degeneration Granules and Vacuoles in the Fibroblasts of Chick Embryos, Bull. Johns Hopkins Hosp., **30**: 81, 1919.

Loeb, L.: Ueber das Waschstum des Epithels, Archiv. Entwicklungsmech., **13**: 489, 1902.

——: The Influence of Changes in the Chemical Environment on the Life and Growth of Tissues, Jour. Amer. Med. Asso., **64**: 726, 1915.

——: Ameboid Movement, Tissue Formation and Consistency of Protoplasm, Amer. Jour. Physiol., **56**: 140, 1921.

——, and M. S. Fleisher: On the Factors which Determine the Movements of Tissues in Culture Media, Jour. Med. Res., **37**: 75, 1917.

——, and W. H. F. Addison: Beiträge zur Analyse des Gewebewachstums, etc., Arch. Entwicklungsmech., **32**: 44, 1911.

——, and C. Hesselberg: Studies on Compensatory Hypertrophy of the Thyroid Gland, Jour. Med. Res., **40**: 265, 1919.

Manley, O. T., and D. Marine: The Transplantation of Ductless Glands, with Reference to Permanence and Function, Jour. Amer. Med. Asso., **67**: 260, 1916.

Marchand, F.: Process der Wundheilung mit Einschluss der Transplantation, Stuttgart, 1901. Also forms Lieferung 16, Deutsche Chirurgie.

Marine, D., and O. T. Manley: Homeotransplantation and Autotransplantation of the Spleen in Rabbits. III. Further Data on Growth, Permanence, Effect of Age, and Partial or Complete Removal of the Spleen, Jour. Exper. Med., **32**: 113, 1920.

Masson, J. C.: Skin Grafting, Jour. Amer. Med. Asso., **70**: 1581, 1918.

Nasu, S.: Beiträge zur Frage der Ueberlebensfähigkeit der Gewebe, Virchow's Arch. Path. Anat., **243**: 388, 1923.

Rous, P.: Parabiosis as a Test for Circulating Antibodies in Cancer, Jour. Exper. Med., **11**: 810, 1919.

Salzer, H.: Zur Frage der Schildrüsentransplantation, Arch. Klin. Chir., **89**: 881, 1909.

Saphir, O.: Endocardial Pockets, Amer. Jour. Path., **6**: 733, 1930.

Shawan, H. K.: The Principle of Blood Grouping Applied to Skin Grafting, Amer. Jour. Med. Sci., **157**: 503, 1919.

Silberberg, M.: Tissue Culture, with Special Reference to Pathology, Arch. Path., **21**: 663, 1936.

Strangeways, T. S. P.: Tissue Culture in Relation to Growth and Differentiation, Cambridge, 1924.

——: Technique of Tissue Culture "in Vitro," Cambridge, 1924.

Wearn, J. T., S. Warren, and O. Ames: The Length of Life of Transfused Erythrocytes in Patients with Primary and Secondary Anemia, Arch. Int. Med., **29**: 527, 1922.

Wolbach, S. B., and P. R. Howe: Tissue Changes Following Deprivation of Fat-Soluble A Vitamin, Jour. Exper. Med., **42**: 753, 1925.

Yoshida, T.: Experimenteller Beitrag zur Frage der Epithelmetaplasie, Virchow's Arch. Path. Anat., **283**: 29, 1932.

12

Tumors

PART I: GENERAL ASPECTS

INTRODUCTION

Although the term tumor in its etymologic sense signifies only swelling, the current usage requires more strict definition. Indeed a tumor, according to present conceptions, may be erosive and destructive in character and show no swelling whatever. A simple definition is that a tumor is an autonomous, progressive, unlimited new growth, the ultimate cause of which is unknown. This definition, however, requires explanation. A tumor is autonomous in that it follows its own laws of growth. Its autonomy is limited in that it derives its nutrition from the host in which it grows. With a few exceptions, any considerable degree of autonomy can exist only if the tumor becomes invasive; it can then grow after transplantation. Complete autonomy is not known and for this reason a tumor is essentially parasitic, but it is not a parasite in the ordinary sense. The new growth is derived from preexisting cells and is thus an offshoot from either somatic or germ cells. The cells of the tumor resemble those of the region of origin, but departures from the original type are frequent. Hyperplasias are in a sense new growths, but the cells resemble fairly closely the cells of origin and the microscopic picture is usually readily identified. The tumor is progressive in growth but not uniformly so, since periods of quiescence or even of regression may interrupt the continuity of progressive enlargement. As a corollary of the progressive growth must be the conception of unlimited growth, but the latter character is of course variable with the type of tumor and fundamentally restricted by the life of the host and its capacity to provide nutrition. Secondary changes such as inflammation and necrosis often seriously interfere with tumor growth. The growth is new not only in the sense of multiplication of cells, but also in the fact that the proliferation may show cell types not in absolute conformity with those from which it originated. In spite of the frequent departure of the form of the cells from normal, tumors may, in some instances, exercise functions like those of the original cells. In the section on Functional Activity, reference is made to the milk-like secretion of tumors of mammary glands, the presence of bile in hepatic tumors and the production of hormones by tumors of endocrine glands. Indeed, metastases and recurrences of tumors of endocrines may produce hormones.

The ultimate cause of tumors, meaning the reason for the growth of new cells which not only proliferate but show departures from normal forms and laws of growth, is not known. As a matter of fact, tumors vary greatly in character and it is possible that no single cause will be found for all. Present studies are largely concerned with conditions that bring about the growth rather than with its primary origin. There are certain predisposing factors, such as age, sex and occupation. There are exciting factors, physical, chemical and biologic, which precede the development of tumors in man and which have been shown in experimental animals to lead to the growth of tumors. Some of these act directly, as painting of tar on the skin, and others operate remotely, for example the induction of cancer of the liver by administration of butter yellow; still others appear to operate through the medium of hormones, for example the induction of carcinoma of the breast by injections of estrogens. Tumors are often looked upon as local manifestations of cell growth but there are factors in the body as a whole, including genetic constitution and perhaps acquired disposition, which play a part in the beginning and development of tumors.

Tumors have been known throughout recorded history. They are mentioned in records of India of about 2000 B.C., and in the cuneiform tablets of the library of Ninevah. Descriptions were given by Hippocrates, Galen and later writers of the Renaissance, but the distinctions of the present time were not recognized. Tumors occur in man, other mammals, birds, amphibia, fish, and reptiles, and are said to affect invertebrates.

The incidence of tumors is of the utmost importance from the viewpoint of public health. In the registration area of the United States there were 1,396,903 deaths in the year 1934, of which 134,428, or about 10 per cent, were ascribed to the various forms of malignant tumors. When the leading causes of death are put into five groups, malignant tumors appear in the fifth place in the decade of 30 to 39 years, are second only to diseases of heart and blood vessels in all succeeding decades up to age 79, when they again drop to fifth place. Certain statistical studies indicate an absolute increase in the incidence of malignant tumors. Since most such figures are based on clinical diagnosis, confirmed by autopsy in only a relatively small percentage and by biopsy principally in only readily accessible parts, it is possible that the increase is only relative and due to improved clinical diagnosis. It may be an absolute increase, however, because of the shift of population to include increasing numbers of older persons (a manifestation of lengthened average life expectancy). Other possibilities may further complicate the interpretations. It seems probable that there is an absolute increase because of the population shift and an apparent increase due to improved diagnosis.

In man and lower animals, tumors are observed most frequently in advanced life. The studies of Pack and LeFevre show that the average age for patients with carcinoma is 53.8 years, whereas those with sarcomas average 38.2 years. In early life sarcomas occur more often than carcinomas and the curve of incidence is gradually and slightly upward. The curve for carcinomas shows a sharp upturn in the decade between 40 and 50 years. Identical types of cancer occur from 2½ to 4 years earlier in females than males. Individual tumors show maximum incidence at variable age periods and there are also sex differences. For example, according to Ewing, the mean patient age for cancer of the scrotum is 47 years and for cancer of the rectum 62 years. Of cancers of the lip, 94 per cent are in males and 81 per cent of cancers of the gallbladder are in females. Malignant tumors of early life progress more rapidly, disseminate more frequently and recur more often after removal than is true of tumors of older life. Sex differences in incidence of cancer in situations other than sex organs is probably largely due to differences in mode of life, exposure to various forms of irritation, differences in metabolism and other factors. Ewing and others believe that many of the tumors which become manifest in later life originated much earlier.

The experimental production of cancer by an irritant such as tar shows that the animals are no more susceptible in old age than in youth and that the time elapsing before the development of the cancer is not materially different. In the Report of the Imperial Cancer Research Fund for 1928-29, it is pointed out that the period of development of tar cancers in mice corresponds to a period of from 10 to 15 years in man. Where irritation can be related to cancer in man, as in dye workers, a period of not less than 2 to 18 years intervenes before the tumor develops. Furthermore the tumors of early life are principally those which seem to be independent of irritation. The assumption seems justified that the tumors which are manifested in late middle and old age have probably had their inception up to 15 years or more before they are sufficiently advanced to be observed. Thus it would seem that age gives opportunity for the tumor to become apparent, in contrast to the view which is commonly held to the effect that aged tissues are especially prone to tumorous change. Nevertheless, tumors may occur at birth and in infancy. The tumor of the retina, called retinoblastoma, has a marked hereditary factor. Aside from this, congenital neoplasms are rare and are derived principally from cells of the nervous system and kidneys. As Wells points out, all these tumors arise in tissues whose carbohydrate metabolism resembles that of malignant tumors, i.e., production of energy principally by glycolysis, as discussed in the section on Metabolism.

It is often said that cancer is preeminently a disease of civilization, yet no analysis with statistical validity has been made to establish this point. Nor is there clear-cut evidence of racial differences in man, except for relatively low incidence of cutaneous carcinoma in colored races. Occupation and habits may play a part, as in the carcinoma of the bladder in aniline workers and the carcinoma of the lip in pipe smokers, and numerous other examples. There appears to be a variation in the incidence of certain tumors in people of different economic levels. For example, tumors of exposed parts may be more frequent in poorer classes than among the well-to-do (Kennaway).

CLASSIFICATION OF TUMORS

From the point of view of both patient and the physician, the most important classification of tumors is into benign and malignant forms. Nevertheless this line of distinction cannot always be sharply drawn and among the malignant tumors there are degrees of malignancy that have an important bearing upon treatment and prognosis. Tumors, like tissues, are of more or less complicated structure, but as a rule have a cell type or types which furnish a basis for classification. These cell types serve to identify a tumor in much the same way as they serve to identify a normal tissue. For example, a papilloma grows from an epithelial surface but has stalks of vascularized connective tissue which support the epithelium of the new growth. It is, in a sense, a mixed tumor, but the epithelium is the significant component. Other tumors, however, may be made up solely of one type of cell, for example, the fibroma which is composed of fibrous tissue cells; nevertheless, these have a vascular supply and often nerves. Most of the classifications of tumors are based upon histologic features and are therefore morphologic in nature. These may refer to the cell type of the tumor itself or to the original germ layer from which the type cell originated.

The earliest of the modern classifications is that of Virchow, into histioid, organoid and teratoid. The histioid tumors include those in which the growth is composed almost entirely of one cell type, as the fibroma. Such a tumor may be regarded as arising from a cell with unipotential character, i.e., with a capacity for forming but one type of cell. The organoid tumors are made up of more than one type of cell and in a general way more or less reduplicate organ forms, as the adenoma with its atypical glandular acini, supporting connective tissue and vascular supply. If such tumors arise from a single cell, that cell must be multipotential. The teratoid tumors include such tumors as arise in certain situations, particularly along the urogenital tract, and produce tissues corresponding to two or more layers of the embryo. The teratoma of the testicle may contain cartilage, intestinal type of tissue, skin-like tissue, nervous tissue, etc. If such a tumor arise from a single cell, that cell must be, like the ovum or the cells of the blastomere, totipotential. This classification can be made to include all tumors, but in many instances is difficult to apply.

Although several classifications, such as that of Adami, are based upon most thoughtful study of the biology of tumor growth, nevertheless, those which are most widely employed represent either the original, or some modification of, the classification proposed by Borst. This is based upon the histology of the tumor. Thus, we recognize connective-tissue tumors, epithelial tumors and mixed tumors. The term connective tissue in this sense is extremely broad, since under it are grouped tumors composed of various types of true connective tissue, those of muscle, those of various types of nervous tissue and those of endothelium.

The nomenclature of tumors is somewhat confused and although that which we adopt cannot be regarded as exact in etymology or descriptive character, yet it is widely employed and can hardly be altered except by making it ponderous. As will be seen subsequently, there are many tumor-like conditions which do not correspond to the definition of tumors given above. In order specifically to indicate that a true tumor of independent growth is meant, the term blastoma is used. Literally this is not fully justified because the cells do not often approach in type those of the blastomere. Nevertheless it has come into common usage. Indeed some use cumbersome terms such as fibroblastoma, lipoblastoma, myoblastoma, etc., in place of fibroma, lipoma, myoma, etc. There are certain faults of development which are nodular or tumor-like, which may become true neoplasms or, so to speak, blastomatous. Thus the capillaries of the liver may fail to regress in one or more places and remain as a nodule of hemangioma (Morse). This in itself is not a true tumor and is not progressive. This kind of fault is called hamartoma. It is also illus-

trated in birth marks. Rarely, the hepatic hemangioma takes on progressive growth and becomes a true tumor; in order to identify the change, it is designated as malignant hemangioma or hemangioblastoma. Sometimes embryonal displacement results in masses whose arrangement resembles that of primitive forms in the species, as the pigmented and hairy nevi; this is called progonoma. Portions of one organ may, in the course of development, be included in another organ, as are adrenal cortical inclusions in the kidney. This embryonal fault is called choristoma. It usually remains quiescent but may occasionally become a neoplasm, the hypernephroma. Tumors may arise at points of junction of embryonal folds or may originate in embryonal cells which have not differentiated for proper development of the organism.

The following arrangement is one of convenience and represents the Borst classification somewhat modified. It follows in some particulars that of Ewing. It serves as a guide both to classification and nomenclature. Any classification at the present time is emphatically one of convenience and cannot be regarded as final. As in all fields of pathology, a system based on cause is the only one which will have both practical and academic value. Until the etiology of tumors is determined and elaborated, no classification can be regarded as fully satisfactory.

A. The Connective-Tissue Tumors.
   I. Connective tissue as a type.
      1. Fibroma—fibrous connective tissue.
      2. Chondroma—cartilage.
      3. Osteoma—bone.
      4. Myxoma—mucoid tissue (like Wharton's jelly).
      5. Lipoma—fat.
      6. Angioma—vessels.
         a. Hemangioma—blood vessels.
         b. Lymphangioma — lymphatic vessels.
      7. Lymphoma—lymphoid tissue.
      8. Chordoma—notochord.
   II. Muscle as a type.
      1. Leiomyoma—smooth muscle.
      2. Rhabdomyoma—striated muscle.
   III. Elements of the Nervous System as a type.

1. Glioma or neuroglioma—neuroglia.
2. Neuro-epithelioma — neuro-epithelium.
3. Neuroma—nerve fibers and cells.

IV. Endothelium as a type.
   1. Endothelioma—endothelium.
      a. Angio-endothelioma.

V. Sarcoma—malignant connective tissue tumors.
   1. Immature forms—of more or less undifferentiated cells.
   2. Mature forms—malignant tumor with differentiated parts like any of the benign forms mentioned above.

B. The Epithelial Tumors.
   I. Papilloma—of surface type of epithelium upon a supporting connective tissue.
   II. Adenoma—glandular epithelium with acinic arrangement.
   III. Carcinoma—malignant epithelial tumors.
      1. Squamous-Cell Carcinoma—epithelium of surface type, with variable degrees of differentiation toward squamous epithelium. Includes also basal cell and intermediate cell (prickle cell).
      2. Transitional-Cell Carcinoma — from transitional epithelium in various places.
      3. Cylindrical-Cell Carcinoma — cylindrical epithelium from glands or surfaces. Includes adenocarcinoma.

C. Mixed Tumors
   I. Simple Mixed Tumors—made up of more than one type of tumor tissue, arbitrarily including monodermal, e.g., osteochondroma, and bidermal, e.g., mixed tumors of parotid and of kidney.
   II. Teratoma—made up of tissues differentiated to represent three layers of embryo, and therefore tridermal.
   III. Embryoma—made up of structures from all three layers of the embryo but in semblance of orderly arrangement like that of the fetus.

This outline will serve as a basis for a systematic study of tumors. Of the groups indicated, the sarcoma and the carcinoma are referred to as malignant. There are two principal features that indicate malignancy, (1) invasion of surounding tissues or structures, and (2) the production of secondary tumors, called metastasis, in more or less remote situations. Malignant tumors tend to recur after removal but this is not an essential feature since it is shared by some of the tumors referred to as benign. Clinically, cachexia is regarded as a phenome-

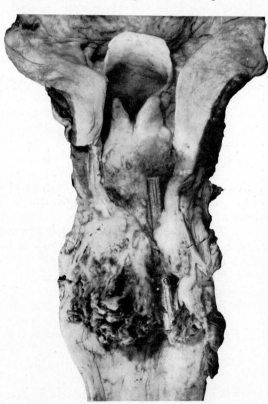

Carcinoma of esophagus about opposite bifurcation of trachea. The rod shows the greatly reduced lumen.

non indicative of malignancy but as will be explained subsequently, this is due to secondary effects of the lesion rather than to production by the tumor of any poisonous or injurious product. Tumors which do not show these characters are commonly referred to as benign. This term, although it has a definite clinical and pathologic significance, is only relative, since no type of tumor can be regarded as absolutely devoid of harmful effect. Truly benign tumors have none of the characters ascribed to malignant tumors, but may produce harmful effects by pressure on important organs which if long continued will lead to pressure atrophy; hollow organs may be obstructed, secretions may be dammed back, nerve trunks and blood and lymph vessels compressed, etc. There are certain tumors, usually classified as benign, which are not strictly so because they exhibit at least one character ascribed to malignancy. For example, the chondroma is likely to recur after removal. The glioma is directly invasive and destructive and frequently recurs after removal. Exceptionally, it may even metastasize. Thus, it has several characters of malignancy, but its structure is so much like other tumors which are benign that it is usually so classified. It is common practice now to use the term cancer to mean all forms of malignant tumor. In scientific parlance, however, it is necessary to specify which kind of malignant tumor or cancer is meant—whether it is sarcoma or carcinoma.

There is considerable discussion as to the possible morphologic changes that may intervene when the normal cell becomes neoplastic. As indicated below, it would appear that certain benign tumors may be transformed into malignant ones. Thus, carcinoma of the colon is often preceded by adenomatous polyps, but the change to carcinoma can only be identified after it has actually taken place. Papillomas develop after painting of the skin of experimental animals with tar, and some but not all may become carcinomas. There is, however, in these instances, no clear cut change in cytology between the two stages of development. Certain human lesions, such as leukoplakia and Bowen's disease of the skin, may become carcinomatous, but in the latter at least, invasion and metastasis may occur without demonstrable changes in the cellular picture of the lesion. During the course of painting with tar many studies of the skin have been made in order to determine just what cellular alterations occur. It has been said that in the intermediate layers of the epidermis there are cytoplasmic and nuclear changes, especially in the form of swelling, but those changes may just as well be a response to irritation as a beginning neoplastic change and there is no proof that these particular cells become

the cells of the carcinoma. Certain lesions and diseases in man that frequently become transformed into carcinoma are often referred to clinically as precancerous. This usage implies that they usually or necessarily do so. This is erroneous, is misleading to the doctor, and may be tragic to the patient. Its only justification would be as a loose generalization.

Transformation of Benign to Malignant Tumors

Most of the experimental studies in animals give no clear indication of the transformation of benign to malignant tumors, probably in large part due to the difficulty of transplanting benign tumors. It is reported, however, that a transplantable adenofibroma of the rat breast showed the development of sarcoma after several generations (Selbie). Ewing states that "transformation of a benign into a malignant tumor occurs in rare instances." Nevertheless, the opinion is widely held that such transformation can and does occur, even although it is not especially frequent. Studies of thyroid tumors by Graham indicate that many of the carcinomas originate in pre-existing benign adenomas. This does not mean, however, that the benign adenoma frequently undergoes such change. The apparent transformation of the fibromyoma of the uterus into sarcoma seems well established, as is true also of fibroadenoma of the breast into carcinoma. Many of the malignant tumors of the testis probably develop from certain elements of the benign teratoma.

The opponents of the idea of malignant transformation suppose that the tumor is malignant from the start and only apparently benign. It is generally agreed, however, that there is less chance of a malignant tumor developing in a benign tumor than of a malignant tumor growing in tissues not otherwise tumorous. In practical experience a tumor is occasionally found which is of benign character throughout most of its extent, but with malignant disease obviously present in a small part. This sort of observation inclines many to the view that there is a hazard of malignant transformation in benign tumors.

MODES OF ORIGIN

The two principal problems involved are: whether a tumor originates in a single cell or in a group of cells; whether it originates from one focus or from several foci. The evidence that the tumor originates in a single cell is entirely inferential, arising, for exam-

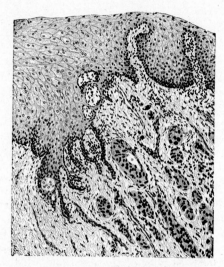

Carcinoma of the esophagus showing downward penetration of interpapillary epithelium.

ple, by studying rates and curves of growth. The same may be said as to the origin in a group of cells but general opinion favors this view. The question will probably not be answered until more is understood of exactly what changes take place in a normal cell to render it a neoplastic cell.

The second proposition concerns the question as to whether a tumor is unicentric or whether it may be multicentric. The former means origin in one group of cells, and may perhaps take place. Nevertheless, by reconstruction of serial sections, it has been found that one small carcinoma of the lip and one of the breast showed several minute foci of origin; hence although a tumor appears grossly to be unicentric, it may not actually be so. Multicentric origin may be observed in one organ or more than one. In the stomach or intestine, for example, multiple polypoid adenomas occur and malignant change can often be demonstrated in several of them. Neurofibromata in the form of multiple neurofibromatosis of von Recklinghausen appear practically simultaneously in

various parts of the skin. Paired organs, such as the breasts, testes and ovaries, may show simultaneous involvement by the same general sort of primary tumor. Lymphosarcoma appears to arise in several members of a chain of lymph nodes, and multiple myeloma of bone marrow also appears to originate in several foci. In some cases a single lymph node or a part of it may be affected first; or in the case of multiple myeloma one point in the bone marrow may appear to be affected before others. Nevertheless, the systemic character of the disease indicates that, when other places are involved, this is not due to metastasis but to separate points of origin.

Multiple Tumors

Two or more different tumors may be present in the body. This is commonly observed in women who frequently have fibromyomas of the uterus and may have another tumor elsewhere. Multiple malignant tumors of different sites are not rare. On the basis of their own and other statistics, Warren and Gates found an incidence of multiple malignant tumors in nearly 4 per cent of persons with malignant tumors. This may be an expression of general susceptibility to tumor growth, thrown into activity by special local factors in two or more situations.

Although tumors arise from pre-existent cells, they must be looked upon as tumors of tissues and organs, and are more or less characteristic in different regions. Thus tumors of the breast are essentially epithelial and grow as adenomas or as carcinomas. Pure connective-tissue tumors of the breast are infrequent. Tumors of the connective tissue septa of the body generally grow as fibromas of various types, including myxoma and lipoma. Epithelial tumors are never primary in these septa. Many examples could be furnished of this general principle of organ and tissue types. Other examples will become evident as the special forms of tumors are studied.

MODES OF GROWTH

There is no doubt that the multiplication of cells in tumor growth is by mitotic division. Amitotic or direct division is described but there is considerable doubt as to whether or not this may be due to pathologic disturbances in the nuclei or to alterations due to fixation and preparation. Mitotic figures are usually typical in every respect but many variations may occur. The usual bipolar mitoses may show hyper- or hypochromatism or may show such large forms as to be called giant mitoses. Distinctly abnormal forms include asymmetrical and multipolar mitoses. In the former a much larger number of chromosomes may migrate toward one centrosome than toward the other. In multipolar mitoses the centrosome apparently divides into several fragments with irregularly placed multiple attraction spheres, of even or uneven number. The resulting asters are not necessarily equal in content of chromosomes. It is supposed by some that the abnormal mitoses result in abnormal cell division but this is not firmly established and it is almost certain that such methods of cell division do not contribute in any material way to the growth of the tumor.

Abortive mitosis, in which there are abnormalities of polarization, irregularities in chromosomes, and degenerations of cytoplasm, are seen particularly in degenerative conditions in tumors. Warren has observed variations from the normal in the angles of mitotic spindles. Nuclear degeneration may produce figures which resemble chromidia, but there is no proof that the cell division is like that of protozoa. Certain observations have indicated that the number of chromosomes is reduced, similar to the reduction in sex cells, and Boveri suggested that this reduction is responsible for unlimited multiplication. Belling, however, found no such reduction. Heiberg and Kemp, and Levine found that in symmetrical division of tumor cells the number of chromosomes is normal and that in atypical mitoses, instead of being reduced, the number may reach 100 or more. Lewis and Strong determined that the tumor cell can multiply without abnormal mitoses and that the abnormalities are coincident rather than fundamental. Mottram observed that abnormalities of mitosis can be caused by agents not cancerogenic and concluded that factors are involved other than those which produce the nuclear changes. Thus there is no satisfactory evidence that tumor cells are like sex cells.

Although the growth of tumors is generally progressive, it may not be continuously so and may even show apparent retrogression. It continues in most cases until surgical removal, or the death of the host. As with other live tissues, tumor cells may be cultivated on artificial media through many generations, extending over years. Animal tumors may be transplanted through many series of the same or, in some instances, closely related species. The reason for the death of the tumor with the death of the host is simply the removal of the source of nutrition. The growth of the tumor from the original group of cells may follow in a general way two different modes. It may be by expansion of the original small mass, whereby the principal but not the sole growth appears in the center of the tumor, often referred to as a centripetal type of growth. Enlargement in this fashion results in compression of surrounding tissues. In part at least, pressure stimulates connective-tissue growth to form a capsule, but the tumor itself also contributes to the capsule. This is a common mode of growth of benign tumors.

Malignant tumors enlarge principally by multiplication of the peripheral cells, an infiltrative or centrifugal type of growth. By infiltration is meant the growth of the tumor cells through tissue spaces, to form buds and elongated projections from the original mass so that the normal tissues are pushed aside much as the tree roots grow into the soil. The tumorous buds and projections enlarge and fuse to destroy the intervening original tissue, with consequent increase in size of the tumor mass. Thus malignant tumors are not likely to be limited by a capsule, grow rapidly and are destructive to surrounding tissues. The penetration of their growth in lymph or blood vascular spaces provides for dissemination or metastasis.

The destruction of neighboring tissues by malignant tumors is probably due to various factors including pressure, interference with blood and lymph supply and perhaps the production of lactic acid by the tumor. Bacterial infection of the tumor may extend to and destroy surrounding tissues. In addition, hyperplasia may occur in neighboring tissues and this may look as if neoplasia had been stimulated. Connective-tissue cells near a carcinoma may seem to be sarcomatous and glandular cells near an adenoma may be hyperplastic, but there is no proof that these cells ever become a part of the tumor. Occasionally, metaplasia is observed in the surrounding cells. There is no good reason to believe that diffusible products of tumors, such as lactic acid, ever initiate new tumors in the surrounding structures.

By the nature of their growth tumors should be spherical, but surface tumors may be eroding ulcers, sessile masses or polypoid. Those which grow freely in viscera are likely to be spherical, but bones, periosteum, the capsules of viscera, ligaments, tendons, fascias, cartilage and skin are resistant to invasion and their position may alter the shape of the tumor. The influence of environment is illustrated by Lucké's study of transplants of a frog carcinoma into the anterior chamber of the rabbit's eye. Growth begins as hemispheric buds which then form a tubulo-papillary structure, as long as the growth is free in the fluid of the anterior chamber. When this growth meets a solid surface, such as iris or cornea, differentiation is lost. If it invades looser structures it again differentiates.

The rate of growth of tumors is highly variable. It may be altered by conditions of nutrition and by limitations imposed by surrounding structures. There are other factors which appear to play a part, because tumors of the same microscopic character appearing in the same organ in different individuals may show different rates of growth. The life history of a particular tumor is often of more value in predicting its rate of growth than are cellular details or type of tumor. There is much more regularity in the growth of transplantable tumors in animals; the rate may approximate but not exceed that of embryonal growth. In occasional instances in man, where restrictions are not imposed by surrounding tissues and the growth is "free," the rate may be exceedingly rapid but again does not exceed that of embryonal growth (Eveleth and Wetzel).

Retrogressive Processes

The cells and tissues of tumors are subject to the same sort of degenerative and other retrogressive changes as are observed in tissues not tumorous. Tumors, for example, furnish some excellent examples of pigmentation. Passive hyperemia within tumors may lead to the deposit of hemosiderin and other blood pigments. The melanoblastoma is an example of formation of pigment in tumor cells. Various tumors may be bile stained in general icterus. Those originating in the liver itself may produce bile pigment. Cloudy swelling is frequent. Fatty degeneration is common, especially in malignant tumors. Fat infiltration is rare, but the lipoma is made up of fat cells, the fat being physically and chemically identical with that of normal fat, but not utilized to any notable degree in metabolism (Wells). Hydropic infiltration may occur, especially when cells are free in edematous fluid. Connective-tissue hyalin and epithelial hyalin are not infrequent. The former occurs in connective-tissue tumors, especially the fibroma and fibromyoma. Epithelial hyalin is seen in both benign and malignant epithelial tumors. Keratohyaline bodies occur in the cytoplasm of epithelial tumor cells, called Russell fuchsin bodies, once falsely supposed to be parasites. Amyloid is sometimes observed, and it is to be remembered that invasive and destructive tumors, e.g., carcinomas, may cause general deposits of amyloid. Colloid is to be found in tumors which originate in the thyroid gland or in the pituitary body, but the iodine content may not be so constant as in the original normal gland structure. The term colloid is often used in reference to a hyalin, which is brown grossly, and to mucinous carcinomas, but this is incorrect because in neither is there true colloid. Mucinous degeneration appears particularly in epithelial tumors. The carcinoma of the intestinal tract, especially that seen in the large intestine, is likely to produce fairly large amounts of mucus, which gives the tumor grossly a gelatinous character. Mucoid is seen particularly in the myxoma where the fibrils are separated by basophilic material. Mucoid degeneration may appear in a considerable number of connective-tissue tumors. Pseudomucin is found in certain tumors. In cystic disease of the ovary it is not uncommon to find fairly large cysts that contain a gelatinous, homogeneous material, pseudomucin, which has some of the properties of mucin but stains with the acid dyes. Glycogenic infiltration is more common in those tumors whose cells are by nature more nearly of embryonal type. Thus, the teratoid type of tumor is likely to be rich in glycogen. On the other hand, those tumors which are made up of cells and tissues more nearly resembling the adult type are likely to show little or no glycogen.

Circulatory disturbances are fairly common and are particularly pronounced in those tumors which are pedunculated. Twisting of the pedicle may lead to obstruction of the outflow of blood and thus induce considerable passive hyperemia. Edema is also common in this type of tumor. It is not to be assumed, however, that all edema seen in tumors is necessarily of mechanical origin, because tumors may be extremely edematous and show relatively little passive hyperemia. Hemorrhage is common in the richly vascularized sarcomata and occurs in other tumors. Passive hyperemia, trauma, degeneration or necrosis in the tumor with involvement of vessel walls, and inflammation, may produce hemorrhage. Necrosis is common more particularly in rapidly growing, malignant tumors. It may result because growth is so rapid that the blood supply is inadequate, or because of ischemia or of complete stasis owing to occlusion of vessels. Such occlusion may be due to pressure by surrounding viscera, or bones, on the growing tumor mass, to thrombosis or embolism of blood vessels, to rupture of vessels, to inflammation, or to twisting of the pedicle of pedunculated tumors. Gangrene may occur in tumors, especially those eroding into the alimentary canal. Tumors are rarely, if ever, the seat of infection by the organisms of the specific granulomata. Suppurative and other simple types of inflammation are observed in tumors when bacteria gain access. This, of course, is more common where tumors erode upon surfaces. Occasionally, a tumor may be invaded by another malignant tumor. Thus, the uterine fibromyoma may be invaded by carcinoma of the uterus.

Inflammation

The tissues in the neighborhood of tumors often show inflammatory reactions of subacute or chronic grade. It is unusual that acute exudative inflammation appears except as the result of infection, but vascular dilatation is not uncommon about the margin of tumors. The subacute infiltration of cells occurs in the neighborhood of invasive tumors rather than in the neighborhood of benign tumors. Thus a rich infiltration of lymphoid cells associated with smaller numbers of plasma and endothelial cells is often found in the margin of carcinoma or sarcoma. In the neighborhood of malignant tumors in certain situations, for example, in the cervix of the uterus and in the large intestine, and sometimes elsewhere, a rich infiltration of eosinophilic cells may appear. There is usually an associated infiltration of the cells just mentioned, but sometimes the eosinophils quite outnumber the other cells. The cause of this subacute reaction and lymphoid infiltration is not known. There are various possibilities. Necrosis in the tumor or surrounding tissues may excite reaction. The presence of the tumor itself may initiate the reaction, because in a restricted sense it is foreign to the surrounding normal tissue. It is also possible that products absorbed from the tumor may irritate the neighboring tissues. The relation of this reaction to resistance will be discussed subsequently. The more chronic type of inflammation, consisting of an overgrowth of connective tissue, is especially prominent around the benign tumors, but may be seen in the form of partial and incomplete encapsulation around malignant tumors, more particularly the sarcomas. That the capsule of benign tumors is entirely the result of chronic inflammation in the neighborhood is not true. Certainly in those tumors made up largely of fibrous connective tissue, such as fibroma, there is little doubt that the tumor itself contributes a considerable part of the capsule. In these benign tumors, there is little reason for believing that necrosis, absorbable products, or local death of the tissues of the host institutes the reaction. Such deposition of connective tissue commonly occurs in places where pressure is exerted, and it is highly probable that the chronic reaction to this type of tumor is due to the pressure instituted by the expansive or centripetal type of growth.

SPECIAL FEATURES OF TUMOR GROWTH

Functional Activity of Tumors

As a general rule, the tumor exhibits no evidence of the functional activity of the cells from which it originates and of which it is built up. The capacity of epithelial and endothelial cells to cover surfaces may be seen in the tumor cells; they may extend to a certain degree over abraded and granulating surfaces. Ameboid activity of living tumor cells is only rarely observed, but phagocytosis by tumor cells of dead tumor cells, erythrocytes, bacteria, fat, tissue fragments, dead leukocytes, pigments, crystals of various kinds and foreign bodies is not uncommon. The capacity of individual cells to retain certain types of function is not uncommon. For example, the melanotic tumors continue to form melanin but this capacity is likely to be lost as anaplasia, that is, dedifferentiation with increased proliferative capacity, becomes more marked. The cells of tumors of the adrenal body may contain lipoids like those of the adrenal, and may contain epinephrine. The cells of lipomata contain fat of normal constitution. Glandular tumors may form secretions. The mucinous carcinomas, especially those of the large intestine, may produce large quantities of mucus, usually not secreted into the gut. Glandular tumors of the liver may contain bile, produced by the endothelial cells and not available for intestinal function. Tumors of the mammary gland may secrete a material like colostrum. A carcinoma of the pancreas is reported to have yielded enzymes like those of the gland itself. The muscle of myomas may contract on stimulation (Bryan and Warren). Tumors of the ductless glands produce internal secretions which function. Certain tumors of the pituitary are associated with gigantism and with acromegaly. Another type appears to be associated with the Cushing syndrome of obesity, hirsutism and hypertension. Tumors of the parathyroids are associated with osteitis fibrosa. Certain thyroid tumors and metastases may contain thyroxin and the maturation factor for tadpoles (Milles). That the thyroid adenoma may be responsible for so-called hyperthyroidism is not definitely established. Tumors of the thymus may be associated with certain polyglandular endocrine disturbances but the effects are not yet well known (see Leyton, Turnbull and Bratton). Tumors of the islets of Langerhans produce insulin, sometimes to such a degree that hypoglycemia occurs. Adrenal tumors, especially in the young, may lead to disturbances in secondary sex char-

acters. Certain tumors of the testis are accompanied by the excretion of a considerable amount of gonadotropic substances in the urine (Twombly, et al.). The arrhenoblastoma of the ovary produces masculinization. The granulosa-cell tumor of the ovary in the young may produce precocious sex development and after the menopause may stimulate irregularly periodic uterine bleeding with endometrial hyperplasia. Melanomas and neurogenic tumors may be accompanied by the presence in the urine of a substance called intermedin, evidently a hormone like that produced in the intermediate portion of the hypophysis. All these phenomena are to be distinguished from the effects of destruction of ductless glands by primary or secondary tumors.

Metabolism. Since they are living cells, tumor cells have metabolic activities. The chemical and physical properties of the tumor cell are considered in the section on Factors Intrinsic to the Cell. The chief problem here is whether or not the metabolism of tumor cells differs significantly from that of their normal prototypes, or in such a manner that the metabolic activity is peculiar to the tumor cell. Studies of carbohydrate metabolism by the Warburg method *in vitro* indicate that about two thirds of energy production of carcinoma occurs by glycolysis and about one third by oxidation, depending on the availability of oxygen. Anaerobic glycolysis is high in malignant tissue, lower in benign tumors and embryonal tissues, and still lower in most of the normal tissues. Aerobic glycolysis remains high in malignant tissues, but not in benign tumors, embryonal tissues and most normal tissues. Furthermore blood draining from malignant tumors *in vivo* shows a decrease of sugar and an increase of lactic acid, but not in sufficient quantity to be demonstrated in systemic blood. The property of aerobic glycolysis is not, however, an identifying characteristic of malignant cells because it is observed in the normal retina, in white blood cells and granulation tissue, and is missing in some of the experimental tumors. (Jackson; Dodds.)

There is little to be said of fat metabolism except that lipomas furnish little or no fat for general metabolism. Phospholipid turnover is high, but this is also true of active normal tissues (Jones et al.).

The protein metabolism has been studied indirectly for the most part and is probably increased. It is indicated that the nucleoprotein metabolism is increased (Kohman and Rusch), but that this is peculiar to the tumor cell is not yet proved. Of great interest is the claim that the amino-acid, glutamic acid, is racemized in malignant tumors, but many studies have contradicted this and it cannot be accepted as valid.

Salt metabolism is not regularly altered except that the content of calcium may be low and that of phosphorus high; as with growing tissues in general the water content is usually high.

The activity of a wide variety of enzymes has been studied extensively. In some instances, certain tumors may show increased activity; for example, proteinase and leukopeptidase have increased activity in butter-yellow tumors of the rat liver, suggesting an alteration of protein metabolism (Maver et al.). In other instances the results are irregular, as is true of arginase (Greenstein et al.). It has not been shown that alterations in enzymatic processes are peculiar to tumor cells. It is reported that blood esterase and liver catalase are reduced, but no generalizations can be made. (See Troescher et al.; Greenstein, Jenrette and White.)

Alterations of general metabolism may be due to changes in the tumor, such as necrosis or infection, and to effects of tumors upon digestive and excretory organs, but it is impossible to ascribe any specific changes to tumors.

Stroma

The connective tissue supporting framework of tumors appears in the form of bands of white fibrous connective tissue, and also in the form of fine fibrils interspersed between the tumor cells. The stroma originates from the connective tissue of the host. It may be scanty and irregularly arranged in anaplastic carcinomas, may form interlacing bands to produce an alveolated structure in other tumors, or may be greater in amount than the epithelium in scirrhous carcinomas. The sarcomas often show a definite framework, but may be so poor in stroma that special stains are required to demonstrate it. In some tumors a part of the stroma may consist of a residuum of the original supporting tissue of the area invaded, but the stroma of tumors is essentially the result of proliferation of the host's connective tissue. Yellow elastic tissue is resistant to destruction by tumors and by special staining may be shown to persist long after all other parent tissues have disappeared. A few observers have noted slight proliferation of elastica along the course of tumor invasion.

Connective tissue may proliferate because of two important mechanisms. The first is a nonspecific fibrous or fibrocellular hyperplasia, seen as a part of the general inflammatory reaction to tumor growth. The other is in the form of a desmoplastic activity of the tumor cell, a propensity to stimulate hyperplasia of connective tissue. As has been mentioned before, collateral hyperplasia of the surrounding tissues may occur in the course of tumor growth. Desmoplastic activity is probably somewhat different from this, in that the proliferation is confined particularly to the connective tissue. This is well illustrated in the scirrhous carcinoma, where marked connective tissue hyperplasia goes hand in hand with the epithelial growth. Metastases from such tumors frequently show quite as much connective tissue hyperplasia as in the original growth, and this is interpreted as indicative of desmoplastic properties on the part of the epithelium. An important question is as to whether or not the stimulating powers of tumor growth may influence the connective tisue to take on malignant properties itself. In experimental and human material, connective tissues adjoining a carcinoma may appear to be sarcomatous, but it is possible and indeed probable that the cells which appear to be elements of a sarcoma are really altered cells of the carcinoma. The stroma of tumors may undergo metaplasia, principally in the form of myxomatous change, but fat, cartilage and bone formation are sometimes observed. The extrusion of tumor products, such as mucus, may excite foreign body reactions in the stroma and in the surrounding tissues.

Blood Vessels

Experimentally, local anemia may favor the growth of tumors, but generalizations cannot yet be made from this fact. Although arteriosclerosis, phlebosclerosis, thrombosis and other vascular changes occur in the neighborhood of tumors, these changes are undoubtedly secondary to the tumor growth rather than the cause of it. The blood vessels of tumors are derived from those of the host. The arteries are like those of the host, but often tortuous and with both dichotomous and irregular branching. They are peculiarly resistant to invasion by the tumor. The veins are like those of the host and vulnerable to invasion. Capillaries grow as they do in the host and form a network in the tumor. In fungating tumors the capillaries proliferate as they do in granulation tissue. Especially in sarcomas, but also in the poorly differentiated carcinomas, blood vascular slits are seen, lined in part by endothelium or completely devoid of it so that the tumor cells constitute the walls. In this restricted sense the tumor may be said to contribute to its own vascular supply. In general, sarcomas are more richly vascularized than carcinomas, but the latter vary from tumors so rich in blood vessels that they pulsate, e.g., thyroid tumors, to those such as scirrhous carcinomas in which the vascular supply may be hard to demonstrate. Benign tumors vary from those made up almost entirely of blood vessels to the dense fibromas with little vascularization.

Nerves may constitute part of the stroma of tumors, but as a rule are remnants of nerves of the original tissue. Sometimes when nerves are interrupted by the tumor, the ends may proliferate in the tumor. (See Ryrie.)

CHARACTERS OF MALIGNANT TUMORS

Invasion. It is probable that nearly all tumors begin originally as a somewhat invasive growth. It is not uncommon, for example, to find simple benign fibroma of the kidney in the early stage, and similar tumors in the skin, which show no capsule or sharp delimitation whatever. Nevertheless, as these tumors increase in size, capsule formation becomes apparent. In a malignant tumor, however, encapsulation is rarely complete except in those instances where the tumor regresses. Experimentally, Loeb has shown that even in these instances, incision of the capsule may permit of renewed invasion by the tumor. Malignant tumors invade largely, if not en-

tirely, by multiplication of peripheral cells, as described above in the section on Modes of Growth. The involvement of various parts of the body depends upon direct extension, metastasis, and implantation upon body surfaces.

The actual demonstration of invasion may fail in certain lesions, which are malignant tumors because of their cytology and

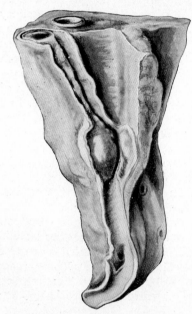

Intravascular tumor growth—a tumor thrombus.

histology. Thus there is the intraepithelial carcinoma of the cervix of the uterus and the *carcinoma-in-situ* of the stomach and the breast. Evidence points to the view that this noninvasive condition is a pre-invasive stage of the tumor, but invasion may not occur for a long time.

Direct Extension. In many instances, malignant tumors grow beyond the limits of the organ originally affected and into surrounding structures. Thus, carcinoma of the uterus may extend directly into the broad ligaments and other structures. Carcinoma of the gallbladder may penetrate directly into the liver. Carcinoma of the tongue may directly invade the floor of the mouth. There are numerous other examples of the same phenomenon. Direct extension may be through tissue spaces, along fascial planes, and through lymph and blood vessels. These factors and the resistance of various tissues in the pathway determine the direction, degree and form of the extension. Lymphatic permeation is really a manifestation of direct extension, but in a restricted sense; it is discussed below. It is important to distinguish between direct extension and metastasis.

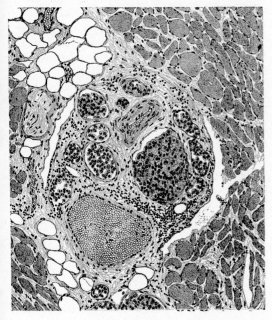

Carcinoma growing in a blood vessel and in surrounding perivascular lymphatics.

Metastasis. This differs from direct extension in that it signifies the transfer of cells or fragments of the original tumor to set up secondary growths in more or less remote position. This transfer is by way of lymphatic or blood vessels. Although there are many exceptions, it is a general rule that carcinomas metastasize through the lymphatics and sarcomas through the blood vessels. Thus the metastases of carcinomas are often local or regional and those of sarcomas widespread. For example mammary carcinoma usually metastasizes to the axillary lymph nodes, carcinoma of the tongue to sublingual or submaxillary lymph nodes, whereas sarcoma of bone metastasizes to lungs and many other structures. The modes of transport through the vessels are by embolism of tumor cells, permeation growth through the vessels and theoretically at least by migration of tumor cells.

That tumor cells or fragments can be carried in lymph and blood, to be deposited in other situations, is unquestionable. The fact that lymph nodes in the drainage areas of cancer show metastases without continuous involvement of intervening lymphatics is conclusive evidence of embolism. The frequency of metastases in the lungs from tumors in distant parts is proof of embolic metastasis through veins. Tumor fragments and cells may be deposited in tissues and then destroyed. Metastasis depends, then, upon lodgment of viable cells, which find suitable conditions for their multiplication. The fact that malignant tumors grow into and along lymphatics and veins explains the origin of the emboli. Carcinomas show a tendency to invade lymphatics, which accounts for their frequent metastasis to lymph nodes. Sarcomas show less tendency to invade lymphatics and metastasize less frequently to lymph nodes. Both types of tumor show growth into minute veins, but usually larger veins are involved before metastasis becomes evident. Sarcomas invade larger veins more often than do carcinomas, except for such epithelial tumors as the chorionepithelioma and renal carcinoma, which are richly vascularzied. Of great importance in entry of tumor emboli into veins is the thoracic duct. This is frequently involved in cases of abdominal, pelvic and sometimes thoracic tumors and this accounts for spread into the venous system. Paradoxical tumor embolism may occur but probably many cases of this nature are really due to actual metastases in the lungs with discharge of emboli into the pulmonary veins. Retrograde embolism may occur in veins but this phenomenon is much more frequent in lymphatics. Obstruction of lymphatics can be caused by tumor, with resultant retrograde flow, which may carry tumor emboli. Often, however, retrograde spread is due to growth of tumor in the vessels.

These principles apply to most metastases. Nevertheless, distribution may be irregular or "bizarre" and not to be explained on the basis of the usual distribution of blood vessels and lymphatics. Batson draws attention to the vertebral and spinal epidural veins which communicate freely with the general venous system and are poorly supplied with valves. Increases in abdominal and thoracic pressure, due to such things as lifting, vomiting, coughing, etc., may divert notable quantities of venous blood into these vertebral veins and carry tumor emboli into them. Thus Batson explains cerebral metastasis of pulmonary and even mammary tumors and bony metastases of prostatic carcinoma.

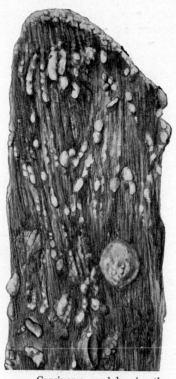

Carcinoma nodules in the pectoral muscle, secondary (metastases) from a cancer of the breast.

Carcinoma may grow along the lumina of lymphatics in a continuous sheet or cord and set up secondary nodules in lymph nodes or other structures. This, of course, is literally direct extension but its importance lies in the fact that it is one of the modes of production of what grossly appear to be metastases. Handley explained metastasis of mammary carcinoma to axillary lymph nodes by this mechanism and went further to explain metastasis to more remote situations such as bones in the same way. He supposed that what appears to be blood vascular metastasis is due to permeation of the perivascular lymphatics. Many other investigators have failed to confirm these observations and it is not likely that the hypothesis explains metastasis as a whole. Gray, in his extensive study of lymphatics and spread of tumors, concludes that permeation is not likely until there is lymphatic obstruction; thus permeation would be a late phenomenon. Nevertheless local extension by lymphatic permeation is not infrequent. When a group of lymph nodes is the seat of metastases, permeation may take place in the intercommunicating lymphatics. Surgical removal of groups and chains of lymph nodes must include the neighboring lymphatics. Metastases and recurrences in skin and other situations may show radiating lines of permeated lymphatics, sometimes visible to the naked eye.

In certain instances, tumor cells have been shown to be motile and estimates indicate that it would take about six weeks for a cell to migrate from carcinoma of the breast to axillary lymph nodes. Motility is not common to tumor cells as a whole, and although motility may account for an occasional metastasis, it is probably of little practical importance.

Malignant tumors vary considerably as to their capacity for metastasis, both as regards types of tumor and individual tumors of the same general type. The less differentiated, or more anaplastic the tumor, the greater the likelihood of metastasis, but there are many exceptions to this rule, so that other factors undoubtedly play a part.

Certain peculiarities of metastasis suggest that the field of implantation is important, either because it is a prepared area or because of inherent factors which favor or inhibit growth. It is well known that lymph nodes in the drainage area of carcinomas are the seat of acute and chronic hyperplasia and it has been suggested that the nodes are thus prepared for successful implantation of tumor emboli or extensions. This hyperplasia is especially marked in connection with ulcerated and infected tumors, where the enlargement may be great without metastasis. As concerns deep-seated carcinomas, it is probable that drainage from necrotic parts of the tumor irritates the nodes. Suspicion is always present that even in these nodes minute foci of tumor may be present and not included in the sections examined. No proof has been furnished that the hyperplasia favors metastasis and it is probable that lymph node metastasis depends upon anatomic relations rather than upon physiologic changes in the nodes.

The distribution of metastases by way of the blood stream varies with different tumors in such a way as to indicate that certain thyroid, prostate, stomach and breast. The Brown-Pearce rabbit tumor grows well when transplanted into the testis, but poorly in subcutaneous tissues. Tissue-culture experiments show that certain chemical and physical factors are essential to the propagation

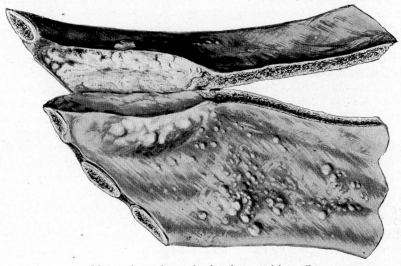

Metastatic carcinoma in the pleura and in a rib.

organs favor and others inhibit the growth of metastases. There must be many emboli in these circumstances and the distribution of the blood should determine their deposit in almost every organ, but metastases are much more common in the liver than in the spleen. This is in part due to large venous drainage into the liver and exclusive arterial supply to the spleen. Nevertheless the melanoblastoma of the choroid of the eye often shows extensive metastasis in the liver, evidently due to arterial transport, with little or none in the spleen. Willis suggests that the susceptibility of the liver, in the light of Warburg's work "depends on the rich carbohydrate content and poor oxygenation of that organ," but this does not explain the frequency of metastasis in the lungs. Carcinomas of prostate, thyroid, breast and to a certain extent stomach have a special predilection for metastasis in bones, an indication that bone marrow furnishes favorable conditions for growth (see Copeland). The fact that when ovaries or adrenals are involved, the condition is usually bilateral, is a further indication of suitability of soil for the implants. Variable degrees of resistance to metastasis are exhibited by spleen, heart and skeletal muscle, kidney, of tumor cells, but the factors which are of significance in the living host have not been identified. Furthermore there are bizarre metastases of individual tumors, which do not seem to follow any general rule.

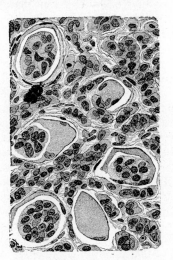

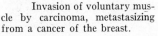

Invasion of voluntary muscle by carcinoma, metastasizing from a cancer of the breast.

Metastases occur in a high percentage of fatal tumor cases, but there is great variation in different types of tumor and in individual members of the same group. In general, malignant tumors in young people metastasize early, as in mammary carcinoma of the pregnant woman. Duration is obviously important. Situation is also significant, not only in relation to veins and lymphatics, but in other obscure ways, for example, lip carcinoma metastasizes earlier than the same type of tumor on the cheek. Sex appears to play a part in that women as a group die earlier of malignant tumors than do men. The general rule is that the more differentiated the tumor the less likelihood of metastasis, or the greater the anaplasia the greater the likelihood of metastasis, but factors such as fibrosis in scirrhous carcinomas, degree of marginal reaction and other conditions appear to modify the rule. The most frequent sites of metastatic tumors are in lymph nodes, liver, lungs, pleura, bones and adrenals. Organs frequently the seat of primary tumors are not often affected by metastasis. As concerns tumor growth there are three groups of organs: (1) those frequently attacked by metastases but much less so by primary malignant tumors, e.g., lymph nodes, liver, lungs, pleura, bone marrow; (2) those commonly the seat of primary tumors but rarely the seat of metastasis, e.g., stomach, breast, pancreas, prostate; (3) those not commonly affected by either primary or secondary tumors, e.g., spleen, heart, skeletal muscle, kidney.

Carcinomatosis or carcinosis is a widespread dissemination of cancer, and may be due to direct invasion of the blood stream by the primary tumor or similar invasion from metastatic nodules in lymph nodes or viscera, and to invasion of the thoracic duct. Tumors of abdominal viscera and of other organs below the level of the diaphragm usually enter the thoracic duct at the receptaculum chyli either by permeation through tributary lymphatics or extension from closely applied lymph nodes. Less frequently thoracic tumors invade the duct, usually due to direct extension or to permeation or embolism through thoracic tributaries. The duct may be a continuous mass of tumor or show discrete plugs at various levels. Soon after this the supraclavicular lymph nodes may be involved especially on the left side, the so-called Virchow or signal node. Not infre-

quently this is the first clinical indication of tumor, particularly in primary carcinoma in the abdomen or elsewhere below the diaphragm. Rarely the supraclavicular node may be involved without disease of the duct, evidently due to lodgment of a tumor embolus in the duct near the node. From the duct, the tumor may be spread by venous drainage into the lungs and thence elsewhere. Furthermore if the duct be obstructed, retrograde lymph flow may occasion dissemination to many parts.

Surface Implantation. The surfaces upon which tumors may be implanted are serous, cutaneous and mucous. Evidence is now ample to show that a tumor which involves a serous surface may be transplanted by the movements of the serous fluid to other parts of the surface and set up other tumor masses. Theoretically, this transfer by means of particles suspended in fluid is an embolic type of metastasis. Of the celomic cavities, the peritoneum shows this phenomenon most often, the pleura next and the pericardium least. Sampson has shown that fragments of ovarian tumors, especially the serous cystadenoma, may be carried in the peritoneal fluid to be deposited upon some part of the peritoneal surface where a low-grade inflammation is excited. The surface cells are destroyed, the tumor cells are entangled in the fibrin and multiply to establish metastases. In the large serous cavities, the tumor may extend through subsurface lymphatics and, especially in the meninges, may extend over the surface. The presence of the metastases may cause adhesion, or excess of fluid presumably due to blockage of lymphatics by tumor. The fact that the fluid is often bloody may be due to blockage or penetration of veins.

There are various reports of implantation of cancer from one epithelial surface to another, such as in the urinary bladder, vagina, vulva, stomach, from renal pelvis or kidney into ureter, tongue to cheek, lip to lip, esophagus to stomach, one part of intestine to another, etc. It is known, however, that in certain cases of transfer from esophagus to stomach, the route was by way of the lymphatics instead of by surface implantation. Certainly the destructive effect of digestive fluids and the low viability of fragments from infected tumor surfaces would hinder rather than favor implantation. Before implantation can be accepted in these situations, Willis points out that consideration should be given to the possibility that there may be a transfer of a carcinogenic agent, that direct permeation of lymphatics or blood vessels has occurred, that embolic metastasis is responsible, or that the two tumors represent multiple origins. Most of the reported cases do not withstand criticism, yet a few are acceptable. Tumor fragments have certainly been transferred from one part of the lung to another via the respiratory tract. Transfer of carcinoma by coitus has not been proved. Transfer from one part to another by

not all, cases the manifestations can be explained otherwise. For example, tumors may obstruct the alimentary tubes; in the esophagus and the stomach this is associated with starvation phenomena and in the intestine with the manifestations of obstruction. Anemia, with its train of dependent symptoms, may be due to prolonged starvation or to repeated bleeding from ulcerated tumor surfaces. The infection of eroded tumor surfaces must be significant. It is possible that the absorption of split protein products from necrotic foci of tumors may produce fever and leukocytosis, but it is not likely that this explains prolonged cachexia. Carcinoma of the stomach is often accompanied by achlor-

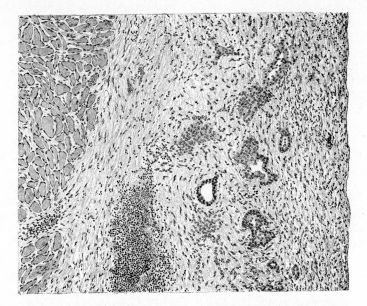

Subcutaneous implantation of adenocarcinoma following operation, probably due to the transfer of tumor cells during operation.

surgical operation is well known. Although experimentally tumor may be transferred from one animal to another by rubbing into abraded surfaces, it has not been accomplished in man. Willis's book gives an excellent presentation of all phases of tumor dissemination.

Cachexia. This term refers to a clinical syndrome of emaciation, loss of weight and strength, anemia, digestive disturbances and other manifestations, which frequently accompanies the presence of malignant tumors. There is usually an implication that the symptoms and signs are due to poisonous or toxic products of the tumor. In most, if

hydria with inadequate digestion, and putrefaction of stomach contents. Faults in absorption of alimentary products may be due to extensive destruction of the liver by tumors and occur occasionally in cases of obstruction of the thoracic duct. In many patients the knowledge of the presence of a malignant tumor produces psychic disturbances with loss of appetite, and inadequate nutrition, rest and exercise.

No proof has been furnished that malignant tumors elaborate any definite substance the absorption of which produces the so-called cachexia. There may be alterations in body metabolism, as pointed out above, but these are not sufficient to account for the prolonged and severe general manifestations.

Death may be due to any of the conditions just enumerated, usually with an associated bronchopneumonia. Sepsis, however, is not a frequent cause of death. Obstruction may develop in various situations as stomach, intestines, ureters, either by tumors of these structures or by pressure or invasion from tumors in the immediate neighborhood. Such obstruction may be caused by benign as well as malignant tumors. Situated in brain or heart, tumors may cause death directly. (See Warren.)

Pathologic Diagnosis of Malignant Tumors. The most important features of malignancy are invasive growth and metastasis. When these can be demonstrated, the diagnosis is established. It is essential, however, for practical purposes of treatment and prognosis that diagnosis be made early, if possible before definite invasion and metastasis have occurred. Critical judgment based on experience is required to determine that departure from normal or hyperplastic tissues which means benign tumor and that further departure which means malignant tumor. Thus, careful gross and microscopic examinations are necessary. In tumor growth the departure from the normal cell and cell arrangement is toward an embryonal type of cell and arrangement. This change is usually referred to morphologically as anaplasia. The greater the degree of anaplasia the more certain the diagnosis of malignancy. In addition to a possible increase of nucleocytoplasmic ratio, a loose arrangement of the cytoplasm with a tendency to basophilia, and changes in the nuclear architecture, mitotic figures are important. Mitoses are likely to be more numerous in malignant than benign tumors, but many may be present in the latter. Abnormal mitotic figures are far more often observed in malignant than in benign tumors. Particularly on the basis of stained fresh tissues, it is said that the nucleolus is larger in proportion to nucleus than is true of normal cells. This variable, however, may be observed in proliferating tissues and in the opinion of many is not thought to be of diagnostic significance. In glandular tumors departure from and loss of cellular polarity is a strong indication of malignancy. Indeed, with increasing experience, it has been possible to diagnose carcinomas microscopically before invasion has occurred, because of pleomorphism, alteration of polarity, loss of differentiation and comparable features. This is called *carcinoma in situ*, or intra-epithelial carcinoma and has been seen in the skin, uterine cervix, stomach and mammary gland. In connective-tissue tumors, rich vascularization, naked vascular slits not lined with endothelium with tumor cells "combed" away from these slits and an immature type of cells indicate malignancy. In many instances the diagnosis requires the intimate correlation of clinical and pathologic data. Age and sex, situation of tumor, duration of disease, metastasis, special phenomena, such as postmenopausal uterine bleeding, digestive disturbances, and other factors must all be given due consideration. Nevertheless, when a diagnosis can be clearly made on microscopic examination, these ancillary facts are of no material aid.

DEGREES OF MALIGNANCY. For prognosis and treatment, it is desirable to determine the relative degrees of malignancy of tumors. The fact that carcinomas of the same organ and same general type vary as to differentiation and anaplasia and that the more anaplasia the greater the degree of malignancy, has long been known. This principle was re-enunciated by MacCarty and applied to carcinomas of the lip, skin and rectum by Broders, to those of the cervix uteri by Martzloff and of the fundus by Mahle, to those of the breast by Greenough, and to other situations by various authors (see Hellwig). Carcinomas of greatest differentiation are put into Grade I, and those of greatest anaplasia into Grade IV. Grades II and III represent intermediate distinctions. For some tumors only three grades are set up. Criteria for the grades are usually established so that the distinctions are not unduly difficult. Some have attached numerical values to various cytologic and histologic features and to others factors such as inflammatory reaction, fibrosis, age, sex, situation, duration, etc., with the idea of establishing a numerical index of malignancy, but it is doubtful that in this intricate biologic problem much if anything has been added. Grading is of aid as regards prognosis and also treatment, especially radiation therapy, for in a general way the greater the anaplasia the greater the sensitivity to irradiation. Experience has shown that there are many exceptions to the rule of radiosensitivity (Stewart) and the individual case must always be given careful consideration. Prognosis and treatment on the basis of grading are really a generality built up on statistical information. Grading represents averages of groups and the individual case may be in either extreme of this group. Thus it is unwise to be too optimistic or too pessimistic because of the grade of the particular tumor. (See Reimann.) These remarks apply to carcinoma because generally speaking the grading of sarcomas has not been satisfactory. Nevertheless, Broders and his associates have graded fibrosarcomas by analyzing the production of collagen, the character of the cells and the mitotic figures but in our opinion this has not yet been adequately confirmed. Furthermore, associated factors, such as situation, time element, invasiveness, etc., are of especial importance in evaluating the malignancy of sarcomas.

Various chemical and other tests have been devised for diagnosis. These are planned (1) to determine the presence in the blood of specific chemical constituents, including salts, amino acids, lipins, glutathione, etc., (2) to detect physicochemical changes in the blood such as surface tension, hydrogen-ion concentration, sedimentation rate of erythrocytes, etc., (3) to determine antigen-antibody reactions and to test changes in enzymatic action, and (4) to detect and assay hormones. The last is of value in respect to certain tumors of endocrines, as discussed under the heading of Function. Some of the others may prove to be of diagnostic aid, but at the present time, there are too many positives in patients without tumors. (See Woodhouse.)

EXPERIMENTAL TRANSPLANTATION OF TUMORS

The experimental studies of tumors in animals are based on observations of (1) naturally occurring tumors, (2) of tumors induced in the animals by various means, and (3) of those which are transplantable from one animal to another. In order to transplant a tumor, the material usually is minced and then injected by syringe, although small fragments can be transplanted through an incision. Various transplantable tumors have been grown in succeeding generations of inoculated animals for many years; it is now agreed that this is due to multiplication of the inoculated cells.

In transplanted material in the new animal host, especially with the larger grafts, the central parts undergo necrosis and the cells which proliferate to form the new tumor are principally those of the periphery. The blood vessels and the connective tissue undergo hyalinization and may entirely disappear, and as the essential tumor cells grow, new blood vessels and fibroblasts are provided from the host tissues. Sometimes the multiplication of new capillaries is especially conspicuous and the reaction is called angioplastic, but in others the reaction is principally on the part of connective tissue and is called fibroplastic. Generally, however, the relation between stroma, blood vessels and essential cells of the tumor is much as was true of the natural tumor.

When a naturally occurring tumor is first transplanted into a group of animals, some do not exhibit new tumors. With succeeding generations of transplants, the number of takes, as they are called, increases considerably. The explanation of this phenomenon is not altogether clear but evidently there is some sort of adaptation of the tumor cells to the new environments. Study of the inoculated tumors shows that their growth is somewhat cyclic and if the transplantation is made when the growth energy is greatest, the chances of success are improved. There is a possibility that there are growth promoting factors, as described by Casey, but that these play a definite part in the cyclic type of growth is not yet established.

Generally speaking, the transplantation of tumors is successful only within the species. Nevertheless it has been found possible to transfer tumor of one mammalian species to young embryos of another but as soon as the embryo attains maturity, tumor growth ceases. A few instances are on record of tumors being transplanted to distinctly different species and finally successful growth attained, as discussed further in the section on Resistance.

Although tumors grow better in young animals than in the old, age is not a deciding factor in success of transplantation. Sex is of relatively little importance except that some experiments show a greater likelihood of takes in females than in males. Diet may play a part but without great regularity. Simple restriction in the amount of food may interfere with the growth of transplantable tumors. A carbohydrate-free diet has been found to reduce the number of successful transplants but this is not true of all tumors. The substitution of lime for other salts in the diet has been found to limit the success of transplantation but if successful the tumor growth will be hastened by return of the natural salts to the diet. Transplantation and growth have been found to be favored in some instances by the subcutaneous injection of cholesterol and of tethelin, of devitalized homologous tumor cells by splenectomy, and by use of homologous tumor emulsion. It is also likely that there are some individual differences within any group of animals subjected to transplantation but exactly why the soil for growth appears to be better in one than in another is not yet known.

That there is a refractory period in the growth of the transplant is not likely. Of course a variable time elapses between the inoculation and the gross appearance of the tumor but this does not of necessity mean that the earlier cells do not begin to multiply at once. The very nature of cell division means that there is an ascending curve of increase in the size of the tumor, but this does not follow a straight line. There is rather a parabolic curve, because each new generation of cells doubles itself if all the new cells divide.

As a rule, transplantable tumors remain true to type throughout their entire existence, although there may be local variations. There are, however, a few instances of alteration of cellular arrangement. When a mixture of sarcoma and carcinoma is inoculated, both may grow. Nevertheless, in certain animals it is found that in some strains one of these tumors will grow and in other strains the other. It would appear then that if the two tumors are to develop side by side, the genetic constitution of the animals must be approximately such that the growth of each component is favored equally.

Spontaneous regression and complete disappearance of implanted tumors may occur. This is usually initiated by degenera-

tion and necrosis, which stimulates the production of connective tissue, so that the final result is a cicatrix. Of interest is the fact that Woglom found no features in the essential cells of the tumor that would distinguish those about to undergo regression.

Explantation

The use of tissue culture in the study of tumors has furnished only a few facts. It has been found that embryonic tissue and neoplastic tissue contain growth promoting factors. Most tumor cells divide by mitosis, but a fowl sarcoma has shown amitotic division. The capacity to grow is not materially different from that of normal cells. The neoplastic cells constitute a new race of cells and inoculation into animals may result in tumor growth. There is nothing in the morphology or metabolism of tumor cells in tissue cultures that specifically distinguishes them from other cells. (See Silberberg.)

RESISTANCE

As with other diseases, factors of susceptibility and resistance have significance in the study of tumors. Susceptibility is in large part hereditary and is discussed subsequently. Immunity is a phenomenon in which various antibodies are demonstrable, but since these have not yet been conclusively shown in respect to tumors, the term resistance is preferred. The evidence of resistance in man, aside from probable hereditary factors, is indirect. Occasionally human tumors regress and this is interpreted by some to mean that the patient has developed resistance, but numerous other factors may really be responsible. Some consider that fibrosis around tumors, infiltration of lymphocytes and other reactive phenomena indicate resistance but final proof has not been offered. Thus the search has been directed principally to tumors in laboratory animals, with special attention to natural resistance, active acquired resistance, passive transfer of resistance and local reactions suggestive of resistance.

Natural Resistance

Natural resistance to inoculated tumors may be observed in animals in which natural "spontaneous" tumors exist. They are thus resistant to one tumor but not to tumors as a group. Transplantation has been studied in reference to age, race, sex and pregnancy. Successful transplants are more frequent in young animals than in those of older age groups. This harmonizes with the view that spontaneous tumors have their beginning much earlier than the time at which they become evident. If this were not true, the internal environmental conditions for successful implantation must be different from those which exist at the time of initiation of spontaneous tumors.

Transplantation into the same species and into the same strain from which the original tumor was taken is more successful than if attempted into other species. Nevertheless in special circumstances the racial barrier may be overcome. Putnocky successfully transplanted the Ehrlich mouse carcinoma, a rapidly growing tumor, into rats. Resistance was induced by injections of minced mouse tissue and mouse carcinoma. The rats with the mouse tumor were resistant to inoculation of rat tumors. DeBalogh was also successful in transplanting the Ehrlich mouse carcinoma to rats. He observed that the architecture was much altered in the subcutaneous growths but remained fairly true to form when inoculated into the kidney. These various phenomena are not yet explained. Greene has successfully transplanted rabbit carcinomas into the anterior chamber of the eye of guinea-pigs, swine, goats and sheep. He has transplanted human carcinoma and sarcoma into the anterior chambers of rabbits and guinea-pigs. These various tumors had attained that degree of autonomy represented by at least local invasion before they were transplantable.

Certain tumors will grow only within the same strain of animals, but the resistance of other strains may be overcome. Warner and Reinhard found that if they irradiated mouse tumors, for which, ordinarily, one strain was highly specific, other strains naturally resistant to it showed takes in a goodly number of animals.

General ill health and poor nutrition interfere with growth of transplants, but this is not so much a factor of resistance as lack of favorable conditions for growth. Although sex is not a factor in subcutaneous transplantation, it is reported that with intracu-taneous inoculation females are more resistant than males (L. Gross). Pregnancy is also a factor. In spite of somewhat divergent reports, the general opinion is that pregnancy is unfavorable to transplantation. It is suggested that nutritional factors are of importance since the tumor requires the same type of nourishment as the embryo and fetus. Indeed it is said that if the number of embryos be large the chance of successful inoculation is less than if the number be small. This is somewhat different from the augmentation of growth of mammary carcinoma in the human female when pregnancy occurs, because the special physiologic activity of the gland probably favors the tumor growth.

Actively Acquired Resistance

Actively acquired resistance is suggested by the fact that animals in which inoculated tumors have regressed are refractory to subsequent inoculation. Nevertheless, it is possible that the reason the tumor regressed is because the animal was naturally resistant and this natural resistance was augmented by the presence of the tumor to the point where the tumor was destroyed. At any rate, it is not a specific resistance because although it is greatest against the same tumor, it is effective in variable degree against others. In certain instances, it has been reported that if in an animal already bearing a tumor a separate tumor is established by intracutaneous inoculation, the regression of the intracutaneous tumor is often followed by regression of the other tumor. (See Saphir and Appel.) This may be an acquired resistance or stimulation of natural resistance. Vaccination with tumor cells, killed by chemical or other means, does not establish resistance. Killed normal cells are also ineffective. Resistance can be excited by injections of live embryo skin and certain normal tissues, but this is only temporary. It is thus evident that the only way in which resistance is acquired is by actual growth of tumor cells in the body. (See Spencer.)

Passive Resistance

The injection of serum from animals that have natural or acquired resistance has not conferred resistance upon other animals. The claims that repeated injection of cells will lead to production of cytolytic immune bodies which kill the tumor cells has not been substantiated. Mann and Welker report the production of a precipitin which reacts specifically with serum of patients with malignant tumors; it is indicative of the presence in the blood of proteins of the tumor. This requires confirmation. There is no indication that the precipitating serum deals in any way with resistance.

Local Resistance

The question of local resistance is not settled. Transplantation of tumors into resistant animals is followed by necrosis of the tumor and an exudative reaction in which there are polymorphonuclear leukocytes, plasma cells and large mononuclear phagocytes. It has been suggested that this is an allergic response, but it is more likely that it is simply a reaction to necrosis of the tumor, a necrosis due to general rather than local factors. Around human tumors there is often a collection of lymphocytes. In this connection Murphy reported that tumors can be inoculated into chick embryos but that this is not possible after spleen and lymph nodes have developed. With his collaborators he reported that reduction of lymphoid tissue and lymphocytes in the circulating blood by means of the roentgen ray resulted in reduction of resistance to inoculation. Increasing the number of lymphocytes by dry heat resulted in increased resistance. The observations have been contradicted by others (Guyer et al.) and it is possible that effects other than alterations in number of lymphocytes are responsible. Although splenectomy favors transplantation, lymph nodes are susceptible to metastasis as is true also of the spleen (Warren and Davis). There is no convincing evidence that local reactions have an important bearing on resistance.

It has been suggested that bacterial infection in the body has an inhibitory effect upon tumor growth and treatment of sarcoma by streptococcal "toxins" is recommended. The clinical results are far from convincing and there has been no real support from animal experiment.

ETIOLOGY OF TUMORS

The behavior of tumors is generally so different from that of infectious diseases that discovery of a specific cause is unlikely. As Ewing puts it, the present information indicates that tumors are conditioned by various factors rather than directly caused by them. Furthermore, tumors are a group of neoplastic diseases rather than a single entity. Ultimately the beginning of a tumor is to be found not merely in factors which excite cellular multiplication but in something that brings about abnormal, unrestrained, autonomous proliferation. Tumor cells are a race of cells set apart by various properties from the normal cells from which they originated, but although various theories as to this independent growth have been offered, none has been established. Studies of experimental and human material have yielded important facts about conditions that surround and influence tumor growth. Some apply to a tumor or group of tumors and not to others. Conditions that operate in experimental animals are not necessarily applicable to man or to other animals. Nevertheless, it appears that the formula, intrinsic factors plus extrinsic factors equals neoplasm, is widely accepted. The values or weighting assigned to each of these factors varies widely; in some instances, for example the retinoblastoma, the intrinsic factor appears to operate alone and in other instances, as, for example, the tar carcinomas of experimental animals, the extrinsic factor may far outweigh any intrinsic factor. In a sense, the intrinsic factor is one that prepares or predisposes and the extrinsic is a realization factor. The discussion which follows is arranged to consider the extrinsic factor first. Probably to be included as intrinsic factors in a certain sense are age, sex and race, as discussed previously. Heredity, cell relations, inherent properties of cells, anaplasia are intrinsic, as in a sense are the actions of hormones, vitamins, etc. The extrinsic factors of especial importance are irritation and parasites. Much of the information collected deals with malignant tumors, and the discussion must follow that line. Certain benign tumors are probably due to excessive or irregularly acting physiologic stimuli (Ingleby) but many are not so explained.

Extrinsic Factors

Irritation. Under this heading are included the possible effects of a single injury and of prolonged or frequently repeated injury. It has been suggested that a single traumatic injury may excite some hypothetical precancerous condition to neoplasia and that cells or cell groups which have been misplaced in embryonal development, supposed especially susceptible to growth stimuli, may actively proliferate to form a tumor. No proof has been furnished in support of these ideas. Nor can they be conclusively applied to any other presumptively precancerous conditions.

to permit of neoplastic growth; the tumor must be at the exact site of injury and must be of a type natural to the affected part. The oft-quoted statement that tumors of the brain are caused by injury to the head is not valid. As a matter of fact, Parker and Kernohan found that brain tumor is as frequent in patients without a history of injury to the head as in those with such history and that a history of comparable injury is even

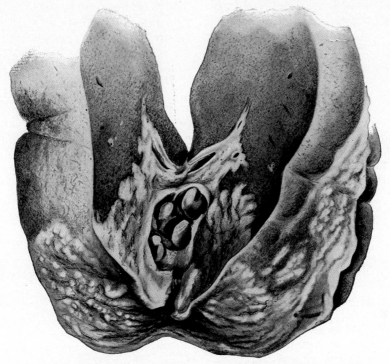

Calculi in gallbladder, with carcinoma of gallbladder directly invading the neighboring liver.

ditions. There is no real evidence, experimental or otherwise, that a single injury directly excites growth of carcinoma, although possibly a succeeding chronic inflammation may indirectly induce it. In a very few instances, sarcoma, especially of bone, may be traced in this way to major trauma to the bone.

Certain criteria are offered as a guide to the question of the initiation of a tumor by a single trauma, but rarely if ever are they met. The injury must have been sufficiently severe to justify its consideration as a possible cause; the affected tissue must be shown to have been free of tumor at the time of injury; adequate time must have elapsed

more frequent in people who are perfectly well than in those with brain tumor. Naturally the problem is one which often enters into law suits; this aspect is well covered by Mock and Ellis.

There is no adequate reason to suppose that a single trauma may excite an existing tumor to accelerated growth. The same holds true for metastasis. The direct injury caused by biopsy does not favor metastasis. Repeated massage, however, has increased the dissemination of metastases in both experimental animals and probably in man. Even though it might be expected that injury could prepare a field so as to determine the site of metastasis, this has not been proved.

Nevertheless, the end results of injury may be of significance. Schrek reports that about 18 per cent of cutaneous carcinomas of legs, arms and scalp develop in pre-existing scars, such as those due to burns, lacerations, surgical operations and in ulcers. Trauma may dislodge epithelium into subcutaneous tissues with subsequent formation of cysts lined by epithelium, but there is little to indicate that these become carcinomatous.

The significance of prolonged irritation has been studied in man and experimental animals, especially as concerns epithelial tumors. There are many examples of this relationship in man. Thus, there is the carcinoma of the lip of smokers, of the thighs and abdomen of the Kashmiri who use Kangri baskets and of the mouth of betel-nut chewers. Carcinoma of the mouth may be associated with jagged teeth, in the skin with chronic inflammations, and in the mucous membranes and skin with chronic ulceration (Knox), and in deeper tissues with persistent draining sinuses. The association of carcinoma of gallbladder and of renal pelvis with calculi is highly suggestive, but often it is impossible to determine which is cause and which is effect. Carcinoma of the esophagus occurs at narrow parts of the tube, and in the pyloric region in the stomach, positions where repeated insults may take place. Chronic infectious granulomata may give rise to tumors, as for example, syphilitic leukoplakia of the tongue, syphilitic lesions of bones, and tuberculosis of the skin in the form of lupus. Carcinoma of the penis is rare in the circumcised. Tumors occur in connection with certain occupations as a definite industrial hazard. Carcinoma of the skin in inadequately protected x-ray workers is a tragic example. The painting of watch dials with radium paint has led to osteogenic sarcoma in the workers, an example of irritative tumor of connective tissue origin (shown experimentally to be due to the alpha rays of radium). (See Martland.) Although carcinoma of the skin may be produced in experimental animals by ultraviolet light (Rusch, et al.), Blum raises some doubt as to the widely accepted view that sunlight actually causes carcinoma of the skin of man. The carcinoma of the lung in the Schneeberg miners is probably due to special irritant factors in the mine dust, perhaps arsenic or more probably radio-active materials. Arsenical keratosis is likely to be complicated by carcinoma especially of basal cell type (Franseen and Taylor). It is said that extremes of heat and cold may be cancerogenic (Haagensen). Occupations which lead to exposure to tar, oils, soot and aniline dyes are notably hazardous. The chimney sweep's cancer of the scrotum is probably due to soot. Similar tumors occur among workers with paraffin and coal tar. Although the statistical evidence is not absolutely convincing, it is generally thought that the workers in anilines are especially subject to bladder tumors. Ferguson and his associates found that the tumors are most often cancers, but may be papillomas or even nonepithelial tumors. Aniline or its derivatives are inhaled, absorbed, circulate in the blood, and act on the bladder, presumably because of a peculiar affinity between agent and cell. The basal layer of epithelium shows the first change. Multiple tumors in the bladder probably represent growth from multiple centra rather than secondary implantation.

There have been many experimental studies of the effects of prolonged irritation, but the mechanism of its operation has not been fully clarified. It is probable, however, that the chronic inflammation produced by irritation is not the sole nor perhaps the principal reason for the development of tumors. Studies have been conducted with lipoid solvents and oils, but, as is true of scarlet red (Eckert, et al.), true neoplasms have not developed, although these produce epithelial hyperplasia. In mice, carcinoma of the breast follows repeated pregnancies in which the animals are not allowed to suckle their young. Ligation of the ducts of the mammary gland is also followed by the development of carcinoma. In both these instances irritation appears to be fundamental. As will be discussed below, parasites may, because of their presence, lead to the development of tumors, presumably because of irritation.

The discovery by Yamagiwa and Ichikawa in 1915, that the repeated application of tar to the skin of mice leads to the development of carcinoma has furnished the background for extensive work along these lines. The studies have been advanced by the fractionation of tar by Kennaway and his associates and others. Many polycyclic hydrocarbons have been developed and synthesized, but the important highlights have been the synthesis of 1:2:5:6-dibenzanthracene and the distillation of 3:4-benzpyrene. Both of these are actively cancerogenic and operate in much shorter periods of time than does tar. The most active of all is methylcholanthrene, which was prepared from a bile acid, desoxycholic acid, and recently from cholic acid. Although it was formerly thought that the phenanthrene nucleus is a necessary constituent, this has been found not to be true. The operation of these hydrocarbons is probably not simply by chronic irritation, but since their action is relatively specific, there are presumably changes brought about in the cells which lead to their development into tumors. There is always a latent period during which the cells become altered in some way and this is true whether the application be frequently repeated or whether there be interruptions in the period of painting. As a rule, the painted area shows no especial sign of disturbance for several weeks and the first indication of alteration is the development of several papillomas. Then some of these become invasive squamous-cell carcinoma.

Various experiments indicate that at some time during the latent period the cells undergo a change which permanently alters their character and that of their descendents. If the area painted with tar be burned with a hot iron four to seven months after starting the experiment, papilloma is produced, but if this be done at seven to 11 months, a carcinoma develops. Scalding of the area will also excite carcinoma. If the painting be done with doses insufficient to cause carcinoma, doses of roentgen rays, in themselves also insufficient to be cancerogenic, will be followed by growth of carcinoma. If a small part of the painted area become carcinomatous and that part is removed a cancer will start in another part. It may be assumed, then, that a change occurs in the cells indicative of a precancerous state, but it is not possible as yet to identify any constant cytological alterations that are specifically indicative of this change (see Cowdry and Paletta).

In addition to the production of carcinoma of the skin by painting with these hydrocarbons, subcutaneous injection leads to development of sarcoma. If injected into viscera, sarcoma or carcinoma may arise. Various tumors of the brain follow injection into the cranial cavity. If insufflated into the trachea, bronchogenic carcinoma may develop. These are all direct applications and the type of tumor depends upon the tissue treated. Somewhat less direct, perhaps, is the induction of leukemia by painting susceptible mice. The various laboratory animals do not all show equal effects. In any case, dosage must be appropriate. (See Cook and Kennaway for general review.)

Tars have been prepared from various vegetable materials, including tobacco, but the degree of their activity is in dispute. It cannot be said from these experiments that the amount of tar produced by smoking is of practical importance. Following studies of products of scarlet red, it was discovered that certain amino-azo compounds produce tumors of the liver either upon subcutaneous injection or feeding. Among these is p-dimethyl-amino-benzene, butter yellow. Fed to rats it produces cirrhosis, hepatoma and carcinoma of the liver. The mechanism of these effects upon an organ remote from the site of introduction is not yet understood, but as far as butter yellow is concerned modification of the diet may greatly or entirely inhibit its effect. Evidently it operates through the medium of enzymes or other substances in the body. (See Caldwell.)

The resemblance of the structural formula of some of the polycyclic cancerogenic hydrocarbons to that of the sex hormones has led to attempts to establish a relationship. As will be indicated in the section on Hormones, estrogenic substances incite carcinoma in secondary sex organs and certain of the hydrocarbons are estrogenic. Nevertheless, in a general way, the better the cancerogenic activity, the less the estrogenic; and the better the estrogenic, the less the cancerogenic.

Substances other than the hydrocarbons such as diodrast, hydrochloric acid and sugars, may lead to the development of sarcoma upon repeated injection, but this does not occur regularly and the action does not appear to be specific.

In spite of the chemical relationship between some of the cancerogenic hydrocarbons and substances in the body, such as bile acids and sex hormones, there is no clear indication that these natural substances in natural amounts are cancerogenic. Nevertheless, extracts of the liver yield substances of the general order of lipids, which produce carcinoma when painted on the skin of the mouse or various tumors upon injection. The amount is said to be somewhat greater in patients with carcinoma than in those without and is rich in the liver of the Bantu natives of the Dutch East Indies and southern Africa, in whom primary carcinoma of the liver is common. (See Kleinenberg et al.; Des Ligneris; Heger; Steiner.)

Parasites. Although it may be true that tumor cells lead a sort of parasitic existence in the host, nevertheless, all the primary or spontaneous tumors are made up of cells which originated within the host. This has no direct bearing on the influence of parasites introduced from without. Tumors may, however, develop in fields of chronic irritation or chronic inflammation produced by parasites. Thus, as has been mentioned, tumors may develop occasionally on the basis of tuberculosis or of syphilis. Tumors may occur in connection with diseases due to higher vegetable parasites such as blastomycosis, and are observed in diseases due to the higher animal parasites such as bilharziasis (Brumpt). In these instances it is unlikely that the parasite operates in any other way than through irritation and chronic inflammation. Certain arguments have been propounded, supposedly in favor of the infectious origin of tumors. Cancer houses and cancer streets have been reported in the older literature, but more careful examination with modern epidemiologic methods shows no basis for support of this hypothesis. Tumors do not occur in epidemic form and in the observations of tumors among lower animals, particularly mice, no evidence can be presented for cage infection or epidemics of any kind. Much time has been spent in studying supposed parasitic inclusions in tumor cells. The Russell fuchsin body has been shown to be simply a form of hyaline degeneration of the cells. The "bird's eye" inclusion, showing a deeply stained central body with a surrounding areola, is chiefly the result of secretory processes. Bacteria, such as *Micrococcus neoformans*, higher vegetable organisms, such as the *Saccharomyces neoformans*, various protozoa and other parasites, have not been shown to have any significance as concerns human cancer. (See Warren.)

Experimentally, Bullock and Curtis have observed production of sarcoma following the implantation of the larval forms of the cat parasite, *Taenia crassicolis*, into rats. This excites inflammation with the production of connective tissue, which in turn becomes sarcomatous. Fibiger was thought to have produced metastasizing carcinoma of the fore-stomach of rats by feeding them a nematode, *Gongylonema neoplasticum*, but it is likely that the deficient diet he used produced the lesions of epithelial hyperplasia of the stomach and that the disease is not malignant (Cramer). Crown gall of plants, such as that due to *Phytomonas tumefaciens*, is probably due to inflammatory proliferation rather than neoplastic growth (see Riker and Berge).

Viruses. The only known tumorous lesion of man which may be transferred by filtrates is the cutaneous wart, but there is no certainty that this is a true neoplasm. Claude and Murphy describe many tumors of the fowl, including the Rous sarcoma, which are transferable by filtrates; Lucké's tumor of the frog is in the same category. The Shope papilloma of the rabbit and certain other tumors and tumor-like conditions can be transferred in the same way. The Shope papilloma becomes transformed into carcinoma, but this is not true of all the papillomas nor does it occur in all animals. The virus certainly induces the papilloma, but whether the virus produces the carcinoma or whether the cells are altered so that other factors bring about the change is uncertain. Indirect evidence points to the virus as the cause of both the papilloma and the carcinoma. Certain changes must take place in the papilloma cells before their conversion into carcinoma cells, even though they are not demonstrable morphologically. There are strains of rabbits in which the virus papilloma does not ordinarily develop into carcinoma, but if the papillomas be painted with tar, the transformation takes place. Conversely the virus may excite malignant change in benign tar tumors. Certainly in both carcinomas and sarcomas due to viruses, the cells become altered to constitute a self-perpetuating group of cells. There is an intricate relationship of virus, cells and host, not yet clearly understood, which produces permanent changes in the character of the cells, transmissible either by filtrates or the cells themselves. (See Rous, et al.; Kidd, et al.) Cells can be destroyed by roentgen rays without injury to the virus, the virus remaining active in the production of tumor. In the chapter on Infectious Diseases there was a brief discussion of the nature of viruses, with the indication that they are obligate parasites. How they operate in the production of tumors is not known but it is difficult or impossible to ascribe this to observable irritation or inflammation. In the sense that they are introduced from without, they should be looked upon as extrinsic factors. It is, however, a far cry from the demonstration that viruses cause certain tumors to a generalization that they cause all tumors or even a large group of tumors.

Intrinsic Factors

The term intrinsic in this connection refers to factors within those cells which become neoplastic, and to factors that originate in the body as a whole. As with the extrinsic factors just discussed, the main problem deals with the mechanisms by which cell growth becomes autonomous and unrestrained. Of the many theories that have been proposed, a few are selected for discussion here. Reference has been made above to the probability that the interaction of intrinsic and extrinsic factors brings about the development of tumors and that the intrinsic factors are in a sense preparatory for the extrinsic or realization factors. The following outline refers first to those factors which are related to the body as a whole. Included in these are the possibility of embryonal displacement of cells, the possibility of alteration of balance between groups of cells, and the influence of endocrines and of vitamins. Secondly are certain properties which are intrinsic in the cells themselves, factors which operate in reversion of the cells toward embryonal forms, and cellular characters of hereditary origin.

Embryonal Theory. Often called the Cohnheim theory, this presupposes that during embryonal life certain groups of cells are misplaced and subsequently may go on to the production of neoplasms. Presumably they retain a power to grow which is excited by some factors within or near them. Reference has been made to the hamartoma, such as the hemangioma, the choristoma, such as the misplaced adrenal cortex in the kidney, and the progonoma, which is represented by the cutaneous nevus. In various circumstances these may become transformed into malignant tumors. The only condition about which there is real information is that the nevus may, because of repeated injury, become transformed into a melanoma. Of interest also are the teratomas, which are masses made up of representatives of all three layers of the embryo. To a certain extent in the ovary and probably to a greater extent in the testis, elements of these masses may become transformed into malignant tumors. Then, too, in positions in which one tissue meets another during embryonal development, there may be a growth of malignant tumors. Thus, carcinoma may develop in the nasolabial folds and the same may be true of remnants of branchial clefts. Remnants of the notochord, situated in the pelvis and at the base of the skull, may become transformed into tumor, the chordoma, which in certain instances may become invasive.

Accessory and supernumerary tissues, such as breast, adrenal, thyroid and parathyroid, may become tumorous. The undescended testis is more likely to show tumor growth than that which has descended normally. The Cohnheim theory fails to explain why these residual structures undergo transformation so that the cells take on unrestrained and autonomous growth. Experimental observations have given no confirmation. The occurrence of occupational tumors and of experimental tumors excited by polycyclic hydrocarbons is not in line with the theory. The observation of early tumors, such as carcinoma of the skin, fail to indicate any embryonal misplacement as a source of origin. A. Fischer proposes a theory not exactly like, but somewhat resembling the Cohnheim theory. He made repeated subcutaneous injections, into the groin, of fragments of normal mammary gland and found that in some instances these fragments become carcinomas. He assumed that this was because the tissue of the mammary gland contained a few isolated cells, which in the unusual environment underwent malignant change. He does not explain fully the realization factor and there has been no confirmation of his results.

Cell Relations. Tissue Tension. In the development and differentiation which produces the various structures of the body, there is evidently a normal balance of growth so that the neighboring elements exercise a restraint one upon another. Two main theories have been offered to account for the loss of tissue tension or tissue balance that occurs in tumor growth. The Thiersch hypothesis supposed that as life advances there is a deterioration of connective tissue so that restraint upon other cells is removed; this permits the cells removed from restraint to multiply beyond natural limits. The Waldeyer theory is that senescence leads to loss of vigor of growth of epithelial cells so that the consequent proliferation of the connective tissue in the immediate neighborhood isolates the epithelial cell masses. These cells become necrotic but enough may remain to form cysts, or if there be certain changes in the connective tissues such as chronic inflammation, malignant proliferation may take place. Both these theories were made at a time when it was supposed that the tumor growth evident in later life was initiated in senescence, whereas modern information indicates that the tumor starts long before it becomes evident.

In contrast to the Cohnheim theory it is possible that postnatal isolation of cell groups may occur in chronic inflammations and in long standing ulcers of epithelial surfaces. Reference has been made to the carcinoma which may take its origin in a chronic inflammation such as tuberculosis of the lung. It has been shown that in chronic ulcers of the skin, epithelial cells become isolated and may grow to produce cancer (Knox). This isolation may represent a loss of normal tissue tension but does not in itself account for malignant proliferation. Burrows and Johnston, basing their conclusions principally on the study of tissue cultures, claimed that there is a driving substance of the cell, which they named archusia; this is ordinarily diffused into the body fluids, but when cell groups are isolated and crowded together it may accumulate and excite inordinate proliferation. This does not explain how the isolation of the cells would prevent the diffusion of this substance into the rest of the body, nor does it explain the concentration in that situation. Tumor-like changes have been observed in tissue cultures of mammary tissue and of monocytes, but there has been no proof that these ever develop into true tumors either in the culture or upon injection into experimental animals. Fundamental to the theory of tissue tension is the proposition that something occurs in the cells of the tumor to render them autonomous. When that takes place the balance of tissue tension is lost, but none of the theories explains the origin of the independent autonomous growth.

Endocrine Influences. Although tumors of endocrine glands may produce secretions which stimulate other glands, there is little evidence that tumors are actually produced in these other glands. The problems that have been studied concern the question as to whether or not endocrines may directly excite tumor growth and whether or not they have an influence on the progress of such growth. The relationships in man are not altogether clear. As a matter of fact, however, although not always the case, mammary carcinoma and prostatic carcinoma are more likely to occur after cessation of sexual activity. Furthermore, it is observed that pregnancy may stimulate mammary carcinoma to active growth. Experimentally the problems have been pursued further. One of the earliest observations was that of Loeb, who found that if in female mice of a strain which frequently develops spontaneous mammary carcinoma, the ovaries are removed early in life, the incidence of carcinoma is strikingly reduced. This does not prevail if the ovariectomy be performed in later life nor does the administration of ovarian extract alter the influence of the ovariectomy. Subsequently it was observed that the prolonged administration of large quantities of estrogen to inbred mice increases the incidence of mammary carcinoma in males of a susceptible strain, but although it does not increase the incidence of females of the same strain, the tumors appear earlier. The reports on resistant strains differ, but the most recent work indicates that estrogens do not produce mammary tumors in such animals. Evidently the estrogens do not overcome hereditary factors of resistance. (See Haagensen and Randall.) It has not been claimed that this is the direct action of the estrogen but rather that the estrogens excite conditions in the mammary gland which favor the subsequent development of carcinoma. This is not true in the rabbit so that it evidently has species limitations.

The synthesis of stilbestrol, a somewhat toxic steroid which has much the same effect as estrogen, has stimulated further experimental work. Repeated injections of this substance will bring about the development of mammary carcinoma. In the male mice of a strain resistant to mammary carcinoma, injections are followed by growth of a tumor of the testis resembling the embryonal carcinoma (Shimkin, et al.). The studies of Lipschütz and his associates show that stilbestrol administered to guinea-pigs incites the growth of fibromyoma, occurring both in the uterus and in other parts of the peritoneal cavity. This action is much more pronounced in female guinea-pigs than in males, but the sex difference is probably a sex-linked factor rather than hormonal. Although the subcutaneous injection of estrogens is followed by development of carcinoma of the breast, the direct application of stilbestrol in pellets will lead to tumors of the breast which recede after the pellets are removed. Thus, although the general action appears to be that of permanent alteration of the cells, that does not seem to be true when the substance is applied directly. The influence of androgens has not been extensively studied as yet but it is of interest that in mammary adenofibroma it is found that estrogens stimulate the epithelial component and that androgens inhibit it (Heiman). The influence of pituitary extracts, however, is such that their administration will inhibit the development of mammary carcinoma in mice of a strain which is highly susceptible (Cramer). Urinary prolans favor the development of carcinoma of the rabbit's uterus but only after there has been a prolonged period of inflammation. It has been found that chemical injury to the fowl testis by certain zinc compounds is followed by growth of a teratoma but it is most effective during the period when the bird is sexually active; this also occurs if anterior pituitary extract be administered. Reference has been made to the resemblance of the structural chemical formula of certain carcinogens and the sex hormones. It is the rule, however, that the higher the cancerogenic activity, the lower the estrogenic activity and the higher the estrogenic activity, the lower the cancerogenic activity.

Vitamins. In the discussion of vitamin deficiencies, reference was made to various cutaneous lesions that may occur, but it has not been shown that any of these leads to the development of tumors. Vitamin A is present in tumors and may aid in diagnosis. A decrease of vitamin A in the body or in the cells is not a necessary prerequisite to tumor formation (Popper and Ragins; Baumann, et al.). The epithelial metaplasia of vitamin-A deficiency has not led to neoplasia. It is said that vitamin-B_1 deficiency may lead to epithelial hyperplasia but no tumor has developed. It is reported that deficiency of pantothenic acid favors an increase in the rate of tumor growth in mice (Morris and Lippincott). Entirely theoretic is Lawrence's suggestion that biotin, by virtue of its avidin-like properties, may influence the development of tumors, but no proof has yet been offered for this assumption.

Vitamin C is taken up readily by various tumors and its addition to the culture medium favors the growth of mouse sarcoma in tissue culture. It is probably of great importance in intracellular metabolism. There is no proof that vitamin D has any direct bearing on tumor growth. Nevertheless, cholesterol may produce tumors upon repeated injection. It is now practically certain that cholesterol plays no part in the development of carcinoma of the skin caused by ultraviolet irradiation. Adamstone reports that destruction of vitamin E in the diet is followed by the development of lymphosarcoma in chicks and suggests that this is due to some alteration of metabolism of anthracene compounds. This has yet to be confirmed. Feeding of extracts of wheat germ oil was reported to have produced sarcoma in rats, but whether it contains vitamin E or not, there are many publications to show that it does not produce tumors of any kind (Ginzton and Connor). Certain vitamins, then, may have an influence on growth of tumors but do not cause them.

Factors Intrinsic to the Cell. The questions involved in this connection concern (1) properties of neoplastic cells that distinguish them from their normal prototypes and (2) origin of factors within the cell that produce autonomous growth. Cowdry's excellent analysis of the subject shows that there are dissimilarities and similarities in the normal and neoplastic cell, but none of these is distinctive. The dissimilarities include: (1) alteration of polarity, (2) alteration in structure of cells with enlargement of cytoplasmic and nuclear components and an increased size of nucleolus out of proportion to that of nucleus (increased nucleolar-nuclear ratio) together with increased water content and decreased viscosity of both cell and nucleus, (3) decreased power of differentiation except for those tumors that originate in embryonal types of cells, (4) decreased dependence of oxygen supply, (5) decreased control of organization, with development of autonomy, (6) more ready transplantability, and (7) increased invasiveness. The similarities include: (1) both may be classified into various types that breed true, (2) increased differentiation is accompanied by decreased multiplication and vice versa, (3) decreased water content inhibits cell division and vice versa, (4) when in undifferentiated state both can multiply indefinitely, (5) motility and invasiveness may occur in both, (6) both may be entered by and support viruses, and (7) both may undergo retrogressive changes. Chemically, malignant tumors may be high in content of cholesterol, cholesterol esters, and phospholipins and low in calcium, but this is not an essential peculiarity. Thus, neither in structure nor in function is there any explanation for the development of a new autonomous race of cells.

Murphy and his associates assume that all cells may have the potentiality to become malignant, and that their growth and differentiation depend upon a balance within them of certain stimulators and inhibitors. The accumulation of stimulator or the reduction of inhibitor might produce conditions that lead to unlimited growth. There are interesting observations in support of this but no final proof.

Another suggestion is that groups of cells may be situated so that they cannot exercise function but may receive nutrition. Thus the vegetative function predominates and a "habit of growth" is formed. Others attribute this to changes in the nuclei. Neither of these theories explains autonomy of growth. Another theory is that in addition to the trephones of Carrel, which stimulate

multiplication, there are the desmones of Fischer, which are supposed to regulate growth. Normal cells use their own desmones; if cells utilize desmones of other cells, abnormal growth takes place.

The fact that tumor cells are a distinct race has led to the suggestion that this is due to mutation. If so, it is unusual in that it is a somatic mutation. Those who support this view look upon the change as gradual rather than the abrupt phenomenon of genetic mutation. Nevertheless, it is likely that changes in genes and chromosomal complex, if they occur in tumors, are secondary and not primary. The theory of mutation is not well supported (Lewis). The conception of dedifferentiation and anaplasia deal with presumably intrinsic changes in the cell.

DEDIFFERENTIATION. ANAPLASIA. The term dedifferentiation is a translation of a German word Entdifferenzierung and indicates a reversal of differentiation back toward embryonal-cell types. The parent cells of the tumor are supposed to have reached mature development and then to have retrogressed in differentiation. This retrogression may vary from the minor degrees observed in the large mononuclear cells of inflammation to marked reversion in tumor cells. In the latter instance the cell has not resumed true embryonal potentialities, since embryonal cells tend to differentiate whereas tumor cells do not. Von Hansemann offered the hypothesis of "anaplasia," a retrogression of differentiation together with increased capacity for multiplication. Beneke doubted that cells can actually revert in the sense of anaplasia, ignoring the morphologic and other evidence in its favor, and proposed the term "kataplasia" to indicate simple loss of function and increase in growth capacity. These theories are not in harmony with the known function of certain tumors and do not explain the origin of the change. By none of these theories is the pathologic character of the cell multiplication adequately explained.

Goodpasture, as a result of the study of senescence and tumor formation in dogs, reached the conclusion that senescence of cells is of the utmost importance in explaining dedifferentiation. Progressive cellular differentiation and multiplication ultimately results in senescence, which in its turn may lead to alterations of structure and function, perhaps with the accumulation of injurious products of metabolism. Many cells die and the remainder may either show no change or lose specialization. As specialization is lost, capacity for growth may increase. Lesser degrees of loss of specialization may be restored by regeneration. With extreme degrees of dedifferentiation, growth capacity becomes dominant and tumor growth may occur. It cannot be said that the biologic characters of tumor cells are satisfactorily explained by these hypotheses of dedifferentiation or anaplasia. Although anaplasia has a broader connotation, the term is often used in a morphologic sense to indicate lack of differentiation in tumors.

Heredity. The part played by genetic constitution in tumors is discussed here on the basis of observations in man and in experimental animals. In either it is recognized that heredity plays but one part in the genesis of tumors and that extrinsic factors may confuse results. The difficulty of studies of hereditary factors in tumors of man, in addition to those just mentioned, is the marked hybridization of the race. Nevertheless there is a familial distribution of tumors that exceeds the likelihood of chance incidence. Neurofibromatosis, cartilaginous exostosis, xeroderma pigmentosum, adenomatous polyposis of the colon, benign cystic epithelioma and retinoblastoma occur in several generations and appear to be hereditary. As Weller points out in his study of retinoblastoma, it is difficult to determine exact mendelian factors and it is likely that predisposition is inherited rather than tumor itself. Some of these conditions are benign and a realization factor operates to excite malignancy. The occurrence of two or more tumors in the same patient is greater than would be expected on the basis of chance alone and points strongly toward a constitutional factor that may well be inherited (Warren and Gates; Tullis).

Studies of twins indicate that hereditary factors are important in determination of comparable situations, type of tumor and age of onset (Macklin). The analysis of the famous cancer family of Warthin by Hauser and Weller adduces further evidence that heredity operates not only in determining the incidence of tumors but also their location, for example, the uterus in one group, and the intestine in another. Waaler made critical studies of 600 cases of cancer in Sweden and found that certain tumors, such as those of breast, uterus and ovaries, follow a distributional pattern indicative of hereditary factors, but that certain others such as carcinoma of the lip do not. In spite of the heterozygous character of man and the extrinsic factors which may operate, it is reasonable to assume that hereditary factors may determine the incidence and situation of cancer, but the mechanisms are not and perhaps cannot be unraveled.

As in man, so in experimental animals, the studies of epithelial tumors yield the greatest information. Although evidence has been gained from other animals, mice are the main source. Slye has observed an enormous number of mice (now over 140,000) as to incidence of tumors, confirmed by autopsy, and has shown convincingly that there is a hereditary factor of susceptibility to spontaneous tumors and that this applies also to the site of growth. Her studies indicate that susceptibility is a simple mendelian recessive. Lynch views the factor as semidominant. Little, however, thinks that a greater homogeneity of genetic constitution obtained by long in-breeding may tell a somewhat different story. It is probable that hereditary factors operate differently in such tumors as mammary and pulmonary carcinomas of the mouse. This indicates a certain complexity of genetic factors not completely clarified by reference to a single or several genes. Nevertheless the evidence points more to a dominant than a recessive trait. In addition, the experiments of Little and his associates favor the idea that extrachromosomal factors are of great importance. His analysis of the mammary epithelial tumors lends support to this view, as does the discovery of his associate Bittner that the milk of female mice of a high mammary cancer stock transmits something to the young that favors the development of mammary carcinoma. This factor is found in the blood also, but it is confined to that one type of tumor and does not apply to carcinoma of the mouse lung. In so far as can be said now, there is a hereditary factor in mice that determines incidence and situation of epithelial tumors. This depends to a considerable degree on chromosomal factors, but exactly how it operates is not settled. In addition, certain extrachromosomal factors play a part. It is of interest that no evidence points to comparable factors in nonepithelial tumors.

Genetic constitution is also studied in reference to transplantable and artificially induced tumors. Transplantable tumors grow better in some strains than in others. Some strains are highly resistant, others are highly susceptible and others in intermediate groups. That this is not a biologic factor of error is shown by selective in-breeding. This can produce families with such genetic uniformity that the percentage of takes is practically constant. (See also Jackson; Wells; Eggers; Blank.)

Evidence has accumulated to the effect that there are strains of animals more susceptible to the effects of tar than are others. This presumably represents the influence of genetic constitution. Nevertheless if dosage be adequate, resistance can be overcome. Thus the extrinsic or realization factor exceeds genetic resistance. Mention has been made of the sarcoma which develops in rats infested with *Taenia crassicollis*. Curtis, Dunning and Bullock have found that susceptibility to invasion of the parasite is heritable. Hence the development of this sarcoma is more likely in susceptibles than in others.

This discussion of heredity makes it evident that direct application to the individual human patient is inadvisable. If the genetic constitution of man were ever to be made uniform, his susceptibilities and resistances might be analyzed so that groups or individuals could be classified. That such homogeneity is desirable is a matter for only the most wise; to put it into practice would be a further problem of no mean proportions. In the meantime, heredity can be accepted as a factor in the etiology of cancer in man, but its exact mode of operation has not been explained.

Summary

In this general discussion of etiology, various hypotheses have been discussed, some well founded and others not. However, a few facts emerge. The tumor cell possesses a totality of characters which distinguish it from its normal progenitor; it becomes an independent autonomous race. Although the intimate nature of this change is not disclosed, it is conditioned by various extrinsic and intrinsic factors. Irritation is the most important of the extrinsic factors, with the possible exception of the viruses. Intrinsic factors include age, sex, race, etc., and particularly genetic constitution.

The formula, extrinsic plus intrinsic factors equals tumor, has been mentioned. There are variables in both of these factors which influence the result. In susceptibles, tumor may be produced by a degree of irritation less than is necessary in the more resistant. Yet irritation may be of sufficient magnitude to effect tumor growth in resistant individuals, as shown with tar carcinomas. Thus the factor of resistance in the equation is reduced or nullified and the factor of irritation becomes predominant. There are tumors, such as the retinoblastoma, in whose development no known factor of irritation operates. In these instances, the extrinsic factor is practically deleted from the equation and the intrinsic factor equals tumor. Hence the summation of the two factors is not always essential, but certainly it operates for most tumors. This is the simplest statement of etiology that can be made. That it does not cover all details is apparent. That it may be changed or abandoned as the result of further research is obvious.

PART II: PATHOLOGY OF SPECIAL TUMORS

CONNECTIVE-TISSUE TUMORS

Introduction

According to classification, the connective-tissue tumors are derivatives of fibrous tissue, cartilage, bone, muscle, vessels, etc., as well as the connective tissue of the central nervous system even though it is of ectoblastic origin. Sometimes more than one tissue is incorporated in the tumor and combined names are used, such as fibromyoma, osteochondroma and the like, the latter part of the name representing the major component. In certain instances, benign tumors may recur after surgical removal; where that is true it will be noted. The type tumor of the benign connective-tissue group is the fibroma.

Benign Tumors

Fibroma. The fibroma is composed essentially of white fibrous connective tissue and may originate in any situation where this type of tissue is found. Such tumors occur in the skin, subcutaneous tissue, fascias of various kinds including sheaths of muscle and nerve, periosteum, in the connective tissue of mucous membranes, and are observed also in solid organs such as the breast, kidney and ovary. The common tumor of the uterus is usually a fibromyoma. Grossly, the tumors vary considerably in size, may reach large dimensions, and may be single or multiple.

cross section is pale. The bulging, somewhat moist, pallid cross section shows whorls of tissue, giving the surface the appearance of "watered silk." If a capsule be present the cross section bulges beyond the capsule. Unusual vascularity, hemorrhage, degenerative and necrotic changes are likely to exhibit their characteristic alterations both upon the outer surface and in the cross section. The soft fibroma is likely to show a gelatinous cross section.

Microscopically, the characteristic cell is the connective-tissue cell, which may appear either as a relatively young connective

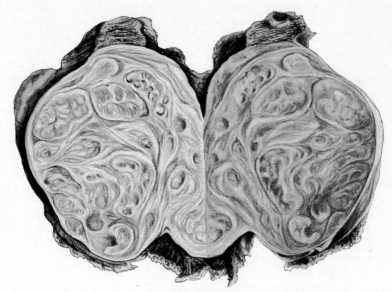

Fibroma of muscle showing encapsulation and the "watered silk" appearance of the cut surface.

In the smaller tumors measuring a few millimeters in diameter a capsule is often not found, but as the tumors increase in size they are definitely encapsulated as a rule. The consistency is variable, but usually the tumor is very firm and is often spoken of as hard fibroma or fibroma durum. Some of the tumors are soft, particularly as the result of edema or degenerative change, and these are referred to as soft fibroma or fibroma molle. This distinction, however, has little practical value in determining the nature of the growth. The tumor cuts with considerable resistance, even when soft, and usually bulges above the cross section of the surrounding tissue. Unless unusually well supplied with blood vessels the tumor both on the outer surface and in the

tissue cell or fibroblast, or the older type with longitudinally striated cytoplasm. The nucleus may be of oval or spindle form, and varies in chromatin density with the maturity of the cell. In any case, the section shows interlacing whorls of parallel cells and fibers which may be cut longitudinally, obliquely or transversely. Mitotic figures are extremely rare. Usually the tumor is poorly vascularized and the larger vessels are carried in fibrous-tissue septa which may divide the tumor into more or less definite lobules. The vessels are likely to follow finer division of the septa, which then appear in the form of a delicate reticulum, and ultimately communicate with very small vessels in the substance of the tumor. The finest vessels appear as vascular slits in the substance of the tumor but are by no means numerous. A few lymph spaces may be found and occasionally also nerve fibers, probably included as the tumor grows. Special stains show the fibroglia fibrils of Mallory. The cellular content of the tumor varies somewhat with its age. The younger tumors are rich in cells and show relatively little collagenous material, but as the tumor ages the collagen increases in amount and the cells are relatively less numerous and arranged compactly. The capsule appears as strands of dense connective tissue, arranged circumferentially about the tumor and usually poor in nuclei. The surrounding tissue is likely to show some degree of compression.

Degenerative changes are not uncommon and the most frequent is hyaline transformation of the collagenous material. Mucoid degeneration may suggest an associated myxoma. Infiltration of small amounts of fat is sometimes observed. Necrosis is fairly frequent in the larger tumors. Calcification is not uncommon. If the tumor be pedunculated, twisting of the pedicle may lead to passive hyperemia, hemorrhage and complete or partial necrosis. Surface tumors are subject to erosion and secondary infection.

Many of the tumors called xanthoma are really fibromata in which the cells are infiltrated with yellow lipoid pigment, but in some instances the pigmented cells predominate and the condition is regarded as a xanthoblastoma.

A fibroma may appear at any time of life but is more frequent in later middle life. The tumors arise insidiously and grow slowly. According to the usual criteria the fibroma is benign in character, but may produce serious disturbance of function owing to compression of, or traction upon, surrounding tissue. The sharp limitation of the tumor makes complete removal simple, but a few cases of incomplete removal have been followed by recurrence.

Combination of the fibroma with other types of tumor is common, such as the fibromyoma of the uterus and the fibro-adenoma of the breast. A fairly common special variety of the fibroma is spoken of as cheloid or keloid. This is most common in the black race, and in the neighborhood of the face and hands where trauma may occur. The origin of the keloid is usually in scars. Grossly, it is a more or less nodular or lobulated mass, projected above the skin and showing the pale, glossy surface of a scar. Although movable, it is not encapsulated. Cross section shows a pale, glossy surface with very little suggestion of whorls. Microscopically, the mass is poor in cells and rich in collagen. Dense heavy bands of fibrils are separated by lines of more cellular material and the overlying epidermis is flattened as is usual in scars. The tendency to recurrence after removal is striking because of the disposition of this tumor to grow in scars, and removal necessarily leaves a scar in its track. Small foci of lymphocytes are often seen in the keloid, suggesting that the lesion is inflammatory rather than neoplastic. Certain authorities look upon it as a hyperplastic scar, but it is tentatively regarded as tumor by most investigators.

NEUROFIBROMA may occur in widespread multiple form to constitute the disease called fibroma molluscum, multiple neurofibromatosis or von Recklinghausen's disease. In this condition the nodules may be distributed along the course of cutaneous or other nerves, or irregularly. The skin over subcutaneous nodules is often pigmented. It often occurs in several members of the same family (Siemens), may be associated with various dysontogenetic defects (Winestine), and with melanoma of nerves or skin. The neurofibroma may also occur as a single or a few discrete tumors. In this form it may be superficial in the skin, or more deeply situated especially in relation to acoustic or other nerves and to periosteum. Solitary or multiple neurofibromas vary in diameter from a few millimeters to several centimeters, are generally globular, firm, pallid, well defined but not always encapsulated, and often show a nerve trunk in intimate relationship. One of the varieties of neurofibroma is the plexiform neurofibroma, which is usually solitary, affects especially face, scalp or buttocks, and gives rise to a plexiform or cirsoid arrangement of bundles of connective tissue and tortuous or coiled nerve fibers. Microscopically, the neurofibroma often resembles the fibroma, but is likely to show many delicate wavy fibrils and small whorls of cells and fibrils. In many neurofibromas, especially those of sensory nerves, particularly the acoustic, there are rows of cells with palisade arrangement of nuclei and an intervening band of parallel wavy fibrils. The tumor is usually benign, except for pressure effects, as of the acoustic neurofibroma. Malignant transformation occurs more especially in the tumors of deep nerve trunks of the extremities, and the outcome is the neurogenous sarcoma (Stewart and Copeland). This is grossly invasive and metastasizes. Microscopically it is like the fibrosarcoma or spindle cell sarcoma, but the wavy fibrils and minute whorls may be seen.

The neurofibroma does not arise from the axis cylinders. Whether it is derived from the supporting connective tissue of the nerves or from the cells of the sheath of Schwann is a matter of controversy (Bailey and Herrmann), but we favor the latter. The cellular picture of the neurogenous sarcoma often resembles that of melanoblastoma and in patients with either tumor, intermedin may be demonstrated in the urine.

Nasal polyps occur as large, soft, pallid, gelatinous, pedunculated masses attached to the lateral walls of the nose near the openings of the accessory sinuses. Microscopically, they are covered by ciliated columnar epithelium and consist of edematous connective tissue, often infiltrated with lymphoid and large mononuclear cells and eosinophils. The connective tissue cells are of spindle form and stellate, and are separated by edema. The mucous glands may become adenomatous in certain polyps or even adenocarcinomatous, and occasionally large cysts of epithelial mucus are encountered. The nature of the lesion and the usual history of nasal inflammation indicate that the polyps are inflammatory. Nevertheless, a true tumor may occur, the juvenile nasopharyngeal fibroma, firm, widely extensive, and composed of both fibrous tissue and elastica.

Chondroma. The chondroma is made up either of hyaline or fibrocartilage. It is often difficult to differentiate it from ecchondrosis or hyperplasia of cartilage. Ecchondroses appear in connection with permanent cartilage, are multiple, of rather limited growth and reduplicate in their structure the cartilage from which they are derived. The chondroma, on the other hand, although it may appear as a multiple tumor, shows the departure from normal in structure and growth which is characteristic of tumors. Not infrequently the term enchondroma is used to distinguish the tumor from the simple hyperplasia. Kettle divides the chondromas into three classes: "(a) Those growing in relation to bones, especially the pelvis, the long bones and the bones of the fingers; (b) in situations where cartilage is normally present, such as the larynx; (c) in organs where cartilage is absent, chiefly the ovaries and testicles and salivary glands." The appearance of a chondroma· may be preceded by local injury. In several instances a distinct hereditary disposition has been noted. Grossly, the chondroma is a dense, solid tumor often lobulated and divided by connective-tissue septa. It cuts with great resistance and shows a firm, pale, glossy cross section in which lobulation is fairly distinct. Microscopically, the tumor shows irregularly disposed spherical or more rarely stellate cartilage cells, in lacunae of varying size and arrangement. The cytoplasm occasionally shows vacuoles. In many tumors the areola about the cells is not clearly defined. The intercellular material may be the usual hyalin or a fibrillated fibrocartilaginous substance; occasionally elastic tissue is present. The vascular supply is carried in the connective tissue septa between the lobules. Various retrogressive changes may take place. Of these, calcification is frequent and this is often followed by ossification. Mucoid degeneration is also common, but whether this is a simple degeneration of the chondroma or a mixture of chondroma and myxoma is hard to decide.

The chondroma may produce serious difficulties as the result of situation. For example, in the pelvic bones it may interfere with labor; in the larynx and trachea it may interfere with respiration. It may completely collapse a lung. Situated in the ovaries, the testes, and in the uterus and even in the breast, the chondroma is usually a part of a teratoma. When the teratoma is malignant, the metastases may contain chondromatous elements. The chondroma itself does not metastasize, but there is a distinct disposition to recur after surgical removal. Malignant transformation produces the chondrosarcoma.

Osteoma. The osteoma is even more difficult than the chondroma to separate from hyperplasia and heteroplasia. Hyperplasia of bone occurs in connection with repeated traumatic insults, and more especially in connec-

tion with inflammation either of the periosteum or of the bone substance itself. In osteomyelitis, extensive and diffuse hyperplasia of
the bone may occur. Similarly, inflammation
of other structures, such as tendons, may
lead to a deposit of bone in or along the tendon, as is well exemplified in rider's bone.
Heteroplastic bone formation, as has been
mentioned in the chapter on Calcification,
may appear in a wide variety of situations,
usually, however, as a result of preceding
chronic inflammation. In addition, a peculiar
form of inflammation of the muscles called
myositis ossificans shows true bone formation.
The true osteoma must therefore arise in situations where it cannot be interpreted as of
inflammatory origin. The pure osteoma is
rare, but may occur in connection with either
long bones, or flat bones such as those of the
head. Deposits of bone in connection with
inflammation are usually referred to as osteophytes. Exostoses are tumor-like projections
from the surface of bones, while enostoses
appear in the substance of the bone or project
into the marrow cavity. Both these and the
true osteomata may be made up of dense
compact bone to form the eburnated variety,
or of spongy bone to form the spongy variety.
Traumatic exostosis may occur at the site of
fractures or in the margins of the alveolar
processes following extraction of teeth.

Osteoma may appear as part of teratoma. Mixtures with other tumors of the
connective tissue group, such as osteofibroma
and osteochondroma, are more common than
pure osteoma. Osteosarcoma occurs in several
distinct varieties, to be discussed in the
chapter on Organs of Locomotion.

The tumorous conditions of teeth and
their anlagen will be discussed in the chapter
on the Alimentary Canal.

Myxoma. The true myxoma is uncommon. The principal component is a mucoid connective tissue, the normal prototype
of which is the Wharton jelly of the umbilical
cord. Epithelial tumors containing mucin are
referred to as mucinous adenomata, mucinous
carcinomata, etc. Connective-tissue mucin,
or mucoid, may appear in inflammatory tissue
and in degenerations of fibroma, lipoma,
chondroma, endothelioma and certain other
tumors. Myxoma may constitute an important part of both teratoid and simple mixed
tumors, and in fact is rarely found as an un-

mixed tumor. The commonest combination
is with chondroma. True myxoma occurs in
subcutaneous and subserous connective tissues, bones, along nerve trunks, in muscle, in
the endocardium, and as a congenital tumor
in or near the umbilicus. Grossly, the tumors
are of variable size and may be pedunculated. They are usually lobulated, pallid,
of soft elastic consistency and may be
only partly encapsulated. They cut easily;
from the soft, bulging, pale, gelatinous

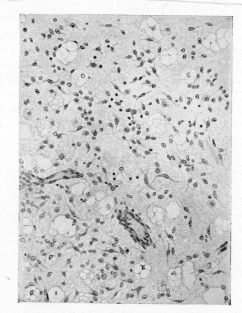

Myxolipoma, showing granular mucoid between the cells.

cross section may be squeezed or scraped
a tenacious, colorless mucoid, soluble in dilute alkali and precipitated by weak acid
solutions.

Microscopically, the characteristic
cells are of spindle form and stellate, with
long interlacing delicate cytoplasmic processes, separated by characteristic basophilic
mucoid, either hyaline or granular. The proportion of cells and mucoid varies even in the
same tumor. Blood vessels are contained in
the septa between lobules and may be much
dilated. Various retrogressive changes, especially hemorrhage, may occur. Mucoid may
usually be differentiated from edema by ordinary stains but in case of doubt the mucicar-
min or thionin stains may be employed. This
is of importance in differentiating between an
edematous fibroma and a true myxoma. The

chemistry of mucoid has been discussed in the chapter on degenerations.

Lipoma. The lipoma, a tumor composed of fat tissue, is of common occurrence. It is derived from a preadipose tissue of mesenchymal origin much as is normal fat. Occasionally it is familial. The most common situation is in the subcutaneous tissue, particularly of the neck and upper parts of the trunk. Nevertheless, such tumors may appear in synovial membranes, along nerve trunks, within the cranial cavity, in the kidneys and other viscera, including the heart. They are sometimes multiple and may even show symmetrical disposition in the body. As a rule of moderate size, they may become extremely large and pedunculated. Excessive growth of fat around the kidneys may form very large perirenal lipomas, and sometimes the whole neck is involved from the face to the shoulders to produce the lipoma annulare colli.

Grossly, small lipomata may have only one lobule but usually the tumor is a well-defined multilobulated tumor, easily removed from the surrounding tissue but with only a thin fibrous capsule. It is soft, elastic in consistency and of the same color as normal fat, except in those instances where a rich admixture of cells of fibrous or other tissues tends to make the color lighter than that of normal fat. It cuts with ease and greases the knife, the cross section being soft, bulging and greasy. Microscopically, the characteristic cell is the large signet-ring cell of adult fat tissue. Certain authorities maintain that the cells of lipoma are larger than those of normal fat tissue, but this is not supported in our experience. Sometimes, embryonal types of fat cells are observed, the cytoplasm studded with small vacuoles and with centrally placed round nucleus. Such cells are likely to be found in the margins of rapidly growing tumors. The septa dividing the tumor into lobules may be of fairly dense connective tissue and support the blood vessels of the tumor. Mucoid degeneration, necrosis and calcification may occur. Occasionally retrogression occurs and serous atrophy of fat is found. Pigmentation may be due to deposits of cholesterol and its esters as in xanthoma.

The chemical composition of the lipoma is like that of normal fat, but it apparently takes no part in fat metabolism of the body. The tumor may even grow in spite of progressive emaciation of the patient.

Pressure upon tubular structures such as esophagus or intestine, growth within these tubes, pressure on the brain in cases of intracranial lipoma, and pressure on nerves may have serious consequences.

The amount of fibrous tissue may be so great as to justify the term fibrolipoma. Combinations with other components are not rare, for example, myxolipoma. There may be a close connection with nerves so that the tumor is tender and painful. Lipoma may be a large component of certain teratoid tumors such as those which may accompany spina bifida. The lipoma is not likely to recur after complete surgical removal. Malignant transformation may take place, but it is likely that most of the liposarcomas are malignant from the start.

Angioma. This is composed of either blood or lymphatic vessels, and is therefore designated as either hemangioma or lymphangioma. It is probably derived from embryonal isolation of mesenchymal tissue and arises by bud-like proliferations of endothelium. It is essentially a hamartoma, although Ewing speaks of it as a tumor. It may become malignant without distinct histologic change, the metastasizing angioma, or may be transformed into an angiosarcoma.

Hemangioma. Localized dilatations of large numbers of blood vessels may occur in connection with granulation tissue, or with varicosities due to stagnation of blood. Sometimes it is difficult to distinguish between these acquired dilatations and true hemangioma. As a rule, the hemangiomata are made up of vessels of capillary character but not necessarily of capillary size. Plexiform angioma, in which the dilated capillaries are elongated and plexiform, is likely to show venules and arterioles but the commoner tumors are more simple in structure. The hemangiomata are usually either of the simple variety, with vessels of small or moderate size, or the cavernous variety with large sinus-like vascular spaces. The simple hemangioma occurs as the birthmark on the skin, more particularly in the face (vascular nevus), but may affect other situations including muscle, viscera and central nervous system. The "port wine" birthmark is said to contain venous blood and the "strawberry" mark arterial blood, but histologically the character is the same. These are to be regarded as simple congenital telangiectases, hamartomatous in type, but they may become blastomatous. They are composed of thin-walled blood vessels, of irregular size and shape, lined by endothelium and separated by a more or less cellular connective tissue. Although not encapsulated they are well defined. They occur in the corium immediately beneath the epiderm. If the intervascular tissue be richly cellular, the cells of endothelial type, the

fibrous connective tissue between. Fibrous septa may divide it into lobules. As with the simple angioma, this form may be combined with endothelial proliferation to form a hemangioendothelioma.

As a rule, the hemangioma is of no importance except for its unsightliness upon the skin. Nevertheless, certain varieties may be serious. It may metastasize without striking alterations in its histology. In certain situations pressure may be serious; paralysis of the legs may be the result of an intraspinal

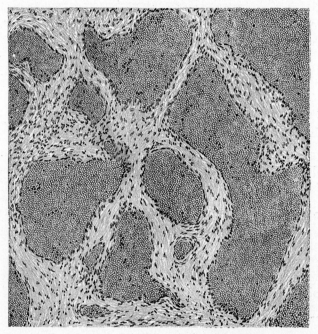

Cavernous hemangioma of the orbit.

lesion is referred to as a hemangio-endothelioma.

The cavernous hemangioma occurs frequently in the liver but may be found in other situations. It is of congenital origin and is hamartomatous (see Moise), but rarely is said to become blastomatous. As usually seen, it appears immediately under the capsule of the liver as a small flat or slightly projecting mass, varying from the usual diameter of a few millimeters up to several centimeters. It is of deep red or purple color, soft, spongy and sharply defined although not always definitely encapsulated. The cross section is spongy and retracts as the blood oozes out. Microscopically, it is made up of vascular sinuses of variable size and shape, with little

hemangioma. One case has been observed in which an angioma of the liver attained enormous size, together with the small amount of remaining liver weighing over 16 kilograms. Hemorrhage from hemangioma of the renal pelvis has led to death.

Lymphangioma. In principle the lymphangioma is like the hemangioma, save that it is composed of lymphatic vessels. The same difficulty arises as to differentiating telangiectases from true angioma. It may appear in the same situations as does the hemangioma. Three forms are described, simple, cavernous, and cystic lymphangioma. The simple forms are likely to occur in the skin as colorless moles. The cavernous lymphangioma is best exemplified by a diffuse mass in the tongue, macroglossia, and a similar condition in the lips, macrocheilia. The cystic lymphangioma is called hygroma. It occurs principally in the neck as hygroma colli cysticum, and rarely in the axilla. It is probably derived from primitive jugular sacs. Present at birth it may extend rapidly. The lymphangioma is usually soft, pale and poorly defined. Diagnosis depends to a considerable degree on the gross appearance in the living patient, because the microscopic appearance may be confused by bleeding into the spaces of the lymphangioma due to operation, or complete drainage of blood from the hemangioma. Lymphangiomas occur also in various viscera.

Dilatation and elongation of lymph vessels in such conditions as elephantiasis are due to obstruction of lymphatic drainage, and accompanied by progressive enlargement and progressive growth of connective tissue; the process is of inflammatory character.

Lymphangiomata may recur after incomplete excision, and occasionally may become malignant. The lymphangio-endothelioma probably originates as such, but may represent the malignant change of a lymphangioma. The mass may obstruct important tubes or may produce serious disturbance because of pressure. (See Walton and McCarthy.)

Lymphoma. The lymphoma is a tumor composed of lymphoid cells. Most tumors of the lymph nodes are either lymphosarcomata or are associated with blood diseases such as leukemia, and at times are difficult to distinguish from granulomata or chronic infection. Indeed a large proportion of the cases called simple lymphoma are probably of infectious origin. The simple lymphoma may appear in any of the subcutaneous chains or even in the deeper nodes, and has been observed in the parotid and other glands and in the viscera. It is slow in growth and after reaching a certain size may remain stationary for many years. Grossly, the tumor may be a single enlarged node, but usually there are several nodes more or less fused together. The tumors are firm and pale and when cut show a smooth, firm, gray surface with no degeneration or necrosis. Microscopically, the architecture of the node is usually obliterated by a diffuse, poorly vascularized proliferation of small lymphocytes, without mitotic figures, but sometimes slightly invading the capsule. The chief danger is from compression of important viscera.

Chordoma. This rare tumor arises from misplaced remnants of the notochord. It is found near the base of the skull, in the region of the cervical vertebrae and near the coccyx. The tumors are usually of little significance but may produce serious symptoms. Grossly, they are soft tumors usually attached to the bone. Like the notochord, the tumors show large globular cells with vesicular cytoplasm, the so-called physaliphora cells, the intercellular substance being a homogeneous mass of mucoid. Careful gross and microscopic study is necessary for the diagnosis, since the myxochondroma and the mucinous carcinoma give somewhat similar microscopic appearances. Recurrence after operation is not uncommon. Chordoma, especially at the base of the skull, may become invasive but only rarely does it metastasize. (See Stewart and Morin; Ramsay; Cappell.)

Myoma. The myomas are tumors composed of muscle. They are of two types, the leiomyoma composed of smooth muscle, and the rhabdomyoma composed of striated muscle and myoblasts. They may be composed entirely of muscle or contain a considerable admixture of connective tissue.

Leiomyoma. Tumors of this type may be found in any position where there is pre-existing smooth muscle, but are particularly frequent in the uterus. They also occur in the stomach, the intestinal tract, the skin, the bladder, in the prostate and not infrequently in the cortex of the kidney. In these situations they are often single and small, although they may attain a diameter of several centimeters so as to obstruct tubular structures. In the uterus, however, the tumors are usually multiple and sometimes grow so that the uterus and its contained tumors weighs several kilograms. The tumors are sharply defined and almost always encapsulated. They are more or less firm, depending in part upon the amount of connective tissue and in part upon the secondary degenerative changes. The color is likely to be somewhat darker than that of the surrounding muscle. They cut with considerable resistance and show a cross section which exhibits the same "watered silk" markings, due to whorls of muscle tissue, as seen in the fibroma. The cross section is softer than that in the fibroma, bulges, and is of the pale red color of muscle. The fibromyoma is often pearly gray in color. Microscopically, the essential cell is the smooth-muscle cell, which is characterized by a fairly rich cytoplasm and a cylindrical vesicular nucleus, long with rounded ends, of the so-called sausage form. Myoglia fibrils can be demonstrated in the cell cuticle by special methods. The cells are

element predominates, because the tumor is essentially a myoma. The term fibroid is incorrect.

As a rule, the leiomyoma is poorly vascularized, but occasionally there is wide dilatation of numerous blood or lymphatic vessels, so that the names lymphangio- and hemangiomyoma are used. In the uterus, epithelial acini may form part of the tumor to constitute the adenomyoma.

Various degenerations may occur. Hyalinization, fatty degeneration and hydropic infiltration may be seen. Edema is

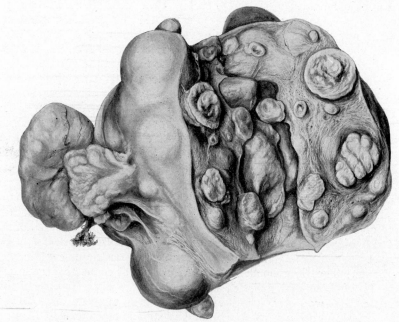

Multiple fibromyomata of the uterus. Note intramural tumor and submucous polypoid tumors. A cystic ovary is present.

arranged in whorls and thus may appear in longitudinal, oblique, or transverse section, in all of which the acidophilic cytoplasm is striking. The character of the cells can usually be made out by ordinary staining methods, but in case of doubt the van Gieson or Mallory connective tissue stain may be employed.

Except in the uterus, the leiomyoma contains but little connective tissue. This is true also of the smaller uterine tumors, but as they enlarge and grow older, connective tissue increases in amount and ultimately may constitute a large part of the nodule. This is called fibromyoma, even if the fibrous

common. Calcification, inflammation, necrosis and hemorrhage are not rare. Necrosis or hemorrhage may lead to cyst formation. When pedunculated, the whole mass may undergo necrosis from twisting of the pedicle. Malignant change sometimes takes place, but this is not common.

RHABDOMYOMA. These tumors may originate in pre-existing striated muscle, when they are called homologous, or may be observed in situations where there is no striated muscle, when they are called heterologous. Although the tumor is a rare tumor under any conditions, the homologous rhabdomyoma has been reported more often in the heart than in other situations. The rhabdomyoma of the heart is practically always congenital and is probably due to embryonal misplacement of muscle fibers or cells. This is supported by the fact that other congenital abnormalities often accompany the tumor, especially tuberous sclerosis of the brain. The lesions in the heart are much more often multiple than solitary. The tumor is fleshy, soft, paler than the surrounding muscle and poorly defined. Microscopically, it is made up of an embryonal type

sacral region and similar tumors of the testis and ovary. Comparable is a tumor which sometimes occurs in the vagina of young children and in the uterus of older women, in which areas of striated muscle are found, the sarcoma botryoides of Pfannenstiel. The rhabdomyoma of the esophagus, the intestinal canal and probably also of the bladder is explained by metaplasia of the original smooth muscle.

MYOBLASTOMA. This occurs particularly in the tongue and lip, although there

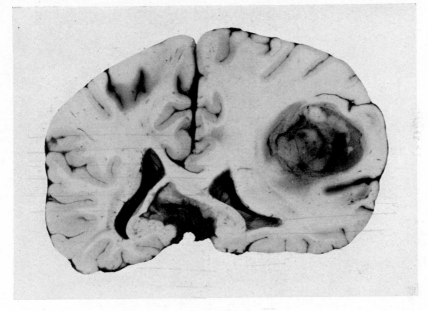

Glioblastoma multiforme of cerebral hemisphere. An illustration of the usual appearance of a glioma.

of muscle cells and striated muscle fibers. The latter are narrow and the transverse striations fairly well separated, with centrally disposed nucleus. Sometimes the fibers show branching. The muscle cells are usually large and often multinucleated. The cytoplasm may be vesicular and often contains tiny rods which resemble the transverse striations in the muscle. Mitotic figures as a rule are infrequent. Rhabdomyoma may also occur in the skeletal muscles, especially of the trunk and extremities. The microscopic picture is much the same. Rhabdomyomatous elements may constitute a small or great part of certain lesions evidently teratoid in character. These include the congenital mixed tumor of the kidney, mixed tumors of the

are occasional reports of it being observed elsewhere. Its incidence is particularly in the third and fourth decades but it may occur as a congenital lesion. Grossly, it is a fleshy, fairly well-defined tumor. Microscopically, muscle fibers are not likely to be found and the mass is made up principally of large cells called myoblasts. These may be multinucleated or have only one nucleus. The cytoplasm is likely to be vesicular and contains the tiny rods indicative of the type of cell.

The rhabdomyoma of the heart is not likely to be malignant. That of skeletal muscle is more often malignant than not. The rhabdomyoma of mixed tumors may take part when those tumors become malignant. The myoblastoma is only rarely malignant.

The subject of muscle tumors is well covered by Geschickter.

Tumors of Nerve Tissues. Tumors of nerve tissues, when regarded in the embryologic sense, should be classified as epithelial, since the nervous system is derived from ectoderm. The cells of the tumors, however, show differentiation in varying degrees and therefore are morphologically unlike epithelium. Few of these tumors show any tendency to metastasize, but many of them are invasive, and by virtue of their situation may produce serious symptoms. It is therefore difficult to regard them as strictly benign, but they usually lack the characters necessary for grouping them as malignant.

GLIOMA. (NEUROGLIOMA). The glioma is composed of neuroglia cells and fibers. It occurs most commonly in the brain, but is also seen in the spinal cord and occasionally in the roots of the cranial nerves. Neuroglia is also found in teratoid tumors. Focalized gliosis, or hyperplasia of neuroglia, is not uncommon and may be confused with glioma. The glioma is usually a solitary tumor varying in size from one to several centimeters in diameter, but may grow to occupy the space of a cerebral hemisphere. It is usually situated in the interior of the brain but may project into the ventricles or upon the outer surface. It is poorly defined and grows by replacing brain tissue; its size may increase intracranial pressure. It is likely to be softer than the brain substance. Its color may be the same as the surrounding substance, but brain markings are obliterated. It is sometimes very pale or, if richly vascularized, is pink or streaked and dotted with red. Hemorrhage is common, as is also necrosis. Cyst formation as the result of hemorrhage or necrosis is frequent, and may also be due to the production of spaces lined by ependyma-like cells.

Microscopically, as pointed out by Bailey and Cushing, the glioma may be composed of a wide variety of cells, and there have been described thirteen types of glioma. The cell type may represent any of the cells which occur in the differentiation of the primary neuro-epithelium to the more mature forms of astrocytes, pineal, choroidal and ependymal cells. Thus, the size and character of the tumor cells vary, and some tumors may contain many glia fibrils and others few

or none. In a general way, the prognosis is better in those tumors where the cells are more highly differentiated. Further details of cell type are given in the chapter on Nervous System. A scattering amount of connective tissue may be present, derived from blood vessels. The blood vessels are of variable size and occasionally angiomatous. Perivascular spaces are found frequently, and sometimes dense masses of glia fibrils surround the ves-

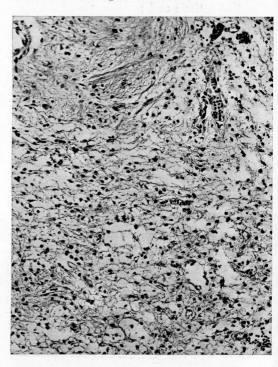

Fibrillary glioma stained by phosphotungstic acid hematoxylin. Note the rich production of fibrils.

sels. Owing to the lack of encapsulation and to destructive and invasive growth, operation is often followed by recurrence. Occasionally, true malignancy is indicated by the occurrence of metastases. The microscopic appearance is not materially altered, and it seems preferable to refer to these as metastasizing or malignant gliomas instead of gliosarcomas. The supposed relation to trauma is not well supported, as indicated previously in the discussion of tumor etiology.

The neuro-epithelioma is a glioma of cellular type, which histologically shows few if any glia fibrils, and an arrangement of cells to form rosettes. The rosette may or may not have a central lumen into which minute rods may project, the primitive rods and cones. From the central portions, cuboidal cells radiate to fuse with the surrounding cell mass. This tumor may occur in various parts of the central nervous system. In the eye it may be bilateral and has a hereditary basis.

NEUROMA. Tumors of nerve tissues are uncommon. Arising from the central nervous system, peripheral nerves and sympathetic system, they may be found in practically any part of the body. They are usually a mixture of nerve cells and nerve fibers. The cellular tumors may be made up in large part, or almost entirely, of cells in any stage of develop-

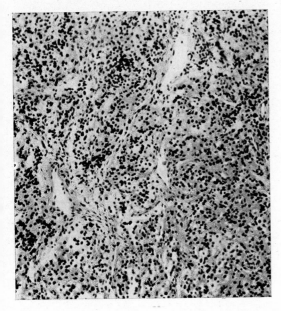

Neuroblastoma of adrenal, to show immature type of cell.

ment from those resembling the primary neuro-ectodermal cells to those of adult type. The cellular tumors are given various names indicating their nature, thus leaving the term neuroma to cover those tumors composed largely of nerve fibers. The cellular tumors are related especially to the sympathetic system with its ganglia, and the adrenal, carotid and coccygeal glands. Bielschowsky outlines the development from sympathicogonia through sympathoblast to the mature ganglion cells. Accordingly there may be the sympathicogonioma, sympathicoblastoma and the ganglioneuroma. The sympathicogonia also gives rise to the phaeochromoblast and the phaeochromocyte, from which the

pheochromocytoma is derived. The sympathicogonioma and sympathiocoblastoma represent divisions of what is often called the neuroblastoma. The pheochromocytoma corresponds to the paraganglioma or chromaffinoma. The neuroblastomatous tumors affect particularly the adrenal in children, and frequently metastasize. The paragangliomas are found in adrenal, retroperitoneal ganglia and carotid. The ganglioneuroma is rarely malignant.

The neuroma is composed principally of nerve fibers. These tumors may originate in nerve trunks or ganglia of various parts of the body. They are usually small, well-defined, fairly firm tumors and when along nerve trunks may be multiple. Microscopically, they may be composed of medullated

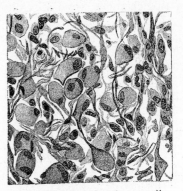

Small section of a ganglioneuroma, showing a cellular portion of the tumor.

or non-medullated nerves, and are called accordingly myelinic or amyelinic. The former occur in the course of peripheral nerves and the latter involve the sympathetic system. They are essentially benign tumors save for their situation, which may lead to pressure symptoms or interruption of impulses. Although some maintain that pure neuroma may occur, it is generally believed that ganglion cells are essential to the proliferation and that adequate search of the tumor would disclose the presence of these cells. Occasionally they are found in considerable numbers. The fibers may be arranged in intricately interlacing bundles which may give the tumor grossly a lobulated appearance, the "plexiform neuroma." Nodular enlargements, presumably tumorous, may be closely approximated along the course of a nerve to constitute the "circoid neuroma." The neuroma is to be distinguished from the neuro-fibroma and from the cellular tumors of the sympathetic system described above. (See Geschickter; Lewis and Geschickter.)

In amputation stumps, a tumor-like growth of nerves may be found, called amputation neuroma or false neuroma. This growth represents an elongation of the nerve fibers due to excessive regeneration, the new fibers interlacing and coiling to form a painful mass. Obviously this is not a true tumor.

Endothelioma. The endothelioma is a tumor derived from the lining cells of blood vessels, lymphatics and serous cavities. The infrequent endothelioma of pleura and peritoneum is sometimes called mesothelioma. The cells of endotheliomas are generally large and round. Formerly tumors containing cells of this character were all called endothelioma and constituted a large group. That group is becoming smaller because the origin of some of its members has been found not to be endothelial. Endothelioma has been described in bones, lymph nodes, pleura and peritoneum, ovaries, uterus, stomach and elsewhere. These are discussed further in the chapters on Systemic Pathology. Nevertheless, a general description follows. The endotheliomas are fairly dense, solid tumors, not well defined, but in the serous cavities may project as nodular or papillary growths. They cut with considerable resistance and show a pale, firm cross section. Derived from lymphatic or from blood vascular endothelium there may be, in some of the tumors, a considerable proliferation of blood vessels even to a point where angiomatous character is apparent, thus giving rise to the terms lymphangio-endothelioma and hemangio-endothelioma. Necrosis is not likely to be marked except in the larger tumors of the serous cavities.

Microscopically, the characteristic cell resembles the endothelial cell. It is large, generally spherical, with a faintly acidophilic cytoplasm. The nucleus is centrally disposed, vesicular and usually has a nucleolus. Mitotic figures are not frequent. The cells are usually spread in rather dense sheets, with little tendency to isolation of individual cells. The connective tissue supporting framework may be so arranged as to divide the tumor into lobules, and proper staining will usually show a certain amount

of stroma between the cells. The cells may be arranged in whorls either independently or around blood or lymphatic vessels. Sometimes the surrounding tissue shows only pressure, and sometimes distinct invasion may appear. The cells of the tumor may be flattened, especially in the cell whorls, so that in cross section they appear to be of spindle form. The diagnosis of endothelioma must be

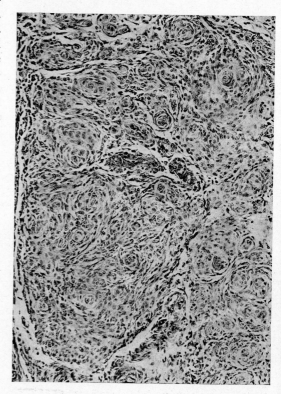

Meningioma of cerebral dura.

made with great caution. In bones, lymph nodes and celomic cavities, metastatic nodules may have an appearance supposedly characteristic of endothelioma, but are identified by further study or autopsy to be secondary (Willis). Nevertheless, in certain situations, especially in bones, the endothelioma behaves as a malignant tumor.

The so-called dural endothelioma has been found to be of other nature. It originates in the arachnoidal villi which naturally extend into the dura, so that grossly the tumor seems to originate in the dura. It is thus of fibromatous nature, but the name meningioma, given by Cushing, has attained wide usage. The psammoma is a meningioma in which there are spherical laminated calcified masses somewhat like pacchionian bodies.

There is dispute as to the occurrence of endothelioma or mesothelioma of the pleura. Some are of the opinion that these tumors are really extensions or metastases to the pleura from primary carcinomas elsewhere in the body (see Willis). Others believe that there is a small group of primary

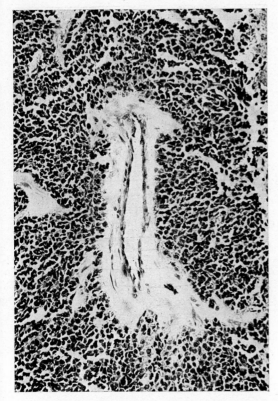

Ewing's endothelial myeloma of the bone.

tumors of the pleura derived from the lining cells (see Klemperer and Rabin; Ewing). We incline to the latter view.

The perithelioma is a tumor which shows sheath-like growth around blood or lymph vessels, supposedly derived from the perivascular endothelium. There is no adequate support for this view, and the peculiarity of arrangement is probably due to nutritional necrosis of those parts of the tumor not near the vessels.

The cylindroma was thought to be endothelial, but is now generally conceded to be epithelial. The cells in various parts of certain tumors are arranged to form cylin-

drical or globular spaces occupied by hyaline material. This may represent a secreted material or hyalinized necrotic cells. Sometimes the material is mucinous. This type of tumor often occurs as a part of the mixed tumor of the parotid.

The cholesteatoma, an unusual tumor of the cerebral meninges and spinal cord, is sometimes regarded as endothelial, but as pointed out in the chapter on diseases of the nervous system is really epithelial.

Giant-Cell Tumor. Although multinucleated giant cells may be observed in both benign and more especially in malignant connective tissue tumors, they are not a necessary or conspicuous feature. There are, however, two lesions in which giant cells regularly occur. These are the giant-cell epulis of the jaw and the giant-cell tumor of bone. The epulis usually appears as a firm, slowly growing nodule in the alveolar process of the jaw and often follows extraction of teeth. It is firm, pale, well defined, cuts with resistance and shows a pale, nonbulging, firm, poorly vascularized cross section. Microscopically, the essential cell is a small spindle cell. In one form of the lesion this is the only cell type. The giant-cell epulis contains the spindle cells and a large number of giant cells, whose condensed or slightly vesicular nuclei are scattered irregularly in the cytoplasm. The epulis is benign and does not tend to recur if completely removed.

The giant-cell tumor of bone arises in the ends of long bones, especially the upper end of the tibia and lower end of the femur. It may occur in spongy bone and rarely in the shaft of long bones. It usually occurs in early adult life. The tumor grows slowly with thinning of the cortex and with little or no new bone formation. Grossly it is a soft, red, jelly-like or friable mass, well vascularized, often hemorrhagic and sometimes necrotic. There is usually no capsule whatever. It cuts readily and shows a soft bulging cross section with the features just noted. Microscopically, the essential cell is a short spindle cell with dense or slightly vesicular nucleus and associated with little formation of collagen. Mitotic figures are usually infrequent. The giant cells are usually large, rounded, and with rich cytoplasm. The slightly vesicular nuclei vary greatly in number from a few to a dozen or sometimes many more. Vascularization is fairly rich but mostly by capillaries. Hemorrhage and necrosis may be slight or marked. In spite of the lack of a capsule and the destruction of bone, these tumors are usually benign and do not recur after thorough curettage. Nevertheless an occasional case shows recurrence and a few are recorded in which metastasis occurred. Jaffe and his associates have set up three grades of this tumor. In grade I, the stromal cells are loosely arranged and the giant cells

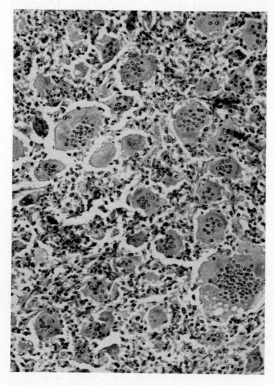

Giant cell tumor of bone.

large and numerous. In grade II, the stromal cells are more compact and sometimes whorled, the giant cells not so large. They claim that grade III is frankly malignant; the stroma is clearly atypical and sarcomatous, the giant cells relatively small and not numerous. This interesting view requires confirmation and is given here as merely tentative.

Malignant Tumors

Introduction and Classification. The malignant connective-tissue tumors are called sarcomata. They may be classified into two great groups, immature and differenti-

ated. In the immature forms there is no clear differentiation of cells to constitute adult types of tissue. In the differentiated forms, structures which resemble fibrous connective tissue, cartilage, bone, muscle, etc., are found. In these, however, there is a variable mixture of undifferentiated cells. Some prefer to name these sarcomatous fibroma, sarcomatous chondroma, etc., but the common practice is to refer to them as fibrosarcoma, chondrosarcoma, etc.

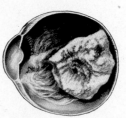

Sarcoma of the eye showing fleshy character and several hemorrhages.

The undifferentiated forms are made up either of spindle cells or round cells. As a rule, the size of the cells is fairly constant within the particular tumor. Thus the names large spindle cell and small spindle cell sarcoma are sometimes used. There are occasional instances of round-cell sarcoma whose derivation cannot be entirely established. Thus, it is sometimes necessary to refer to a small round-cell sarcoma or a large round-cell sarcoma. Tumors formerly included in this group have now been shown to be tumors of lymphoid apparatus or even carcinomas.

Sarcomas as a group exhibit the features of malignancy, namely, invasive and destructive growth, metastasis and recurrence after removal. As has been pointed out earlier, metastasis is usually but not exclusively by way of the blood vessels. Generally speaking, the immature forms of sarcoma, as is true of carcinoma, are more malignant than the differentiated forms. Nevertheless the latter must be thought of as distinctly malignant lesions. As will readily be understood, sarcomas can originate in any part of the body where connective tissues exist.

In early life, sarcomas are somewhat more frequent than carcinomas. Nevertheless, when sarcomas are viewed as a group they are more frequent in middle and advanced life than in early life. Frequently there is a history of the rapid assumption of growth by a tumor that has previously grown slowly, but many of these tumors grow rapidly from the time that they are first noticed.

Gross Morbid Anatomy. As the name indicates, the sarcoma is a fleshy tumor. It is usually bulky but may be small. It is more or less adherent to surrounding structures, and the overlying skin or other parts show distended vessels. Capsule formation is absent or incomplete. The immature forms are of soft consistency, pink in color, poorly defined, partly encapsulated, and show distended superficial blood vessels. They cut with about the resistance of living muscle, and show a bulging, soft, somewhat friable, bleeding, pallid, pink or red cross section, in which small and large blood vessels can be seen; necrosis and hemorrhage are commonly present. The more highly differentiated forms vary from the consistency of fibroma to that of bone, are less well vascularized and usually less subject to secondary degenerative changes. Reactive inflammation of the surrounding parts is mild subacute or chronic.

Microscopic Appearance. Although each sarcoma has its individual characters, there are certain features common to practically all. These include particular characters of cells, of cellular arrangement, of stroma and of vascularization. The essential cells are usually immature and thus the cytoplasm is likely to be only slightly acidophilic or even basophilic. Cell outline may be obscure and the tumor sometimes appears to be made up of masses of syncytial character. The nuclei are large and vesicular. Mitotic figures, both typical and atypical, bipolar or multipolar, are common in freshly fixed material. Multinucleated cells are often seen. The supporting framework is supplied in part by the host, but inasmuch as the tumor cells are of the connective-tissue type they furnish the greater part of the fibrils. The term stroma usually refers to that part of the connective-tissue support furnished by the tumor cells. The stroma may occur as dense bands which ramify through the tumor or even divide it into alveoli, or as fine reticular fibrillae between the tumor cells. The presence

and character of the stroma were formerly thought to be of importance in differentiation of carcinoma from sarcoma, and in identifying different types of sarcoma, but this view no longer holds, since fine stroma may be demonstrated by special methods in many types of malignant and nonmalignant growth. The blood vessels are derived ultimately from the host, which certainly provides all the more important vessels. New capillaries grow by endothelial multiplication from the smaller branches. Communicating with these are vascular slits within the tumor, bordered principally by the essential cells of the tumor

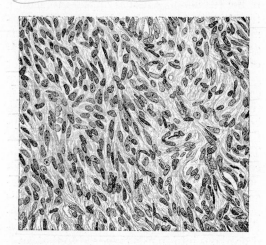

Spindle-cell sarcoma showing cell type.

itself, and only occasionally showing an isolated lining endothelial cell. The development of vascular slits is one of the most important items in the diagnosis of sarcoma. In the spindle-cell tumors, the cells are often arranged at an angle to the vascular slit, parallel rows of cells and nuclei in the form of a wide palisade ranging from the vessel as though they had been "combed." The more gross indications of invasiveness are seen in sections which include the surrounding tissue.

Retrogressive Changes. In spite of the rich vascularization of most of the immature tumors, necrosis is common. It usually occurs in small areas, although the greater mass of the tumor may be involved. Consistent with the vascularization, hemorrhage is frequent. Other retrogressive changes are seen in the more mature forms, such as hyaline and mucoid degeneration in the fibrosarcoma. Owing to the rapid growth of sarcomas, the surrounding tissues may be more or less devitalized, thus removing local resistance to growth; erosion on skin surfaces and into body tubes is common, resulting in infection and inflammation of the tumor, with further necrosis, sloughing and even gangrene.

Histogenesis and Etiology. Although malignant tumors as a class grow principally by centrifugal growth, many of the sarcomata show both centrifugal and centripetal growth; in other words, all the cells appear to be active in enlarging the tumor. Sometimes the reactive inflammation in the surrounding tissues appears to show a transition between normal surrounding connective tissue and sarcomatous cells. It is generally believed that such transformation of cells does not occur, and that the tumor grows entirely by multiplication of its own cells. Injuries of various kinds may precede the manifestations of sarcoma, as blows on a bone preceding bone sarcoma, or chronic inflammation leading to cutaneous sarcoma. The significance of injury is no clearer in connection with sarcomas than with carcinomas. It is possible, however, that the organization of hemorrhage following injury may progress to sarcoma. As has been mentioned before, injection of carcinogenic hydrocarbons into tissues may lead to the development of sarcoma. Reference has also been made to the development of sarcoma of the liver incident to infestation by *Taenia crassicollis*. Sarcomas may also be induced by filterable viruses, the most striking example being the Rous sarcoma of the fowl. Sarcoma occasionally develops in the base of tuberculous ulcers of the skin and it is said that tuberculous lymphadenitis may become sarcomatous. Mention has also been made of the sarcomatous transformation of Hodgkin's disease. Congenital sarcomas are almost certainly due to embryonal cell isolations, misplacements or faults of development, and it is possible that these phenomena play a part in adult sarcomata. These suggestions are all hypothetical and subject to much further investigation.

Spindle-Cell Sarcoma. The spindle-cell sarcomas are commonly found in the bone, periosteum, subcutaneous connective tissue and in the fascias, muscle and tendon sheaths. More rarely they are observed in the

uterus, ovaries, breast, testis, thyroid and other situations in the body. This tumor typifies the fleshy character of sarcomas. There are, however, various gradations between the spindle-cell sarcoma and the fibrosarcoma so that, on the one hand, very firm tumors may be encountered and, on the other, soft tumors, with intermediate grades between.

Microscopically, the cells may be large, small or intermediate; the oatcell sarcoma with a short broad spindle form is

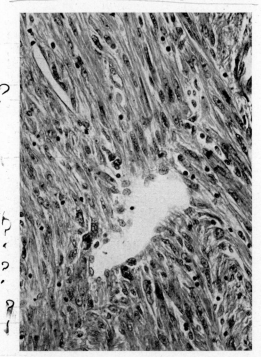

Spindle-cell sarcoma showing vascular slits, lined mainly by tumor cells and "combing" of the cells. Numerous mitotic nuclei.

unusual. Extremes are easily recognized, but intermediate types of cells are divided according to personal preference of the observer. The differentiation into large and small spindle-cell sarcoma is of little practical value. Nevertheless, it is stated that the tumors arising from fibrous connective tissue are likely to show small cells, while those originating from periosteum and smooth muscle are more likely to show large forms. The cells are of elongated spindle form, rich in cytoplasm, arranged closely together with a small amount of collagen between. The nuclei are large, vesicular and of long ellipsoid form. The cells are arranged in bundles of various size which ramify irregularly through the tumor, sometimes giving rise to a whorled appearance of the cross section, and in the microscopic section showing cells cut in various planes. If this fact be not borne in mind, the tumor may appear to be made up of both round cells and spindle cells. Vascularization is usually rich and typical "combing" of cells is very common. Large spindle-shaped, multinucleated giant cells are often observed in the large spindle-cell sarcoma, but are not so frequent in the small-

spindle form sarcoma certain special types. This depends upon cell character and arrangement. Thus, the neurogenic sarcoma, the liposarcoma, the fibrosarcoma and the fascial sarcoma can be identified.

Small Round-Cell Sarcoma. Most of the tumors of this category are really lymphosarcoma but occasionally a tumor is encountered in the connective tissue of muscles, fascias and in certain other situations made up entirely of small round cells of uniform size. Usually the cytoplasm is scanty

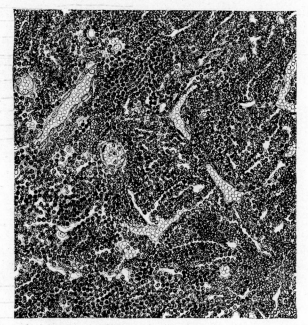

Small round-cell sarcoma.

cell variety. A fine stroma may be provided by the spindle cells but is never very rich. Occasionally, however, masses of dense connective tissue fibrils may divide the tumor into more or less distinct nodules. In epithelial organs, it is very difficult to state whether the spindle form cells are of connective tissue origin or are epithelial in character, and the diagnosis of sarcoma in certain situations is often open to considerable doubt. The difficulty of distinguishing histologically between granulation tissue and sarcoma has led to mistakes in diagnosis, but the intimately intermingled inflammatory changes in the former usually indicate its nature. As the sarcomas have been more completely studied, it has been possible to separate out from the

and the nucleus large, round and vesicular. Although well vascularized, secondary changes, particularly necrosis, are likely to be extensive, and hemorrhage is a frequent complication. A fine reticulum may be demonstrated between the cells but is usually very scanty. Not infrequently, however, the tumors may be alveolated by the growth of fairly dense connective tissue septa. The tumors of this order are usually highly malignant, as would be expected from the undifferentiated type of cell which comprises them.

Large Round-Cell Sarcoma. This also is a rare tumor and occurs in much the same situations as the small round-cell sarcoma. It is much more likely to be alveolated and is not so highly malignant. Formerly included in this category were the embryonal carcinoma of the testis and certain carcinomas of the thyroid. In any event, the diagnosis small round-cell sarcoma or large round-cell sarcoma usually indicates an inability to identify the exact type of the tumor.

Fibrosarcoma. In clinical and pathologic features, this type of tumor stands midway between the fibroma and the spindle-cell sarcoma. It is invasive but grows comparatively slowly; although circumscribed, a capsule is poorly developed or absent. Microscopically, it differs from the spindle-cell sarcoma in a distinctly richer content of

sarcoma, or cartilage cells may appear in extremely immature form, with great irregularity in size, poorly defined areolae and scanty hyaline or fibrillar matrix. The degree of malignancy cannot be entirely predicated on cellular differentiation, because a tumor that is so well-differentiated that it has the microscopic appearance of chondroma may be markedly invasive and destructive.

Osteosarcoma. Among the various tumors that may originate in bone are forms of sarcoma which appear to be derived from cells which have to do with bone formation. The production of bone in the tumors varies

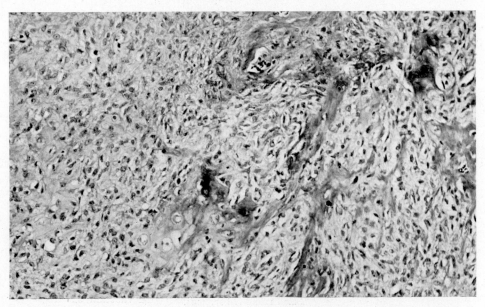

Low-power drawing of an osteosarcoma.

collagen fibers, either diffusely scattered or arranged in bands. The cells are more condensed but larger than those of the fibroma; multinucleated cells are occasionally present. Mitotic figures are not common. "Combing" of cells about thin-walled vascular slits can usually be made out. Metastasis may occur late in the course of the tumor but is not likely to be widespread. The diagnosis of malignancy is often difficult in those tumors which approach more closely to the fibroma.

Chondrosarcoma. Grossly, this may resemble chondroma or may be distinctly fleshy. It is invasive but usually grows slowly. Microscopically, it may occur as a form combining chondroma and spindle-cell

from practically none to a moderate amount. Thus they are preferably called osteogenic sarcomas. This serves to distinguish them from others that take origin in cells of the marrow, lymphocytes, endothelial cells and blood vessels, as well as those derived from cartilage and fat. The osteogenic sarcomas arise in medulla, subperiosteum and periosteum, may be telangiectatic, sclerosing and in the form of fibrosarcoma. They occur principally in early life and may affect any part of the bone. The cells may be spindle form or round. The tumor has the characteristic structure and vascularization of sarcoma in general. Some show the formation of irregular trabeculae and islands of bone; others show the production of osteoid, a bone-like tissue poor in lime salts. Combinations may occur to form the osteochondrosarcoma and the myxo-osteochondrosarcoma. Among the osteogenic sarcomas, the more cellular forms metastasize early and widely; viscera and soft tissues are involved more often than bones. Sometimes roentgenograms of the chest may disclose pulmonary metastases by the time the original tumor becomes clinically evident.

Myxosarcoma. This malignant form of the myxoma is found in the same situations as the myxoma, namely subcutaneous and subserous connective tissues, intermuscular septae, nerves, bones (marrow) and meninges. A congenital form with admixture of lipoma, fibroma and spindle cell sarcoma occurs. The immature forms often show mucoid degeneration, which forms confusing pictures. The myxosarcoma is highly invasive and metastasizes widely. The histologic picture is that of a highly cellular myxoma, well vascularized and with irregular sized large spindle cells, characteristic perivascular arrangement and numerous mitotic figures. Much more common are the forms in which chondromatous or chondro-osteomatous elements are also present.

Liposarcoma. Although this may appear anywhere that lipoma does, nevertheless, Ewing states that the particular situations are intermuscular, periarticular, perineal regions and mediastinum. It may grow slowly or rapidly and at the beginning is encapsulated. Microscopically, it is characterized by the appearance of cells varying from spindle form to round form. In the cytoplasm are numerous tiny droplets of fat, the cells in many instances resembling the embryonal type of fat cell. Many of the highly undifferentiated cells contain no fat. In the intermuscular form, myxomatous cells often appear, thus constituting the myxoliposarcoma. Liposarcomatous elements are also found in the mixed sarcomata of the retroperitoneal region. Primary liposarcoma of bone is uncommon but is highly malignant; metastasis occurs in other parts of the skeleton and sometimes in the soft tissues (Stewart; Rehbock and Hauser).

Angiosarcoma. This term is usually applied to a sarcoma provided with numerous, wide, vascular spaces. The angioma is, however, more an embryonal fault of development than a true blastomatous tumor. Malignant changes rarely occur, but when they do they are often accompanied by no important change in the histology. Malignant forms, probably originating as such, are seen in the form of angio-endotheliomas, the endothelium originating in perivascular spaces, and not in the endothelium of the vessels concerned. Vascular sarcomas are likely to show necrosis of cells remote from the vessels, leaving a sheath of cells around the vessels; these are often incorrectly called perithelial angiosarcomas, but are simple vascular sarcomata with secondary necrosis. The use of the term "angiosarcoma" has little justification on morphologic or genetic grounds, for the tumors to which it is applied are either sarcomas with secondary necrosis, or endotheliomas of particular form.

Myosarcoma. The leiomyoma of the uterus or intestinal canal may become transformed into leiomyosarcoma, although Ewing is of the opinion that most of these are malignant from the start. Grossly, the tumor is red, soft, often necrotic and hemorrhagic, clearly invasive and often accompanied by metastasis. Microscopically, the cells are irregular as to shape and size, with large or hyperchromatic nuclei and often multiple nuclei. Usually some fairly typical smooth-muscle cells with their elongated nuclei ("sausage shaped") are present. Vascularization is rich and there may be large cavernous blood vascular spaces; "combing" is usually evident. There are rare cases of metastasizing leiomyoma, in which the original tumor and the metastases show no significant departure histologically from the ordinary leiomyoma.

The rhabdomyoma may become transformed into a rhabdomyosarcoma, but this is more true if situated in skeletal muscle than elsewhere. Invasion and metastasis occur. Microscopically there are many cells of myoblast type and the fibers are scanty and often fail to show transverse striation.

Malignant Tumors of the Hematopoietic System. These include the lymphosarcoma, the chloroma and various forms of the myeloma, which will be taken up in connection with special diseases of the hematopoietic system.

EPITHELIAL TUMORS

Introduction

Epithelium in its growth derives support from connective tissue, and nutrition from blood vessels. Tumors composed of epithelium require supporting tissue and vascular supply, and as the epithelial proliferation progresses the connective tissue and blood vessels must grow accordingly. If support and nutrition are not sufficient, degenerations or necrosis occur. Epithelium may derive nutrition as it penetrates lymphatic and tissue spaces, but extensive tumor growth cannot occur in this way. As surface epithelium proliferates beyond the surface, it becomes folded above the surface and, as it grows, connective tissue support and vascular supply are provided. A papillary tumor arises in this fashion. Proliferation of epithelium of ducts and glands forms acinic spaces often of irregular size and shape; supporting tissues also proliferate in different degrees. The adenoma is formed thus. Solid growth in the form of masses or bundles of cells occurs principally in the malignant epithelial tumors, but this also cannot progress independently of support and nutrition. The epithelial tumors then are really combinations of epithelium, connective tissue and blood vessels. They are sometimes called fibro-epithelial, but such a term is supererogatory since from all points of view the epithelium is the essential tumor element.

In the more undifferentiated epithelial tumors, the cells may not be readily identified as epithelial. Sometimes this identification is inferential, but certain features, when present, are of aid. These include the presence of intercellular bridges, keratinization, intracellular mucin, intracellular hyalin, and the absence of fine stroma between the individual cells.

Secondary changes, such as fatty and other forms of degeneration are not uncommon. In the rapidly growing tumors, more particularly those which are malignant, necrosis is common and widespread due to the failure of the blood supply to keep pace with the epithelium and perhaps to other factors. Infection and inflammation occur, since many of the tumors are superficial and others may erode upon surfaces.

There is often much difficulty in distinguishing between a blastomatous growth of epithelium and hyperplasias. The latter occur as the result of inflammation and may produce papillary outgrowths resembling true papillomata. In the margins of ulcers of the skin, of the intestinal canal, etc., the epithelium may undergo hyperplasia and infiltrate a short distance into deeper tissues. This may go on to actual tumor formation, but the exact stage of transition is impossible to define with exactness, and confusion is easily possible. Inflammation of glands may produce microscopic pictures closely resembling certain forms of adenoma.

Benign Epithelial Tumors

Papilloma. This type of tumor grows characteristically from surface epithelium, but may also originate in epithelium lining glandular ducts and acini; papillomata may even appear upon serous surfaces and are then covered with endothelium. The cores or papillae made up of supporting connective tissue may be large or small, broad and flat or long and narrow, nonbranching, simply branching or branching to form multiple divisions. This connective tissue is continuous with that of the region from which the papilloma arises, and may be either moderately or richly vascularized. The base may be coextensive with the tumor or the latter may represent a polypoid mass attached by a single, more or less narrow, peduncle. The "hard" papilloma is covered with stratified squamous epithelium; the "soft" papilloma is covered with either transitional, simple, or stratified columnar epithelium. These old terms, hard and soft, are being displaced by more exact terminology such as squamous-cell papilloma, transitional-cell papilloma, etc. The color and consistency of the tumor depend upon the thickness and density of the covering epithelium and the vascularization of the papillae, as well as incidental secondary changes.

Microscopically, the papillary arrangement is usually clearly indicated, but since the section is but one plane of a branching mass extending in two planes, or three diameters, various papillae may be cut obliquely or transversely to show isolated islands of connective tissue surrounded by epithelium. Stratified squamous epithelium may show various degrees of keratinization up to marked hyperkeratosis in which thick, horny masses of keratinized cells project from the apices of the papillae. In the interstices of the tumor a concentrically laminated mass of keratinized cells may form the so-called epithelial "pearls." The intermediate cells may show the inclusion of hyaline globules, the so-called Russell fuchsin bodies. Cell bridges may be much more prominent mous papillomas. Mitotic figures may also appear in this form of papilloma.

The squamous-cell or transitional-cell papillomas appear on skin surface, mouth, pharynx, larynx, esophagus, vagina and neighboring parts of cervix uteri, urinary bladder, renal pelvis. The cylindrical-cell papillomas may be found in the nose, stomach, intestinal canal, gallbladder, uterus and

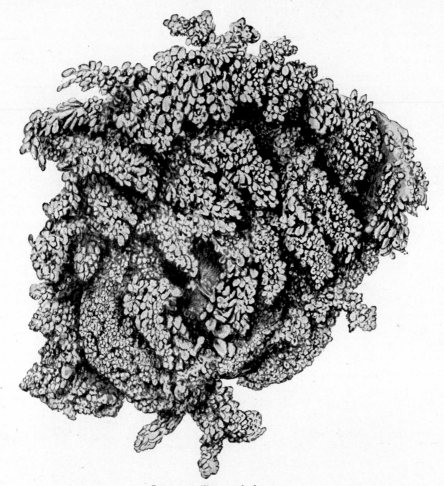

Large papilloma of the anus.

than in normal epithelium. Mitotic figures may be found in strictly benign tumors; any supposition that their axes are differently placed than in malignant papillomata is not sufficiently well founded to be of diagnostic import. The simple or stratified columnar epithelial papillomata may show ciliated cells, goblet mucinous cells or various types of cellular degenerations. Desquamation seems more frequent in these than in squa- fallopian tubes. Metaplasia may determine the appearance of squamous papillomas in places normally covered with columnar epithelium. The superficial position and projection of papillomas subject them to trauma; injury and infection are common and may predispose to malignant change.

Malignant transformation of a papilloma is usually indicated by infiltrative growth of the epithelium about the base. The

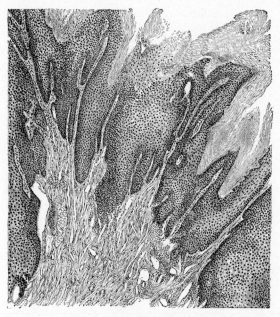

Low-power drawing of a squamous papilloma, showing fine connective tissue villi covered by stratified squamous epithelium with superficial hyperkeratosis.

peritoneum. This may show no clear microscopic evidence of malignancy, but usually invasive proliferation of epithelium is found. The papilloma of the urinary bladder may recur repeatedly after excision and yet show no histologic evidence of malignancy. On the other hand, the growth may be so atypical and invasive that a diagnosis of papillary carcinoma may be made without hesitation. The production of papillary growths in cysts and glandular spaces will be referred to in discussing adenoma.

Irritative and inflammatory hyperplasias may closely resemble papilloma, and in the individual instances may be quite indistinguishable from true tumors. Thus, papillary outgrowths may be observed in the neighborhood of chronic catarrhal inflammations and around ulcers. The nasal polyp may be papillary and is probably of inflammatory origin. There is still some doubt as to whether the cutaneous wart is inflammatory or neoplastic. The acuminate condyloma, or venereal wart, occurs on the external genitalia as a papillary growth of epithelium due to irritation such as that of gonorrhea. Molluscum contagiosum may produce pedunculated tumor-like masses, undoubtedly of viral ori-

papilloma of ovarian cystoma is infiltrative early in its course, breaks through the ovary and extends widely over the surface of the

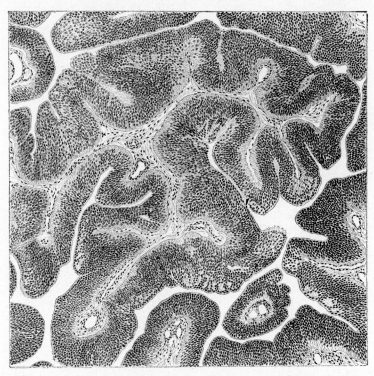

Papilloma of the urinary bladder—transitional epithelium.

gin, with curious, large, vesicular epithelial cells containing the so-called molluscum bodies. Cutaneous horns and other types of hyperkeratosis are not likely to be confused with true papillomata. Irritants may produce papilloma as is the case with papilloma of the bladder in aniline workers. (See Becker on benign tumors of skin.)

Adenoma. The adenoma is a tumor which in its growth reduplicates glandular tubules or acini or both. As with epithelial growth elsewhere, there is a certain amount of connective-tissue supporting framework. This sometimes is differentiated to form a

In certain situations it appears that inflammation may play an important part in the development of true tumorous adenomas, and it is well known that gland-like proliferation may occur in connection with inflammation of glandular tissues and organs. Thus, adenomatous proliferation in the breasts is not uncommon in chronic inflammation, and most of the cases of adenoma of the liver show an associated and perhaps causative chronic inflammatory process, cirrhosis of the liver. Grossly, the adenoma may be intraglandular or polypoid in form. The intraglandular forms appear as rounded nodules

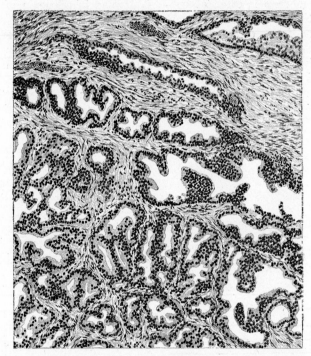

Adenoma of the prostate, showing papillary infolding of lining epithelium.

tunica propria and practically always shows the formation of a basement membrane. Adenomata are practically always derived from tissues in which there is pre-existing glandular substance, although certain forms appear which are undoubtedly due to embryonal displacement or faults in development. Probably the commonest situations are in the prostate, the thyroid gland, and the female breast. They are not uncommon in the skin where they arise from sweat glands or oil glands, in the kidney, the adrenals, the pancreas, intestines and uterus.

which may be more or less lobulated; they are practically always circumscribed and usually encapsulated. The polypoid forms may be flat or elevated, round or lobulated, and attached either by a broad base or a small peduncle; they are frequent in the colon and may affect other surfaces. The consistency depends upon the amount of admixture of connective tissue but as a rule these tumors are fairly firm. They cut with moderate resistance and the cross section may be simply dull, flat, slightly bulging, sometimes with gray stroma and yellowish-white nests of acini; if the acini are sufficiently large, the cross section is spongy. Microscopically, the tumor may be a solid adenoma, a tubular adenoma, in which the acini are of tubular form, or an alveolar adenoma in which well-developed acini appear. The solid forms, in which there are cell masses with only slight differentiation into acini, are more likely to be seen in connection with adenoma of the liver, the adrenal, sebaceous glands and sometimes the thyroid gland. The acini of the adenoma usually lack uniformity in size, and are frequently more irregular in outline than are normal acini. The identification of an intact basement membrane is often of considerable aid in distinguishing between truly benign and malignant forms of adenomatous tumors.

The connective tissue is usually moderate in amount and does not show any characters that would distinguish it as blasto-

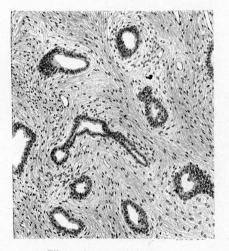

Fibro-adenoma of the breast.

matous. It may be richly or only moderately vascularized. In the breast, however, it is likely to be rich in amount, and the usual adenoma of the gland is so rich in fibrous tissue that the term fibro-adenoma or even adenofibroma is justified. The lining cells of the spaces may be low or high, cuboidal or columnar, and usually are in a single layer but may show a certain amount of multiplicity and stratification. Certain authorities maintain that the presence of multiple layers of epithelium in the acini indicates a disposition to malignant change, but according to Kettle and numerous others, this view is not

justified. Nevertheless, it seems reasonable to suppose that when the epithelium grows in multiple layers, is thrown up into folds, or constitutes solid masses within the acinic space, epithelial growth must be regarded as going on more actively than in other simpler forms of this tumor. Malignant change, to form adenocarcinoma, may be indicated by penetration of the basement membrane, or by pleomorphism of the cells and disturbance of their polarity. Functional activity may persist so that bile may be formed in adenoma of the liver, colloid is commonly formed in adenoma of the thyroid, and mucin is formed in adenoma of the gut and other mucous membranes. The production of secretory products by the cells of the adenoma may dilate the acinar spaces to form cysts, and the adenoma then becomes a cystadenoma.

The cystadenoma, then, is an adenoma in which the accumulation of fluid in the spaces has led to cystic dilatation. The cystadenoma may be either a true tumor or may be the result of tumor-like fault in embryonal development, as manifested in the congenital cystadenoma of the kidney and similar processes in the liver and in certain other situations. Cystadenoma may occur in any situation in which adenoma occurs, but among the most common is the cystadenoma of the ovary. Here two important types are found, namely, the pseudomucinous glandular cystadenoma and the papilliferous serous cystadenoma. In the former there are numerous cystic spaces, which contain pseudomucin. Microscopically, there is a delicate, poorly developed, supporting framework, with the large glandular spaces surrounded by more or less flattened, low, cuboidal or almost squamous epithelium. The papilliferous cystadenoma shows the formation of papillae extending out from the lining of the cystic spaces. These papillae branch in an intricate fashion so that they largely fill up the cyst space. The content of these cysts other than the papillae is usually a thin serous fluid.

Papilla formation in various types of adenoma is fairly common. This may be exhibited in the form of dense, flat papillae as seen in the intracanalicular adenofibroma of the breast, where the large, dense papillary masses of connective tissue fill up the entire lumen, leaving simply narrow strips of double layers of epithelium from apposed sides of the acini. The papilliferous cyst-adenoma of the ovary is one of the best examples of very intricate branching of papillae within an adenomatous growth. In this case, it is accompanied by cyst formation. Many adenomata show papillae without true cyst formation. In this case, it appears that the epithelium lining the acini grows to such an extent that it can no longer lie flat along the

differentiated being the squamous-cell carcinoma. From transitional epithelium arises the transitional-cell carcinoma. Carcinomas derived from cylindrical and cuboidal epithelium may be of differentiated form, the adenocarcinoma. Completely undifferentiated forms develop usually in glandular organs and the name given is carcinoma simplex. Whereas the benign epithelial tumors show more or less co-ordinate growth of epithelium and connective tissue, in the malignant forms

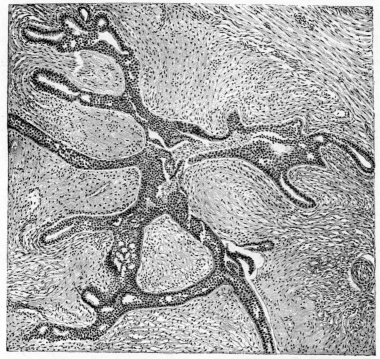

Intracanalicular adenofibroma of the breast. The bulbous connective tissue papillae distort the outline of the large acinus.

outer circumference of the acinus. It then folds inward to produce papillary ingrowth into the acinar spaces. Only where the papilla formation is marked, is it customary to add the name papilliferous to specify the type of growth.

Malignant Epithelial Tumors

Introduction. A malignant epithelial tumor is a carcinoma. Sometimes such a term as malignant adenoma is used, but the lesion is a carcinoma even though its malignancy may not be marked. Carcinomas are classified according to cell type. Thus there are forms of epidermal carcinoma, the most

the epithelium usually outstrips the connective-tissue growth; these tumors are essentially epithelial as represented by multiplication, invasion, and metastasis of epithelial cells. The amount of associated connective-tissue growth determines the consistency; hard cancers are called scirrhous cancers and the adjective may be used as a noun by changing the spelling to scirrhus; soft cancers are referred to as medullary. Scirrhous and medullary are used especially to indicate gross characters, but are also associated with well-defined histologic characters. Carcinomas are invasive and poorly defined. From the point of view of invasion and metastasis the epidermoid carcinomas are not so highly malignant as the cylindrical-cell carcinomas. The role of inflammation and irritation in the development of tumors has been discussed, but nowhere is it so well illustrated as in the growth of carcinoma. Ulcers of the skin, such as chronic leg ulcers, cutaneous ulcers in wearers of the Kangri basket, ulcers of tongue or lip due to irritation of teeth or smoking, etc., are likely to be complicated

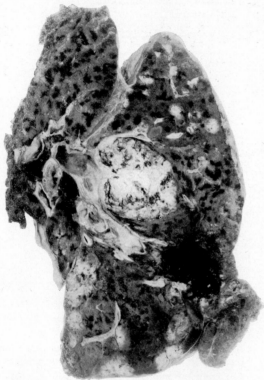

Bronchogenic carcinoma of lung with metastases in lung. Atelectasis just distal to main tumor.

by the development of epidermoid carcinomas. Chronic gastric and intestinal ulcers may be the basis for cylindrical cell carcinomas. The experimental sudan-oil, tar and spiroptera tumors have already been discussed. The situation, time of occurrence and history of human carcinoma stresses the importance of avoiding chronic irritation.

Carcinoma is a disease of advanced life, occurring particularly between 40 and 60 years of age; this does not exclude the possibility of its occurrence in later or earlier life. Indeed carcinoma of the new born has been reported, but care should be taken in these instances to exclude mixed tumors. Ac-

cording to Borst, carcinoma occurs in females more often than males in the proportion of six to four, owing to the incidence of carcinoma of the breast and of the uterus.

The mode of metastasis of carcinoma is by the lymphatic vessels, either by permeation or by embolism. Certain carcinomas, however, grow in intimate relation with blood vessels, as certain thyroid carcinomas and the chorionepithelioma; these are more likely to metastasize by the blood stream, the emboli lodging first in the lungs and there setting up secondary growths. It is generally believed that benign epithelial tumors may become malignant epithelial tumors, and this possibility is of importance in the management of the benign forms. The carcinoma usually follows the type of epithelium from which it originates, as in the epidermoid and glandular forms, and the same rule holds true when it is derived from a pre-existent benign tumor.

The epithelial cells may undergo mucinous, colloid, hyaline and fatty degeneration, calcification and necrosis. As the result of fatty degeneration, especially when associated with necrosis, a more or less viscid, opaque, granular fluid can be scraped from the cross section, the "cancer milk." The connective tissue often shows mucoid or hyaline degeneration. Uninfected carcinomas show much marginal reaction in the form of cellular infiltrates of lymphoid, large mononuclear and plasma cells.

As compared with the sarcoma, the carcinoma shows no capsule, is less vascular, less subject to hemorrhage, more subject to necrosis; its metastases are characteristically by the lymph stream and therefore tend to be regional rather than widespread.

Epidermoid Carcinoma. The term "epidermoid" does not necessarily refer to skin, because tumors of this general order may arise from any surface covered by stratified squamous epithelium. Included in the group are the squamous-cell carcinoma which may be in various degrees of differentiation, the basal-cell carcinoma, and the intermediate-cell carcinoma. The tumors may occur as ulcers, as nodules or as papillary masses. Striking examples are found in the lip, tongue, esophagus, anus, and in the skin surfaces, more particularly of exposed parts. In a single section it is often possible to see transitions from normal surface epithelium to true tumor growth. The deeper interpapillary epithelium is first seen to be growing deeper parts. The extension is in three diameters, so that a single section may cut numerous strands more or less transversely,

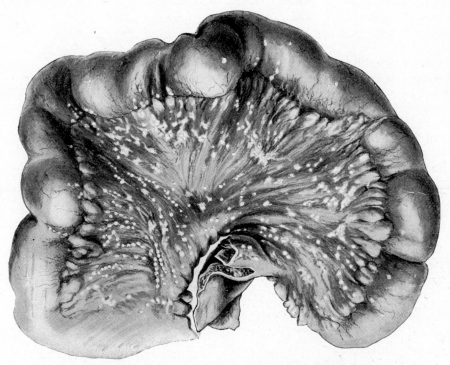

Multiple metastatic nodules of a carcinoma of intestine in the lymphatics of the mesentery.

deeply into the corium; solid masses of cells are formed, from which branching columns penetrate more deeply and extend into the

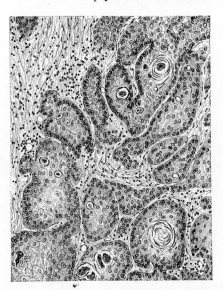

Squamous cell carcinoma showing nests of cells, differentiation and pearl formation.

thus giving the appearance of isolated islands of cells. It is true that isolated islands may be formed as the tumor extends through lymphatics and tissue spaces, but in the primary tumor most of the cell masses are interconnected. The growth tends to form layers of basal, intermediate and squamous cells. In the cutaneous tumors and in certain of those originating from transitional epithelium, keratinization is well marked. The keratinization is central in the mass, i.e., away from the peripheral basal cells, and thus the flat horny cells are deposited in concentrically laminated cell whorls or epithelial "pearls." A tumor rich in keratinized epithelium and pearls is often called acanthoma. Hyaline inclusions in the cells are not uncommon and cell bridges are often well displayed. On the other hand, squamous-cell carcinomas may show no pearl formation and relatively little keratinization. The cells show the usual characters of stratified squamous epithelium. The intermediate cells and to a less extent the basal cells may show chromatic disturbances of nuclei. Mitotic figures are not more frequent in the basal than in the intermediate cells, but are likely to be multipolar and atypical. Many of these tumors originate as ulcers or become ulcerated, and acute or chronic inflammation is common. In certain situations, as the cervix uteri, the cellular infiltrate may be made up largely of eosinophils. Necrosis may or may not be extensive. In the cervix uteri and sometimes in other situations, there may be much central necrosis of the cell masses instead of keratinization. In various situations the pearls may become necrotic; they may also serve as bodies around which foreign-body giant cells form.

The basal-cell carcinoma is common in exposed parts of the skin of elderly people,

Rarely a tumor is found, made up almost entirely of intermediate cells with intercellular bridges, with few basal cells and no keratinization. It is called intermediate epidermoid carcinoma or prickle-cell carcinoma.

None of these tumors is highly malignant. The squamous forms are graded in order of malignancy depending upon degree to which keratinized cells are formed. The basal-cell forms are of a low order of malignancy and are radiosensitive. Many believe that the basal-cell tumors are derived from hair matrix and sebaceous glands (Haythorn). Often, however, there are mixtures of basal-cell and squamous-cell forms. Thus, it is difficult to conceive of these as entirely separate and distinct varieties, with different points of origin.

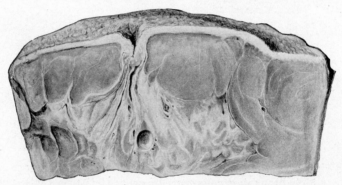

Scirrhous carcinoma of breast, showing retraction of surrounding structures, notably the nipple, dense character of tumor and cyst formation.

especially about the face and hands. Of the same nature is the rodent ulcer of the foot or other skin surface. The basal-cell carcinoma begins insidiously either as a small ulcer or area of thickening of the skin with a tendency to ulcerate. It progresses and erodes slowly. Microscopically it is made up of small cells, round, cuboidal, or polyhedral, with a resemblance to basal cells of the epiderm. The cytoplasm is often basophilic, the nuclei small and dense, mitotic figures present but not frequent. Invasion is observed but is not likely to be extensive. The benign cystic epithelioma or acanthoma adenoides cysticum is similar grossly, but, microscopically, although the cell type is much the same, is found to be sharply circumscribed and lobulated, the lobules containing small cyst-like spaces.

Transitional-Cell Carcinoma. This is most frequent in the urinary bladder, but may occur in renal pelvis and ureter. It probably is preceded in many instances by papilloma. It often shows trabeculae resembling the stalks of papilloma and may be grossly papillary in structure. Thus it can be called a papillary carcinoma, the term papilliferous (papilla bearing) being reserved for adenomatous or cystic tumors in which papillae grow. The small cell or oat-cell carcinoma of the bronchus is sometimes called transitional cell, but this is not correct; the tumor probably arises from intermediate cells or "reserve" cells of the bronchial mucosa.

Cylindrical-Cell Carcinoma. This general group of tumors may be derived from epithelium of glands or ducts, or from surfaces covered by cylindrical or cuboidal epithelium. Grossly, it may be of scirrhous, medullary or mucinous type. Microscopically there are two principal forms, adenocarcinoma and carcinoma simplex.

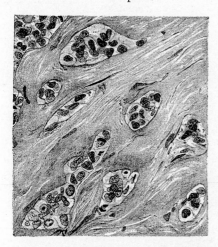

Scirrhous carcinoma of the simplex type.

Carcinoma Simplex. The carcinoma simplex is diagnosed by its microscopic appearance. It occurs in glandular organs and in surfaces covered by columnar epithelium. The cells of the tumor are arranged in solid masses, nests and cords, supported by variable amounts of connective tissue. The margins often show very clearly the extension through lymphatics. The individual epithelial cells are no longer cylindrical, but are spheroidal or polyhedral with moderately acidophilic, finely granular cytoplasm and occasional cell inclusions. The nuclei are vesicular and fairly large; normal and abnormal mitotic figures are present and sometimes multinucleated cells are seen. There is practically no intercellular reticulum. The cells are irregularly placed, and no arrangement of marginal basal cells or formation of acini can be discovered. Fatty and other types of degeneration occur, and it is not uncommon to find necrosis in the center of cell masses or involving a large part of the tumor. In the scirrhous varieties the connective tissue is rich and in the medullary forms poor. In either case, it is usually poor in cells and rich in collagenous fibers. The scirrhus is usually densely fibrous and the connective tissue

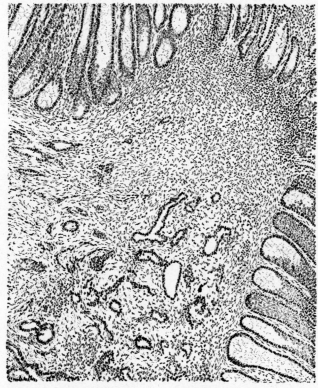

Adenocarcinoma of the pylorus, showing hyperplastic glands and deep situation of acinus-like cancer nests.

often hyalinized. The epithelium is present as narrow cords or bands of cells, and the cells are often smaller than their normal prototype. A scirrhus may at any time become cellular and grow rapidly, but the integral part the connective tissue plays is shown by the fact that often the metastases are quite as fibrous as the original tumor. The connective tissue of the scirrhus tends to contract so as to produce a slowly growing, dense mass with little necrosis, moderately invasive, firmly adherent to and producing retraction of the surrounding parts. Such tumors cut with leathery resistance and show a dense retract-

Adenocarcinoma. Tumors of this group may originate in any variety of cylindrical epithelium. Grossly, they have no features to distinguish them unless cysts are formed; otherwise they do not differ from the carcinoma simplex, except that the latter is more often a scirrhus than is the adenocarcinoma. The cells are more highly differentiated in that they are arranged with a tendency to form more or less characteristic acini. Tumors occur which are generally of the simplex form, but which show small acini here and there; if these can be made out clearly they are referred to as adenocar-

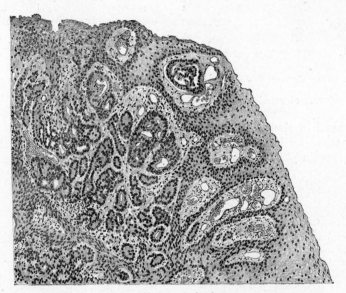

Adenocarcinoma of the breast.

ing, pearly gray cross section, often showing small yellow areas of epithelial masses. Metastasis is usually late and scanty. The medullary carcinomas grow more rapidly, invade deeply, metastasize early and widely. They are massive, ill defined, soft tumors which cut with ease, showing a soft bulging. moist, necrotic or hemorrhagic cross section. The knife will scrape from the cut surface a viscid, granular, cloudy yellow fluid, "cancer juice or milk," made up of liquefied cells and tissues. Although a scirrhus may become softer and even of medullary type, the reverse is not observed. Reactive inflammation with infiltration of mononuclear cells is common. Eosinophils may be numerous in certain situations, particularly in the alimentary canal.

cinoma. The adenocarcinomas may be graded on the basis of degree of differentiation of acini, those with great differentiation being regarded as more malignant than those in which acini are poorly developed; the carcinoma simplex is often grouped with these as a grade of high malignancy. The acini are of irregular outline and size, the cell lining tends to be multiple, with a disposition to fill the acinus. Solid columns of cells extend from the acini through tissue spaces. The basement membrane is incomplete or often absent. The cells are like simple or stratified columnar epithelium. Mitotic figures are frequent, often abnormal and multipolar, and with lack of uniformity in equatorial plane. If they arise from places where ciliated epithelium exists, the tumor cells may be ciliated. Carcinoma of the rectum are particularly likely to show mucinous goblet cells. Papilla formation may be extensive within the acini, giving rise to the name papilliferous adenocarcinoma. Necrosis is common, reactive inflammation almost constant, and acute inflammation resulting from erosion frequent.

Cyst formation in adenocarcinoma is by no means rare, the cysts containing papil-

fering in that the acini are filled and more or less distended with hyaline or granular basophilic mucin. It is unusual to find much mucin within the cells. Distention may flatten the lining cells. Desquamation of more or less degenerate cells is common, and the picture of a small cystic space filled with mucin, with few or no lining cells, and with centrally disposed, clumped, desquamated cells in the mass of mucin, is common.

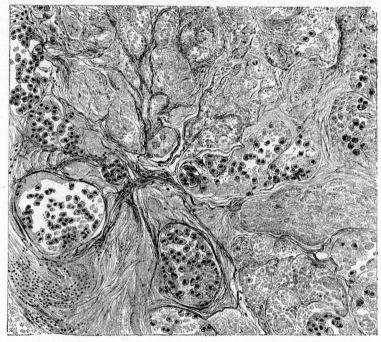

Mucinous carcinoma of the colon, showing acini with desquamated cells and masses of mucin in acinus-like structures free from cells.

lary outgrowths or various kinds of fluid. Carcinomas of the colon are especially prone to the formation of multiple cysts filled with mucin. These are often called colloid carcinomas because of the brown color and gelatinous consistency of the mucin. It is obvious that the correct term is mucinous carcinoma. Grossly, such tumors are poorly defined, of variable size, and of relatively soft elastic consistency. They cut with ease and show a soft, friable, gelatinous cross section either with little tissue definition, or of cystic character, the loculi measuring a few millimeters in diameter, and containing viscid or semisolid mucin. Microscopically, the picture is fundamentally that of adenocarcinoma, dif-

Regression of carcinoma may occur as the result of irradiation or spontaneously. The tumor cells undergo degeneration and necrosis and a diffuse growth of connective tissue occurs. Irradiation produces rapid necrosis of cells with pyknosis, karyorrhexis and karyolysis (see Loeb). Tumor cells may become multinucleated. Sometimes phagocytosis of destroyed cells is observed and in more extensive destruction, especially as the result of thrombosis of vessels, foreign-body giant cells are found. The changes in spontaneous retrogression are slower and less pronounced. Fibrosis proceeds from the margins and is essentially organization and cicatrization. Such appearances are quite different from those of the scirrhous cancer, which shows large bands of connective tissue and is a progressive lesion.

SPECIAL EPITHELIAL TUMORS

Introduction

In this group are placed certain tumors whose cell character does not correspond to ordinary adult epithelium. They are therefore difficult to classify with the groups of tumors as given in our outline. In each instance, however, the cells from which they arise originate in embryonal epithelium. The same is true of tumors of the nervous system; in this instance the tumors show cell types in more or less close resemblance to adult cells, not of mature epithelial character.

great amounts as to hide the nucleus. By special stains, figures resembling meissnerian corpuscles can be found, as well as sensory nerves with tiny end bulbs in contact with the cells of the nevus. Foot and others believe that the cells are derivations of the sheath of Schwann and therefore that the nevus is of the same nature as the neurofibroma. Laidlaw pointed to the resemblances between cutaneous nevi and the tactile bodies of reptiles and amphibia, especially as concerns elevation, pigmentation and groups of tactile elements in the corium. He expressed the view that the nevus represents a link of transition in phylogenetic scale from the pigmented tactile corpuscles of reptilian type to the hairy tactile organs of mammalian type. Thus the nevus would be a progonoma. Further indica-

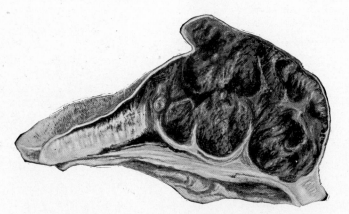

Cross section of melanoblastoma of the scalp.

Melanoma. Melanoblastoma. The exact origin of the cells of the pigmented nevus or mole is not settled, but it is discussed here because of our belief that it is ultimately derived from neuro-ectoderm. The pigmented nevus of the skin is flat or slightly elevated, sometimes papillary, well defined, pale yellow or dark brown, and is sometimes hairy. It occurs as a birthmark or appears later at times when growth of hair is noteworthy, as at puberty and late middle life. Microscopically, the upper corium contains many cells, uniform in size, round, with a moderate amount of cytoplasm and a round, fairly vesicular nucleus. These are arranged as cordlike, or more commonly, spherical masses, devoid of capsule. Some or many of the cells contain fine dark-brown granules of melanin in the cytoplasm, sometimes in such

tion of the ectodermal origin is the fact that patients with malignant transformation of the nevus contain intermedin in the urine (Ferguson) and that the cells respond to the dopa reagent, mentioned in our discussion of melanins, as do the basal cells of the epidermis. Ewing employs the term melanoma to indicate the malignant tumors of this order, in contradistinction to the benign pigmented mole. Many emphasize the neoplastic nature by using the term melanoblastoma. The mole usually remains quiescent throughout life. Ewing believes that in those instances of malignant transformation following a single injury, or excision, most of the moles were already neoplastic. Repeated injury or prolonged irritation is a more probable cause of malignancy, but sometimes this occurs without notable cause. When malignant, it is an invasive, widely metastasizing tumor. According to Peller, melanoma constitutes 4.1 per cent of the malignant tumors of the skin. When the nevus becomes malignant, it usually increases in size and depth of pigmentation. The cells, instead of being uniform in size and form, become notably pleomorphic, variable as to size and shape and may contain many mitotic figures; vascularization often increases. Metastasis is usually by blood-vascular routes, but sometimes transmission is also through the lymphatics. The metastatic nodules are often widespread and appear in almost any organ of the body. They are usually multiple in the organ, vary as to size and many are not pigmented. Microscopically, the metastases often show a good deal of uniformity of cell type rather than the pleomorphism of the original melanoblastoma. The dopa reaction is positive in the cells.

Melanoblastoma may arise in the choroid coat of the eye. Some of these tumors are composed of round cells and some of spindle cells. Removal of the eye may give good results, but metastases may grow years after the enucleation. Metastasis is observed most often in the liver, which may become enormously enlarged by the nodules, usually so deeply pigmented as to be practically black. Metastasis also occurs in bone marrow and in other organs. (See Callender and Wilder.) Melanoma also occurs in the large intestine but for the most part this is at the ano-rectal junction and the tumor is derived from the skin. Only rarely are melanomas found elsewhere in the large intestine. A pigmented tumor of the adrenal is also described and it is reasonably certain that the pigment is melanin, but the exact point of origin and the nature of the cells which produce the melanin are not known. This may metastasize widely. There are also rare cases of melanoma of the meninges of brain or cord derived from chromatophores that accompany the blood vessels. In the chapter on Pigmentation, reference has been made to the fact that in cases of melanoma the urine often contains a precursor of melanin which becomes black either on standing or by the addition of oxidizing agents, because of transformation of the precursor into melanin. The reader is referred especially to the article by Dawson for a survey of the origin and clinical and pathologic features of melanoma.

Chorionepithelioma. This tumor is derived from the covering cells of the chorionic villi. The cells which take part in the tumor growth are the cuboidal cells of Langhans and the syncytium, both of which are derived from trophoblast and thus geneti-

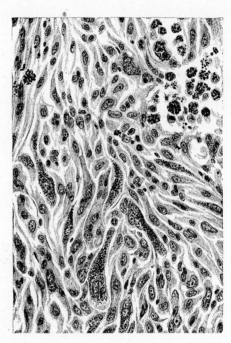

Metastatic melanoblastoma of liver. Pigment appears in fine granules in tumor cells and in coarser granules in phagocytic large mononuclear cells.

cally similar to ectoblastic epithelium. The tumor usually develops several months after delivery of a hydatidiform mole, abortion, miscarriage or normal pregnancy, but may occur earlier. It may arise from residual chorionic villi in the placental site or from villi or villus cells which become lodged in uterine veins. Occasionally villus cells may be transported to neighboring veins, as those of the vagina, and set up tumor growth there. Chorionepithelioma may even appear as part of teratoid tumors in the testis. The common variety of the tumor appears as a soft, red, spongy, often hemorrhagic tumor projecting into the cavity of the fundus uteri. Cross section shows definite penetration of the mass into the uterine wall. Microscopically, it shows irregular masses of cuboidal cells, with small vesicular or solid nuclei and finely granular or somewhat vesicular edematous cytoplasm containing glycogen; intermingled are multinucleated cell masses representing the chorionic syncytium. The cytoplasm of the multinucleated cell masses is usually vesicular and may contain much fat; the nuclei are usually dense rather than vesicular. Mitotic figures are more common in the cuboidal than in the multinucleated cells. The blood vessels are numerous and often cavernous; masses of tumor cells are

carcinoma is to be distinguished from the malignant hydatidiform mole or chorio-adenoma. The latter represents the invasive stage of the mole wherein, with preservation of the connective tissue part of enlarged and multiple cystic villi, the epithelium prolif-erates extensively and invades the uterine sinuses and musculature. Destruction and penetration of the uterus may occur but metastasis is rare. (See Schmitz and Hueper.)

Adamantinoma. This tumor is found principally in the jaws, especially the lower

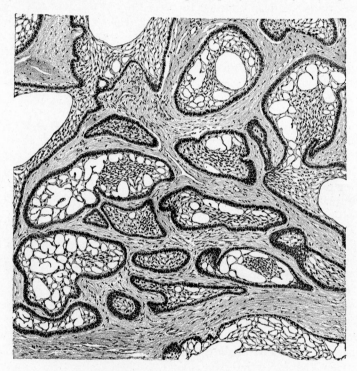

Cystic type of adamantinoma.

often found in the latter. Uterine curettings may contain retained placenta, which histo-logically shows masses of cells similar to those of the chorionepithelioma. The diag-nosis in these cases is simply retained pla-centa, unless there is great irregularity of cell growth with fairly rich vascularization, or definite penetration of muscularis. The intra-vascular position of much of the chorionepi-thelioma determines local extension to neigh-boring parts, particularly the vagina, and metastasis through the blood stream, most often to the lungs, rarely to the heart or other viscera.

The chorionepithelioma or chorio-

jaw, but occurs also in the pituitary and rarely in the tibia. Those of the jaw may be solid or cystic, may attain large size, are locally invasive and may recur after removal but rarely show distant metastases. Grossly they may be bony-hard, solid, firm, spongy or cystic. Microscopically, they show cell nests and masses, the marginal cells resembling ameloblasts. These differentiate centrally either to spindle and stellate cells or to form intermediate prickle cells and keratinized epithelium. Sometimes the central cells are cuboidal. With a loose central arrangement of the cells, cystic spaces occur and this phe-nomenon accounts for the grossly cystic forms. The adamantinoma is supposed to originate from misplaced cells of the dental groove or from the enamel organ, and the character of the tumor favors this assumption. Those in the hypophysis may be parts of a mixed tumor or may represent displacement of epithelium potentially like that of the dental groove, but those in the tibia are unexplained. (See McFarland and Patterson.)

Hypernephroma. In the course of development of the adrenal, cortical substance may be misplaced and be found in postfetal life in the kidney, along the urogenital canal, in the lower surface of liver and in the pancreas. The remnants or rests, representing a choristoma, usually remain quiescent throughout life. Rarely, however, such a rest may be transformed into a malignant tumor, the hypernephroma. This occurs in the kidney as a mass several centimeters or more in diameter, of bright yellow color, confined on its outer aspects by the capsule of the kidney but invading renal substance; it is soft, cuts readily and shows a bulging, soft, yellow cross section, mottled with extensive necrosis and hemorrhage. Microscopically, it has numerous delicate or broad trabeculae of well-vascularized connective tissue, from which grow strands or cords of large polygonal or round cells with markedly vesicular cytoplasm and a central, small vesicular nucleus. Mitotic figures are usually infrequent. The invasion of the kidney may be followed by extension along renal veins into the inferior vena cava. Metastasis occurs first in the lungs and then may be more widely distributed.

It has been found that many of the tumors formerly classified as hypernephroma are really renal carcinomas derived from epithelium of the kidney. The renal carcinoma may originate in renal adenoma or perhaps from cysts of the kidney. The gross description is the same as that of hypernephroma. Indeed, the microscopic appearance may be the same, but if a search, which may require numerous blocks of the tissue, is made, acinic or tubular structures will be found as well as groups of cells resembling renal epithelium. Extension into veins and route of metastasis are the same as described for hypernephroma. Further discussion appears in the chapter on Urinary System.

MIXED TUMORS

Introduction

Mixed tumors include a wide variety of tumors which do not conform to those already considered in that they contain several tissue or cell types instead of only one main tumorous element. There may be mixtures of several different connective tissues, or of connective tissues and epithelial structures, in which the connective tissue plays a greater part than that of support, or there may be representatives of practically all the tissues of the body. Some of these have been mentioned in the foregoing discussions but have not been classified. These tumors, then, represent adult tissues of types which take origin in one, two or three germinal layers of the embryo, and may be classified as mono-, bi-, and tridermal mixed tumors. We prefer, however, a simpler classification in which those representing one or two layers are called mixed tumors and those representing all three layers are called teratoid tumors or teratomas. It is of interest to speculate as to whether these tumors originate in single cells or cell groups of blastoderm or original embryonal layers, or arise from cells in which varying degrees of differentiation have occurred. If the first supposition be true, the simpler mixed tumors are the derivatives of multipotential cells. In so far as concerns these tumors the problem has not been solved, but in the teratomata, the common situation in sex glands would make it seem probable that aberrations in germinal cells may lead, by development from totipotential cells, to the multiple tissues in the tumors. As has been indicated earlier, there is little experimental evidence relating to the question. Mixed tumors vary considerably as to recurrence and metastasis and in this relation only the individual tumor types can be discussed. Malignancy may develop in mixed tumors that are primarily benign. If this occur, the metastases may be made up of only one or two elements, or all of the constituents, of the primary tumor. Rarely, a primary malignant tumor may be mixed to form a combined carcinoma and sarcoma, a point to be discussed subsequently. The field of mixed tumors is so large and individual cases show such great variations, that it is possible only to indicate some of the more important features.

Mixed Tumors

Arbitrarily we include here those tumors composed of tissues representing derivatives of only one or two embryonal layers. These comprise tumors already described, as for example, such simple mixtures as osteochondroma and more complex forms as the fibromyxolipoma or liposarcoma. Two forms of the mixed tumor, the mixed tumors of salivary glands (especially parotid) and embryonal mixed tumors of the kidney, deserve special consideration.

Mixed Tumors of the Salivary Glands. This type of tumor may occur in any of the salivary glands, in the lachrymal glands, in the gums and in certain other situations, but are most common in the parotid gland. They occur in adult life, usually grow

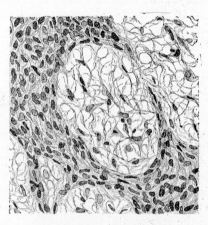

Small section of a mixed tumor of the parotid gland with epithelial type cells and mucoid tissue.

slowly as firm, in the early stages movable, sometimes nodular, tumors, varying in size from the usual diameters of 1 or 2 cm. to very large size. As they enlarge they become increasingly adherent to surrounding structures. When excised they are fairly well circumscribed but as a rule, only partly if at all encapsulated. They are firm, pale, and often resemble chronically enlarged lymph nodes; they cut with considerable resistance and show a slightly bulging, moist, pale cross section usually free from necrosis. Microscopically, there are several elements present, all but one of which can be regarded as mesoblastic. A ground substance of connective tissue may show fibromatous, myxomatous,

chondromatous and sometimes other elements. Supported on this are numbers of round cells of moderate size, with moderately chromatic nuclei and fairly dense cytoplasm. Mitotic figures are rare. These cells may be simply in masses, or may be arranged to form acinus-like structures, which may contain mucin or mucoid; they may also be arranged to form tubular spaces containing hyaline cylinders, thus exhibiting cylindromatous character.

Removal of the encapsulated forms is usually successful, but removal of the partly or unencapsulated forms may be followed by repeated recurrence and malignant change may ultimately occur. The nature of these tumors is disputed. The idea that the essential cells are endothelial has been generally abandoned, because in many respects they may exhibit epithelial characters, including intercellular bridges and pearl formation. The tumor may be seen to arise from parotid gland ducts and acini, but it is possible that others may arise from branchial cleft inclusions. Investigations now point toward the tumors as purely epithelial. Ewing is satisfied that the cartilage and mucoid tissue may be derived from epithelium. Zymbal regards the presumptively mesoblastic tissue as a metaplasia from epithelium and has shown by tissue culture that mucoid and cartilage-like structures may develop. Thus it is probable that the tumor is not a mixed tumor but wholly epithelial in origin and to be referred to as epithelial tumor of salivary-gland type.

Embryonal Mixed Tumors of the Kidney. These tumors are fairly common, usually appear in the first three years of life and may attain enormous size, diameters of 35, 37, and 40 cm. having been reported. They are almost always intrarenal but may be entirely extrarenal. They are large, fairly dense, usually encapsulated, smooth or lobulated tumors, sometimes with large single or smaller multiple cysts. Upon section, the surface is usually fleshy, bulging, moderately vascularized and may show necrosis and hemorrhage. Microscopically, the picture varies in different parts of the tumor. The most constant feature is the presence of medium-sized round or oval cells with fairly dense cytoplasm, frequently containing glycogen, and a small, slightly vesicular nucleus. These fuse with areas of spindle cells, which predominate in some tumors. In the cellular masses there are acinar or tubular areas, surrounded by cuboidal or cylindrical cells, which may be separate from or fused with the surrounding less-differentiated cells. The spindle cells often show the characters of sarcoma. Intermingled in the tumor are areas of other types of tissue, not all of which are necessarily present in each tumor, namely cartilage, smooth muscle, embryonal striated muscle, fat, edematous and myxomatous con-

blue, painful and exquisitely tender. Microscopically, it is an angioneuromyoma, made up of a mixture of vascular tubes, smooth muscle, nonmedullated nerves and the large round or polyhedral cells arranged in masses or sheets. Rarely, the tumor may occur in other situations than those mentioned. It may be somewhat invasive, but metastases have not been reported. (See Blanchard; Murray and Stout.)

Mixed Carcinoma and Sarcoma. The difficulty in diagnosis of a carcinosarcoma lies principally in the interpretation of spindle cells intermingled or associated with

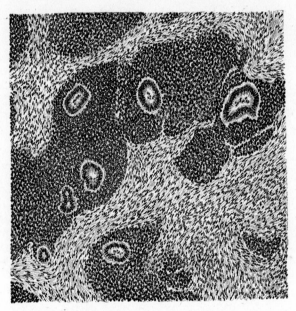

Embryonal mixed tumor of the kidney with spindle cells, round cells and tubular structures.

nective tissue, and rarely other types of tissue. It seems probable that these tumors originate in renal blastema, the cells differentiating to form the various tissues and cells of the tumor. Although the histologic picture is often characteristic of malignancy, metastasis is rare. When it occurs it is most common in the liver, but it may appear in the lungs and other organs.

Glomangioma. The cutaneous glomus is made up of specialized arteriovenous anastomoses, nerve fibers and large round "epithelioid" cells. These structures are found in the corium of the skin of various parts of the body, especially the digits and also under the nails. The tumor which may develop is small,

cells that are obviously epithelial. If a carcinosarcoma exists, it must be due to development from cells which have the potentiality of producing both epithelium and connective tissue, or to a carcinoma which produces sarcoma or a sarcoma which produces carcinoma. Various studies show that epithelial cells may assume spindle form and that a large portion of a carcinoma may consist of such cells (Martin and Stewart). This fact has probably led to the confusion of these spindle cells with connective-tissue cells. Saphir and Vass analyzed reports of 153 cases of supposed carcinosarcoma and found that not more than four could be accepted. Other confusing features include marked anaplasia of epithelial cells, a reaction of surrounding connective tissue that may be mistaken for sarcoma, and a rich infiltration of lymphocytes suggestive of lymphosarcoma. There is no real support for the view that the tumor arises from multipotential cells, or that carcinoma can be transformed into sarcoma or the reverse. Experimentally, inoculation of sarcoma and carcinoma results in development of one or the other, or both, depending upon

Teratomata

The teratomata include certain true tumors and progressively growing tumor-like embryonal inclusions, in which representatives of all three embryonal layers are present in disorderly fashion. The latter group shades into the group of monsters, but monsters are characterized by a more orderly arrangement of tissues and organs (see Willis). In their undeveloped forms they represent the condi-

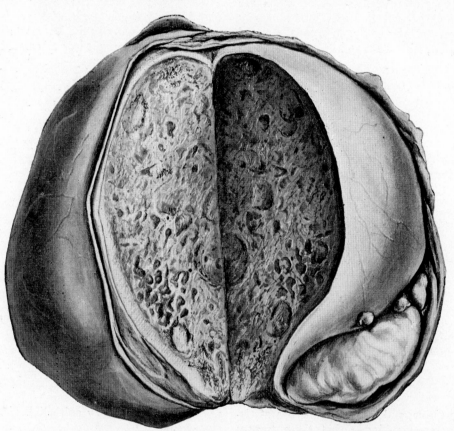

Teratoid tumor of the testis, exact size, showing variable character of cut surface.

the soil provided, as has been discussed above. It is reported that a transplantable carcinoma was transformed into a sarcoma in the thirty-fifth generation but this may well be due to the confusion mentioned in reference to human tumors. If true carcinosarcoma exists at all, it is rare.

Carcinoma and sarcoma may originate in neighboring points and fuse to form a combination of the two, a "collision" tumor. Furthermore, a benign connective-tissue tumor may be invaded by a carcinoma either directly or by metastasis.

tion spoken of earlier as hamartoma. The blastomatous tumors of teratoid nature contain immature cell forms and are often malignant. The fetal inclusions show mature cells, tissues and organoid forms. They differ from the monsters not only in the disorderly arrangement of tissues, but also in that their individual tissues are prone to true blastomatous proliferation and malignancy. It can readily be seen that with all three layers of the embryo partaking in the production of the tumors and tumor-like masses, the possible combinations are almost innumerable.

Fundamentals of classification may serve as a guide in individual tumors, but only a few of the more common varieties can be discussed. As has been indicated, the teratomata may be classified as immature forms with relatively undifferentiated cells and tissues, which are younger than those of the host, the so-called embryoma, or as adult coetaneous forms in which the cells and tissues are mature and of the same relative age (either from the point of view of actual age—fetal inclusions—or that of differentiation) as the host. Since many of the tumors arise in sex glands, the classification into genital and extragenital varieties is of importance.

Teratoma of Testis. This tumor is fairly common in the adult testis, and is said to be more frequent in undescended than descended testes. The mature type of teratoma contains a variety of cells and tissues, such as connective tissue, mucoid tissue, cartilage, bone, epithelium of almost any variety, glands, gastric mucosa, various components of the nervous system, etc. Malignant changes in any of the elements of the tumor may be observed and the metastases may be carcinoma, sarcoma, or represent several elements of the original tumor. Grossly, the tumor may attain considerable size, but is usually observed and removed fairly early in its course. Circumscribed, often encapsulated, it may grow within the testis destroying it or may push it aside. It is a bulky, usually nodular, tumor and although sometimes cystic rarely shows the dermoid cysts so common in the ovary.

There is also a group of tumors of the testis, discussed further in the chapter on Genital System, which is classified microscopically as embryonal carcinoma or seminoma, adenocarcinoma, and chorionepithelioma. These tumors probably are forms of teratoma, in which one element outgrows all others. Grossly, they are likely to be soft, fleshy, well vascularized, variable as to size, often showing necrosis and hemorrhage. Metastasis may be early and widespread, especially in the case of chorionepithelioma.

Ovarian Teratoma. The teratoid tumors of the ovary may be solid or cystic. The solid forms are rare, are unilateral, and both grossly and microscopically resemble the mature and partly mature forms described in

the testis. The cystic forms, much more common, are the so-called dermoid cysts, or more specifically complex dermoid cysts.

Complex Dermoid Cysts. These are mature forms of teratoma and are properly called cystic teratomata. They may occur at any time of life but are most frequently encountered in middle age. They may be unilateral, bilateral, single or multiple, and may vary markedly in size. The common, large

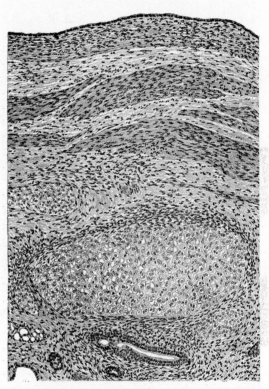

Teratoid tumor of ovary showing smooth muscle, connective tissue, cartilage and gland structures.

monolocular cyst usually shows a capsule and a moderately thick wall, which often at one point shows extra thickness. Upon opening the cyst a semifluid, oily or buttery, pale yellow or white, grumous mass is found, containing long interlacing hairs, which usually grow from the thickest part of the cyst wall. Microscopically, the wall shows a lining of skin with epiderm, papillary corium, sweat and sebaceous glands and hair follicles. The deeper parts of the wall show mature tissues and organoid forms, the total of which in various tumors includes practically all the tissues of the body except the sex glands.

Cartilage, bone, teeth, various epithelial structures, ganglion cells, neuroglia, etc., are common but organs such as liver, kidneys, pancreas are rarely present. Malignant change is not common. Similar tumors may occur in other situations, more particularly in body fissures and in the region of the branchial clefts of the neck.

Simple Dermoid; Epidermoid Cyst. The cystic teratoma must be distinguished from the simple dermoid, which may occur in a variety of situations, as a result of trauma or faulty development, the cysts containing grumous, buttery material and lined with skin but without mixed elements in the surrounding tissues. Epidermoid cysts may be of the same origin, but are surrounded only by epiderm instead of skin. Obstruction of sebaceous glands, rarely of sweat glands, produces cysts which often project on the skin surface and contain sebaceous material; the names often applied are atheroma cutis or atheromatous cysts of the skin, or sebaceous cysts.

Sacral Teratoma. This condition, by no means common, is much more a fault of development (of the body fissures) than a true tumor. It appears as a nodular mass projecting from the region of the sacrum and coccyx, sometimes displacing the rectum anteriorly. Upon section it is usually spongy or cystic. It differs from the teratomata considered previously in that the tissues and organs composing it are much more mature. Rudimentary extremities, legs, arms, toes, fingers, may be formed occasionally. Malignant change may involve any element. (See Meister.)

Epignathus. This projects forward from the pharynx, and may either be a complex teratoid mass with organs and organoid forms resembling the sacral teratoma or be much more mature, showing fairly well developed organs and parts of extremities. The latter variety might with justice be classified with the monsters rather than with teratomata. True teratomata and dermoids also occur in the pharynx.

Monsters

In the development of the embryo and fetus a variety of conditions may determine abnormalities. These may be of little functional import and not incompatible with apparently normal life, or more severe and lead to shortened life, or so marked as to lead to intrauterine or early postnatal death. Some of the minor abnormalities, such as extra fingers and toes, are hereditary, but most others have no such basis. Only the more severe abnormalities are included in the term monsters. These may affect single individuals or be double monsters. In single individuals, the important monstrosities are connected with faulty development of the various body fissures, particularly facial (cleft-palate, harelip), branchial, urogenital and neural. In the last group are included cranioschisis and acrania due to faults near the cephalic pole, rhachischisis along the area of the spinal canal, and spina bifida at the caudal pole. The double monsters may be symmetrical or asymmetrical. The former include twin fetuses joined together at the cephalic poles (craniopagus), at the thoracic portion (thoracopagus), or at the caudal poles (ischiopagus). These may appear in extremely varied patterns. The asymmetric forms include numerous types of parasitic fetus attached to various parts of the body or included within the body. This group shades into the epignathi and sacral teratomata. Monster formation must be regarded as a pathologic alteration of development of ovum and embryo, and the discussion of the etiology is therefore far reaching. The complete discussion of the forms of monsters is a catalogue of descriptive terms, and cannot be included in a book of this scope. The reader is referred to such works as those of Ballantyne, Hirst and Piersol, and most particularly Schwalbe for details of etiology and morphology.

Cysts

Introduction. The cyst is a sac with connective tissue or other type of wall, containing fluid or semifluid material. Many cysts have no relation whatever to tumors and are included here simply for convenience; many tumors, however, contain cysts even to such an extent as to be called cystic tumors; certain cysts by proliferation of elements in their walls may give rise to tumors. Cysts may be monolocular with only one sac, or multilocular with several sacs. They vary considerably in origin and may be classified as congenital or acquired. Our discussion is necessarily much restricted, but will be further developed in the sections on Systemic Pathology.

Congenital Cysts. These may be due to persistence of ducts established in embryonal life, which normally disappear, or to faulty development of glandular organs. Persistent tubes or ducts, which normally should completely disappear, may show interrupted closure because of disappearance only of parts; secretory or other products may then accumulate and the tube remnant become cystic. Included in these are thyrolingual cysts in the midline of the neck, branchiogenic cysts in the region of the branchial clefts, vitello-intestinal cysts near the umbilicus and urachal cysts in the lower abdominal cavity. Numerous types of cyst are found in relation to both male and female genital organs, due to persistence of remains of the wolffian body, paroöphoron, Gaertner's duct, muellerian duct, etc. Congenital cysts of glandular organs are best exemplified in congenital polycystic kidney and liver. The congenital cystic kidney is usually considerably enlarged, made up of multiple cysts of diameters of a few millimeters to a centimeter or more, thin walled, containing colorless or pale yellow fluid, or colorless, yellow or brown hyaline material. The cysts of the liver are multiple, of moderate size, usually contain clear, colorless fluid and often appear to be dilatations of lymphatics. There is rarely a so-called cystic diathesis in which both kidneys and liver are cystic.

Acquired Glandular Cysts. These develop in pre-existing glands or ducts. There are two forms, the retention cyst and the follicular cyst. The retention cyst occurs as the result of occlusion of a duct or ducts. The corresponding dilatation behind the obstruction may be temporary, if the obstruction be removable, or permanent. If temporary, the subsequent changes in the gland depend upon duration. In general, obstruction leads to atrophy and disappearance of the parenchymatous cells, with more or less extensive replacement fibrosis. It is of interest that in the pancreas the islets of Langerhans survive long after the disappearance of the acinar cells. It is of further interest that the secretory pressure in glands may be so great as to produce large cysts, the contents of which, more or less different from the normal secretion, may be under extremely high physical pressure. This pressure probably induces an inflammatory fibrosis. Retention cysts occur in the cutaneous glands, especially the sebaceous cyst, in salivary glands ("ranula" of sublingual glands), pancreas, kidney, liver and other organs. Similar cystic accumulations occur in the gall bladder, chronically inflamed fallopian tubes, etc. Follicular cysts occur in glands without ducts and are well represented in the thyroid and ovary.

Cysts in Solid Organs. These are due to necrosis and softening of localized foci. Anything which can produce localized necrosis may produce these cysts, the most common being vascular occlusion or hemorrhage. The best examples are in the brain, where a focus of necrosis due to vascular occlusion undergoes liquefaction necrosis, and is surrounded by a fibrous and neuroglial capsule to produce a cyst. The same phenomenon may follow a hemorrhage, the cyst contents in this case being tinged brown by blood pigment, as are also the walls of the cyst. Ducts may rupture into solid organs, secretions accumulate, and become organized with the formation of cysts. Cysts of this general group are often called pseudocysts.

Parasitic Cysts. Although small cysts may be formed by the fibrous tissue deposit around *Trichinella spiralis* in muscle, the only large parasitic cyst in man is that of the cysticercus stage of *Taenia echinococcus*. The adult form occurs in the dog, the feces of which contain the ova. Transferred to the intestinal canal of man, the cysticercus stage is built up in the liver or more rarely in other viscera. Usually one large cyst is formed containing fluid and daughter cysts. The major cyst has a wall made up of concentric hyaline laminae surrounded by fibrous tissue of the host. Fluid from the cyst usually contains hooklets from the scolices of the worm, but sterile cysts are sometimes encountered. Old cysts may contain only a pale brown or yellow gelatinous material. Occasionally, the daughter cysts project outward from the primary cyst to form a multiloculated cyst.

Neoplastic Cysts. In the consideration of certain epithelial tumors, particularly of adenomatous character, it has been pointed out that distention may occur to form cysts, with or without papilla formation, and sometimes with special contents, as in the mucinous carcinomas. Tumors may also exhibit necrotic cysts or hemorrhagic cysts in much the same form as they occur in solid organs. The glioma is not infrequently cystic, probably due to necrosis, but in certain instances possibly because of the ependymal character of the cells.

REFERENCES

Adamstone, F. B.: Relation of Vitamin E to Substances of the Anthracene Group, Arch. Path., 31: 722, 1941.

Albrecht, E.: Die Grundprobleme der Geschwulstlehre, Frank. Zeitschr. f. Path. Anat., 1: 221, 1907.

Bailey, P.: Histologic Atlas of Gliomas, Arch. Path. and Lab. Med., 4: 871, 1927.

——, and H. Cushing: A Classification of the Tumors of the Glioma Group, etc., Philadelphia, 1926.

——, and J. D. Herrmann: The Role of the Cells of Schwann in the Formation of Tumors of the Peripheral Nerves, Amer. Jour. Path., 14: 1, 1938.

deBalogh, E.: Investigations on a New Heterologous Tumor, "Budapest 1938," Successfully Propagated in Hungarian White Rats, Amer. Jour. Cancer, 39: 45, 1940.

Bashford, E. F.: Heredity and Disease, Proc. Roy. Soc. Med., 2: General Reports, 63, 1909.

——: The Immunity Reaction to Cancer, ibid., 3: Therap. Section, p. 69, 1910.

Batson, O. V.: The Role of the Vertebral Veins in Metastatic Processes, Ann. Int. Med., 16: 38, 1942.

Baumann, C. A., E. G. Foster, and P. S. Lavik: The Effect of Certain Carcinogens on Vitamin A in the Liver, Jour. Nutr., 21: 431, 1941.

Becker, S. W.: Benign Epidermal Neoplasms, Arch. Derm. and Syphilol., 26: 838, 1932.

Belling, J.: The Number of Chromosomes in the Cells of Cancerous and Other Human Tumors, Jour. Amer. Med. Asso., 88: 396, 1927.

Beneke, R.: Ueber physiologisches und pathologisches Wachstum, Berl. klin. Wochenschr., 42: 1133, 1186, 1905.

Bielschowsky, M.: Neuroblastic Tumors of the Sympathetic Nervous System, Section XXIV, Vol. III, p. 1085; Penfield, W.: Cytology and Cellular Pathology of the Central Nervous System, New York, 1932.

Bittner, J. J.: Possible Method of Transmission of Susceptibility to Breast Cancer in Mice, Amer. Jour. Cancer, 39: 104, 1940.

——: The Preservation by Freezing and Drying in Vacuo of the Milk-Influence for the Development of Breast Cancer in Mice, Science, 93: 527, 1941.

Blanchard, A. J.: The Pathology of Glomus Tumours, Canad. Med. Asso. Jour., 44: 357, 1941.

Blank, F.: The Role of Genetics in Cancer, Ohio State Med. Jour., 37: 947, 1941.

Blum, H. F.: Sunlight and Cancer of the Skin, Jour. Nat. Cancer Inst., 1: 397, 1940.

Borst, M.: Die Lehre von den Geschwülsten, Wiesbaden, 1902.

Borst, M.: Echte Geschwülste, Aschoff's Pathologische Anatomie, Vol. 1, Jena, 1921.

Boveri, T.: The Origin of Malignant Tumors, Baltimore, 1929.

Broders, A. C.: Carcinoma-Grading and Practical Application, Arch. Path. and Lab. Med., 2: 376, 1926.

——, R. Hargrave, and H. W. Meyerding: Pathological Features of Soft Tissue Fibrosarcoma, with Special Reference to the Grading of Its Malignancy, Surg., Gynec. and Obst., 69: 267, 1939.

Brumpt, E.: Rôle des Bilharzies dans la Production de Certains Cancers, Etude Critique a Propos d'un Cas Nouveau, Ann. de Parasitol., 8: 75, 1930.

Bryan, C. S., and S. Warren: Functional Activity of Smooth Muscle Tumors of the Uterus, Proc. Soc. Exper. Biol. and Med., 47: 356, 1941.

Bullock, F. D., and M. R. Curtis: Further Studies on the Transplantation of the Larvae of Taenia Crassicollis, etc., Jour. Cancer Res., 10: 393, 1927; see also Jour. Cancer Res., 12: 326, 1928.

Burrows, M. T.: Studies on the Nature of Growth Stimulus in Cancer, Jour. Cancer Res., 10: 239, 1926.

——, and C. G. Johnston: The Action of Oils in the Production of Tumors, with a Definition of the Cause of Cancer, Arch. Int. Med., 36: 293, 1925.

Caldwell, G. T.: Chemical Carcinogenic Agents, Jour. Urol., 42: 651, 1939.

Cappell, D. F.: Chordoma of the Vertebral Column, with Three New Cases, Jour. Path. and Bact., 31: 797, 1928.

Carrel, A.: Essential Characteristics of a Malignant Cell, Jour. Amer. Med. Asso., 84: 157, 1925.

——, and A. H. Ebeling: The Transformation of Monocytes into Fibroblasts through the Action of Rous Virus, Jour. Exper. Med., 43: 461, 1926.

——, and A. H. Ebeling: The Fundamental Properties of the Fibroblast and the Macrophage. IV. The Malignant Fibroblast of Jensen Sarcoma, Jour. Exper. Med., 48: 285, 1928.

Casey, A. E.: The Experimental Alteration of Malignancy with an Homologous Mammalian Tumor Material, Amer. Jour. Cancer, 21: 760, 776, 1934.

——: Specificity of Enhancing Materials from Mammalian Tumors, Proc. Soc. Exper. Biol. and Med., 31: 663, 1934.

Chambers, H., G. Scott, and S. Russ: On the Action of X-rays upon the Transplantation of a Spontaneous Carcinoma of the Rat, Jour. Path. and Bact., 23: 384, 1919-20.

Claude, A., and J. B. Murphy: Transmissible Tumors of the Fowl, Physiol. Rev., 13: 246, 1933.

Cook, J. W., and E. L. Kennaway: Chemical Compounds as Carcinogenic Agents. Second Supplementary Report: Literature of 1938 and 1939, Amer. Jour. Cancer, 39: 381; 521, 1940.

Copeland, M. M.: Skeletal Metastases Arising from Carcinoma and from Sarcoma, Arch. Surg., 23: 581, 1931.

Coplin, W. M. L.: A Basis for the Prevention of Cancer, Jour. Amer. Med. Asso., 78: 1523, 1922.

Cowdry, E. V.: Properties of Cancer Cells, Arch. Path., 30: 1245, 1940; see also F. X. Paletta, E. V. Cowdry, and C. E. Lischer: Comparison of Methylcholanthrene Hyperplastic Epidermis with Benign Hyperplastic Epidermis in Healing Wounds, Cancer Res., 1: 942, 1941.

Cowdry, E. V., and F. X. Paletta: Changes in Cellular, Nuclear, and Nucleolar Sizes during Methylcholanthrene Epidermal Carcinogenesis, Jour. Nat. Cancer Inst., 1: 745, 1941.

Cramer, W.: Papillomatosis in the Forestomach of the Rat and Its Bearing on the Work of Fibiger, Amer. Jour. Cancer, 31: 537, 1937.

——: The Prevention of Spontaneous Mammary Cancer in Mice by Anterior Pituitary Hormone, Amer. Jour. Cancer, 40: 431, 1940.

Curtis, M. R., W. F. Dunning, and F. D. Bullock: Genetic Factors in Relation to the Etiology of Malignant Tumors, Amer. Jour. Cancer, 17: 894, 1933.

Cushing, H.: The Meningiomas (Dural Endotheliomas), etc., Brain, 45: 282, 1922.

Dawson, J. W.: The Melanomata, Their Morphology and Histogenesis, Edinburgh Med. Jour., 32: 501-732, 1925.

Des Ligneris, M. J. A.: The Production of Benign and Malignant Skin Tumours in Mice Painted with Bantu Liver Extracts, Amer. Jour. Cancer, 39: 489, 1940.

——: Precancer and Carcinogenesis, ibid., 40: 1, 1940.

Dodds, E. C.: Recent Biochemical Research in Cancer with Special Reference to the Metabolism of the Normal and Malignant Cell, Amer. Jour. Cancer, 15: 2765, 1931.

——: A Study of Specificity in Relation to Hormone and Other Biological Relations, Harvey Lectures, Baltimore, Williams and Wilkins, 30: 119, 1936.

Eckert, C. T., Z. K. Cooper, and M. G. Seelig: Scarlet Red as a Possible Carcinogenic Agent: An Experimental Study, Arch. Path., 19: 83, 1935.

Eggers, H. E.: The Etiology of Cancer, Arch. Path., 12: 983, 1931; 13: 112; 296; 462, 1932.

Eveleth, M. S., and N. C. Wetzel: Rapid Growth of a Bronchiogenic Carcinoma, Cancer Res., 1: 721, 1941.

Ewing, J.: Neoplastic Diseases. A Treatise on Tumors, 4th ed., Philadelphia and London, Saunders, 1940.

Fender, F. A.: Liposarcoma. Report of a Case with Intracranial Metastasis, Amer. Jour. Path., 9: 909, 1933.

Ferguson, R. S., G. H. Gehrmann, D. M. Gay, L. W. Anderson, and V. D. Washburn: Symposium on Aniline Tumors of the Bladder, Jour. Urol., 31: 121, 1934.

Fibiger, J.: Untersuchungen über die Nematode (Spiroptera, sp. 26.) und deren Fähigkiet papillomatöse und carcinomatöse Geschwulstbildungen, etc., Zeitschr. Krebsforsch., 13: 217, 1913; 14: 295, 1914; see also Jour. Cancer Res., 4: 367, 1919.

Fischer, A.: Factors of a Growth Regulatory Nature in Tissue Cells, Amer. Jour. Med. Sci., 173: 562, 1927; see also Klin. Wochenschr., 7: 48, 1928; The Theory of the Developmental Physiology of Malignant Tumors, Amer. Jour. Cancer, 31: 1, 1937.

Foot, N. C.: Concerning the Histology of Melanoma, Amer. Jour. Path., 8: 309; 321, 1932.

Franseen, C. C., and G. W. Taylor: Arsenical Keratoses and Carcinomas, Amer. Jour. Cancer, 22: 287, 1934.

Geschickter, C. F., and M. M. Copeland: Recurrent and So-called Metastatic Giant Cell Tumors, Arch. Surg., 20: 713, 1930.

Geschickter, C. F.: Tumors of Muscle, Amer. Jour. Cancer, 22: 378, 1934.

——: Tumors of the Peripheral Nerves, Amer. Jour. Cancer, 25: 377, 1935.

Ginzton, L. L., and C. L. Connor: Crude Wheat-Germ Oil as a Factor of Tumor Formation in Rats, Amer. Jour. Cancer, 38: 90, 1940.

Goldstein, H. I.: I. Goldstein's Heredo-familial Angiomatosis with Recurring Familial Hemorrhages (Rendu-Osler-Weber's Disease), Arch. Int. Med., 48: 836, 1931.

Goodpasture, E. W.: An Anatomical Study of Senescence in Dogs, with Especial Reference to the Relation of Cellular Changes of Age to Tumors, Jour. Med. Res., 38: 127, 1918.

Graham, A.: Malignant Tumors of the Thyroid, Ann. Surg., 81: 30, 1925.

Gray, J. H.: Relation of Lymphatic Vessels to Spread of Cancer, Brit. Jour. Surg., 26: 462, 1939.

Greene, H. S. N.: Familial Mammary Tumors in the Rabbit, Year Book of Pathology and Immunology, Chicago, Year Book Publishers, 1940; p. 63.

——: Heterologous Transplantation of Mammalian Tumors. I. The Transfer of Human Tumors to Alien Species, Jour. Exper. Med., 73: 475, 1941.

Greenough, R. B.: Varying Degrees of Malignancy in Cancer of the Breast, Jour. Cancer Res., 9: 453, 1925.

Greenstein, J. P., W. V. Jenrette, G. B. Mider, and J. White: Chemical Studies on the Components of Normal and Neoplastic Tissues. V. The Relative Arginase Activity of Certain Tumors and Normal Control Tissues, Jour. Nat. Cancer Inst., 1: 687, 1941.

——, and J. White: The Liver Catalase Activity of Tumor-Bearing Rats and the Effect of Extirpation of the Tumors, Jour. Nat. Cancer Inst., 2: 283, 1941.

Gross, L.: The Influence of Sex of Mice on Acquired Resistance to a Transplantable Sarcoma, Cancer Res., 1: 880, 1941.

Guyer, M. F., F. E. Mohs, and E. M. Shebesta: Effects of Artificially Induced Lymphopenia in Cancer-Resistant and Cancer-Susceptible Rats, Arch. Path., 19: 66, 1935.

Haagen, E.: Die Bedeutung der Monozyten bei der experimentelle Tumorerzeugung, Deutsch. med. Wochenschr., 54: 92, 1928.

Haagensen, C. D.: Occupational Neoplastic Disease, Amer. Jour. Cancer, 15: 641, 1931.

——, and H. T. Randall: Production of Mammary Carcinoma in Mice by Estrogens, Arch. Path., 33: 411, 1942.

Hamilton, A.: Discussion of the Etiology of So-called Aniline Tumors of the Bladder, Jour. Indust. Hygiene, 3: 16, 1921.

Handley, W. S.: Cancer of the Breast and Its Operative Treatment, Ed. 2, New York, Hoeber, 1922.

v. Hansemann, E.: Die mikroskopische Diagnose der bösartigen Geschwülste, Berlin, 1902.

——: Was ist Anaplasie? Berl. Klin. Wochenschr., 44: 1850, 1909.

Harvey, W. F., and T. D. Hamilton: Carcinosarcoma. A Study of the Microscopic Anatomy and Meaning of a Peculiar Cancer, Edinburgh Med. Jour., 42: 337, 1935.

Hauser, I. J., and C. V. Weller: A Further Report on the Cancer Family of Warthin, Amer. Jour. Cancer, 27: 434, 1936.

Haythorn, S. R.: Studies on the Histogenesis of the So-called "Basal Cell Carcinoma," Amer. Jour. Cancer, 15: 1969, 1931. See also Spies, A. W.: Adenoid Cystic Carcinoma. Generalized Metastases in

Three Cases of the Basal Cell Type, Arch. Surg., **21:** 365, 1930.

Heiberg, K. A., and T. Kemp: Ueber die Zahl der Chromosomen in Carcinomzellen beim Menschen, Virchow's Arch. Path. Anat., **273:** 693, 1929.

Heiman, J.: The Effect of Androgens and Estrogens on Spontaneous Benign Mammary Tumors in the Rat, Amer. Jour. Cancer, **40:** 343, 1940.

Hellwig, C. A.: The Scientific Basis of Biopsy in Tumors, Arch. Path., **14:** 517, 1932.

Hieger, I.: The Examination of Human Tissue for Carcinogenic Factors, Amer. Jour. Cancer, **39:** 496, 1940.

Hirst, B. C., and G. A. Piersol: Human Monstrosities, Vols. 1-4, Philadelphia, 1891-1893.

Hoffman, F. L.: The Mortality from Cancer Throughout the World, Newark, N. J., 1915.

Hosoi, K.: Multiple Neurofibromatosis (von Recklinghausen's Disease) with Special Reference to Malignant Transformation, Arch. Surg., **22:** 258, 1931.

Howard, W. T., and O. T. Schultz: Studies in the Biology of Tumor Cells, Monographs of Rock. Inst. Med. Research, No. 2, 1911.

Ingleby, H.: Etiology of Benign Tumors, Arch. Path., **19:** 303, 1935.

Jackson, H., Jr.: Certain Biological Aspects of Cancer, Medicine, **7:** 345, 1928.

Jaffe, H. L., L. Lichtenstein, and R. B. Portis: Giant Cell Tumor of Bone. Its Pathologic Appearance, Grading, Supposed Variants and Treatment, Arch. Path., **30:** 993, 1940.

Jones, H. B., I. L. Chaikoff, and J. H. Lawrence: Phosphorus Metabolism of Neoplastic Tissues (Mammary Carcinoma, Lymphoma, Lymphosarcoma) as Indicated by Radioactive Phosphorus, Amer. Jour. Cancer, **40:** 243, 1940.

Kennaway, E. L.: Occupational Mortality: The Registrar-General's Decennial Supplement, England and Wales, 1931, Amer. Jour. Cancer, **36:** 110, 1939.

——, and B. Sampson: Tumors of the Skin and Mammary Gland Caused by Pyrogenous Products of Cholesterol, Jour. Path. and Bact., **31:** 609, 1928; *see also* Cook, J. W., I. Hieger, E. L. Kennaway, and W. V. Mayneord: Production of Cancer by Pure Hydrocarbons, Proc. Roy. Soc., London, Series B., **111:** 455, 1932.

Kettle, E. H.: The Pathology of Tumors, London, 1916.

Kidd, J. G.: The Course of Virus-Induced Rabbit Papillomas as Determined by Virus, Cells and Host, Jour. Exper. Med., **67:** 551, 1938.

——, and P. Rous: A Transplantable Rabbit Carcinoma Originating in a Virus-Induced Papilloma and Containing the Virus in Masked or Altered Form, Jour. Exper. Med., **71:** 813, 1940.

Kingery, L. B.: The Etiology of Common Warts, Jour. Amer. Med. Asso., **76:** 440, 1921.

Kleinenberg, H. E., S. A. Neufach, and L. M. Schabad: Further Studies of Blastomogenic Substances in the Body, Cancer Res., **1:** 853, 1941.

Klemperer, P., and C. B. Rabin: Primary Neoplasms of the Pleura. A Report of Five Cases, Arch. Path., **11:** 385, 1931.

Knox, L. C.: Epithelioma and the Chronic Varicose Ulcer, Jour. Amer. Med. Asso., **85:** 1046, 1925; Trauma and Tumors, Arch. Path., **7:** 274, 1929.

Kohman, T. P., and H. P. Rusch: Relative Metabolic Activities of Normal and Tumorous Liver Nucleoproteins Indicated by Radiophosphorus, Proc. Soc. Exper. Biol. and Med., **46:** 403, 1941.

Laidlaw, G. F., and M. R. Murray: Melanoma Studies. A Theory of Pigmented Moles. Their Relation to the Evolution of the Hair Follicles, Amer. Jour. Path., **9:** 827, 1933.

——: Addenda to a Theory of Pigmented Moles, Amer. Jour. Path., **10:** 319, 1934.

Laurence, W. L.: Induced Biotin Deficiency as Possible Explanation of Observed Spontaneous Recessions in Malignancy, Science, **94:** 88, 1941.

Levine, M.: Studies in the Cytology of Cancer, Amer. Jour. Cancer, **15:** 211, 1931.

Lewis, D., and C. F. Geschickter: Tumors of the Sympathetic Nervous System: Neuroblastoma, Paraganglioma, Ganglioneuroma, Arch. Surg., **28:** 16, 1934.

Lewis, M. R., E. S. G. Barron, and R. E. Gardner: Comparison of the Reducing Power of Cancer Tumors and Tumors Produced by Filterable Viruses, Proc. Soc. Exper. Biol. and Med., **28:** 684, 1930-31.

——, and L. C. Strong: A Study of Spontaneous Tumors of the Mouse by the Tissue Culture Method, Amer. Jour. Cancer, **20:** 72, 1934.

Lewis, W. H.: Normal and Malignant Cells, Science, **81:** 545, 1935.

Leyton, O., H. M. Turnbull, and A. B. Bratton: Primary Cancer of the Thymus with Pluriglandular Disturbance, Jour. Path. and Bact., **34:** 635, 1931.

Lipschütz, A., R. Thibaut, and L. Vargas, Jr.: The Fibromatogenic Action of Specific Urinary Estrogens (Metahormones) in the Guinea Pig, Cancer Res., **2:** 45, 1942.

Little, C. C.: A Review of Progress in the Study of the Genetics of Spontaneous Tumor Incidence, Jour. Nat. Cancer Inst., **1:** 727, 1941.

Loeb, L.: On Transplantation of Tumors, Jour. Med. Res., **6:** 28, 1901.

——: Internal Secretions as a Factor in the Origin of Tumors, ibid., **40:** 477, 1919.

——: The Etiology and Biology of Cancer, Ann. Int. Med., **4:** 669, 1930-31.

Lucké, B.: Frog Carcinoma, Year Book of Pathology and Immunology, Chicago, Year Book Publishers, 1940; p. 66.

Lynch, C. J.: Symposium on Etiology of Tumors. Hereditary Factors, Arch. Path., **21:** 716, 1936.

Mabrey, R. E.: Chordoma: A Study of 150 Cases, Amer. Jour. Cancer, **25:** 501, 1935.

MacCarty, W. C.: Biological Conception of Neoplasia, Amer. Jour. Med. Sci., **157:** 657, 1919; Sistrunk, W. E., and W. C. MacCarty: Life Expectancy Following Radical Amputation for Carcinoma of the Breast, Ann. Surg., **75:** 61, 1922.

Macklin, M. T.: Tumours in Monozygous and Dizygous Twins (Report of 19 New Cases), Canad. Med. Asso. Jour., **44:** 604, 1941.

——: Is the Increase in Cancer Real or Apparent? Amer. Jour. Cancer, **16:** 1193, 1932.

Mahle, A. E.: The Morphological Histology of Adenocarcinoma of the Body of the Uterus in Relation to Longevity, Surg., Gynec. and Obst., **36:** 385, 1923.

Mann, L. S., and W. H. Welker: A Specific Precipitin Antiserum for Carcinoma Protein, Amer. Jour. Cancer, **39:** 360, 1940.

Markwald, E.: Cysten, Ergeb. d. allg. Path. u. Path. Anat., **2**: 286, 1895.

Martin, H. E., and F. W. Stewart: Spindle-cell Epidermoid Carcinoma, Amer. Jour. Cancer, **24**: 273, 1935.

Martland, H. S.: The Occurrence of Malignancy in Radio-Active Persons, Amer. Jour. Cancer, **15**: 2435, 1931.

Martzloff, K. H.: Carcinoma of Cervix Uteri, etc., Bull. Johns Hopkins Hosp., **34**: 141, 184, 1923.

Maver, M. E., G. B. Mider, J. M. Johnson, and J. W. Thompson: The Comparative Proteinase and Peptidase Activities of Rat Hepatoma and Normal and Regenerating Rat Liver, Jour. Nat. Cancer Inst., **2**: 277, 1941.

Maximow, A.: Ueber krebsähnliche Verwandlung der Milchdruse in Gewebskulturen, Virchow's Arch. Path. Anat., **256**: 813, 1925.

——: Tissue Culture of Mammary Gland, Anat. Rec., **27**: 210, 1924.

McConnell, G.: The Experimental Production of Epithelial Proliferation, Jour. Amer. Med. Asso., **49**: 1498, 1907.

McFarland, J., and H. M. Patterson: Adamantinomata. A Review of One Hundred and Ninety-Six Cases Reported in the Medical and Dental Literature, Dental Cosmos, **73**: 656, 1931.

McGowan, J. P.: On Rous, Leucocytic and Allied Tumors in the Fowl, London, 1928.

Meister, W.: Kritische Betrachtungen zur Entstehung der angeborenen Steissgewächse unter Zugrundelegung zweier beobachteter Fälle, Virchow's Arch. Path. Anat., **288**: 286, 1933.

Milles, G.: A Principle Accelerating Growth and Maturation Demonstrated in Metastases of a Tumor of the Thyroid Gland, Arch. Path., **17**: 631, 1934.

Minot, G. R., and R. Isaacs: Lymphoblastoma (Malignant Lymphoma); Age and Sex Incidence, Duration of the Disease, and the Effect of Roentgen-Ray and Radium Irradiation and Surgery, Jour. Amer. Med. Asso., **86**: 1185, 1926.

Mock, H. E., and J. D. Ellis: Trauma and Malignancy, Ibid., **86**: 257, 1926.

Moise, T.: The Origin of Hemangiectases, Bull. Johns Hopkins Hosp., **31**: 369, 1920.

Morris, H. P., and S. W. Lippincott: The Effect of Pantothenic Acid on Growth and Maintenance of Life in Mice of the C3H Strain, Jour. Nat. Cancer Inst., **2**: 29, 1941.

Mottram, J. C.: Production of Epithelial Tumours by a Combination of Beta Radiation and Painting with Benzpyrene, Amer. Jour. Cancer, **32**: 76, 1938.

——, and S. Russ: Observations and Experiments on the Susceptibility and Immunity of Rats toward Jensen's Rat Sarcoma, Proc. Roy. Soc., London, **90**: 1, 1919 (series B).

Murphy, J. B.: The Lymphocyte in Resistance to Tissue Grafting, Malignant Disease and Tuberculous Infection. An Experimental Study, Monograph Rockefeller Inst. for Med. Research No. 21. New York, 1926.

——: The Effect of a Growth-Retarding Factor from Normal Tissues on Spontaneous Cancer of Mice, Ibid., **60**: 305, 1934.

——, and E. Sturm: A Factor from Normal Tissues Inhibiting Tumor Growth, Jour. Exper. Med., **60**: 293, 1934.

Murray, J. A.: Cancerous Ancestry and the Incidence of Cancer in Mice, Fourth Sc. Rep. Imp. Cancer Res. Fund, 1911, p. 114, Proc. Roy. Soc., Series B, **84**: 42, 1911-12.

Murray, M. R., and Stout, A. P.: The Glomus Tumor. Investigation of Its Distribution and Behavior, and the Identity of Its "Epithelioid" Cell, Amer. Jour. Path., **18**: 183, 1942.

Noble, R. L., and J. B. Collip: Regression of Oestrogen Induced Mammary Tumours in Female Rats Following Removal of the Stimulus, Canad. Med. Asso. Jour., **44**: 1, 1941.

Oertel, H.: On the Mechanism of Cancer Development, Canad. Med. Asso. Jour., **23**: 183, 1930.

Pack, G. T., and R. G. LeFevre: The Age and Sex Distribution and Incidence of Neoplastic Diseases at the Memorial Hospital, New York City, Jour. Cancer Res., **14**: 167, 1930.

Parker, H. L., and J. W. Kernohan: The Relation of Injury and Glioma of Brain, Jour. Amer. Med. Asso., **97**: 535, 1931.

Peller, S.: Malignant Melanoma Cutis, Cancer Res., **1**: 538, 1941.

Popper, H., and A. B. Ragins: Histologic Demonstration of Vitamin A in Tumors, Arch. Path., **32**: 258, 1941.

Putnoky, J.: On the Immunity Reactions of a Heterotransplantable Mouse Carcinoma Propagated in Rats for Seven Years, Amer. Jour. Cancer, **32**: 35, 1938.

Ramsey, T. L.: Sacrococcygeal Chordoblastoma, Arch. Path. and Lab. Med., **5**: 232, 1928.

Rehbock, D. J., and H. Hauser: Liposarcoma of Bone. Report of Two Cases and Review of Literature, Amer. Jour. Cancer, **27**: 37, 1936.

Reimann, S. P.: The Issues at Stake in the Grading of Tumors, Arch. Path., **8**: 803, 1929.

Ribbert, H.: Das Karzinoma des Menschen. Bonn, 1911.

——: Geschwulstlehre, Bonn, 1914.

Riker, A. J., and T. O. Berge: Atypical and Pathological Multiplication of Cells Approached through Studies on Crown Gall, Amer. Jour. Cancer, **25**: 310, 1935.

Robertson, H. E.: "Endothelioma" of the Pleura, Jour. Cancer Res., **8**: 317, 1924.

Rous, P.: The Virus Tumors and the Tumor Problem, Amer. Jour. Cancer, **28**: 233, 1936.

——, and W. F. Friedewald: The Carcinogenic Effect of Methylcholanthrene and of Tar on Rabbit Papillomas due to a Virus, Science, **94**: 495, 1941.

Roussy, G., and M. Wolf: Le Cancer, An Extensive and Admirable Discussion of All Phases in Nouveau Traité. de Medicine by Roger, Widal and Teissier, Vol. 5, Paris, 1922.

Rowntree, L. G., A. Steinberg, G. M. Dorrance, and E. F. Ciccone: Sarcoma in Rats from the Ingestion of a Crude Wheat-germ Oil Made by Ether Extraction, Amer. Jour. Cancer, **31**: 359, 1937.

Rusch, H. P., B. E. Kline, and C. A. Baumann: Carcinogenesis by Ultraviolet Rays with Reference to Wavelength and Energy, Arch. Path., **31**: 135, 1941.

Russ, S., H. Chambers, G. Scott, and J. C. Mottram: Experimental Studies with Small Doses of X-rays, Lancet, **50**: 692, 1919.

Ryrie, G. M.: On the Significance of Nerve Fibres in Human Malignant Neoplasms, Jour. Path. and Bact., **36**: 13, 1933.

Sampson, J. A.: Implantation Peritoneal Carcinomatosis of Ovarian Origin, Amer. Jour. Path., 7: 423, 1931.

Saphir, O., and A. Vass: Carcinosarcoma, Amer. Jour. Cancer, 33: 331, 1938.

——, and M. Appel: Regression of Primary Brown-Pearce Testicular Carcinoma and Metastases Following Intracutaneous Transplantation with Homologous Tumor, Amer. Jour. Cancer, 38: 55, 1940.

Schlegel, M.: Die Missbildungen der Tiere, Ergeb. d. allg. Path. u. Path. Anat., 19(2): 650, 1921.

Schmitz, H., and W. Hueper: Malignant Chorionepithelioma Uteri, Jour. Amer. Med. Asso., 95: 1413, 1930.

Schrek, R.: Cutaneous Carcinoma. III. A Statistical Analysis with Respect to Site, Sex and Pre-existing Scars, Arch. Path., 31: 434, 1941.

Schwalbe, E.: Die Morphologie der Missbildungen des Menchen und der Thiere, Jena, 1913.

Selbie, F. R.: A Transplantable Mammary Fibroadenoma of the Rat Showing Sarcomatous Changes, Brit. Jour. Exper. Path., 22: 156, 1941.

Shimkin, M. B., H. B. Grady, and H. B. Andervont: Induction of Testicular Tumors and Other Effects of Stilbestrol-Cholesterol Pellets in Strain C Mice, Jour. Nat. Cancer Inst., 2: 65, 1941.

Siémens, H. W.: Aetiologisch-dermatologische Studien ueber die Recklinghausen'sche Krankheit, Virchow's Arch. Path. Anat., 260: 234, 1926.

Silberberg, M.: Xanthome und Xanthoblastome, Virchow's Arch. Path. Anat., 254: 63, 1925.

——: Tissue Culture, with Special Reference to Pathology, Arch. Path., 21: 663, 1936.

Slye, M.: Some Misconceptions Regarding the Relation of Heredity to Cancer and Other Diseases, etc., Jour. Amer. Med. Asso., 86: 1599, 1926.

——: Some Observations in the Nature of Cancer, etc., Jour. Cancer Res., 11: 135, 1927.

——: The Relation of Heredity to Cancer, ibid., 12: 83, 1928.

Spencer, R. R.: Tumor Immunity, Jour. National Cancer Inst., 2: 317, 1942.

Steiner, P. E.: The Production of Tumors with an Extract from Human Liver, Cancer Res., 1: 750, 1941.

Stewart, F. W.: Primary Liposarcoma of Bone, Amer. Jour. Path., 7: 87, 1931.

——: Radiosensitivity of Tumors, Arch. Surg., 27: 979, 1933.

——, and M. M. Copeland: Neurogenic Sarcoma, Amer. Jour. Cancer, 15: 1235, 1931.

Stewart, M. J., and J. E. Morin: Chordoma, A Review with Report of a New Sacrococcygeal Case, Jour. Path. and Bact., 29: 41, 1926.

Sturm, E., and J. B. Murphy: Further Observations on Experimentally Produced Sarcoma of the Chicken, Jour. Exper. Med., 47: 493, 1928; Mackenzie, R. D., and E. Sturm: Some Factors Determining the Localization of Chicken Tumor Agent, Jour. Exper. Med., 47: 345, 1928.

Symmers, D.: The Metastasis of Tumors, Amer. Jour. Med. Sci., 154: 225, 1917.

Treves, N., and G. T. Pack: The Development of Cancer in Burn Scars, Surg., Gynec. and Obst., 51: 749, 1930.

Troescher, E. E., and E. R. Norris: Micro Blood Esterase Determination Applied to Studies of Rats Bearing Adenocarcinoma, Jour. Biol. Chem., 132: 553, 1940.

Tullis, J. L.: Multiple Primary Malignant Lesions, Jour. Lab. and Clin. Med., 27: 588, 1942.

Twombly, G. H., H. M. Temple, and A. L. Dean: Clinical Value of the Ascheim-Zondek Test in the Diagnosis of Testicular Tumors, Jour. Amer. Med. Asso., 118: 106, 1942.

Verocay, J.: Zur Kenntniss der "Neurofibrome," Beitr. Path. Anat. u. Allg. Path., 48: 1, 1910.

Visscher, M. B., R. G. Green, and J. J. Bittner: Characterization of Milk Influence in Spontaneous Mammary Carcinoma, Proc. Soc. Exper. Biol. and Med., 49: 94, 1942.

Voegtlin, C.: Biochemistry of Malignant Tissues, Physiol. Rev., 17: 92, 1937.

Volkmann, J.: Ueber eine eigenartige Hodengeschwulst bei einem Kinde mit Traubenmolen und chorionepitheliomartigen Wucherungen, Virchow's Arch. Path. Anat., 229: 362, 1921.

Waller, G. H. M.: Ueber die Erblichkeit des Krebses, beurteilt nach dem von Norwegischen Krebskomitee gesammelten Material, Oslo, 1931—abstracted in Editorial, Jour. Amer. Med. Asso., 98: 1656, 1932.

Warburg, O.: Ueber den Stoffwechsel der Tumoren, Berlin, 1926.

——: The Metabolism of Carcinoma Cells, Jour. Cancer Res., 9: 148, 1925.

Warner, S. G., and M. C. Reinhard: Effect of X-Rays on a Tumor of Known Genetic Constitution, Proc. Soc. Exper. Biol. and Med., 42: 673, 1939.

Warren, S.: The Immediate Causes of Death in Cancer, Amer. Jour. Med. Sci., 184: 610, 1932.

——: The Angle of the Mitotic Spindles in Malignant Cells, Amer. Jour. Path., 9: 781, 1933.

——, and A. H. Davis: Studies on Tumor Metastasis. V. The Metastases of Carcinoma to the Spleen, Amer. Jour. Cancer, 21: 517, 1934.

——, and O. Gates: Multiple Primary Malignant Tumors. A Survey of the Literature and a Statistical Study, Amer. Jour. Cancer, 16: 1358, 1932.

Warren, S. L.: The Bacterial Flora of Cancer of the Breast, Amer. Jour. Med. Sci., 171: 813, 1926.

——, and H. E. Pearse: The Repeated Inoculations of Animals with So-Called "Cancer Organisms," Ibid., 171: 820, 1926.

Watson, W. L., and W. D. McCarthy: Blood and Lymph Vessel Tumors. A Report of 1,056 Cases, Surg., Gynec. and Obst., 71: 569, 1940.

Weber, F. P.: Periosteal Neurofibromatosis, with a Short Consideration of the Whole Subject of Neurofibromatosis, Quart. Jour. Med., 23: 151, 1930.

Weller, C. V.: Intrinsic Factors in the Etiology of Neoplasms, Amer. Jour. Cancer, 30: 39, 1937.

——: The Inheritance of Retinoblastoma and Its Relationship to Practical Eugenics, Cancer Res., 1: 517, 1941.

Wells, H. G.: The Fats and Lipoids of Malignant Renal Hypernephromas, Jour. Med. Res., 17: 461, 1907-08.

——: The Fat Metabolism of Lipomas, Arch. Int. Med., 10: 297, 1912.

——: The Influence of Heredity on the Occurrence of Cancer, Jour. Amer. Med. Asso., 81: 1017, 1103, 1923.

——: The Influence of Heredity on the Occurrence of Cancer in Animals, Ann. Int. Med., 4: 676, 1930-31.

——: The Nature and Etiology of Cancer, Amer. Jour. Cancer, 15: 1919, 1931.

Wells, H. G.: Adipose Tissue, a Neglected Subject, Jour. Amer. Med. Asso., **114**: 2177, 1940.

——: Occurrence and Significance of Congenital Malignant Neoplasms, Arch. Path., **30**: 535, 1940.

Wilder, H. C., and G. R. Callender: Malignant Melanoma of the Choroid, Amer. Jour. Ophth., **22**: 851, 1939.

Williams, W. R.: The Natural History of Cancer, New York, 1908.

Willis, R. A.: The Spread of Tumours in the Human Body, London, 1934; The Structure of Teratomata, Jour. Path. and Bact., **40**: 1, 1935.

Winestine, F.: The Relation of von Recklinghausen's Disease (Multiple Neurofibromatosis) to Giant Growth and Blastomatosis, Jour. Cancer Res., **8**: 409, 1924.

Woglom, W. H.: The Study of Experimental Cancer (Crocker Foundation), Columbia Univ. Press, New York, 1913.

Woglom, W. H.: The Regression of Spontaneous Mammary Carcinoma in the Mouse, Jour. Cancer Res., **7**: 379, 1922.

——: Experimental Tar Cancer, Arch. Path and Lab. Med., **2**: 533; 709, 1926.

Wolff, J.: Die Lehre von der Krebskrankheit, Jena, 1913.

Wood, F. C.: Immunity in Cancer, Jour. Amer. Med. Asso., **85**: 1039, 1925.

Woodhouse, D. L.: The Chemodiagnosis of Malignancy, Amer. Jour. Cancer, **40**: 359, 1941.

Yamagiwa, K.: Ueber die künstliche Erzeugung von Teercarcinom und Sarkom, Virchow's Arch. Path. Anat., **233**: 235, 1921.

Zweifel, P., and E. Payr: Die Klinik der bösartigen Geschwülste, Leipzig, 1927.

Zymbal, W. E.: Histologische und experimentelle Untersuchungen über die Geschwülste der Speicheldrusen, Beitr. Path. Anat. u. Allg. Path., **91**: 113, 1933.

PART TWO

SYSTEMIC PATHOLOGY

13

The Cardiovascular System

HEART

PERICARDIUM

Congenital Anomalies

Congenital abnormalities of the peri-cardium are unusual. The pericardium may be entirely absent in cases of ectopia cordis. Defective development of the pericardium may result in absence of part of the parietal layer, usually of the left side and anterior portions, so that the left lung and heart lie in a common cavity. Diverticula and failure of attachment to the central tendon of the diaphragm are also reported. (See South-worth and Stevenson.)

Degenerations

Degenerations of the pericardium occur usually as a part of inflammations. The only common infiltration is by fat, occurring in connection with obesity, of little practical significance and not to be confused with fat infiltration of the myocardium. Atrophy of subepicardial fat is common in long standing wasting diseases and is often an associated condition in atrophies of the heart. The reduction in amount of fat is usually accompanied by an infiltration of fluid producing the so-called serous atrophy of fat. The fat in the heart grooves is of deep yellow color, soft and of translucent, gelatinous character, and the overlying epicardium flaccid and wrinkled.

Circulatory Disturbances

Circulatory disturbances are common.

Hyperemia and Edema. Active hyperemia appears as a part of inflammation. Passive hyperemia is usually the result of failure of the myocardium, but may result from mediastinal tumors or inflammations, with pressure upon pericardial veins. The most important sequence is accumulation of edematous fluid within the sac, called hydropericardium, or hydrops pericardii. The fluid is of low specific gravity, poor in cells and does not clot, although small fibrin flakes sometimes form after withdrawal. The pericardium normally contains 20 to 50 cc. of clear, straw colored, limpid fluid, of the nature of lymph, but a pathologic diagnosis

349

of hydropericardium is not made unless the amount of fluid is 100 cc. or more. It is not uncommon to find 400 or 500 cc. of fluid, and amounts up to 2000 cc. and more are reported. Williamson finds that fluid injected in the pericardial sac accumulates first along the diaphragmatic surface, pushing down the left lobe of the liver, then about the great vessels at the base of the heart; only when the fluid is large in amount is the anterior wall of the heart covered. The small amount of fluid normally in the pericardium exerts no pressure. When excesses are present in amounts sufficient to compress incoming veins, there is a decrease in arterial pressure

veins and also inhibits cardiac diastole. The resultant "cardiac tamponade" is rapidly fatal.

Hemorrhage into the tissues of the pericardium may appear as petechiae in death from asphyxia or convulsions, in tuberculous pericarditis, pericarditis due to hemolytic bacteria, tumor involvement of the pericardium and such hemorrhagic diseases as scurvy and purpura, and blood may also leak into the pericardial fluid.

Hemopericardium, indicating the presence of free and unmixed blood, is due to direct trauma, to rupture of pericardial vessels, especially when they are the seat of aneu-

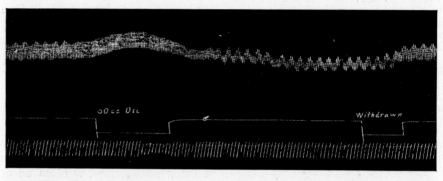

Tracing of blood and pulse pressure in experimental hydropericardium in the dog. The signal line is also the base line. Time in two seconds. Note after the primary rise the fall in mean arterial and pulse pressure following injection of 30 cc. olive oil into the sac, with restoration to normal upon withdrawal of fluid.

and an increase in venous pressure, due to damming back of blood from the lungs and reduced inflow into the left heart. Vasoconstriction may maintain systemic pressure for a considerable period. Extremely slight increase in intrapericardial pressure may reduce arterial pressure profoundly and decreases may elevate arterial pressure (Lewis). Increased intrapericardial pressure may affect the heart muscle and its rhythm by a relative anoxemia of the myocardium (Katz, Feil and Scott). Katz and Gauchat find that pulsus paradoxus, accompanying excess pericardial fluid, is due to alteration of normal variations of intrapericardial pressure. The pressure effect of pericardial inflammatory exudates is augmented by the coincident myocardial degenerations. In hemopericardium from rupture of an aneurysm or the heart wall, the intraventricular or intra-aortic pressure is communicated directly to the pericardial sac; this compresses intrapericardial pulmonary

rysm, rupture of the heart and of the large vessels communicating with it. The effects are noted above.

Pneumopericardium is usually due to injury, but occasionally may result from entry of air from lungs or pleura. Inflammation or hemorrhage or both often accompany it.

Inflammation

Acute Pericarditis. Pericarditis may be acute or chronic. The causes of acute pericarditis include infectious diseases, particularly rheumatic fever, acute tonsillitis, chorea, pyemia, extension from neighboring foci of inflammation, such as pleura, mediastinum and myocardium, and infected wounds. The pericardium may also be affected in the terminal infectious states of various chronic diseases. Acute fibrinous pericarditis sometimes occurs in uremia; it is a chemical inflammation because so far it has not been found to be due to infection. Acute pericarditis may be fibrinous, fibrinoserous, fibrinopurulent, purulent and hemorrhagic. There is often localized nonbacterial acute fibrinous pericarditis over myocardial infarcts. Acute fibrinous pericarditis is often manifested by a pericardial friction rub, but the inflammation soon becomes fibrinoserous and the separation of the two surfaces eliminates the rub. When seen in its earliest stage,

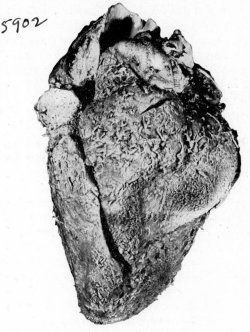

Acute fibrinous pericarditis, the shaggy heart, or cor villosum.

acute fibrinous pericarditis may be localized but it soon involves the entire sac. The surface loses its gloss and a thin film of sticky fibrin, arranged in irregular bands and of light yellow color, is seen. This is sometimes called the "bread and butter" pericardium, because of its fancied resemblance to the appearance of the butter after a bread and butter sandwich is pulled apart. Increase in the amount of fibrin produces the "shaggy heart" or "cor villosum." As the fibrin is separated from the exudate, the movements of the heart whip it into thin, gray villi and heavier bands, which occasionally are arranged spirally about the heart, the heavier bands being near the base. Microscopically, hyperemia of the pericardium is seen with a moderate infiltration of leukocytes, lympho-

cytes and other cells of acute inflammation in the interstitial tissues, and even in superficial parts of the subepicardial fat. The endothelium has disappeared or remains as a few swollen, degenerate cells. On the surface is a mass of fibrin in heavy bands and fine reticular mesh, enclosing leukocytes, lymphocytes and other migrating cells, and occasionally also bacteria. Organization begins very early and is often well marked within 24 hours of the clinical onset. This is the dry or plastic pericarditis of the clinicians. It is soon accompanied by an increasing amount of fluid exudate. The fluid is disposed as in hydropericardium, but is a cloudy, limpid fluid of relatively high specific gravity, contains cells of the exudate and tends to clot upon aspiration. The fluid is often present in quantities of 400 or 500 cc. and may materially exceed those amounts. This is the so-called pericarditis with effusion. The mechanical effects of the fluid are essentially those of hydropericardium, referred to above.

If the pericarditis be the result of pyemia, or other infection with pyogenic organisms, extension from neighboring suppurations or wounds, the process rapidly becomes purulent. There may be little fibrin present at any period of a purulent pericarditis, and if present early may be subsequently reduced by the lytic action of cellular and bacterial enzymes. The pus may be thin and limpid or thick and viscid, depending upon the amount of exuded fluid. This is sometimes called "pyopericardium." Microscopically, the appearance of the pericardium is much the same as in fibrinous pericarditis, except for the smaller amount of fibrin and the large number of leukocytes and pus cells. Infection by gas-forming organisms may lead to pneumopericardium in addition to the suppurative process.

The exudate of acute pericarditis may be hemorrhagic in tuberculous pericarditis, in that due to hemolytic bacteria, in the irritation of the pericardium due to invasion of malignant tumors, and when pericarditis occurs in hemorrhagic diseases such as scurvy, purpura or hemophilia. Acute pericarditis is usually a part of some infectious disease, and therefore likely to be accompanied by degenerations of parenchymatous viscera and inflammatory changes in various situations. If the pericarditis be primary, which is most probable as the result of infected wounds, it may extend to surrounding structures such as pleura, lungs, mediastinum, lymph nodes and rarely to the myocardium.

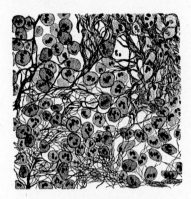

Leukocytes and fibrin in acute fibrinous pericarditis.

Chronic Pericarditis. The outcome of an acute pericarditis may be either chronic pericarditis or cicatrization. Chronic pericar-

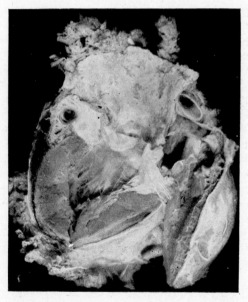

Organizing acute fibrinous pericarditis with adhesion. Note the adhesion of parietal pericardium over the flap of left ventricle.

ditis may be localized or widespread, in which case adhesions are likely to be present. A rare form of chronic pericarditis is the nodular variety, in which tiny nodules a millimeter or so in diameter, firm, opaque, and covered by endothelium, are distributed on the epicardium, especially along the coronary sulci. Extremely common are the so-called milk plaques, or soldier spots. Rare in early life, they are more frequently found as age advances. The epicardium, especially over the anterior surface of the myocardium, shows an area of fibrous thickening and opacity with a smooth surface, fairly well defined from the surrounding epicardium. The plaques may be multiple and widely distributed. They vary from a few millimeters to several centimeters in diameter, but do not exceed 2 mm. in thickness. Usually the heart shows other chronic disease, e.g., in the valves. Some plaques appear to be chronic inflammatory tissue and others merely scars, but in any event they are probably the outcome of a preceding inflammatory process (Nelson).

Fibrous adhesions between the visceral and parietal pericardium may occur as a part of chronic adhesive pericarditis or may be the scars of a preceding acute pericarditis. Pure chronic adhesive pericarditis is not frequent but it occurs in connection with rheumatic heart disease, tuberculous pericarditis, and some of the cases of so-called Pick's syndrome. In some instances the adhesion between parietal and visceral pericardium becomes more and more extensive and ultimately results in obliteration of the sac to constitute "synechia pericardii." The connective tissue may become hyalinized and sometimes calcified; in occasional instances the latter is extensive. Ordinarily adhesions produce no functional effects. In spite of former views to the contrary, pericardial adhesion does not of itself produce cardiac hypertrophy even when extensive mediastinal fibrosis is also present. When hypertrophy occurs there is some reason for it other than pericardial adhesion.

The fused layers become much thickened, more especially as the result of healing of purulent or tuberculous pericarditis. The resultant rigidity limits diastolic expansion of the heart and in this way exercises a compressive effect, referred to as pericardial constriction or constrictive pericarditis. There are various symptoms and signs of myocardial insufficiency, due principally to reduced inflow of blood to the heart. Probably the first sign to be manifest is ascites but there are also dyspnea on exertion, cyanosis, increased venous pressure, low pulse pressure and passive hyperemia of the viscera together with roentgenologic signs of fixation of the heart and limitation of diastolic excursion (Beck).

Serous pericarditis, such as that which may accompany chronic tuberculous pericarditis, is classified as chronic by the Criteria Committee of the New York Heart Association, but in our opinion this is an acute component of the chronic disease because it is an exudative inflammation.

Pick's syndrome, or pericardial pseudo-cirrhosis, includes adherent pericardium, adherent pleura and capsular fibrosis of the liver. Its cause is unknown. It may be accompanied by the same physiologic disturbances as have been noted above in connection with pericardial constriction.

Tuberculosis. Tubercles may be found in the pericardium as a part of disseminated miliary tuberculosis; there is often little or no inflammation of the membrane. In contrast, tuberculous pericarditis shows marked inflammation, which may be acute or chronic. It is usually the result of extension from lungs, pleura, mediastinal lymph nodes or bones. An acute fibrinous pericarditis may occur, but more commonly the process is chronic with increased connective tissue, often adherent, with remnants of fibrin and with fairly extensive caseation. Tubercles may be evident grossly or may require microscopic demonstration. Sometimes there is a large amount of serous exudate which may be blood tinged, or even distinctly hemorrhagic. Fibrin may be rich in amount and there may be slight hemorrhage. Rarely, the exudate is purulent. Tubercle bacilli are rarely demonstrated in the exudate by staining, but the material produces tuberculosis upon injection into guinea pigs.

Syphilis. Gummata rarely occur in the pericardium. Possibly some forms of pericardial fibrosis may be syphilitic. Other granulomata are rare.

Tumors

Primary tumors, including fibroma, lipoma, angioma, and sarcoma are very rare. Secondary tumors are also unusual. They may be due to extension from the secondary nodules in the myocardium, or to extension from primary or secondary tumors in the mediastinum and especially from broncho-genic carcinoma of the lung. Very rarely they may be implanted in the scanty blood vessels of the pericardium.

Parasites

In man, the echinococcus cyst is the only parasitic infestation of importance in the pericardium; it is rare.

ENDOCARDIUM

Congenital Anomalies

When there are gross anomalies of the heart as a whole, the endocardium is correspondingly altered. There are, however, other anomalies. Delicate fibrous cords may be found in the ventricles stretching from one point to another. In the lateral wall of the right atrium, similar cords may be found which not infrequently constitute an interlacing mesh, spoken of as the Chiari network. (See Helwig.) Fenestration of the cusps of the semilunar valves is not infrequent but occurs more often in the aortic than in the pulmonic valve. The perforations are tiny, with rounded edges that appear near the commissures between the free border and the line of closure. Supernumerary cusps or leaflets are occasionally encountered, especially in the semilunar valves. These abnormalities are without functional significance but occasionally supernumerary leaflets in mitral or tricuspid valves may result in insufficiency. Bicuspid aortic and pulmonic valves must be distinguished as to whether they are congenital or acquired. They are more frequent in the aortic valve than the pulmonic. In the aortic valve, two cusps may be fused in the course of development of the heart. In the situation of what should have been the commissure there is a vertical raphe, rounded, hemicylindrical in character, which extends down the aortic wall of the sinus of Valsalva to the bottom of the sinus. An acquired bicuspid aortic valve due to preceding inflammation is characterized by the fusion of two cusps; the raphe in this instance lies in the floor of the sinus of Valsalva, extending from the wall to the line of fusion of the cusps, expanding as it approaches the cusp. (See Koletsky.) Distinctions of this sort are supported by microscopic examination which shows peculiarities of distribution of elastica in the two different forms. Congenital bicuspid aortic valve leads to no functional disturbance except that occasionally a very faint diastolic murmur may be heard. Acquired fusion leads to stenosis.

Degenerations

Cloudy swelling and fatty degeneration of the endothelium may occur as a part of acute infectious diseases, poisoning by chloroform or phosphorus, and accompany inflammations of the endocardium. Calcification is common as the sequence of chronic inflammations and endocardial sclerosis. Amyloid sometimes infiltrates the subendothelial connective tissue, particularly of the right side of the heart.

Circulatory Disturbances

Circulatory disturbances of importance include thrombosis and embolism. Embolism is of little significance as concerns the endocardium except that there are occasional instances of acute endocarditis that appear to be due to lodgment of emboli in blood vessels of the valves. The most frequent thrombosis is that which is a part of acute endocarditis. Marantic thrombosis of the auricular appendages is not uncommon. It forms an adherent, mottled, red and gray thrombus, enmeshed in the pectinate muscles, often filling the appendage and sometimes extending into the atrium. A massive thrombus, due to old or recent mural endocarditis, may accumulate to constitute a large ball attached to the wall by a pedicle. This is especially likely to occur in the left atrium and may be of such size as to produce obstruction. It is referred to as the ball-valve thrombus. Thrombosis in the ventricles is most frequent toward the tip of the ventricle where the mottled mass is enmeshed in the columnae carneae. This may be the result of prolonged dilatation of the heart or a localized dilatation due to recent or remote infarction. Because of degeneration, fragments of the thrombi may break loose to lodge as emboli in other organs.

Endocardial Sclerosis

By this term is meant a fibrous thickening of the endocardium which may or may not be accompanied by atheroma and is not due to preceding inflammation. A lesion of this sort is particularly common in the an-

terior leaflet of the mitral valve. Even in early life there may be a thickening situated in the middle of the leaflet and accompanied by fatty change. As age advances, this disturbance becomes more conspicuous. A similar condition is rarely found in the tricuspid leaflets. Rarely if ever does it occur in the aortic or pulmonic cusps. Occasionally fibrous thickening is found in localized areas of the mural endocardium but it is usually difficult to say that this is not the result of a preceding inflammation or an underlying infarct. There has been much discussion of a condition called calcific sclerosis of the aortic valve but in our opinion this is the result of preceding inflammation and is discussed further under the heading of Aortic Stenosis. The involvement of aortic cusps by extension of syphilitic disease from the aorta is inflammatory rather than sclerotic.

Inflammation

Endocarditis may be acute, subacute, chronic and recurrent. It may affect valves, mural endocardium and chordae tendineae. It is so predominantly valvular that the term

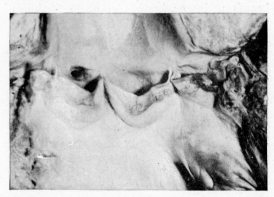

Acute verrucous and vegetative endocarditis of aortic valve.

endocarditis, unless qualified as mural or chordal, means valvulitis. It is classified etiologically into rheumatic and bacterial. The anatomic classification is the one selected as the basis of discussion.

Acute Endocarditis. Anatomically, this is divided into verrucous and vegetative forms. Verrucous endocarditis is usually of rheumatic origin, but may occasionally be due to bacterial infection. Vegetative endocarditis is almost always due to bacterial infection. Ulceration may occur in acute vege-

acute veg.

15884 ē ulc. of some of valvula

vesicular nuclei and centrally disposed chromatin from which delicate strands extend to the nuclear membrane. In the cases of septicemia, polymorphonuclear leukocytes predominate and vascular thrombosis is more common. In endocarditis minima, the lesion is only slight.

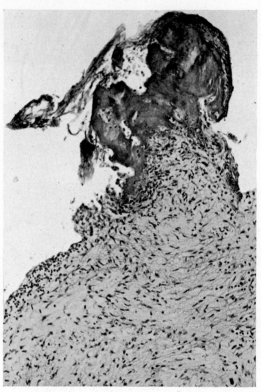

Acute rheumatic valvulitis, to show character of verruca and inflammation in endocardium.

tative endocarditis and the lesion is then called acute ulcerative endocarditis. Ulceration rarely occurs except as a complication of vegetative endocarditis.

ACUTE VERRUCOUS ENDOCARDITIS. This is the characteristic and typical form of acute rheumatic endocarditis, but it may occur occasionally in septicemias and also in that form often called toxic endocarditis or endocarditis minima. The verrucae are minute, pale yellow, soft, sessile, loosely adherent, sometimes superficially lobulated nodules, less than a millimeter in diameter, situated along the line of closure of the leaflet, sometimes extending more widely on the leaflet. Rheumatic verrucae are early covered by endothelium and as usually seen at autopsy are associated with a chronic valvulitis. Septicemic verrucae tend to be larger, softer and more widespread. The verrucae of endocarditis minima are extremely minute, usually few in number and occur in connection with deaths from chronic exhausting diseases. Microscopically, verrucae are made up principally of fibrin in coarse and fine strands, sometimes with a few leukocytes and mononuclear cells and platelets. Rheumatic verrucae contain bacteria only when there is complicating infection. The underlying tissue, in the rheumatic case, shows edema, hyperemia, infrequent vascular thrombosis, a few lymphocytes and occasionally leukocytes, and the so-called Aschoff cells with their

In the earlier discussion of rheumatic fever it was indicated that the process begins in the substance of the leaflets and that the endothelial surface becomes the seat of these minute thrombi as the deeper lesion spreads to the surface. The impact of closure probably determines the situation along the line of closure. It is probable that the same principle applies to septicemic endocarditis, where bacteria may gain entrance to capillaries or infected emboli lodge in larger vessels. In the former instance, verrucae are likely to occur; and in the latter, massive vegetations.

VEGETATIVE AND ULCERATIVE ENDOCARDITIS. The situation of the larger thrombi of acute vegetative endocarditis varies more widely than that of the acute verrucous

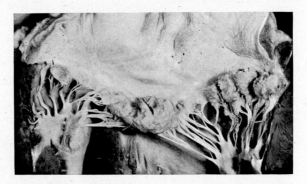

Acute vegetative endocarditis of mitral valve.

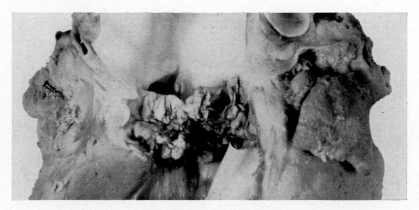

Acute vegetative endocarditis of aortic valve, due to pneumococcus.

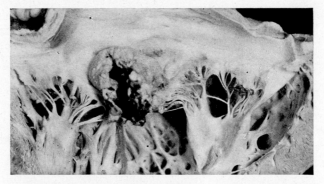

Acute ulcerative endocarditis of mitral valve with perforation. A sheet of black paper behind the leaflet indicates the extent of the perforation.

form. Smaller masses may be found along the line of closure. Larger masses may be found near the middle of the line of closure; they may originate near the middle of the substance of the leaflet or may appear to spread laterally upon the leaflets from a point of origin at or near a commissure. Such lesions occur upon otherwise normal or upon previously diseased leaflets. The vegetations, if multiple, may attain a diameter of 5 or 6 mm. Sometimes a vegetative mass may attain a diameter of 1 or 2 cm., in which case there are likely to be several small vegetations 1 or 2 mm. in size closely associated. Usually sessile and firmly attached, the vegetations may occasionally be pedunculated. The color may be some shade of yellow, or mottled red and yellow, but is usually dark red or mottled light and dark red. The nodules are fairly firm but friable and the outer surface finely or coarsely lobulated. If superficial necrosis has occurred, the resulting ulcer has a shaggy friable base upon which a fresh currant-jelly clot may adhere. If ulceration penetrate into the valve substance, a leaflet aneurysm may result. If the ulceration perforate the leaflet, small dark-red or yellow vegetations appear around the perforation on both surfaces of the leaflet. In the case of perforated semi-lunar cusps the vegetations may be massive in the sinuses of Valsalva. In the case of atrio-ventricular leaflets the vegetations may extend to the chordae tendineae and to the mural endocardium. Without ulceration, extension of acute vegetative endocarditis beyond the limits of the leaflets may occur and in either instance the process may occasionally invade the myocardium to produce abscesses.

Microscopically, the thrombus shows fibrin masses and mesh, much as in the verrucous form. More red blood cells and blood pigment give the darker color of these nodules as compared with verrucae. Polymorphonuclear leukocytes are abundant as are also clumps of bacteria. Even without ulceration, foci of necrosis are common within the exudate. The substance of the leaflet shows hyperemia, mononuclear cell infiltrations, edema, and polymorphonuclear leukocytes as in acute exudative inflammation, at first external to the elastic lamina and later penetrating more deeply. In the event of ulceration of the leaflet, necrosis is observed and

polymorphonuclear leukocytes increase in number. Thrombosis of the leaflet vessels is much more common in vegetative than in verrucous endocarditis. Fibrin strands may be found in the leaflet in continuity with fibrin of the vegetation. Proliferation of connective tissue is only slight, but in rare instances granulation and organization may result in complete healing and cicatrization.

Recurrent Endocarditis. This term implies that superimposed on a preceding chronic or acute endocarditis there is a fresh acute endocarditis of essentially the same nature. It is particularly exemplified in rheumatic endocarditis because, not uncommonly, acute verrucous endocarditis may be found upon a valve already the seat of more or less marked chronic endocarditis. Recovery from acute bacterial endocarditis results in cicatrization of the leaflet and rarely a new bacterial endocarditis may be superimposed. More or less continuously recurrent is subacute bacterial endocarditis.

Subacute Bacterial Endocarditis. (ENDOCARDITIS LENTA.) This is subacute in that the disease often runs a prolonged course over several months but is not true subacute inflammation. The term endocarditis lenta, meaning slow endocarditis, expresses both the clinical course and the anatomic nature of the disease. It is a disease in which vegetations are formed and become organized, to be followed by the production of new vegetations, so that ultimately the mass may be large, composed superficially of vegetations and more deeply of granulation tissue and cicatrization. It rarely occurs upon a valve that is otherwise normal. In from 50 to 80 per cent of the cases the preceding disease is rheumatic. It is said that it may be superimposed on syphilitic valvular disease but in all probability the syphilitic valvular disease is accompanied by and complicated by rheumatic disease. It may occur upon the basis of congenital defects of valves. The valvular lesions vary greatly in degree. The vegetations are fairly firm, moderately friable, usually of pale yellow color occasionally mottled with red, and of variable size from less than a millimeter to more than a centimeter. They are not situated directly on the leaflet, for there is an intervening mass of tissue, softer toward the vegetation and firmer toward the valve, and endothelialized well up toward the vegetation. Extension from the mitral leaflets to the chordae tendineae is frequent, and sometimes to the atrial endocardium. Aortic valve lesions often extend to the ventricular aspect of the mitral leaflet and sometimes to the ventricular endocardium. Microscopically, the vegetation is more often of vegetative than of verrucous type. This merges through granulation tissue to the underlying endocardium.

The disease has bacterial and abacterial stages. In the true abacterial phase, there are no living bacteria in the circulating blood, and according to Libman none in the vegetations. *Streptococcus viridans* (alpha) is the most frequent invader (Libman), but others including the influenza bacillus may be recovered. *S. haemolyticus* (beta) is recovered in a few cases. Organisms may be found in the vegetations when not recoverable from the blood. The portal of entry is thought to be most often from the upper respiratory tract (Weiss). Clawson and Bell believe the lesion to be determined by factors of virulence and resistance, and that it differs only in degree from other forms of endocarditis, but Von Glahn and Pappenheimer concluded that it is a new infection superimposed on unhealed rheumatic endocarditis.

In the morbid anatomic diagnosis of endocarditis, it is important to remember that normally the free edges of the atrioventricular leaflets are somewhat thick and nodular, and that in the semilunar valves the corpora Arantii may be of considerable size. In infancy and early childhood the atrioventricular valves may also be the seat of fairly soft fleshy masses (noduli Albini), remaining after the condensation of connective tissue in the rest of the valve. Not infrequently the atrioventricular leaflets of infants show small, dark red, nodular masses. The exact nature of these is subject to differences of opinion; some regard them as small hematomas; others as dilated persistent blood vessels and still others as true angiomas.

Indeterminate Endocarditis. A type of vegetative endocarditis is described in which the lesions are larger than verrucae and smaller and flatter than vegetations of acute or subacute bacterial endocarditis. They are distributed irregularly on various parts of the valve flaps, without relation to the lines of closure. Bacteria are not found on blood culture or in the vegetations. Microscopically they are rich in fibrin and likely to show marked organization. This is the form that may be found in disseminated lupus erythematosus. It also occurs in the disease called clinically atypical verrucous endocarditis or Libman-Sacks disease (*see* Gross and Friedberg).

SEQUELS OF ACUTE AND SUBACUTE ENDOCARDITIS. Emboli of various sizes may be discharged from the vegetations. In subacute and in septicemic varieties of endocarditis, cutaneous petechiae are common. Infarcts occur in viscera, and, depending on bacterial content of the emboli, may suppurate. Menin-

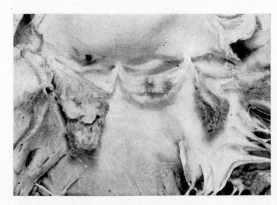

Endocarditis lenta or subacute bacterial endocarditis of aortic valve.

gitis, productive endarteritis and embolism are described in the brain (Winkelman and Eckel). Mycotic aneurysms may occur. The endocarditis may extend to mural endocardium, but only rarely to aorta, to myocardium or pericardium. Functional disturbance of the orifice is unusual except with large vegetations or perforations. Being an infectious disease, acute endocarditis is accompanied by degenerations of parenchymatous viscera, splenic hyperplasia, anemia, etc., and nephritis, which in endocarditis lenta is often focal glomerulonephritis. Recovery of patients with bacterial endocarditis may possibly permit cicatrization, but the rheumatic forms often go on to a genuine chronic endocarditis.

ETIOLOGY. As noted above, the etiologic classification of endocarditis divides it into rheumatic and bacterial forms. Anatomically the acute rheumatic form is a verrucous type of endocarditis. Nevertheless, a true bacterial endocarditis may be superimposed occasionally. Bacterial endocarditis is principally vegetative or ulcerative and may be due to hemolytic streptococci. *S. viridans* is associated especially with endocarditis lenta. The other bacteria, to be mentioned subsequently, cause vegetative and ulcerative endocarditis. It is said that endocarditis may occur in fetal life due to transfer of organisms from maternal blood. Gross's study leads to the conclusion that there are no inflammatory residua in defects of valves observed at birth, and that the deformities are due to fetal abnormalities. Acute endocarditis is uncommon in infancy but occurs in childhood and increases in frequency in the second and third decades. According to Buday, endocarditis lenta has its peak in the third decade, syphilitic disease of the endocardium in the fourth decade, and chronic endocarditis in the fifth decade. In general, endocarditis affects males and females about equally but mitral stenosis is somewhat more frequent in females than males, whereas syphilitic involvement of the aortic valve is more common in males.

The exciting causes of endocarditis may be discussed from the point of view of the diseases with which it is associated, the bacteria concerned, the influence of trauma, the participation of the vessels within the leaflets and cusps, and factors concerned with virulence of organism, resistance of host, and allergic phenomena.

Rheumatic valvular disease is not in itself primarily or fundamentally bacterial. Bacteria may be found as secondary invaders but they do not excite the original lesion.

Pneumonia, osteomyelitis, septicemias and pyemias resulting from wounds and infections incident to childbirth, etc., typhoid fever, scarlatina, diphtheria, measles, variola, influenza, tuberculosis, gonorrhea and other infectious diseases may be complicated by endocarditis. About 4 per cent of cases of pneumonia develop endocarditis, but in only about half these instances is the pneumococcus found, other bacteria recovered probably being secondary invaders (Locke). The endocarditis which accompanies the other infectious diseases shows the causative organism of the general disease in some instances and what appear to be secondary invaders in others. Gonococcal endocarditis must show the presence of gonococci in the blood or

lesion to be accepted as such. The endocarditis of epidemic meningitis practically always reveals meningococci.

There is almost no limit to the variety of microorganisms which may be associated with endocarditis. The more common among these are identified by Thayer, in ascending order of severity, as follows: *Haemophilus influenzae, Streptococcus viridans, Neisseria gonorrhoeae, Staphylococcus albus, Staphylococcus aureus, Diplococcus pneumoniae, Streptococcus haemolyticus.* Various other organisms have been recovered, including *Brucella abortus (melitensis)* and higher organisms such as actinomyces. Even fungi have been encountered, producing a mycotic endocarditis (see Wikler, et al.).

There are certain forms of acute endocarditis, which are found in the terminal stages of prolonged exhausting disease, such as carcinoma and tuberculosis; these do not appear to be due to bacteria. Bacteria may occasionally be present in the vegetations but are not thought to be causative. Included in these lesions is endocarditis minima, with very tiny vegetations.

TRAUMA to the endocardium may be direct or indirect and the few observations which have been made indicate that there is no genuine endocarditis but simply an endocardial thrombus which heals and cicatrizes. It has been supposed that the snapping together of valves in closure may cause the primary injury that results in endocarditis, but histologic study of rheumatic valvulitis indicates that the inflammation is primary in the substance of the leaflets and the same is probably true of other forms. The vegetations then are secondary. Experimentally trauma does not produce endocarditis, but the supposed trauma to leaflets resulting from intravenous injections of particulate matter such as potato particles and charcoal is followed by endocarditis when bacteria or toxic bacterial products (Fulci) are introduced into the blood. The injection of bacteria alone will produce endocarditis but without regularity or high frequency (see Fulci; Fox). Rosenow reports a fairly high frequency following injection of bacteria, due to embolism in the leaflet vessels, but this type of lesion is not common in man. It is doubtful that the injection of particulate matter produces trauma to the leaflets. The experiments of Semsroth and

Koch and others indicate that the use of such materials induces a functional sensitization of the reticulo-endothelial cells of endocardium and myocardium so that there is an inflammatory response to bacteria and bacterial products.

The question of elective localization of streptococci has been discussed in the chapter on Infectious Diseases. There is no convincing evidence that organisms have a special affinity for endocardium. The structure of endocardium, its relatively scanty vascularization, and the physiologic closure of valves, all probably enter into the determination of the deposit of bacteria in and on endocardium.

called allergy, which if in the form of increased reactivity especially of the mesoblastic tissues has been named hyperergy. In the discussion of rheumatic fever in the chapter on Infectious Diseases, the theory of hyperergy was discussed as probably the most reasonable explanation of the effects of rheumatic fever, whether in the heart or elsewhere. (*See* Karsner for general discussion of endocarditis.)

Chronic Endocarditis. Fibrosis of the endocardium, especially with deformity of valves, may be due to chronic inflammation or to cicatrization. The cicatrization may be due to healing of an acute or chronic endocarditis. Chronic endocarditis is due

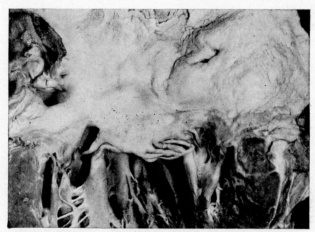

Chronic rheumatic endocarditis, with involvement of leaflets, chordae tendineae and atrial endocardium.

Resistance and Virulence. It is well known that several of the organisms concerned in endocarditis vary considerably in virulence. It is also well known that the human body both constitutionally and at various periods in life varies in resistance. An organism of low virulence may, in a state of low resistance of the body, excite general phenomena and local inflammations as severe as those induced by an organism of high virulence in a highly resistant body. Clawson and Bell emphasize this relation in endocarditis and assume with good reason that local and general manifestations may depend to a large extent upon factors of virulence and resistance, especially in the explanation of subacute bacterial endocarditis. Resistance may vary from time to time, as is indicated in those alterations of tissue reactivity usually

chiefly and perhaps solely to rheumatic disease. Morphologically, the usual criteria of chronic inflammation may not be found, but often the history of the patient can only be explained on the basis of a gradually progressive valvular deformity. Microscopically, however, the fibrosis may be accompanied by the infiltration of lymphocytes, plasma cells and large mononuclear cells common to chronic inflammation in any organ. Furthermore, the fact that the extent of the deformity is greater than could be explained by cicatrization of the tiny acute rheumatic verrucae points toward the view that there is a progressive chronic inflammation. The deformity may be slight, moderate or marked. Most important are thickening, stiffening and fibrous adhesion of leaflets, and retraction of leaflets and chordae tendineae. Density and retraction may progressively increase and cause progressive symptoms. The adhesion and thickening produce obstruction in the valve orifice; the retraction permits regurgitation. The leaflet in chronic endocarditis shows fibrous, often somewhat nodular, thickening most marked near the edge; the remainder of the leaflet is moderately or markedly thickened but may show little change. Sometimes the free edge may be thin and pliable but is usually involved in the fibrosis of the line of closure. The aortic cusps may show a curling of the free border inward toward the sinus of Valsalva. Adhesion between adjacent cusps is often just below the free borders near the commissures, so-called submarginal adhesion. The blood vessels which grew into the leaflets during the acute inflammation may persist as grossly visible vessels especially on the atrial surface of the anterior mitral leaflet. Calcification may occur in the ring of the valve, at the base of the leaflets, at the region of adhesions at the free border; it may be extensive in calcific disease of the aortic valve discussed under aortic stenosis. Chronic mural and chordal endocarditis show the same processes, modified by the situation of these structures.

Microscopically, the valve leaflets and cusps show dense fibrosis often with hyalinization, infiltration of lymphocytes and large mononuclear cells, vascularization well out toward the free border, rarely necrosis and sometimes calcification; usually the endothelial covering is intact.

Recovery from acute bacterial endocarditis is infrequent, but occasionally irregularly disposed scars with deformities not so characteristic as encountered in rheumatic disease, indicate the cicatrization of healed acute bacterial disease. Chronic rheumatic disease does not invariably lead to progressive and marked deformity. Frequently in people of middle and advanced life lesions of valves are discovered at autopsy. They were not suspected clinically because the deformity is so slight that there were no functional disturbances. All the features of chronic rheumatic valvulitis are present but in only minor degree. The age of the patient in comparison to the time rheumatic fever probably occurred and the absence of microscopic evidence of active chronic inflammation points to healing of a chronic lesion that has pro-

gressed for only a limited time. This inactive valvulitis is often called healed nondeforming endocarditis.

Certain features vary slightly in different valves, necessitating brief consideration of lesions and effects in each area. In the following discussion, consideration is given especially to chronic valvular disease in both its morphologic and functional aspects. Acute endocarditis may produce comparable functional disturbances but they are naturally of relatively short duration.

Mitral Stenosis. In this condition the size of the mitral orifice may be moderately reduced or so greatly contracted that its diameter does not exceed a few millimeters. Fibrous adhesions at the junction of the two leaflets may be slight or extensive; the leaflets are thickened more particularly toward the line of closure. The chordae tendineae show thickening, adhesion to one another and shortening, together with fibrosis of the tips of the papillary muscles. The fusion of the leaflets may progress to form the "funnel shaped" valve, or they may become relatively fixed as a dense rigid diaphragm in the center of which is a narrow orifice, the "button hole" valve. Calcification of the ring is frequent and calcareous deposits may be found near the free border of the leaflets themselves. The rigidity of the leaflets and an associated retraction may cause an accompanying insufficiency; it may be that retraction of the chordae tendineae contributes to insufficiency. Not infrequently fresh verrucae are found along the line of closure or bacterial infection may lead to superimposed mycotic endocarditis. When calcareous masses project through the surface of the leaflets, acute vegetations may form over them.

Production of mitral stenosis in the circulation model is followed by a fall of systemic and pulse pressure and an elevation of venous pressure. In man, the gradual development of the stenosis causes a diastolic accumulation of blood in the atrium with resultant hypertrophy. This induces increasingly active atrial systole so that the defect is compensated. Nevertheless, the hypertrophy may ultimately be ineffective or the stenosis may be so great that no degree of hypertrophy can compensate. Minor degrees of inadequate compensation over a considerable period of time lead to increased pulmonary venous

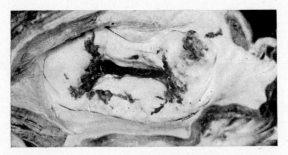

Mitral stenosis viewed from above. A "button hole" mitral with calcification and vegetations. Rheumatic fever.

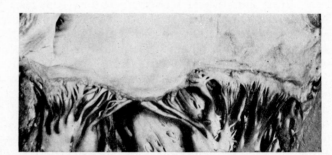

Chronic and acute rheumatic endocarditis. Note the verrucae along free edge of larger leaflet and along line of closure of smaller leaflet.

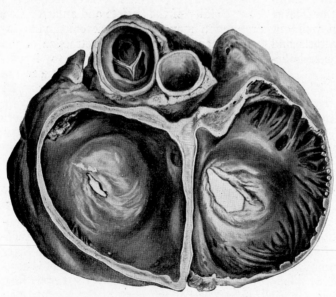

View from above of chronic valvular endocarditis with stenosis of aortic, mitral (button hole) and tricuspid orifices.

pressure and ultimately to increased pulmonary arterial pressure with consequent hypertrophy of the right ventricle. The passive hyperemia of the lungs may be marked and the lungs are spoken of as being the seat of brown induration. Probably because of the intercommunicating spiral arrangement of cardiac muscle there may be slight hypertrophy of the left ventricle. Only when there is congestive failure of the heart accompanied by dilatation of the tricuspid ring does generalized passive hyperemia occur. There may be accompanying thrombosis in the left atrial appendage and sometimes this extends into the atrium itself.

Clinically, mitral stenosis occurs in early and later middle life; it is more frequent in women than in men. Statistically it leads to death earlier than is true of aortic stenosis. It may give little in the way of clinical manifestations and often is observed first on a routine examination of the heart. The murmurs are usually soft and heard in mid-diastole, late diastole, or as presystolic murmurs merging with the first sound of the heart. The pulse is usually normal but may become arrhythmic if auricular fibrillation occurs. Blood pressure is usually normal but the pulse pressure may be somewhat reduced. The roentgenogram is likely to show an alteration in the configuration of the left border of the heart due to enlargement of the pulmonary conus. The oblique views show enlargement of the left atrium. The electrocardiogram usually shows right ventricular preponderance incident to hypertrophy of the right ventricle.

Mitral insufficiency occurs with or without mitral stenosis. In either case, it is due to retraction of the leaflets, chordae tendineae or both. Minor degrees of mitral insufficiency are common. The leaflets show slight thickening and retraction, usually of inflammatory origin. Mechanically, the atrial pressure rises and the mean arterial pressure falls. The increase in atrial pressure is probably due to transfer of hydrodynamic pressure from the ventricle rather than to any large regurgitation of blood. Consequently, unless the myocardium fails, there is not likely to be serious pulmonary hyperemia or elevation of pulmonary arterial pressure. The tension in the atrium may induce slight hypertrophy, but the latter is rarely marked.

The high atrial pressure increases the initial tension in the ventricle and may even lead to increased output and slight hypertrophy. Moderate degrees of mitral insufficiency produce little alteration of circulation and only slight or no hypertrophy of left atrium and ventricle. Dilatation of these chambers may finally occur with stasis, primarily in the pulmonary and ultimately in the general circulation.

Relative insufficiency of the mitral orifice may result from failure of the myocardium, with consequent stretching of the ring and sometimes of the papillary muscles. The first prevents apposition of leaflets and the second allows them to override into the atrium with leakage.

Clinically there may be no symptoms, and often the systolic murmur is discovered only during some routine physical examination. Enlargement of the left atrium may be demonstrated by physical examination and the roentgenogram.

Aortic Stenosis. Although vegetations on the aoritic cusps may produce

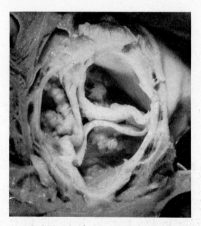

Rheum + syph. 15886

Calcific stenosis of aortic valve, viewed from above. Calcific masses conspicuous on aortic aspect of the cusps.

stenosis, chronic valvular disease is the more frequent cause. Chronic rheumatic aortic valvulitis, by virtue of fusion of commissures and rigidity of the cusps, often causes variable degrees of stenosis, in association with mitral disease. In addition, calcific disease of the aortic valves may produce profound stenosis. For years this condition was thought to be sclerotic in origin, but numerous studies have shown that it is originally inflam-

c̄ subacute 14553

matory in so many of the cases that the rest are probably of the same nature; furthermore, the inflammation is like that of chronic rheumatic disease (Karsner and Koletsky; Hall and Ichioka). In this condition the cusps are thickened and rigid, usually more so at the base than at the free border; adhesions vary from moderate to marked, so much so that the acquired bicuspid state is fairly common. In the cusps and often projecting above the level of their surfaces are calcific nodules, a millimeter or more in diameter, closely approximated and likely to be

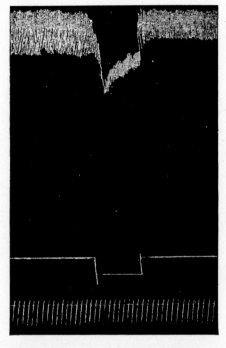

Tracing of aortic stenosis in the dog, produced by means of a slip ligature about base of aorta. Signal line is also base line. Time in two seconds. Note fall in mean pressure and amplitude.

especially conspicuous at the base of the cusps and the adjacent parts of the sinuses of Valsalva.

Aortic stenosis produces hypertrophy of the heart which is especially marked when the lesion is calcific disease. Calcific stenosis affects men more often than women and, although observed at any time from the second decade onward, has its highest incidence in the sixth decade. In the circulation model, and in animal experiments, aortic stenosis produces a fall in mean blood pressure and pulse pressure. Intraventricular pressure rises sharply and the ejection pressure is increased. The period of ejection is prolonged but the amount of blood discharged is normal save when the stenosis is marked. The length of systole and diastole remains about normal. Clinically there is usually a loud systolic murmur at the aortic area transmitted to the neck, often accompanied by a corresponding thrill. The pulse is small and rises slowly, the "*pulsus parvus et tardus.*" Physical examination and roentgenogram show marked cardiac enlargement and fluoroscopy may demonstrate "dancing" shadows of the calcareous masses in the valve. The mean blood pressure may be high or normal and, in some cases, the pulse pressure is reduced. The electrocardiogram shows left ventricular preponderance in most cases and various types of arrhythmia in some. Because of rigidity and shortening of the cusps, there may be an associated aortic insufficiency.

Aortic Insufficiency. This may be caused by dilatation of the ring accompanying marked dilatation of the heart. It may be due to acute endocarditis, or to chronic valvulitis of rheumatic origin because of retraction and rigidity of the cusps, but here there is usually an associated stenosis. Occasionally it may be caused by rupture of a diseased cusp, the result of great muscular effort or trauma; rupture may occur occasionally in a normal valve (Howard). Nevertheless the most frequent cause of aortic insufficiency is syphilis. This operates either by dilatation of the ring because of syphilitic aortitis or by extension of the aortitis to affect the cusps. In the former, the cusps may enlarge and for some time effect adequate closure. In the latter, the commissures are widened because that part of the cusps near them becomes flattened back against and adherent to the walls of the sinuses of Valsalva. In an early case, Saphir and Scott found this to be due to a productive inflammation extending from the aortic wall to involve the cusp, and because of fibrosis the part of the cusp near the commissure becomes adherent. Jason, however, in a study of advanced cases, attributed the change to a destructive inflammation and reparative fibrosis. The cusps usually are diffusely but moderately thickened, often retracted and show a curling of the free border toward the ventricle. Other deformities of the cusps may be found. Sometimes the endocardium of the septum immediately below is thickened and shows pockets with openings toward the valve, but this is of no functional importance (Saphir).

The circulation model shows a marked fall in diastolic pressure with little or no drop in systolic pressure; thus there is increased pulse pressure. In experimental animals there is a fall in mean pressure and increase in amplitude of the pulse, with a striking tendency for return of systolic pressure toward

enlargement and the roentgenogram shows elongation of the heart; the fluoroscope shows wide amplitude of pulsations in the aortic arch. The systolic blood pressure is normal or increased, whereas the diastolic pressure is considerably or greatly reduced. When systolic pressure is increased it may be due to the increased systolic discharge and may be augmented by hypertension. Wiggers draws attention to the fact that pressure falls during the latter part of systolic ejection and that this may account in part for the drop in diastolic arterial pressure. The peripheral pulse shows a rapid rise fol-

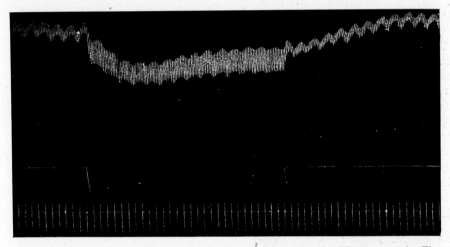

Tracing of aortic insufficiency in the dog, produced with the Wiggers cannula. The signal line is also the base line. Time in two seconds. Note the fall in mean pressure and the increase in amplitude. Vasoconstriction tends to increase mean pressure and, after termination of insufficiency, elevates general pressure level.

normal. The significant physiologic observations include enlargement of the left ventricular chamber in diastole due to back flow of blood and of pressure. This increased diastolic intraventricular pressure results in high initial tension and augmented systolic discharge, together with prolongation of systole.

Clinically, syphilitic aortic insufficiency occurs in early middle life and more often in males than females. There is usually a history of syphilis, with inadequate or no treatment; the serologic tests are positive in about 85 per cent of the cases. Pallor, capillary pulsation manifested in the nail beds, collapsing pulse and sometimes mental disturbances are noted. A diastolic murmur, sometimes musical, usually replaces the aortic second sound. There is marked cardiac

lowed by a rapid fall—the collapsing, Corrigan, or water-hammer pulse. The rapid rise is due to increased ejection at the beginning of systole. The fall occurs in the latter part of systole (before diastole) and is due to decrease in the amount ejected. The changes are intensified by the time the pulse reaches the peripheral arteries, such as the radial. Wiggers attributes capillary pulsation to essentially the same mechanism.

Valves of the Right Side of the Heart. The most common affection of these is a relative tricuspid insufficiency, which usually occurs as the result of dilatation of the right ventricle and atrium. This diminishes the muscular support of the ring and chordae tendineae, so that the leaflets do not appose. This accounts in large part for the venous stasis of decompensated hearts. **Acute**

15886

tricuspid valvulitis occurs in association with acute endocarditis of the left heart but is unusual. We have observed minute vegetations in septicemias. Gonococcal endocarditis commonly shows lesions of both left and right side of the heart (Thayer). Chronic lesions are nearly always associated with a chronic lesion of the left side. In our experience, chronic tricuspid valvulitis produces stenosis much more often than insufficiency, but they are likely to be combined.

Pulmonary insufficiency is uncommon but occurs as the result of dilatation of the ring in decompensation, acute or chronic endocarditis, aneurysms or rupture of cusps, congenital anomalies, but only rarely if ever, as a result of arteriosclerosis of the pulmonic aorta. The principle causes of pulmonic stenosis are lesions due to endocarditis, acute or chronic, and congenital stenosis of the conus, ring, or root of the pulmonic aorta. We have observed two cases of pulmonic stenosis, as the result of bulging of saccular aneurysms of the root of the systemic aorta and of the aortic sinus of Valsalva. The principles of circulatory disturbance must be much the same as those in the left side of the heart; such studies as have been made confirm this view.

Tumors

Vascular hamartoma may occur in valves and tiny papillary structures are seen occasionally. Myxoma or fibromyxoma may grow from the endocardium, especially of the left atrium. Whether this is actually neoplasm or organization of thrombus with myxomatous changes is not settled. When large, it produces functional effects like those of mitral stenosis. Metastasis of malignant tumors into the endocardium is rare, but metastasis in the myocardium may extend into the endocardium.

MYOCARDIUM

Introduction

In presenting this phase of the subject of heart disease, time and space will be conserved by including certain abnormal conditions of the heart as a whole, because many of the diseases of the myocardium are intimately related to the entire organ.

Congenital Anomalies

The heart develops from a primary tube which becomes tortuous to form the S-shaped tube, and develops septa and valves to form the four-chambered organ. At any time in this period of development, interruptions, alterations and inflammatory lesions may occur to produce an anomalous heart. These may be so slight as to be of no functional importance, or on the other hand may seriously cripple the heart or be incompatible with life. The heart may be absent (acardia), or rudimentary (hemicardia); it may project through the anterior body fissure (ectopia cordis). It may be transposed in position so that the greater ventricle is to the right and the apex points to the right (dextrocardia). This may be associated with complete transposition of the viscera, or with transposition of the great vascular trunks. A pathologic, rather than anomalous, dextrocardia may be caused by lesions of the chest such as pleural effusions, adhesions, tumors, etc., but the chambers are not transposed.

Developmental defects at the foramen ovale are common (see Patten). These vary from minor abnormalities in the primary and secondary septa as they form the interatrial septum, patency of the foramen demonstrable only by probe and of no functional significance, to wide and easily visible patency. The larger patencies constitute the so-called interatrial septal defect, which may lead to hypertrophy, especially of the right side of the heart, with various clinical manifestations of heart disease and death from congestive failure. (See Tinney; Bedford, Papp and Parkinson.) There may also be deficiencies of the interventricular septum. Thus trilocular and even bilocular hearts may be formed. Congenital atresias of orifices may be due to developmental faults. One of the more serious anomalies that may permit survival into adult life is the TETRALOGY OF FALLOT. In this are found congenital pulmonic stenosis, defect of the interventricular septum, right ventricular hypertrophy and a shift of the root of the aorta a little to the right of its natural position, called dextroposition of the aorta.

Depending upon the direction of the blood in patencies of the septa, these openings may give rise to venous arterial shunts or arterial venous shunts (Abbott and Dawson). Although there is divergence of views, it is probable that the cyanosis of cardiac anomalies is due to inflow of venous blood into the systemic circulation. This cyanosis (morbus caeruleus) may be marked, slight or absent, depending upon the amount of un-

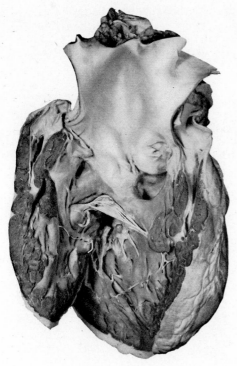

Patent interventricular septum at upper portion, viewed from right ventricle. The heart is the seat of the tetralogy of Fallot. Note hypertrophy of right ventricle and rotund papillary muscles. The aorta is far enough to the right so that it was opened with the pulmonary artery.

aërated blood. The right heart is the seat of hypertrophy variable in degree. Extensive discussion is provided by Abbott, Mönckeberg and Schwalbe.

Degenerations

Cloudy Swelling. Cloudy swelling of the myocardium occurs in many acute infectious diseases such as diphtheria, scarlet fever and others, may be the result of poisons such as phosphorus, arsenic, chloroform, iodoform, ether, alcohol, and may be due to anemia, either acute or chronic, primary or secondary. It is of importance to note that these agents cause general cloudy swelling, and that the affection of the heart is only a

part of a more widespread, similar lesion. Grossly, the heart may be dilated and the muscle is likely to be soft, flabby and cloudy. The cross section bulges, shows a cloudy brown or boiled appearance and is more friable than normal. Microscopically, the muscle fiber cells are swollen, show diminution or loss of transverse striation, and may contain acidophilic granules. A pathologic diagnosis must take into account the length of time the individual has been dead, because postmortem changes may very closely simulate those of cloudy swelling. There are no constant changes clinically, but often low blood pressure, cardiac dilatation, rapid rate and sometimes arrhythmia may be associated. The nature and cause of the arrhythmia are not clearly understood.

Fatty Degeneration. This is due to essentially the same causes as those of cloudy swelling, operating over a longer time or with greater intensity. Grossly, the heart is soft and flabby and has a dull, opaque appearance. If the fatty degeneration be diffusely scattered throughout the heart, the muscle has a dull yellow color; if the fat be irregularly distributed in the muscle, the so-called "tigroid" or "tabby cat" appearance is produced. This tigering is often seen better through the endocardium of the right ventricle than that of the left, and is likely to be more prominent in the papillary muscles than in the columnae carneae. It is seen best through the endocardium as short, parallel, transverse lines of yellow color, about a millimeter in width and separated about a similar distance from adjacent lines. Microscopically, the change is satisfactorily demonstrated only by the use of special stains such as osmic acid, Sudan III or Scharlach R. For this purpose, formalin fixation must be employed. As with cloudy swelling, there is no constant clinical picture. Low blood pressure, rapid or slow heart, and sometimes cardiac arrhythmia are observed. Garvin reports a case in which fatty degeneration was the only lesion found in death from myocardial insufficiency; this, however, is rare.

Fat Infiltration. This is fairly common, especially in obese patients. The subepicardial fat is usually increased in amount but the demonstration of true infiltration is found on transverse section; the normal sharp line of demarcation between fat and myocardium is obscured and lines of fat tissue extend into the myocardium. The lesion is more common in the right than in the left ventricle. Microscopically, the fat tissue extends from the subepicardial tissue downward between the muscle bundles, the fiber cells of which are often atrophic. Moderate degrees of fat infiltration have no apparent functional significance but it may be marked enough to produce dyspnea on exertion, and Saphir and Corrigan report cases in which it seemed to be the only reasonable cause of death.

Other Degenerations. Hyaline degeneration in its simple form is not likely to affect the myocardium except in the interstitial tissues and in the blood vessels. Zenker's hyaline is referred to below in connection with necrosis. Amyloid may be found in the secondary form in both the vessels of the heart and under the endocardium. The heart is occasionally included among the mesoblastic tissues affected in primary amyloidosis. Indeed one case is reported in which it appeared to be the cause of death (Binford). Calcification may occur in foci of necrosis, or of extensive fibrosis, and in coronary arteries. Metastatic calcification affects the heart, particularly in the right side.

Segmentation of Myocardium. Practically never in infancy, rarely before the twentieth year and increasing in frequency as age advances, the myocardium may show numerous transverse fractures of the muscle fibers microscopically. Lateral enlargement between fractures is slight or absent and neighboring reactive inflammation never observed. It is usually stated that segmentation occurs in the line of the intercalated disks, and that a slightly different condition called fragmentation shows fractures of the fibers between, and not necessarily involving the disks. The studies of Saphir and Karsner, as well as of others, show that the fractures are in the intercalated disks in both, the differences in appearance being due to differences in number and conformation of the disks under various conditions. Aschoff attributes the change to postmortem decomposition, but we found that it can be produced in rabbits by suddenly elevating intraventricular pressure and producing dilatation, and that animals can live for at least 48 hours with the lesion. The heart of segmentation may be soft, flabby, and dilated, but there are no gross characteristics.

Necrosis. This is most likely to appear as a sequence of degeneration, as a part of acute myocarditis of infectious diseases, or as the result of occlusion of branches of the coronary arteries. In the last instance, it is massive coagulation necrosis, to be considered under circulatory disturbances. In the others, it appears as foci either of hyaline or granular necrosis, or as Zenker's hyaline necrosis with lateral swelling and rupture of fibers.

Circulatory Disturbances

General anemias may be acute or chronic. In the former, such as occurs follow-

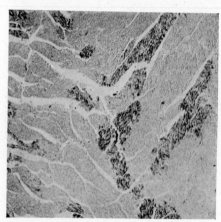

Foci of hyaline necrosis of myocardium of dog, due to experimental coronary occlusion.

ing large hemorrhage, the heart is pale, grayish-red or grayish-yellow, but differs from the heart of fatty degeneration in that it remains firm. Profound anemias from repeated smaller hemorrhages or as the result of exhausting diseases or chronic blood diseases, lead to more or less widespread fatty degeneration. Local anemia or ischemia of the myocardium is due principally to reduction in the size of lumen of the coronary arteries or to occlusion. If the occlusion be sudden, the region supplied by the vessel undergoes infarction; if reduction progress gradually the affected area shows atrophy of muscle and consequent fibrosis.

Infarction. This is usually due to occlusive thrombosis in coronary arteries. The thrombus forms in vessels that are al-

Effort + myocardial infarction JAMA 128:775 '45

in mural hemorrhage

ready the seat of disease, especially arteriosclerosis. Occlusion may also be due to hemorrhage from capillaries which grow in the arteriosclerotic wall (Wartman). Occlusion is also reported as being due to embolism into the coronaries, from valvular disease, mural thrombus or lesions within the coronaries themselves. In our experience it is infrequent and when it does occur it is usually an infected embolus with consequent

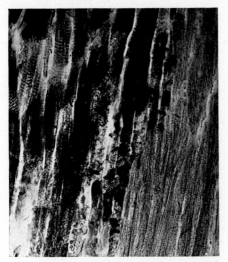

Photomicrograph of hyaline and granular necrosis in experimental myocardial infarct of the dog.

abscess formation. (See Garvin and Work.) Others, however, maintain that bland embolic occlusion of the coronaries is not rare (Hamman). It is said that the gradual occlusion of coronary arteries by arteriosclerosis may result in infarction but we have not observed this. Nor have we seen infarction without organic occlusion, as reported by others (Gross and Sternberg). In the human heart it is possible also to observe occlusion by thrombosis without resulting infarction. This appears to depend upon the establishment of collateral circulation through arteries 40 micra or more in diameter. Although it has been thought that anastomoses of this sort develop as a result of age, it now appears that the development is due to occlusion of other branches of the arteries, principally because of arteriosclerosis. Without such narrowing or occlusion the anastomoses do not develop. (See Schlesinger, et al.; Blumgart, et al.) With this exception, it is generally true that the size of

the infarct depends upon the size of the artery occluded. It is often said that the site of election for occlusion is in the left descending ramus about 2.5 cm. from its origin, but the studies of Schlesinger and Zoll indicate that this situation predominates to only a slight degree and that, in general, occlusions are not significantly more numerous in the left than in the right coronary arteries. Nevertheless, infarcts are more frequent in the left ventricle and septum than elsewhere, but they do occur in the right ventricle and in the atria (Cushing, et al.) Experimentally, Blumgart and associates found that if occlusion be maintained for from 5 to 20 minutes, infarction does not occur, but after a duration of 25 minutes infarction results.

The course of events in myocardial infarction of the human heart is much the same as described for experimental infarction in the chapter on Disturbances of Circulation. It may be a recent, white or yellowish white infarct, or may show stages from that on to complete cicatrization. It preserves the general conical form of infarcts but this is modified by the distribution of the coronary arteries and the conformation of the heart wall. The apex is toward the epicardium and the base toward the endocardium. Usually, however, there is a thin layer of preserved muscle underlying the endocardium, probably because of nutrition of this part of the wall through the thebesian vessels (Wearn). The overlying epicardium often shows acute fibrinous pericarditis. When cicatrization occurs following large infarcts, the wall of the heart is much thinned. This may result in bulging of the outer surface of the wall, the myocardial aneurysm. Anatomically, this is divided into true aneurysm, as just described, and a localized enlargement of the ventricular chamber without bulging of the outer wall, spoken of as false aneurysm. As a matter of fact, in the latter condition there is probably bulging in life due to the intraventricular pressure. A large fresh infarct may rupture with the production of hemopericardium or it may perforate the interventricular septum. In the earlier stage of infarction, mural thrombosis is only occasionally observed, but after cicatrization with local bulging takes place, such thrombosis is common. In many instances, coronary thrombosis occurs in patients who have hyperten-

Duguid, J.B. Am. J. Path + Bact — What is interpreted as arteriosclerosis in coronaries is often recanalized thrombus 58:207 '46

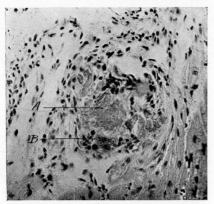

Experimental myocardial infarct of the dog, showing at A necrotic muscle, and at B, foreign body giant cell as part of the process of organization.

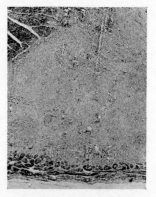

Low power photomicrograph of cicatrized myocardial infarct of the dog, showing triangular outline with base toward endocardium and layer of surviving muscle under endocardium.

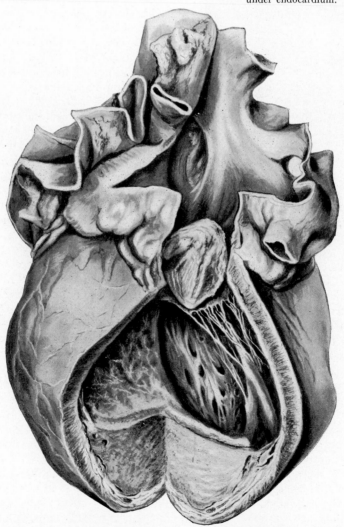

Partial aneurysm of left ventricle due to old coronary occlusion. The apex of the left ventricle is thin and made up largely of scar tissue, and within the ventricle is a large mottled thrombus.

sion, and thus there is an associated cardiac hypertrophy. Nevertheless, even in those who do not have hypertension, hypertrophy may occur and is probably due to diastolic stretching, the result of destruction of part of the cardiac wall.

In addition to the larger regions of fibrosis which follow obvious infarction, the myocardium frequently shows smaller foci of fibrosis. These are often referred to as myocardial scars. It is now apparent that they are due to occlusion of smaller branches of the coronary arteries, either sudden or gradual. This results in atrophy or necrosis of a small region of muscle and consequently fibrosis follows. It is possible, however, that in the myocardium of old rheumatic disease some of the scarring is due to destruction of the muscle in the course of the acute rheumatic myocarditis.

The clinical manifestations of myocardial infarction include cardiac pain, referred to subsequently, fall of blood pressure, pericardial friction rub, leukocytosis, fever and increased sedimentation rate.

FUNCTIONAL EFFECTS OF CORONARY OCCLUSION. In experimental animals the effects of ligation of branches of the coronary arteries are roughly proportional to the size of the occluded artery. On the basis of a fairly large occlusion, Wiggers sets up the results as immediate and delayed. The immediate effects may be ectopic beats, tachycardia and ventricular fibrillation and death, or there may be hypodynamic beat with low blood pressure and small pulse. If the animal survive, the circulation may return to normal, but death from congestive failure is likely to occur one to three months later. The result of the occlusion in the animal is infarction, but, even before morphologic changes take place, functional disturbance in the ischemic muscle is observed. Tennant and Wiggers report a decrease or absence of contractility within a minute after occlusion of an artery. Electrocardiographic changes are much like those in man.

The direct transfer of experimental results to man is not justifiable. The animal's heart is essentially normal at the start of the experiment. In man, however, various degrees of arteriosclerosis almost always precede the occlusion and this may have produced deterioration of the myocardium so

that occlusion of a relatively small artery may cause death. In contrast, the arteriosclerosis may bring about establishment of a collateral circulation of such extent that occlusion of a fairly large branch may not produce serious disturbance (Blumgart, Schlesinger and Zoll). The physiologic effects in man follow closely those seen in experimental animals, including the irregularities of beat, drop in blood pressure and ventricular fibrillation. Electrocardiographic changes are variable depending upon the size of the ischemic region and also its position in reference to the conduction system. These are described in the books on medicine and on physiology. Pain will be discussed in the next paragraph. Death may be immediate, delayed a few hours or longer, or the patient may survive the attack. Indeed he may live several or even many years. Repetition of the attacks is more and more likely to be fatal. In fatal cases, the heart at autopsy may or may not show infarction depending on whether or not sufficient time for the infarct to become manifest had elapsed after the occlusion occurred.

Angina Pectoris. This is a clinical syndrome which includes substernal oppres-

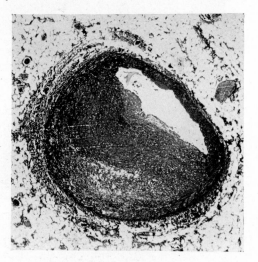

Marked arteriosclerosis of left descending ramus of coronary artery, with narrow, eccentrically placed lumen.

sion, precordial pain which often radiates as a referred pain to the left arm and shoulder, ashen pallor and a sense of impending death. It is due to an absolute or relative ischemia of parts of or the whole myocardium. Thus a coronary occlusion means a localized ischemia. Nevertheless, pain may occur without organic occlusion and sometimes seems to be due to coronary arterial spasm. In its action the muscle utilizes great quantities of oxygen; coronary flow may not be sufficient to provide enough oxygen, with resultant relative anoxemia, especially when, as in exercise, the utilization of oxygen is vastly increased. This accounts for the "angina of effort." Relative ischemia is favored by coronary arteriosclerosis, by syphilitic aortitis with reduction in size of coronary ostia, by aortic stenosis, anemias, etc. (See Blumgart, et al.; Wilson and Johnston.)

Inflammation

Acute Myocarditis. This term is sometimes loosely employed, but to the pathologist indicates a condition in which there

suppurative myocarditis. It is a common accompaniment of acute infectious disease, particularly diphtheria, scarlatina, typhoid fever, pneumonia, influenza, and septicemias or pyemias. It also occurs in connection with chronic disease such as duodenal ulcers, ulcerative colitis and malignant tumors. There is dispute as to the effects of exophthalmic goiter, but Weller reports it in that condition and Goodpasture has produced it by the use of thyroxin and chloroform. There have been many experimental studies which have thrown little or no light on the human disease. Nevertheless, it has been produced in animals by the use of adrenalin, nicotine, strophanthin, digitalis, diphtheria toxin and other agents. In man, it is likely that the disease is due principally to bacterial products and perhaps injurious substances of metabolic origin.

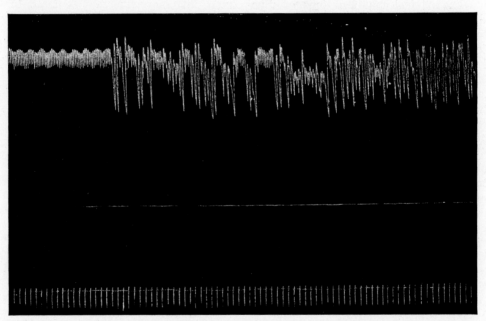

Tracing of cardiac arrhythmia in the dog, incident to experimental acute myocardial necrosis produced by multiple injections of 95 per cent alcohol into the myocardium. The injections were made before this tracing was made, so that the arrhythmia follows a period of normal mechanism. Time in two seconds.

is, associated with muscle degeneration or necrosis, an infiltration into the interstitial tissues of cells usually found either in acute or subacute exudative processes. In the heart, a differentiation between acute parenchymatous and acute interstitial myocarditis does not seem justifiable. The lesion might be more properly referred to as an acute non-

Grossly, the heart of acute myocarditis shows the soft, flabby, pallid, sometimes yellow, opaque muscle seen in cloudy swelling and fatty degeneration, but not infrequently in greater degrees. Microscopically, the muscle fibers show a variety of changes varying from simple cloudy swelling to fatty degeneration and granular and hyaline necrosis.

Necrosis is often in small, irregularly disposed foci, about which the cellular infiltration may be greater than in other places. Sometimes vacuolar degeneration is seen. Unless necrosis is present, the nuclei show little change, except perhaps for slight pyknosis. The more severe degenerative changes are especially common in diphtheria. The cellular infiltrate of the interstitial tissue may consist of lymphocytes, leukocytes, plasma cells, and ultimately a growth of connective tissue. Inflammatory edema may be present and occasionally hemorrhage is encountered. Eosinophils are frequently encountered, sometimes in large numbers. The acute myocarditis of rheumatic fever shows much the same changes plus the occurrence of Aschoff

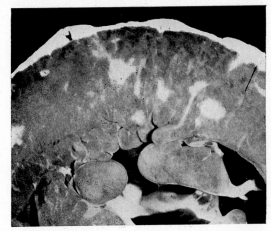

Fibrosis of wall of left ventricle in an old rheumatic heart.

nodules. The heart of acute myocarditis often dilates, and sometimes to such an extent that thrombosis occurs in the chambers of the heart either on the right or the left side.

Functionally, extreme weakness of the circulatory mechanism and various types of arrhythmia may appear. Wiggers quotes certain authors as having described degenerative and infiltrative changes in the transmission bundles, which may explain certain cases of arrhythmia. Circulatory failure may be pronounced and, more especially in diphtheria, may lead to sudden death. The circulatory failure in diphtheria is apparently not of vasomotor origin, but it is possible that a shock-like loss of fluids into the tissues may cause inadequacy of atrial filling, with low pressure in spite of vasoconstriction. Acute

myocarditis may lead to death, or, in the event of recovery, may lead to chronic fibrosis. Apparently complete recovery may follow cases which occur in early life.

ACUTE SUPPURATIVE MYOCARDITIS. This is usually referred to as abscess of the myocardium. It is most commonly a part of a pyemia or septicemia, although it may be a direct extension from acute valvulitis or suppurative pericarditis. Streptococci, staphylococci, pneumococci, and rarely gonococci may be recovered. The abscesses are likely to be multiple, with a diameter of only 2 to 3 mm. and surrounded by a zone of hyperemia or hemorrhage. They occur most commonly in the lower three-fourths of the left ventricle, especially in the subepicardial muscle, and in the papillary muscles. Large, infected emboli may produce infected infarcts. Microscopically, there may be a centrum of necrotic tissue, often containing a bacterial mass, surrounded by the usual cells of the abscess, or the cells infiltrate the necrotic area to produce the typical, focalized collection of pus. Rarely, healing occurs with cicatrization, but as a rule the patients die of the underlying septicemia or pyemia. Possible complications include extension to produce acute pericarditis, rupture of papillary muscle with valvular insufficiency, ulceration into endocardium with possible subsequent embolism.

ACUTE ISOLATED MYOCARDITIS. This occurs usually in early middle life, with insidious onset, signs of myocardial insufficiency and death after the lapse of several months. It is not associated with inflammation of the endocardium or pericardium, and no cause has been found. Grossly the heart shows hypertrophy, often great, and a flabby pale yellow myocardium. Microscopically, two forms have been described. In both, degeneration of muscle may be marked. In one there is a more or less extensive infiltration into the interstitial tissues of lymphocytes, large mononuclear cells, polymorphonuclear leukocytes and sometimes eosinophils. In the other there are granulomatous lesions with cells of the exudate, fibroblasts and multinucleated giant cells, but neither tuberculosis nor syphilis has been proven to be a cause. (*See* Saphir for review of myocarditis.)

Myocardial Fibrosis. This may be observed as a diffuse fibrosis of the myocardium or in a focalized form. The diffuse form is seen in those conditions where more or less widespread fibrosis of various organs of the body occurs. This is likely to be associated with chronic processes such as chronic alcoholism, gout, lead poisoning, syphilis, tuberculosis, and is secondary to senile atrophies of parenchymatous tissues, and to arteriosclerosis. The disease responsible for the fibrosis may cause hypertrophy of the heart; an associated hypertension is common. Upon gross examination the heart is enlarged and the muscle extremely firm. Tangential section of the myocardium shows parallel fine lines of retraction which gives

carditis does not occur, or if it does it is rare. The name "myocardosis" has been suggested to cover the clinical manifestations of decreased cardiac reserve, cardiac failure and even arrhythmias, where there is no valvular, vascular, or renal disease to explain the condition, but in these cases the underlying condition is either myocardial fibrosis or coronary arterial disease, perhaps accompanied by acute degenerations.

Granulomata. The most important are syphilis and tuberculosis, although others such as actinomycosis may occur. Gumma formation in the heart is uncommon in congenital syphilis (Williams) and not frequent

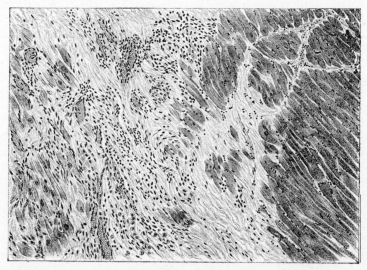

Cicatricial type of myocardial fibrosis.

the coarsely striated appearance of tough beef.

The focalized form of myocardial fibrosis is usually cicatricial in character, following either small necroses incident to acute myocarditis, or atrophy or necrosis of the myocardium due to diminished nutrition. Focalized atrophies are particularly likely to occur with arteriosclerosis of the coronary arteries. The fibrosis is patchy in character, appearing as small or large scars throughout the myocardium. Such foci are particularly likely to be seen in the left ventricle, more especially near the apex and in the septum, but they may appear in the right ventricle or even in the atria. The fibrosis of chronic rheumatic heart disease may be a true progressive chronic myocarditis; but otherwise, with the possible exception of syphilis, chronic myo-

in acquired syphilis. In the latter the gummas occur near the base of the heart and may interrupt the conduction system to produce heart block. Warthin claimed that diffuse chronic myocarditis is common in syphilis and set up criteria for the anatomic diagnosis. These include focal and diffuse infiltration of small and large mononuclear cells, edematous or mucoid connective tissues, and diffuse fibrosis. Although it is possible that syphilis may produce myocardial disease, even with sudden death, there is nothing to distinguish it morphologically from similar disease in nonsyphilitic hearts (Saphir).

Tuberculosis of the myocardium is rare and may extend from tuberculous pericarditis, be a part of disseminated miliary tuberculosis or occur as conglomerate tubercles, especially in connection with massive tuberculosis of the mediastinal lymph nodes. (See Gouley, Bellet and McMillan.)

Abnormalities of the Size of the Heart

Hypoplasia. The heart may be small because of hypoplasia. In this condition, the heart is small in all dimensions but otherwise normal. As compared with the normal weight of approximately 250 grams in women and 300 grams in men, the heart of hypoplasia frequently weighs as little as 200 grams. It is likely to be associated with hypoplasia of the arterial system generally, and may be found in status thymolymphaticus and in chlorosis.

Atrophy. This is distinguished from hypoplasia in that it is a reduction in size of a heart that has attained full growth. It occurs in connection with wasting diseases such as tuberculosis and malignant tumors and in prolonged severe anemias. It is frequent in old age, probably because of decreased nutrition of the heart brought about by coronary arteriosclerosis. The heart may weigh 200 grams or less. There is general reduction in size, but the valves are of about normal dimensions. The coronary arteries do not share in the decrease of size and therefore become tortuous. The subepicardial fat may be the seat of serous atrophy. The myocardium is usually firm, because its connective tissue does not undergo comparable atrophy. The color of the muscle, especially in young individuals, is fairly normal, and the condition is spoken of as simple atrophy. More particularly in older individuals, brown atrophy occurs. In this condition the muscle is of deep brown color. This is because the pigment persists in spite of the muscular atrophy and is therefore relatively increased in amount; there may possibly be an absolute increase. Karsner, Saphir and Todd found that, in atrophy, all the fibers undergo reduction in size, even to complete disappearance of some of the small fibers, and that the nuclei are small and more closely approximated to each other than normal. The atrophic heart is usually adequate to meet the mode of life of the individual, but certainly shows a decrease in reserve power.

Hypertrophy: Increase in Size. The heart may be increased in general size because of hypertrophy or dilatation or both. HYPERTROPHY OF THE HEART signifies an increase in the bulk of cardiac muscles as indicated by its absolute weight and the ratio of heart-body weight. The physiologic basis for cardiac hypertrophy is an increase in the diastolic volume of the chambers, a diastolic stretching of the muscle. This may be due to mechanical disturbances in circulation such as may be caused by valvular disease, by disturbances in systemic circulation such as hypertension, alterations in pulmonary circulation and perhaps nervous influences. It may also be due to disease of the myocardium, including infarction, and to various degenerations. In addition to idiopathic congenital hypertrophy referred to below, occasional cases of hypertrophy of the adult heart are observed without known cause (Levy and Von Glahn).

The lesions of the endocardium of importance are especially chronic valvular disease. Nevertheless, hypertrophy is also observed in association with subacute endocarditis and also with acute forms which last for several months. The stresses thrown upon the heart by valvular insufficiency and stenosis have been discussed in connection with chronic valvular disease. Not all valvular disease, however, produces notable hypertrophy of the heart, this being particularly true of mitral insufficiency. Particular valve lesions may lead to hypertrophy, predominantly in one chamber or on one side of the heart. This is associated with a lesser degree of hypertrophy of the other chambers, because of the spiral arrangement of the muscles. Such hypertrophies occur without any general circulatory disturbance. The relative degrees of hypertrophy of the right and left ventricle can be determined by separation of the two by such methods as those described by Lewis and by Herrmann.

HYPERTENSION, or elevated blood pressure, is a common cause of cardiac hypertrophy. Hypertension may be secondary to such conditions as obesity, hyperthyroidism, menopause, arteriovenous fistula, certain adrenal tumors and perhaps other endocrine disturbances. It occurs in glomerulonephritis, particularly the chronic form. A common variety not associated with these various conditions is called essential hypertension. There is evidence that it is hereditary (Ayman). It is more common in males than females, in negroes than whites, runs a prolonged course and terminates either by failure of the hypertrophic heart, cerebral hemorrhage or renal insufficiency. Goldblatt's work indicates that essential hypertension, like the renal form, is dependent upon renal influences. Anatomically, arteriolar sclerosis of the kidneys is the most frequent and probably the earliest lesion (Moritz and Oldt). It involves other arterioles and may be widespread. In non-hypertensives, it may be found in various situations but is rare in the kidney. It may exist for a long time without disturbance of renal function, but when it arises in earlier life periods, the kidneys are often injured. Whether the widespread arteriolar disease is due to the hypertension or due to the basic cause of the renal arteriolar disease is not known but the latter view is probably true. The experimental studies of Goldblatt and his associates have clearly indicated that in the dog, monkey, rabbit, rat, goat and sheep, reduction of the circulation in the kidney by the application of an especially devised clamp to the renal artery produces a persistent hypertension identical with chronic (essential) hypertension in man. Although nervous influences may determine temporary variations in pressure, they are not primarily responsible for this type of disease. Adrenal cortical activity plays a necessary but undetermined part. The part played by the hypophysis and by the carotid sinus is still uncertain. Evidently, impaired circulation through the kidney results in the elaboration of a product, presumably renin. The action of renin on a globulin in the blood plasma, referred to as prehypertension or hypertensinogen, results in the formation of a pressor substance, called hypertensin or angiotonin. Certain investigators, including Dock and Cox, question the part played by renal circulatory disturbance as related to hypertension, but the evidence offered is for the most part indirect.

As pointed out in the chapter on Disturbances of Circulation, an increase of circulating fluid causes an enlargement of the vascular bed, including the heart, and especially in connection with arteriovenous communications, is associated with hypertrophy. The so-called beer drinker's cardiac hypertrophy is probably not due to an increased amount of circulating fluid, because that is readily reduced, but is due to other influences, perhaps the alcohol. There has been much discussion about the influence of athletic sports and of hard muscular work upon hypertrophy of the heart. Certain clinical studies support the view that athletics and hard work produce hypertrophy of the heart and others contradict this view. Although the weight of the heart is likely to be more or less parallel to the amount of skeletal muscle, there is no satisfactory evidence adduced by postmortem examination of the heart to show that athletics or hard muscular work produces a true hypertrophy.

Numerous conditions in the chest may induce resistance in the pulmonic circuit. These include chronic diseases of the lung, such as chronic tuberculosis, emphysema, bronchiectasis, and extensive organized pneumonia. Prolonged pleural effusion, empyema, pneumothorax, and pleural tumors may produce resistance in the pulmonary circulation, as is true also of mediastinal tumors, aneurysm and marked kyphosis and scoliosis of the spine. Mitral stenosis is also a common cause. The hypertrophy of the heart in these conditions is especially marked in the right ventricle, often called *cor pulmonale*. Pulmonary arteriosclerosis often accompanies the hypertrophy of the heart, but in our opinion this is due to the underlying disease rather than to pulmonary hypertension. There are rare cases of right ventricular hypertrophy without demonstrable cause (de Navasquez, et al.).

Hypertrophy of the heart may complicate exophthalmic goiter, possibly as the result of the tachycardia which is often present in this disease, but this assumption is not established. Paroxysmal tachycardia may also be associated with hypertrophy, but again it is not clear that the tachycardia itself is the cause of hypertrophy, and we have observed it in an atrophic heart. That drugs which increase the rate of the heart, such as alcohol, nicotine, coffee and others lead to hypertrophy is open to question, and even if such hypertrophy be demonstrated, it is not clearly proved that the hypertrophy is due to the rapid rate.

CONGENITAL IDIOPATHIC HYPERTROPHY of the heart is a condition that occurs in infants and young children, without demonstrable cause. In certain cases the enlargement may be brought about by degeneration and atrophy with progressive fibrosis, not a true hypertrophy (Kugel and Stoloff). Many cases are the cardiomegalic form of glycogen disease, described in the chapter on Degenerations and Infiltrations. Hypertrophy may be due to renal diseases and disturbances of pulmonary circulation even in young children. Hence, thorough gross and microscopic study of autopsy material is required before a case can be accepted as idiopathic. Occurring during the time of growth, hypertrophy in childhood is accompanied by increase in number of fibers as well as increase in their size.

MORBID ANATOMY. The chief criterion of hypertrophy of the heart is increased weight. The thickness of the walls cannot be depended upon for diagnosis, because dilatation may thin the wall of a hypertrophic heart to a measurement less than normal, and stoppage in systole may result in a wall thicker than normal. Arbitrarily, a heart 600 grams or more in weight is called *cor bovinum*. The muscle of hypertrophy is firm and of more reddish tinge than normal. Fibrosis, a common accompaniment, increases firmness and degenerations decrease it. The papillary muscles and columnae carneae are likely to be large and rotund. The endocardium and valves, especially of the left side, may be somewhat thickened and opaque because of fibrosis. The coronary arteries grow in length and increase somewhat in diameter in consonance with the growth of the heart. Two forms of hypertrophy are described, concentric and eccentric. In the former, the walls are thick and the chambers reduced in size; in our opinion this does not exist in life and its presence is due to postmortem rigor of the myocardium. Eccentric hypertrophy shows increased weight and enlarged chambers. The enlargement of the chamber may well be a part of the hypertrophy in the sense that the factors which induce hypertrophy cause a certain amount of dilatation. Nevertheless great hypertrophy may exist without any increase in transverse diameter of the heart in the living patient by roentgen-ray study. Dilatation, due to degeneration of the muscle, is frequent toward the end of the patient's life.

The microscopic appearance was described in the chapter on Progressive Tissue Changes. The fibers increase in width and length; they approach uniformity because this increase affects especially fibers that were originally of relatively smaller size (Karsner, Saphir and Todd). The nuclei are characterized by increase in transverse diameter and squaring of the ends.

Physiologically, the muscular power of the heart is increased, and circulation is maintained. The heart is said to be in a state of compensation. The reserve, however, is probably reduced. Congestive failure of the heart ensues when the contractile power no longer maintains adequate circulation. This may be due to degenerations incident to infectious diseases. It may also occur when there is inadequacy of the response to the stimulus which induces hypertrophy; in other words there is a limit to hypertrophy. Shipley and Wearn have found that as the fibers grow, the capillary supply per unit of volume does not keep pace and is relatively reduced, thus limiting the progress of hypertrophy and ultimately leading to myocardial failure.

Dilatation of the Heart. In dilatation, the chambers of the heart are enlarged and the walls reduced in thickness. Normally the heart shows little alteration of volume except for the accommodation of variations in blood volume, as discussed in the chapter on Disturbances of Circulation. Dilatation of the heart may be passive, secondary or tonogenic, or it may be active, primary or myogenic. The former occurs as the result of increased volume of the blood in the chambers without an accompanying intrinsic disease of the myocardium. This is due particularly to valve defects and to increased peripheral resistance. Transient increases in blood volume in the chambers are followed by recovery. Lasting increases lead to hypertrophy. Primary myogenic dilatation is due to disease of the myocardium. This may be in the form of degenerations due to acute infectious diseases, local or general anemias, and coronary sclerosis and occlusion. The dilatation of a hypertrophic heart may be apparently tonogenic, when the limit of hypertrophy is reached, for in certain of these cases no intrinsic myocardial disease is found to explain the dilatation. The same may be true when stresses are thrown upon the hypertrophic heart, which exceed its reduced reserve. The hypertrophic heart may undergo dilatation as the result of any of the causes given above for primary myogenic dilatation. The chamber of the heart upon which special stress is thrown usually shows the predominant dilatation. Thus, in mitral stenosis, the left atrium is the seat of especial dilatation. In systemic hypertension, the left ventricle is the principal region of dilatation. In general dilatation, which is usually myogenic, the right atrium shows a greater degree of dilatation than the other chambers. In some instances the dilatation may be in part sec-

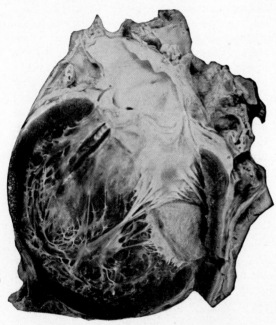

Dilated heart with enlargement of chamber and flattening of columnae carneae and of papillary muscles. Note also the anomalous cord-like fibrous trabeculae.

ondary and in part primary. For example, in pneumonia there may be an increased resistance in the pulmonary circulation which causes right ventricular dilatation, and to this is added the degeneration of the myocardium incident to the acute infectious disease.

The dilated heart is enlarged and usually of globular form. In secondary forms the muscle is soft, flabby and dark red. In primary forms the muscle shows various types of degeneration, anemia or necrosis. The chambers are enlarged as indicated above. In the ventricles the especial feature of dilatation is flattening of the columnae carneae and papillary muscles. Microscopically, the muscle fibers are narrowed because of attenuation. The nuclei may share in the attenuation. There may be no notable degenerative

change in the muscle or there may be cloudy swelling, fatty degeneration or necrosis. The principal effects of dilatation are fall in mean systemic pressure and in pulse pressure, associated with passive hyperemia of the viscera, with all the attendant changes incident to passive hyperemia, both functional and morphologic. The passive hyperemia has as its anatomically important sequels not only stagnation of blood in the vessels but edema, pigmentation, hemorrhage, parenchymatous degeneration, catarrhal inflammation and fibrosis. These may all give symptoms and signs referable to particular regions. Thus, there may be edema and bronchitis in the pulmonary area. There may be digestive disturbances due to changes in the various digestive glands. There may be disturbances of renal function somewhat resembling nephritis. Cardiac edema has already been discussed in the chapter on Disturbances of the Circulation. Of great physiologic importance are cardiac cyanosis and cardiac dyspnea.

Cyanosis. The blue tinge of skin and certain mucous membranes is an important sign of cardiac decompensation. Of importance in explaining this type of cyanosis is the fact that capillaries, particularly in the lungs, are widely distended with blood and the systemic circulation is slowed. In addition, the lungs are likely to show various degrees of edema. The slowed pulmonary circulation, the dilated capillaries and the presence of fluid within the alveoli all operate to reduce interchange of gases. If the hyperemia be prolonged, fibrosis of the alveolar walls may occur with further interference with interchange. There is an increase of carbon dioxide in the systemic blood so that the mean level of oxygen unsaturation of the capillary blood is elevated sufficiently to produce the cyanosis (see Lundsgaard and Van Slyke; Meakins and Long).

Cardiac Dyspnea. This varies from shortness of breath on exercise, to dyspnea at rest, and orthopnea. The mechanisms are not fully known. From the viewpoint of pathologic anatomy, there must be a reduction of vital capacity because of the passive hyperemia in the lungs with enlargement of capillary bed. This in itself reduces alveolar volume and in addition edema is often present as an additional factor. In prolonged passive hyperemia there may be a reduction in elasticity due to the accompanying fibrosis. The physiologic mechanisms are not fully explained. Shortness of breath on exercise probably is due to reflex stimulation rather than to changes in the blood. The dyspnea at rest is probably to be explained by an integration of various factors including "(a) reflexes from the lungs, (b) fixed acid acidosis with inadequate compensatory reduction of CO_2, and (c) anoxia both anoxemic and stagnant." Orthopnea is a condition in which the dyspnea is more marked when the patient is recumbent than when sitting up. There are various theories to explain this but none has been established. Cardiac asthma is a paroxysmal dyspnea which usually occurs at night and is brought on by distention of the abdomen, coughing and emotional stresses. Again there are various theories as to cause, none of which is wholly satisfactory. (See Wiggers.)

Alterations of Position of the Heart

These may occur from congenital conditions already referred to or from pathologic conditions in the heart itself in various types of hypertrophy or dilatation. Tumors of the chest, pleural exudates, intrathoracic adhesions, curvature or angulation of the spine, may push or pull the heart out of normal position. Distention of the abdomen by pregnancy, ascites, tumors, distention of gut by gas, may elevate the diaphragm and move the heart into a transverse position. Bodily habitus as in long narrow or broad short torsos may show the heart in more vertical or more transverse position.

Rupture of the Heart

As pointed out by Krumbhaar and Crowell, most cases of spontaneous rupture of the heart are due primarily to coronary disease, which may produce numerous minute areas of fibrosis, may produce infarction and partial or complete aneurysm. Death in these cases is usually due to hemopericardium. Rarely, if ever, does either degeneration or abscess lead to rupture. Traumatic injury of the heart may lead to death from hemopericardium, or, if the pericardium be sufficiently torn, from acute anemia. Infection from such wounds is usually confined to the pericardium but may involve the myocardium. Indirect injury may cause contusion of the wall of the heart and produce symptoms and signs somewhat resembling those of infarction (Moritz and Atkins).

Tumors

Those of the endocardium and pericardium have been discussed. Kaufmann mentions among benign tumors the occurrence of fibroma, angioma, lipoma, leiomyoma, and particularly myxoma which is likely to occur in the left atrium and often is covered by a thrombus. Rhabdomyoma oc-

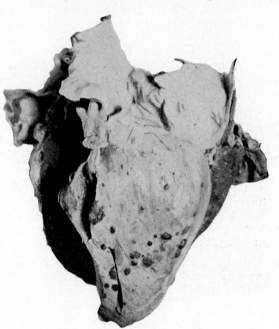

Multiple metastases of melanoblastoma of skin to myocardium and pericardium.

curs as single or multiple tumors, probably congenital in origin, and may be accompanied by tuberous sclerosis of the brain (Farber). Sarcoma may also originate in the myocardium (Weir and Jones). Primary tumors of the myocardium are rare. Metastatic sarcoma is not uncommon but secondary carcinoma is more unusual, occurring particularly in carcinomatosis. Melanoma metastasizes to the heart in a considerable percentage of the cases. Direct invasion of the peri- and myocardium may follow carcinomas of esophagus, lung, thymus and the mediastinal lymph nodes. Leukemia may show diffuse or focal infiltration of the myocardium. The occurrence of congestive failure in a patient with a malignant tumor suggests the possibility of metastasis to the heart (Scott and Garvin).

Parasites

Of the cysticerci observed in the heart, the echinococcus cyst is the most important. It may rarely lead to rupture of the heart. Sarcosporidia, common in lower animals, may occur in man (Hewitt).

Foreign Bodies

Foreign bodies, particularly metallic objects such as shot and needles, sometimes enter the heart apparently by transport in the circulation, or in the case of needles by direct wandering in the body.

Cardiac Arrhythmias

This field is so large and is covered so admirably in texts on medicine as well as such special texts as those of Lewis, Hirschfelder, Lamson, MacKenzie, Neuhof, Wiggers and others, that only the pathologic basis of arrhythmias will be mentioned here. This pathologic basis is both functional and morphologic and is concerned particularly with irritability and conductivity. Such alterations may be due to infectious or toxic agents which produce no lesion of the conduction system demonstrable by present histologic methods and little change of significance in the myocardium. There may be tachycardia and bradycardia, sinus arrhythmias, atrial flutter and fibrillation, partial and complete heartblock. Autopsy may show only acute or chronic myocarditis without lesion of the bundles and it is conceivable that such anatomic lesions may alter the irritability and conductivity of the myocardium, but how they operate is problematic. Acute degenerative and inflammatory lesions of the nodes and bundles are sometimes demonstrable. These may lead to increased excitability and perhaps to increased conductivity after the same fashion that acute inflammations produce increased nervous excitability. They may on the other hand be sufficiently destructive to produce depression or complete suppression of excitability and conductivity.

Autopsy may disclose various lesions of the atrioventricular node, the bundle of His and its branches. These include inflammatory processes including abscess and fibrosis. Ulceration secondary to bacterial endocarditis and the extension of calcification from calcific disease of the aortic valve are reported. Probably most important is infarction, although occasionally a gumma is found. Nevertheless there are certain cases in which block is characteristic clinically but without demonstrable morphological lesions grossly or microscopically (Krumbhaar).

VASCULAR SYSTEM

ARTERIES

Congenital Anomalies

The evolution of the arteries is through such a series of developments and atrophies that frequent minor and major anomalies are to be expected. It is remarkable that they are not more common than they are found to be. Fetterolf describes anomalies in origin, position and branching of fifty arteries in a large anatomical material and this undoubtedly does not exhaust the list. Such alterations are of the utmost importance to the surgeon but are rarely of functional significance except by accident.

A most important anomaly is persistent patency of the ductus arteriosus. Minor degrees of patency may be of no significance, but the larger openings produce a series of disturbances which may lead to diagnosis and successful surgical operation. Eppinger and Burwell have found that as much as 45 to 75 per cent of the left ventricular discharge may be shunted into the pulmonary artery. With this there is evidently a transfer of pressure as indicated by hypertrophy of the right ventricle. Transposition of the great vessels occurs with, or independently of, situs inversus viscerum and may be complete or partial (McMeans).

Hypoplasia of aorta and larger vessels is usually accompanied by hypoplasia of the heart. It sometimes occurs in cases of chlorosis, pernicious anemia, hemophilia, and status thymolymphaticus, but there is no proven etiological relationship. The aorta is not only reduced in size but usually has an abnormally thin wall. The condition may apparently predispose to acute aortitis. The associated conditions and symptoms are discussed by Abbott.

Various anomalies of the aortic arch, even to complete obliteration, with or without patency of the ductus arteriosus, occur, most of which are not compatible with life beyond a few days. Coarctation of the aorta, a persistence of the fetal aortic isthmus, is often survived until middle life. The result is higher blood pressure above the stenosis, manifest in the upper extremities. There is hypertrophy of the arteries which take off from the arch and development of a collateral circulation, especially through the internal mammary and intercostal arteries; the hypertrophy of the latter may cause notching of the ribs, visible in roentgenograms. The proximal aorta usually has a thin wall susceptible to rupture and consequent sudden death. (See Evans; Lewis.)

Degenerations

Cloudy Swelling. There is little doubt that toxic agents, infectious diseases and local inflammations may produce cloudy swelling of endothelium and of muscularis, and that the latter may have some physiological influence upon arterial tension, but the most significant of the degenerations from the viewpoint of pathologic anatomy is fatty degeneration or lipoidosis of the intima. It is most common in children, dead of acute infectious disease, in the form of longitudinal, narrow, slightly elevated yellow streaks along the posterior wall of the aorta. Microscopically, the fat is in the form of minute droplets within the connective-tissue cells, in tissue spaces and sometimes within phagocytes, the whole mass often constituting stellate figures. The sequence of this change is unknown, but it may possibly be a forerunner of arteriosclerosis. Fatty degeneration of the media of smaller arteries may be observed in many infectious diseases.

Pigmentation of the endothelium of smaller arterioles may be observed in malaria. Hyalin is particularly common in the central arterioles of the spleen, but occurs in numerous other small arteries and is seen in glomerular capillaries of the kidney in such acute infections as diphtheria and scarlatina. Amyloid is common in arterioles and capillaries.

Necrosis of the arteries is most frequently a part of arteriosclerosis, but as the result of either toxic agents or acute infectious diseases, small necrotic areas may occur in either the media or intima. It is particularly common in the media as the result of syphilitic mesarteritis. It is said to occur also as the result of embolic or thrombotic occlusion of vasa vasorum. Idiopathic cystic medial necrosis of aorta and disseminated medial necrosis of the aorta, in which considerable lengths of the media show necrosis of muscle and elastica together with mucoid degeneration, are not rare. This lesion is of importance in reference to rupture of the aorta and dissecting aneurysm. (See Moritz.)

Calcification is most common in the intima as a part of arteriosclerosis and may follow fatty degenerations, hyaline transformation and necrosis. It occurs in the media of medium sized arteries, more especially of the lower extremities, in old age, as the senile or Mönckeberg type of arteriosclerosis, to be discussed subsequently. Calcification of the arteries also occurs as part of so-called metastatic calcification.

Atrophy occurs normally in the retrogression of arteries which function only in fetal life. It may be a part of senile changes. It occurs from disuse, as following amputations or occlusion.

Hypertrophy may occur in arteries which participate in collateral circulation and as the result of the increased pressure of hypertension.

Inflammation

Acute Inflammation. This is usually secondary to lesions elsewhere. Acute periarteritis occurs when local inflammation extends so as to involve the adventitia. It may extend further into the vessel and lead to rupture, unless circulation has been shunted by occluding thrombosis. The hemorrhage may be local, producing a hematoma or false aneurysm, or the blood may pour into a cavity or on a body surface. Acute inflammation of the media and intima is commonest in small arteries, and is described especially in meningeal arteries in the course of various forms of acute meningitis. Acute inflammations primarily involving the intima are usually due to lodgment of infected emboli. These may occlude and subsequently produce abscesses or may result in mycotic aneurysms. Acute endarteritis of the aorta and pulmonary artery is usually the result of extension of an acute endocarditis from aortic or pulmonic leaflets, and the lesion may also be embolic. The presence of pre-existing chronic disease of the aorta, such as sclerosis, appears to predispose to acute lesions (see Rappaport).

In addition to these manifestations, acute arteritis, localized or widespread, may occur in a so-called primary form, in which the causes are unknown or ill-defined. The lesions include degenerative, necrotizing, exudative, proliferative, organizing and mixed forms (Karsner).

Periarteritis Nodosa. This is one of the forms of acute arteritis of unknown cause which exhibits degeneration and necrosis, exudation and ultimately organization. It affects the entire thickness of the wall, but the exudation may be especially prominent in the adventitia and periarterial structures. It occurs at almost any period of life, often runs a prolonged course, and affects particularly the renal, coronary, small abdominal, cerebral and other small arteries. Its distribution is highly irregular. Grossly, the lesions may appear as nodules varying in size from one to several millimeters, firm, pinkish-yellow or occasionally red in color, projecting along the course of the arteries and often associated with small hemorrhages, surrounding necrosis and infarcts.

Microscopically, there is edema and necrosis of the media together with cellular exudation, which, however, is especially pronounced in the adventitia. Extension to the intima may cause thrombosis. The destruction of the wall is responsible for small aneurysms, hemorrhages and false aneurysms. The cellular exudate consists of polymorphonuclears, lymphocytes, plasma cells and is more or less rich in eosinophils. Various hypotheses have been proposed as to the cause. It is said to be due to a variety of infective agents including streptococci and also to a filterable agent. There is some evidence to support the view that it is an allergic manifestation (Kline and Young). The term polyarteritis acuta nodosa is more descriptive than is periarteritis nodosa. (See Motley.) Clinically there is a great variety of symptoms and signs depending upon the distribution of the arterial disease.

Chronic Inflammations. There are several different forms of chronic inflammation of arteries.

ARTERIOSCLEROSIS is included in this category because it is a progressive disease associated with fibrosis and other incidental changes. We agree with the conclusions published in the Comptes Rendus of the International Society of Geographic Pathology that the correct term is arteriosclerosis rather than atherosclerosis. This will be discussed before the other forms of chronic inflammation. Thorel defines arteriosclerosis in the broader sense as including all those pathologic alterations of the arteries which lead to thickening of the wall, particularly of the intima, and which in their development exhibit degenerative processes, such as fatty and mucoid degenerations, with their sequences. Included in Thorel's conception are calcification (also in the media), and in addition hyperplastic alteration of the connective tissue and elastic elements of the intima and perhaps also inflammatory proliferative growth of the connective tissue of the intima. All these are interrelated in a more or less complex fashion.

The discussion will be directed first to simple intimal arteriosclerosis, in which there is usually a sequence of fibrosis, hyalinization, atheroma and calcification. The primary change is in the intima but exactly what first takes place has not been finally determined. Suggestions as to the nature of the earliest lesion include small tears of the elastica or connective tissue, fatty degeneration such as has been mentioned above, local degeneration or necrosis due to disease of the vasa vasorum, acute inflammatory lesions of the intima including fibrin formation, toxic necrosis of the intima or of its endothelium, and infiltration of lipoids.

We accept the assumption that the first lesion is damage in the lower intima with splitting of the elastic fibers, some destruction of fibrous connective tissue and even of muscle, and deposit of lipoids. In response to this injury connective tissue is formed in excess to produce intimal plaques. At autopsy these plaques project into the lumen of the vessel, but that this is true in life is open to some question. This fibrous overgrowth is succeeded by hyalinization and, either before or coincident with hyalinization, there may be mucoid degeneration of the connective tissue. Grossly, the plaques now assume a pale blue translucent appearance, instead of a dull gray opaque appearance of the fibrous plaque. The next change, commonly called atheroma, is really a fatty necrosis of the thickened intima. The plaques now become yellow in color and soft in consistence. Microscopically, there are found fat globules, lipoid globules and fatty acid and lipoid crystals. The necrotic region may become very much softened and the plaque appears as a fluctuating mass with semifluid, yellow, granular contents. This is sometimes incorrectly referred to as the atheromatous abscess. The superficial intima may become involved in the process and slough, leaving the atheromatous ulcer which may serve as the basis of thrombus formation. Calcareous deposits occur either in the hyaline material or the atheromatous masses and occasionally may be succeeded by true ossification. Calcified plaques may also project through the intima and produce marked roughening of the wall of the vessel with possible thrombus formation.

without being accompanied by any serious lesion of the aorta, and vice versa.

ETIOLOGY. Arteriosclerosis is more common in males than females and becomes increasingly frequent as age advances. Nevertheless it occurs in both sexes, it may be seen in comparatively early life and occasionally is only slight or absent in old people. Thus it is not dependent upon sex, nor is it a necessary accompaniment of age. We cannot agree that it is a natural involutionary process of aging and look upon it as a disease initiated by some form of injury to the arterial wall followed by the sequence of changes outlined above. Some claim that habits of life are important and it is attributed on the one hand to hard physical work and on the other to sedentary life. As a matter of fact, it occurs in persons of all occupations. Attention has been directed to various articles in the

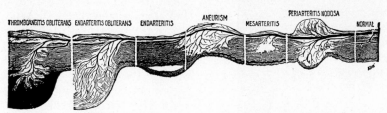

Schematic drawing of various types of arterial lesions. From Hirschfelder, Diseases of Heart and Aorta.

When the plaques are large, atrophy of the media immediately under them often occurs.

In the aorta, the disease is likely to extend throughout, but the more advanced lesions are usually in the distal portion near and at the bifurcation, whereas the proximal part for several centimeters beyond the root may be relatively unaffected. Affecting medium sized or small arteries, the same condition may produce the type of lesion now commonly called endarteritis deformans, in which the lumen is deformed by the projecting plaques, or produce endarteritis obliterans in which the plaque formation entirely occludes the vessel. Endarteritis deformans is important in that it predisposes to thrombosis, which is especially significant in coronary and cerebral arteries, as well as those of the extremities. As a rule, the disease in the aorta is accompanied by similar lesions in smaller vessels, but this is not necessarily the case. The process may be confined to coronary vessels, to renal vessels, to cerebral vessels

diet, with the thought that metabolic disturbances are significant, but no convincing evidence has been adduced. Nor has there been real proof to incriminate various poisons, except that the disease is frequent in chronic lead poisoning. Coffee, tea, nicotine and alcohol have been considered but the available evidence is against their being causative. Nicotine may induce arterial spasm, but there is no proof that this causes arteriosclerosis. The disease accompanies such chronic diseases as gout, nephritis and chronic rheumatic affections, but the relationship is not known. It has been suggested by von Balo that acidosis, which may occur in these diseases, can produce the primary injury to the arterial wall, but this is based on experimental observations of vascular disease in animals, not comparable to human arteriosclerosis.

Arteriosclerosis is certainly more common in diabetics than in others. It is supposed that this is due to imbibition of lipoids from the blood and that the lipoids initiate the

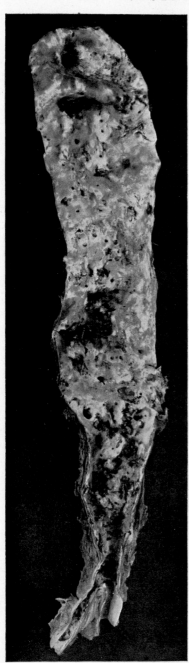

Simple arteriosclerosis, showing fibrous and hyaline plaques, atheroma, and at the bifurcation, stiffening by calcification. Army Medical Museum 13121.

sults in a rich deposit of cholesterol and its esters in the aortic intima. Duff has pointed out in detail the fact that this lesion is not comparable to human arteriosclerosis and in his own experiments showed that injury to the wall precedes the deposit of the lipoids. Hueper reports that administration of various macromolecular compounds results in their deposit in the aorta and other organs, but does not claim to have produced arteriosclerosis. Dragstedt and his associates find that the aorta of depancreatized diabetic dogs shows chronic arterial lesions and attribute this to abnormal fat metabolism incident to inadequate amounts of lipocaic. The arterial disease does not closely simulate human arteriosclerosis. The fact remains, however, that diabetics usually have arteriosclerosis and that the lesions are rich in cholesterol and its esters. While, in our opinion, there is not adequate reason to assume that the disease is initiated by the diabetes, yet when arteriosclerosis is established it is probable that diabetes can augment and accelerate it.

There are differences of opinion concerning the part played by hypertension. In some instances plaques are found at the ostia of intercostal and abdominal arteries, a place where the wall is naturally thin. It is supposed that intra-aortic pressure is poorly withstood and causes injury which excites sclerosis. This explanation may be valid, but often arteriosclerosis is extensive with little or no involvement at these points; at the best it does not explain sclerosis in other situations. Furthermore patients die of marked prolonged hypertension yet show but little arteriosclerosis at autopsy. Experimental results have not given support to hypertension as a cause. By suspending rabbits head down repeatedly, Klotz observed thickening of the arteries of the neck but this was hypertrophy rather than sclerosis. Pearce showed that lesions in the rabbit's aorta following injections of adrenalin are not like arteriosclerosis of man and are due to injury of the walls rather than to the evanescent hypertension. Although the dog is not a suitable subject for study of simple intimal arteriosclerosis, this disease has not been found by Goldblatt in a large number of animals hypertensive for months or years. Evidence concerning the effects of high pressure in the

injury. It appears to occur especially in diabetics on a high fat diet. Experimental prolonged feeding of cholesterol in large quantities to herbivora, especially the rabbit, re-

pulmonary artery is not convincing. Hypertension is probably not a cause of arteriosclerosis, but may perhaps augment and accelerate that which is present.

Cholesteatosis of the aorta, due to feeding cholesterol, is accelerated by castration (Löwenthal), thyroidectomy, splenectomy (Shapiro) and administration of posterior pituitary extracts (Moehlig and Osius). It is inhibited by administration of testosterone propionate or estradial benzoate to female rabbits but not to males (Ludden, et al.). No clear application of these various observations to human arteriosclerosis can be made.

In summary, it is probable that no single cause will be found for arteriosclerosis. It appears that several factors must operate. It is our opinion that of the various factors, infectious diseases play a prominent part. This, however, does not explain the progressive character of the disease. It is not known whether the initial lesion develops after recovery from the infection, whether there must be repeated infections, or whether there must be an element of chronicity following the acute infection. It is probable that nutritional or toxic disturbances, either acute or chronic, which may produce degenerations elsewhere, also operate upon the arteries, and further that the accompanying degenerative arterial lesion requires more chronic derangement in order for the lesion to become progressive. The rôle of increased blood pressure, if any, has not been determined but it is possible that established arterial disease may be augmented by this factor. Important references are the book edited by Cowdry and the Comptes Rendu of the International Society for Geographic Pathology, and the studies of Rosenthal.

The clinical manifestations of arteriosclerosis depend principally upon the special organs affected, for example, brain, heart and kidney. The atrophies of tissues consequent to gradual reduction in lumina of arteries may be of great importance. The predilection of sclerotic arteries for thrombosis is of especial significance in the organs mentioned as well as others, including mesenteric arteries and those of the extremities. The resulting infarction or ischemic necrosis is often serious and may be fatal. Intimal arteriosclerosis may rarely cause aneurysm, cylindrical or fusiform rather than saccular, but syphilitic vascular disease must be excluded before this diagnosis can be accepted (Korns). In advanced life, the disease of the aorta may cause diffuse dilatation and corresponding increase of aortic blood volume, which can reduce speed of circulation. The volume and the rigidity of the wall account for an increase of systolic pressure without corresponding elevation of diastolic pressure. This is only a systolic hypertension and is probably of little or no significance.

Senile arteriosclerosis is often called Mönckeberg arteriosclerosis, although previous writers had described it. The condition is common in old age and affects particularly such arteries as the femoral, radial, temporal and dorsalis pedis. Other than this the cause is not known. The early change is usually fatty degeneration of the middle layers of the musculature and elastica of the media, which may be associated with necrosis. There is then calcification in the same situation. This may be in small nodules or more commonly in partial or complete rings, which give the so-called "corduroy" artery, or continuous calcification by fusion of the rings producing the "pipestem" artery. Rarely, ossification is observed. There is discussion as to whether or not it should be regarded as arteriosclerosis, but it is included in the general definition we have accepted. Thorel is of the opinion that it is not essentially different from intimal sclerosis. The intima of the affected arteries may or may not show some stage of sclerosis. This is in addition to that simple increase in thickness of intima which Thayer and Fabyan have shown to accompany old age. Severe degrees of peripheral senile sclerosis may be associated with little sclerosis in the aorta. Medial calcification occurs in the aorta almost solely as an extension from intimal disease.

Endarteritis Obliterans or Deformans. This has been referred to in discussing simple intimal arteriosclerosis and is the same disease in smaller vessels. The lesion, however, occurs in both its deforming and obliterating stages as a purely productive process with growth of connective tissue and without atheroma or calcification. The normal prototype of this condition is seen in the obliteration of umbilical and hypogastric arteries and ductus arteriosus. Similarly, the obliterated diseased artery becomes converted into a fibrous cord. Much the same appearance may be produced by organization of a thrombus.

DIFFUSE ARTERIOLAR SCLEROSIS. Sometimes called arteriocapillary fibrosis of Gull and Sutton and diffuse hyperplastic sclerosis, the changes in the arterioles have been clarified by Moritz and Oldt. The intima may show endothelial hyperplasia, hyalinization and reduplication of elastic lamellae. The media is the seat of increased collagenous tissue and hypertrophy of the smooth muscle in variable degrees. The lesions are irregularly distributed in the affected arteriole and accompanied by uneven reduction of the caliber of the lumen. It is found in the arterioles of the kidney, liver, brain (especially meninges), gastro-intestinal tract, skeletal muscle, adrenal, pancreas and other organs. It is so frequent in the spleen as to be of little significance. The only organ in which it can be diagnosed grossly is the kidney, as described in the chapter on Urinary System. In all these situations the disease is more frequent and more severe in hypertensive than in nonhypertensive subjects, but this difference is especially pronounced in the kidney, where arteriolar sclerosis is almost constant among the hypertensives and rare among the nonhypertensives. The sclerosis may be complicated by superimposed acute necrotizing or exudative arteriolitis and these acute forms may rarely occur as an independent disease. The cause of arteriolar sclerosis, of its acute complications and of acute arteriolitis, is not yet known.

Thrombo-Angiitis Obliterans. This is an inflammatory lesion of arteries and veins with both acute and chronic phases, probably of unknown infectious origin, occurring more especially in Polish, Galician and Russian Jews and attacking the lower more often than the upper extremities. According to Buerger's studies, it originates as a red thrombus in the vessel with marginal foci of leukocyte infiltration, often succeeded by "giant cell foci," resembling miliary tubercles. Organization and canalization of the thrombus are accompanied by fibrosis of media, in which are also found occasional giant-cell foci. The chronic inflammatory process of the vessel walls may involve surrounding tissues and accompanying nerve trunks. The disease may be progressive involving several extremi-

ties. Ischemic necrosis of the extremities usually results.

Other diseases leading to necrosis of the extremities include endarteritis obliterans, either primary or as a complication of senile arteriosclerosis. Raynaud's disease, which in the earlier stages shows temporary anemia of the parts or sometimes cyanosis (acro-asphyxia) often induced by exposure to cold, is probably due to spasm of the blood vessels, is not necessarily associated with definite morphological changes in the vessels and does not always lead to necrosis.

Ischemic necrosis of the extremities is more frequent in lower than upper extremities. It may become infected by saprophytes with the production of gangrene. The "dry gangrene" of the surgeons is ischemic necrosis (infarction) and the "wet gangrene" a true gangrene. This is usually due to thrombosis in an artery the seat of senile arteriosclerosis but may follow endarteritis obliterans, or other forms of arterial disease. It affects males more often than females and is a disease principally of the sixth and seventh decades. Diabetics are prone to it, but there is no significant difference between the arterial lesions of diabetics and non-diabetics (see Hines). It is said to occur in ergotism.

Syphilis. Although gumma formation may occur in arteries, the two most important lesions are syphilitic (luetic) mesaortitis and syphilitic inflammation of smaller arteries. Syphilitic mesaortitis is sometimes called Döhle-Heller disease because those authors established its relation to syphilis. The lesion probably begins as a chronic endarteritis of the vasa vasorum of the adventitia together with perivascular infiltration of lymphocytes and a few plasma cells. This extends into the media, with local destruction of elastica and muscle, followed by cicatrization and secondary effects upon the intima. It affects males much more commonly than females, usually occurs in the fourth and fifth decades of life and in untreated or neglected cases leads to death about twenty years after the initial infection. Warthin, however, has found the lesion within eighteen months of the primary infection. Symmers and Wallace conclude quite properly that the production of syphilitic aortitis "is favored by certain other factors among which age, sex, the length and character of antisyphilitic treatment, in-

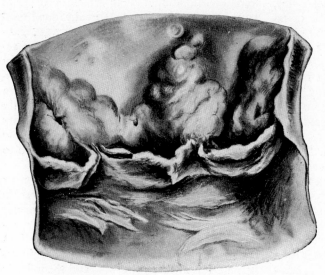

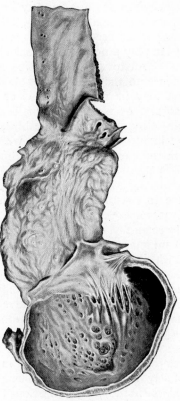

Syphilitic mesaortitis above aortic valves, showing hyaline plaques and retraction of intima, with thickening and retraction of valves, and widening of commissures.

Syphilitic mesaortitis and dilatation of arch of aorta. Aortic valves are thickened and retracted, commissures are widened and heart much dilated.

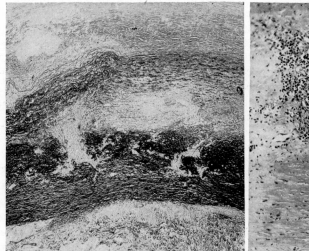

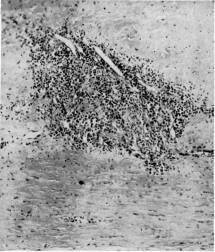

Syphilitic mesaortitis. At left is specimen stained for elastica showing interruption of elastica. At right is a hematoxylin-eosin preparation, showing perivascular cellular infiltration. Army Medical Museum 46837, 28475.

tercurrent disease, especially infections such as acute rheumatic arthritis, alcoholism, and occupations necessitating prolonged physical strain play a not unimportant rôle."

Anatomically the lesion is usually localized to the ascending aorta or the arch, but may be more extensive or localized in thoracic or abdominal portions. There are projecting patches of pale blue, translucent, hyalinized thickened intima with little or no atheroma or calcification. Within or between the patches there is retraction of the intima producing stellate or parallel depressed lines, due to contracting cicatrices in the media. Transverse section of the media may show the small foci of fibrosis. Due to interruption of muscularis and elastica, the affected part is usually dilated and in about 30 per cent of the cases accompanied by aneurysm. Dilatation of the aortic ring is extremely common. The involvement of aortic valve with widening of commissures and deformities of the cusps has been described in the section on aortic insufficiency. The ostia of the coronary arteries may be much reduced in size or completely occluded. Microscopically, the intima shows fibrosis, hyalinization and, uncommonly, atheroma and calcification, corresponding to the gross appearance. The media shows irregularly disposed perivascular (vasa vasorum) collections of lymphoid and plasma cells. There may be a few large mononuclear cells and occasionally when necrosis occurs the lesion resembles miliary gumma. Sometimes giant cells are observed. The muscularis and elastica are definitely interrupted by the lesion. Surrounding it is usually dense fibrous connective tissue in more or less stellate arrangement, often in association with retraction of the intima. The adventitia may be fibrotic and usually shows similar perivascular lymphoid and plasma cell infiltration. *Treponema pallidum* may be demonstrated within the lesion and in the nearby portions of the vessel. Similar lesions are described in congenital syphilis.

"The early symptoms and signs of syphilitic aortitis are a positive Wassermann reaction, precordial pain, slight dyspnea, attacks of paroxysmal dyspnea, angina pectoris, cardiac hypertrophy, increased pulsation of the vessels of the neck and signs of dilatation of the aorta" (Longcope). Physiologically, the effects are much the same as those of aortic arteriosclerosis, until aortic insufficiency due to dilatation of the ring or retraction of the leaflets supervenes.

The arteries of the base of the brain may be involved by syphilis. The arteries are thick, stiff, semitranslucent vessels "like cooked macaroni." Microscopically, the entire thickness of the wall shows a subacute granulomatous inflammation in which spirochetes have been demonstrated. Warthin found definite syphilitic mesarteritis in carotid, subclavian, iliac, femoral and pulmonary arteries, usually of slight degree and only demonstrable microscopically, but occasionally grossly visible and even with aneurysm formation. In addition to disease of the ostia of the coronary arteries noted above, Moritz has described a few instances of chronic syphilitic inflammation of the proximal 10 to 12 mm. of these arteries.

Tuberculosis of the arteries may occur primarily as a tuberculous periarteritis or as a tuberculous endarteritis. The former is common as the result of extension of a tuberculous lesion where the adventitia is first affected, followed by subacute or chronic inflammation of the entire wall and thrombotic occlusion of the vessel. The vessel is converted into a fibrous cord; vessels so converted form some of the trabeculae in tuberculous cavities of the lung. The disease may, however, lead to such weakening of the wall with or without the formation of aneurysms, that rupture occurs. Similar aneurysms of the aorta are reported as the result of tuberculous mediastinal lymph nodes. These aneurysms differ from those of syphilis in that the latter are due to stretching of a cicatrized wall rather than a wall, part of which is destroyed by inflammatory destruction as in tuberculosis. Extension of the lesion into arteries may discharge bacilli into the blood stream with a consequent disseminated miliary tuberculosis. In cerebral and other similar arteries infarction may follow occlusion. Tuberculous endarteritis is rare but has been observed in the aorta upon either a normal or a sclerotic intima. It is characterized by the appearance of miliary or small conglomerate tubercles. The lesion may be seen in medium sized arteries, in which it is more likely to be an accompaniment of, than a cause of, disseminated miliary tuberculosis.

Aneurysms

An aneurysm is a permanent, more or less circumscribed dilatation of an artery due to some lesion of its wall. There are two great divisions, true aneurysms and false or spurious aneurysms. The wall of the true aneurysm contains portions of two or more of the coats of the artery. Included in this group are primary or spontaneous aneurysms, traumatic,

to general dilatation, elongation and tortuosity of the artery, the tortuosity being accentuated by local points of dilatation; it is seen principally in temporal arteries.

Of especial importance are aneurysms of the aorta. They are due principally to disease of the media, because this is the coat that offers resistance to the internal distending pressure. Cylindrical and fusiform aortic

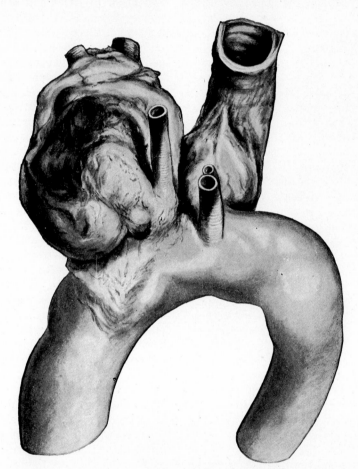

Saccular aneurysm of the aortic arch with compression of trachea.

dissecting, embolic and erosive aneurysms. False aneurysms are due to rupture of the arterial wall, the formation of a hematoma which becomes encapsulated and communicates with the artery. This is true of most of the cases of arteriovenous communications. Congenital aneurysms may occur in the circle of Willis and in persistent ductus arteriosus.

True aneurysms are classified as to whether they are fusiform, cylindrical, saccular, or cirsoid. The cirsoid aneurysm is due

aneurysms may rarely be due to marked intimal arteriosclerosis because of atrophy of the underlying media. They may also be due to syphilis. In these forms some part of all three coats constitutes the wall of the aneurysm. We have seen localized dilatations of the arch in intimal arteriosclerosis but no saccular forms. Saccular aneurysm of the arch and thoracic aorta is due to syphilitic mesaortitis; if there are exceptions they are exceedingly rare. Kampmeier's study of 633 cases, showed 214 in the ascending, 205 in the transverse and 147 in the descending portion of the arch and only 30 in the descending thoracic aorta. In 23 instances more than one aneurysm was found.

The saccular aneurysm begins as a localized dilatation of the wall, due to the destructive disease of the media. As the dilatation proceeds, the media becomes more and more atrophic until in the convexity of the

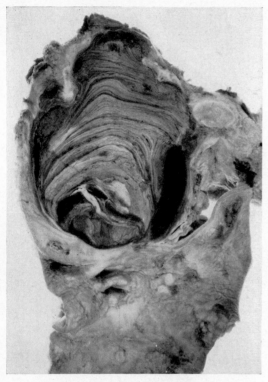

Saccular aneurysm of the arch of aorta. Note laminated thrombus. The bone in upper left of specimen is sternum, which is eroded. The aortic intima shows the wrinkling of syphilitic mesaortitis.

sac, it disappears and the wall is constructed of connective tissues of adventitia and intima. This becomes so densely collagenous that it is like cicatricial tissue. The result may be compression of surrounding structures. There are two additional features of importance, formation of laminated thrombus and erosion. In the diffuse forms, thrombosis is absent or only local, and caused by the roughening of the diseased walls, but in the saccular forms thrombosis is common. With the formation of the sac there are present a roughened wall and a somewhat slowed and disturbed circulation, so that a thin film of thrombus is de-

posited, whose surface conforms to the chord of the arc of the saccular dilatation. As the sac dilates in all directions, a larger arc with greater concavity is formed, leaving a space between the flatter thrombus and the dilating wall. Consequently another thrombus is deposited between the original thrombus and the wall of the aneurysm. This is repeated as dilatation progresses and finally results in the formation of a laminated thrombus whose youngest members are nearest the wall of the aneurysm. Since the wall itself is made up largely of dense fibrous connective tissue, organization of the clot does not proceed very rapidly and the thrombus is almost never extensively adherent to the wall of the aneurysm. It is probable that a thrombus which fills the sac inhibits the continued enlargement of the sac. It probably damps the pulsating pressures within the sac. Furthermore, the surface of the thrombus at the neck of the sac is much smaller than that of the interior of the sac. Thus the distending force of the arterial pressure would be exercised against a relatively small surface, so that the total effect would be less than if it operated upon the entire wall of an open sac.

In addition to compression of surrounding structures, a saccular aneurysm may erode them. Saccular aneurysms of the aorta may erode vertebral column, sternum and ribs. They may extend into trachea, esophagus, pleural cavities and occasionally pulmonary artery. Rupture into these structures and through the anterior thoracic wall may be the result. The mechanism of erosion is not fully understood and various theories have been offered. Our present view is that the pressure causes atrophy of the neighboring structure and a low-grade chronic inflammation. The fibrous tissues so produced become incorporated in the fibrous wall of the sac and as further dilatation ensues, this poorly nourished tissue gives way. When the spine is eroded, the bones are destroyed to a greater extent than are the intervertebral disks. The vascularity of the bone would permit of more inflammatory reaction than in the relatively avascular cartilage; in addition, small hemorrhages in the bone increase the rate of destruction.

Saccular aneurysms of the abdominal aorta may be syphilitic, but some, probably half, are not. We think that among the latter the medial injury may be due to infectious diseases or to local infections. Saccular aneurysms occur in popliteal, femoral, iliac, carotid, subclavian, innominate and other arteries. Those in branches from the proximal aorta are usually syphilitic. Those of the arteries of the extremities may be due to medial sclerosis, to infections and to trauma. Congenital aneurysms of the circle of Willis are often saccular.

from about 60 to 85 per cent of the cases. Saccular aneurysms of other regions produce local signs and symptoms, depending on situation.

Hemorrhage from rupture of an aneurysm may occur into viscera or body cavities. In the pleural or pericardial cavities, it may produce death by interference with function of the contained organs or death may result from loss of blood. Sometimes the hemorrhages may be in the form of slight leakage

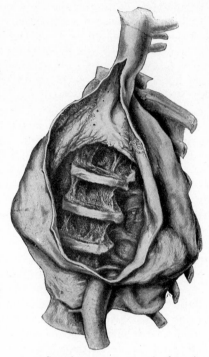

Saccular aneurysm of thoracic aorta eroding vertebrae. Note the resistance of the intervertebral discs.

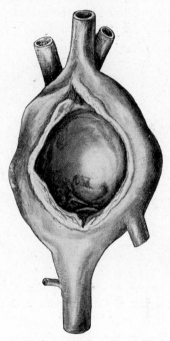

Fusiform aneurysm of popliteal artery.

ANEURYSM OF THE PROXIMAL AORTA usually develops clinically from 10 to 20 years or more after the initial syphilitic infection, but rare cases are observed earlier. Negroes are affected more than whites and males more often than females. The symptoms include dyspnea, cough, hoarseness, pain, dysphagia and palpitation. The signs include tracheal tug, thrill, diastolic impact at aortic area, percussible thoracic tumor and characteristic roentgen-ray observations. There may be inequality of the pulse in the two upper extremities. True aneurysm does not produce hypertrophy of the heart. The serologic tests for syphilis are positive in

and infiltration of surrounding tissues and this often warns of larger hemorrhage. Erosion on skin surfaces or into surfaces communicating with the exterior such as trachea, esophagus and gut may be followed by fatal hemorrhage when rupture occurs. In these situations trauma, infection or digestion may aid in the rupture. Rupture to form arteriovenous communication is referred to in that connection.

True traumatic aneurysms result from traumatic influences which rupture either adventitia alone or adventitia and media, so weakening the wall that distention occurs. Swallowing of bones and foreign bodies of various kinds, as well as stab wounds, fractures, bullet wounds and other similar accidents may produce the lesion. These are usually saccular in form and tend to early rupture.

Dissecting aneurysms represent a penetration of blood along the media of an artery, with or without communication with the lumen. Most frequent in the aorta, there is usually a transverse tear in the intima and inner half or two-thirds of the media, situated transversely in the arch near its beginning or end. The blood usually lies between the middle and outer thirds of the media. The dissection may be long or short in extent and

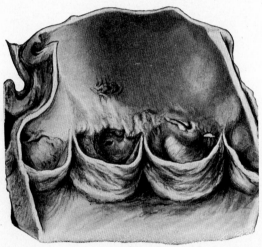

Small aneurysms of the aorta due to healed acute endarteritis.

may penetrate into pleura, pericardium or abdomen. In some instances there is a communication with a distal part of the lumen, and the aneurysm may become lined with endothelium. Intimal arteriosclerosis is common but may be only slight. The lesion is rare in syphilitic aortitis. The lesion probably starts as some variety of idiopathic medial necrosis, discussed above. Indeed it is likely that hemorrhage occurs from the vasa vasorum of the diseased media and extends along the course of the necrosis. The rupture into the lumen is probably secondary to poor nutrition of the inner layers of the media consequent upon the hematoma. The disease occurs in hypertensives and this may favor rupture. (See Tyson.)

Embolic and Mycotic Aneurysms. The simple embolic aneurysms are due to lodging in small vessels of hard particles such as small pieces of calcified arteries or valves or calcified thrombi, which because of their density penetrate into the wall of the vessel and lead to local dilatation. Such a condition is reported more particularly in the vessels at the base of the brain. The infected embolic aneurysms are also often called mycotic aneurysms. They are likely to be multiple and occur in such infections as rheumatic fever, scarlet fever, septicemia, typhoid fever and pneumonia. In the majority of cases endocarditis is associated with these infections. Infected emboli may lodge in small vessels or upon the bifurcation of larger vessels and produce inflammation and weakening of vascular walls, so that local dilatation occurs. Of similar nature are small aneurysms of the aorta due to infected emboli in the vasa vasorum, leading to acute suppuration of the media. (See Stengel and Wolferth.)

Erosive aneurysms are somewhat similar to the mycotic aneurysms. They are found in the sinuses of Valsalva and neighboring parts of the aorta, as the result of extension from acutely diseased heart valves, and development of an ulcerative type of acute endarteritis with destruction of intima and underlying media.

False or Spurious Aneurysms. A puncture wound of an artery as the result of shell, bullet or stab wounds, or erosion into the artery by some foreign body, may produce a localized hemorrhage or hematoma. The lesion of the vessel may close and the hematoma undergo organization and absorption. If, however, the wound of the vessel wall remains open, organization proceeds as usual, forming a sac around the hematoma. Since it communicates with the vessel, it is usually referred to as a form of aneurysm.

Arteriovenous communications are usually of traumatic origin and due to simultaneous wounds of both vessels (see Pemberton). It is possible, however, for an aneurysm of an artery to rupture into a vein and thus establish a communication, or very rarely for a local dilatation of a vein to penetrate into an artery. An intermediate sac may also be formed through the production of a false aneurysm. If there be a sac between the artery and vein in the course of the communication, the condition is called *varicose aneurysm*. If there be no such intermediate sac, the condition is referred to as *aneurysmal varix*. Fairly large communications between reasonably large vessels cause direct shunting of a considerable volume of blood. Lewis and Drury point out that this leak causes low diastolic pressure, large pulse pressure, water hammer or collapsing pulse, and that con-

appear to be aneurysms grossly are either minute dissecting aneurysms, between intima and media, or minute hematomata communicating with the ruptured sclerotic artery. Similar gross appearances may be produced by capillary hemorrhages into the perivascular spaces.

Tumors

The angioma may be arterial in character and occurs in skin and in the cerebral or spinal meninges. It may resemble cirsoid aneurysm. The glomangioma, a mixed tumor derived from the cutaneous glomus, has been described in the chapter on Tumors. It is doubtful that sarcoma ever originates in the arteries. Except for tiny vessels, arteries in contrast to veins are extraordinarily resistant to invasion by malignant tumors. The adventitia may be involved, but invasion further into the media is rare. Tumor emboli may lodge in the pulmonary arteries, where they may or may not grow. In the former case a tumor thrombus forms, usually associated with blood thrombosis. The tumor may remain within the lumen or invade the wall to produce a larger metastatic mass.

Foreign Bodies and Parasites

The foreign bodies are usually swallowed and may erode the aorta from the esophagus or as in one of our cases lodge in the stomach and erode the gastric arteries. Needles and fish bones are the commonest. In man the only parasite of importance which may invade arteries is the *Taenia echinococcus*.

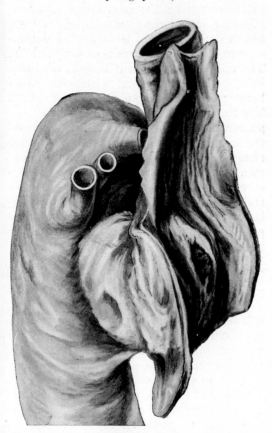

Aneurysm of persistent ductus arteriosus with erosion into esophagus.

secutive changes in the circulation bring about capillary pulsation and differences in arm-leg systolic pressure. Cardiac enlargement is common. This is probably due to increased cardiac filling the result of augmentation of the effective venous pressure, a so-called adjustment dilatation; hypertrophy contributes in only slight degree to the enlargement.

The term MILIARY ANEURYSM refers to small fusiform or saccular aneurysms of small arteries, particularly of the brain substance or more rarely of other situations such as the gut or lungs. However, such aneurysms are extremely rare, if they occur at all. What

Rupture

Rupture of arteries may be spontaneous or traumatic. Spontaneous rupture is due usually to disease of the wall. In the aorta, idiopathic medial necrosis is the most frequent forerunner. In other arteries the usual cause is extension of infectious processes into the arterial wall, as, for example, tuberculosis or abscess. Spontaneous rupture sometimes occurs in the thin wall of the aorta proximal to coarctation. The spontaneous ruptures may be transverse, longitudinal, irregular or spiral. The spontaneous rupture of cerebral arteries is preceded by arteriosclerosis, which may be of only slight degree when hypertension exists. Traumatic rupture may be caused by indirect injury, crushing wounds and severance by projectiles and cutting instruments.

VEINS

Degenerations

The veins may show a variety of retrogressive changes, such as cloudy swelling and necrosis, when they are in the field of an inflammatory process. Aside from this, the simple degenerations are uncommon. Fatty degeneration may occur but is unusual. Amyloid is found much less frequently in small veins than in small arteries. Calcification is most likely to occur in connection with varicosities of veins but may also be observed as a part of metastatic calcification. Minute hemorrhages may be observed in the walls of large veins as a part of asphyxia or in such blood diseases as pernicious anemia and acute leukemia. Atrophy of veins occurs normally in the disappearance of such blood vessels as the umbilical vein. In this process, there is a proliferation of the connective tissue of the intima with occlusion of the lumen and subsequent conversion of the vein into a fibrous cord. Similar conversion of veins into fibrous cords may occur pathologically when veins are the seat of thrombosis. Although thrombosis of veins may occur as the result of trauma and interruption of continuity of the lining membrane, and may be produced experimentally by painting the outer wall of the vein with corrosives such as silver nitrate, nevertheless, in human medicine thrombosis is most commonly the result of inflammation either extending through the wall of the vein or originating within the vein.

Inflammation

Acute Phlebitis. Acute inflammations of the smaller veins are a practically constant accompaniment of any localized inflammatory reaction. Of importance are the inflammations of larger veins. The cause is usually extension of neighboring inflammation into the vein. Thus abscesses in various regions may cause phlebitis. Infection may be implanted in the lining of veins in septicemias or because of retrograde embolism. It is rare for any inflammation of a vein to occur without associated thrombosis. Thus, most instances of phlebitis are really thrombophlebitis. It is important, clinically and otherwise, to distinguish between thrombophlebitis and that thrombosis which is common in varicose veins sometimes called phlebothrombosis. Whether originating within or outside the vein, the process rapidly involves all the structures of the wall, and in the majority of instances it is impossible to distinguish an endo- or periphlebitis. The wall of the vein is infiltrated with this inflammatory exudate and as the endothelium becomes involved, thrombosis rapidly ensues. The thrombus furnishes an excellent field for growth of bacteria and extension of the inflammatory process. This may then continue along the course of the vein. Examples are seen in the case of suppurative mastoid disease with involvement of the jugular vein and the venous sinuses of the head. Similarly, acute suppurative appendicitis may produce thrombophlebitis of radicals of the portal vein, called pylephlebitis. In certain instances where resistance is high, the thrombosis of the infected vein may undergo organization. In other cases the extension of the inflammation into the thrombus converts this into a mass of pus, from which emboli may be transmitted to other parts of the body or from which bacteria may gain entrance to the blood stream.

The consequences of embolism from the infected thrombi depend upon the situation of the primary disease. Thus, if the lesion be in the portal circulation, emboli become lodged in the smaller divisions of the portal vein in the liver and may produce multiple abscesses of the liver. If the primary process be in the general circulation, other than the portal system, emboli may lodge in the pulmonary artery and produce abscesses of the lung. From the abscesses in the liver or in the lung, access may be had to the arterial circulation and a general pyemia develop. With either pyemia or septicemia, acute endocarditis may occur and serve as an additional focus for dissemination of bacteria.

Grossly, the vein the seat of an acute thrombophlebitis is usually somewhat distended and firm. When opened, the lumen is found to be filled with the thrombus which has undergone more or less extensive suppuration. Upon removal of the somewhat adherent thrombus the lining wall is found to be rough and more or less necrotic. Microscopically, the entire vein wall is infiltrated with leukocytes and other cells of the acute inflammatory exudate, associated with edema and necrosis. The inflammatory exudate infiltrates not only the walls of the vein but also the thrombus contained within it.

Chronic phlebitis may or may not be associated with thrombosis. It may be secondary to such chronic infections as tuberculosis or syphilis, secondary to localized or general dilatations of the veins to be described subsequently, or may be a part of thrombo-angiitis obliterans. Any variety of chronic thrombophlebitis shows fibrosis of the entire wall of the vein with atrophy of the muscle and with greater or less degree of organization of the thrombus.

PHLEBOSCLEROSIS differs from arteriosclerosis in that only rarely are there intimal plaques of thickening, hyalinization and calcification formed. It is diffuse or localized and the fibrosis involves both intima and media with disorganization of the normal structure (see Hauswirth and Eisenberg).

PROGRESSIVE THROMBOPHLEBITIS is a slowly extending process with involvement of new places as the older become quiescent. Except for the fact that the first lesion usually follows trauma, nothing is known of the etiology (see Lipschitz).

Granulomata. Tuberculosis. In the involvement of veins by tuberculosis, it is often possible to distinguish sharply between a tuberculous periphlebitis and a tuberculous endophlebitis; the former is probably much more common. Thus, in the enlargement of a tuberculous focus the process may extend along the adventitia of veins, producing a chronic periphlebitis. Sooner or later the involved vein becomes thrombosed and subsequently organized. Such structures are particularly in evidence in the trabeculae of tuberculous cavities of the lung. Tuberculous endophlebitis may be due to lodgment of tubercle bacilli within veins, or may be due to the extension of tuberculosis through the wall of the vein with involvement of the intima. In the former case, small, rather flat, discrete, subintimal tubercles are observed. In the latter, the tubercles are less numerous and project into the lumen of the vein after involvement of media and intima. Benda

states that even although pulmonary tuberculosis is much more common in the upper lobe of the lung, tuberculous endophlebitis is more often observed in the lower lobe. This serves as a focus of dissemination of tubercle bacilli since thrombosis, although it occurs, is likely to be slow in development.

Syphilis. The veins in the neighborhood of primary or secondary lesions of syphilis show infiltration of lymphocytes and plasma cells either around the veins, in the adventitia or in the walls of the veins themselves. The same picture may be found in the organs of congenital syphilis (Ekehorn). This may be preceded by a chronic proliferation of connective tissue, rather moderate in degree. Sometimes the smaller veins in the neighborhood of the larger lesions, in addition to showing round cell infiltration, may also show thrombosis and subsequently obliteration. Occasionally, larger veins may show a nodular periphlebitis, due to syphilis, with the microscopic picture of round cell infiltration and sometimes giant cell formation, and there may also be a localized proliferation of the intima of large veins. Gumma may involve a large vein but practically never originates within the vein itself. There is nothing in veins comparable to syphilitic mesarteritis.

Other Granulomata. The leprous nodule may involve the wall of veins in its growth, producing a chronic inflammation and ultimately occlusion of the vein. Actinomycosis and glanders involve the veins in very much the same fashion as do acute suppurative processes.

Enlargement of Veins

Enlargement of veins may occur because of hypertrophy of the vein or because of dilatation. Physiologic hypertrophy occurs most particularly in the pregnant uterus. Pathologic hypertrophy occurs when the veins take part in collateral circulation. Thus, when the portal circulation is interfered with by cirrhosis of the liver, drainage from the portal area is aided by collateral circulation through abdominal veins communicating directly with the inferior vena cava, through drainage into the azygos veins by way of the gastric and esophageal veins, and through the epigastric and internal mammary veins. The resultant increase of volume and pressure leads to enlargement of the lumen and hypertrophy of the musculature. (See Lehmann.)

Dilatation of the veins may be either diffuse, when it is commonly called phlebectasia, or circumscribed, when it is called varix. A cirsoid form is also described but is difficult to differentiate from a combination of phlebectasia and varix. These dila-

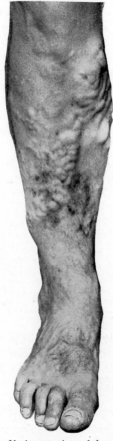

Varicose veins of leg.

tations may be the result of hypertrophy as indicated above and are very commonly the sequence of some condition which interferes with drainage of venous blood from a part. There are other instances in which dilatation of the vein appears to be due to some inherent weakness within the wall of the vein or to lack of support by surrounding structures. Thus, repeated pregnancies, or the thrombosis following typhoid fever, may lead to varicose veins of the leg; chronic constipation with straining at stool leads to hemor-

rhoids. Cirrhosis of the liver may lead to anal hemorrhoids, to a dilatation of superficial veins around the umbilicus, often called the caput Medusae, and to dilatation of veins at the lower end of the esophagus, sometimes referred to as esophageal hemorrhoids. It is often difficult to explain the dilatation of veins of the pampiniform plexus, more common in the male but often occurring in the female, referred to as varicocele, except by supposing inherent weakness of the veins. Simple phlebectasia may occur as cylindrical or fusiform dilatation of the veins. Commonly, however, this is associated with varicosities or localized dilatations which are the venous prototype of aneurysms. Thus, great tortuosity of the veins ensues and adjoining varicosities may communicate. The vein wall loses its elasticity and is sometimes thickened by fibrosis. The interior may show plaque-like thickening of the intima. Local or widespread thrombosis may follow. Microscopically, there is found fibrosis of all the walls of the vein with atrophy or even complete disappearance of musculature and with interruption or disappearance of elastica. There is often infiltration of lymphoid and plasma cells, more particularly in the adventitia. If thrombosis be present for sufficient length of time, organization will occur.

Dilatations of veins may give no symptoms whatever, or may be distinctly painful. The latter is commonly true of anal hemorrhoids where infection is common and subacute or acute inflammation is likely to occur. Repeated attacks of acute inflammation lead to chronic inflammation of these veins. Thrombosis, of course, is more common when infection or inflammation has occurred. In the veins of the leg, infection or further extension of the disease due to trauma is not uncommon, and the general disturbance of circulation of the extremities may in part account for the troublesome trophic ulcers of the leg. Rupture of the veins of anal hemorrhoids is not likely to be extensive and the consequent hemorrhages are usually small but frequently repeated. It is only rarely that severe hemorrhage occurs in this situation. In the esophageal veins, however, rupture may be fatal. In favorable circumstances the thrombi undergo organization and may subsequently become calcified, and if the vein is in a deep-seated position, the phlebolith may produce confusing roentgenograms.

The dilatation of veins is due in large part to the pressure within them. Veins that are not well supported are more likely to show dilatation than those surrounded by viscera or muscle. It is at least possible that the rings around the valve may dilate more slowly than the rest of the vein and therefore produce a point of relative obstruction to circulation. The effect of damming back of blood varies with different individuals, in some producing varicosity and in others not. It is probable that low grade acute or chronic inflammations may account for the weakening of the vein wall and the consequent local or general dilatation. Yet it is also probable that constitutional differences in resistance of the veins play an important part in determining the development of varicosity.

Tumors

Aside from angiomata in which veins may play a part, other PRIMARY tumors are extremely rare but are said to include endothelioma, myoma, angio- and other forms of sarcoma.

Veins are of great importance in the dissemination of malignant tumors, which in their growth invade and grow through the walls of the veins. Tumor and blood thrombi are formed. The tumor may extend by growth along the veins, or tumor fragments are dislodged to constitute emboli, thus providing for hematogenous metastasis. Because of their richer vascularization, sarcomata metastasize in this way more frequently than carcinomata.

Parasites

The most important are the three species of schistosomas, namely *S. hematobium*, *S. mansoni* and *S. japonicum,* which are found in perivesical and perirectal veins and arteries. The vessels usually show no lesion but in occasional instances may show marked intimal proliferation. Echinococcus cysts of the liver may break into hepatic veins and lead to new cysts in heart or lungs. Foreign bodies may erode into veins as into arteries.

LYMPHATIC VESSELS

Inflammations

Acute Lymphangitis. Acute lymphangitis is very common and may be caused by bacterial infection from wounds of various kinds. It may also arise as a primary lesion, may be associated with such infections as syphilis and gonorrhea, and may follow the skin reactions to poisonous plants or the bites and stings of insects. Warthin recognizes three types: simple, purulent, and proliferative.

Simple lymphangitis is more truly a perilymphangitis. Thus, there is edema and cellular infiltration in the outer wall of the lymphatic with, as a rule, only cloudy swelling of the lining endothelium. The lymph within the vessel may remain fluid, or coagulate to constitute a thrombolymphangitis. A complete restoration to normal may follow the subsidence of the inflammation. At its height, the lymphangitis causes the red line commonly seen extending up extremities as the result of infected wounds. The line is somewhat tortuous and usually terminates at a regional lymph node. The surgeon sometimes differentiates between a reticular lymphangitis in which there is localized swelling and redness, and a "tubular" lymphangitis as described above. The purulent form shows infiltration of leukocytes through the wall of the lymphatic, and swelling and desquamation of the endothelium. The lumen of the vessel is likely to be filled with pus which may be coagulated to form a purulent thrombolymphangitis. In those vessels provided with valves, the swelling between the valves may give the lymphatic a beaded appearance. Abscesses may form at any point in the course of the lymphatic but are particularly likely to develop in the lymph nodes into which the vessels drain. Acute proliferative lymphangitis may be seen in connection with gonorrhea or in the acute stages of syphilis. The wall of the vessel is considerably thickened by the formation of fibroblasts, sometimes associated also with proliferation of the lining endothelium. There is likely to be edema and a slight degree of cellular exudate in the outer wall of the lymphatic and in the surrounding structures.

Chronic Lymphangitis. This may be due to chronic infections, to prolonged absorption through the lymphatics of injurious material, to invasion by malignant tumors and to the presence in the lymphatics of parasites such as the filariae. The walls are thickened and the vessels become much more prominent than normal because of the fibrous overgrowth, and the process may become so advanced as to obliterate the vessel completely. In the earlier stages, the swollen endothelial cells may be prominent in histologic sections and may be mistaken for invading tumor cells. The condition is common in serous surfaces, particularly the visceral pleura where the anatomic lobules may be sharply marked out by the gray, opaque lines of lymphatic vessels. This is especially frequent in various forms of pneumonokoniosis, in chronic tuberculosis, and chronic emphysema. If the network of the lymphatics be sufficiently intricate, no serious results are observed but if the process involve a large draining lymphatic or a plexus of lymphatics, lymph may be dammed back into the tributary vessels with the production of edema.

Tuberculosis. As pointed out in the section on granulomata, lymphatic vessels offer a favorable situation for the growth of tubercles. Tuberculous involvement is therefore common. It may occur as miliary tubercles within the wall of the lymphatic or the tuberculous process may occupy both lumen and wall, converting the lymphatic into a more or less caseous nodular mass. The latter process is seen particularly well in perivascular and peribronchial tuberculosis of the lungs. The former variety, in which discrete miliary tubercles are easily observed, is especially well seen in tuberculous involvement of the lymphatics of the intestine and mesentery.

Syphilis. In the neighborhood of the chancre an acute proliferative type of lymphangitis is likely to be observed, and the same may be true in the neighborhood of secondary lesions. In late syphilis a general fibrosis of many lymphatics may be observed. These acute and chronic forms of lymphangitis associated with syphilis are not characteristic of that disease in gross or microscopic appearance. Only rarely are gummata found in the walls of larger lymphatics.

Dilatation

Owing to the extreme complexity of communication between smaller lymphatics, obstruction must be very extensive, or must operate upon a large vessel, in order to produce a damming back of lymph and dilatation of the vessels. Such obstruction may be due to disease of the lymphatic itself such as a chronic obliterative lymphangitis, occlusion by tumor growth, pressure from without by tumors or cicatricial tissue, enlarged lymph nodes, etc., or may be due to presence within the lymphatic of parasites, the most striking example being the *Filaria sanguinis hominis.* The dilatation may be diffuse, is sometimes localized with aneurysm-like sacs and sometimes produces fairly large lymph cysts. In peripheral parts, obstruction to the main lymphatic drainage is likely to give rise to marked cutaneous and subcutaneous edema of chronic type. This constitutes elephantiasis, observed particularly in the lower extremities and scrotum. With the chronic edema there is likely to be overgrowth of connective tissue, not only in the lymphatics but in the surrounding tissue; and not infrequently the skin itself is considerably thickened by the fibrous overgrowth. The congenital forms of elephantiasis are of the nature of tumor-like anomalous growth of the lymphatics; the acquired form as observed in nontropical latitudes may be due to any of the causes given above. In the tropics the most frequent cause is filariasis. If the dilated vessels rupture, the condition known as lymphorrhagia ensues. Lymph may leak into peritoneum, pleura, pericardium, bladder, kidney and other structures. If the lymph be rich in fat, the fluid assumes chylous characters.

Tumors

The so-called benign tumor of greatest importance is the lymphangioma. As has been mentioned in the chapter on Tumors, it is difficult to say whether these tumors are to be regarded as true neoplasms or simply as anomalies of development. In those forms which occur later in life it is equally difficult to distinguish true lymphatic neoplasm, and dilatation and hyperplasia in pre-existing lymphatics. The congenital forms are more likely to be of cystic character, as well exemplified in macrocheilia, macroglossia and the congenital cystic tumor of the neck, the so-called hygroma colli cysticum. Those tumors appearing as moles, warts and nevi are less likely to be cystic in character. It is probable that endothelioma may originate from the endothelium of lymphatic vessels, and sometimes there is observed a combination of endothelial growth and lymphatic proliferation referred to as the lymphangio-endothelioma. As is well known, the lymphatic vessel serves as a mode of transmission of malignant tumors, more particularly the carcinoma. The growth of carcinoma through lymphatic vessels is commonly ob-

in the walls of the duct. Dilatation of the thoracic duct may occur as the result of pressure from thoracic tumors or aneurysms of the aorta, or from lesions within the duct such as thrombosis, tuberculosis and tumor involvement. The dilatation of the duct itself is not easily recognizable, but the receptaculum chyli may be so distended as to constitute a mass palpable through the abdominal wall. Associated symptoms of importance are chylous ascites, chylous hydrothorax and hydropericardium, and chyluria.

Malignant tumors may invade the receptaculum chyli and thence metastasize through the thoracic duct and blood stream. Tumors

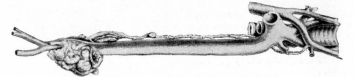

Drawing of tuberculosis of retroperitoneal lymph nodes and of the thoracic duct.

served and may or may not be associated with a chronic lymphangitis.

Thoracic Duct

This largest lymphatic of the body may be anomalous, as exemplified by the presence of two ducts, or may be represented by a lymphatic plexus. Anomalies of termination are fairly frequent so that the outlet may be double or may enter into almost any of the large veins of the upper thorax and the neck. It is supposed by some that the fat of fat embolism may gain access to the circulation through the lymphatic ducts; whether or not this be true, it is certainly possible that the amount of fat draining into the blood through the thoracic duct may seriously augment that which gains entrance to the circulation directly. The thoracic duct is subject to the same type of acute and chronic inflammations as described above for the other lymphatics. It is commonly the seat of tuberculosis and probably serves in a certain percentage of cases for the entrance of tubercle bacilli into the blood stream, thus constituting a common cause of disseminated miliary tuberculosis. Syphilitic gumma of the thoracic duct is occasionally observed, and Warthin states that in congenital syphilis there is usually a large number of spirochetes

of abdomen and thorax may invade and grow in the duct and subsequently be disseminated in the same manner.

REFERENCES

Abbott, M. E.: Atlas of Congenital Cardiac Disease, New York, Am. Heart Assn., 1936.

—— and W. T. Dawson: The Clinical Classification of Congenital Cardiac Disease, Internat. Clin., Series 34, Vol. 4, 156, 1924.

Aschoff, L.: Pathologische Anatomie, Ed. 5, Leipzig, 1921.

Ayman, D.: Heredity in Arteriolar (Essential) Hypertension: A Clinical Study of the Blood Pressure of 1,524 Members of 277 Families, Arch. Int. Med., 53: 792, 1934.

von Balo, J.: Die mit Ammoniumhydroxydvergiftung erzeugbare experimentelle Arteriosklerose, Frankfurt. Zeitschr. f. Path., 52: 205, 1938.

Beck, C. S.: Acute and Chronic Compression of the Heart, Amer. Heart Jour., 14: 515, 1937.

Bedford, D. E., C. Papp, and J. Parkinson: Atrial Septal Defect, Brit. Heart Jour., 3: 37, 1941.

Beitzke, H.: Zur Entstehung der Atherosklerosis, Virchow's Arch. Path. Anat., 267: 625, 1928.

Benda, C.: Die Gefässe, in Aschoff, L.: Pathologische Anatomie, 5th ed., Leipzig, 1921.

Binford, C. H.: Primary Amyloid Disease of the Myocardium and Blood Vessels: Report of a Case with Death from Myocardial Failure, Arch. Path., 29: 314, 1940.

Blalock, A.: Experimental Hypertension, Physiol. Rev., 20: 159, 1940.

Blumgart, H. L., M. J. Schlesinger, and D. Davis: Studies on the Relation of the Clinical Manifestations of Angina Pectoris, Coronary Thrombosis, and Myocardial Infarction to the Pathologic Findings, Amer. Heart Jour., **19**: 1, 1940.

Blumgart, H. L., M. J. Schlesinger, and P. M. Zoll: Angina Pectoris, Coronary Failure and Acute Myocardial Infarction, Jour. Amer. Med. Asso., **116**: 91, 1941.

——, D. R. Gilligan, and M. J. Schlesinger: Experimental Studies on the Effect of Temporary Occlusion of Coronary Arteries. II. Production of Myocardial Infarction, Amer. Heart Jour., **22**: 374, 1941.

Buday, L.: Statistisches über Endokarditiden und Klappenfehler, Frankfurt. Zeitschr. Path., **38**: 450, 1929.

Buerger, L.: The Circulatory Disturbances of the Extremities; Including Gangrene, Vasomotor and Trophic Disturbances, Philadelphia, Saunders, 1924.

Clawson, B. J., and E. T. Bell: A Comparison of Acute Rheumatic and Subacute Bacterial Endocarditis, Arch. Int. Med., **37**: 66, 1926; The Heart in Syphilitic Aortitis, Arch. Path. and Lab. Med., **4**: 922, 1927.

Comptes rendus de la IIme. Conference de la Société Internationale de Pathologie Géographique, Utrecht, Oosthoek, 1934.

Cowdry, E. V.: Arteriosclerosis. A Survey of the Problem. A Publication of the Josiah Macy Jr. Foundation, New York, 1933.

Criteria Committee of the New York Heart Association: Nomenclature and Criteria for Diagnosis of Diseases of the Heart, New York, Ed. 4, 1939.

Cushing, E. H., H. Feil, E. J. Stanton, and W. B. Wartman: Infarction of the Cardiac Atria: Clinical, Pathological and Experimental Studies, Brit. Heart Jour., to be published in 1942.

Dock, W., and A. J. Cox, Jr.: The Vascular Bed of the Kidney in Hypertension, Trans. Asso. Amer. Phys., **56**: 305, 1941.

Dragstedt, L. R., D. E. Clark, O. C. Julian, C. Vermeulen, and W. C. Goodpasture: Arteriosclerosis in Pancreatic Diabetes, Surgery, **8**: 353, 1940; see also Arch. Surg., **44**: 260, 1942.

Duff, G. L.: Experimental Cholesterol Atherosclerosis and its Relationship to Human Arteriosclerosis, Arch. Path., **20**: 81; 259, 1935.

——: The Nature of Experimental Cholesterol Arteriosclerosis in the Rabbit, Ibid., **22**: 161, 1936.

Ekehorn, G.: Die syphilitische Vasculitis der Nebelgefässe beim Neugeborenen, Virchow's Arch. f. Path. Anat., **242**: 93, 1923.

Eppinger, E. C., and C. S. Burwell: The Mechanical Effects of Patent Ductus Arteriosus on the Heart and Their Relation to X-ray Signs, Jour. Amer. Med. Asso., **115**: 1262, 1940.

——: The Effects of the Patent Ductus Arteriosus on the Circulation, Jour. Clin. Investigation, **20**: 127, 1941.

Evans, W.: Congenital Stenosis (Coarctation). Atresia and Interruption of the Aortic Arch. A Study of Twenty-eight Cases, Quart. Jour. Med., **26**: 1, 1933.

Farber, S.: Congenital Rhabdomyoma of the Heart, Amer. Jour. Path., **7**: 105, 1931.

Fetterolf, G.: Variations in the Arteries of the Human Body, Univ. Penna. Med. Bul., **21**: 323, 1909.

Fox, H.: Ein Beitrag zum Studium den experimentelle Endocarditis, Centralbl. Allg. Path., **24**: 529, 1913.

Fulci, F.: Experimentelle Versuche ueber die Existenz einer Endocarditis durch bacterielle Toxine, Beit. Path. Anat. u. Allg. Path., **44**: 349, 1908.

Garvin, C., and J. L. Work: Coronary Embolism. Report of Three Cases, Amer. Heart Jour., **18**: 747, 1939.

Garvin, C. F.: Fatty Degeneration of the Heart Causing Myocardial Insufficiency, Arch. Int. Med., **66**: 603, 1940.

Goldblatt, H.: Experimental Hypertension Induced by Renal Ischemia, Harvey Lectures, Baltimore, Williams & Wilkins, vol. 33, 1937-38.

——, H. A. Lewis, and J. R. Kahn: The Pathogenesis and Treatment of Hypertension. Experimental Observations, Nelson's Loose Leaf System of Medicine, 1942.

Goodpasture, E. W.: The Influence of Thyroid Products on the Production of Myocardial Necrosis, Jour. Exper. Med., **34**: 407, 1921.

Gouley, B. A., S. Bellet, and T. M. McMillan: Tuberculosis of the Myocardium: Report of Six Cases with Observations on Involvement of Coronary Arteries, Arch. Int. Med., **51**: 244, 1933.

Gross, H., and W. H. Sternberg: Myocardial Infarction without Significant Lesions of Coronary Arteries, Arch. Int. Med., **64**: 249, 1939.

Gross, L.: The Blood Supply to the Heart, New York, 1921.

——, and C. K. Friedberg: Nonbacterial Thrombotic Endocarditis: Classification and General Description, Arch. Int. Med., **58**: 620, 1936.

Gross, P.: Concept of Fetal Endocarditis: A General Review with Report of an Illustrative Case, Arch. Path., **31**: 163, 1941.

Hall, E. M., and T. Ichioka: Etiology of Calcified Nodular Aortic Stenosis, Amer. Jour. Path., **16**: 761, 1940.

Hamman, L.: Coronary Embolism, Amer. Heart Jour., **21**: 401, 1941.

Hauswirth, L., and A. A. Eisenberg: Disseminated Venofibrosis (Phlebosclerosis): Its Clinicopathological Significance, Arch. Path., **11**: 857, 1931.

Helwig, F. C.: The Frequency of Anomalous Reticula in the Right Atrium of the Human Heart "Chiari Network," Report of Eight Cases, Amer. Jour. Path., **8**: 73, 1932.

Herrmann, G. R.: Experimental Heart Disease; III. Methods of Dividing Hearts; with Sectional Proportional Weights and Ratios for 200 Normal Dogs' Hearts, Amer. Heart Jour., **1**: 213, 1925-26.

Hewitt, J. A.: Sarcosporidiasis in Human Cardiac Muscle, Jour. Path. and Bact., **36**: 133, 1933.

Hines, E. A., Jr., and N. W. Barker: Arteriosclerosis Obliterans. A Clinical and Pathologic Study, Amer. Jour. Med. Sci., **200**: 717, 1940.

Hirschfelder, A. D.: Diseases of the Heart and Aorta, Philadelphia and London, 1918.

Howard, C. P.: Aortic Insufficiency Due to Rupture, by Strain of a Normal Aortic Valve, Jour. Amer. Med. Asso., **84**: 1952, 1925.

Hueper, W. C.: Macromolecular Substances as Pathogenic Agents, Arch. Path., **33**: 267, 1942.

Jason, R. S.: Insufficiency of the Aortic Valve Due to Syphilis; A Study of Its Genesis, Arch. Path., **32**: 409, 1941.

Kampmeier, R. H.: Saccular Aneurysm of the Thoracic Aorta: A Clinical Study of 633 Cases, Ann. Int. Med., **12**: 624, 1938.

Karsner, H. T.: The Pathology of Endocarditis —A Summary Review, Jour. Amer. Med. Asso., **96**: 411, 1931.

Karsner, H. T.: Primary Inflammation of Arteries, Ann. Int. Med., 11: 164, 1937.

——, and J. E. Dwyer: Studies in Infarction. IV. Experimental Bland Infarction of the Myocardium, Myocardial Regeneration and Cicatrization, Jour. Med. Res., 34: 21, 1916.

——, and S. Koletsky: Calcific Sclerosis of the Aortic Valve, Trans. Asso. Amer. Phys., 55: 188, 1940.

——, O. Saphir, and T. W. Todd: The State of the Cardiac Muscle in Hypertrophy and Atrophy, Amer. Jour. Path., 1: 351, 1925.

Katz, L. N., and H. W. Gauchat: Observations on Pulsus Paradoxus (with Special Reference to Pericardial Effusions), Arch. Int. Med., 33: 371, 1924.

——, H. S. Feil, and R. W. Scott: The Electrocardiogram in Pericardial Effusion; II. Experimental. Amer. Heart Jour., 5: 77, 1929-30.

Kaufmann, E.: Lehrbuch der speciellen pathologischen Anatomie, Berlin, 1911; see also English translation by Reimann, S. P., Philadelphia, 1929.

Kaufmann, L.: Zur Frage der Aorta Angusta, Jena, 1919.

Kline, B. S., and A. M. Young: Normergic and Allergic Inflammation, Jour. Allergy, 6: 247, 1934-35.

Klotz, O.: Experimental Production of Arteriosclerosis, Brit. Med. Jour., 2: 1767, 1906.

Koletsky, S.: Congenital Bicuspid Aortic Valves, Arch. Int. Med., 67: 129, 1941.

——: Acquired Bicuspid Aortic Valves, ibid., 67: 157, 1941.

——: Congenital Bicuspid Pulmonary Valves, Arch. Path., 31: 338, 1941; see also Year Book of Pathology and Immunology, Chicago, Year Book Publishers, 1941, p. 123.

Korns, H. M.: Ueber das atherosklerotische und Kombinationsaneurysma, Virchow's Arch. Path. Anat., 279: 512, 1930-31.

Krumbhaar, E. B.: Adams-Stokes Syndrome, with Complete Heart Block, without Destruction of the Bundle of His, Bull. Ayer. Clin. Lab., 6: 38, 1910; also in Arch. Int. Med., 5: 583, 1910.

——, and C. Crowell: Spontaneous Rupture of the Heart, a Clinicopathological Study, etc., Amer. Jour. Med. Sci., 170: 828, 1925.

Kugel, M. A., and L. Gross: Gross and Microscopical Anatomy of the Blood Vessels in the Valves of the Human Heart, Amer. Heart Jour., 1: 304, 1925-26; see also Ibid., 3: 433, 1927-28.

——, and E. G. Stoloff: Dilatation and Hypertrophy of the Heart in Infants and in Young Children, Amer. Jour. Dis. Child., 45: 828, 1933.

Lamson, P. D.: The Heart Rhythms, Baltimore, 1921.

Lehmann, E.: Ueber Aetiologie, Pathogenese und histologische Struktur von Varizen, Frankfurt. Zeitschr. Path., 33: 300, 1926.

Levy, R. L., and W. C. Von Glahn: Further Observations on Cardiac Hypertrophy of Unknown Etiology in Adults, Trans. Asso. Amer. Phys., 52: 259, 1937.

Lewis, T.: Lectures on the Heart, New York, 1915; Clinical Disorders of the Heart Beat, London and New York, 1914.

——: Material Relating to Coarctation of Aorta of Adult Type, Heart, 16: 205, 1931-33.

——, and A. N. Drury: Observations Relating to Arterio-Venous Aneurism, Heart, 10: 301, 1923.

Libman, E.: A Consideration of the Prognosis in Subacute Bacterial Endocarditis, Amer. Heart Jour., 1: 25, 1925-26.

——: Characterization of Various Forms of Endocarditis, Jour. Amer. Med. Asso., 80: 813, 1923.

Lipschitz, M.: Zur Frage der Thrombophlebitis migrans, Deutsch. Med. Wochenschr., 55: 744, 1929.

Locke, E. A.: Pneumococcus Endocarditis, Boston, Med. and Surg. Jour., 191: 913, 1924.

Löwenthal, K.: Die experimentelle Atherosklerose bei Omnivoren, Frankfurt. Zeitschr. Path., 34: 145, 1926.

Longcope, W. T.: Syphilitic Aortitis: Its Diagnosis and Treatment, Arch. Int. Med., 11: 15, 1913.

Ludden, J. B., M. Bruger, and I. S. Wright: Experimental Atherosclerosis: IV. Effect of Testosterone Propionate and Estradiol Dipropionate on Experimental Atherosclerosis in Rabbits, Arch. Path., 33: 58, 1942.

Lundsgaard, C., and D. D. Van Slyke: Cyanosis, Medicine, 2: 1, 1923.

Mackenzie, J.: Diseases of the Heart, London, 1914.

McMeans, J. W.: Incomplete Transposition of the Great Vessels in a Girl of 16, Bull. Internat. Asso. Med. Mus., 7: 53, 1918.

Meakins, J., and C. N. H. Long: Oxygen Consumption, Oxygen Debt, and Lactic Acid in Circulatory Failure, Jour. Clin. Invest., 4: 273, 1927.

Moehlig, R. C., and E. A. Osius: The Pituitary Factor in Arteriosclerosis. Its Experimental Production in Rabbits, Ann. Int. Med., 4: 578, 1930.

Mönckeberg, J. G.: Herzmissbildungen. Ein Atlas Angeborener Herzfehler in Querschnitten mit besonderer Berücksichtigung des Atrioventrikularsystems, Jena, 1912.

Moritz, A. R.: Syphilitic Coronary Arteritis, Arch. Path., 11: 44, 1931.

——: Medionecrosis Aortae Idiopathica Cystica, Amer. Jour. Path., 8: 717, 1932.

——, and M. R. Oldt: Arteriolar Sclerosis in Hypertensive and Non-hypertensive Individuals, Ibid., 13: 679, 1937.

——, and J. P. Atkins: Cardiac Contusion: An Experimental and Pathologic Study, Arch. Path., 25: 445, 1938.

Motley, L.: Periarteritis Nodosa with Report of a Case Showing Unusual Features and Apparent Recovery, Jour. Amer. Med. Asso., 106: 898, 1936.

de Navasquez, S., J. R. Forbes, and H. E. Holling: Right Ventricular Hypertrophy of Unknown Origin; So-called Pulmonary Hypertension, Brit. Heart Jour., 2: 177, 1940.

Nelson, A. A.: Pericardial Milk Spots, Arch. Path., 29: 256, 1940.

Neuhof, S.: Clinical Cardiology, New York, 1917.

Pardee, H. E. B.: Disease of the Coronary Arteries, Med. Clin. N. Amer., 4: 1491, 1920-21.

Patten, B. M.: Developmental Defects at the Foramen Ovale, Amer. Jour. Path., 14: 135, 1938.

Pearce, R. M., and E. M. Stanton: Experimental Arteriosclerosis, Jour. Exper. Med., 8: 74, 1906.

Pemberton, J. de J.: Arteriovenous Aneurysm, Arch. Surg., 16: 469, 1928.

Rappaport, B. Z.: Primary Acute Aortitis, Arch. Path. and Lab. Med., 2: 653, 1926.

Rosenow, E. C.: Experimental Infectious Endocarditis, Jour. Infect. Dis., **11**: 210, 1912.

Rosenthal, S. R.: Studies in Atherosclerosis: Chemical, Experimental and Morphologic, Arch. Path., **18**: 473, 660, 1934.

Saphir, O.: The Effect of Certain Metabolic Changes Upon the Aorta of Rabbits and Guinea Pigs, Amer. Jour. Path., **1**: 403, 1925.

——: Involvement of Medium-Sized Arteries Associated with Syphilitic Aortitis, ibid., **5**: 397, 1929.

——: Endocardial Pockets, ibid., **6**: 733, 1930.

——: Syphilitic Myocarditis, Arch. Path., **13**: 266, 436, 1932.

——: Myocarditis: A General Review, with an Analysis of Two Hundred and Forty Cases, Arch. Path., **32**: 1000, 1941; **33**: 88, 1942.

——, and M. Corrigan: Fatty Infiltration of the Myocardium, Arch. Int. Med., **52**: 410, 1933.

——, and H. T. Karsner: An Anatomical and Experimental Study of Segmentation of the Myocardium and Its Relation to the Intercalated Discs, Jour. Med. Res., **44**: 539, 1924.

——, and R. W. Scott: The Involvement of the Aortic Valve in Syphilitic Aortitis, Amer. Jour. Path., **3**: 527, 1927.

Schlesinger, M. J., and P. M. Zoll: Incidence and Localization of Coronary Artery Occlusions, Arch. Path., **32**: 178, 1941.

Schwalbe, E.: Die Morphologie der Missbildungen des Menschen, etc., Jena, 1913.

Scott, R. W., and C. F. Garvin: Tumors of the Heart and Pericardium, Amer. Heart Jour., **17**: 431, 1939.

Semsroth, K., and R. Koch: Studies on the Pathogenesis of Bacterial Endocarditis: II, Arch. Path., **10**: 869, 1930.

Shapiro, S.: The Influence of Thyroidectomy, Splenectomy, Gonadectomy and Suprarenalectomy upon the Development of Experimental Atherosclerosis in Rabbits, Jour. Exper. Med., **45**: 595, 1927; *see also* Endocrinology, **11**: 279, 1927.

Shipley, R. A., L. Shipley, and J. T. Wearn: The Capillary Supply in Normal and Hypertrophied Hearts of Rabbits, Jour. Exper. Med., **65**: 29, 1937.

Southworth, H., and C. S. Stevenson: Congenital Defects of the Pericardium, Arch. Int. Med., **61**: 223, 1938.

Stengel, A., and C. C. Wolferth: Mycotic (Bacterial) Aneurysms of Intravascular Origin, Arch. Int. Med., **31**: 527, 1923.

Symmers, D., and G. H. Wallace: The Etiology of Syphilitic Aortitis, Jour. Amer. Med. Asso., **46**: 397, 1916.

Tennant, R., and C. J. Wiggers: The Effect of Coronary Occlusion on Myocardial Contraction, Amer. Jour. Physiol., **112**: 351, 1935.

Thayer, W. S.: On the Cardiac Complications of Gonorrhea, Johns Hopkins Hosp. Bull., **33**: 361, 1922.

——, and M. Fabyan: Studies on Arteriosclerosis,

With Special Reference to the Radial Artery, Amer. Jour. Med. Sci., **134**: 811, 1907.

Thorel, C.: Pathologie des Krieslauforgane des Menschen, Ergeb. Allg. Path. u. Path. Anat., **17**:(2): 90, 1915; **18**(1): 1, 1915.

Tinney, W. S., Jr.: Interauricular Septal Defect, Arch. Int. Med., **66**: 807, 1940.

Tyson, M. D.: Dissecting Aneurysms, Amer. Jour. Path., **7**: 581, 1931.

Von Glahn, W. C., and A. M. Pappenheimer: Relationship between Rheumatic and Subacute Bacterial Endocarditis, Arch. Int. Med., **55**: 173, 1935.

Warthin, A. S.: Diseases of the Lymphatic Vessels, Osler and McCrae's Modern Medicine, Philadelphia and New York, 1915, Vol. IV, p. 579.

——: Syphilis of the Medium and Smaller Arteries, New York Med. Jour., **115**: 69, 1922.

——: Sudden Death due to Exacerbation of Latent Syphilitic Myocarditis, Amer. Heart Jour., **1**: 1, 1925.

Wartman, W. B.: Occlusion of the Coronary Arteries by Hemorrhage into Their Walls, Amer. Heart Jour., **15**: 459, 1938.

——: Factors Concerned in Narrowing or Occlusion of Coronary Vessels, Publication 13, Amer. Asso. Adv. Sci., 1941.

Wearn, J. T.: The Role of the Thebesian Vessels in the Circulation of the Heart, Jour. Exper. Med., **47**: 293, 1928.

Weir, D. R., and B. C. Jones, Jr.: Primary Sarcoma of the Heart, Amer. Heart Jour., **22**: 556, 1941.

Weiss, H.: Relation of Portals of Entry to Subacute Bacterial Endocarditis, Arch. Int. Med., **54**: 710, 1934.

Weller, C. V., R. C. Wanstrom, H. Gordon, and J. C. Bugher: Cardiac Histopathology in Thyroid Disease, Amer. Heart Jour., **8**: 8, 1932; *see also* G. Rake and D. McEachern: A Study of the Heart in Hyperthyroidism, ibid., **8**: 19, 1932.

Wells, H. G.: Chemical Pathology, 5th ed., Philadelphia, 1925.

Wiggers, C. J.: Physiology in Health and Disease, Philadelphia, Lea and Febiger, 3d ed., 1939.

Wikler, A., E. G. Williams, E. D. Douglass, C. W. Emmons, and R. C. Dunn: Mycotic Endocarditis. Report of a Case, Jour. Amer. Med. Asso., **119**: 333, 1942.

Williams, J. W.: Multiple Gummas of the Heart in the New Born, Amer. Jour. Path., **6**: 573, 1930.

Wilson, F. N., and F. D. Johnston: The Occurrence in Angina Pectoris of Electrocardiographic Changes Similar in Magnitude and in Kind to Those Produced by Myocardial Infarction, Amer. Heart Jour., **22**: 64, 1941.

Winkelman, N. W., and J. L. Eckel: The Brain in Bacterial Endocarditis, Arch. Neurol. and Psychiatr., **23**: 1161, 1930.

Winternitz, M. C., R. M. Thomas, and P. M. LeCompte: The Biology of Arteriosclerosis, Springfield, Ill., Thomas, 1938.

14

The Hematopoietic System

INTRODUCTION

The hematopoietic, hemopoietic, or as Krumbhaar prefers the hemolytopoietic, system of adult life comprises the spleen, lymph nodes, bone marrow, the reticulo-endothelial apparatus, and the liver. The liver is considered in a special chapter. The thymus gland is discussed in the chapter on Ductless Glands. Brief consideration will be given the anemias, polycythemias and leukemias here.

THE BLOOD

Anemia is a general disease in which there is a reduction in the total amount of blood, in the content of hemoglobin or in the number of erythrocytes in circulation. Usually the reduction in number of erythrocytes is regarded as the indication of anemia. Dependent upon the size of the erythrocytes and the amount of hemoglobin in the blood, it is possible to separate three forms, namely, hypochromic and microcytic, hyperchromic and macrocytic, and orthochromic and normocytic. Other combinations may also be observed. The hypochromic microcytic is the most common form and is usually due to some well-defined cause, although rarely cases without identifiable cause occur. Pernicious anemia is a hyperchromic macrocytic anemia, but secondary forms may also show this type of blood picture. As indicated below, the conditions of origin of pernicious anemia are recognized but the exact cause is unknown. A comprehensive presentation of the anemias, and other diseases of the hematopoietic system, is given by Kracke. For convenience, the anemias will be discussed as secondary and primary.

THE ANEMIAS

Secondary Anemias

Included in this group are anemias, the cause of which can usually be identified. Anemias of this order may be due to hemorrhage, which may be single and large or small and multiple, to acute and chronic infectious diseases, to the various causes of purpura, including certain drugs, and to malignant tumors because of their interference with nutrition or because of erosion and hemorrhage. Anemias may also be due to destruction of bone marrow, as for example, by primary or secondary tumors and the lymphoblastic diseases. Acute poisonings, such as by carbon monoxide, or chronic poisoning, such as by lead, may lead to anemia. Various parasites may do the same. These include the forms of hookworm, *Ankylostoma duodenale* or *Necator americanus* as well as *Balantidium coli*. *Diphyllobothrium latum* (fish tapeworm) infestation may also be included in the group, although the pathogenesis of the anemia is not entirely known. Parasites in the blood itself, especially the *Plasmodium malariae*, are important causes. Various factors may be involved in the production of secondary anemia, including the destruction of blood cells, the depression of bone marrow activity and the actual loss of blood.

Hemorrhage. The abrupt loss of from 15 to 20 per cent of the blood is likely to result in collapse, weakness, nausea, blurred vision, pallor, sweating and low blood pressure. Immediately after the hemorrhage there is a simple anemia but subsequently it may be a hypochromic microcytic anemia. Very soon there is an increase in the total number of leukocytes and platelets of the blood. The plasma volume begins to increase immediately and the total volume is restored in about 72 hours. At first the plasma is poor in protein but in a few hours the globulin and albumin become normal in amount and ratio. Reticulocytes appear almost immediately and persist in relatively high proportion until the total red-cell volume is restored. Depending upon various conditions, complete restoration occurs in from four to six or eight weeks. (See Ebert, Stead and Gibson.) Repeated small hemorrhages give rise to a chronic type of anemia and may be caused by the bleeding from ulcers of the gastro-intestinal tract, from eroding malignant tumors, from the bleeding of anal hemorrhoids and other similar conditions. This also is a hypochromic microcytic anemia but commonly shows anisocytosis and poikilocytosis, and sometimes polychromatophilia.

Infection. Anemia is a common accompaniment of various acute infectious diseases and in some instances may be profound. It is probably due in part to destruction of erythrocytes and in part to depression of the bone marrow. Ordinarily the anemia is normochromic but if the infection be prolonged it may be hypochromic, either with or without decrease in the size of the erythrocytes. Chronic infections, such as tuberculosis, syphilis, undulant fever, subacute bacterial endocarditis, ulcerative colitis, or chronic pyelonephritis, produce an anemia which is usually markedly hypochromic. Microcytosis may or may not be present.

The anemia of chronic glomerulonephritis appears to be due principally to depression of the bone marrow (Brown and Roth). This anemia is usually moderate but may be marked and is ordinarily a hypochromic microcytic anemia. The anemia due to destruction of bone marrow by primary or secondary tumors is ordinarily a microcytic hypochromic anemia and nucleated erythrocytes may appear in large numbers. There is often a leukopenia, and immature forms of the granulocyte series may be found. The anemias produced by various poisons are generally due to destruction of blood and are said to be of hemolytic character. As a rule, these anemias are orthochromic normocytic, but the hypochromic microcytic type may be observed. Anisocytosis, poikilocytosis and microcytosis may occur, and reticulocytes may be numerous. Included are lead poisoning, characterized by the appearance of basic stippling of the erythrocytes, and poisoning by phenylhydrazine, the sulfonamide drugs and others.

Infestation by intestinal parasites, such as the hookworm, may be accompanied by a moderate degree of simple orthochromic normocytic anemia. The malarial parasite does not often produce a great degree of anemia in spite of the destruction of cells by the parasite. With a moderate reduction in the number of erythrocytes there may be a considerable reduction of hemoglobin, a hypochromic anemia. It is possible also that bone-marrow depression plays a part in this disease. In contrast, the anemia of *Diphyllobothrium latum* infestation shows a macrocytic hyperchromic anemia and the disease closely resembles pernicious anemia clinically, as does the blood picture. In addition to a presumptive hemolytic substance produced by the worm, there probably is also a depression of bone marrow together with a delay in maturation of the cells.

Primary Anemias

These are forms in which the exact mechanism of development of the anemia may be known but the ultimate cause obscure. They may be placed in three categories, (1) those the result of decreased formation of blood, (2) those the result of blood destruction, and (3) those of uncertain cause and pathogenesis. Among those due to decreased formation of blood are anemias resulting from deficiency of a hematopoietic factor such as is found in liver and liver extract, the anemia of sprue and in part at least that due to *Diphyllobothrium latum*. A second group includes anemias due to negative iron balance such as chlorosis, microcytic hypochromic anemia and "idiopathic" hypochromic anemia. A third group includes hypoplastic (aplastic) anemia, either idiopathic or due to poisoning by benzene and other agents.

There are various anemias due to destruction of blood such as the forms of hemolytic icterus and those due to certain poisons. The anemias of uncertain cause and pathogenesis include sickle-cell anemia and the erythroblastic anemias of infancy and childhood. It is obviously impossible to discuss all these and certain illustrative forms have been selected.

Pernicious Anemia. Patients with this disease may show little or no wasting but usually the skin is of a lemon-yellow tint, perhaps due to the presence of bile pigment in the blood plasma. Associated with the blood changes are chronic glossitis, gastric achylia accompanied by atrophy of the gastric mucosa, and because of lesions of the spinal cord, acro-ataxia and acroparesthesia. The red cells in the circulating blood are markedly decreased in number but usually increased in size. The hemoglobin is not reduced in proportion to the reduction in number of cells and the color index is accordingly one or more. The stained blood film shows anisocytosis, with predominance of large forms, poikilocytosis, polychromatophilia and sometimes basic stippling. Nucleated forms are common, especially the macroblasts. Reticulocytes appear in response to treatment. Leukopenia, with an absolute decrease in the number of polymorphonuclears, is nearly always present. A hemorrhagic tendency may be associated with reduction in number of platelets and quantity of prothrombin. The pathologic anatomy is discussed subsequently in a separate section.

Pernicious anemia is most frequent in the fifth decade and about twice as common in males as females. It is a disease largely of the white race in temperate zones. A hereditary basis is suggested by the studies of Stamos. The studies of Whipple, Minot and Murphy, Castle, Sturgis, Peabody, and others have shown that the disease is due to a deficiency, of digestive or metabolic origin, whereby substance or substances necessary for the maturation of erythrocytes are not available. This material is present generally in mammals and is not species specific. It apparently is the product of the action of an intrinsic factor in the gastric juice and an extrinsic factor provided principally by the meat of the diet. The intrinsic factor, at least in vitro, acts as an enzyme. Its absence accompanies gastric achylia, but it is not HCl nor pepsin; indeed it is certainly independent of HCl. The blood-maturing substance is found in storage depots, especially liver and kidney. Treatment by injection of liver extracts or by feeding of liver and extracts is thus a substitution therapy. The efficacy of hog stomach is probably due to the formation of blood-maturing substance *in situ* by action of gastric juice upon stomach muscle. Blood destruction is apparent in the active disease, but is not evident in the remissions. Whipple points out that pigment-building substances are amply available and thus concludes that the deficiency is in the stroma-forming materials. The destruction of cells during relapse is probably related to the stroma deficiency.

THE ANEMIA OF SPRUE is almost identical with that of pernicious anemia but the other clinical manifestations differ so that a distinction can usually be made. The anemia due to infestation by *Diphyllobothrium latum* has been referred to above.

FUNCTIONAL ASPECTS. These have been studied in connection with the secondary anemia due to hemorrhage and with pernicious anemia. Reference has been made above to the restoration of blood following acute massive hemorrhage. In addition, nitrogen metabolism is increased, together with associated destruction of protein. The regeneration of plasma proteins and erythrocytes is favorably influenced by high protein diets and the feeding of liver, muscle and kidney (Whipple).

In pernicious anemia an increase of nitrogen metabolism sometimes occurs. Purin output is usually low but may be increased in remissions presumably because of destruction of nucleated erythrocytes and other cells. There may be a slight decrease of plasma proteins, but the cellular protein is increased because of the larger size of the erythrocytes. Study of the lipids has been directed toward possible changes that might render the cells especially susceptible to hemolysis, but the results have been negative (Bloor and MacPherson).

There are indications that in addition to faults of maturation of erythrocytes, hemolysis is also a part of the disease. There is an increase of iron in the body as indicated by the large amounts of hemosiderin in the liver and sometimes in other organs. Furthermore, there is phagocytosis of erythrocytes by reticulo-endothelial cells, especially those of the bone marrow (Peabody and Brown). Blood destruction is indicated by the presence of bile pigment in the blood and of urobilinogen in the urine. Dobriner and Rhoads find that the urine contains coproporphyrin I and urobilin in relapse, which disappears after remission sets in. Whipple does not deny the hemolytic character of pernicious anemia. He thinks, however, that, in addition, the presence of hemoglobin may stimulate the bone marrow to overproduction of pigment.

SYMPTOMS. Clinically the main symptoms of anemia are ready fatigue, weakness and faintness, shortness of breath and dizziness. Pallor and loss of weight are variable. Other symptoms and signs depend upon the special effects of certain of the forms of the disease. Thus in pernicious anemia there may be sore tongue, loss of appetite, nausea, vomiting and tingling of the extremities, etc.

Hypochromic Anemias. CHLOROSIS. This is a disease of adolescent girls and young women, formerly called green sickness. The anemia is of the hypochromic microcytic type but is usually not severe and not likely to show abnormal forms of cells. It occurs in families but apparently because of habits rather than heredity. Disorders of appetite are observed but gastric analysis gives variable results. Menstrual disorders are common but, unless the bleeding is far beyond normal, have no bearing on the cause of the disease. Although the disease is relieved by the administration of iron, it is probable that it is the result more of disorder of iron metabolism in the processes of hematopoiesis than due to simple lack of iron in the body. (See Heath and Patek; Alsted.)

Hypochromic anemias may be due to loss of blood and various causes outlined in the discussion of secondary anemias.

AN IDIOPATHIC HYPOCHROMIC ANEMIA, hypochromic microcytic in type and frequently accompanied by gastric achlorhydria, has also been described. It is possible that it is due to remote blood loss coupled with iron and other deficiencies, including perhaps the vitamin-B complex. There is some doubt that it is an entity.

Hypoplastic Anemia. Also called aplastic anemia, this probably includes a variety of conditions, the common character of which is that they are refractory to treatment. This form of anemia may occur in connection with other diseases, such as profound infections and the leukemias. The condition is represented also in benzol poisoning. In a general way, the hemoglobin is reduced out of proportion to the reduction in erythrocytes. There may be anisocytosis, poikilocytosis, polychromatophilia, and occasionally nucleated erythrocytes appear. The bone marrow may be markedly hypoplastic and fatty or may look like normal marrow. Intermediate grades of change occur, but in none is there clear evidence of arrest of maturation of red cells.

Hemolytic Jaundice. Hemolysis may take place in a variety of circumstances and may be accompanied by variable degrees of jaundice. The term hemolytic jaundice, however, is usually restricted as Tileston points out, "to a form of jaundice usually chronic, in which diminished resistance of red cells to hypotonic salt solutions is a conspicuous feature, while bile pigment is present in the stools and absent from the urine. Enlargement of the spleen and anemia complete the picture."

The disease is said to be of two forms, congenital and acquired, but some authorities doubt that the acquired form actually exists. The congenital or familial form of the disease is hereditary and probably transmitted as a mendelian dominant but is not sex-linked. The disease may affect any race, age and sex but most commonly occurs in early adult life. There may be relatively inactive periods, which may be interrupted by crises of anemia and jaundice. The anemia is moderate except in the crises, when it may be profound. The reduction in number of erythrocytes is accompanied by a greater decrease of hemoglobin, so that the color index is less than one. Peculiar to the disease is the appearance of the so-called spherocytes, cells which are reduced in transverse diameter and with loss of biconcave form, but the cell volume is approximately normal (see Haden). Striking is the fragility of the erythrocytes in hypotonic salt solutions, due to the presence of spherocytes. Except for an increase in the crises the leukocytes are usually normal. Cholelithiasis is a fairly frequent accompaniment.

The spleen is usually much enlarged, red, firm and shows chronic fibrous capsulitis. Microscopically, there is marked hyperemia and pigmentation. Erythrocytes and fragments of them are taken up by macrophages. The connective tissue is only slightly increased. The cord cells of the liver, the sinus endothelium of lymph nodes and the renal convoluted tubular cells are likely to show hemosiderosis. There is usually considerable hyperplasia in the bone marrow, both erythroblastic and myeloblastic. It is of interest that splenectomy usually furnishes relief.

Kracke refers to acquired hemolytic anemia as characterized by "sudden onset in an adult who has not shown evidence of hemolytic anemia during childhood." The blood picture differs in that the anemia is of simple type, there are few if any spherocytes, and the fragility of the cells is not increased. The disease may arise in patients with syphilis, tuberculosis, malaria, Hodgkin's disease, and certain diseases of the liver, but that they are the cause of the hemolytic icterus is not certain. It is possible that cases of this sort have familial hemolytic icterus in latent form, which is excited to activity in later life. (See Dameshek and Schwartz.)

In connection with this discussion, mention should be made of spirochetosis icterohemorrhagica, spirochetal jaundice, or Weil's disease. This has been described in the chapter on Infectious Diseases. As a rule there is a moderate anemia, sometimes with leukocytosis and usually accompanied by jaundice. The pathologic lesions include hemorrhages in various parts of the body, principally in the lung; the viscera are likely to be icteric. Necrosis is found in the liver and in the convoluted tubules of the kidney. The spleen is not enlarged grossly but microscopically may show phagocytosis of erythrocytes by macrophages, and sometimes large or small hemorrhages. (See Jeghers, Houghton and Foley.)

Sickle-Cell Anemia. A familial and hereditary disposition to the formation of sickle and stellate forms of erythrocytes occurs in negroes and occasionally in whites. This trait may be demonstrated by incubating sealed fresh blood films or by intravital staining with cresyl blue, but when anemia develops, the sickling is usually evident without especial treatment of the film. The anemia may be profound and when it occurs in early life is often fatal. Although the anemia is normochromic there are various indications, such as bilirubinemia and increased fragility of the erythrocytes, showing that it is hemolytic in character. In crises of the anemia, various immature cells of both the erythrocyte and the leukocyte series may appear in the circulating blood. Hemosiderosis is found in various organs. Hyperplasia of erythroblastic and leukoblastic centers occurs in the bone marrow. The spleen in the earlier stages is somewhat enlarged and microscopically shows distention of the sinusoids with blood, especially around the malpighian corpuscles. Later the spleen may become small, firm and somewhat nodular; in addition to the diffuse siderosis there are foci of dense fibrosis in which iron and calcium salts are found, siderotic nodules, but these are not peculiar to this disorder. (See Diggs; Ham and Castle.)

A familial and hereditary anomaly is observed in the occurrence of *elliptical erythrocytes*, often called ovalocytes. This occurs principally in whites but is occasionally observed in negroes. Anemia is infrequent but when it occurs is of macrocytic type. (See Wyandt et al.)

Anemias of Childhood

These vary from the physiologic anemia of the first month to various profound and fatal anemias. In the first chapter, reference was made to hemorrhagic disease presumably due to deficiency of vitamin K. Erythroblastosis fetalis was discussed in reference to Rh factor of the blood, and anemia is one of the features. Cooley's erythroblastic anemia is probably quite different from erythroblastosis fetalis. It originates in late infancy and exhibits a hemolytic type of anemia. It occurs in Mediterranean peoples and has a familial distribution. The patients usually show mongolian facies, hypochromic anemia with deformity of erythrocytes, and the presence of reticulocytes and nucleated erythrocytes. The bone marrow is markedly hyperplastic and in the skull may extend through the inner table. The spleen is enlarged in the earlier stages and small and fibrotic in later stages. Hemosiderosis may be marked in liver, spleen, pancreas and other organs. The disease runs a chronic course and ends in death. Whipple and Bradford suggest that the disturbance is a racial alteration of metabolism with deficient maturation of erythrocytes.

Von Jaksch's anemia, or pseudoleukemia infantum is characterized by enlarged spleen and liver and marked increase of leukocytes in the blood together with slight or moderate anemia. There is doubt that this is a disease entity.

The acute hemolytic anemia of Lederer, probably of infectious origin, is a rare form of anemia of early life. The anemia may be of macrocytic, normocytic or microcytic type and is often accompanied by a considerable degree of leukocytosis. The spleen, liver and lymph nodes are enlarged. Hyaline thrombosis of arterioles and capillaries occurs in lymph nodes and spleen, sometimes with tissue necrosis. (See Josephs.)

Purpura

This is a condition in which hemorrhages occur in the skin, mucous membranes and elsewhere, either spontaneously or as the result of slight trauma. Purpura may be either symptomatic (secondary) or idiopathic. The symptomatic forms occur in various infectious diseases, the hemorrhagic or "black" forms of smallpox, scarlatina, measles, diphtheria, etc. It may complicate chronic diseases such as nephritis, malignant tumors, tuberculosis, leukemia and pernicious anemia. Drugs, such as iodine, mercury, antipyrine, chloral, etc., may produce purpura. Mechanical purpura may occur in prolonged passive hyperemia, convulsions, pertussis and asphyxia. Constriction of a part may produce cutaneous hemorrhages, especially when there is increased permeability of capillaries, as in scarlatina and scurvy (Rumpel-Leede Phenomenon). Schönlein's purpura, associated with rheumatic fever, and Henoch's purpura, with abdominal pain, vomiting and diarrhea, are probably due to streptococcal infections.

Idiopathic thrombocytopenic purpura of Werlhoff is a disease usually of early adult life which affects women more often than men. Although it may occur in families, there is no assurance that it is hereditary. There is decrease of the number of thrombocytes (platelets) in the blood, but occasionally this is also true of symptomatic cases. Whether the thrombocytopenia is a coincidence in a widespread disturbance of clotting or is but one of a peculiar combination of factors is unknown. Prothrombin, antithrombin, coagulation time and clotting time are essentially normal, but the clot fails fully to retract and the bleeding time is prolonged. The blood shows a reduction in number of thrombocytes to 100,000 or less and often a hypochromic anemia. The bone marrow is normal save for a slightly increased number of megakaryocytes and normoblasts. The spleen may show hyperplasia and necrosis of follicles. Nickerson and Sunderland report megakaryocytes, probably transported from bone marrow, in spleen and other organs. These changes, together with hemorrhages, constitute the pathologic anatomy of the disease. The suggestion that the disease is due to production by the spleen of a substance that destroys platelets has not been confirmed (Colmer and Mersheimer; Paul). Correct diagnosis is important because of relief of the disease by splenectomy; sometimes the platelets are restored to normal numbers but this is not always true. (See Wiseman, Doan and Wilson.)

Pathologic Anatomy of Anemias

The most severe changes are found in pernicious anemia, but other anemias may, if severe, show somewhat similar changes. At autopsy on a case of pernicious anemia, the state of nutrition and the color of the muscle may be excellent, in contrast to the pallor of the body. The skin and body fat usually have a lemon-yellow tint. The blood is watery and the postmortem clots are of small size. Petechiae may be found in various regions. The parenchymatous viscera are the seat of cloudy swelling and often fatty degeneration, and the yellow tigering of the myocardium is common.

In the liver, cloudy swelling and fatty degeneration are common, but the most significant change is hemosiderin pigmentation, visible both grossly and microscopically and in both instances demonstrable by the potassium ferrocyanide and hydrochloric acid test. Microscopically, the pigment is found to be present in the form of minute granules within the liver cells throughout the lobules, and careful examination may show similar granules within some of the endothelial cells lining the sinusoids. It is rare for any secondary anemia to show such extensive pigmentation. In severe and prolonged anemias the liver may regain to a limited extent its function as an erythroblastic organ, and foci of marrow-like cells are found.

The kidneys may show cloudy swelling and fatty degeneration and sometimes hemosiderin pigmentation of the tubular epithelium. The spleen of cases of pernicious anemia is often slightly enlarged at autopsy, but only infrequently palpable clinically (Bigg). Pigmentation may be demonstrable but is much more a feature of primary than of secondary anemia. Microscopically, the arterioles, sinusoids and follicles appear normal, but the pulp contains a larger number of red cells than is usual. Small granules of hemosiderin may be found within phagocytic endothelial cells and not infrequently in extracellular position. In addition, phagocytes may be encountered containing whole red blood corpuscles or their fragments. In secondary anemias the phagocytosis of red blood corpuscles may be more prominent but pigmentation is not likely to be so marked. If the cause of the secondary anemia be an infectious disease or the case constitute one of the forms of splenic anemia, the spleen may show an acute or chronic hyperplasia. Occasionally, in pernicious anemia the microscopic examination of the spleen may reveal small islands of myelocytes and also of nucleated red cells. The lymph nodes show no characteristic changes, but the hemal lymph nodes may show definite hyperplasia and also considerable phagocytosis of red blood corpuscles and of pigment.

The grossly visible changes in bone marrow of pernicious anemia are seen best in long bones; in these the hyperplasia of the red marrow extends well into the shafts, as is well exemplified in humerus, tibia and femur. The marrow of spongy bones, e.g., sternum, ribs and vertebrae is compact and deeper red than normal. Microscopic studies are made of biopsy material obtained by puncture of a patient's sternum, by smear and by microscopic section of marrow. In sections, the cellular marrow is much increased in amount and shows hyperplasia of all elements, especially the erythrocyte series. There are many normoblasts, with occasional megaloblasts and microblasts. Immature forms of erythrocytes are found and there is phagocytosis of pigment and of erythrocytes by macrophages, as demonstrated by Peabody and Brown.

In pernicious anemia, there is often an acute glossitis. The stomach shows atrophy of the mucosa or a true chronic atrophic gastritis. In 1 or 2 per cent of the cases, carcinoma of the stomach occurs, principally in the pyloric portion. The spinal cord may show multiple small hemorrhages. Of greater significance is combined degeneration of, or occasional large hemorrhages of, lateral and posterior tracts, discussed in the chapter on the Nervous System.

In both secondary and primary anemias the capacity of the hemoglobin for carrying oxygen and carbon dioxide is not materially altered, but the quantity of these gases conveyed must be reduced in proportion to the absolute content of hemoglobin. Thus, as is pointed out by Lundsgaard and Van Slyke, cyanosis is not observed in severe anemias. There is very little tendency for anemics to show the symptoms of anoxemia. This is believed by Fahr and Ronzone to be due to a compensatory mechanism which includes increased systolic output and minute volume of the blood, with increased blood velocity due to lowered viscosity and "increased effective cross section of the vascular tubing."

Myelophthisic Anemia

This is due to destruction of, or crowding out of, bone marrow by various lesions. Thus the anemia which commonly accompanies leukemia may be the result of replacement of erythroblastic centers by the hyperplasia of the myeloid centers. Malignant tumors, such as myeloma, and extensive metastases of other tumors to the marrow, may destroy so much marrow as to cause anemia. Osteosclerotic anemia is due at least in part to crowding of marrow by proliferated bone. The Albers-Schönberg type of this disease, or osteopetrosis, is familial, occurs in infancy and childhood. The "marble bones" are dense and subject to fracture because of their fragility. The anemia is hypochromic and the disease appears to be due to a faulty differentiation of osseous and hematogenic tissues (Clifton, et al.). There may be a slight leukocytosis and a relative lymphocytosis. Extramedullary hematopoiesis may occur in liver, spleen and lymph nodes (Chapman). Other forms of osteosclerotic anemia include thickening of bone due to inflammation and tumors, and a diffuse sclerosis in adults without demonstrable cause. (See Mettier.)

HEMOPHILIA

Pratt defines this as a "hereditary constitutional anomaly limited to the male but transmitted by the female, characterized by a tendency to bleed from trivial cuts and bruises, and by a marked delay in the coagulation of the blood." It is transmitted as a recessive, sex-linked character. The clot, when formed, is normal in all respects and there is no alteration of any of the constitu-ents of the blood which normally take part in clotting. There is, however, in normal blood plasma a globulin fraction, which upon addition to hemophilic blood brings about a normal clotting time (see Pohle and Taylor). Custer and Krumbhaar find that the hematopoietic system shows normal regenerative ability; in the bone marrow there is a large number of megakaryoblasts and megakaryocytes. The remarkable transmission through females to males has been thoroughly studied, running through many generations without a well authenticated case in a female. Somewhat similar is *hereditary pseudohemophilia*, which occurs in both males and females and is transmitted by either sex. It differs further in that although the clotting time is normal, the bleeding time is prolonged; clot retraction is normal; there is no demonstrable change in platelets. (See Fowler.)

POLYCYTHEMIA

Harrop defines polycythemia as "that condition in which there is an increased number of erythrocytes per unit of the circulating blood." Temporary polycythemia may be due to factors such as dehydration. Persistent polycythemias are divided into secondary or symptomatic forms, often called erythrocytosis, and polycythemia vera.

The symptomatic forms include those associated with high altitudes, emphysema and other chronic diseases of the lungs, conditions which interfere with expansion of the lungs, agents such as epinephrine and carbon monoxide, congenital heart disease, especially congenital pulmonic stenosis, and acquired heart disease, particularly mitral stenosis. Pulmonary arteriosclerosis, syphilitic and nonsyphilitic, is found in a vaguely defined variety of the disease described by Ayerza as "cardiacos negros." The erythrocytosis of poison-gas pulmonary irritation and that of infectious disease probably results from dehydration.

Polycythemia vera, or rubra vera, erythremia, Vaquez-Osler disease and other terms are applied to a syndrome of chronic cyanosis, or erythrosis (Lundsgaard and Van Slyke), splenomegaly and polycythemia, of unknown cause. It occurs in middle life, affects males and females about equally, and is thought by some to have a constitutional basis. It is considered by many to be "a primary excessive erythroblastic activity of the bone marrow" (Weber), which Harrop believes to be due to reduced pulmonary permeability for gases, consequent lowered oxygen tension in the bone marrow, increased viscosity of the blood with reduced flow through the lungs and a chronic anoxemia manifested especially in the central nervous system. The erythrocytes, normal as to size, morphology and staining, may reach twice the normal number in the circulating blood. The red-cell mass is increased, in contrast to no increase in secondary polycythemia (Haden). There is a definitely lowered coefficient of oxygen utilization. The reticulocytes are not often in excess, but the resistance of erythrocytes to hypotonic salt solutions may be increased. The platelets are usually increased in number and megakaryocytes may appear in the blood. The leukocytes may be normal or considerably increased in numbers. An increase in the number of myelocytes may suggest a relation to myeloid leukemia, but this is not established. The increase of blood volume may be manifest in various organs and tissues.

The spleen is considerably increased in size, weight and firmness. The capsule is smooth, thick and opaque, the trabeculae prominent, and the organ sometimes shows infarction. The enlargement is due to the reservoir function of the spleen rather than to hematopoietic activity. The liver is large, due to increased blood content, and may rarely show associated cirrhosis or portal thrombosis. The bone marrow shows hyperemia, marked erythroblastic hyperplasia, many megakaryocytes, and sometimes myeloblastic hyperplasia. With distention of the vascular system, varices may occur in esophagus, intestine and elsewhere. Hemorrhage may occur from rupture of varices and does not seem to depend upon a hemorrhagic disposition of the blood. The increased number of platelets and the increased viscosity of the blood probably play a part in the occasional occurrence of vascular thrombosis. This causes coronary and cerebral arterial occlusions and may be responsible for ulcers of duodenum and stomach.

THE LEUKEMIAS

Leukemia is a general disease of the hematopoietic system, which affects particularly those parts which have to do with the production of white blood cells. The circulating blood contains an increased number of white blood cells, although there are phases or forms of the disease in which the number of cells in the blood is not increased, and even decreased. These aleukemic states may occur early in the disease, as stages of remission, terminal events or throughout the course. The primary difficulty appears to be in either the formation or the maturation of the white cells or both. The morbid anatomic changes are found principally in the spleen, lymph nodes, bone marrow and liver, but other organs may also be affected. For the sake of classification and discussion, two principal forms of leukemia are recognized, namely, the lymphoid or lymphatic leukemia, sometimes called leukemic lymphadenosis, and the myeloid or splenomyelogenous leukemia, sometimes referred to as leukemic myelosis. To these may be added a third form, monocytic leukemia. These are further subdivided into acute and chronic varieties. It must be recognized, however, that border line cases occur in which it is difficult to say positively whether the disease is myeloid or lymphoid, acute or chronic. Furthermore, certain forms occur which suggest further subdivision of the disease. The acute leukemias are usually observed in childhood and early adult life, but not exclusively. The chronic forms occur in early and later middle life. Males are more often affected than females. The discussion given below must be regarded as representing typical forms of the disease, in which distinctions are not difficult.

Chronic Lymphoid Leukemia

This variety is less frequently observed than is the myeloid form. The onset is gradual with progressive loss of strength and signs of anemia. The patient usually notices enlargement of the superficial lymph nodes, although this may be much delayed. In addition to the general symptoms of anemia there may be gastro-intestinal symptoms, and in many cases there are short periods of fever with exacerbation of general symptoms and signs. The physical examination shows en-

not discussed under acute

largement of the superficial lymph nodes and often of important groups of deeper lymph nodes, associated with enlargement of the spleen. The white blood cells commonly range between 60,000 and 100,000 per cmm., but may reach 1,000,000 or more. From 80 to 90 per cent or more of these cells are lymphocytes and of these the vast majority are small lymphocytes. Although the polymorphonuclear cells are reduced in proportion, it is unusual that they are reduced in absolute number. Myeloid cells may sometimes be found, but if so only in small numbers. There may or may not be an anemia which, in more moderate degrees, is usually hypochromic, but in the more severe degrees

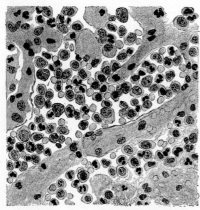

Infiltration of liver in lymphoid leukemia.

may show a high color index with anisocytosis, poikilocytosis and nucleated erythrocytes. The blood is increased in volume and in viscosity and in those cases where the number of lymphocytes is extremely large, may have a pale yellow color.

The pathologic anatomy is fairly characteristic. Grossly, the lymph nodes of the body are usually enlarged throughout. They are pale, firm, and usually are discrete within each group. The tonsils and the lymphadenoid tissue of the intestines, as well as other lymph nodes, may be affected. Rarely, the thymus is involved (Major).

Microscopically, the architecture of the lymph nodes is obscured by multiplication of lymphocytes, although the follicles may be clearly defined. In the more chronic cases a slight fibrosis may appear. Mitotic figures are unusual and vascularization is not abnormal. The spleen is moderately or con-

siderably enlarged, weighing usually from 500 to 1,000 grams, although in our experience two spleens of over 2,000 grams have been observed.

The connective tissue of the spleen is increased more particularly in the capsule and trabeculae. The cross section is relatively firm and sometimes shows considerably enlarged follicles, although this is by no means constant. Infarcts are sometimes found. Microscopically, the more or less marked fibrosis is observed, the follicles may or may not be enlarged, and the pulp shows a very marked increase of lymphocytes throughout.

The bone marrow may or may not be seriously involved. In more severe cases the marrow of the shafts of long bones may be grossly of distinctly gray or reddish-gray color. Microscopically, this shows islands of hyperplastic lymphogenic tissue, associated in the more severe cases of anemia with some hyperplasia of the erythroblastic centers.

Although more common in acute lymphoid leukemia, nevertheless, the chronic form may show lymphomata in various organs, .particularly liver, kidneys and lungs. These are lymphoid nodules varying from microscopic size to grossly visible tumor-like masses exceeding a centimeter in diameter. These nodules are only fairly well circumscribed, relatively soft and with a slightly bulging, gray cross section. Microscopically, they are poorly vascularized masses of lymphocytes which grow through connective tissue spaces pushing apart the parenchymatous elements. They are infiltrative rather than destructive and apparently originate in minute pre-existing lymphoid aggregates. Somewhat similar nodules may appear in the skin. If the anemia be pronounced there may be cloudy swelling and fatty degeneration of the parenchymatous viscera. A disposition to hemorrhage into the organs is less pronounced in chronic than in acute lymphoid leukemia.

Lymphosarcoma-cell leukemia is in reality lymphosarcoma with the appearance of cells of sarcomatous type in the blood. When this occurs, the disease runs a rapid course. (See Bethel; Wiseman.) The condition is also called leukosarcoma. Many doubt that this should be included in the group of leukemias.

Chronic Myeloid Leukemia

This is a disease of the hematopoietic system, characterized by an increase in the number of circulating myelocytes and cells of the myeloblastic series. The disease is of gradual onset, with progressive loss of flesh and strength, and abdominal swelling due to enlargement of the spleen. Hemorrhage, gastro-intestinal disturbance, respiratory

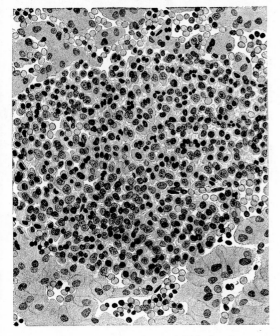

Infiltration of liver in myeloid leukemia.

symptoms such as dyspnea and cough, fever and other symptoms and signs may be present. Examination of the blood shows as a rule 100,000 to 500,000 white blood cells but counts of 1,000,000 to 1,500,000 and more have been recorded. Of these cells from 50 to 90 per cent are myelocytes, polymorphonuclear leukocytes and a small number of transition forms between the two. The cytoplasmic granulation of these cells is principally neutrophilic although there is a distinct increase in the basophilic cells and an absolute but not always a relative increase in the eosinophilic cells. Of these granular forms, the adult type of leukocyte usually preponderates over the myelocytes and myeloblasts, but collectively there is an enormous absolute increase in number. Although the lymphocytes may be proportionately reduced, nevertheless, they are considerably increased in absolute numbers and there is a relatively large proportion of large lymphocytes. Anemia is usually fairly well marked and is usually hypochromic. In the more severe anemias the red blood cells may show anisocytosis and poikilocytosis. Regardless of whether or not there is an anemia, nucleated erythrocytes are almost always found. The number of platelets is also increased. There is an increase in volume and in viscosity of the blood (see Minot, Buckman and Isaacs).

The most striking features of the pathologic anatomy are changes in the spleen and bone marrow. The spleen is usually enormously enlarged attaining weights of 2,000 and 3,000 grams and even up to 10,000 grams. The organ is large, dark red and, depending upon the duration of the disease, shows increase of connective tissue, sometimes with adhesions to surrounding organs. The capsule may be thin and tense but usually is thick, dense, opaque, and sometimes hyalinized, and the trabeculae and other connective tissues of the spleen are also increased. The cross section usually shows no follicles but a definite increase of connective tissue with a general gray or yellowish-gray tint to the red color of the pulp. The latter is of normal or firm consistency and may show numerous small foci of necrosis, as well as infarcts. Microscopically, the spleen is converted into a myeloblastic organ. The follicles are small and often cannot be made out at all. The pulp shows large numbers of myelocytes and leukocytes of the various orders. Lymphocytes are usually present but may be obscured by the granular cells. Nucleated red blood corpuscles are sometimes found but usually not in large numbers. Megakaryocytes, sometimes exhibiting phagocytosis, are also found. Pigmentation is not increased.

The bone marrow shows an enormous myeloblastic hyperplasia. The marrow in the shafts of the long bones has a semisolid or diffluent consistence and is of grayish-yellow color, so much resembling pus that the bone marrow is often spoken of as pyoid. Microscopically, the bone marrow is made up principally of myelocytes and leukocytes, but nongranular cells are also encountered which for the most part are myeloblasts. Lymphogenic foci are usually absent. Erythroblastic activity is present but not marked. The megakaryocytes are large and numerous. There is little phagocytosis of cells and fragments and little or no pigmentation; mitotic figures may be prominent, more especially in the myeloblasts. The liver is usually considerably enlarged, sometimes attaining a weight of 5,000 grams or more. The organ is firm, with somewhat rounded edges and tense capsule and in cross section sometimes shows, even grossly, minute foci of gray color representing infiltration in the periportal spaces. Microscopically, the periportal spaces usually are much enlarged by a rich infiltrate of myelocytes and of leukocytes. In addition, all the blood spaces show large accumulations of these cells. This engorgement of capillaries by blood rich in myelocytes and leukocytes is practically constant throughout the body. The skin sometimes shows focal infiltrates grossly similar to those of lymphoid leukemia. In myeloid leukemia, however, the rule is for diffuse infiltration of tissue rather than the formation of tumor-like nodules as in lymphoid leukemia. If the accompanying anemia be pronounced, there is cloudy swelling and fatty degeneration of the parenchymatous viscera. In spite of poor extravascular clotting, thrombosis may be observed in various situations, sometimes with infarction.

Acute Leukemia

Lymphoblastic Leukemia. Acute leukemia runs a course of a few weeks or several months, generally much shorter than is observed in the chronic forms. Symptoms develop rapidly and are severe. Fever is often a prominent feature. Hemorrhages are common. Although it may occur in older persons it is usually a disease of children or young adults. Leukemias as a whole affect males and females in the ratio of 2 to 1, but this sex difference is not striking in childhood. The number of white cells in the blood does not often attain that seen in chronic leukemias and is often in the neighborhood of 40,000 to 80,000 per cu. mm. Of these 80 to 90 per cent are large mononuclear cells with nongranular cytoplasm. It is frequently difficult to decide whether they are lymphoblasts, myeloblasts or more primitive forms. Many cases show no increase in total white count or even a decrease, but the blood film shows many blast forms.

At autopsy the organ involvement may be like lymphoid or myeloid leukemia, but usually both systems are involved in variable degree. Except for the fact that fibrosis of spleen, lymph nodes and liver is less marked in the acute forms, tissue sections throw little light on whether the leukemia is acute or chronic. Sections show the mononuclear cell hyperplasia, but the determination of cell type is even more difficult than in blood films. Thus in many cases with complete study no distinction of the form of leukemia can be made and the diagnosis of acute leukemia is the limit of differentiation.

Monocytic Leukemia

This disease affects both sexes and may occur in any life period from childhood to old age, but the number of authenticated cases so far reported is not sufficient for statistical analysis.

The course may be acute or chronic, and in general the clinical manifestations are like those of other leukemias. The number of white blood cells increases gradually in the course of the disease and rarely exceeds 100,000. Monocytes constitute about 60 or 70 per cent of the white cells. These are identified by the minute, numerous azurophile granules in the cytoplasm and the specific staining properties with neutral red and Janus green. There is moderate anemia and sometimes thrombocytopenia. Enlargement of lymph nodes and spleen is common but not great. Tissue sections show disruption of architecture of these organs with marked hyperplasia of large cells of monocyte type, sometimes with indented or bizarre nuclei. Multinucleated cells may be fairly numerous. Similar hyperplasia may occur in liver and bone marrow as well as in the connective tissues of other organs. Although there has been controversy as to the existence of monocytic leukemia as a disease entity, modern studies leave no doubt that it constitutes the third variety of the leukemias. (See Doan and Wiseman.)

Other Forms

A few cases have been reported, in which the predominance of special types of the cells appears to justify designation as eosinophilic, basophilic or plasma-cell leukemia, but it is likely that these are variants or special forms of myeloid leukemia.

Chemistry

More definite information has been yielded by the study of myeloid than by that of lymphoid forms. The spleen, lymph nodes, and bone marrow of myeloid leukemia, if placed upon gelatine plates, show definite proteolytic activity. Bone marrow of lymphoid leukemia may act in the same way, but probably because of myeloid cells since lymph nodes and spleen are not proteolytic. In this disease the blood shows no excess of products of protein decomposition, but in the blood of myeloid leukemia there is an increase of noncoagulable nitrogen, in large part proteoses. Nuclear destruction, in part at least due to the action of enzymes, may result in the increase of uric acid, purine bases and phosphoric acid in the blood and urine, together with increases of proteoses and amino-acids due to associated cytoplasmic destruction. Charcot-Leyden crystals, probably derived from the nucleoproteins, may occur in the blood and various tissues. In concordance with these facts metabolism is also more increased in myeloid than in lymphoid leukemia. Clotting of the blood is likely to be delayed and incomplete, especially in myeloid leukemia. No satisfactory explanation is to be offered except that in one case Whipple found an excess of antithrombin. The whole problem of the chemistry of these diseases is admirably discussed by Wells.

Nature of Leukemia

The exciting cause of human leukemia is not known. In some cases traumatism precedes the appearance of symptoms and may possibly furnish a portal of entry for an infectious agent, but if so no such agent has been identified. Schmeisser, Ellerman and others have clearly demonstrated the transmissibility of fowl leukemias. Filtrates can transfer the disease, but as Opie points out, no bacterial causes have been demonstrated. In the fowl, the same filtrate can produce either myeloid or lymphoid leukemia, thus indicating that the disease represents alterations of reaction rather than of cause. Lymphoid leukemia of the mouse, which corresponds much more closely to the human form, is transferred by cells, but so far filtrates have not been effective. Richter and MacDowell consider that in spontaneous mouse leukemia there is an inherited susceptibility, apparently a mendelian dominant factor. Furth and his associates have shown, however, that cell inoculaton is successful in strains not naturally susceptible.

Leukemia is a part of a system disease whether lymphoid, myeloid or monocytic. Aleukemic phases are common to all these forms. The term leukosis covers all the manifestations and may be specified as lymphoid, myeloid or monocytic leukosis, with or without the changes in the blood characteristic of the leukemic phases. This conception is valuable but does not answer the question as to whether the disease represents a hyperplasia or a tumorous or tumor-like condition.

In the outline of experiments given above certain features are like those of experimental tumors. Filtrates are effective in fowl leukemias but not in those of mice. In mice there is an apparently heritable susceptibility to spontaneous leukemias, but the disease is produced by inoculation regardless of strain. In the mouse it is necessary to inoculate viable leukemic cells, and the disease in the inoculated animals represents a multiplication of the inoculated cells. Furthermore if the cells be transplanted into subcutaneous tissues a localized tumor, without leukosis, develops, and the cells from this tumor inoculated into the blood give rise to a leukosis. Subcutaneous injection of the filterable agent of fowl leukemia is followed by local tumor formation. Büngeler has found that the cells of a leukemia produced by indol administration show a shift from the oxidative to glycolytic type of metabolism observed in tumor cells. The accumulated evidence points strongly toward the neoplastic nature of experimental leukemias. In man, the cell masses in the tissues often appear to be invasive and there are instances in which the leukemia is accompanied by the presence of neoplastic nodules in other situations, which are comprised of cells like those of the leukemia. Nevertheless, human leukemia has not been shown to be transmissible and certain cytologic features differ from those of tumor cells. Studies of metabolism of the leukemic cells give conflicting results, but at least some behave more like immature normal cells than like tumor cells. Although we favor the view that human leukemia is neoplastic, it cannot be said that the results in experimental animals can be directly transferred to interpretation of the disease in man.

Leukemoid Reactions

The blood may show pictures resembling those of myeloid, lymphoid and monocytic leukemias. This is usually of short duration and may occur in the course of acute infectious diseases, tuberculosis, syphilis, Hodgkin's disease, various forms of anemia, tumors metastatic to bone marrow, osteosclerosis and other conditions. Extramedullary hematopoiesis is sometimes observed in spleen, liver, lymph nodes and other situations. (See Hill and Duncan.)

AGRANULOCYTOSIS— NEUTROPENIA

This condition is characterized by a prolonged, severe reduction in number of leukocytes and their precursors in the blood, and a tendency to succumb to bacterial infection. The lymphocytes and monocytes may be reduced in absolute number. A slight hypochromic anemia may be present. Local infections, as for example in the mouth, show little or no leukocytic reaction, progress rapidly and may be markedly necrotic. The spleen and lymph nodes may be enlarged, principally by hyperplasia of reticulo-endothelial cells, with associated circulatory disturbances. The bone marrow shows a variable picture, but especially important is the lack of maturation of the granulocyte series, particularly at the stage of myeloblasts (Darling, Parker and Jackson). The disease occurs especially in whites, females, middle life and the better social classes. Bacteria are secondary invaders rather than causative. Many cases are due to drugs which contain the benzene ring, operating probably through intermediate and end products of the benzamine group. Jackson states, however, that at least 44 per cent of the cases are without known cause. (See Kracke.)

Extraneous Substances in the Blood

The dissolved pigments of the blood include particularly bilirubin, but others such as methemoglobin also occur. Solid pigments include the pigment granules of malaria and more rarely crystals of bilirubin, and also carbon particles which gain access presumably through lymph nodes. Substances such as uric acid, urates, glycogen, sugar, creatinine, etc., may, under various conditions, accumulate in pathologic amounts in the blood. Embolism, fatty, gaseous, and due to amniotic fluid, has been discussed in the chapter on Disturbances of Circulation.

Parasites

The most important and common is the *Plasmodium malariae* which has its asexual cycle in the human blood and perhaps under certain circumstances may go through a sexual cycle. Others of importance include the *Filaria sanguinis hominis*, the *Distomum hematobium*, various forms of trypanosomes, especially that of African sleeping sickness, and larval forms of the *Trichinella spiralis*. Spirilliform parasites include particularly the spirillum of recurrent fever and the *Treponema pallidum* of syphilis. Various bacteria may appear in the circulating blood.

THE SPLEEN

Congenital Anomalies

Very rarely, in association with general malformations, the spleen may be absent; this may even occur in individuals who are otherwise normal, without interfering with growth and development. Congenital variations in size also occur. A certain amount of lobulation of the spleen, particularly in the form of linear depressions in its margin, is not uncommon. Accessory spleens are not rare, appearing as small globular bodies, especially in the gastrosplenic ligaments. These resemble lymph nodes but have the characteristic color of the spleen and participate in the pathological processes of the spleen. Histologically, their structure is characteristic. In malformations where the abdominal cavity is not closed, ectopia of the spleen may be observed.

Alterations of Position

The spleen may be pushed upward by swellings within the abdominal cavity such as are produced by ascites, abdominal tu-

PLATE XI

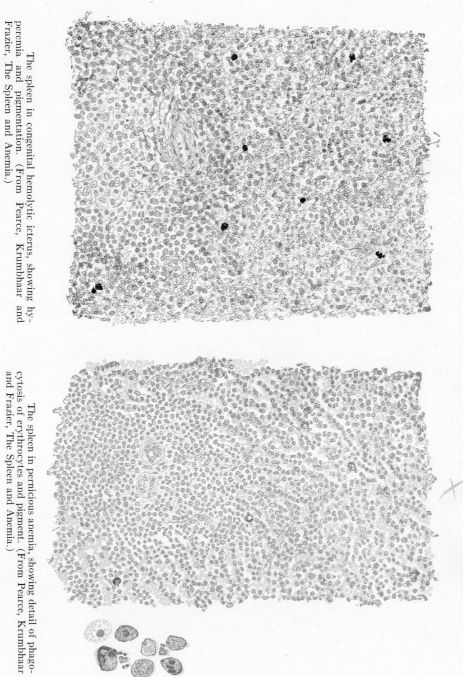

The spleen in congenital hemolytic icterus, showing hyperemia and pigmentation. (From Pearce, Krumbhaar and Frazier, The Spleen and Anemia.)

The spleen in pernicious anemia, showing detail of phagocytosis of erythrocytes and pigment. (From Pearce, Krumbhaar and Frazier, The Spleen and Anemia.)

mors and pregnancy. The spleen may be pushed or pulled downward by the weight of considerable enlargement, or its ligaments may be stretched by tight lacing and by conditions such as ascites, tumors and pregnancy, which after their removal leave relaxed ligaments. Such floating spleens usually become the seat of passive hyperemia and become chronically enlarged. Sometimes the pedicle becomes twisted and the spleen strangulated. Adhesions may fix the organ in abnormal position.

Retrogressive Processes

Of the various degenerative and infiltrative processes of the spleen, secondary amyloid is the most important. This may be an isolated occurrence in the spleen but is more commonly associated with amyloid of other organs, and in any case is due to the usual causes of amyloid. Two grades of amyloid exist, namely, that involving the follicles, the sago spleen, and the more diffuse form sometimes called the bacony or lardaceous spleen. In the former the spleen is moderately enlarged and firm, usually without thickening of the capsule. The cross section is firm, of red color, and shows small glassy hyaline areas, corresponding in size to enlarged follicles, which transmit the underlying red color of the organ. Special stains such as iodine or the iodine and sulfuric-acid process, demonstrate the characteristic reaction in the foci of the amyloid. In diffuse amyloid the spleen is likely to be larger although it rarely exceeds a weight of 500 to 600 grams. The appearance is much the same as in the sago spleen, except that in the cross section the glossy or gelatinous character is considerably more diffuse. Similarly, the reaction to the special stains is also diffuse. Microscopically, the amyloid is found in the central arterioles and in the substance of the follicles, associated with reduction in number of cells. In the diffuse forms, in addition to the follicular involvement, the hyaline material occurs also in the reticular substance and the walls of the vascular sinuses. Tubercles may also be present.

Hyaline degeneration of the central arterioles of the spleen is very common and in people past middle life is almost constant. This is differentiated from amyloid by the fact that it is confined to the arterioles, and also by special staining. Hyalin may also appear in the capsular substance and in the trabeculae as well as in the reticular connective tissue.

The usual necrosis of the spleen is that of infarction. Rarely, however, multiple necroses occur, originally called *Fleckmilz*. These are multiple, small or large, irregularly outlined foci of necrosis widely distributed and sometimes associated with identifiable infarcts. The condition is reported in uremia, arteriosclerosis, pernicious anemia and other conditions (see Schmeisser and Harris). Necrosis of the centers of the malpighian bodies occurs in the hyperplasias of acute infectious diseases and in status thymolymphaticus. Atrophy is found in old people and in those dead of prolonged chronic diseases. The organ is small, firm, pale and shows a relative or absolute increase in connective tissue of pulp and capsule. Various pigmentations of the spleen are common. Hemosiderin is practically always present in small amounts in adult spleens, occurs in larger quantities in cases of secondary and primary anemia and is often seen around the borders of infarcts. Hematoidin is likely to appear within the necrotic tissue of infarcts. Malarial pigment is common also. Calcification may result from necrosis as of infarction, occurs in tuberculosis, in arteriosclerosis, in the formation of phleboliths and as a part of syphilitic involvement to be described subsequently.

Circulatory Disturbances

Anemia of the spleen is usually the result of a general anemia. Unless enlarged because of blood destruction, the organ is usually somewhat reduced in size, of firmer consistence than normal and pallid both on the outer and cut surfaces. The relationship of the spleen to anemias offers problems along the line of blood formation, blood destruction, iron metabolism, influence upon the bone marrow and lymph nodes, etc., but for these the reader is referred to Pearce, Krumbhaar and Frazier.

Active hyperemia of the spleen is a common occurrence physiologically, especially during the process of digestion. It also occurs pathologically in connection with a wide variety of acute infectious diseases and is in part responsible for the enlargement of the

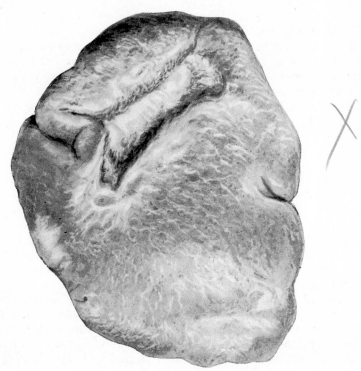

Large healed infarct of spleen.

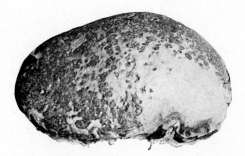

Chronic hyperplasia of spleen (malaria)
with   chronic   hyalocapsulitis   (zuckerguss).
Army Medical Museum 30190.

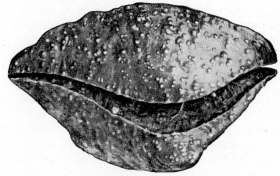

Miliary tubercles of spleen projecting in capsule.

spleen noted in these conditions, both clinically and pathologically.

Passive hyperemia, incident to chronic heart and lung disease, local passive hyperemia due to disease of the liver, and due to portal hypertension, is also extremely common. In cases of passive hyperemia of short duration, the organ is moderately enlarged, of moderate consistence and with a tense capsule. The cross section is of dark red color, bulges and bleeds freely. There is no important change in connective tissue incident to the hyperemia, but the follicles are usually obscured by the soft red pulp. Microscopically, the organ is characterized by a rich content of erythrocytes and a minor grade of hemosiderin pigmentation. The follicles are of normal or somewhat reduced size. As the duration of hyperemia increases, connective-tissue overgrowth becomes more conspicuous and the spleen correspondingly firmer. The organ may attain a weight of 200 or 300 grams or more, and shows a somewhat thickened, opaque, slate-colored capsule. The organ cuts with increased resistance and shows a fairly firm, dark red or purple cross section (cyanotic induration) which becomes a brighter red color upon exposure to the air. It bulges slightly and bleeds slightly. The follicles may or may not be visible. The trabeculae are increased in size and are visible grossly as irregular bands of dense connective tissue. Microscopically, the connective-tissue hyperplasia is particularly apparent in capsule and trabeculae but also involves the reticular substance. Large quantities of blood are present and hemosiderin pigmentation may be conspicuous. Later stages of passive hyperemia are likely to show a somewhat shrunken spleen, due particularly to the contraction of the hyperplastic connective tissue, representing a cyanotic atrophy. The organ is normal or reduced in weight with a thick, opaque, slate colored capsule and a retracting, firm, dark red or somewhat slate colored cross section with extreme prominence of the connective tissue trabeculae. Certain special forms of passive hyperemia of the spleen will be considered subsequently with the splenomegalies.

Embolism of the splenic arteries and its branches occurs particularly as the sequence of valvular disease of the heart, but may be due to any of the other causes of arterial embolism. The main branch of the splenic artery may be occluded, followed by complete necrosis of the spleen.

Infarction. Smaller infarcts of the spleen follow the usual course of the process. At first they are swollen, dark red, hemorrhagic, solid, conical areas which subsequently undergo necrosis and decolorization to become white infarcts. As the process advances, the central substance becomes more and more necrotic and there is reactive fibrosis in the margin, and shrinkage of the entire focus. Microscopically, the connective tissue architecture of the spleen may be apparent in the infarct even after necrosis is well advanced. In the earlier stages necrosis is associated with extensive hemorrhage in the area, and in the later stages the necrosis may be accompanied by a considerable deposition of hematoidin. Ultimately, the infarcts may be converted into dense fibrous scars which are sometimes confused with congenital lobulations of the organ. If the embolism be of infectious nature, abscesses of the spleen occur.

Hemorrhages of the spleen are likely to occur in connection with the enlargement incident to acute infectious diseases. Grossly, they appear in the spleen as irregularly disposed and shaped, dark red masses. Sometimes the spleen may rupture, with serious or fatal hemorrhage into the abdominal cavity. This occurs only rarely in connection with acute infectious diseases, such as malaria, and is usually caused by traumatic injury.

Thrombosis of the splenic vein may be due to inflammatory lesions along the course of the vein, such as ulcer of the stomach, tumors, inflammatory lesions of the pancreas; may be due to compression or other involvement by tumors and is likely to occur as the result of twisting of the pedicle of a floating spleen. This produces considerable enlargement of the spleen of the order described above in connection with the more acute forms of passive hyperemia. Emboli and thrombi within the spleen may undergo organization and calcification, to form phleboliths. These are hard, pearly, well defined nodules, 1 to 2 or 3 mm. in diameter. Most of the calcified nodules in the spleen, however, are obsolete tubercles. (See Sweany.)

Hyperplasia

Acute Hyperplasia. This is sometimes referred to as acute hyperplastic splenitis and as acute splenic tumor. Although not constantly present, it is one of the commonest postmortem indications of acute infectious disease. The response to various infections is different in degree and in certain special characters. The hyperplasia is believed to follow the acute hyperemia of the spleen in infectious diseases. The spleen of acute hyperplasia may attain weights of 500 or 600 grams or more but in other instances may be enlarged only slightly beyond the normal. In moderate degrees the organ is firm but the more severe cases show a soft, pulpy consistency. The capsule is thin and tense. The organ cuts with normal resistance and shows a bulging red, bluish-red or reddish-gray, pultaceous or pulpy cross section, from which a considerable amount of diffluent material may be scraped. The firm spleen shows a relatively firm cross section. The swelling of the pulp is likely to obscure all markings by follicles or connective tissue trabeculae. Microscopically, the connective tissue is normal in amount but may appear to be reduced because of the increase in cellular content. In many cases the follicles are of normal size but in others, more especially in diphtheria and scarlatina, when occurring in childhood, the follicles are somewhat enlarged because of hyperplasia affecting particularly the secondary nodules which may also be the seat of a small amount of necrosis. The pulp shows a rich or moderate content of blood and a considerable increase in the number of lymphocytes and endothelial cells, the latter originating for the most part from the endothelium of the sinuses. Polymorphonuclear leukocytes may be present in considerable numbers, especially in septicemia and pyemia. Fatty degeneration of the hyperplastic endothelial cells may also be present. The large mononuclear cells are likely to be phagocytic for fragments of other cells, particularly lymphocytes and red blood corpuscles, nuclear fragments and hemosiderin. Phagocytosis is often prominent in typhoid fever. Hemorrhage into the substance of the spleen may also occur, especially in plague and anthrax. Small foci of necrosis of the pulp are not uncommon, especially in the later stages of acute hyperplasia, which probably accounts for the softer consistence of the organ in later stages. Typhoid fever and plague produce the most constant and greatest acute hyperplasia of the spleen. Other diseases which may produce considerable enlargement, but may also produce little noticeable change, include anthrax, acute miliary tuberculosis, septicemia, and pyemia. Scarlatina, diphtheria and pneumonia are not likely to produce great enlargement, although in the last disease the spleen may be larger after the crisis than before. Following recovery, the spleen may be completely restored to normal, although in most cases it seems likely that there is some residuum in the form of fibrosis of the capsule and trabeculae and perhaps hyalin of the central arterioles. Evans divides the acute hyperplasias into a red and a gray variety, the former occurring in typhoid fever with marked hyperemia of the spleen and the latter in such diseases as pneumonia and septicemia where there is marked cellular hyperplasia. The distinction is not constant. (See Goldzieher.)

ABSCESS of the spleen is most commonly the result of infected emboli but may also be due to extension from neighboring processes such as gastric ulcer, perirenal abscess, abscess of pancreas, pylephlebitis and infection of traumatic hemorrhage. The gross and microscopic features do not differ from those observed elsewhere.

Chronic Hyperplasia. Although the term splenomegaly is sometimes applied to acute hyperplasia, it is, as a rule, limited to the chronic hyperplasias. Chronic hyperplasia of the spleen may be due to such chronic infectious diseases as syphilis, tuberculosis, malaria, kala-azar and other tropical diseases; may be due to blood diseases such as leukemia; may be due to passive hyperemia including that incident to cirrhosis of the liver, and may be a part of certain diseases whose nature is not well known but which almost constantly exhibit enlargement of the spleen. In the early stages, the chronic enlargement may be due very largely to the hyperplasia of the cellular content of the spleen with a moderate involvement of the connective tissue, but in the later stages the connective tissue predominates and the cellular part may be the seat of considerable atrophy. The more common forms of spleno-

PLATE XII

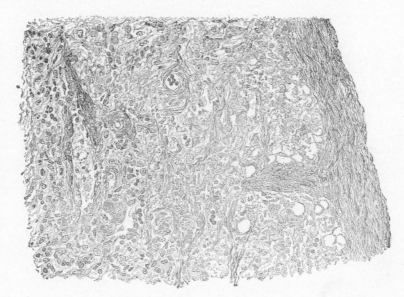

Reticular hyperplasia of spleen in early Banti's syndrome (fibroconnective splenomegaly). (From Pearce, Krumbhaar and Frazier, The Spleen and Anemia.)

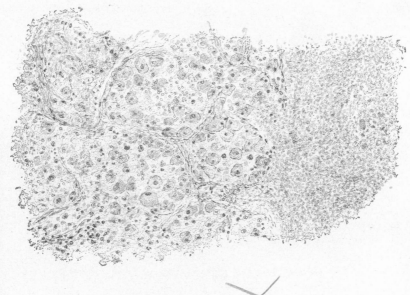

Alveolar arrangement of characteristic cells in the spleen of Gaucher's disease. (From Pearce, Krumbhaar and Frazier, The Spleen and Anemia.)

megaly show only moderate enlargement. The organ has a thick, dense, slate colored, opaque capsule. It is firm, cuts with increased resistance and shows a nonbulging, light or dark red, firm cross section with preponderance of connective tissue. Microscopically, there is a considerable overgrowth of connective tissue which in some instances affects principally the capsule and trabeculae, in others principally the connective tissue of the reticulum, and in others, both. The follicles may or may not be enlarged. The central arterioles are usually the seat of hyaline change. The lymphocytes are usually increased and, in addition, in special forms of splenomegaly other cell characters are observed. These will be considered under the heading of the separate diseases which appear to be worthy of mention.

The spleen may contain the so-called Gamna or Gandy-Gamna nodules, now usually referred to as siderotic nodules. There are minute foci, sometimes 3 or 4 mm. in diameter, which microscopically show necrosis, giant cells, eosinophils, crystals and pigment, which chemically are made up of calcium and iron (Kalkeiseninkrustation) and a surrounding zone of hyperemia. The critical studies of Reimann and Kurotchkin show that the nodules are not characteristic of splenomegaly and that they occur in other spleens and other tissues. They may well be the result of focal hemorrhages.

Splenomegaly

Malaria. In the more acute forms of the disease, enlargement of the spleen may be that of acute hyperplasia, characterized by the presence microscopically and even grossly of the malarial pigment. The parasites may also be discovered in the blood. The chronic splenomegaly of long standing malaria constitutes the so-called "ague cake." The organ may be considerably enlarged, attaining weights of 1,000 grams or more. It is firm, and shows a thick, opaque, slate-colored capsule which is sometimes adherent to the surrounding structures. The organ cuts with distinctly increased resistance, and shows a firm, nonbulging, brownish-red or brown cross section in which the trabeculae are prominent. Microscopically, in addition to the fibrosis of capsule and trabeculae, there may be moderate fibrosis of the reticulum and there

is almost constantly a considerable number of minute, dark-brown granules which do not give the iron reaction. These are for the most part in large mononuclear cells but may be found in extracellular positions. (See Photakis.)

Kala-azar, an infectious disease of Oriental tropical countries, caused by the *Leishmania donovani*, shows recurring fever, gradual loss of flesh and strength, secondary type of anemia and enlargement of spleen and liver. The careful studies of Meleney make it apparent that the pathologic changes are essentially due to proliferation of cells of the reticulo-endothelial apparatus in liver, spleen, lymph nodes and bone marrow, resulting from invasion by the parasite. The organisms enter the cells and multiply. Capillary endothelium may be invaded and react; even the parenchymatous cells of the liver may contain parasites. The spleen is large, firm as the result of endothelial hyperplasia and hyperemia rather than of fibrosis, and dark red. The follicles are small and the special feature is the large number of invaded endothelial cells, both mononuclear and multinuclear, whose cytoplasm is filled with large numbers of organisms. These are minute bodies, about the size of a blood platelet, with clear cytoplasm and usually two very minute chromatin masses.

Blood Diseases. The spleen of leukemias and of the more common varieties of anemia has been described in the section on diseases of the blood. The spleen of the so-called splenic anemia simply shows the picture of a chronic splenomegaly without any special features. As a matter of fact, splenic anemia is probably not a separate disease entity. Chronic splenic enlargement may also accompany infantile types of anemia and hemolytic jaundice. The spleen may also be enlarged, fibrotic and pigmented in hemochromatosis.

Follicular Lymphoblastoma. This affects both spleen and lymph nodes. The spleen may be enormously enlarged, firm, not especially fibrotic and show large follicles in the cross section, sometimes several millimeters in diameter. Microscopically, there is marked hyperplasia of the central large cells of the follicles. Ultimately, the condition becomes lymphosarcoma (See Baehr and Klemperer; Gall, et al.)

Banti's Syndrome. This has been described as an association, clinically, of enlarged spleen, hypochromic anemia, leukopenia, hepatic cirrhosis, ascites, and hemorrhage from esophageal varices. Formerly considered a disease entity, it has been found to be a group of symptoms and signs which do not necessarily occur in all cases. The names congestive splenomegaly and fibrocongestive splenomegaly are more suitable in the light of present knowledge.

Hypertension in the portal circulation and in the splenic vein may be due to hepatic cirrhosis, including that due to schistosomiasis, and a group of extrahepatic lesions such as thrombosis of the veins from infection or injury, scars, compression by tumors and congenital stenosis of the splenic vein. Of these, cirrhosis of the liver is the most frequent. The splenic vein is usually enlarged and tortuous, especially at the hilum of the spleen. The organ is large, red, firm, with fibrosis of pulp and capsule. Microscopically, there are diffuse fibrosis, reduction in size of follicles, dilated sinuses filled with blood and sometimes hemorrhages near the follicles, diffuse hemosiderosis and siderotic nodules. (See Thompson.)

Splenomegaly in the Lipidoses. A variety of primary and secondary disturbances of lipoid metabolism may be associated with splenomegaly, such for example as Gaucher's disease and Niemann-Pick disease. These and other diseases of somewhat similar nature will be discussed with the reticuloendothelial system since disturbances of this group of cells play a prominent, although not exclusive, part in the lesions.

Hodgkin's disease has been considered in the chapter on Infectious Granulomata. In addition to the general phenomena in the lymph nodes and circulating blood, the spleen is likely to be slightly or moderately enlarged but may uncommonly attain a weight of 1,800 grams or more. It may escape involvement or in some rare cases appear to be the only organ attacked. The capsule is usually tense and smooth, but its thickness and opacity depend upon the stage of the disease and the degree of fibrosis, which increases as the disease progresses. Similarly, the consistency may be normal or extremely firm. The character of the cross section also varies with the degree of fibrosis, in the later stages, showing considerable overgrowth of the trabeculae and reticular tissue. It may be mottled gray because of foci of cell hyperplasia, and gross areas of necrosis may occur (porphyry spleen). Microscopically, the condition is characterized by variable degrees of fibrosis throughout the spleen, usually with reduction in the size of the follicles and diminution in distinctness of their outline. Irregularly distributed are foci of variable size, made up of typical mononuclear and multinuclear giant cells, lymphocytes, plasma cells and in many cases a considerable number of eosinophils. Small foci of necrosis are likely to be encountered and pigmentation is common. The granuloma may extend into blood vessels.

Infectious Granulomata

Syphilis. Congenital syphilis may show some chronic hyperplasia of the spleen, principally due to connective tissue overgrowth involving capsule, trabeculae and reticular substance. Gummata may also be encountered in congenital syphilis. *Treponema pallidum* is often present in large numbers in the congenital lesion. In the secondary stage of syphilis the spleen may show a moderate acute hyperplasia. In later syphilis gummata may be encountered, but the more common change is a chronic hyperplasia due principally to overgrowth of connective tissue in which occasionally treponemas may be demonstrated. The thick capsule may show hyalinization.

Tuberculosis. In addition to the acute hyperplasia which may accompany acute disseminated miliary tuberculosis, the spleen is frequently the seat of tubercles of various forms and sizes. Acute miliary tuberculosis of the spleen is usually a part of disseminated miliary tuberculosis. The organ is moderately or considerably enlarged, with a tense, thin, translucent capsule through which the miliary tubercles may be visible. The consistence may be firm but sometimes is soft and diffluent. In the cross section the miliary tubercles appear as minute or larger, definitely rounded, solid, gray or pale yellow nodules which can easily be picked out on the point of a knife. They are to be distinguished from follicles because of the fact that follicles are of more definitely gray color and less sharply circumscribed. In later stages the tubercles may be encapsulated as a part of chronic miliary tuberculosis. Microscopically, the spleen is likely to show all the features of acute hyperplasia and in addition the presence of typical miliary tubercles with minute necrotic centers and surrounding zones of epithelioid, lymphoid cells and giant cells. Not infrequently they develop within the

majority of instances, tuberculosis of the spleen can be easily demonstrated as secondary to tuberculosis in some other situation. There are cases, however, in which the primary focus is either not demonstrated or in such a state of quiescence as to be overlooked or regarded as insignificant (Winternitz).

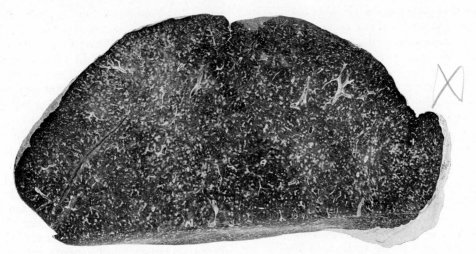

Cross section of spleen, the seat of acute miliary tuberculosis. Army Medical Museum 2713.

follicles. More particularly in children, acute or subacute tuberculosis of the spleen shows the presence of large numbers of small or larger conglomerate tubercles with extensive caseation of the centers. This closely resem-

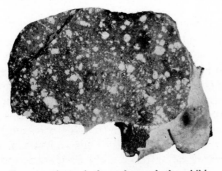

Cross section of the spleen of the child, showing multiple conglomerate tubercles.

bles tuberculosis of the spleen as it occurs in monkeys. The same condition may affect adults and appears to be more common in negroes than in whites. Very rarely a large solitary tubercle, the so-called tuberculoma, may be observed in the spleen. In by far the

Tumors

Of the primary benign tumors of the spleen, the hemangioma is the most common. This is usually cavernous. It may appear as a uniform, more or less marked enlargement of the spleen or may be grossly of nodular character. Cases also occur in which the hemangioma is simply a small nodule within the otherwise normal spleen. Grossly, there is usually some overgrowth of connective tissue of capsule and trabeculae. The spleen is large and of spongy consistence; upon cutting, it bleeds freely and loses considerable weight. Microscopically, the character of cavernous hemangioma is clearly distinguishable. (See Pines and Rabinovitch.) Benign tumors are rare and include fibroma, chondroma, and osteoma. Primary sarcoma of the spleen is rare, but spindle-cell forms, reticulo-endothelial sarcoma, and angiosarcoma have been observed. Of particular importance is the fact that in certain cases of lymphosarcoma the spleen may be the seat of considerable enlargement. Metastatic tumors, both carcinomas and sarcomas, are by no means rare.

Cysts of the spleen are not common.

Large blood-filled cysts may result from traumatism. Lymphatic cysts are said to occur and polycystic disease has been reported. The capsule may show small herniations with extrusion of splenic pulp into them. Dermoid cysts and also epidermoid cysts have been observed (Shawan).

Parasites

The most important metazoan parasite in human medicine is the echinococcus which may produce cysts of considerable size in the spleen. Cysticerci and pentastomum may occur.

Capsule of the Spleen

The acute inflammations of the capsule designated as acute capsulitis or perisplenitis are usually a part of local or general peritonitis, but may follow abscesses in the spleen and bland or septic infarction. Healing may produce fibrous adhesions to the diaphragm, abdominal wall and neighboring viscera, i.e., a chronic adhesive perisplenitis. Chronic fibrous perisplenitis may be the sequence of acute inflammations, but is more commonly the result of attacks of acute hyperplastic splenitis or due to chronic hyperplasias, tumors, parasites, etc. The fibrous thickening is accompanied by increasing opacity so that the underlying color of the spleen is poorly transmitted and the capsule appears to be slate colored. Hyaline degeneration of the thickened capsule is common and may be in the form of small, projecting nodules or a smooth, extensive mass. The clear, translucent, pearly gray or pale-blue sheet resembles icing on a cake and is referred to as the "iced," "sugar coated," or "zuckerguss" spleen. This occurs often in chronic syphilitic hyperplasia but is not confined to that disease. Calcification may be extensive and ossification may occur.

Suppuration in the neighborhood of the spleen such as subdiaphragmatic abscess or that originating in neighboring organs is referred to as parasplenitis.

The functional alterations of diseases of the spleen have not been included because of limitations in knowledge of normal and altered functions. What is known is well covered by Perla and Marmorsten.

LYMPH NODES

Introduction

Since the parenteral absorption of substances in solution and the transport of particulate matter in the body is through the lymphatic vessels, the lymph nodes are in direct line of attack by injurious materials. Particulate substances may be retained permanently within the lymph nodes or may pass on into the blood circulation. Substances in solution pass through the lymph nodes and gain access to the general body circulation. The cells and tissues of the lymph nodes react variously to the passage of irritant substances of differing character. The pathologic alterations, therefore, are practically always secondary to some condition in the region drained by the lymph node or nodes concerned. Certain other conditions, however, are regarded at present as primary in lymph nodes, because their mode of origin has not been determined. These, however, are infrequent in proportion to the secondary lesions and include such conditions as Hodgkin's disease, lymphoma, lymphosarcoma, Gaucher's disease, etc.

Retrogressive Conditions

Pigmentation of the lymph node is common, particularly in the mediastinum where coal pigment is deposited from the lungs. Similarly, other dusts such as silica, lime, iron, vegetable dusts, etc., also occur. This is seen primarily in the sinuses either free or within macrophages but later is found in the pulp cells. It may lead to considerable fibrosis of the nodes. Inflammatory or necrotic lesions of the node, particularly such as occur in tuberculosis, may produce adhesion to and then rupture into surrounding structures. Rupture into a vein may be followed by anthracosis (or siderosis, etc.) of other organs, especially liver and spleen. The pigment of tattooed skin is transported to regional lymph nodes sometimes in considerable quantities. Nodes draining regions of hemorrhage may be pigmented with hemosiderin, either transported as such, or formed by destruction of transported erythrocytes within the node. The pigment of skin in Addison's disease may also be transported to lymph nodes.

Cloudy swelling and fatty degeneration may appear in the lymph nodes, usually as the result of inflammatory lesions of various degrees. These are evident only on microscopic examination and particularly in the endothelial cells of the sinuses. Amyloid infiltration occurs as a part of general amyloidosis. It occurs along the connective tissues and the walls of capillaries and arterioles. It may be so extensive as to lead to marked atrophy of the essential cellular components. Hyaline degeneration may appear in the blood vessels of the nodes but is more commonly a part of chronic inflammation of the nodes, particularly that due to tuberculosis. It is essentially a connective tissue hyalin due to transformation of bands of connective tissue, and has been referred to as von Recklinghausen's hyalin. Calcification of the lymph nodes occurs particularly as the result of calcification of tuberculosis foci or under other conditions where necrosis is present. It is sometimes observed in carcinomatous nodes. Passive hyperemia is not uncommon, and more especially when there is inflammation, hemorrhage may be observed. Edema also occurs, more particularly in acutely hyperplastic or inflamed nodes. After puberty, the nodes undergo a gradual regression throughout life and in old age show distinct atrophy. The atrophy is a simple decrease of the cellular element with a relative and sometimes absolute increase of connective tissue. Not infrequently there is a fat substitution of the atrophic areas by an ingrowth through the hilum, a condition likely to be well exemplified in the retroperitoneal nodes of obese individuals.

Hyperplasias and Inflammation

Acute Hyperplasia. Acute hyperplasia of the lymph nodes, or acute hyperplastic lymphadenitis, occurs under conditions somewhat similar to those which affect the spleen. Although there may be no exudation, nevertheless this type of reaction to irritants is broadly regarded as of inflammatory nature. If the primary lesion be focalized, the affection of the lymph nodes is usually confined to the group which drains the diseased region. Thus, injuries and infections of the lower extremities are likely to be accompanied by acute hyperplasia of the lymph nodes of the groin, and those of the upper extremities affect the epitrochlear and axillary lymph nodes. Lesions of the mouth and throat affect the draining nodes of the neck. The condition may be produced by irritants in solution, but even when bacteria are present the lesion of the lymph node does not necessarily pass beyond the stage of hyperplasia. If, however, the organisms be sufficiently virulent and survive in the lymph nodes, abscess formation or acute suppura-

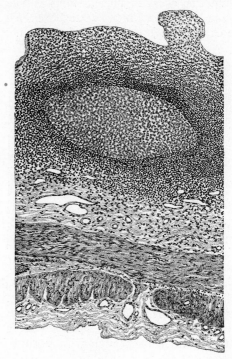

Acute hyperplasia of intestinal lymph node.

tive lymphadenitis may occur. There is usually a certain degree of lymphangitis but this may be sufficiently mild to escape detection. The node is large, soft, red from hyperemia, and with a tense capsule. It cuts with slight resistance and shows a bulging, pink or red, soft cross section from which the pulp can easily be scraped. Hemorrhage is sometimes present also.

Microscopically, the node shows enlargement of the follicles, often with an increase in the size of the secondary nodules. These central cells may show mitotic figures and especially in young individuals a certain amount of necrosis, granular or hyaline. The pulp is usually hyperemic and shows increase in the number of endothelial cells which are swollen, sometimes degenerated; macrophages contain red blood corpuscles, cell debris and bacteria. As with the spleen, certain types of acute hyperplasia may show special features. Thus, in typhoid fever there are many macrophages. In hyperplasia secondary to regions of suppuration, polymorphonuclear leukocytes may be found. In anthrax, hemorrhage and extensive necrosis often occur, as is true of bubonic plague. Other special forms of hyperplasia and inflammation occur in such diseases as tularemia and granuloma inguinale, as described in the chapter on Infectious Granulomata.

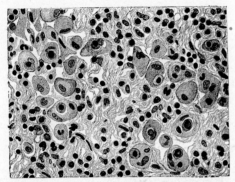

Acute hyperplasia of lymph node in typhoid fever, showing phagocytic endothelial cells.

Hyperplasia may be local, as just described, or widespread. Local enlargement may occur in the neck in diphtheria and scarlatina, in the abdomen in typhoid fever and in the groin in connection with genital infections. ACUTE MESENTERIC LYMPHADENITIS, especially in nodes draining the lower ileum, occurs in young people and clinically may be confused with appendicitis. It may accompany appendicitis or occur independently in cases of visceroptosis, chronic constipation, diseases of the gallbladder and malignant tumors in the abdomen (Foster). Widespread hyperplasia of superficial nodes is observed clinically in many of the acute infectious diseases, such as scarlatina, measles, diphtheria, varicella, smallpox and acute infectious mononucleosis. Usually the deeper nodes and the lymphoid apparatus of the intestine are also affected. In the early stage of syphilis, the inguinal nodes are hyperplastic and in the secondary stage this is often widespread, as indicated subsequently.

Acute Suppurative Lymphadenitis. This is most likely to occur in the nodes which drain regions of suppuration. The node is large, soft, pale yellow or hyperemic, and fluctuant. Pus is discharged upon incision. Microscopically, the abscess formation begins with a collection of leukocytes either within the pulp or rarely within the follicles, followed by central necrosis and extension of the leukocytic infiltration until an abscess is formed. This may enlarge to involve the capsule with consequent suppuration in neighboring structures. Sinuses may be produced by pointing into any of the body surfaces.

Chronic Hyperplastic Lymphadenitis. This is due to prolonged absorption of low-grade irritants by the lymph nodes such as may be observed in infections of low virulence, carious teeth, catarrhal inflammations, chronic skin lesions, and in tumors in the drained area, etc. Chronic hyperplasia may also follow any of the acute hyperplasias or even be the sequence of acute suppuration, or tumor involvement, and of course is likely to accompany chronic infections. In the state of enlargement, the node is large, pale, firm, and has a thickened capsule. It cuts with increased resistance and shows a firm, nonbulging or retracting, pale gray cross section. Microscopically, there is an increase in the connective tissue of the capsule and of the node itself, and not uncommonly an enlargement of the follicles and a general increase of lymphoid cells of the pulp. Endothelial hyperplasia of the sinuses may or may not be present. Hyaline degeneration of the connective tissue increases in amount and the adenoid tissue is reduced, and the nodes may then become a small indurated mass. In some instances, fat infiltration proceeds from the hilum of the node. Depending upon the cause and its localization, the chronic lymphadenitis may be confined to a few nodes or a chain of nodes, or, as in the case of syphilis, may be widespread.

Tuberculosis. Tuberculosis of lymph nodes is extremely common and can practically always be shown to be secondary to a primary focus in the region drained. There are, however, occasional cases where the primary focus is concealed or has disappeared, in which circumstances the lymph node tuberculosis appears to be primary. Occasionally, in cases of this sort, a great number of lymph nodes of the body are involved. Affecting the lymph nodes, tuberculosis may appear as a miliary form, as a diffuse cellular hyperplasia, or as caseous conglomerate tuberculosis. In the miliary form of the disease, the tubercles are usually multiple and there is an associated acute or chronic hyperplasia of the nodes. The tubercles are frequently characteristic, with necrotic centers, epithelioid and giant cells and a surrounding layer of lymphoid cells. Commonly, however, the tubercles appear simply as masses of epithelioid cells surrounded by a thin condensed rim of lymphoid cells. The tubercles are likely to coalesce and form larger masses and when the

a fairly common occurrence. It probably originates as a miliary tuberculosis with rapid coalescence of the miliary tubercles to form a large and caseous mass. The node is large, either soft or firm, depending upon the consistence of the caseous material, and shows a thickened capsule. The condition often extends through the capsules of nodes so as to produce more or less marked coalescence in a chain or group. Coalescence of groups of tuberculous mesenteric nodes is referred to as tabes mesenterica. The cross section shows the typical appearance of case-

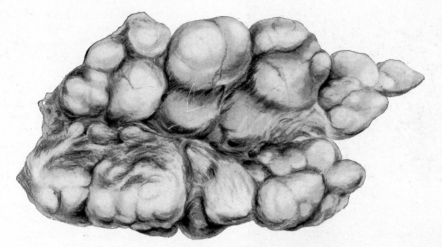

Conglomerate tuberculosis of axillary lymph nodes.

conglomerate form appears there is usually an acute perilymphadenitis. If the condition persist and the advance be not too rapid, the tubercles may be surrounded by fibroblasts and connective tissue.

In diffuse tuberculosis of the lymph nodes there is an irregular cellular hyperplasia which consists of endothelial cells intermingled with lymphoid and plasma cells. Giant cells may also be present. It is likely to be chronic and lead to gradual enlargement of the nodes over a long period of time, subsequently followed by fibrosis and contraction. If the process be focal in the nodes the later stages may show rims of connective tissue around the foci. It is usually limited to a group of nodes but may be generalized throughout the body. Such cases must be differentiated from Hodgkin's disease, lymphosarcoma, Gaucher's disease and other similar conditions.

Conglomerate caseous tuberculosis is

ous material. It is usually firm, yellow or yellowish-gray, more or less homogeneous, dry and friable. In some cases the caseous material is soft or semifluid. Microscopically, the caseous focus is surrounded by a rim of epithelioid and lymphoid cells which are often intermingled. There may also be giant cells, and not infrequently daughter tubercles are seen in the surrounding areas. Extension of the caseation into the surrounding tissue may lead to rupture through the skin, through the bronchi or through other neighboring structures, establishing a chronic sinus. This type of tuberculosis is common in the cervical lymph nodes of childhood, in the mediastinal nodes and in the mesenteric and retroperitoneal nodes. Cervical nodes may become infected through lesions of the mouth such as ulceration due to carious teeth, and especially through the tonsils. These foci of entrance may show no or very little tuberculosis in spite of the fact that the cervical nodes may be extensively involved. The mediastinal nodes are usually involved through the lungs where the primary lesions may be absent or so slight as to escape observation. Infection of mesenteric nodes may be due to lymphatic transmission from the thorax or the result of tuberculous enteritis. As indicated in the chapter on Infectious Granulomata infection of cervical and mesenteric nodes by bovine

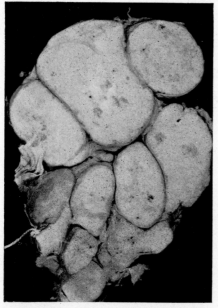

Cross section of caseous conglomerate tuberculosis of lymph nodes, showing necrosis and fusion. Army Medical Museum 30441.

tubercle bacilli is decreasing in frequency. The portals of entry for the tubercle bacilli may also serve for the establishment of secondary infections and subsequent suppuration.

Syphilis. In the secondary stages of syphilis the lymph nodes are likely to be enlarged throughout the body, especially evident in the superficial nodes and due to a low-grade acute or subacute hyperplastic lymphadenitis, sometimes with a granulomatous type of reaction (Michelson and Rusten). In the later stages this becomes a chronic hyperplasia, with subsequent reduction in size of the nodes and increased density with atrophy of the adenoid material. Gumma of the lymph nodes is but rarely observed. A few weeks after the primary infection, the lymph

nodes of the groin may become very considerably enlarged to constitute the so-called syphilitic bubo. This is an acute hyperplastic lymphadenitis with a considerable multiplication of fibroblasts. *Treponema pallidum* is present microscopically and may be demonstrated by experimental inoculation into animals. The condition may regress with a chronic fibrosis of the node or secondary infection may be established and suppuration occur.

Hodgkin's Disease. This forms fairly large tumor-like masses in the lymph nodes, most commonly in the neck, but affects other groups such as those of the axilla, thorax, retroperitoneum, mesentery and inguinal region. Gross examination shows that the individual nodes are moderately or considerably enlarged and except in rare instances are discrete and separated from one another by loose connective tissue. Except in the early stages, the nodes are firm, pale or pink in color, with a somewhat thickened capsule. The cross section may bulge slightly, is usually moist, of pale gray or pink color, and may show minute foci of necrosis. Microscopically, the very early stage shows a hyperplasia involving secondary nodules of the follicles and the lymphoid tissue of the pulp. The endothelium of the sinuses also shows hyperplasia and there may be some infiltration of polymorphonuclear and eosinophilic leukocytes. Very soon, however, the architecture of the nodes is completely obliterated by the marked hyperplasia of connective tissue and cells. The connective-tissue hyperplasia is slight in the early stages but progresses throughout the course of the disease, so that in the later stages there may be relatively few other cells remaining. The characteristic cell masses are made up of lymphocytes, plasma cells, endothelial cells, the peculiar mononuclear or multinuclear giant cells of Hodgkin's disease (Sternberg or Dorothy Reed cells) eosinophils, and very rare neutrophilic leukocytes. Small foci of necrosis are not uncommon. The more general phases have been discussed in the chapter on Infectious Granulomata. Hodgkin's disease or lymphogranulomatosis, the leukemias, lymphosarcoma and other similar conditions constitute a large group which may be included in the category of lymphomatoid diseases (Krumbhaar).

PLATE XIII

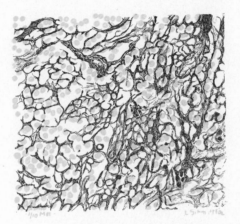

Section of lymph node of Hodgkin's disease, specially stained to show connective tissue hyperplasia. (Longcope.) The connective tissue is stained blue.

Leukemia. In the lymphoid form, general enlargement of the lymph nodes is practically constant. Superficial and deep nodes are involved but large tumor-like masses such as are seen in Hodgkin's disease are not common. The nodes in the acute form are likely not only to be large but to show a tense capsule and are of about normal consistency. The cross section bulges, and is of gray or pinkish-gray color. In the chronic forms the appearance, grossly, is much the same except that in the later stage the nodes are likely to be firmer because of fibrous overgrowth. In either form the nodes remain discrete and are not likely to show necrosis. Microscopically, the process represents a hyperplasia of lymphoid elements extending out from the follicles. This progresses until the architecture of the node is entirely obliterated by the mass of lymphoid cells. The reticulum in the early stages is fine and delicate but as time passes, connective-tissue overgrowth becomes more and more prominent and in very chronic cases may constitute a large part of the node. Vascularization is present but not likely to be prominent. Lymphoid cells may appear in the capsule as if invasion were occurring. Enlargement is not often encountered in myeloid leukemia, but occasionally it may be widespread. The nodes are moderately firm and show a slightly bulging, moist, grayish red cross section. Microscopically, this is found to be due to a myeloid metaplasia of the node or only of parts of it, in which are found the cells characteristic of bone marrow.

The diagnosis of lymphoid leukemia of the lymph nodes is in part determined by the condition of the blood. Enlargement of the lymph nodes occurs identical in all respects with that seen in lymphoid leukemias, except that the blood changes are not present. In such cases the condition is referred to as lymphoid leukosis. It is difficult to say that this condition represents an entity separate and distinct from leukemia. It may be an early stage of the process or may represent an intermission, but there are cases on record in which no important blood changes have been encountered at any time, and which must be regarded as certainly not leukemic. Clinical and microscopic features vary greatly (Baldridge and Awe).

Tumors

Lymphosarcoma. This, the most important malignant tumor of the lymph nodes, may arise in any lymphoid aggregate, whether in nodes or other structures. It affects males about twice as often as females, and occurs at almost any time of life but is most frequent in the fifth and sixth decades. Its course is comparatively slow, and fatal. The first sign clinically is usually enlargement of a group of nodes, followed by the usual symptoms of malignant tumor. It is likely to appear first in neck, groins, axilla, or tonsils. Then other groups, including those of mediastinum, abdomen and intestines, may be affected and the disease may involve various organs, especially those where tiny lymphoid aggregates are naturally present, such as liver, lung, kidney, bone marrow and skin. Many speak of this as metastasis, but it seems probable that this secondary involvement is due to the more widespread operation within the lymphoid system of whatever excited the original growth. We look on lymphosarcoma as a system disease.

Lymphosarcoma shows a distinct tendency to invade through the capsule of the node and into the surrounding tissues, so that within groups of nodes fusion is likely to be marked, and the individual nodes or groups are not freely movable because of the invasion of and adhesion to surrounding parts. Grossly, the nodes are moderately or markedly enlarged, and although individuals of a group may be clearly made out, there is likely to be a greater or less degree of fusion. Owing to fairly rich vascularization the nodes are likely to be of pink color. The cross section is soft, bulging, pink in color and shows slight or sometimes extensive necrosis. Microscopically, two forms of tumor are recognized, in both of which the architecture is obliterated. In the lymphosarcoma, or malignant lymphocytoma, the cells correspond in size and form to the mature small lymphocyte.

In reticulum-cell sarcoma, or retotheliosarcoma, the cells are larger, often angular in outline and correspond to reticulo-endothelial cells with their intimately connected reticulum fibrils. In both forms the cells may or may not be uniform in size and shape, are round or oval with a moderate amount of cytoplasm and have round or oval, somewhat vesicular nuclei. Multinucleated cells occur in both forms. Mitotic figures are frequent. Vascularization is fairly rich in the form of small vessels and some of these are without independent walls. Reticular connective tissue is present either as a delicate network or, in prolonged cases, as a diffuse fibrous overgrowth. Reference has been made to the occurrence of lymphoid or lymphosarcoma-cell leukemia in a small percentage of cases, and accompanying this, acceleration of the course of the disease. It is said that reticulum-cell sarcoma has preceded or accompanied monocytic leukosis. (See Callender; Sugarbaker and Craver.)

Endothelioma. This is uncommon, but when it occurs it may involve groups of nodes such as the cervical or axillary or may be systemic with the involvement of large numbers of lymph nodes. Invasion of the capsule is not so likely to occur as in the lymphosarcoma but in the later stages may be very apparent. Vascularization is less marked in these tumors and the color is likely to be pallid. Necrosis is not uncommon. Ewing finds that this condition is likely to develop upon a pre-existing granulomatous involvement of some sort. Microscopically, the condition is characterized by the presence of solid sheets of large round cells, at first in the sinuses of the nodes and later invading more widely. The cytoplasm is rich and may be somewhat vesiculated, the nuclei relatively small and vesicular. The massing of the cells in sheets may give the tumor a somewhat alveolated appearance, but there is not likely to be great fibrous tissue overgrowth or fibrous trabeculae except in later stages. Mitotic figures may be observed.

Secondary Tumors. Metastasis to lymph nodes is common, especially in carcinoma. As a rule, the microscopic character of the metastasis is like that of the primary tumor, as to degree of differentiation and desmoplastic properties. It is unusual for a carcinoma metastatic in lymph nodes to show a lower degree of differentiation than the original neoplasm. The growth appears first in the sinuses of the nodes, gradually invades, and may even penetrate through the capsule. Considerable connective-tissue growth may sometimes occur, with such secondary changes as hyalin and calcification. Secondary sarcomas also reduplicate the appearance of the original tumor. These may appear primarily in the lymphoid sinuses, or may be found within the pulp of the nodes because of blood vascular transmission. Chloroma is especially likely to affect lymph nodes and produce considerable enlargement. The involvement is uniform throughout the nodes and may sometimes invade the capsule. It is characterized grossly by the green tint of the node and microscopically by the myeloid cells.

Parasites

Those mentioned as occurring in the lymph nodes include the echinococcus, cysticerci and, more particularly in the mesenteric lymph nodes, the *Trichinella spiralis*. The lodgment of *Filaria sanguinis hominis* in the larger lymphatic vessels and also in the nodes is the cause of that chronic form of edema known as elephantiasis.

Hemolymph Nodes

These are usually embedded in fat near large blood vessels and are found in the prevertebral retroperitoneal region, near renal vessels, about the brim of the pelvis, the root of the mesentery and sometimes in the omentum. They are small, red, mottled or pale nodes, whose color can be seen best by transmitted light. They differ from lymph nodes in that the capsule is thicker and there are blood sinuses instead of lymph sinuses, although the latter may also be present. Little is known of their pathologic changes, but Warthin points out that they have an important part in hematopoiesis, especially in blood destruction. In infections of various kinds they show acute hyperplasia, well marked in the sinuses where endothelial phagocytosis of erythrocytes is prominent. Hemosiderosis may be marked. In secondary anemias the nodes may show marked myeloid metaplasia, but in pernicious anemia blood destruction is the most conspicuous feature. The hemal nodes may show lymphoid hyperplasia in lymphoid leukemia, and myeloid metaplasia in myeloid leukemia. Symmers reports a hemangiolymphoma of hemal nodes, which may give rise to local or selective subperiosteal metastases.

BONE MARROW

Retrogressive Processes

The bone marrow may undergo a marked hyperplasia in infancy and childhood as a result of severe anemias. Cells of the bone marrow may show cloudy swelling and fatty degeneration when inflammation occurs. Probably the most significant change in the bone marrow is the so-called "gelatinous degeneration." This may be acute or chronic and is the sequence of prolonged exhausting diseases such as chronic tuberculosis, malig-

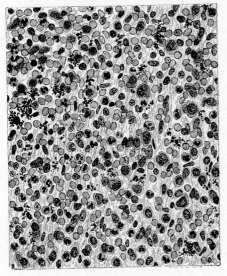

Malarial pigmentation and hyperplasia of bone marrow.

nant tumors, and chronic nephritis, poisoning by metals such as lead, mercury and arsenic, and inanition in early or late life. (See Michael.) It may be incident to exhaustion of marrow following the hyperplasias of anemias and leukemias and is one of the bone marrow lesions of hypoplastic anemia. Grossly, the marrow has a yellow or pinkish-yellow color, is somewhat reduced in volume, and shows a gelatinous, semi-translucent appearance. Microscopically, there is reduction in the blood forming constituents and in the fat, the connective-tissue cells becoming transformed into stellate and spindle cells with a matrix between, which closely resembles mucoid. Toxic agents such as benzol and mustard gas (Krumbhaar) may markedly depress the bone marrow. Simple atrophy of the marrow may be due to exhausting diseases, to the advancement of osteosclerosis and to irradiation and may occur in the aged. With the simple atrophy there is usually an accompanying fibrosis. Anemias of all varieties may be accompanied by hemosiderin pigmentation of the bone marrow. Malarial pigmentation may be prominent. Anthracosis, and also pigmentation of the marrow may occur in the neighborhood of secondary malignant melanoma. Small foci of necrosis, which may be visible to the naked eye, may appear in the bone marrow as the result of certain infectious diseases such as typhoid fever, pneumonia, smallpox, plague, septicemia, etc.

Hyperplasia

Associated with the leukocytosis of acute infectious diseases, the bone marrow may be hyperplastic. Hyperplasias of this sort are usually not severe and the marrow is restored to normal when the exciting disease disappears. More pronounced hyperplasias accompany the anemias and leukemias. Although in response to the first stimulus, the reaction is likely to take place in all the elements of the bone marrow, nevertheless, as time goes on, one or more groups of elements may predominate and the hyperplasia may therefore be erythroblastic, leukoblastic or in some cases lymphoblastic. Further subdivisions are possible because of predominance of particular types of cells. Thus, there may be a normoblastic or a megaloblastic type of erythroblastic hyperplasia. Similarly, the leukoblastic hyperplasia may show predominance of the neutrophilic, eosinophilic, basophilic or myeloblastic types. The erythroblastic hyperplasia may be confined to those situations in which red marrow is normally present or may be so extensive as to involve marrow which is normally fatty, thus appearing in the shafts of long bones. The milder forms of hyperplasia occur in secondary anemias, but both in these forms when severe, and in pernicious anemia, erythroblastic hyperplasia may be pronounced. The neutrophilic leukoblastic hyperplasias are especially common in connection with leukocytosis. It is only when the primary infection is prolonged and severe that hyperplasia extends into the shaft of the long bones. A preponderance of the nongranular myeloblasts may be observed sometimes in cases of prolonged leukocytosis, but is more characteristically observed in cases of leukemia. Eosinophilic hyperplasia may be observed in trichinosis. Lymphoblastic hyperplasia may be observed in lymphoid leukemia and in status lymphaticus. These are described in detail by Dickson and have been referred to in the previous discussion of diseases of the blood. Considering the bone marrow as a whole, these changes represent hypertrophy because there is associated increase in the fundamental activity of the bone marrow, but in considering cell groups there is no reason to believe that the functional capacity of individual cells is increased, and it therefore seems desirable to refer to these changes as hyperplasia rather than hypertrophy. The hyperplasias of the anemias and leukemias are essentially chronic in character except when those diseases are acute. In addition, however, the bone marrow may show chronic hyperplasia principally in the form of an overgrowth of connective tissue, associated sometimes with infiltrations of lymphocytes and plasma cells. Such conditions may accompany certain chronic diseases such as chronic pulmonary tuberculosis, chronic nephritis, cirrhosis of the liver, etc. (See Jaffe.)

Inflammation

In addition to the fact that hyperplasia is often associated with infections, bacteria may enter the marrow and produce inflammation. Thus, in septicemias small abscesses may arise in the marrow, sometimes visible grossly. There is seldom if ever any noteworthy depression of function of the marrow. Healing results in the formation of small scars. Such diseases as typhoid fever, pneumonia, smallpox and plague are likely to show in the bone marrow small foci of necrosis surrounded by hyperemia, edema and fairly rich fibrin formation. In the immediate neighborhood, phagocytosis of corpuscles by endothelial cells may be prominent and after the lesion has healed, hemosiderin pigmentation is likely to be observed. In typhoid fever there may be little or no necrosis and the lesion be represented simply by local accumulation of endothelial cells, phagocytic for bacteria and cell debris similar to the lesions observed in the liver and spleen.

Abscess formation in the marrow, as indicated above, is of little direct significance so far as function of the marrow is concerned.

Nevertheless, extension is likely to occur involving the bony substance leading thus to an osteomyelitis, as described in the chapter on Organs of Locomotion. Although other organisms occur, the staphylococcus is most frequently associated with this condition.

Granulomata. Tuberculosis of the bone marrow commonly accompanies an acute disseminated miliary tuberculosis. Microscopically, the miliary tubercles have the usual form. The marginal zone of lymphocytes may be somewhat richer in plasma cells than is ordinarily the case in other tissues. The most serious involvement by tuberculosis is that which includes not only the marrow but also the bone. This is likely to occur in the ends of long bones, more especially in childhood, and also in spongy bones such as the bodies of the vertebrae. It is an important cause of amyloid disease.

Only rarely do gummata appear in the bone marrow. In Warthin's cases of late syphilis, "premature and excessive osteoporosis of the bone and fatty atrophy of the marrow characterize the majority of cases. In a small number of cases, the lymphoid marrow was found to be increased."

In Hodgkin's disease the bone marrow not infrequently shows nodules of essentially the same character and cell composition as seen in lymph nodes and spleen.

Tumors

It is only rarely that primary benign tumors occur in the bone marrow. Occasional cases of hemangioma, chondroma and fibroma have been reported. The primary malignant tumors include lymphosarcoma, multiple myeloma, endothelial myeloma and chloroma. Craver and Copeland found involvement of the marrow in 10 per cent of cases of lymphosarcoma. They call it metastasis, but we look upon it as a part of a system disease.

Multiple Myeloma. Although this may occur at any time of life, including childhood, the peak of incidence is in the sixth decade. Males are affected about twice as often as females. Patients complain of pain in involved bones and the x-ray shows punched-out areas of decreased density when the nodules destroy bone. There may be deformities of the thorax and spine due to destruction of bones. The urine may contain Bence-Jones protein. Hyperproteinemia is often marked, usually because of increase of globulins, but other proteins may predominate (Gutman, et al.). This may be accompanied by rouleaux formation of erythrocytes. Hypercalcemia is associated with increase in phosphorus, which is practically peculiar to this disease. There is a hypochromic anemia and the blood films may show myelocytes and a form of cell resembling the plasma cell.

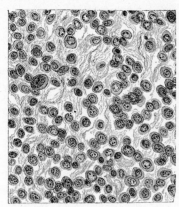

Multiple myeloma with cells of myelocyte type.

The disease terminates fatally in two or three years but may last longer.

    Grossly, the tumors appear in the marrow as nodules of variable size, soft or firm, translucent or opaque and of gray or red color depending on vascularization and hemorrhage. Microscopically, the cell type is uniform, and the tumor is usually made up of cells which morphologically are plasma cells. When tumors of other cell types occur, the cells are probably derivatives of the plasma cell (Ewing). Vascularization may be rich, but stroma is usually scanty. Invasion and destruction of bone are often observed. Although it is said that a primary tumor may precede multiple tumors, and that myeloma may originate in soft tissues, these statements cannot be accepted, because the roentgen ray does not detect the tumors of the marrow unless bone has been destroyed; hence additional tumors cannot be excluded. For the most part, the tumor is multicentric in origin and especially affects spongy bone such as skull, spine, ribs and pelvis; long bones may also be involved. Metastases may occur in soft tissues, such as liver, spleen and kidneys. The amyloidosis of multiple myeloma may

be related to the hyperproteinemia, yet it is usually distributed as is primary amyloidosis. Renal insufficiency may be observed, the kidneys showing hyaline masses in the glomerular capillaries and also hyaline casts which appear to be made up of Bence-Jones protein. (See Donhauser and de Ronville; Batts; Tarr and Ferris.)

    Endothelial Myeloma. Often called Ewing's tumor of bone, this affects usually the shaft of a long bone in early life; it may occur also in spongy bone. The roentgen ray shows enlargement of the shaft so that the bone becomes fusiform in outline. Microscopically, the tumor is likely to invade both bone marrow and bony substance. It is made up of sheets of cells sometimes in an alveolated arrangement, sometimes poorly and sometimes well vascularized and with relatively little reticulum. The cells in some tumors show solid cytoplasm and in others the cytoplasm is somewhat vesicular. Metastases to other parts are distinctly unusual. As with the myeloma and chloroma, the endothelioma itself shows no tendency to bone formation. As indicated in the chapter on tumors, it is probable that certain cases supposed to be endothelioma are really metastatic tumors. Roentgen treatment is effective for a time, but the tumor recurs.

    Chloroma. Closely related to the multiple myeloma is the tumor called chloroma or sometimes chloromyeloma. This invades bone from the bone marrow in much the same manner as does myeloma, but more commonly involves the lymph nodes in addition to metastases in other organs. It is characterized grossly by a pale green color. Microscopically, the tumor is made up of cells with granular cytoplasm, either neutrophilic or eosinophilic and sometimes mixtures with one or the other form predominating. Basophilic cells do not occur. Alterations of the blood are very common, particularly in the form of a mild anemia or moderate increase of the cells of the myelocyte series, or both. Kandel, as a result of the study of a large series of cases, concludes that there is an inevitable association with myeloid leukemia and it is thus a variant of that disease with the myeloblast as the type cell of the tumor. Some prefer the term "chloroleukemia."

    Secondary Tumors. Any type of malignant tumor may metastasize into the marrow of bones. Most common, however, is carcinoma and especially those forms originating in the prostate, thyroid, and breast. Many other carcinomas metastasize to bone but with less frequency. Sarcomas of soft tissues may metastasize to bone, but sarcomas of bone only rarely metastasize to other bones. Metastases in bones may be destructive only, when they are called osteolytic, or they may excite bone formation when they are osteoplastic. If the marrow be widely destroyed there may be an associated myelophthisic anemia. Pathologic fractures may result from bone destruction.

THE RETICULO-ENDOTHELIAL SYSTEM

Introduction

The reticulo-endothelial system consists of two groups of cells with similar functions, but not of necessity genetically related. According to Aschoff the system is comprised of (a) the RETICULUM cells of the splenic pulp and of the follicles and pulp cords of lymph nodes and other parts of the lymphatic apparatus, and (b) the RETICULO-ENDOTHELIAL or endothelial cells of the lymph-node sinuses, the blood sinuses of the spleen, the capillaries of the liver lobules, especially the Kupffer cells, and the capillaries of bone marrow, adrenal cortex and hypophysis. Quantitatively most of these cells are found in the hematopoietic tissues. They are mononuclear cells of mesoblastic origin, grouped together because of similarity in phagocytic activity, reaction to vital dyes, and certain functional manifestations displayed normally and pathologically. The restricted inclusiveness of the name to the organs noted above is somewhat artificial, as similar cells are observed in other parts of the body, but the term is now widely used. The activity in these cells has been much clarified by the use of vital dyes by Aschoff and his associates, Maximow, Foot, Sabin and her coworkers and many others, as covered in the reviews by Sacks, by Jaffe, and by Aschoff.

Discussion centers about the identity of the various cells concerned, especially those cells fixed as reticulum and vascular endothelium, the wandering cell of the tissues called tissue histiocyte by Aschoff and clasmatocyte by Sabin, and the large mononuclear cell of the blood generally called monocyte. Mallory thinks that the latter two forms may arise from vascular endothelium, but others do not finally accept this view. Lewis and Lewis think that the monocyte and clasmatocyte are interrelated. Sabin prefers to regard them as separate functional entities. Doan and Wiseman regard the blood and tissue monocyte as identical. They consider the mononuclear phagocyte of the tissues to be of two orders, the monocyte, derived from mesenchymal reticular tissues and the clasmatocyte, derived from endothelium.

The place of the reticulo-endothelial system in hematopoiesis is not settled. Hypotheses that these cells give rise to granulocytes and lymphocytes and indirectly to erythrocytes, are generally regarded as without adequate proof. Phagocytosis of blood cells, particularly erythrocytes, is observed in anemias, hemolytic jaundice and acute infectious diseases. It is more probable that the erythrocytes are previously damaged than that there is an excessive primary functional activity on the part of the reticulo-endothelial system. Iron bearing pigments are found in the cells of this system in the diseases enumerated and in severe nutritional disturbance. Whether this pigmentation is due to intracellular digestion of the erythrocytes, transformation of absorbed hemoglobin or taking up of pigment produced in the plasma is not certain. The relation of this system to bilirubin formation has been referred to in the chapter on Pigmentations, but it may be said that endothelial cells are capable of forming bilirubin and that probably they are entirely responsible for its formaton. The cells of the reticulo-endothelial system phagocytose platelets and appear to play a part in thrombocytopenic purpura. This view is supported by the favorable results of splenectomy.

Monocytosis is the term usually applied to an increase in number of the large mononuclears, principally monocytes, in the circulating blood. It is presumed that this increase is due to stimulation of the reticulo-endothelial system. The phenomenon may be observed in malaria, kala azar, brucelliasis, endocarditis lenta, certain anginas and some of the septicemias. The significance of monocytes in the circulating blood, especially in regard to the ratio of lymphocytes has been established in tuberculosis (see Sabin). In animals an increase in number of monocytes appears to be related to susceptibility and in man and animals such increases, especially with decreases of lymphocytes, are associated with unfavorable progress of the disease, whereas favorable progress is indicated by decrease of monocytes with increase in lymphocytes. Sabin believes the monocytes to be precursors of the epithelioid cells of the tubercle.

Often included in this general category is acute glandular fever or *acute infectious mononucleosis*. Occurring principally in childhood and youth, the disease is febrile, often with enlargement of cervical and other lymph nodes, sore throat and the presence of slight or moderate leukocytosis with a relative increase in large mononuclear cells. The cells are probably derivatives of lymphocytes rather than monocytes. Notable is the appearance of heterophile antibodies in the blood. The lymph nodes show acute hyperplasia, especially in secondary nodules of the follicles, and often macrophages containing cell fragments. Several organisms have been recovered, including *Listerella monocytogenes* (Pons and Julianelle) and a virus is reported (Nettleship) but no exact cause has been identified. (See Berstein.) Monocytic leukemia was discussed with the leukemias.

Cells of this system play a part in the local lesions of the *infectious granulomata*, especially tuberculosis, leprosy, rhinoscleroma, sporotrichosis, blastomycosis, Hodgkin's disease, granuloma inguinale and to a lesser extent in syphilis.

Many studies point to the part played by the system in inflammation (see Maximow on mesenchymal reactions). Gay maintains that the cells are important in local immunity. The relation to antibody formation in general has been studied by the so-called blockading of the system by the use of particulate matters, with or without splenectomy (see Cannon, et al.). It is stated that small amounts of blockading material stimulate the liberation of antibody whereas large amounts tend to depress it. That these experiments indicate activity within the endothelial cells rather than influence upon phenomena of absorption has yet to be settled.

Lipidoses

These include a wide variety of local and widespread hyperplasias of reticuloendothelial cells associated with the presence within them of lipids. Thannhauser divides them into cholesterosis, cerebrosiderosis and sphingomyelinosis. In the first group are the xanthomatoses, characterized by the presence of cholesterol and its esters. These forms may be primary essential, secondary and local. The primary diseases may be hypercholesterolemic, including such conditions as xanthelasma of the eyelids, xanthomas of tendons and blood vessels and that form associated with hepatic cirrhosis; or normocholesteremic, including disseminated xanthomatosis of skin, of serous membranes, of bones and the condition called Schüller-Christian syndrome. Secondary xanthomatosis, due to hypercholesterolemia include a familial form of hepatosplenomegaly, xanthomatosis in diabetes mellitus, in glycogen disease and lipoid nephrosis. Localized xanthomatosis occurs in chronic inflammations, tumors and certain other conditions. Selected for discussion are Schüller-Christian syndrome (cholesterosis), Gaucher's disease (cerebrosiderosis) and Niemann-Pick disease (sphingomyelinosis). These differ in the nature of the lipid concerned and in other respects. Gaucher's disease and Niemann-Pick disease affect females especially and Schüller-Christian syndrome males. In Gaucher's disease, skeletal involvement is uncommon, but when it occurs is usually widespread. In Schüller-Christian syndrome, involvement of bones is the rule, especially at the base of the skull. In Niemann-Pick disease, the marrow may be involved but the bone is not likely to be affected. Rowland and others have taken the view that the presence of the lipids is due to infiltration but Thannhauser and Magendantz, and Thannhauser, hold that there is an intracellular disturbance of metabolism, inherent in the cells and not dependent on changes in the blood.

Schüller-Christian Syndrome

This is one of the primary xanthomatoses, as mentoned above. It affects children principally but may occur in adults. The condition is more common in males than in females and does not show a familial distribution. The principal manifestations are defect in membranous bones of the skull, exophthalmus and diabetes insipidus; disseminated xanthomatosis of the skin may also occur. Headache, drowsiness, pain in affected bones, fever and other symptoms occur. The spleen and liver are often enlarged. The blood shows a marked anemia and a slight leukocytosis, sometimes with a relative increase in eosinophils. The cholesterol level of the blood is normal. In the affected tissues there is a deposit of cholesterol and its esters, phospholipid and neutral fats. Nodules occur, varying from a few millimeters to a centimeter or more in size, increasing in firmness with the progress of the disease and of bright or dull yellow color. The lesion in the skull appears to start in the meninges and then invades the tables, sometimes with complete penetration. The defects are plainly visible in the roentgenogram. Occasionally other spongy bones are involved. The diabetes insipidus is probably due to secondary effects upon the hypothalamic region. The exophthalmus is due principally to nodular deposits in the orbit. Similar nodules may be found in the ethmoid air cells, the mediastinum, omentum, retroperitoneal regions, adrenals, kidneys, heart, etc. Generally, however, the lymph nodes, spleen and liver are more diffusely involved. The capillary endothelium of the brain and the ganglion cells may show a few foamy cells. The cells show a conspicuous vesicularity of the cytoplasm and may be multinucleated. As the disease progresses, fibrosis takes place and in the late stages there may be a few or no foam cells. This growth of the connective tissue is often granulomatous in character. The disease may produce characteristic nodules in the skin, with papular or hemorrhagic eruption (Lane and Smith). Although there is a unity of the basic morphology of the disease, the clinical manifestations may be so varied that it is looked upon as a syndrome rather than a disease entity. (See Rowland.)

Gaucher's Disease

This occurs in an acute form in children and occasionally in a more chronic form in adults. In the former it usually terminates fatally in an average of 6 months after it becomes evident, but in adults it may run a prolonged course of several years, often without serious disability. It is more common in females than males, often has a familial distribution and affects the Jewish race especially. In later stages there may be a hypochromic anemia with a slight degree of leukopenia. The lesions contain a lipid in the group of cerebrosides, determined to be kerasin. The deposits occur especially in spleen, lymph nodes, liver and bone marrow. The spleen is usually moderately or considerably enlarged and shows the changes most markedly, although in some instances the bone marrow is particularly affected. The bones may be irregularly decalcified ("cotton wool" appearance to roentgen ray) and the lower ends of the femur may be enlarged (flask-like). The chronic splenomegaly is characterized microscopically by the presence of many large mononuclear and sometimes multinucleated cells, rich in cytoplasm and with dense nuclei often wrinkled in outline. In ordinary stains the cytoplasm is not vesicular but special stains show the presence of the lipid. These cells are usually round but may be elongated and even fibrillated. It is generally agreed that they are derived from reticulo-endothelium.

Niemann-Pick Disease

This is also called lipoid histiocytosis (type Niemann-Pick). It occurs in infancy and childhood, principally in the Jewish race, is familial, and runs a rapid course usually terminating fatally in the first two years of life. Spleen and liver are much enlarged, the skin is often pigmented yellowish-brown, emaciation progresses and idiocy may develop. Grossly, the spleen is firm and of salmon-pink color and in the cross section may show mottling of pale yellow and gray areas. Microscopically, it is characterized by the presence of many large cells, usually with only one nucleus and a foamy cytoplasm described as containing mulberry-like vacuoles. In frozen sections the cells do not stain positively for lipid until after mordanting with potassium bichromate. The lipid is a diaminophosphatide, sphingomyelin, but neutral fat and other lipids may be present. The cells are principally reticulo-endothelial, but endothelial cells may also be affected. The foamy cells are found in many situations including spleen, liver, lymph nodes, adrenal, kidney, lung, pancreas, endocrine glands, bones and marrow, aorta and adventitial cells of loose connective tissue. They may be present in the brain to resemble Tay-Sachs amaurotic idiocy, but Thannhauser considers the two diseases to be separate. (See Bloom.)

There are descriptions of typical cases, but variations from type are not infrequent both clinically and as to exact lipid concerned. Furthermore, there are reticulo-endothelioses without lipid deposits such as Litterer-Siwe disease, which occurs in infants and young children, with hepatosplenomegaly, enlarged lymph nodes, osseous defects and cutaneous petechiae or purpura (see Abt and Denenholz).

Tumors

The principal primary tumor is the reticulum-cell sarcoma discussed with the lymphosarcomas. This may rarely be associated with monocytic leukemia.

REFERENCES

Abt, A. F., and E. J. Denenholz: Litterer-Siwe's Diseases, Amer. Jour. Dis. Child., **51:** 499, 1936.

Alsted, G.: Chlorosis. Essential Juvenile Iron Deficiency Anemia, Amer. Jour. Med. Sci., **201:** 1, 1941.

Aschoff, L.: The Reticulo-Endothelial System, Lectures on Pathology, New York, 1924.

Baehr, G., and P. Klemperer: Giant Follicle Lymphoblastoma; Benign Variety of Lymphosarcoma, New York State Jour. Med., **40:** 7, 1940.

Baldridge, C. W., and C. D. Awe: Lymphoma: A Study of One Hundred and Fifty Cases, Arch. Int. Med., **45:** 161, 1930.

Batts, M., Jr.: Multiple Myeloma: Review of Forty Cases, Arch. Surg., **39:** 807, 1939.

Berstein, A.: Infectious Mononucleosis, Medicine, **19:** 85, 1940.

Bethell, F. H.: Lymphogenous (Lymphatic) Leukemia, Jour. Amer. Med. Asso., **118:** 95, 1942.

Bigg, E.: Spleen Size in Pernicious Anemia, Ann. Int. Med., **14:** 277, 1940.

Blankenhorn, M. A.: The Bile Content of the Blood in Pernicious Anemia, Arch. Int. Med., **19:** 344, 1917.

Bloom, W.: The Histogenesis of Essential Lipoid Histiocytosis (Niemann-Pick's Disease), Arch. Path., **6:** 827, 1928.

Bloor, W. R., and D. J. MacPherson: The Blood Lipoids in Anemia, Jour. Biol. Chem., **31:** 79, 1917.

Brown, G. E., and G. M. Roth: The Anemia of Chronic Nephritis, Arch. Int. Med., **30:** 817, 1922.

Büngeler, W.: Die experimentelle Erzeugung von Leukämie und Lymphosarkom durch chronische Indolvergiftung der Maus, Frankfurt Zeitschr. Path., **44:** 202, 1933.

Callender, G. R.: Tumors and Tumor-like Conditions of the Lymphocyte, the Myelocyte, the Erythrocyte and the Reticulum Cell, Amer. Jour. Path., **10:** 443, 1934.

Cannon, P. R., R. B. Baer, F. L. Sullivan, and J. R. Webster: The Influence of Blockade of the Reticulo-Endothelial System on the Formation of Antibodies, Jour. Immunol., **17:** 441, 1929.

Castle, W. B., W. C. Townsend, and C. W. Heath: Observations on the Etiological Relationship of Achylia Gastrica to Pernicious Anemia. III. The Nature of the Reaction between Normal Human Gastric Juice and Beef Muscle Leading to Clinical Improvement and Increased Blood Formation, etc., Amer. Jour. Med. Sci., **180:** 305, 1930.

Chapman, E. M.: Osteosclerotic Anemia, ibid., **185:** 171, 1933.

Clifton, W. M., A. Frank, and S. Freeman: Osteopetrosis (Marble Bones), Amer. Jour. Dis. Child., **56:** 1020, 1938.

Colmer, M. L., and W. L. Mersheimer: Relation of Splenic Extract to Etiology of Essential Thrombopenia, Arch. Surg., **43:** 422, 1941.

Cooke, J. V.: Acute Leukemia in Children, Jour. Amer. Med. Asso., **101:** 432, 1933.

Craver, L. F., and M. M. Copeland: Lymphosarcoma in Bone, Arch. Surg., **28:** 809, 1934.

Custer, R. P., and E. B. Krumbhaar: The Histopathology of the Hemopoietic Tissues in Hemophilia, Amer. Jour. Med. Sci., **189:** 620, 1935.

Dameshek, W., and S. O. Schwartz: Acute Hemolytic Anemia (Acquired Hemolytic Icterus, Acute Type), Medicine, **19:** 231, 1940.

Darling, R. C., F. Parker, Jr., and H. Jackson, Jr.: The Pathological Changes in the Bone Marrow in Agranulocytosis, Amer. Jour. Path., **12:** 1, 1936.

Dickson, W. E. C.: The Bone Marrow. A Cytological Study, London and New York, 1908.

———: The Bone Marrow, Internatl. Clinic, **17(2):** 299, 1907.

Diggs, L. W.: Siderofibrosis of the Spleen in Sickle Cell Anemia, Jour. Amer. Med. Asso., **104:** 538, 1935.

Doan, C. A., and B. K. Wiseman: The Monocyte, Monocytosis and Monocytic Leukosis: A Clinical and Pathological Study, Ann. Int. Med., **8:** 383, 1934.

Dobriner, K., and C. P. Rhoads: Metabolism of Blood Pigments in Pernicious Anemia, Jour. Clin. Invest., **17:** 95, 1938.

Donhauser, J. L., and W. H. deRouville: Multiple Myeloma, with Special Reference to Soft Tissue Metastasis, Arch. Surg., **43:** 946, 1941.

Ebert, R. V., E. A. Stead, Jr., and J. G. Gibson, 2d: Response of Normal Subjects to Acute Blood Loss, with Special Reference to the Mechanism of Restoration of Blood Volume, Arch. Int. Med., **68:** 578, 1941.

Ellermann, B.: The Leucosis of Fowls and Leucemia Problems, London, 1922.

Ewing, J.: Neoplastic Diseases, Philadelphia and London, Saunders, 4th ed., 1940.

Foot, N. C.: The Endothelial Phagocyte. A Critical Review, Anat. Record, **30:** 15, 1925.

Foster, A. K., Jr.: Mesenteric Lymphadenitis: Report of Twenty-four Cases with Tabulation Showing Relation to Appendicitis and Other Diseases; Need of Better Understanding of the Mesenteric Lymph Nodes, Arch. Surg., **38:** 131, 1939.

Fowler, W. M.: Hereditary Pseudo-Hemophilia, Amer. Jour. Med. Sci., **193**: 191, 1937.

Furth, J.: Transmission of Myeloid Leukemia of Mice. Its Relation to Myeloma, Jour. Exper. Med., **61**: 423, 1935.

——, H. R. Seibold, and R. R. Rathbone: Experimental Studies on Lymphomatosis of Mice, Amer. Jour. Cancer, **19**: 521, 1933.

Gall, E. A., H. R. Morrison, and A. T. Scott: The Follicular Type of Malignant Lymphoma; A Survey of 63 Cases, Ann. Int. Med., **14**: 2073, 1941.

Goldzieher, M. A.: The Structure of Infectious Splenic Swelling, Arch. Path. and Lab. Med., **3**: 42, 1927.

Gutman, A. B., D. H. Moore, E. B. Gutman, V. McClellan, and E. A. Kabat: Fractionation of Serum Proteins in Hyperproteinemia, with Special Reference to Multiple Myeloma, Jour. Clin. Invest., **20**: 765, 1941.

Haden, R. L.: Mechanism of Increased Fragility of Erythrocytes in Congenital Hemolytic Icterus, Amer. Jour. Med. Sci., **188**: 441, 1934.

——: The Red Cell Mass in Polycythemia in Relation to Diagnosis and Treatment, Trans. Asso. Amer. Physicians, **53**: 139, 1938.

Ham, T. H., and W. B. Castle: Relation of Increased Hypotonic Fragility and of Erythrostasis to the Mechanism of Hemolysis in Certain Anemias, Trans. Asso. Amer. Physicians, **50**: 127, 1940.

Harrop, G. A.: Polycythemia, Medicine, **7**: 291, 1928.

Heath, C. W., and A. J. Patek, Jr.: The Anemia of Iron Deficiency, Medicine, **16**: 267, 1937.

Hill, J. M., and C. N. Duncan: Leukemoid Reactions, Amer. Jour. Med. Sci., **201**: 847, 1941.

Jackson, H.: The Relation of Amidopyrin and Allied Drugs to the Etiology of Agranulocytic Angina, Amer. Jour. Med. Sci., **188**: 482, 1934.

Jaffé, R. H.: Reticulo-endothelial System: Its Rôle in Pathologic Conditions in Man, Arch. Path. and Lab. Med., **4**: 45, 1927.

——: The Bone Marrow, Jour. Amer. Med. Asso., **107**: 124, 1936.

Jeghers, H. J., J. D. Houghton, and J. A. Foley: Weil's Disease: Report of a Case with Postmortem Observations and Review of Recent Literature, Arch. Path., **20**: 447, 1935.

Josephs, H. W.: Anemia of Infancy and Early Childhood, Medicine, **15**: 307, 1936.

Kandel, E. V.: Chloroma. Review of the Literature from 1926 to 1936 and Report of 3 Cases, Arch. Int. Med., **59**: 691, 1937.

Kracke, R. R.: Diseases of the Blood and Atlas of Hematology, 2d ed., Philadelphia, Lippincott, 1941.

Krumbhaar, E. B.: A Classification and Analysis of Clinical Types of Splenomegaly Accompanied by Anemia, Amer. Jour. Med. Sci., **150**: 227, 1915.

——, and H. D. Krumbhaar: The Blood and Bone Marrow in Yellow Cross Gas (Mustard Gas) Poisoning, Jour. Med. Res., **40**: 497, 1919.

——: Functions of the Spleen, etc., Physiol. Rev., **6**: 160, 1926.

——: The Lymphomatoid Diseases, Jour. Amer. Med. Asso., **106**: 286, 1936.

Lane, C. W., and M. G. Smith: LXXXIV.—Cutaneous Manifestations of Chronic (Idiopathic) Lipoidosis (Hand-Schüller-Christian Disease). Report of Four Cases, Including Autopsy Observations, Arch. Dermat. and Syph., **39**: 617, 1939.

Lederer, M.: Three Additional Cases of Acute Hemolytic (Infectious) Anemia, Amer. Jour. Med. Sci., **179**: 228, 1930.

Lewis, M. R., and W. H. Lewis: The Transformation of White Blood Cells into Clasmatocytes (Macrophages), Epithelioid Cells, and Giant Cells, Jour. Amer. Med. Asso., **84**: 798, 1925.

Lundsgaard, C., and D. D. Van Slyke: Cyanosis, Medicine, **2**: 1, 1923.

Major, R. H.: A Thymus Tumor Associated with Acute Lymphatic Leukemia, Johns Hopkins Hosp. Bull., **29**: 206, 1918.

Mallory, F. B.: The Principles of Pathologic Histology, Philadelphia, 1914.

Maximow, A. A.: A Text-Book of Histology, Philadelphia, 1930.

Meleney, H. E.: The Histopathology of Kala-Azar in the Hamster, Monkey and Man, Amer. Jour. Path., **1**: 147, 1925.

Mettier, S. R.: Hematologic Aspects of Space Consuming Lesions of the Bone Marrow (Myelophthisic Anemia), Ann. Int. Med., **14**: 436, 1940.

Michael, P.: Gelatinous Degeneration of the Bone Marrow, Jour. Path. and Bacteriol., **33**: 533, 1930.

Michelson, H. E., and E. M. Rusten: II. The Superficial Lymph Glands in Early Syphilis, Arch. Derm. and Syphil., **25**: 457, 1932.

Minot, G. R., and Buckman, T. E.: Certain Aspects of Polycythemia, Jour. Amer. Med. Asso., **80**: 1954, 1923.

——, and R. Isaacs: Lymphoblastoma (Malignant Lymphoma): Age and Sex Incidence, Duration of the Disease, and the Effect of Roentgen-ray and Radium Irradiation and Surgery, Ibid., **86**: 1185, 1926.

——, and W. P. Murphy: Treatment of Pernicious Anemia by a Special Diet, Ibid., **87**: 470, 1926.

Nettleship, A.: On Infectious Mononucleosis, Proc. Soc. Exp. Biol. and Med., **49**: 116, 1942.

Nickerson, D. A., and D. A. Sunderland: The Histopathology of Idiopathic Thrombocytopenic Purpura Hemorrhagica, Amer. Jour. Path., **13**: 463, 1937.

Opie, E. L.: Experimental Study of the Leucemias and Lymphomata, A Review, Medicine, **7**: 31, 1928.

Paul, J. T.: The Effect of Splenic Extracts from Cases of Essential Thrombocytopenic Purpura on the Platelets and Hematopoietic Organs of Rabbits, Jour. Lab. and Clin. Med., **27**: 754, 1942.

Peabody, F. W.: The Pathology of the Bone Marrow in Pernicious Anemia, Amer. Jour. Path., **3**: 179, 1927; *see also* C. A. Doan, Jour. Exper. Med., **43**: 289, 1926.

——, and G. O. Broun: Phagocytosis of Erythrocytes in the Bone Marrow with Special Reference to Pernicious Anemia, Amer. Jour. Path., **1**: 169, 1925.

Pearce, R. M., E. B. Krumbhaar, and C. H. Frazier: The Spleen and Anemia, Philadelphia, 1918.

Perla, D., and J. Marmorston: Natural Resistance and Clinical Medicine, Boston, Little, Brown, 1941; Chap. 28, The Spleen and Resistance, p. 763.

Photakis, B. A.: Veränderungen der Milz bei Malaria, Virchow's Arch. Path. Anat., **271**: 194, 1929.

Pines, B., and J. Rabinovitch: Hemangioma of the Spleen, Arch. Path., **33**: 487, 1942.

Pohle, F. J., and F. H. L. Taylor: The Use of a Globulin Substance Derived from Beef Plasma as a

Local Hemostatic in Hemophilia, Jour. Clin. Invest., 17: 677, 1938.

Pons, C. A., and L. A. Julianelle: Isolation of Listerella Monocytogenes from Infectious Mononucleosis, Proc. Soc. Exper. Biol. and Med., 40: 360, 1939.

Pratt, J. H.: Purpura and Hemophilia, Osler and McCrae's Modern Medicine, Philadelphia and New York, 1915, Vol. IV, p. 687.

Reimann, H. A., and T. J. Kurotchkin: The Relationship of Fungi to Chronic Splenomegaly of Unknown Origin, Amer. Jour. Med. Sci., 181: 107, 1931.

Richter, M. N., and E. C. MacDowell: Studies on Leukemia in Mice, I. The Experimental Transmission of Leukemia, Jour. Exper. Med., 51: 659, 1930; MacDowell, E. C., and M. N. Richter: Studies on Mouse Leukemia, II. Hereditary Susceptibility to Inoculated Leukemia, Jour. Cancer Res., 14: 434, 1930; Potter, J. S., and M. N. Richter: Mouse Leukemia, VIII. Continuity of Cell Lineage in Transmission Lines of Lymphatic Leukemia, Arch. Path., 15: 198, 1933.

Rowland, R. S.: Xanthomatosis and the Reticulo-Endothelial System: Correlation of an Unidentified Group of Cases Described as Defects in Membranous Bones, Exophthalmos and Diabetes Insipidus (Christian's Syndrome), Arch. Int. Med., 42: 611, 1928.

Sabin, F. R., C. A. Doan, and C. E. Forkner: Studies on Tuberculosis, Jour. Exper. Med., 52: Supplement No. 3, Dec., 1930.

Sacks, B.: The Reticulo-Endothelial System, Physiol. Rev., 6: 504, 1926.

Schmeisser, H. C.: Leukemia of the Fowl: Spontaneous and Experimental, Johns Hopkins Hosp. Reports, Series 17, Baltimore, 1915.

——, and L. C. Harris, Jr.: Multiple Necroses of the Spleen (Fleckmilz), Amer. Jour. Path., 14: 821, 1938.

Shawan, H. K.: Epidermoid Cysts of the Spleen, Arch. Surg., 27: 63, 1933.

Stamos, H. F.: Heredity in Pernicious Anemia, Amer. Jour. Med. Sci., 200: 586, 1940.

Sturgis, C. C., and R. Isaacs: Desiccated Stomach in the Treatment of Pernicious Anemia, Jour. Amer. Med. Asso., 93: 747, 1929. See also Sturgis, C. C.: Middleton Goldsmith Lecture of the New York Pathological Society, October 18, 1930, Lancaster, 1931.

Sugarbaker, E. D., and L. F. Craver: Lymphosarcoma: A Study of 196 Cases with Biopsy, Jour. Amer. Med. Asso., 115: 17, 112, 1940.

Sweany, H. C.: On Nature of Calcified Lesions, with Special Reference to Those in the Spleen, Amer. Jour. Roentgenol., 44: 209, 1940.

Symmers, D.: Primary Hemangiolymphoma of the Hemal Nodes; an Unusual Variety of Malignant Tumor, Arch. Int. Med., 28: 467, 1921.

Tarr, L., and H. W. Ferris: Multiple Myeloma Associated with Nodular Deposits of Amyloid in the Muscles and Joints and with Bence-Jones Proteinuria, Arch. Int. Med., 64: 820, 1939.

Thannhauser, S.: Lipidoses: Diseases of the Cellular Lipid Metabolism, Oxford Medicine, New York, Oxford Univ. Press, 1940; Chapter VII-A, p. 214.

——, and H. Magendantz: The Different Clinical Groups of Xanthomatous Diseases; A Clinical and Physiological Study of Twenty-two Cases, Ann. Int. Med., 11: 1662, 1938.

Thompson, W. P.: The Pathogenesis of Banti's Disease, Ann. Int. Med., 14: 255, 1940.

Tileston, W.: Hemolytic Jaundice, Medicine, 1: 355, 1922.

Warthin, A. S.: A Case of Ayerza's Disease, etc., Trans. Asso. Amer. Phys., 34: 219, 1919, p. 67.

——: The New Pathology of Syphilis, Harvey Lectures, Philadelphia, Lippincott, 1917-19.

——: Diseases of the Lymphatic System, Osler and McCrae's Modern Medicine, Philadelphia and New York, 1915, Vol. IV, p. 729.

——: A Contribution to the Normal Histology and Pathology of the Hemolymph Glands, Jour. Med. Res., 6: 3, 1901.

——: The Changes Produced in the Hemolymph Glands of the Sheep and Goat by Splenectomy, Hemolytic Poisons and Hemorrhage, ibid., 7: 435, 1902.

Weber, F. P.: Polycythemia, Erythrocytosis, and Erythraemia (Vaquez-Osler Disease), London, 1921. See also Quart. Jour. Med., 2: 85, 1908.

Wells, H. G.: Chemical Pathology, Philadelphia, 5th ed., 1925.

Whipple, G. H.: Hemoglobin Regeneration as Influenced by Diet and Other Factors. Nobel Prize Lecture, Jour. Amer. Med. Asso., 104: 793, 1935.

——, and W. L. Bradford: Racial and Familial Anemia of Children Associated with Fundamental Disturbances of Bone and Pigment Metabolism (Cooley, von Jaksch's), Amer. Jour. Dis. Child., 44: 336, 1932.

——, F. and S. Robscheit-Robbins, and G. B. Walden, Blood Regeneration in Severe Anemia, XXI. A Liver Fraction Potent in Anemia Due to Hemorrhage, Amer. Jour. Med. Sci., 179: 628, 1930.

Winternitz, M. C.: Tuberculosis of the Spleen, Arch. Int. Med., 9: 680, 1912.

Wiseman, B. K.: Lymphatic Leukemia. Important Facts Additive to Its Clinical and Hematologic Recognition, Jour. Amer. Med. Asso., 118: 100, 1942.

——, C. A. Doan, and S. J. Wilson: The Present Status of Thrombocytopenic Purpura with Special Reference to Diagnosis and Treatment, ibid., 115: 8, 1940.

Wyandt, H., P. M. Bancroft, and L. O. Winship: Elliptic Erythrocytes in Man, Arch. Int. Med., 68: 1043, 1941.

15

The Respiratory System

THE NOSE

Congenital Anomalies

In cases of marked facial or cranial malformation the nose may be markedly deformed, cleft or absent. Stenosis or atresia of the posterior nares, absence of septum, absence or deformity of one or more turbinal processes, and deviation of septum occur. Clefts of the floor of the nose and anterior nares occur with cleft palate and harelip.

Circulatory Disturbances

Active hyperemia, particularly in the vascular turbinal processes, occurs as the result of irritants of various kinds, gaseous, particulate and organismal. This may or may not be the preliminary stage of an inflammation. Passive hyperemia occurs in connection with congestive failure of the heart, as well as with local interferences with venous drainage. Hemorrhage from the nose, or epistaxis, may be due to trauma, to active or passive hyperemia, to acute or chronic inflammation, to tumors, particularly the nasal polyp, to anemias and leukemias and to such hemorrhagic diseases as scurvy and hemophilia; it may be a prodromal sign of or accompany certain acute infectious diseases. Ulcers of various kinds including those of syphilis, tuberculosis, etc., may lead to hemorrhage. In extremely rare cases typhoid ulcers may appear in the nose and lead to hemorrhage. Hemorrhage may also represent vicarious menstruation. It may occur in chronic hypertension. Only in case of chronic ulcers, tumors and the hemorrhagic diseases is epistaxis likely to be serious.

Inflammation

Acute inflammations may be catarrhal, purulent, ulcerative and fibrinous. Acute inflammations of the nose may be accompanied by similar inflammations of adjacent mucous membranes, such as those of the accessory sinuses, conjunctiva, and middle ear. The most frequent example is the common cold. This is an upper respiratory infection due to a filterable virus. Mudd and his colleagues demonstrate that exposure of the body surface to cold leads to reflex vasocon-

440

striction and ischemia of the nose and pharynx, which possibly reduces local resistance. The first change commonly observed in the mucous membrane is hyperemia, followed rapidly by the pouring out of a considerable amount of serous or seromucous secretion. This subsequently becomes yellow and thick because of increased content of leukocytes and mucin. In the stage of serous exudation, the mucosa shows cloudy swelling of the epithelium and increase in mucin in the glandular cells, together with an infiltration of lymphoid cells into the tunica propria. Subsequently the degenerative change becomes more marked, desquamation of surface epithelium occurs, and the membrane becomes infiltrated with polymorphonuclear leukocytes. Local inflammations, with or without involvement of adjacent structures, may also be due to inhalation of irritant gases, to inhalation of large quantities of dust, and to inhalation of protein dust to which the individual is hypersusceptible, as exemplified by hay fever, etc.

Acute purulent rhinitis may be secondary to an acute catarrhal rhinitis, because of the activity of the pyogenic bacteria. It may also be primarily due to pyogenic bacteria, gonococci, or foreign bodies. It may occur in various acute infectious diseases. It is likely to be accompanied by purulent infection of the accessory air sacs. Rarely it may lead directly to meningitis, or more commonly, indirectly by way of the accessory air sacs.

The most important cause of fibrinous rhinitis is the diphtheria bacillus. This may produce an acute or chronic diphtheritic rhinitis. The latter may apparently produce no symptoms other than the viscid discharge, but serves as a focus for dissemination of diphtheria bacilli to other individuals. Fibrinous inflammations may also be caused by other organisms such as the streptococcus and pneumococcus.

Inflammations of the nose often extend to the accessory air sacs and by way of the eustachian tube to the middle ear and mastoid.

Chronic inflammations may be of the hypertrophic or the atrophic variety. In the former, the mucosa is thickened either by fibrous overgrowth or lymphoid cell infiltration, or both, in the tunica propria. It may be

diffuse throughout the nose or especially prominent in the turbinal bodies. It is not uncommonly associated with polyp formation. The discharge from the nose may be serous, mucous or purulent. Chronic atrophic rhinitis may be primary or may follow the hypertrophic form. There is considerable atrophy of the surface epithelium, often with loss of cilia and further metaplasia to form flat cells, atrophy of the glandular epithelium and the formation of a dense connective tissue in the tunica propria. The contraction of the connective tissue may lead to considerable shrinkage of the turbinal bodies. The discharge from the nose is usually thin and serous in character.

Ozena or fetid chronic atrophic rhinitis is a form of the disease characterized by foul odor and the formation of crusts. It occurs especially in wide-faced individuals. The mucosa and glands are atrophic and the surface epithelium shows metaplasia to a stratified squamous form. Believed by some to be due to a special organism, the so-called *Bacillus ozenae*, this organism is now considered to be a proteus bacillus and the odor probably due to stagnation and putrefaction of secretions. Syphilis is believed by some to be the cause but this is not constantly proved; the condition, however, is common in congenital syphilis.

Infectious Granulomata

Tuberculosis of the nose is not common but may occur in two main forms, the proliferative or the ulcerative. The latter is likely to occur in patients who are otherwise tuberculous, and may complicate tuberculosis of the pharynx and of the larynx. The proliferative type may extend from the skin through the anterior nares, or may be apparently primary. Tuberculosis of the nose is most common in the cartilaginous portion of the septum, but may also appear in the turbinal processes and even involve the bony substance. It is usually unilateral and produces no important symptoms other than obstruction to the nose and a slight secretion. The proliferative form is characterized by multiple miliary tubercles which may be restricted to a small area or may appear as a large tuberculoma.

Microscopically, the tubercles show a rich lymphoid infiltration, a moderate number of epithelioid and giant cells and relatively little disposition to caseation. The demonstration of tubercle bacilli or the infection of animals by the material is essential to the positive diagnosis of tuberculosis, for syphilis presents confusing gross and histologic pictures and is much more common in the nose than is tuberculosis. Rarely, tuberculosis of the nose of the proliferative variety, and sometimes of the ulcerative variety, may produce the symptoms and signs of ozena.

Syphilitic involvement of the nose is common. Congenital syphilis may give rise to a chronic atrophic rhinitis with foul-smelling discharge, a syphilitic ozena. There also occurs a form in which primarily there is papule formation, particularly upon the septum, followed by ulceration. The ulcers may perforate the septum and destroy a large portion of cartilaginous and bony substance. This is the usual cause of the "saddle nose" of congenital syphilis. Although chancre may appear upon the exterior of the nose it is extremely rare in the interior. Secondary lesions may involve the nose. Of greatest importance, however, is gumma within the nose which involves particularly the septum and originates usually in the periosteum or perichondrium. The breaking down of the gumma leads to ulceration which often perforates the septum. The process may give rise to pain, to foul discharge, to obstruction and to hemorrhage which may be severe. Extensive ulceration may produce the "saddle nose" of acquired syphilis.

Glanders may affect the human nose in the same manner as that of the horse. It produces a nodular growth which tends to break down and form ulcers with a yellow necrotic base. These may invade cartilage and bone with perforation of the septum. The glanders bacillus can be isolated from the profuse secretion. The mass is grossly granulomatous in character, and histologically is made up of lymphoid cells, leukocytes, and endothelial cells with distorted cytoplasm and nuclei, as described in the chapter on Infectious Granulomata. Central necrosis occurs and when ulceration follows, the picture of leukocyte infiltration becomes more pronounced.

Leprosy may affect the nose, where it is observed as the cutaneous type of leproma.

This often becomes ulcerated. Ulceration may become severe and lead to perforation of the septum and even to the production of a saddle-nose. Acid-fast bacilli are found in smears from the nose and the histologic picture shows a low-grade chronic granuloma with the typical lepra cells.

Rhinoscleroma originates usually in the posterior part of the nose and leads to a dense cellular infiltration which may extend anteriorly, but more commonly invades the pharynx and the posterior part of the mouth. The bacillus of rhinoscleroma may be recovered from discharges or identified in the material. Microscopically, the granuloma is fairly characteristic, being made up of lymphoid and plasma cells in the midst of which are numerous Mikulicz cells.

Tumors

Although true tumors and granulomas of the nose may be polypoid, they differ from the lesion called nasal polyp.

Nasal polyps, usually as an accompaniment of chronic rhinitis or sinusitis, may be sessile or may be pedunculated. The latter are attached to the lateral wall of the nose near the orifices of the accessory sinuses. They may vary in size, sometimes reaching a length of several centimeters and a width of a centimeter or more. They are smooth of surface, soft and of gelatinous character. Microscopically, loose connective tissue is separated by edematous fluid, often associated with infiltrations of neutrophilic and of eosinophilic leukocytes. Polyps probably originate as a productive inflammation, which by some is thought to be hyperergic. In some instances glandular acini are numerous enough to suggest a true adenoma and in others the mass may be angiomatous. Generally, however, they are merely masses of edematous connective tissue covered by columnar epithelium which may show metaplasia.

Benign tumors of the nose include chondroma, osteofibroma, osteoma, and dermoid cysts. These, however, are comparatively rare.

The sarcomas include particularly the round-cell sarcoma, the spindle-cell sarcoma, and angiosarcoma. The round-cell sarcoma is the most common and is likely to begin in the posterior part of the nose or in the soft palate, rapidly extending posteriorly and anteriorly. Carcinoma simplex, adenocarcinoma and even squamous cell carcinoma may occur in the nose. The adenocarcinoma is often made up of cuboidal cells suggesting origin from the basal cells of the mucosa. Highly anaplastic, richly cellular tumors, containing principally round cells are encountered and are believed to be epithelial. Sometimes called lymphoepithelioma (Ewing), or transitional cell carcinoma, this tumor is usually a carcinoma simplex. Metastasis of nasal carcinoma rarely extends beyond the lymph nodes of the neck.

Accessory Air Sacs

These are usually involved together with the nose in acute and chronic inflammations. Although sphenoid and ethmoid cells may be attacked, the antra of Highmore and the frontal sinuses are more frequently involved. Usually they drain well and no further trouble results. If drainage be poor the infected secretion remains and may lead to hydrops (seromucous secretion), or to empyema, both of which are commoner in the antra than in the frontal sinuses. Ash classifies the inflammations as infectious, allergic and combined. He notes the infrequency of suppurative inflammation and draws attention to marked increase of stroma in chronic inflammations; there may be hyperplastic lymphoid nodules and sometimes cystic dilatation of pseudo-glands which may become abscesses.

Tumors are much the same as in the nose.

Parasites

Of the parasites, *Rhinosporidium seeberi,* although uncommon outside of India, is of importance. These endosporulating organisms are found in inflammatory polypoid structures situated usually upon the septum at the junction of bony and cartilaginous portions (Caldwell and Roberts).

LARYNX AND TRACHEA

Congenital Malformations

Various cartilages as well as the entire larynx may be hypoplastic or absent. There may be atresia of the larynx, and also membranous bands leading to stenosis. Outpouching of the ventricle of the larynx may be apparent upon external examination of the neck. The trachea may be the seat of stenosis or atresia, the latter occurring usually at the upper end and often with an esophageal fistula. Occasionally, there are two main bronchi to the right lung. Failure of complete obliteration of the branchial clefts may produce external fistulae, branchiogenic cysts or fistulae between the skin surface and either pharynx or trachea.

Circulatory Disturbances

Passive hyperemia due to general or local causes is of particular importance in producing chronic catarrhal inflammation. Dilated veins may rupture and produce hemorrhage. Edema of the larynx may be due to passive hyperemia, to local irritation or inflammation. It produces difficulty of respiration and may lead to death from asphyxia. The process is found in the lower surface of the epiglottis, the vocal cords and the tissues over the upper margins of the laryngeal cartilages. The submucous connective tissue is especially involved and the affected areas are swollen, soft, doughy and either pale or red, depending on whether or not inflammation is present.

Inflammation

The causes of acute catarrhal inflammation are essentially the same for the larynx and trachea as for the nose, and are often secondary to catarrhs of the nose and pharynx. The process accompanies numerous acute infectious diseases. It occurs in the trachea and bronchi in pertussis, and microscopically bacilli morphologically identical with the Gengou bacilli are found enmeshed between the epithelial cilia. Acute catarrh of the larynx may also be due to prolonged and strenuous use of the vocal organs. The acute catarrhs of the larynx produce hoarseness or aphonia. The gross and histologic pictures are characteristic of acute catarrhal inflammation. Chronic catarrhs are much more likely to be hypertrophic than atrophic.

Acute fibrinous inflammation of the larynx is usually diphtheritic, usually secondary to diphtheria of the fauces or nose but occasionally primary. Similar inflammations may be due to measles, typhoid fever and other infections. It produces marked difficulty in respiration and even asphyxial death. The fibrinous pseudomembrane covers false and true vocal cords, extends down into the larynx and not infrequently also into the trachea and bronchi. It is usually more firmly adherent in the larynx than in the trachea. It is gray or yellow, smooth or slightly roughened, fairly dense but friable.

Microscopically, it is made up of a fibrin net extending as far down as the base-

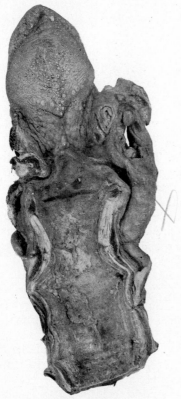

Erosions and inflammation of trachea and bronchi due to "mustard gas" inhalation. Army Medical Museum 2792.

ment membrane and enmeshing leukocytes, lymphocytes, desquamated and necrotic epithelium and various bacteria including the diphtheria bacillus. True croup, due to fibrinous laryngitis, must be distinguished from spasmodic croup, occurring in children in paroxysms of relatively short duration and believed to be due to spasmodic stenosis of the glottis.

Acute purulent laryngitis is usually due to ulceration, such as may accompany tuberculosis, syphilis, typhoid fever, to trauma or to extension from neighboring suppurations. It may be limited to the mucous membrane or be complicated by suppurative perichondritis.

Infectious Granulomata

Tuberculosis of the larynx is practically always secondary to pulmonary tuberculosis. The disease may involve the larynx as multiple, small, superficial ulcers, most frequent in the lower part of the epiglottis or as deeper ulcers of the larynx itself, especially about the posterior superior part of the organ. In other cases they are larger, solitary or few in number, deep, with necrotic or caseous base, and irregular, somewhat undermined margins; miliary tubercles may be seen in the base or near the margins. Hoarseness or aphonia are caused either by ulceration of the vocal cords or catarrhal inflammation secondary to the ulcers. Deep penetration may produce a tuberculous perichondritis. Multiple small tubercles, or tuberculous granulation tissue, originating in deeper connective tissue may produce nodules which project into the lumen of the larynx. Looper and Schneider show that tuberculosis of the larynx is secondary to pulmonary tuberculosis. Infection is carried to the larynx by the sputum but may be transferred by blood or lymph vessels.

Multiple miliary tubercles are not rare in the trachea, usually associated with a chronic catarrhal inflammation. Superficial or deep ulcers also occur.

Syphilis. In the secondary stages of syphilis, the larynx may be affected either by papules or superficial ulcers similar to those observed in the mucous membranes elsewhere. These usually heal without leaving subsequent scarring of any significance. In late syphilis, the lesion may be either a diffuse submucous inflammation of gummatous character, or single, and sometimes multiple nodular gumma, usually beginning within the deeper connective tissue. The gummata are usually small and flat because of necrosis and ulceration, but may project into the larynx sufficiently to produce obstruction. The gummatous ulcers are moderately deep, usually with sharp indurated margins, although in some cases, particularly when secondary infection occurs, the margins may become ragged and undermined. Syphilitic lesions are usually in the upper part of the larynx, not infrequently involving also the base of the epiglottis, but the lower part of the larynx may also be attacked. The vocal cords may be the seat simply of a secondary inflammation or may be in part, or entirely, destroyed by the ulcerative process. Hemorrhage is usually slight but may be severe and even fatal. The deeper ulcers may extend into the cartilage and sometimes into the surrounding tissues of the larynx. Healing of the process, either spontaneously or under treatment, may

Tumors

Squamous Cell Papilloma. The commonest tumor is the squamous cell papilloma which usually originates near or in the anterior commissure of the vocal cords. It may be either single or multiple, either sessile or pedunculated. It constitutes a small, red, moderately firm mass with the usual mulberry-like surface. Microscopically, the supporting connective tissue may be either in broad or in very delicate bands, usually fairly well vascularized and covered with stratified squamous epithelium. The design of the

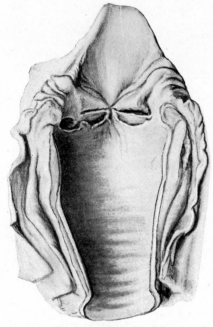

Syphilitic ulcer of larynx involving vocal cords.

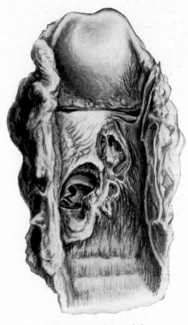

Ulcerating gummata of larynx and upper part of trachea.

lead to serious contraction of the scar so as to distort the larynx, or if the process extend into the surrounding tissue may lead to displacement of the larynx. Islands of epithelium between scarred areas may proliferate to form polypoid outgrowths.

Syphilis may involve the trachea in much the same fashion as the larynx and there is sometimes an extension from the larynx. Cicatrization may lead to distortion of the tube.

Leprosy may produce nodular and ulcerative lesions in the larynx and the scar formed after healing may constrict or distort the organ. Glanders, rhinoscleroma, and actinomycosis occasionally involve the larynx.

papillae may be so intricate that pearl formation is observed. If placed in fixative promptly, mitotic figures may be seen. The benign growth, however, shows no invasion of the papillary supporting framework or of the underlying laryngeal tissue. It is especially common in singers and others who use the voice a great deal and frequently originates upon a basis of chronic inflammation. It tends to recur after excision.

Polypoid tumors, also fairly common, may have as base a fibroma, a chronic inflammatory type of connective tissue or an adenomatous proliferation of mucous glands. They are covered by stratified squamous epithelium when originating in the false or true vocal cords, or by columnar epithelium in those parts of the larynx where columnar epithelium occurs normally. The epithelial covering usually shows a fairly straight line of basement membrane. Amyloid infiltration sometimes occurs as an isolated process in the larynx, where it may diffusely involve the connective tissue under the mucous membrane or may occur in a nodular, tumor-like form, the so-called amyloid tumor.

Carcinoma of the larynx may originate directly from the surface, from glandular epithelium, or be a malignant change in a squamous papilloma. It is often a projecting nodular ulcerated mass, or may be almost entirely an eroding tumor. The vocal cords are likely to be primarily involved when the process is derived from a squamous papilloma. The projecting forms may give rise to serious obstruction of the larynx whereas the ulcerative forms may produce principally hoarseness, aphonia and cough. Microscopically, it is usually squamous cell carcinoma but there may be extensive proliferation of connective tissue producing a scirrhous type of growth. Although a combination with tuberculosis and syphilis is possible, it is extremely unusual, and in one of our cases foreign-body giant-cell formation about the cancer pearls was confused with a granuloma. Metastasis is late and usually involves only the cervical lymph nodes. Submaxillary nodes may be involved and in some cases wide dissemination occurs. Cylindrical-cell carcinoma originating in the surface and glandular epithelium is extremely rare. When sarcoma occurs, which is also extremely rare, it is usually a spindle-cell sarcoma which may be of nodular form. Various forms of small round-cell sarcoma are also reported. It is probable that many of the latter are really lymphosarcomata originating in pre-existing lymphoid tissue of the larynx.

Tumors of the trachea are very uncommon. Among the benign forms are included ecchondrosis of the tracheal rings, ecchondroma of the submucous tissue, osteoma probably originating upon the same basis (see D'Aunoy and Zoeller). Of the malignant tumors which are also extremely rare, carcinoma is most frequent (Breslich), appearing usually as the squamous-cell carcinoma, probably originating in islands of squamous epithelium either of congenital origin or as the result of metaplasia following injury. Sarcoma is also rare (Weinberg). Secondary tumors are decidedly unusual. In our experience the most common secondary invasion is direct extension of carcinoma of the esophagus into the trachea or bronchi.

Foreign Bodies

Foreign bodies include particles of food which gain entrance to the larynx, more especially in individuals with paralysis of throat muscles and in the insane, or due to carelessness on the part of children. Fragments of tumors of the tongue and of the larynx itself may produce obstruction. Very rarely, calculi are observed in the ventricles, forming in accumulated secretion. The muscular tissue of the larynx may be invaded by *Trichinella spiralis*.

BRONCHI

Inflammation

Acute catarrhal bronchitis is due to essentially the same causes as those given for acute rhinitis and acute laryngitis. The mucous membrane is thick, velvety, red and obscures the underlying muscle markings. The exudate upon the surface may be thin and serous, seromucous, or mucopurulent, depending upon the severity and duration of the disease. Except in infants, children and the aged, it usually runs a limited course and leads to recovery. When affecting the extremes of life, or complicating such diseases as measles or pertussis, it may extend into the smaller bronchi and bronchioles to produce the so-called capillary bronchitis or bronchiolitis. Occasionally this may lead to death from suffocation because of the accumulation of exudate in the bronchioles but is more often of importance because it may be the preliminary stage of a bronchopneumonia. Whereas in the larger bronchi there is an accumulation of exudate and desquamated epithelium upon the surface, in the smaller bronchi and bronchioles a similar amount of exudate may reduce the lumen considerably. Acute fibrinous bronchitis is usually the result of extension downward from a laryngeal diphtheria.

The microscopic examination shows the usual picture of acute fibrinous inflammations which in the smaller bronchi may extend laterally and involve the peribronchial lymphatics. A fibrinous bronchopneumonia may be produced either by aspiration or by direct extension. A fibrinous bronchitis of the smaller bronchi and bronchioles may result from extension of a fibrinous pneumonia into the bronchi. Very rare cases of acute fibrinous bronchitis of unknown origin are reported. They extend widely throughout the bronchi and produce fibrinous casts of the tubes. Acute purulent bronchitis may follow acute catarrhal bronchitis, usually because of infection by pyogenic bacteria. Acute gangrenous bronchitis may follow any of the forms enumerated. This is due to invasion by saprophytic organisms. The process invades the wall of the bronchi, with subsequent necrosis, and produces by its destruction of cartilage and muscle, as well as the sloughing out of necrotic material, a local or widespread acute dilatation or bronchiectasis.

Chronic Bronchitis. This is usually catarrhal. It may be due to repeated attacks of acute bronchitis, to prolonged exposure to irritant dusts and gases, or to prolonged passive hyperemia. It is a common accompaniment of chronic ulcerative tuberculosis, and of bronchiectasis. Grossly, the mucosa is usually thick, dense, often red and sometimes pallid. The thickening usually obscures the bands of muscle and sometimes the rings of cartilage. In some instances the mucosa is thinned and translucent. It is covered with a thick, tenacious, mucinous or mucopurulent exudate, and sometimes, more especially when due to passive hyperemia, intermingled with blood. Microscopically, there is a rich infiltration of lymphoid cells in the epithelial and connective tissues, usually with a considerable overgrowth of fibrous connective tissue, and in the cases due to chronic passive hyperemia there may be interstitial hemorrhage and hemosiderin pigmentation. The mucous glands are either the seat of marked mucoid degeneration or may be atrophic.

Bronchial asthma is characterized by paroxysmal attacks of dyspnea, especially expiratory and accompanied by wheezing. The sputum often contains the Curschmann spirals of mucus, desquamated epithelium with moving cilia, mononuclear eosinophils and sometimes Charcot-Leyden crystals. Some of the cases can be shown to be due to hypersusceptibility to inhaled, ingested or injected proteins, but some are apparently due to inhalation of large quantities of insoluble dusts or to chronic inflammations of the upper respiratory tract, incident to such abnormalities as deflected nasal septum, nasal polyps, enlarged tonsils, etc. When it occurs in early life it is usually due to ingestion of foods, such as milk or eggs, later either to foods or bacterial infection and, in middle age or later, to bacterial infection. With the bacterial infection there is some hypersusceptibility to the bacterial proteins, although it is possible that the absorption of bacterial products may stimulate bronchial muscle to spasm. Asthma due to parenteral injections of proteins such as horse serum may occur at any time of life, as is true also of that due to inhalation of pollens and animal effluvia. There is evidently constriction of the bronchial muscle together with edema and secretion of mucus.

Autopsy on a case of bronchial asthma may show nothing distinctive, but if the disease be prolonged there are certain associated lesions. These occur especially in medium-sized bronchi and include mucinous degeneration of lining epithelium, hyaline thickening of the basement membrane, hypertrophy of the muscle and mucinous degeneration of the glands. Fibrosis in variable degrees may be found in all coats. The bronchi may be occluded with plugs of mucin in which Curschmann spirals and Charcot-Leyden crystals may be found. There is usually a cellular exudate of lymphocytes, polymorphonuclear leukocytes, large mononuclear cells and variable numbers of eosinophils. This may be present in the wall of the bronchus, around the glands and in the mucus in the lumen. Bronchiectasis, saccular or diffuse, may be associated and there may be foci of atelectasis of the lungs. If there be emphysema or other chronic pulmonary disease, the right heart may be hypertrophic. The anatomic features of status thymolymphaticus, discussed in the chapter on Ductless Glands, are said by some to be present, but not by others. (See Thieme and Sheldon; Craige.)

Bronchial Stenosis

Obstruction to the flow of air to the bronchial system may be due to lesions in the bronchial wall, pressure from without, and foreign substances or tumors in the lumen.

The bronchial wall may be reduced in caliber by scars of old ulcers, particularly those of syphilitic and tuberculous nature, and by tumors involving the walls. Either acute or chronic inflammations of the bronchial wall may be so marked as to produce complete occlusion of small divisions. Pressure from without may be the result of disease of the lymph nodes including anthracosis, tuberculosis and tumor involvement, tumors of the mediastinum and of the lung, tumors of the esophagus, and aneurysms of the aorta. The lumen may be seriously reduced by secretion and exudate originating within the bronchial tree.

A variety of foreign bodies may be aspirated. If not dislodged they may lead to inflammation because of bacterial contamination and may result in ulceration or in perforation with subsequent inflammation of the surrounding tissue. Bronchial perforation from aneurysms, abscess, gangrenous foci or tuberculosis of the lungs, anthracosilicotic or tuberculous lymph nodes, tumor masses in the lung or lymph nodes, or esophageal carcinoma may lead to the presence in the bronchi of blood, pus, caseous material, necrotic tissue, tumor masses, or swallowed food. Partial obstruction may lead to alveolar emphysema; complete obstruction usually causes local atelectasis because of absorption of air in the lung.

Bronchiolitis fibrosa obliterans is a rare disease, which occurs more often in the young than in the old. It may be due to irritant gases, to acute infectious diseases or have no discernible cause. The bronchioles are the seat of acute fibrinous exudate, but fibrosis soon begins in the walls and progresses into surrounding tissues (La Due).

Bronchiectasis

Bronchiectasis, permanent dilatation of the bronchi, may be saccular or cylindrical, congenital or acquired, diffuse or focalized. It may be of spindle form or, if a series of sacs be present, it may be varicose. The more acute forms of bronchiectasis are due to destructive disease of the wall such as acute purulent, or acute gangrenous bronchitis. The usual chronic forms of bronchiectasis are commonly associated with a chronic catarrhal bronchitis which may undergo secondary changes following the dilatation. The diffuse

form of bronchiectasis is usually cylindrical in character and affects the lower lobes of the lungs particularly. The involved lung is nodular to the touch and upon section shows the dilated bronchi, which contain secretion or exudate, depending upon the nature and duration of the disease. In the saccular variety the sacs are usually small, but may attain considerable size; the lesions are usually confined to one or both upper lobes.

Microscopically, the dilated bronchi show a more or less severe chronic bronchitis. The mucous membrane usually shows a chronic atrophic catarrh, although occasional cases occur in which the catarrh is hypertrophic, sometimes with the formation of folds of thickened mucous membrane. The connective tissue is infiltrated with lymphoid and plasma cells and in the later stages shows considerable fibrous hyperplasia. In some instances, more particularly in the saccular form, the epithelium may show metaplasia with the formation of squamous epithelium. In the advanced cases there may be marked atrophy of the epithelium and of the glands and also of muscle and even of cartilage, so that the tube or sac is formed of a fibrous wall lined by flattened epithelium. The material within the bronchi may be simply a thick viscid mucus, mucopurulent material or pus. The movement of this material is limited by the enlargement of the bronchus and is susceptible to invasion by saprophytic organisms, and the mass and the breath have a foul odor. With suppuration and with rich invasion of saprophytic bacteria, ulceration and even perforation of the bronchial wall may occur.

Erb's studies indicate that bronchiectasis originates in an acute respiratory infection. This may involve bronchi as an ulcerative lesion, with destruction of muscle and elastic tissue of the bronchial wall and penetration of inflammation into the surrounding lung tissue. This is replaced by a granulation tissue, which in turn becomes fibrous tissue co-extensive with the destroyed area. As this process goes on, there is epithelial regeneration often with some degree of squamous metaplasia. Dilatation is often observed before there is any contraction of the fibrous tissue. The process is favored by the obstruction of foreign bodies, enlarged lymph nodes, swollen mucosa and inspissated exudate. Infection by pyogenic bacteria and especially fusospirochetal organisms is destructive and augments the process. In addition to disease originating in the walls, conditions outside the bronchi, such as local or general collapse of the lung, and destructive disease in the neighborhood may favor bronchiectasis (see Ogilvie). Local dilatations may be caused by retraction of scar tissue.

The congenital forms of bronchiectasis are of two main varieties. In the one form there is failure of development of the alveolar sacs associated with enlargement of the members of the bronchial tree. This is usually a cylindrical enlargement with little or no inflammation of the bronchi. It is ordinarily discovered only accidentally, rather than because of any symptoms, and as a rule is limited to one lobe although it may be more widespread. In the other form such as that described by Koeckert, the alveoli show complete failure of development and the bronchus grows out from the primary tube as an extremely thin-walled, cyst-like mass replacing an entire lobe or an entire lung. It is therefore a balloon-like distention of an improperly developed large bronchus. It is lined by cylindrical epithelium, and shows in its wall isolated areas of cartilage and of muscle. When extensive, the condition may be incompatible with life.

Infectious Granulomata

Tuberculosis. Miliary tubercles in the mucous and submucous tissues of the bronchi are not uncommon but are more likely to appear in cases of chronic ulcerative tuberculosis than in other varieties of the disease. The work of Reichle and Frost indicates that the involvement of the bronchial lining is principally due to extension from the neighboring tissue through the spaces between the cartilages, although organisms may also be deposited upon the bronchial surface. The miliary or small conglomerate tubercles may break down to form small ulcers. In caseous bronchitis the wall may or may not show tubercles, but the lumen is partly or completely filled with an exudate made up of lymphoid, large mononuclear and desquamated epithelial cells, which rapidly becomes caseous. This is especially common in cases of caseous pneumonia with involvement of small bronchi and bronchioles. It may, however, occur in larger bronchi, to form an occluding caseous gelatinous mass. When the larger bronchi are involved, the epithelium is often desquamated in places, the connective tissue is the seat of subacute or chronic inflammation, and miliary tubercles may be seen. Affecting smaller bronchi, the lesion may become fibrotic and sometimes completely encapsulated. Obstruction of bronchi by a caseous mass or by fibrotic stenosis, may prevent outlet from cavities and this can apparently delay healing.

Syphilis may affect the smaller bronchi and main bronchi in essentially the same way as the trachea. The same is true of other granulomata.

LUNGS

Congenital Malformations

The most significant malformations affecting the lungs are those which really originate in the bronchi. Variations in the number and arrangement of lobes are not uncommon and accessory inferior lobes upon either or both sides are frequent. Occasionally, faults in development in alveoli are observed and we have seen one case in which throughout both lungs almost all the alveoli were sacs 1 mm. or more in diameter, supported on an excess of connective tissue. One case was observed in our laboratory in which there was complete absence of one lung and death was due to lodgment of a peanut in the main bronchus of the opposite lung. Accessory portions of lungs may be found in various parts of the thorax and indeed in the upper part of the abdomen.

Atelectasis

This term means collapse of an entire lung or part of the lung. The term collapse is often restricted to those cases in which it is known that the alveoli have previously been air-containing. A lung the seat of atelectasis is reduced in size, and increased in specific gravity and consistence. The gray color of the normal lung is due in large part to the content of air, while in atelectasis the color is dark red because of the relative increase in blood content. Since the lung does not expand and collapse as in normal respiration, a certain amount of stagnation of blood occurs and the color may be blue or purple. The organ is flabby, airless and of leathery consistence. If the condition persist for a considerable time there may be an overgrowth of connective tissue so that the density and firmness and resistance to cutting increase considerably.

Microscopically, the principal change is marked reduction in size of the alveoli accompanied as a rule by an increased amount of blood in the capillaries, veins and sometimes in the arteries. When of longer duration this may be accompanied by hemosiderin pigmentation. Fibrosis begins in the supporting connective tissue of the lungs, and with atrophy and disappearance of alveolar epithelium there may be fibrous replacement of the alveoli. The same description applies to local areas of atelectasis, usually due to complete obstruction of a bronchus. The passive hyperemia may lead not only to pigmentation and fibrosis but also to edema and in some instances to a hypostatic bronchopneumonia. Atelectasis may be found in the newborn as the result of failure of air to gain access to the alveoli. Judging from appearances at autopsies, it seems probable that several weeks elapse before the lungs are entirely expanded, for in infants it is common to find small areas of atelectasis in an otherwise well distended lung.

The most important form of atelectasis in postfetal life is that due to compression. Usually this is the result of accumulation of fluid or air in the pleura, including the transudate of edema, inflammatory exudates and air which may gain access through rupture of the lung, or by traumatic perforation of the thoracic wall. Tumors in the pleura, tumors of the mediastinum, thoracic aneurysm and extreme enlargement of the heart may also compress the lung. Deformity of the thorax, such as that produced by kyphoscoliosis of the thoracic spine, may lead to moderate degrees of compression atelectasis. The same is true of deformity of the thorax due to the diaphragm being pushed upward by such conditions as ascites, gaseous distention of the stomach and intestines and abdominal tumors and swellings. Localized areas of acquired atelectasis are usually due to obstruction in the bronchial tree, such as may be due to foreign bodies, exudates and inflammatory swelling of the mucous mem-

branes, etc. The air in the atelectasis tends toward, but does not reach, gaseous equilibrium with venous blood and quantitatively is ultimately entirely absorbed by the blood (Coryllos and Birnbaum).

The important functional significance of atelectasis is seen in reduced vital capacity and in failure or reduction of gas interchange in the affected part of the lung. Owing to the large factor of safety in functional capacity of the lung, important manifestations due to these changes are not observed unless the collapse is extensive. The fact that a considerable part of the lung tissue may be destroyed in chronic disease, and in experimental work as much as five-sixths of the lung may be removed, the condition being compatible with normal life in both instances, indicates the great reserve capacity of these organs. In compression atelectasis the return of blood to the left atrium is somewhat reduced, so that in the general circulation there may be a fall in mean systemic arterial pressure and in pulse pressure.

Acute Massive Atelectasis. Since attention was drawn to this condition, as massive collapse of the lung, by W. Pasteur, it has been found to be a not uncommon postoperative complication. It may complicate peritonitis and the paralyses of diphtheria. Anatomically there is collapse of the air cells of the lung, usually unilateral but sometimes bilateral, extensive and often involving an entire lung. The heart and mediastinum are displaced toward the affected side. It is probably due to a vagal reflex which may cause an excess of bronchial secretion, muscular spasm or edema of the bronchi. Plugging of the tubes by secretion has been observed at autopsy. (See Scott; Lee.)

Emphysema

Broadly this term indicates an increase in the air capacity of the lung or parts of it. Acute pulmonary emphysema is exemplified in the lungs of guinea-pigs in anaphylactic shock. It is observed in man in some cases of anaphylactic death, death from drowning, traumatic and other forms of asphyxia. The lungs are distended and pale, and except for anaphylactic types are compressible. The alveoli are distended, with little or no rupture. Interstitial emphysema, an acute process, is considered later. In chronic emphysema distention is accompanied by rupture of alveolar walls to produce vesicles which may attain considerable size. The principal forms of chronic emphysema are substantive emphysema, senile emphysema and complementary emphysema.

population. There is no conclusive evidence as to its cause. Kountz and Alexander divide the various theories of cause into mechanical and degenerative. The fact that expiration is passive gives rise to the idea that obstruction in the bronchi, such as may be produced by

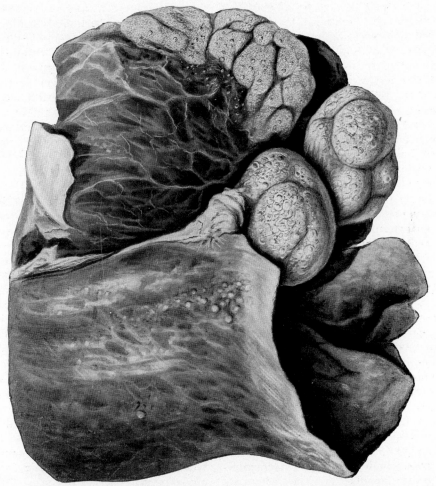

Emphysema of lungs showing well marked bullous emphysema at the margins.

Chronic Pulmonary Emphysema.
This is also called chronic substantive, chronic essential, large lung and, incorrectly, hypertrophic, emphysema. It occurs most commonly in middle-aged males. It is observed in connection with chronic bronchitis, asthma, chronic pulmonary tuberculosis, workers in irritant dusts and gases, and may occur in connection with kyphosis and other forms of fixation of the chest. It is not more frequent among glass blowers and players of wind instruments than among the general

exudate or spasm, results in less air being expired than is inspired, thus leading to alveolar distention. In contrast, it is supposed that forced inspiration may stretch the alveolar walls, or that with fixation of chest, due to calcification of costal cartilages or to kyphosis, the lungs are kept in the inspiratory position with consequent prolonged alveolar distention. Theories concerning degenerative changes in the lungs are based largely upon the occurrence of emphysema following respiratory infections, but this view is hardly tenable because the inflammations are local and the emphysema general. It is possible, however, that the emphysema of Ayerza's disease is due to nutritional deficiency as the result of arteriolar disease. Vague constitutional factors may be of importance. The reduction of elasticity may just as well be the result as the cause. Reduction of elasticity increases with age (Metz) and may account for the age incidence of emphysema.

Upon gross examination the lung is large, spongy, of cottony consistency, resists compression and is pale because of the great content of air, relatively reduced amount of blood and separation of anthracotic foci. The enlarged air spaces may be plainly visible. The anterior and inferior sharp margins may show bullae, from a few millimeters to several centimeters in diameter, due to fusion of alveoli, and blebs due to separation of pleural layers by infiltrated air. The larger bullae may not communicate with bronchi, resist high external pressure and may contain only nitrogen. The organ cuts with normal or slightly increased resistance and shows a pallid, relatively dry cross section in which individual alveoli are easily visible. Microscopically, the alveoli are large and their walls thin. Projecting into the margins of the vesicular spaces are small spurs representing the remnants of ruptured alveolar walls. Fibrosis of interstitial connective tissue can often be discerned in the less distended parts and special stains show reduction in the amount of elastica. Chronic catarrhal bronchitis is a frequent accompaniment. Interference with circulation may be marked, so that in the terminal stages passive hyperemia may be severe both grossly and microscopically, and there may be the usual changes accompanying passive hyperemia.

The chest of such patients is large and shows reduced motility. This factor, together with the reduced elasticity of the lungs, results in an increase in the dead space and a decrease of vital capacity. This leads to deficient ventilation within the lungs, which may be in part compensated for by increase in the rate of respiration. The alveolar air contains unusually large quantities of carbon dioxide and the same is true of the blood. As Scott has shown, the patients are resistant to increases in carbon dioxide in inspired air, and whether or not this be due to altera-

tion in sensitivity of the respiratory center, it can be stated very simply that the blood may show much more carbon dioxide without respiratory symptoms than in normal individuals. In discussing polycythemia it was pointed out that such alteration of ventilation in the lung may lead to increase in the circulating red cells and an increase in their individual size. The limitation of expansion and collapse of the lungs and the loss of pulmonary elasticity remove definite aids to pulmonary circulation. Stagnation is further favored by the obliteration of pulmonary capillaries. These factors lead to hypertrophy of the right heart, or cor pulmonale. Even with mechanical adequacy of circulation the reduction of the capillary bed results in a reduced gas interchange in the pulmonary blood, producing an increase in content of carbon dioxide.

Senile Emphysema. This is a small-lung type of emphysema occurring in aged individuals, and due primarily to atrophy of the alveolar walls. With the atrophy and weakening of the walls, normal respiratory pressures apparently are sufficient to produce rupture. Owing to the decrease in capillary content the lung is likely to be pale and because of the fusion of the alveoli by rupture of their walls, they may be clearly visible to the naked eye. Sometimes the large-lung type of emphysema is referred to as hypertrophic emphysema and the small-lung type as atrophic emphysema. Since the underlying condition in both is atrophy of the alveolar walls the term hypertrophic should be abandoned.

Complementary Emphysema. Sometimes the lung near atelectatic foci is emphysematous. Often, however, chronic diseases of the lungs such as tuberculosis, tumor, etc., with destruction of the lungs, are accompanied by local or widespread emphysema. Anatomically, this is like the chronic emphysema described above and probably is due to the same essential causes. This is often called compensatory emphysema, but it is incorrect to think that emphysema can be compensatory when there is reduction of elasticity and obliteration of much of the capillary bed.

Interstitial Emphysema. Air may enter the interstitial tissues of the lungs as the result of tearing of the alveoli by needle punctures, rib fractures, stab and bullet wounds and other trauma. Especially in childhood, violent coughing, as in pertussis or other acute respiratory infections, may have the same effect. The air is present in bubbles of various sizes situated in the interstitial tissue and underneath the pleura between the anatomic lobules. Sometimes it extends into the mediastinal connective tissues and may follow the cervical fascias up into the neck. In some cases it extends down over the chest and even as far as the abdominal wall. Emphysema of the thoracic wall may follow wounds and puncture by needles in aspiration of the pleura; this may be due to entry of air into the wound from the exterior and does not necessarily mean that the lung has been punctured. Wounds of the bronchi, and of the trachea as in tracheotomy, may cause interstitial emphysema. There are rare cases of mediastinal emphysema without demonstrable cause (see Caldwell).

Circulatory Disturbances

Vascular Disease. Primary thrombosis of veins and arteries occurs. Embolism is referred to below. The pulmonary arteries may show lesions in rheumatic fever and syphilis. Pulmonary arteriosclerosis is common but not necessarily related to generalized arteriosclerosis. It is present in most cases of mitral stenosis and often occurs in such diseases as chronic bronchitis, chronic emphysema and other chronic diseases of the lungs. It occurs in rare instances without known cause. (See Brenner.) Right ventricular hypertrophy does not always occur, and, in our opinion, pulmonary hypertension is not an important cause of the sclerosis (Karsner, Simon and Fujiwara). Arteriolar disease in the form of sclerosis, or more acute lesions with or without thrombosis, is rare. There is an accompanying pulmonary hypertension and right ventricular hypertrophy. The chronic disease is the anatomical basis of Ayerza's disease. (See Kaump and Dry.)

Active Hyperemia. The inhalation of irritant gases and dusts, inert or protein (in hypersensitives), the early stages of inflammation, and reduction of barometric pressure may produce active hyperemia. Asphyxia may produce active hyperemia with petechiae or larger hemorrhages. If the lung be compressed by fluid in the thorax and this is rapidly removed, the inflow of blood into the lungs is accelerated and active hyperemia results. This may lead to edema of the lungs, which in occasional instances is so severe as to be fatal.

Passive Hyperemia. Examination of the lungs at autopsy practically always shows a considerable accumulation of blood in the dependent parts of the lower lobes. This is a relatively acute form of passive hyperemia incident to failure of the circulation shortly before death. The affected portions of the lung are dark red or purple, somewhat firmer and less crepitant than normal. If the condition persist for a considerable length of time there may be small hemorrhages into the alveoli, edema, and sometimes a bronchopneumonia, referred to as hypostatic bronchopneumonia.

Much more important pathologically and clinically are those forms of passive hyperemia which are of considerable duration and involve the entire lung. Outstanding among the causes of this condition is mitral stenosis, which may produce prolonged passive hyperemia. Other valvular lesions are of importance only when the heart or the valve orifices dilate. In the early stages, the lung is large, dark red or purple in color, somewhat firmer and with less crepitation than normal. Microscopically, the capillaries as well as veins are distended with blood. Small hemorrhages, edema, and hemosiderin pigmentation in macrophages may accompany the passive hyperemia. The more chronic forms are characteristically described as "brown induration." The color is caused by deposit of hemosiderin in the lung, and the increased consistence by overgrowth of connective issue. Grossly, the lung does not collapse readily when the thorax is opened, is large, firm and of reddish-brown or "brick red" color. It cuts with increased resistance and shows a firm, dark red or reddish-brown, freely bleeding, moist cross section. Microscopically, there is distinct overgrowth of connective tissue involving the alveolar walls and the other interstitial supporting connective tissue framework. Capillaries and veins are filled and distended with blood. Many macrophages containing hemosiderin, "heart-failure cells," are found in the alveoli and often in the surrounding lymphatics. Free erythrocytes are also found and there is usually marked edema. Occasionally the alveoli contain concentrically laminated, radially striated corpora amylacea. Arteriosclerosis of the larger and smaller divisions of the pulmonary artery is common. Sometimes the pulmonary capillaries show small saccular dilatations projecting into the air spaces. Rupture of these probably accounts for blood streaked sputum or expectoration of blood.

Clinically, shortness of breath on exertion, dyspnea and reduced vital capacity occur. These are all contributed to by the slowed circulation, the distention of capillaries, the fibrosis of alveolar walls and the frequent presence of edema.

Pulmonary Edema. The fluid in the alveoli may be transudate or an inflammatory exudate. The transudates are usually due to passive hyperemia. This results principally from cardiac disease but may also be due to pulmonary disease or to compression from substances in the pleural cavity; not infrequently it accompanies nephritis; and it may be produced experimentally by injections of large quantities of adrenalin and by neuropathic disturbances of pulmonary circulation (Luisada). Circulation may be so altered following rapid withdrawal of fluid from the pleura as to cause pulmonary edema. Irritant gases also produce edema and this has been found to be especially true of certain war gases such as phosgene and chlorpicrin. When due to passive hyperemia, it is possible that there is a combination of high pressure in the pulmonary capillaries and increased permeability of their walls owing to reduced nutrition. In other instances, it appears that increased permeability is of considerably greater importance, especially where toxic factors are concerned. The lung of edema is large, pallid, pits upon pressure and sometimes is so firm as to suggest consolidation. Upon cutting, considerable frothy fluid pours out from the wet cross section, and may occupy parts of the bronchial tree. Depending upon the degree of associated hyperemia, the fluid may be colorless, salmon colored or red. In lesser degrees of edema it is necessary to press upon the lung to express the edema fluid. The histologic character of the fluid in the alveoli depends upon its content of protein and the method of fixation. It may appear either as a delicate hyaline sheet of faintly acidophilic material or as a finely granular acidophilic material. It may partly or completely fill the alveoli and extend into the infundibuli and the bronchi. Minute air bubbles are sometimes observed.

The presence of edema reduces the vital capacity and interferes with interchange of gases in the alveoli. The fact that it so commonly appears as a terminal event suggests that it is the direct cause of death. Certainly, if edema be extensive, the functional disturbance is great, but the experiments of Winternitz and Lambert make it seem probable that much larger amounts of fluid than are ordinarily observed are necessary in order to produce death.

Inflammatory edema appears in the early stage, and may also appear at any time during the course, of lobar pneumonia. It is also commonly present around areas of bronchopneumonia, and of abscess, gangrene, or other inflammatory conditions in the lung. Histologically, it may be designated as inflammatory because of its position in reference to definitely inflammatory conditions, but may show no other characteristic features. Because of its larger protein content it is likely to stain more deeply than the noninflammatory forms. When fibrin is present, the inflammatory character is evident.

Hemorrhage. Blood may appear in the lungs because of aspiration from hemorrhages in the upper respiratory tract, or from blood in the stomach which has been vomited and aspirated. Perforation of aneurysms into bronchi is a common cause of blood in the lungs. Hemorrhage may occur into the pulmonary tissue as the result of traumatism and the destruction of lung substance by inflammatory or tumor involvement. When pneumonia complicates hemorrhagic or "black" infectious diseases, the exudate may be of hemorrhagic character. Passive hyperemia, asphyxia, and the hemorrhagic diseases such as purpura may lead to hemorrhage in the lung. Of great practical importance is that variety due to erosion of blood vessels by chronic ulcerative tuberculosis, where hemorrhage may be severe and fatal.

Pulmonary Embolism. There are two chief varieties of pulmonary emboli; one in which a large branch of the pulmonary artery is occluded and the other in which small branches are occluded to produce either local

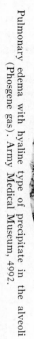

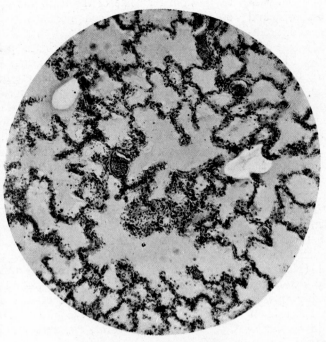

Pulmonary edema with hyaline type of precipitate in the alveoli (Phosgene gas). Army Medical Museum, 4992.

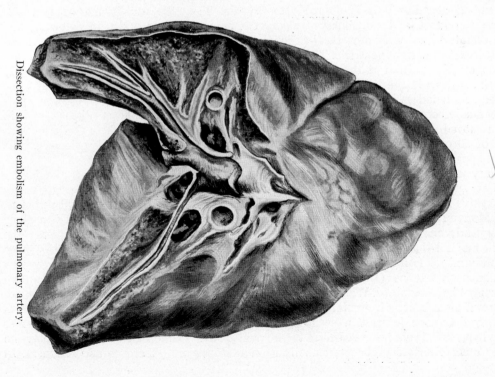

Dissection showing embolism of the pulmonary artery.

circulatory disturbance or infarction. The former is a common cause of death following septic or aseptic operations, traumatism with subsequent bland or septic thrombosis, and infective inflammation with associated thrombosis, in various parts of the body (see Mc-Cartney). A large embolus, liberated by dislodgment or disintegration of a venous thrombus, may pass through the heart and lodge in a trunk of the pulmonary artery. The same general effect may be produced by the lodgment of multiple emboli in smaller arteries. Death may ensue immediately, within the course of a few hours, or after the course of 18 or 24 hours, and occasional cases of embolism recover (Schumacher and Jehn; Mann). Immediate death is usually associated with medium-sized emboli rather than a single large embolus and is thought by some to be due to cardio-inhibitory reflex, although this view is disputed (Hall and Ettinger). Later death, usually associated with a large embolus, is probably due to anoxia of the brain or of the heart itself (Mendlowitz). It is accompanied by a shock-like fall of blood pressure and special electro-cardiographic signs. Death following a temporary period of improvement results from various factors, contributed to largely by ultimate cardiac insufficiency. To demonstrate large emboli at autopsy it is desirable to examine the heart and pulmonary trunks before removal from the body, the incision being started in the right ventricle. The large embolus originates from a thrombus in a long vein, such as in the lower extremity or the iliacs. As it lodges in the pulmonary artery, it usually becomes coiled to be occlusive. When removed and uncoiled it may have a length of 50 cm. or more. It has the usual mottled appearance of the original thrombus. Secondary red clots appear distally and sometimes proximally. The lungs usually show passive hyperemia and edema.

MULTIPLE SMALL EMBOLI, many or few, are frequently encountered at autopsy, even more in medical than in surgical cases, and are readily mistaken for primary thrombi in the pulmonary arteries (Belt). The origin often cannot be ascertained. When numerous, the general disturbance of circulation in the lung may determine infarction, even when passive hyperemia is not present. Unless there is some other circulatory change, embolism leads only to a localized region of hyperemia and edema, a condition that may well be responsible for some of the temporary post-operative pulmonary complications (Cutler and Hunt).

Pulmonary emboli originate principally in veins and in the right heart. It is rare for them to originate in the left heart, to be transferred through a patent foramen ovale (paradoxical embolism). The larger emboli are derived principally from thrombi in varicose veins in the lower extremities, from iliac veins and from vena cava. Thrombophlebitis in these vessels is also a source. Smaller emboli may come from these veins or from those of the pelvis or other situations. Surgical operations, fractures, or traumatic injury often precede the embolism but cases occur without such a history. In some instances, the venous thrombosis is due to direct injury of the veins. In some, it appears that getting out of bed dislodges thrombi that have formed during a period of rest after operation.

Embolism by fat, air, amniotic fluid and fragments of tumors has been discussed in the chapter on Disturbances of Circulation.

Pulmonary Infarction. At autopsy, infarcts of the lung are almost always hemorrhagic. They are usually moderate in size not exceeding 3 or 4 cm. in diameter, and occur most commonly in the lower lobes although larger infarcts and infarcts in other position are not infrequent. They are usually due to emboli whose source can readily be ascertained, but occasional cases occur, particularly in chronic heart disease and in chronic kidney disease, where the lesions appear to be due to thrombosis primary in the pulmonary artery.

Our studies of embolism in the dog indicate that infarction does not occur unless there is additional circulatory disturbance, such as passive hyperemia. Embolism alone leads to localized hyperemia and edema. The capillaries of the lung branch directly from arterioles and form an extraordinarily rich plexus of large capillaries susceptible to dilatation. Thus collateral circulation is sufficient to maintain nutrition, unless interfered with by other circulatory disturbance (Karsner and Ash). The bronchial arteries play no significant part (Ghoreyeb and Karsner). In man, pulmonary infarction rarely occurs unless there is passive hyperemia due to cardiac incompetency, or lesions of the pleura. Sometimes, a multitude of emboli may so disturb circulation that infarction occurs without passive hyperemia of the whole lung; sometimes when there is occlusion of the main artery to a lobe, a small infarct may be found in the periphery. The process of infarction has been described in the chapter on Disturbances of Circulation.

The usual infarct of the lung is hemorrhagic, solid, well defined, near the periphery, bulging on the outer surface, and generally of conical form. The cross section also shows a generally triangular area, truncated by the margin of the lung, with a red, slightly bulging, firm, relatively dry and sometimes friable surface. Microscopically, the alveoli are filled with blood, fresh or in various stages of degeneration and necrosis. The pulmonary tissues are slightly or extensively necrotic, depending on the duration of the lesion, and may be present as mere shadows or entirely absent. Thrombosis of vessels within the infarct is frequent. As a rule, the patient dies of his general disease while the infarcts are still hemorrhagic. Nevertheless, survival permits the development of decolorized, white infarcts of the lung, but the progress is slower than in the more solid organs. Encapsulation may occur and even complete cicatrization without residua of necrosis. With appropriate methods of study, such healed infarcts, and probably cicatrized foci of hyperemia and edema due to embolism, are not infrequent (Castleman; Hampton and Castleman). Infected emboli may produce abscesses or infected infarcts; infection may also occur in bland infarcts.

Inflammations

These may be acute or chronic. The acute forms are exudative and vary from fibrinoserous to suppurative and the formation of abscess. Except when suppurative, the term pneumonia is usually applied to inflammations of the lungs. The typical forms of pneumonia are lobar pneumonia, lobular or bronchopneumonia, and interstitial pneumonia. They run a fairly characteristic clinical course and have fairly distinctive anatomic lesions. Nevertheless, there are many instances in which the disease departs from type, both clinically and anatomically. Sometimes these are called atypical pneumonias and sometimes the term pneumonitis is used. Pneumonias are also classified etiologically, depending on the cause, be it certain bacteria, strains of bacteria, virus or some other organism. The following discussion is largely on an anatomic basis and is partly etiologic.

Lobar Pneumonia. This is a more or less self-limited infectious disease with its principal anatomic manifestations in the lungs. It is usually of abrupt onset but may be preceded by a period of cough or coryza. Invasion is frank and the disease rapidly reaches its acme or fastigium, which remains for a period usually of seven to eleven days to be followed in half the cases by crisis and in the other half by lysis. Convalescence may be interrupted by a variety of complications.

The onset is often accompanied by chill and pain in the chest, followed by fever, leukocytosis, rapid respiration and other respiratory changes, physical signs, at first of moisture in the lungs and then of consolidation. When crisis occurs the temperature rapidly falls, often with signs of collapse, and the exudate disappears. In order to render more clear the discussion of etiology and secondary effects, the morphology of the disease will be presented. Three stages are recognized in the lungs: engorgement, hepatization and resolution. Two substages of hepatization are recognized, red and gray. Resolution may be delayed, the exudate may become organized, or abscess or gangrene supervene.

THE STAGE OF ENGORGEMENT is not often observed at autopsy except as part of the process of extension of the pneumonia. The involved portion is not so sharply defined as in the later stages of hepatization. The diseased region is large, soft, red and flabby. Blood flows from the red, smooth, moist, cross section and a considerable amount of edematous fluid can be expressed. Microscopically, the capillaries and other blood vessels are markedly engorged. The alveoli and bronchioles are practically filled with edematous fluid with a few strands of fibrin, together with only a few cells, including large mononuclears, desquamated lining cells, lymphocytes, polymorphonuclear leukocytes and erythrocytes. Bacteria may also be present.

THE STAGE OF HEPATIZATION includes red hepatization and gray hepatization, but it must be understood that the stage of red hepatization is of very short duration, probably rarely lasting more than one or two days and merging rapidly into gray hepatization. Often sharp distinction between the two is impossible and mixtures are observed.

Red Hepatization. Grossly, this stage practically always shows a fibrinous exudate upon the pleura, especially over the consolidated part of the lung. Although the consolidation is lobar in distribution and affects the right lower lobe more commonly than other lobes, nevertheless, it is common to find more than one lobe involved and the process extending to a limited degree into adjacent lobes. The involved portion is large, firm, and of red, gray, or mottled color, and often shows the indentations of ribs. Crepitation is entirely absent except that the margins may sometimes contain air. The lung cuts with somewhat reduced resistance and the cross section is red, gray or mottled, and relatively dry. The dryness is not absolute, but if the cross section be gently scraped with a knife, the consolidated part shows much less moisture than the surrounding lung; this difference is slightly less marked in red than in gray hepatization. Another important feature is that the cross section is finely granular. Tiny plugs of exudate project because they do not retract as do the alveolar walls.

In gray hepatization, the acute fibrinous pleurisy is more advanced and is likely to show early organization. In addition, at this stage, there may be a moderate amount of fluid in the pleural cavity.

Microscopically, the differentiation between the exudate of red and gray hepatization is usually readily recognized, but intermediate stages exist in which an exact diagnosis is not possible. In the earlier stages of red hepatization, exudation is most pronounced in the bronchioles where desquamation of epithelium, infiltration of lymphocytes, a few leukocytes, and large mononuclear cells, together with a moderate number of red blood corpuscles enmeshed in a fluid and fibrinous exudate, are prominent. During this stage the alveoli may show little more than fluid exudation, but rapidly the same type of exudate as that seen in the bronchioles involves the infundibula and the air cells. Even in the same section, various stages of this process may be observed. Bacteria may be demonstrated in considerable numbers. The smaller blood vessels and capillaries are the seat of intense hyperemia. The bronchi may or may not be involved in the process, but typically, they show no important lesion. In this stage of consolidation the cells are not densely packed in alveoli or bronchioles.

In the stage of gray hepatization the cellular content of the exudate is vastly increased, so much so that the exudate is packed tightly within the alveoli. The cells are principally polymorphonuclear leukocytes although a considerable number of small and large mononuclear cells may still be present. These cells may show phagocytosis of bacteria and cell fragments but not to any great extent. Red blood corpuscles, present in the stage of red hepatization in moderate numbers, are practically absent in gray hepatization except as shadow cells. The involvement is fairly uniform through the alveoli and the smaller members of the bronchial tree—more uniform than in red hepatization. At this time bacteria are numerous. The arrangement of the fibrin in the alveoli is more or less characteristic in both stages although the appearance is more pronounced in the later stage. The strands are arranged irregularly but show a general disposition to radiate out from a point in the alveolar wall. The fibrin in adjacent alveoli communicates through small pores or holes in the wall, the pores of Cohn, thus giving the fibrin mass a double fan or hourglass arrangement. Miller believes the pores to be the result of desquamation of lining cells from the adjacent parts of neighboring alveoli.

In the later stages of hepatization, the fibrin tends to contract and in the microscopic section is separated from the alveolar walls. The polymorphonuclear leukocytes are reduced in number and the large mononuclear cells are increased in number; many of these phagocytose and destroy bacteria. These macrophages are much more actively phagocytic than the already degenerated leukocytes. (See Robertson.)

RESOLUTION is characterized by the solution of the exudate. In the earlier stages the lung is still consolidated but is soft and

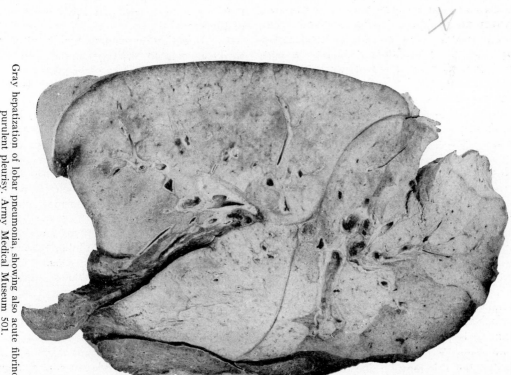

Drawing of red hepatization to show the cellular character of the exudate and the fibrin.

Gray hepatization of lobar pneumonia, showing also acute fibrino-purulent pleurisy. Army Medical Museum 501.

flabby instead of firm. The pleural exudate is reduced in amount and loose adhesions may be present as the result of organization. The color of the mass is gray or yellow and in either case may be mottled with red. The lung cuts easily but the cross section instead of being dry and granular is smooth and moist, and from it can be expressed a considerable amount of granular or somewhat slimy, semifluid remnants of the exudate. This may resemble pus grossly but is not pus. The lung substance is still friable. As the exudate is removed, partly by expectoration of the softened mass and more largely by absorption, the lung gradually contains more and more air. The exudate is finally removed and save for moderate hyperemia lasting over a few weeks, the lung is restored to normal. Microscopically, there is necrosis of the leukocytes of the exudate and solution of the fibrin. Macrophages are numerous and have taken up not only bacteria but also fragments of cells and of fibrin. Fat is present in moderate amounts. Pneumococci are recoverable both in sputum and from the exudate but are not numerous in the histologic section. The epithelium of the bronchioles and of the alveoli is renewed during the process of resolution. As far as can be determined by histologic methods the ultimate restoration is absolutely to normal. The stage of resolution is practically coincident with the crisis or beginning lysis of the clinical disease.

CAUSES OF LOBAR PNEUMONIA. Although pneumonia may spread fairly widely in given localities it is not likely to occur in great epidemics. It is more frequent in cities than in the country and in closely inhabited areas than in places where the population is dispersed. Indoor life in crowded conditions and in fact crowding under almost any conditions, such as in institutions and in army encampments, appears to predispose to the disease. Occupations which lead to considerable variations in temperatures predispose. It may affect any period of life but is more common between 30 and 50 years. It attacks males more frequently than females, probably because of occupational and other influences rather than because of sex. Negroes appear to be more susceptible than whites but this may be due to hygienic conditions rather than to racial differences.

The disease is likely to follow exposure to cold and alcoholism. In these conditions there may be factors that favor aspiration of organisms and mucus, and perhaps alteration of inflammatory reaction so that emigration of leukocytes is inhibited. (See Pickrell.) Probably similar mechanisms are effective in the pneumonia which sometimes follows general anesthesia, although this is more often bronchopneumonia than lobar pneumonia. In certain instances, trauma, especially of the chest, seems to predispose to lobar pneumonia. Coryza precedes about half the cases, but others show abrupt onset with little in the way of prodromal symptoms.

The exciting cause of typical lobar pneumonia in the great majority of cases is the *Diplococcus pneumoniae*. Similar clinically, but often less so anatomically, are pneumonias due to *Streptococcus haemolyticus, Staphylococcus aureus,* Friedländer's bacillus and other organisms. That due to Friedländer's bacillus often shows destruction of pulmonary tissue, frequently leads to abscess formation and may become chronic (Julianelle). This form and that due to type III pneumococcus will show a sticky mucinous form of exudate in the cross section of the lung.

Infection by pneumococci is not necessarily associated with pneumonia. In Finland's study of 3,682 cases of pneumococcus infection, about 15 per cent failed to show pneumonia. Of those who had lobar pneumonia, about 80 per cent were due, in descending order of frequency, to the six types, I, III, II, V, VIII and VII. The type distribution in pneumococcal bronchopneumonia or atypical pneumonia, and in the pneumonias of childhood, is somewhat different. Infection with type III is the most virulent and it is generally stated that type VIII is of low virulence. Positive blood cultures are reported more frequently in lobar than in the atypical pneumonias and predicate a high mortality rate regardless of the extent of the pneumonia.

PATHOGENESIS AND DISTRIBUTION. The fact that pneumococci are harbored in the throats of many otherwise normal people suggests that the same organisms may be transferred to the lungs and cause pneumonia. The types found in throats, however, do not correspond in rate of incidence to those found in pneumonia and are different biologically. Ordinarily these organisms are not virulent forms and do not produce disease in the host or in others. Nevertheless, after contact with pneumonia patients, or in crowded areas and institutions where endemics are under way, apparently healthy persons may harbor virulent organisms in the throat occasionally. The transfer from person to person is probably by droplet infection. The dose of organisms required for infection of experimental animals varies considerably as to species and individuals, and there is no means of knowing the dose necessary for infection of man. Inoculation into the nose of animals rarely produces pneumonia; the organisms must be introduced into the lungs.

Gunn states that it is now generally conceded that lobar pneumonia is the result of infection by the intrabronchial route. There is not adequate support for the hypothesis that lobar pneumonia is primarily a septicemia with secondary localization of the inflammatory process in the lungs. The work of Stillman and Branch with mice indicates that septicemia may develop from intrapulmonic implantation and further, that certain factors of resistance may determine the localization of the inflammation in the lung.

Experimental investigation shows that in animals the earlier lesions arise near the hilum of the lung and thence spread to involve the entire lobe. There can be no doubt that in experimental animals interstitial and lymphatic involvement is somewhat more prominent than in man. The early phases of pneumonia in man progress so rapidly and the difficulty of obtaining material at this time is so great, that it has been impossible to confirm a definite similarity between these early stages in man and the early stages in animals. Blake and Cecil interpreted their results with experimental pneumonia in monkeys as indicative of a primary interstitial infection and inflammation near the hilum, which progress by way of the lymphatics to involve the whole lobe. Robertson and his associates found in the dog an inflammation near a terminal bronchus, at first as a peribronchial and perivascular exudative and hemorrhagic inflammation with interstitial involvement. As the process advances radially from this focus, it is pre-ceded by a zone of edema, rich in bacteria, in alveoli and peritrunkal lymphatics. This is transformed into an exudative pneumonia involving the lobe. The dispersion of bacteria is at first through the tissues, but soon they appear in edematous fluid and are disseminated as the edema progresses. It is thus possible that the edema is produced as bacteria are distributed over respiratory surfaces, or that it is a reactive process which provides a fluid culture medium for the organisms. The flow from lymphatics near the pleura is toward the pleural lymphatics and this may well account for pleural inflammation.

It is likely that the advancing zone of edema, containing many organisms, accounts also for the spread of the disease in the human lung. It may be that factors of dosage, virulence and resistance are responsible for variations in spread, so that in some cases an entire lobe is quickly consolidated and in others several days may elapse before central consolidation extends to the periphery.

RESOLUTION. When the disease has progressed for some time, as a rule seven to eleven days, the exudate usually but not constantly begins to dissolve. This is quite independent of whether clinically there is crisis or lysis of the disease. Solution occurs in the exudate because of enzymes and does not affect the living tissues which, as elsewhere, are resistant to enzyme action. The exudate in the consolidated lung shows increased hydrogen-ion concentration (Lord) and contains the products of protein disintegration including a variety of amino-acids, thus showing that protein breakdown has occurred. Lord has shown that there is liberated from the cells a proteolytic enzyme capable of digesting coagulated protein and probably also capable of splitting peptone to amino-acid nitrogen, the latter activity operating over a wider range of pH concentration than the former. Avery and Cullen demonstrate enzymes in pneumococci, which act as protease, peptonase, lipase, invertase, amylase and inulase. The quantitative relation between the enzymes of the exudate and those of the pneumococci is not determined, but it seems probable that those of the exudate are of more importance. Increasing acidity of the exudate may limit the activity of the proteolytic enzymes but also to be considered is the presence of antienzyme in the blood.

With solid exudate the access of plasma is probably restricted and if, as Kline and Winternitz maintain, the circulation through the consolidated lung be diminished, there is additional reason for decreased supply of antienzyme and accordingly more free activity of the enzymes. Although the question is not finally settled, the fact that hydrogen-ion concentration is greater in the pneumonic lung than in other tissues points toward poor circulation. Kline believes that intratracheal injection of serum delays resolution, further indicating that resolution is favored by decreased access of antienzyme. Lord and Nye find that at pH 6.8 to 5.1 the pneumococcus is rapidly killed and is injured at pH 6.8 to 7.4. The increased acidity of the consolidated lung is in part due to growth of the pneumococci, which here as in culture, build up an acidity which is fatal to the organism. It is possible that immune bodies play a part. As noted above, macrophages are numerous in the stage of resolution and play a part in breaking down and removal of the exudate. (See Gunn; Robertson.)

PHYSIOLOGY. It is well known that in pneumonia the blood pressure is diminished and venous distention may be prominent. Cardiac dilatation is common, especially manifest in the right side. Probably this is due largely to degeneration or inflammation of the myocardium, but increased resistance to circulation in the consolidated lung may determine the more marked dilatation of the right heart. The carbon-dioxide combining power of the blood is usually somewhat reduced. There is, however, considerable difference of opinion and perhaps of observation concerning the oxygen content of the blood, but it appears to be true that certain cases show a decreased oxygen content and can be benefited by the administration of oxygen in the respired air (Lundsgaard). In these cases, it seems probable that the fault is not directly connected with the oxygen combining power of the blood. The pneumococcus can produce methemoglobin in the blood, but usually the acid content of the blood is not great enough to permit of this being a serious factor. The well-known retention of chlorine before crisis was shown by Peabody to be true of both sodium and calcium, but not of potassium and magnesium. Sunderman, Austin and Camac dem-

onstrated that the depression in electrolytes as a whole is followed by prompt return to normal after crisis except that the NaCl returns more slowly. The protein values are also depressed but return promptly when fever disappears. The output of organic acids is high, as is true also of ammonia, but there is little disposition to acid intoxication (see Hastings, et al.).

IMMUNITY. Immune sera have been produced in animals by the use of pneumococci, their carbohydrates, and autolysates. The type specificity of these sera has proved useful in treatment and in the laboratory identification of types of organism. The detection and titration of immune bodies in the serum of pneumonia patients aids in directing treatment. In recovering pneumonia patients Sia, Robertson and Woo found a definite increase of pneumococcidal, opsonic, agglutinating and mouse-protecting antibodies in the blood serum and infer that these are of importance in resolution of the exudate and recovery of the patients. Experimentally, local immunity appears to develop before general immunity. Gunn believes this to be due to the activity of the macrophages. Except for the temporary passive immunity due to immune sera, there has been little or no success in development of active immunity by vaccination or otherwise.

The recurrence of pneumonia is common, varying in different statistics from 13 to 31 per cent. Indeed, multiple attacks have been observed suggesting some sort of constitutional susceptibility to the disease. The fact that the convalescent patient has immune bodies in his blood evidently does not confer a durable resistance. How long this lasts is not certain, except that recurrences are infrequent before about a year has elapsed. The type of pneumococcus found in the recurrence may be the same as, or different from, that of the original attack. Nor is there evidence of local resistance, because the same or a different region of the lung may be affected. The recurrences are likely to show more extensive pulmonary involvement and be more atypical than the first attack. (See Finland and Winkler; Ruegsegger and Cockrell.)

COMPLICATIONS. Pneumonia being a general infectious disease, it is to be expected that cloudy swelling and even fatty degeneration of the parenchymatous viscera may occur. Zenker's necrosis may occur in the diaphragm and is perhaps a cause of respiratory failure (Wells). When pneumococcal septicemia develops, the prognosis is poor. Acute bacterial endocarditis is not rare in these cases. The septicemic cases are also those in which methemoglobin formation occurs. An important complication is the development of empyema as a sequel of the acute fibrinous pleurisy; this is discussed in connection with the pleura. The pleurisy may extend to pericardium and upper peritoneum. Pneumococcal meningitis may be a complication of, or a sequel of, pneumonia or may occur independently.

The complications within the lung itself include, especially, organization of the exudate, gangrene, and abscess formation. Organization of a small part of the exudate is not uncommon but only rarely does organization become coextensive with the original pneumonic process. Insofar as resolution depends upon enzymatic processes, it is possible that restoration of circulation during resolution can provide excess of antienzyme to such a degree that resolution is retarded. Into the unresolved exudate, new capillaries and fibroblasts grow from the alveolar walls. The fibroblasts grow along the scaffolding of the fibrin. Thus, the lines of organization are likely to radiate out from the general situation of the pores of Cohn and parallel the lines of fibrin in the exudate.

The production of abscess depends upon invasion by pyogenic organisms, such as staphylococcus or streptococcus. The abscesses may be single or multiple, usually the former, and are not so extensive as the original consolidation, usually being much smaller. Both grossly and microscopically, the abscess is characterized by pus formation, which leads to extensive destruction of pulmonary tissue. It is a serious and usually fatal complication, although cures have been reported by postural and surgical treatment.

Gangrene presupposes the occurrence of some necrosis in the course of the disease and subsequent to this the invasion of saprophytic organisms. The investigations of Kline indicate that pulmonary gangrene is commonly due to the activity of fusiform bacilli and spirochetes similar to those of Vincent's angina, often associated with a considerable number of other organisms. Gangrene may lead to rapid death or may become subchronic in course, somewhat resembling tuberculosis of the lungs.

Neither abscess nor gangrene necessarily depends upon pre-existing pneumonia, as they may occur independently of this process. Gangrene may occur on the basis of tuberculosis, tumors, and sometimes arises without any determinable pre-existing cause. Depending upon the situation, whether it is near the pleura or not, course of the disease, and cause of the disease, gangrene may be complicated by pleurisy which, in the earlier and less severe cases may be a simple acute fibrinous pleurisy or may become suppurative. Chronic adhesive pleurisy is likely to be found in the chronic cases of gangrene. The gross appearance of gangrene and of the abscess may at times be somewhat confusing, but practically always the foul odor and the brown or green necrotic tissue of gangrene are sufficient for the diagnosis. The odor also aids in the clinical differentiation of these diseases. Microscopically, both processes show extensive destruction of lung substance, surrounded by reactive inflammation. In the abscess, however, the suppurative character of the reaction is more pronounced and the exudate much richer in polymorphonuclear leukocytes. The subject of pneumococcal pneumonias is well covered by Heffron.

Bronchopneumonia. In its narrowest sense, this term is applied to those forms of pneumonia which extend from a bronchitis to involve small portions of the lungs immediately adjacent to a bronchiole. The pneumonic process, therefore, is likely to be lobular in character. In its broadest sense, the term is commonly employed to cover all forms of pneumonia not suppurative and not lobar in character. It is not a specific disease as is lobar pneumonia but may be caused by a wide variety of agents, either infectious or simply irritative. In the commoner infective forms the general symptoms of infectious disease accompany the inflammation. The same complex of general symptoms may, but does not necessarily, accompany the irritative forms. The causative organisms include a wide variety such as staphylococcus, streptococcus, pneumococcus, Friedländer's bacillus, other mouth organisms, colon bacillus, and others which may cause infection in any situation. On the other hand, the process may be more or less specific, as in pneumonic plague.

With the exception of certain special forms of bronchopneumonia to be mentioned subsequently, the disease appears to attack the extremes of life, namely infancy, childhood and old age, but is not especially more common in males than females and shows no particular racial predisposition. Failure of

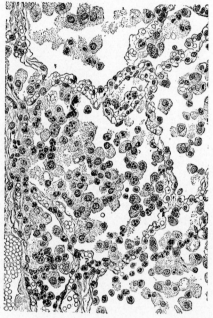

Early bronchopneumonia in which most of the cells are desquamated alveolar epithelium.

the circulation predisposes to that especial form known as hypostatic bronchopneumonia. The disease is often preceded by a more or less prolonged bronchitis, and as a rule the same organism which causes the bronchitis causes the bronchopneumonia. It complicates a number of acute infectious diseases such as measles, pertussis, influenza, diphtheria and less frequently scarlet fever and other infections. It may also result from irritating gases such as chlorine, ammonia, nitrogen tetroxide, bromine and certain of the war gases, particularly that known as mustard gas. These are sometimes referred to as chemical pneumonias. We have shown that, in the rabbit, prolonged inhalation of

high concentrations of oxygen will lead to bronchopneumonia. Lobular types of pneumonia may also accompany septicemia, in which case the organisms are brought to the lung by the blood stream, thus causing exudation into the alveoli without necessarily involving the bronchioles.

Thus, bronchopneumonia may be primary or secondary, the latter being the forms that are complications of or sequels of other disease. Terminal pneumonia is a clinical term used to denote a pneumonia, usually bronchopneumonia, developing in the last stages of some other disease.

The commoner types of bronchopneumonia show patchy areas of consolidation, particularly in the lower lobes of the lung, usually bilateral and sometimes extending widely throughout all the lobes. Occasionally the patches are coextensive with physiologic or anatomic lobules, but as a rule this distinction cannot be made out and the foci are irregularly distributed, usually rather poorly defined, varying in diameter from 5 to 15 mm. or more, and associated with hyperemia and often edema of the lungs. The bronchioles and usually the bronchi are the seat of an acute catarrhal inflammation, the exudate of which may be distinctly purulent in character. The foci of consolidation are easily palpable in the unopened lungs and in the cross section project slightly as generally rounded, poorly defined, moist, fairly firm foci, from which the exudate may readily be expressed as slimy or mucopurulent or distinctly purulent drops. Even in those instances where fibrin appears in the exudate the cross section is not so dry as in lobar pneumonia. In the earlier stages the patches are pink or red whereas in the later stages they become yellow or gray in color. Acute fibrinous pleurisy is not constant but may be observed more especially in those cases where the consolidation approximates the pleura. Empyema may also accompany bronchopneumonia, apparently more commonly in those cases due to the *Streptococcus haemolyticus* than to other organisms. Acute fibrinous pleurisy is frequent in mustard gas pneumonias but not so common in other irritative forms. It is not rare for foci of bronchopneumonia to become confluent so that they occupy a considerable portion of or an entire lobe. The gross confusion with lobar pneumonia is usually obviated by noting the moist non-granular character of the cross section, and the fact that in adjacent lobes and in other lobes there are patches of bronchopneumonia.

Microscopically, the exudate is usually seen to be patchy in character involving smaller or larger groups of alveoli, although in the confluent forms this cannot be made out. Hyperemia is likely to be prominent. The bronchi and bronchioles show catarrhal inflammation with desquamation of epithe-

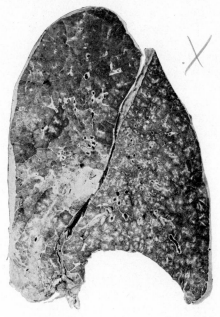

Bronchopneumonia, acute interstitial pneumonia and acute emphysema in influenzal pneumonia. Army Medical Museum 3130.

lium, and catarrhal exudate within the lumen. In the more severe cases, exudation of polymorphonuclear leukocytes is found in the bronchiolar and bronchial walls and the exudate within the lumen is distinctly purulent. Within the alveoli the earlier and simpler stages show principally lymphoid cells, desquamated alveolar cells and macrophages. Leukocytes appear in small numbers. This differs from the early stage of lobar pneumonia principally in distribution and in the more widespread affection of bronchi. In addition, fibrin does not appear so early or in such great quantities, and in many bronchopneumonias it is entirely absent. Whereas in lobar pneumonia, edema is prac-

tically constant in the early stages, it may be absent in bronchopneumonia. In bronchopneumonias due to pneumococcus and diphtheria bacillus, fibrin may be fairly conspicuous, and in the latter condition involves not only the alveoli but frequently also the peribronchial and perivascular lymphatic spaces. In the later stages of bronchopneumonia, polymorphonuclear leukocytes appear in greater and greater numbers but rarely entirely blot out the mononuclear cells. The lung intervening between the consolidated parts may show nothing other than hyperemia or may show edema with a moderate amount of desquamation of lining cells. In the early stages of bronchopneumonia the associated bacteria are richer in the bronchioles than in the alveoli, but as the process extends they are found in great numbers in the alveoli. In certain cases, more especially the pneumonic form of plague and also in hemolytic streptococcus pneumonias, hemorrhage is a prominent feature both grossly and microscopically. With recovery the exudate undergoes resolution in essentially the same way as in lobar pneumonia. In bronchopneumonias also there may be organization of the exudate and the disease may be complicated by the occurrence of abscess or gangrene.

The primary bronchitis and bronchiolitis may extend into the alveoli either by continuity along the epithelial surface, or by contiguity through the bronchial walls and interstitial tissues, to neighboring alveoli. In the former the involvement is principally in the physiologic lobules, whereas in the latter it is more irregular. It is difficult as a rule, however, to distinguish these processes in any given section, and certainly in the later stages both types of process play a part.

Clinically, bronchopneumonia usually comes on insidiously, frequently following prolonged bronchitis. The period of fastigium or acme is of irregular duration, sometimes being relatively short and sometimes prolonged. Crisis is very unusual, most of the cases tending toward convalescence after a variable period of lysis. Certain special forms and those secondary to other diseases develop slowly or rapidly and are likely to end fatally.

Hypostatic Bronchopneumonia. This is a common terminal event in patients who die from chronic or acute heart disease where there is passive hyperemia in the lung. The passive hyperemia affects particularly the lower and posterior parts of the lung and accordingly the pneumonia is likely to appear there. Passive hyperemia of the lung, as elsewhere, is likely to predispose to catarrhal inflammation which may be directly excited by bacteria of various kinds. Hypostatic pneumonias are usually bilateral but not very extensive. Grossly, the red, hyperemic, edematous, bloody, lower posterior parts of the lung are found to contain easily palpable nodules which in the cross section are solid, poorly defined, projecting masses, which may be of the same color as the surrounding hyperemic lung or of lighter gray or deeper red color. In the later stages, the color may be gray or yellowish-gray. Sometimes these foci become confluent to form fairly large patches of consolidation. The bronchi are the seat of subacute catarrhal inflammation but the pleura is not often affected. Microscopically, the exudate is patchy in distribution and shows involvement of bronchi, bronchioles and alveoli. In both early and later stages there is likely to be a greater amount of edema and diapedesis of red blood corpuscles than in the ordinary bronchopneumonia. In the later stages hematogenous pigmentation may be conspicuous, which also is true if the preceding hyperemia has been of long duration.

Aspiration Pneumonia. Many pneumonias are due to aspiration of infectious material from positions higher up in the respiratory tract, but this term is usually applied to those pneumonias where large particles of infectious material are drawn into the bronchi. These include particularly food particles and particles of exudate, especially of pharyngeal inflammations. The material aspirated passes down through the bronchial tree and lodges in some distal part. The respiratory surface, tributary to the bronchus or bronchiole affected, may show simply atelectasis after the absorption of the contained air but as infective agents are commonly present, and closing off of a number of alveoli favors the growth of bacteria, infection extends through a more or less conical area immediately under the pleural surface, establishing a pneumonia which in the earlier stages is similar to other forms of bronchopneumonia save for the peculiar subpleural disposition and the likelihood of subsequent suppuration. Overlying these foci there is an acute fibrinous pleurisy which may become purulent. The cross section shows the generally triangular outline with the base toward the pleura. The triangular mass is well defined, elevated above the rest of the cross section, red in the early stages, and gray and yellow in the later stages. When suppuration ensues it may extend laterally so as to increase the area involved and blot out the triangular shape and the clear definition. Lipid pneumonia is discussed later.

Influenza. This is a systemic disease with special manifestations in the upper respiratory tract. Two closely related viruses, A and B, have been identified as the cause. *Haemophilus influenzae* is often present, but whether it is a symbiont or an incidental accompaniment is not certain. Following a brief incubation period, rarely more than three days, the onset is rapid with cough, sore throat, fever, headache and pains in muscles. Blood pressure is usually low and in severe cases vasomotor collapse may occur. The leukocyte count is normal or low unless complications occur. There may be albuminuria, presumably due to cloudy swelling of the kidneys. Vomiting may occur and in some cases diarrhea is the chief complaint. Disturbances of the central and peripheral nervous system as well as of the special senses may accompany or follow the disease. Rarely, scarlatinoid or macular eruptions occur. Immunity, if it occurs at all, is of short duration. This summary is preliminary to the discussion of postinfectious pneumonias, because pneumonia is a frequent accompaniment or sequel of influenza. (See Shope.)

Postinfectious Pneumonia. In diphtheria, pneumonia may develop as the result of aspiration of exudate, producing a bronchopneumonia with considerable fibrin in the exudate and sometimes fibrin in the interstitial tissues and lymphatics. The predominating organism under these circumstances is the diphtheria bacillus. This does not exclude, however, the possibility of development of pneumonia in diphtheria, nasal, pharyngeal or laryngeal, due to other organisms. In such instances the character of the exudate depends to a certain extent upon the

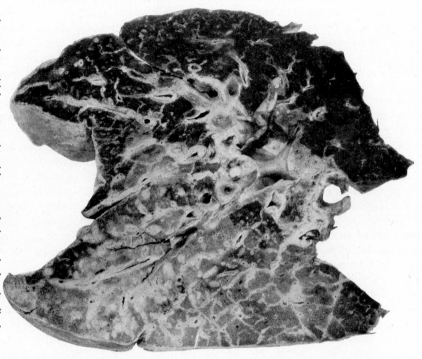

Acute interstitial pneumonia with many foci cut in longitudinal section. Army Medical Museum 606.

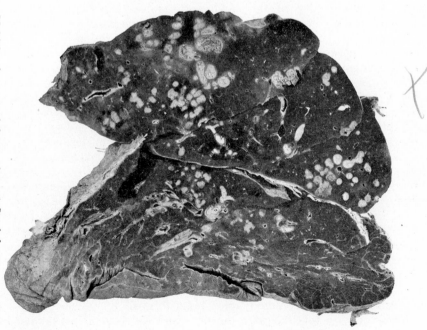

Multiple abscesses of lungs, due to *Staphylococcus aureus*. Army Medical Museum 1141.

organism involved, except that pneumococcus bronchopneumonias may or may not show fibrin formation. L. W. Smith points out that in pertussis the complicating diffuse bronchopneumonia shows a mucopurulent exudate and hyperplasia of the tracheobronchial lymph nodes is common. Pneumococci, staphylococci and tubercle bacilli are found, but in a considerable number of cases pertussis bacilli predominate. Prolonged pneumonia may be accompanied by chronic bronchiectasis. In pneumonias following measles and influenza the pneumonic process is practically always due to organisms which must be regarded as secondary invaders. In measles, the severity is somewhat greater and in influenza the pneumonias are fatal in a considerable proportion of cases.

Much of the information which we now have concerning pneumonia following measles and influenza has been the result of studies conducted during the World War I. In this country admirable work was contributed by various commissions appointed by the Army to study these epidemic diseases. Extensive publications have been made by the commissions headed by MacCallum and by Opie (see also Lucksch, and Jordan). The bacteria recovered were principally *Streptococcus haemolyticus*, but pneumococcus and staphylococcus were frequently encountered; in civil life, staphylococci have been often found (Michael). The morphology of the pneumonia varies considerably whether it follows measles or influenza. In our experience this type of disease showed more commonly than is otherwise observed a combination of lobar pneumonia and bronchopneumonia. There is a striking tendency to interstitial and intra-alveolar hemorrhage as well as to acute emphysema. As a dominant feature of the pathologic picture, many cases show the so-called acute interstitial pneumonia in which the exudate, made up principally of leukocytes, accumulates in perivascular and peribronchial situations forming nodules which to the naked eye are two to three millimeters in diameter, white or pale yellow in color, projecting above the cross section of the lung, sometimes with a fine central depression representing the small bronchus or bronchiole. Without careful examination the picture may be confused grossly with that of miliary tuberculosis.

Wolbach's studies indicated that the early change in postinfluenzal pneumonias is an acute alveolar emphysema, in which the alveoli are lined by hyaline fibrin. Between these areas of emphysema there may be various types of consolidation, and as secondary invaders, such as streptococcus or pneumococcus, manifest their activities, the character of the pneumonia may materially change, thus producing various types of discrete or confluent bronchopneumonia, interstitial pneumonia and even lobar pneumonia. In his series of influenzal pneumonias this feature was constant. Others, including MacCallum, have expressed the view that although this may be constant in influenzal pneumonias, nevertheless, it is frequent in other postinfectious pneumonias, notably those following measles. It cannot therefore be regarded as pathognomonic of postinfluenzal pneumonia. Acute emphysema is probably due to partial obstruction of bronchi and bronchioles by epithelial swelling and exudate. Complete obstruction is followed by regions of atelectasis, a change especially common in the pneumonias of childhood. In MacCallum's experience the acute interstitial pneumonia is most likely to be associated with *Streptococcus haemolyticus*. He points out further that pneumonias similar to those seen following measles and influenza may arise without these diseases as preliminaries and spread in infectious form.

The pneumonias of childhood and infancy may show the fusion of alveolar cells with the production of multinucleated cell masses. The same phenomenon is observed in poison-gas pneumonias. The formation of giant cells is without known cause and does not justify a special term such as giant-cell pneumonia (Moore and Gross). The pneumonia that may occur in rheumatic fever has been discussed in the chapter on Infectious Diseases.

Acute Interstitial Pneumonia. In the preceding section it is pointed out that acute interstitial pneumonia may occur in postinfectious pneumonias. Nevertheless, acute interstitial pneumonia may arise otherwise than as the sequence of acute infectious diseases. It may extend from suppurative lesions of neighboring structures such as the pleura, mediastinal lymph nodes, tissues of the neck and the vertebrae. In these latter instances, the process extends along peribronchial and perivascular lymphatics and interalveolar tissues, forming long and somewhat branching, more or less purulent, white or yellowish-white lines 2 or 3 mm. or more in diameter. These may extend inward from the pleura constituting the so-called pleurogenous pneumonia, or may extend outward from the hilum of the lung. In the postinfectious form, the lines are not so continuous and are more likely to be observed in cross section where they constitute slightly projecting white or yellowish-white masses, sometimes showing the central depression of a bronchiole from which pus may be expressed. In either case the surrounding alveoli are likely to be involved by the inflammatory process. The bronchi are also involved in the inflammation and may be more or less occluded by swelling and exudate, thus leading to foci of atelectasis. Bronchiolar inflammation may lead to narrowing of the lumina, bronchiolitis obliterans, which may become permanent by cicatrization. The peritrunkal lymphatics usually contain exudate. The alveoli become involved by contiguity and contain fibrinoleukocytic exudate (see MacCallum.

Atypical Viral Pneumonia. Often called pneumonitis, this is an infectious disease, met most often in young people. The onset is usually abrupt, with high fever, severe headache and marked cough with but little or no sputum. The physical signs of pneumonia are not marked but the roentgen ray shows fairly extensive bronchopneumonia especially in the lower lobes. After a few days the fever subsides only to recur after a brief interval followed as a rule by recovery after a course of two or three weeks. Not uncommon are pleurisy, venous thrombosis of the extremities and involvement of the peripheral nerves, described in the chapter on Nervous System as a neuronitis.

In the few autopsies on such cases, it appears that the picture in the lungs is one of red, moist, lobular consolidation associated with a purulent bronchitis. Microscopically, the exudate in the alveoli is edematous, the most numerous cells being large mononuclear forms, some of which are phagocytic, erythrocytes, a few leukocytes, but practically no fibrin. The bronchi also contain exudate of the same nature but richer in polymorphonuclear leukocytes. There is no regular association with pneumococci or other bacteria. Undoubtedly these pneumonias are of viral origin, but the identification of the virus or viruses is difficult. In one form it could be transferred only to the mongoose (Weir and Horsfall). Certain other viruses have also been recovered in different epidemics. (See Reimann and Havens; Hesdorffer and Duffalo; Goodpasture; Adams.)

Abscess. As indicated above, abscess of the lung may be a sequel of lobar or bronchopneumonia. It may occur in pyemia and may be the result of infection of a bland infarct. It may also follow aspiration of infected material, foods, etc. It sometimes is observed without preceding history of infection. It may be of short duration or prolonged over many months. There has been much discussion of its occurrence as a postoperative complication. It is thought by some to be due to pulmonary embolism, and Holman and Mathes have shown that the focus of hyperemia and edema can become infected. Others think that the aspiration of material from the throat, especially with the relaxation of epiglottis during inhalation anesthesia, produces the abscess (Cutler; Longacre and Herrmann). Our experience leads to the opinion that either process may operate.

Chronic Interstitial Pneumonia. It is hardly proper to include in this category of progressive fibrosis of the lung the final cicatrization of destructive processes such as infarcts, abscesses, gangrene, wounds, conglomerate and cavitating tuberculosis, as well as the organization of different forms of pneumonia. The term may well be applied to the fibrosis incident to chronic passive hyperemia of the lung, such as accompanies mitral stenosis, the so-called brown induration, and the fibrosis seen in connection with chronic bronchitis, bronchiolitis and arteriolitis. Especially noteworthy are those forms observed in pneumonoconiosis, especially silicosis, and in connection with chronic tuberculosis, the so-called fibroid tuberculosis. In silicosis, there are numerous fibrous nodules scattered throughout the lungs, firm, poorly defined, of variable size and colored in different degrees by the associated anthracosis. In fibroid tuberculosis, the region affected is firm and cuts with increased resistance. The cross section shows masses of irregular outline, and interlacing bands of thickened trabeculae, dense, of fundamentally gray color, and retracted in variable degree. Deeply anthracotic foci are frequent.

Microscopically, the fibrosis is relatively acellular and often hyalinized, with collections of lymphocytes and other mononuclear cells. Fibrous thickening of the pleura is more common in connection with fibroid tuberculosis than with silicosis except when there is associated tuberculosis. Atkinson and others report that comparable degrees of chronic interstitial pneumonia or pneumonitis may be nontuberculous.

Lipid Pneumonia. This is due to aspiration of oily substances such as mineral oils, cod-liver oil and milk. Mineral oils are used in nose drops and as laxatives; the former constitute a particular hazard. The lesion occurs in children and adults and may be preceded by exhausting diseases, malignant tumors, nervous disease, insanity and anything that may inhibit the cough reflex. The disease in the lung may be acute but is more often chronic. The lesions are found especially in the lower lobes and near the hili as pale yellow or gray, firm, well- or poorly defined nodules, discrete or coalescent, often surrounded by a zone of bronchopneumonia. Fluorescence with the longer ultraviolet wave lengths gives colors which are fairly characteristic of the different oils concerned. Microscopically, the early inflammation differs with different oils, showing numerous polymorphonuclears with cod-liver oil and many macrophages with mineral oil. The oils are taken up by macrophages which often fuse to form giant cells. These may be within alveoli and in surrounding tissues. Connective tissue proliferates to form nodular granuloma-like masses. Degradation of the oils may occur and cod-liver–oil droplets may show a margin of acid-fast hyalin. (See Graef; Cannon; Wolman and Bayard.)

Infectious Granulomata

Many of the infectious granulomata may involve the lung, but in adult life the one of outstanding importance is tuberculosis. Actinomycosis, glanders and syphilis may also affect the adult lung. Syphilis, however, is of considerably more importance in the fetal lung than in the adult lung. Our discussion of the granulomata will be more specifically directed toward tuberculosis and syphilis than the other granulomata.

Tuberculosis. The modes of entry of the tubercle bacillus have been discussed in the chapter on Infectious Granulomata. The primary infection, usually in childhood, sets up the primary complex of a small conglomerate tubercle and tuberculosis of satellite lymph nodes. The destructive disease of adult life may be due to superinfection or in some instances to reinfection. It is also possible for the primary infection to extend rapidly and produce widespread destructive tuberculosis in the child's lungs. In both childhood and adult life the human variety of the bacillus is the chief invader, but occasional instances, due apparently to the bovine form, have been reported.

The reaction to tubercle bacilli is in the form of exudation, proliferation or both. The tubercle must be regarded as principally proliferative, although in the earlier stages there is slight exudation. In contrast to this, however, is the other form of involvement of the lung, namely, tuberculous pneumonia which primarily and principally is exudative in character. The determination of reaction on the part of the lung involves the question of virulence and dosage of tubercle bacilli, as well as sensitization and local or general resistance. The fact that the wax of tubercle bacilli, and other foreign bodies, may produce nodules practically identical with the tubercle, suggests the possibility that the more intense exudative reactions are in response to products of the organism. Nevertheless, in tuberculous pneumonia large numbers of organisms are present, and it may well be that dosage of organism is of equal importance with its soluble products.

Three modes of dissemination within the lung are recognized, namely, by the blood stream, by the lymphatic stream, and by the air passages. In order to simplify the discussion these will be taken up in the order mentioned. It must be noted, however, that the direct local invasion of the tuberculous process is of the greatest significance and probably represents the most frequent mode of spreading of the disease.

HEMATOGENOUS TUBERCULOSIS. This occurs in the lungs as disseminated miliary tuberculosis. It is usually due to penetration into a pulmonary artery of lesions within the lung or mediastinal lymph nodes. Occasionally it may be carried from other parts of the body, especially male genitalia, by way of the thoracic duct. It may be disseminated in one lobe, several lobes or the entire lung. As a rule, the disease is acute. The lungs are large and hyperemic. The pleura may show miliary tubercles or acute tuberculous pleurisy. Palpation discloses innumerable fine nodules. The cross section shows these to be of fairly uniform size, widely and evenly distributed.

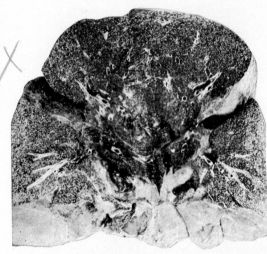

Acute miliary tuberculosis of lung. Army Medical Museum 2779.

They are discrete, gray or pale yellow, well defined, projecting spherical nodules, 1, 2 or 3 mm. in diameter. The process may be confined to the lung but is commonly associated with a similar condition in other viscera, particularly the liver, spleen and kidney. Microscopically, the nodules may be single miliary tubercles, with the usual histologic character of centrally disposed epithelioid cells surrounded by lymphoid cells, and frequently fairly numerous Langhans giant cells. More common, however, is the finding that the tubercles, which grossly appear as discrete single masses, are histologically made up of fusion of one, two, three or more true miliary tubercles. In either case, caseation may be present but is likely to be more conspicuous in the latter. The tubercles, of course, are interstitial in situation but apparently have no predilection for a site near the bronchioles or

smaller blood vessels. Whether the tubercles originate within a capillary where the bacilli are deposited, or whether the bacilli migrate or are carried either into neighboring lymphatics or into the alveolar spaces is not definitely known. Reaction in the surrounding aveoli is limited in amount, but occasionally slight desquamation and infiltration of lymphocytes and even polymorphonuclears may be observed. Bronchitis is not a prominent factor.

If the patient survive a sufficient length of time the miliary tuberculosis may become chronic. Grossly, the distribution is the same but hyperemia is likely to be less marked. The nodules are commonly somewhat larger than in the acute form, sharply circumscribed and firm. Microscopically, they are characterized by distinct connective-tissue formation in the margins, which may be loose masses of fibroblasts, or thin but dense connective-tissue capsules. Anatomically, the quantitative destruction of alveoli does not appear to be extensive, but clinically, reduction of vital capacity is often a very striking phenomenon. This may be due in part to the tuberculosis, and contributed to by the hyperemia which is common in the acute form.

LYMPHOGENOUS TUBERCULOSIS. The extension of tuberculosis in the adult lung through the lymphatic tracts cannot be regarded as finally established, and indeed many regard the form described under this name as hematogenous in origin. It forms a distinct variety anatomically and tends to be located principally in perivascular and peribronchial lymphatics. This may, however, be due to interstitial deposition of organisms from the vascular tree and subsequent extension into the neighboring lymphatics. Extension through lymphatics may be favored by tuberculosis of hilic lymph nodes, so marked as to block the lymphatics and cause retrograde flow of lymph; the extension, however, is more by direct progression of the tuberculosis in the vessels than by transport of bacilli in the lymph. The involvement of the perivascular and peribronchial lymphatics (often called peritrunkal) may be confined to one lobe or involve several lobes.

Usually there is a pre-existent tuberculosis, either chronic ulcerative, or conglomerate caseous in the lung, or massive tuberculosis of the hilic lymph nodes. Cross section of the lung shows that, what seem to be nodules a centimeter or more in diameter upon external palpation, are made up of staphyloid (like a bunch of grapes) clusters of tubercles, each tubercle being about 1, 2 or 3 mm. in diameter. The individual members of the group are fairly well-defined, projecting, gray or yellowish-gray masses, which upon close

monia. The walls of the bronchi may be infiltrated and tubercles appear in the lining membrane. The same may be true in regard to the smaller blood vessels. It is unusual for this process to become chronic in character, and therefore it is uncommon to find a connective tissue reaction of any significance either grossly or microscopically. This peribronchial or perivascular tuberculosis repre-

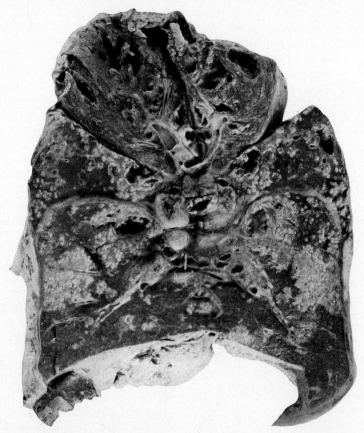

Chronic ulcerative tuberculosis of upper lobe showing trabeculation and ramifications. Small chronic cavities in middle and upper part of lower lobes. Peribronchial and perivascular tuberculosis of middle and lower lobes. Tuberculous acute fibrinous pleurisy. Conglomerate tuberculosis of peribronchial lymph nodes.

inspection reveal a minute point of central depression, corresponding to a small blood vessel or bronchiole. The masses of tubercles are commonly found in the center of the lung rather than near the periphery. Microscopically, there are fused miliary tubercles in the perivascular or peribronchial lymphatics. Neighboring hyperemia is prominent and indeed, alveoli in the immediate neighborhood may show the exudate of tuberculous pneu-

sents an extremely common form of extension of the disease in association with chronic ulcerative tuberculosis of the lung. It must not be confused with tuberculous pneumonia whose picture is distinctive.

AEROGENOUS TUBERCULOSIS. Under this heading must be included that form of tuberculosis which is common in the adult, namely, conglomerate tuberculosis in the apex of the lung followed either by cicatrization and calcification, or by extension and cavity formation. In addition must be included those forms in which tuberculosis is disseminated from a pre-existing focus, by aspiration of tuberculous material, into more remote parts of the bronchial tree, usually near the surface of the lung. Quantities of tuberculous material, particularly from a cavity, may be aspirated into a smaller bronchus, and, largely because of atelectasis in the region supplied, a tuberculous focus of conical form with the base under the pleura, develops. This may be a mass of small conglomerate or discrete miliary tubercles, or may be a massive caseous tuberculous pneumonia. Overlying it there is almost always an acute miliary tuberculosis of the pleura or an acute fibrinous tuberculous pleurisy, and sometimes a chronic adhesive tuberculous pleurisy. In cross section, the conical outline with the base under the pleura is usually characteristic.

The commonest form of pulmonary tuberculosis in the adult is that which runs one of two courses in the apex of the lung. Rather than enter again into the argument which has been discussed in the general pathology of tuberculosis, we will assume that this is air borne.

The primary or so-called Ghon tubercle is usually formed in the lung near the hilum or under the outer surface in a band area lateral to the hilum. Satellite lymph node or nodes are also involved, the whole constituting the primary complex. The primary tubercle is likely to become encapsulated and ultimately calcified and the lesion in the lymph nodes calcified. In contrast to the usual position of the primary tubercle, the disease in adult life affects the upper lobe near or at the apex and is much less likely to become fibrous, encapsulated or calcified than is the original lesion. Why the apex, and more particularly the right apex, is selected is unknown. If the limited excursion of the upper part of the thorax has any influence, the same influence should be found in other infections. If the light specific gravity of the tubercle bacillus is of any significance, both apices should be infected with equal frequency, and such a hypothesis assumes that the infection is blood borne. That circulation is less in the upper lobe and therefore resistance diminished has yet to be proved. The fact that the main bronchus to the right upper lobe comes off fairly directly from the trachea might explain lodgment in the right upper lobe but does not satisfactorily explain lodgment in the apex.

It may safely be assumed that on gaining access to the apex the growth of the tubercle follows the usual course, namely, primary involvement of the lymphatics with the development of a tubercle which, with the multiplication of the organisms, increases in size, both by direct growth and the formation of daughter tubercles, and subsequently a conglomerate tubercle of moderate size is formed. In favorable cases the reaction of connective tissue is sufficiently great to provide a capsule of fibrous tissue around the tubercle and thus limit its growth. As has been pointed out in the section on calcification, the caseous mass within the center of the tubercle is a favorite site for calcification. Thus, these so-called healed tubercles may show either a caseous center or a completely calcified center.

Microscopically, in these later stages, little that is characteristic of the tubercle remains; there is simply the caseous or calcified center surrounded by dense connective tissue. In the more recent cases, however, the inner layers of the capsule may show lymphoid infiltration. Such healed tubercles, however, are not functionally healed because tubercle bacilli may be recovered by inoculation into animals, although rarely found by histologic methods within the mass.

Cavity Formation. In the less favorable cases the tubercle continues to grow with only a moderate amount of capsule formation and, at any time, hematogenous or lymphogenous or even aerogenous dissemination may occur to other parts of the lung. These accidents, however, are not common until the local process has become so extensive that it invades a bronchus and discharges its contents into this bronchus to be coughed up and expectorated. This leaves a tuberculous cavity communicating with a member of the bronchial tree. The rich bacterial content of the upper respiratory tract may thus infect the cavity, producing secondary infection. The organisms of secondary infection include particularly the staphylococcus and *Micrococcus tetragenus*, although the streptococcus, pneumococcus, Friedländer's bacillus and even various forms of yeasts may contaminate the cavity. As the local process extends, a chronic obliterative bronchitis occurs in the bronchi within the lesion and a thrombosis, with subsequent organization, in the blood vessels. These constitute fairly resistant dense masses of connective tissue, not readily susceptible to the destructive action of the tubercle bacillus, and they consequently remain as trabeculae or spurs within the cavity. After the secondary infection the cavity may continue to enlarge considerably, but apparently with the secondary infection the growth of connective tissue becomes more rapid and the fibrosis of the wall of the cavity more extensive. Thus is constituted the cavity of CHRONIC ULCERATIVE TUBERCULOSIS.

Grossly, the cavity may vary considerably in size from a diameter of 1 or 2 cm. to a size coextensive with the entire upper lobe. It may be generally spherical or may ramify irregularly through various planes in the lobe. The wall is fairly well outlined and under the pleura may be coextensive with the connective tissue of that organ. In most cases the surrounding lung substance is likely to show various forms of tuberculous pneumonia, peribronchial and perivascular tuberculosis and numerous small conglomerate or miliary tubercles. When the lesion is sufficiently near the surface so that the pleura constitutes part of the wall of the cavity, the pleura is markedly thickened by fibrous and often hyalinized connective tissue, and shows chronic fibrous adhesions with obliteration of that part of the pleural cavity. In more deeply situated cavities the pleura may not be involved or may show acute fibrinous pleurisy, miliary tuberculosis of the pleura or a chronic fibrous pleurisy.

The thickness of the cavity wall varies from a millimeter to several millimeters. It is made up of dense fibrous connective tissue, which may show hematogenous pigmentation and commonly shows a considerable concentration of anthracotic pigment. The inner surface of the wall is usually rough and irregular because of the persistence of connective tissue septa and the trabeculae formed by obliterated blood vessels and bronchi. The latter may extend through the cavity as dense heavy bands suggesting the stalactites and stalagmites of underground caves. The color of the lining may be dark red, because of granulation tissue; yellow, because of the

presence of pus; or gray because of caseation. The contents may be cheesy or caseous or purulent in character, not uncommonly mixed with variable amounts of blood. Sometimes the presence of saprophytic organisms gives a foul odor. The associated tuberculous pneumonia, localized miliary or conglomerate tubercles, peribronchial tuberculosis or other similar processes, may be confined to the upper lobe but as a rule extend in greater or lesser degree into the other lobes. Although the cavity may be in one lung only, the various forms of extension may be observed in both lungs. Microscopically, the wall of the cavity is made up of dense connective tissue which may show varying degrees of hyalinization. The inner layers of the wall usually show granulation tissue associated with varying degrees of infiltration of polymorphonuclear leukocytes, depending upon the severity of the secondary infections. In the milder forms of infection, lymphoid cells and epithelioid cells may be prominent. It is rare to find actual tubercle formation within the connective tissue of the cavity wall. The process is identified particularly by finding tubercles or other tuberculous processes in the immediate neighborhood. The inner layers toward the cavity may or may not contain considerable numbers of tubercle bacilli. The contents of the cavity, however, are usually fairly rich in tubercle bacilli.

The fibrosis of the cavity wall may apparently be the starting point of a diffuse fibrosis of the neighboring tissue, wherein dense bands of connective tissue radiate throughout the lobe, or extend more widely in the lung. Sometimes chronic miliary or small conglomerate tubercles are associated with the process. The condition is slowly progressive in character and constitutes CHRONIC FIBROUS (OR FIBROID) TUBERCULOSIS, more common in late middle than in earlier life. Microscopically, there are found heavy bands of fibrous tissue, often with finer fibrosis of alveolar walls and not infrequently showing more or less fibrotic miliary and small conglomerate tubercles. There is destruction of alveolar substance in the progress of the disease. Often small spaces approximating the size of an alveolus are found lined by cuboidal epithelium. Whether these are old alveoli with pseudometaplasia of the lining epithelium or new spaces budding from bronchioles as an abortive regeneration is not known.

In association with chronic ulcerative tuberculosis there is almost constantly a chronic catarrhal bronchitis and this may be responsible for complementary emphysema in portions of the lungs. More particularly in the neighborhood of the cavity, the bronchitis is definitely tuberculous in character with tubercles in the lining membrane. More rarely, as mentioned in the section on diseases of the bronchi, there may be an extensive caseous tuberculous bronchitis. Within the extending tuberculous process the bronchitis may be catarrhal or tuberculous, but in either case the exudate is likely to fill up the lumen, and granulation tissue grow out from the wall of the bronchus so as to convert the tube into a fibrous cord. The blood vessels usually undergo thrombosis fairly early and this is followed by organization and cicatrization. On the other hand, the outer layers of vessel walls may be destroyed by the advancing tuberculosis without thrombosis. Aneurysms may or may not form, but in either case the weakened walls may rupture, especially when there is increased pulmonary pressure such as occurs in coughing, followed by severe or fatal hemorrhage. Such vascular lesions are more common in chronic ulcerative tuberculosis, but may also occur in small foci of conglomerate tuberculosis and in tuberculous pneumonia. Fatal hemorrhages are likely to occur only in connection with chronic ulcerative tuberculosis. Most of the blood is expelled by coughing, but some is aspirated into the lungs and may fill a large part of the bronchial tree. Death is due to asphyxia from filling of the bronchial tree by blood rather than from the amount of blood lost; the patient "drowns in his own blood." Sometimes hemoptysis is the first clinical manifestation of tuberculosis and the lesion is found only by the roentgen ray as a "minimal lesion." In cases of pulmonary tuberculosis with hemorrhage, the prothrombin level may be low and clotting in the ruptured vessel delayed. In such cases, vitamin K may be beneficial (see Savacool; Sheely).

TUBERCULOUS PNEUMONIA. Although the presence of tuberculosis may apparently predispose to various forms of bronchopneumonia, that form which is designated as tuberculous pneumonia is due to the tubercle bacillus. The organisms are numerous in the exudate and are probably transmitted through the air passages. Two forms are recognized although they are not necessarily connected and not always sharply distinguishable.

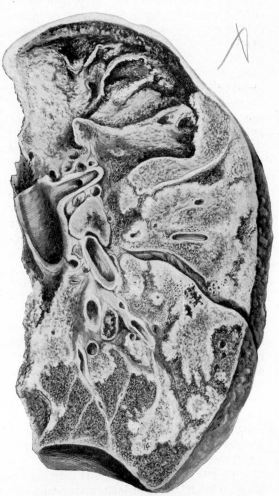

Chronic ulcerative tuberculosis of upper lobe, extensive caseous pneumonia of lower part of upper lobe and lower lobe, and conglomerate tuberculosis of peribronchial lymph node.

Gelatinous tuberculous pneumonia is exudative in character. It rarely involves large parts of the lung, usually being present as a smaller involvement in the neighborhood of chronic ulcerative tuberculosis or tuberculous caseous pneumonia. Grossly, the involved portion is poorly defined and of irregular outline, 2 or 3 cm. or more in diameter. The lung is not densely consolidated but of gelatinous consistency. The cross section is smooth, nongranular, moist, semitranslucent and of pale gray or reddish-gray color. A moderate amount of slightly cloudy colorless fluid can be expressed from it. A few miliary and small conglomerate tubercles may be observed in the consolidated areas. Microscopically, the alveoli show moderate capillary hyperemia, edema sometimes with fibrin, and considerable desquamation of lining cells. The cells are largely desquamated alveolar cells and macrophages, lymphoid cells, a few polymorphonuclear leukocytes and an occasional red blood cell. Special staining usually shows a considerable number of tubercle bacilli. The smaller bronchi are involved in the same type of process.

Caseous tuberculous pneumonia may be the sequence of gelatinous tuberculous pneumonia or apparently may arise quite independently. There is no reason to suppose that gelatinous pneumonia necessarily progresses to caseous pneumonia. The latter process, however, is more distinctly destructive of pulmonary tissue than exudative in character. Grossly, it may involve only a small part of the lung near chronic ulcerative or other form of tuberculosis. Not infrequently, however, it may be lobar in extent. Grossly, the affected part of the lung is consolidated and of dense consistence. In the more extensive forms, the overlying pleura may show acute fibrinous pleurisy or a more definitely tuberculous form of pleurisy. The lung cuts readily and shows a slightly bulging, gray or yellowish-gray, dry, nongranular cross section in which the alveolar markings are more or less obliterated. Tubercles are not usually found in this consolidated portion. The mass is distinctly friable. It may resemble gray hepatization of lobar pneumonia but is distinguished because of the nongranularity of the cross section, by the great friability and by the obliteration of various lung markings. The color is darker in deeply anthracotic lungs. Frequently, the caseous material breaks down and discharges into bronchi so as to leave single or multiple small cavities, lined by caseous material but only rarely showing a fibrous wall. Microscopically, the mass is made up of caseous material showing shadows of exudate, of alveolar walls and of septa. Smaller bronchioles and smaller blood vessels are usually destroyed by the process. The larger bronchioles and bronchi show as a rule chronic catarrhal or tuberculous bronchitis. Blood vessels in the neighborhood of the consolidation may show fairly extensive thrombosis. The process may not be uniform in a given microscopic preparation, but shows in certain areas an exudative form of pneumonia similar to that seen microscopically in gelatinous pneumonia, but usually much richer in cells. Tubercle bacilli are likely to be numerous in the consolidated mass. The cavities appear microscopically as places in which the caseous material has dropped out, and there is almost never any secondary infection and reaction as seen in the chronic ulcerative tuberculosis. Sections taken from the margins of the tuberculous pneumonia are likely to show miliary and conglomerate tubercles.

Especially in children, tubercle bacilli may also cause a bronchopneumonia of exudative type indistinguishable grossly and microscopically from ordinary bronchopneumonia. Upon special staining these areas show large numbers of tubercle bacilli. Lesions of this sort are probably responsible for fairly rapid extensions and regressions of the local disease clinically and roentgenologically, the so-called "epituberculosis." (See Reichle.)

Syphilis. This disease affects the lungs of the new born and infants much more commonly than it does the adult lung. In the former, it may appear either as single or multiple gummata or more often as the so-called white pneumonia or pneumonia alba. The gummata have the usual gross and microscopic appearances and may be found in association with pneumonia alba. In the latter condition, large or small parts of the lung are consolidated and in the cross section show either a glossy gray or a dull gray or even cheesy appearance. Microscopically, the most characteristic feature is incomplete or entirely deficient development of the alveoli. In some cases, there are found only sprouts of bronchioles lined by cuboidal epithelium. In others, the alveoli are present as spaces smaller than normal. Around the bronchi and blood vessels in the septa and between the alveoli, there is a mass of connective tissue whose cellular constitution varies from short spindle cells resembling somewhat those of the mesoblast, and often with multiple processes, larger fibroblasts and adult connective tissue. The alveoli, except for their small size, may be normal but usually contain desquamated epithelium which rapidly undergoes fatty degeneration, macrophages and lymphocytes. The connective tissue mass must be regarded as a direct evolution from mesoblastic tissue, which has not been displaced by the growing alveoli because their develop-

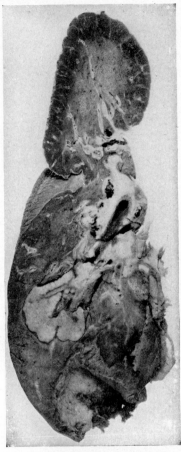

Gumma of lung in acquired syphilis. Note fibrosis in margin of gummatous area.

ment has been interrupted by the syphilitic process. Blood vessels often show distinct thickening of their walls, which may go on to complete obliteration. This, then, is rather a failure of development than a true pneumonia.

The gumma is the most characteristic syphilitic lesion of the lung in acquired syphilis. It is rare and is observed especially in the middle and upper part of the lower lobe. The lesion is usually single, 1 or 2 cm. in diameter, well defined, shows fibrosis either throughout or in the margin and has little

tendency to caseation, although cavitation is said to occur. Fibrosis may extend radially from the gumma toward the pleura and produce retraction to form the rare, so-called pulmo lobatus. Clinically and roentgenologically, a diffuse fibrosis of the lung is found in syphilitics, but diffuse lesions of this sort are not frequently confirmed by autopsy. Many are found to be tuberculosis or tumor. Nevertheless more or less diffuse fibrosis may be found, with the evidence pointing toward syphilis as a cause. In the earlier stages there is diffuse fibrosis associated with infiltration of lymphocytes and plasma cells. These cells may be formed into vascularized miliary nodules, sometimes with giant cells, the miliary syphiloma. These may deform the alveoli. Peritrunkal distribution of the cellular infiltration may be associated with vasculitis and bronchiolar obliteration. The later cicatricial stage of this lesion shows no characteristic features and is diagnosed only inferentially because of syphilitic disease in other viscera (Herxheimer; Denman). Syphilis may affect the pulmonary artery as a syphilitic mesarteritis, or presumably as an obliterating arteriolitis (Karsner).

Other Granulomata. GLANDERS may produce small nodules which resemble tubercles, but with a tendency to suppuration. There may be single or multiple abscesses, or foci of bronchopneumonia sometimes caseous in type. There is usually a primary focus in the nose or elsewhere.

Actinomycosis may affect the lung either as the result of aspiration from involvement of nose or mouth, or direct infection from esophagus or other neighboring organs, or extremely rarely by blood metastasis. The lesion in the lung does not differ materially from that elsewhere, except that in the margin of the actinomycotic nodule there is likely to be a certain amount of reactive pneumonia. As pointed out in the chapter on Infectious Granulomata, infections by streptothrix and by blastomyces and other higher vegetable organisms may produce more or less diffuse consolidation and destruction of the lung, sometimes resembling tuberculosis, usually chronic in character and identified by finding the organism concerned.

Tumors of Bronchi and Lungs

Benign tumors usually originate in the bronchi and include adenoma, papilloma, fibroma, lipoma, chondroma and osteoma. The principal effect is obstruction in the bronchus. Although all are infrequent, BRON-CHIAL ADENOMA is by no means rare. It occurs

acinic differentiation. Although slightly invasive locally, metastasis does not occur.

Of the malignant tumors, sarcoma is much more rare than carcinoma. The sarcoma is usually single, occupying either a large part of a lobe or sometimes invading the entire lung. It is usually a massive, infil-

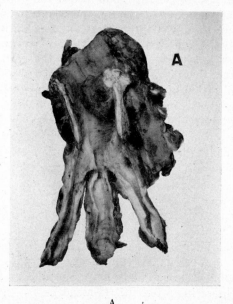

A.

Adenoma of secondary bronchus. Note nodule in larger bronchus near top of specimen.

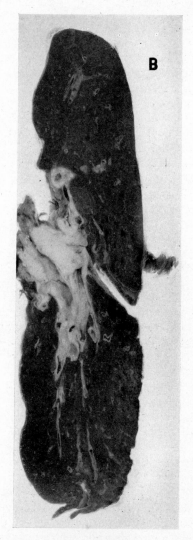

B.➤

Bronchiogenic carcinoma involving main stem bronchus to lower lobe of lung. Note reduction in size of lumen near margin of bronchus. Pleura shows tag of adhesion. Surgical specimen.

more often in females than in males and between 20 and 40 years of age. The lesion usually arises in one of the larger bronchi, grows slowly in polypoid or sessile form, leads to cough, sometimes with slight hemoptysis, and may produce secondary atelectasis, bronchiectasis and pneumonia. The final diagnosis depends on bronchoscopic biopsy. Microscopically, there are groups of uniform small cuboidal or columnar cells sometimes with

trating tumor which microscopically appears as either a spindle-cell sarcoma or a small round-cell sarcoma, and occasionally shows polymorphous forms of cells. Nodules of lymphosarcoma are usually multiple. In addition, there may be sarcoma combined with more differentiated elements to constitute more especially chondrosarcoma and osteosarcoma. We have observed one chondrosarcoma which replaced an entire lung.

Primary carcinoma of the lung originates in the bronchial epithelium; thus it is more properly called bronchogenic carcinoma. It is not rare and constitutes about 10 per cent of malignant tumors observed at autopsy; it is less frequent, however, in the general population. Nevertheless it is much more often recognized than was formerly true. There is much discussion as to whether this is an absolute increase, or a relative increase due to improved diagnosis and to the increased average length of life. The greatest incidence is in the sixth decade; males are more often affected than females; the right lung is attacked more often than the left and bilateral involvement is rare. Clinically, there is a variety of symptoms, cough, dyspnea, slight hemoptysis, pain, anemia, etc. The roentgenograph is usually characteristic, and biopsy diagnostic.

Grossly, classification is based on distribution of the disease in the lung. We prefer the simple classification into four forms, a nodular mass near the hilum, a diffuse infiltrative form, a peripheral form and miliary carcinosis. These may represent, in part, different stages of the same process. In our experience, the hilic form is the most frequent. In this there is found near the hilum of the lung a poorly circumscribed, infiltrating mass of tumor tissue, showing variable degrees of necrosis, poorly vascularized, more or less friable and often associated with constriction of larger members of the bronchial tree. It appears to affect the middle and lower lobes more extensively than the upper lobes but may invade widely throughout the entire lung. Extensions may be seen for a comparatively short distance along the bronchi and blood vessels.

In the diffuse infiltrating form, the lesion at the hilum is not so striking and tumor masses are found, irregularly distributed throughout the lung, poorly vascularized, pallid and necrotic, of irregular size, sometimes fusing to form large masses.

In miliary carcinosis there are innumerable nodules a few millimeters in diameter, usually situated along the course of the lymphatic vessels. In this form it is particularly important to rule out a primary focus in some other organ. Depending upon the involvement of the bronchi there may be more or less widespread areas of atelectasis. Foci of bronchopneumonia are not uncommonly a terminal accident. Usually the pleura is free from involvement, but in the more extensive and peripheral tumors there may be chronic adhesive pleurisy and occasionally definite involvement of the pleura by tumor. The peribronchial and mediastinal lymph nodes are frequently involved. About 10 per cent show no metastasis and 20 per cent show metastasis limited to the thoracic cavity, in which involvement of the hilic lymph nodes is the most common. The remaining cases show more widespread metastasis which involve in the approximate order of frequency, the regional lymph nodes, liver, kidney, lung, pericardium, abdominal lymph nodes, pleura, brain, adrenals, bone, cervical lymph nodes and heart.

Microscopically, the tumor may be squamous cell carcinoma, small cell or reserve cell carcinoma, adenocarcinoma, and a carcinoma simplex which often shows great cellular pleomorphism. The small-cell carcinoma is composed of small spindle cells (so-called oat cells) and small round cells, often somewhat alveolated by connective tissue bands, and with little or no reticulum. Of practical importance is Koletsky's observation that the squamous-cell carcinoma metastasizes later and less widely than the other forms, thus making it favorable for surgical removal. There is no conclusive evidence that carcinoma of the lung originates elsewhere than in the bronchi (Karsner and Saphir). Except for the dusts of the Schneeberg cobalt mines, no definite cause for bronchiogenic carcinoma has been discovered. (See Fried; Matz; Rosahn; Ochsner and de Bakey; Menne and Anderson.)

Secondary tumors of the lung may occur by direct extension as from the pleura or mediastinal lymph nodes. Much more commonly, however, secondary tumors arise as the result of blood vascular transmission. Lymphatic transmission also occurs as is seen probably in the frequent involvement of the lung secondary to carcinoma of the breast. Tumor cells borne in the venous blood are especially likely to lodge in the pulmonary capillaries, their first point of obstruction in the circulation. Therefore, the metastasis of various forms of sarcoma is extremely common, as is also that from thyroid carcinomas, hypernephroma and chorionepithelioma. Secondary involvement from carcinoma may occur as the result of a generalized carcinomatosis in which metastasis is largely by the blood stream, and may also be secondary to cancer metastases in the liver which involve the blood vessels and are then transmitted to the lungs.

The nodules vary in size from minute points to fairly large masses exceeding several centimeters in diameter, fairly uniform in size, more or less compressing the surrounding lung tissue, rather rarely occluding important members of the bronchial tree, and showing the characters of the primary tumor. Occasionally, secondary extension of the tumor occurs through the lung, particularly by the lymphatics, and may thus be deposited in the mediastinal lymph nodes or by retrograde extension involve the subpleural lymphatics, sometimes producing the so-called "cancer en cuirasse."

Lymphosarcoma, Hodgkin's disease and lymphomas of leukemia may develop from the tiny lymphoid aggregates of the lung.

Parasites

In addition to such higher vegetable parasites as cause granulomatous lesions, aspergillus and certain forms of mucor are reported. Of the animal parasites monolocular or multilocular echinococcus cysts occur. In Japan and China an important infestation is that of *Distomum pulmonale* or *Paragonimus Westermanni*. *Endamoeba histolytica* may gain access by direct extension from hepatic abscess. Echinococcus cyst may also occur (Arce).

PLEURA

Hydrothorax

Hydrothorax is essentially an edema of the pleural sac and may be caused by general conditions which lead to edema, such as heart failure and kidney disease, or local causes such as intrathoracic tumor or aneurysm, or inflammatory processes which may interfere with drainage of the blood or lymph. The fluid is clear, light yellow in color, limpid, of low specific gravity (about 1014), contains only a few endothelial cells and is not likely to clot upon standing. Ordinarily it collects in the lower and posterior parts of the pleural sac, but the distribution may be materially altered by pre-existing fibrous adhesions. These may be so widespread as to produce a sacculated form of hydrothorax, which may be supradiaphragmatic, under the thoracic wall, or interlobar, depending upon the position of the adhesions. In these cases the fibrous bands which constitute the adhesions may also show considerable edema.

The fluid may be mixed with fat in fine or coarse emulsion, more especially when the hydrothorax is due to tumors or similar masses in the thorax, which not only compress veins but also compress the thoracic duct. The fatty material presumably gains access through leakage from the thoracic tributaries of the ducts. When compression is confined to the thoracic duct alone or when there is traumatic rupture of the duct, the material in the thorax may be practically pure chyle. A certain amount of fat may also be present when the hydrothorax occurs in lipemic individuals. When fat is contributed by fatty degeneration of cells in sufficient quantities to produce cloudiness or milkiness of the fluid, there is usually extensive tumor involvement of the pleura. The degree of cloudiness and the separation of fat upon standing depend essentially upon the type of emulsion. Excluding those cases in which the fat is due to fatty degeneration of cells or to lipemia, we apply to all others, in agreement with Blankenhorn, the name chylous hydrothorax, in which the fluid may vary considerably in degree of milkiness. We thus do away with the older terms pseudochylous and chyliform, used to represent lesser degrees of milkiness.

The lung shows degrees of atelectasis depending upon the amount of fluid. It is small, firm, reduced in air content and the seat of passive hyperemia which gives it a dark red or a slate-blue color. The negative pressure of the pleura remains normal and the atelectasis is due to decreased expansion because of filling of the sac. Only in those portions where the lung is actually immersed in the fluid and subject to its hydrostatic pressure is there a true compression atelectasis. When atelectasis is marked, the lung lies in the upper part of the chest more or less flattened against its hilum and the spinal column. Fibrous adhesions may alter the position. The physiologic effects will be discussed after presenting the morbid anatomy of other conditions in which the contents of the pleura are increased.

Hemothorax

This term is usually restricted to the presence of considerable quantities of free blood within the pleura. Such hemorrhage may be due to penetrating wounds of the thoracic wall, tearing of the lung by wounds, by needle punctures, or by fractured ribs, rupture of intrathoracic aneurysms and destructive processes such as tuberculosis and malignant tumors. Small hemorrhages into the substance of the visceral and parietal pleura are observed following death from asphyxia, certain poisons such as phosphorus, arsenic and mercuric chloride, severe infectious disease, the various hemorrhagic diseases, and following death from heart failure. As a rule, this is limited to petechiae but occasionally considerable leakage may occur into the pleural cavity.

Inflammation

Although strictly this should be referred to as pleuritis, nevertheless, common

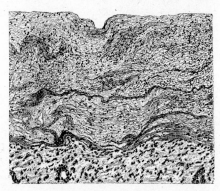

Acute fibrinous pleurisy.

usage accepts the term pleurisy. Acute pleurisy may be fibrinous, fibrinoserous, purulent, putrid, and hemorrhagic. Occasionally, bacteria gain access to the pleura from some unknown portal of entry. There are, however, many cases of fibrinoserous pleurisy in which bacteria are not ordinarily recoverable by the usual cultural methods, and no definite point of origin can be detected clinically. By injection into guinea pigs, however, many of these can be shown to be tuberculous in character.

Acute pleurisy may develop in the course of pyemia and septicemia and various enteric infections, in which the organisms can usually be recovered from the pleural fluid. Presumably also blood borne are those pleurisies which occur in various acute infectious fevers. In some of these no organisms are recoverable.

The most important cause of acute pleurisy, however, is direct extension from

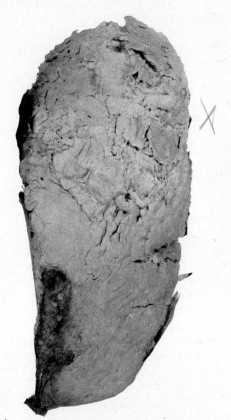

Acute fibrinous pleurisy in late stage, more truly acute fibrinopurulent. Army Medical Museum 501.

neighboring inflammation, the most striking example being the pleurisy which accompanies lobar pneumonia. Extension to the pleura may also occur from other types of pulmonary inflammation, from inflammation of the mediastinal lymph nodes, the pericardium, the peritoneum, especially where the latter inflammation is secondary to liver or spleen abscess or ulcer of the stomach. Extension may also occur from inflamed ribs and vertebrae and from infection entering through carcinomas or other destructive lesions of esophagus, stomach and bronchi.

Acute fibrinous pleurisy such as occurs in acute infectious diseases of various kinds, lobar pneumonia and tuberculous caseous pneumonia, shows, upon the hyperemic visceral and parietal pleura, a layer of fibrin varying from a thin, yellow butter-like film in the less severe and earlier cases to a thick, rough, gray, shaggy mass in the more severe and long standing cases. In the latter the movements of the lungs are likely to whip the fibrin into fairly heavy bands.

(about 1020-1023), rich in proteins of various kinds, and likely to coagulate upon standing. The fluid contains flakes of fibrin, desquamated endothelium, which may be more or less degenerate, and cells of the exudate, particularly polymorphonuclear leukocytes and lymphocytes.

Empyema. Acute purulent pleurisy, sometimes called pyothorax and usually called empyema, may represent an alteration of a fibrinous or fibrinoserous pleurisy or may originate as a purulent process. It may occur as the result of direct infection from wounds, as a part of pyemia and septicemia

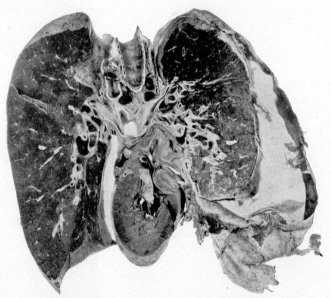

Section of thoracic viscera including left parietal pleura in a case of acute empyema, showing position of fluid in left pleura and atelectasis of left lung. Small foci of bronchopneumonia are visible as dark areas in right lung. Army Medical Museum 16359.

Microscopically, there is the usual picture of fibrinous exudate enmeshing a few cells of exudative character. In the earlier stages there is swelling of the endothelium, followed by desquamation and disappearance. Organization begins early in the process. This becomes an acute fibrinoserous pleurisy when a considerable amount of serous exudate is poured out, thus constituting "the pleurisy with effusion" of the clinician. At autopsy, this diagnosis is not made unless the fluid in the pleural cavity exceeds 200 cc. in amount. As withdrawn upon thoracentesis, the fluid is usually light yellow in color, turbid, of relatively high specific gravity

and may complicate various inflammations of the lungs, more particularly those due to streptococcus. In the earlier stages the pus is free in the pleural cavity, but there is apparently a rapid organization about the margin so that the pus tends to become more or less localized in certain parts of the pleura. The pus is usually found under the thoracic wall in the lower part of the chest but may be observed overlying the diaphragm or between the lobes of the lung. The causative organisms are usually identified readily in the earlier stages of the process but as it becomes more chronic they are difficult to find.

Acute putrid or gangrenous pleurisy may be the result of gangrene of the lungs or the introduction of organisms ordinarily saprophytic through wounds of the thoracic wall. If gas-forming organisms be present, there may be considerable accumulation of gas in the pleural cavity. As with empyema, provided the patient survives the acute stage of the process, encapsulation can progress fairly rapidly.

Acute hemorrhagic pleurisy may be seen where pleurisy occurs in connection with the various diseases mentioned as producing petechiae of the pleura, but of outstanding importance are tuberculosis and malignant tumors of the pleura. In this condition, as in hemothorax, bile pigment may be found provided the blood remains a sufficient length of time in the pleural cavity.

Local Sequences of Acute Pleurisy. It is probable that minor grades of acute fibrinous pleurisy may recover with complete restitution to normal, or there may be simply a fibrous scar. If extensive, however, the granulation proceeding from both layers of the pleura results in the formation ultimately of fibrinous adhesions between the two layers. This is to be regarded as a cicatrizing non-progressive condition which presumably has no functional significance, because respiration may go on normally in spite of complete obliteration of the pleural sac. It is usual to distinguish chronic fibrous pleurisy in which there is simple thickening of the layers of the pleura, chronic adhesive pleurisy and chronic obliterative pleurisy. For the most part these represent scars, but more particularly in connection with chronic tuberculosis of the lung and with tumors of the pleura or the lung, the condition may be progressive, and is then to be regarded as a true chronic inflammation. In hydrothorax the fluid can be removed readily by lymphatic absorption if the causative condition be cured. The same is true if an acute fibrinoserous pleurisy terminates early in its course. If very extensive and of long duration, the processes of organization going on in the pleura may so interfere with lymphatic drainage that natural removal is slow and sometimes incomplete. The purulent exudate of empyema may remain for extremely long periods of time after encapsulation has occurred, thus giving rise to prolonged absorption of the products of bacterial activity and protein decomposition. Occasionally, such conditions burrow through the thoracic wall, usually in the intercostal spaces but occasionally through the ribs, and drain spontaneously, but as a rule surgical intervention is necessary. If the exudate remain in situ for long periods, either with or without drainage, the secondary inflammatory processes of the pleura and in the compressed lung may by contraction lead to considerable deformity of the affected side of the chest.

Chronic Pleurisy. As has been mentioned, many of the so-called forms of chronic pleurisy represent merely cicatrization. There are, however, chronic forms which are definitely progressive and these are most commonly observed in chronic tuberculosis of the lung. In addition to adhesions, the pleura may become enormously thickened attaining a thickness of 8 to 10 mm. or more. This is primarily a chronic progressive fibrosis which, however, usually shows an extensive hyalinization and frequently calcification. Rarely heteroplastic bone formation is observed.

Pneumothorax. Air may gain access to the thoracic cavity either by wounds of the thoracic wall or by rupture of the lung into the pleural cavity, such as may occur in chronic ulcerative tuberculosis or other forms of tuberculosis of the lung, abscess, gangrene, tearing of the lung by fractured ribs or by exploratory needles, suppurative types of pneumonia, infected infarcts; and it is said to occur from rupture of an emphysematous lung or a normal lung with an extreme expiratory effort in coughing, etc. Gas-forming bacteria may also lead to the presence of gas in the pleural cavity. External wounds which remain open may lead to the so-called open pneumothorax. Ruptures of diseased lungs may close down leaving a closed pneumothorax, or the tissues around the opening may operate in a valve-like fashion so that air enters during inspiration and cannot be expelled completely during expiration. Communications of this general kind, valve-like or not, are often called bronchopleural, or pulmonopleural fistulas. Infection occurs rapidly and as usually seen the condition is a pyopneumothorax. The presence of organisms ordinarily saprophytic may transform this into a gangrenous pyopneumothorax. Clinically, the condition is distinguished, in addition to other features, by the fact that the fluid level is horizontal, because the collapse of the lung brings it above the level of the fluid and the latter remains in the bottom of the pleural sac.

At autopsy, it is important to differentiate between air in the pleura as the result of postmortem collapse of the lung and that which is there antemortem. For this purpose the skin of the chest may be dissected so as to form a cup-like depression into which water is placed. A small cut through the intercostal muscle permits air to bubble through this fluid. Without disfiguring the skin a needle may be plunged through the thoracic wall, and if a lighted match or taper be held above it the escape of air or gas will extinguish it. Examination of the gas usually shows that it may be either normal air, or the oxygen may be reduced by absorption and the carbon dioxide increased over that of outside air. In putrid pneumothorax the carbon dioxide may be very rich, and, more especially with the anaerobes, there may be enough hydrogen and methane produced to render the gas combustible.

Pneumothorax may be complicated by an interstitial emphysema of the lung, either following the rupture of diseased lungs or by the same trauma that caused the pneumothorax. Similarly, interstitial emphysema of the thoracic wall may occur, usually localized but sometimes extending up in the neck and down over the abdomen. Exploratory needle punctures may be followed by interstitial emphysema of the thoracic wall if air be in the pleura or be introduced during the puncture. This does not presuppose puncture of the lung since the air in the pleura may gain access to the subcutaneous structures during expiratory effort.

Tuberculosis of the Pleura. Tubercle bacilli may produce either tubercles or an exudative or productive type of inflammation in the pleura. The former is referred to as tuberculosis of the pleura and the latter as tuberculous pleurisy. Tuberculosis of the pleura usually occurs as miliary tuberculosis and is either a part of a miliary tuberculosis of the lung or a disseminated miliary tuberculosis. The tubercles appear as minute discrete gray or yellowish-gray nodules projecting slightly above the surface of the pleura but covered by endothelium. In cattle, the so-called "perlsucht" disease is not uncommon.

This is a chronic productive type of tuberculosis, leading to the formation of sessile and sometimes pedunculated nodules several millimeters or a centimeter or more in diameter. They are usually firm, definitely fibrotic and on section show a variable amount of central caseation. Conditions approaching this are rarely found in man.

Tuberculous pleurisy may be acute fibrinous or more commonly an acute fibrinoserous pleurisy with a large quantity of fairly clear fluid which is sometimes tinged with blood. These forms are recognized anatomically, as a rule, by identification of extensive tuberculosis in the lung. The assurance that they are definitely tuberculous, however, must depend upon the presence of miliary tubercles in the pleura or the demonstration of tubercle bacilli in the exudate, which usually is done by animal inoculation. Sometimes in these conditions, there is extensive tubercle formation, not only of discrete miliary tubercles but of conglomerate tubercles. Chronic tuberculous pleurisy may be a chronic fibrous, a chronic adhesive, or chronic obliterative process. In many instances this is assumed to be tuberculous because of its intimate relation to chronic tuberculosis of the lung. On the other hand, the lesion may show, in the thickened pleura, definite tubercle formation and sometimes extensive caseation. The great thickenings of the pleura in chronic pleurisy are usually tuberculous when not a part of chronic empyema, and the appearance of hyalinization and calcification is more common in the tuberculous form.

Other granulomatous lesions such as syphilis and actinomycosis are practically always secondary to the effects of these diseases in the lung, the mediastinal contents, or the thoracic wall.

Postmortem examination of the pleura often shows near the apex of the lung a localized, densely fibrous thickening of the pleura, 1 or 2 cm. in diameter, irregular in outline and somewhat retracted. If these be associated with adhesions they are probably of tuberculous origin, but careful study of the nonadherent forms gives no satisfactory evidence of previous tuberculosis (Bessin).

Tumors

Primary benign tumors are extremely uncommon and may include fibroma, lipoma, angioma, chondroma, and osteoma. Primary sarcomas are also unusual and may be spindle-cell sarcoma, lymphosarcoma, or various forms of combined sarcoma, such as the fibrosarcoma and chondrosarcoma.

The so-called pleural endothelioma or mesothelioma usually occurs in the pleural sac near the base of the lung as a flat often nodular mass, involving both parietal and visceral pleura. Extensive fibrosis is common and may result in the formation of locules, which contain serous or bloody fluid or inflammatory exudate. Microscopically, the tumor cells are large round cells in nests of various size and often arranged as acini or tubular structures. Tumor nodules are often found in mediastinal lymph nodes and in more remote parts of the body. Robertson concludes that many cases are carcinoma, either squamous or more often adenomatous; sarcoma; or unclassified, and in the last group he thinks that most of the instances are secondary carcinomas. Klemperer and Rabin report several tumors of the pleura which are truly primary. It is rare however to find tumors which on microscopic examination justify the term endothelioma or mesothelioma.

Secondary tumors of the pleura are usually extensions from primary or, more commonly, secondary tumors of the lungs, but occasionally metastases occur extensively in the pleura with but little involvement of the lungs.

Physiologic Alterations Due to Increased Pleural Contents

Increases of fluid and solid contents may produce bulging of the chest without altering the normal negative pressure of the pleura. By reducing the normal curvature of the diaphragm, a moderate increase of pleural content leads to a restriction in the respiratory outward movement of the costal margin, whereas greater increases may lead to an inward instead of an outward movement (Hoover). Both experimentally and clinically, large quantities of fluid may accumulate in the pleura without altering the negative pressure. Nevertheless, the weight of the column of fluid exerts pressure on that part of the lung which is immersed and contributes to the bulging of the intercostal spaces and chest. Injection of fluid into the dog's pleura produces a marked fall in systemic blood pressure, due in part to compression and perhaps kinking of the intrathoracic vena cava, and in part to reduction of circulation through the lungs incident to diminution of respiratory aid to the pulmonary circulation and to actual compression of the lungs; perhaps in extreme cases there is compression of the pulmonary veins. Thus, there is deficient filling of the left and ultimately of the right atrium. Reduction of vital capacity varies with the degree of collapse of the lung.

The closed nonvalvular pneumothorax operates in essentially the same way as do pleural fluids. Ventilation and gas interchange are not seriously interfered with. In open pneumothorax there is atmospheric pressure in the affected side, so that the mediastinum moves toward the healthy side in inspiration and away from it in expiration, thus limiting the exchange of air. Dyspnea may be severe, the blood showing reduction of oxygen and increase of carbon dioxide. This is due not only to the diminished lung excursion, but may also be contributed to by blowing air from the normal lung into the diseased side and sucking it back again in inspiration. Closure of the pneumothorax restores the oxygen and carbon dioxide content of the blood practically to normal. In valvular pneumothorax the inspiration of air into the pleura establishes atmospheric pressure which may be markedly increased during expiration. The mediastinal contents are pushed toward the healthy side and the diaphragm depressed. Except for the compression of normal lung its respiratory action is not decreased, because with the pressure in the diseased side, the mediastinum moves toward the healthy side in expiration and away from it in inspiration. The pathologic physiology of open pneumothorax is admirably discussed by Graham.

REFERENCES

Adams, J. M.: Primary Virus Pneumonitis with Cytoplasmic Inclusion Bodies: Study of an Epidemic Involving Thirty-two Infants, with Nine Deaths, Jour. Amer. Med. Asso., 116: 925, 1941.

Arce, J.: Hydatid Disease (Hydatidosis): Hydatid Cyst of the Lung, Arch. Surg., 43: 789, 1941.

Ash, J. E.: Sinusitis from the Viewpoint of the General Pathologist, Trans. Amer. Acad. Ophth., 44: 304, 1939.

Atkinson, D.: The Nontuberculous Pulmonary Fibroses, Amer. Jour. Med. Sci., 170: 693, 1925.

Avery, O. T., H. T. Chickering, R. Cole, and A. R. Dochez: Acute Lobar Pneumonia, Monograph Rockefeller Inst. No. 7, 1917.

——, and G. E. Cullen: Studies on the Enzymes of Pneumococcus, I, II, III, Jour. Exper. Med., 32: 547, 571, 583, 1920.

Belt, T. H.: Autopsy Incidence of Pulmonary Embolism, Lancet, 1: 1259, 1939.

Berry, F. B.: Lobar Pneumonia-Analysis of 400 Autopsies, Med. Clin. N. Amer., 4: 571, 1920-21.

Bessin, A.: Ueber die knorpelähnlichen Pleuraschwielen, Virchow's Arch. Path. Anat., 280: 837, 1931.

Blake, F. G., and R. L. Cecil: Studies on Experimental Pneumonia I, II, III, IV, Jour. Exper. Med., 31: 403, 445, 499, 519, 1920.

Blankenhorn, M. A.: Chylous and Pseudochylous Effusions, Arch. Int. Med., 32: 129, 1923.

——: The Causes of Turbidity in Milky Ascitic Fluids, Ibid., 32: 140, 1923.

Brenner, O.: Pathology of the Vessels of the Pulmonary Circulation, Arch. Int. Med., 56: 211, 457, 724, 976, 1189, 1935.

Breslich, P. J.: Squamous Cell Carcinoma of the Trachea, Jour. Cancer Res., 14: 144, 1930.

Bullowa, J. G. M.: The Management of the Pneumonias, New York, Oxford Univ. Press, 1937.

Caldwell, G. T., and J. D. Roberts: Rhinosporidiosis in the United States: Report of a Case Originating in Texas, Jour. Amer. Med. Asso., 110: 1641, 1938.

Caldwell, H. W.: Spontaneous Mediastinal Emphysema, Jour. Amer. Med. Asso., 116: 301, 1941.

Cannon, P. R.: The Problem of Lipid Pneumonia. A Brief Review, Jour. Amer. Med. Asso., 115: 2176, 1940.

Castleman, B.: Healed Pulmonary Infarcts, Arch. Path., 30: 130, 1940.

Cole, R.: Pneumococcus Infection and Lobar Pneumonia, Harvey Lectures, Philadelphia, Lippincott, 1913-14, p. 85.

Coryllos, P. N., and G. L. Birnbaum: Studies in Pulmonary Gas Absorption in Bronchial Obstruction. III. A Theory of Air Absorption in Atelectasis, Amer. Jour. Med. Sci., 183: 347, 1932; see also Y. Henderson and M. C. Henderson, Arch. Int. Med., 49: 88, 1932.

Craige, B., Jr.: Fatal Bronchial Asthma: Report of Seven Cases, Arch. Int. Med., 67: 399, 1941.

Cutler, E. C.: The Experimental Production of Abscess of the Lung, Amer. Jour. Dis. Child., 38: 683, 1929.

——, and A. M. Hunt: Postoperative Pulmonary Complications, Arch. Int. Med., 29: 449, 1922.

D'Aunoy, R., and A. Zoeller: Primary Tumors of the Trachea: Report of a Case and Review of the Literature, Arch. Path., 11: 589, 1931.

Denman, H. C.: Syphilis of the Lung. Report of a Case with Autopsy Findings, Ann. Int. Med., 5: 895, 1932.

Erb, I. H.: Pathology of Bronchiectasis, Arch. Path., 15: 357, 1933.

Ewing, J.: Lymphoepithelioma, Amer. Jour. Path., 5: 99, 1929.

Finland, M.: The Significance of Specific Pneumococcus Types in Disease, Including Types IV to XXXII (Cooper), Ann. Int. Med., 10: 1531, 1937; see also Arch. Path., 23: 801, 1937.

Finland, M., and A. W. Winkler: Recurrences in Pneumococcus Pneumonia, Amer. Jour. Med. Sci., 188: 309, 1934.

Fried, B. M.: Primary Carcinoma of the Lung. A Clinical and Pathological Study, Medicine, 10: 373, 1931.

——: Allergic Inflammation of the Lungs: The Pathogenesis of Lobar Pneumonia, Arch. Path., 18: 865, 1934.

Ghoreyeb, A. A., and H. T. Karsner: A Study of the Relation of Pulmonary and Bronchial Circulation, Jour. Exper. Med., 18: 500, 1913.

Goodpasture, E. W., S. H. Auerbach, H. S. Swanson, and E. F. Cotter: Virus Pneumonia of Infants Secondary to Epidemic Infections, Amer. Jour. Dis. Child., 57: 997, 1939.

Graef, I.: Studies in Lipid Pneumonia. I. Lipid Pneumonia due to Cod Liver Oil. II. Lipid Pneumonia due to Liquid Petrolatum, Arch. Path., 28: 613, 1939.

Graham, E. A.: Alterations of Intrapleural Pressure and Their Significance, Medicine, 3: 417, 1924.

Gunn, F. D.: Changing Concepts in Lobar Pneumonia, Arch. Path., 24: 835, 1937.

Hall, G. E., and G. H. Ettinger: An Experimental Study of Pulmonary Embolism, Canad. Med. Asso. Jour., 28: 357, 1933.

Hampton, A. O., and B. Castleman: Correlation of Postmortem Chest Teleroentgenograms with Autopsy Findings, with Special Reference to Pulmonary Embolism and Infarction, Amer. Jour. Roent. and Radium Ther., 43: 305, 1940.

Hastings, A. B., J. M. Neill, H. J. Morgan, and C. A. L. Binger: The Acid-base Balance in Pneumonia, Proc. Soc. Exper. Biol. and Med., 21: 66, 1923-24.

Heffron, R.: Pneumonia with Special Reference to Pneumococcus Lobar Pneumonia, New York, The Commonwealth Fund, 1939.

Herxheimer, G.: Zur Aetiologie und pathologischen Anatomie der Syphilis, Ergeb. Allg. Path. u. Path. Anat., 11(1): 1, 1907.

——: Zur pathologischen Anatomie der kongenitalen Syphilis, Ibid., 12: 499, 1908.

Hesdorffer, M. B., and J. A. Duffalo: American Q Fever. Report of a Probable Case, Jour. Amer. Med. Asso., 116: 1901, 1941.

Holman, E., and M. E. Mathes: The Production of Intrapulmonary Suppuration by Secondary Infection of a Sterile Embolic Area. An Experimental Study, Arch. Surg., 19: 1246, 1929.

Hoover, C. F.: The Diagnostic Significance of Inspiratory Movements of the Costal Margins, Amer. Jour. Med. Sci., 159: 633, 1920.

zu Jeddeloh, B.: Untersuchungen zur Histologie chronischer Stauungslungen. Gleichzeitig ein Beitrag zur normalen Histologie der Lunge, Beitr. Path. Anat. u. Allg. Path., 86: 387, 1931.

Jordan, E. O.: Epidemic Influenza—A Survey, Chicago, 1927.

Julianelle, L. A.: The Pneumonia of Friedländer's Bacillus, Ann. Int. Med., 15: 190, 1941.

Karsner, H. T.: The Pathological Effects of Atmospheres Rich in Oxygen, Jour. Exper. Med., 23: 149, 1916.

——: Productive-cicatricial Syphilitic Disease of the Pulmonary Artery, Arch. Int. Med., 51: 367, 1933.

——, and J. E. Ash: Experimental Bland Infarction of the Lung, Jour. Med. Res., 27: 205, 1912-13.

Karsner, H. T., and A. A. Ghoreyeb: The Circulation in Experimental Pulmonary Embolism, Jour. Exper. Med., 18: 507, 1913.

——, and O. Saphir: Small Cell Carcinomas of the Lung, Amer. Jour. Path., 6: 553, 1930; see also W. Boyd, Notes on the Pathology of Primary Carcinoma of the Lung, Canad. Med. Asso. Jour., 23: 210, 1930.

——, M. A. Simon, and T. F. Fujiwara: Relation of Experimental Pulmonary Arterial Hypertension to Arteriosclerosis, Arch. Path., 31: 585, 1941.

Kaump, D. H., and T. J. Dry: Pulmonary Arteriolar Sclerosis: A Clinicopathologic Study, Arch. Int. Med., 61: 1, 1938.

Keilty, R. A.: Primary Endothelioma of the Pleura, Amer. Jour. Med. Sci., 153: 888, 1917.

Klemperer, P., and C. B. Rabin: Primary Neoplasms of the Pleura: A Report of Five Cases, Arch. Path., 11: 385, 1931.

Kline, B. S.: Experimental Study of Organization in Lobar Pneumonia, Jour. Exper. Med., 26: 239, 1917.

——: Pulmonary Abscess and Pulmonary Gangrene, Jour. Amer. Med. Asso., 90: 2008, 1928.

——: Spirochetal Pulmonary Gangrene, Ibid., 77: 1874, 1921.

——: Experimental Gangrene, Jour. Infect. Dis., 32: 481, 1923.

——, and S. S. Berger: Spirochetal Pulmonary Gangrene Treated with Arsphenamine, Jour. Amer. Med. Asso., 85: 1452, 1925.

——, and M. A. Blankenhorn: Spirochetal Pulmonary Gangrene, Ibid., 81: 719, 1923.

Koeckert, H. L.: Fetal Bronchiectasis, Amer. Jour. Dis. Children, 17: 95, 1919.

Koletsky, S.: Primary Carcinoma of the Lung. A Clinical and Pathologic Study of One Hundred Cases, Arch. Int. Med., 62: 636, 1938.

Kountz, W. B., and H. L. Alexander: Emphysema, Medicine, 13: 251, 1934.

LaDue, J. S.: Bronchiolitis Fibrosa Obliterans: Report of a Case, Arch. Int. Med., 68: 663, 1941.

Lee, W. E.: Acute Massive and Partial Collapse of the Lungs, Bull. Ayer Clin. Lab. Penna. Hosp., 9: 5, 1925.

——: Postoperative Pulmonary Complications, Ann. Surg., 79: 506, 1924.

Longacre, J. J., and L. G. Herrmann: Experimental Studies on Pulmonary Suppuration, Arch. Surg., 30: 476, 1935.

Looper, E. A., and L. V. Schneider: Laryngeal Tuberculosis: A Study of Five Hundred Patients, etc., Jour. Amer. Med. Asso., 91: 1012, 1916.

Lord, F. T.: The Relation of the Pneumococcus to the Production of Acid in Fluid Culture Mediums and the Reaction of the Pneumonic Lung, Ibid., 72: 1364, 1919.

——: The Relation of Proteolytic Enzymes to Hydrogen Ion Concentration. An Explanation of Resolution, Jour. Exper. Med., 30: 379, 1919.

——: Pneumonia, Cambridge, 1922.

——, and R. N. Nye: Studies of the Pneumococcus, I, II, III, IV, Jour. Exper. Med., 35: 685, 689, 699, 703, 1922.

Lucksch, F.: Pathologic Anatomy of Influenza: A Review Based Chiefly on German Sources, Arch. Path., 5: 448, 1928.

Luisada, A.: The Pathogenesis of Paroxysmal Pulmonary Edema, Medicine, 19: 475, 1940.

Lundsgaard, C.: Anoxemia in Lobar Pneumonia, Medicine, 4: 345, 1925.

MacCallum, W. G.: The Pathology of the Pneumonia in the United States Army Camps During the Winter of 1917-18; Monographs of the Rockefeller Inst., N. 10, 1919.

Mann, F. C.: Pulmonary Embolism, an Experimental Study, Jour. Exper. Med., 26: 387, 1917.

McCartney, J. S., Jr.: Pulmonary Embolism: A Report of 73 Cases, Arch. Path. and Lab. Med., 3: 921, 1927.

Matz, P. B.: The Incidence of Primary Bronchiogenic Carcinoma, Jour. Amer. Med. Asso., 111: 2086, 1938.

Mendlowitz, M.: Experimental Pulmonary Embolism, Jour. Thoracic Surg., 8: 204, 1938-39.

Menne, F. R., and Anderson, M. W.: Bronchiogenic Carcinoma. Incidence in the Pacific Northwest, with a commentary on Eighty-four Cases, Jour. Amer. Med. Asso., 117: 2215, 1941.

Metz, G. A.: Zur Pathogenese des Lungenemphysems, Krankheitsforschung, 9: 1, 1931.

Michael, M., Jr.: Staphylococcus Aureus Pneumonia with Special Reference to its Occurrence as a Complication of Influenza, Jour. Amer. Med. Asso., 118: 869, 1942.

Miller, W. S.: The Alveolar Pores of Pneumonia, Jour. Exper. Med., 42: 779, 1925.

Moore, R. A., and P. Gross: Giant Cells in Inflammation of the Lung in Children, Amer. Jour. Dis. Child., 40: 247, 1930.

Mudd, S., S. B. Grant, and A. Goldman: The Etiology of Acute Inflammations of the Nose, Pharynx and Tonsils, Ann. Otol., Rhinol. and Laryngol., 30: 1, 1921.

Ochsner, A., and M. DeBakey: Carcinoma of the Lung, Arch. Surg., 42: 209, 1941.

Ogilvie, A. G.: The Natural History of Bronchiectasis: A Clinical, Roentgenologic and Pathologic Study, Arch. Int. Med., 68: 395, 1941.

Olitsky, P. K., and J. E. McCartney: Studies on the Nasopharyngeal Secretions from Patients with Common Colds, Jour. Exper. Med., 38: 427, 1923.

Opie, E. L., F. G. Blake, J. C. Small, and T. M. Rivers: Epidemic Respiratory Disease, St. Louis, 1921.

——: The Pathologic Anatomy of Influenza Based Chiefly on American and British Sources, Arch. Path., 5: 285, 1928.

Peabody, F. W.: The Oxygen Content of the Blood in Lobar Pneumonia, Jour. Exper. Med., 18: 7, 1913.

Pickrell, K. L.: The Effect of Alcoholic Intoxication and Ether Anesthesia on Resistance to Pneumococcal Infection, Bull. Johns Hopkins Hosp., 63: 238, 1938.

Reichle, H. S.: Resolving Exudates in Pulmonary Tuberculosis of Childhood, Amer. Jour. Dis. Child., 45: 307, 1933.

——, and T. T. Frost: Tuberculosis of the Major Bronchi, Amer. Jour. Path., 10: 651, 1934.

Reimann, H. A., and W. P. Havens: An Epidemic Disease of the Respiratory Tract, Arch. Int. Med., 65: 138, 1940.

Robertson, H. E.: "Endothelioma" of the Pleura, Jour. Cancer Res., 8: 317, 1924.

Robertson, O. H.: Recent Studies on Experimental Lobar Pneumonia. I. Pathogenesis, Jour. Amer. Med. Asso., **111**: 1432, 1938.

——, and M. Hamburger: Studies on the Pathogenesis of Experimental Pneumococcus Pneumonia in the Dog., Jour. Exper. Med., **72**: 275, 1940.

——, and M. Hamburger: The Mechanism of Interlobar Spread in Experimental Pneumococcus Pneumonia in the Dog, Trans. Asso. Amer. Phys., **55**: 209, 1940.

Rosahn, P. D.: Incidence of Primary Carcinoma of the Lung: A Review of Yale Autopsy Protocols, 1917 to 1937, Arch. Path., **29**: 649, 1940.

Ruegsegger, J. M., and S. L. Cockrell: Recurrence in Pneumonia, Jour. Lab. and Clin. Med., **26**: 1262, 1941.

Savacool, J. W.: Prothrombin Studies in Pulmonary Tuberculosis, Amer. Jour. Med. Sci., **201**: 830, 1941.

Schumacher, E. D., and W. Jehn: Experimentelle Untersuchungen über die Ursache des Todes durch Lungenembolie, Zeitschr. Ges. Exper. Med., **3**: 340, 1914.

Scott, R. W.: Observations on the Pathological Physiology of Chronic Pulmonary Emphysema, Arch. Int. Med., **26**: 544, 1920.

Scott, W. J. M.: Postoperative Massive Collapse of the Lung, Arch. Surg., **10**: 73, 1925; *see also* W. J. M. Scott, and E. C. Cutler: Jour. Amer. Med. Asso., **90**: 1759, 1928.

Sheely, R. F.: Prothrombin Deficiency in Pulmonary Tuberculosis. Clinical Relation and Significance in Hemoptysis, Jour. Amer. Med. Asso., **117**: 1603, 1941.

Shope, R. E.: Recent Knowledge Concerning Influenza, Ann. Int. Med., **11**: 1, 1937.

Sia, R. H. P., O. H. Robertson, and S. T. Woo: A Study of the Mechanism of Recovery from Lobar Pneumonia, Jour. Exper. Med., **48**: 513, 1928.

Smith, L. W.: The Pathological Anatomy of Pertussis, etc., Arch. Path. and Lab. Med., **4**: 732, 1927.

Stillman, E. G., and A. Branch: Susceptibility of Rabbits to Infection by Inhalation of Virulent Pneumococci, Jour. Exper. Med., **44**: 581, 1926.

Sunderman, F. W., J. H. Austin, and J. G. Camac: Studies in Serum Electrolytes, I. Concentration of Electrolytes and Non-Electrolytes in the Serum during Lobar Pneumonia, Jour. Clin. Invest., **3**: 37, 1926-27.

Thieme, E. T., and J. M. Sheldon: A Correlation of the Clinical and Pathologic Findings in Bronchial Asthma, Jour. Allergy, **9**: 246, 1938.

Van Allen, C. M., W. E. Adams, and L. S. Hrdina: Bronchogenic Contamination in Embolic Abscess of the Lungs, Arch. Surg., **19**: 1262, 1929.

——: Embolism in Bronchogenic Infection of the Lung, Ibid., **19**: 1279, 1929.

Weinberg, T.: Sarcoma of the Trachea, Amer. Jour. Cancer, **37**: 201, 1939.

Weir, J. M., and F. L. Horsfall, Jr.: The Recovery from Patients with Acute Pneumonitis of a Virus Causing Pneumonia in the Mongoose, Jour. Exper. Med., **72**: 595, 1940.

Wells, H. G.: Waxy Degeneration of the Diaphragm: A Factor in Causing Death in Pneumonia and in Other Conditions, Arch. Path. and Lab. Med., **4**: 681, 1927.

Winternitz, M. C., and R. A. Lambert: Edema of the Lungs as a Cause of Death, Jour. Exper. Med., **29**: 537, 1919.

——, G. H. Smith, and F. P. McNamara: Epithelial Proliferation Following the Intrabronchial Insufflation of Acid, Jour. Exper. Med., **32**: 205, 1920.

——, I. M. Wason, and F. P. McNamara: The Pathology of Influenza, New Haven, 1920.

Wolbach, S. B.: Comments on the Pathology and Bacteriology of Fatal Influenza Cases, etc., Johns Hopkins Hosp. Bull., **30**: 104, 1919.

Wolman, I. J., and A. B. Bayard: Experimental Aspiration Pneumonia: Fluorescence and Pathology, Amer. Jour. Med. Sci., **202**: 542, 1941.

16

The Alimentary Canal

MOUTH

Congenital Malformations

The commonest malformation is harelip (cheiloschisis) which is often combined with cleft palate (anathoschisis). These are due to failure of union of the nasal process and the maxillary processes which go to form the lower part of the face. The middle third of the upper lip and the premaxillary part of the upper jaw are contributed by the nasal process. Since harelip is due to failure of fusion of nasal and maxillary processes, it occurs at the outer margin of the middle third of the upper lip and may be single or double. There may be only a slight indentation of the lip, or the fissure may extend upward and communicate with the anterior nares. Median harelip is extremely rare. In the more extensive cases of unilateral or bilateral harelip there is an associated cleft palate, the fissures in the latter extending to either side of the intermaxillary bone, which provides the incisor teeth, and often accompanied by altered or incomplete development of these teeth.

When it occurs in the posterior part of the hard palate, the fissure is median because the palatal plates are provided by the maxillary processes. Fissures of the lower lip are rare. The development of the lips may

489

proceed too far toward the median line, leaving only a small opening (microstomia), or there may be a failure of development laterally, leaving a wide mouth fissure sometimes extending nearly to the ears (macrostomia). Numerous other more severe faults of development which occur are usually incompatible with life. These are treated in the texts on embryology and congenital malformations.

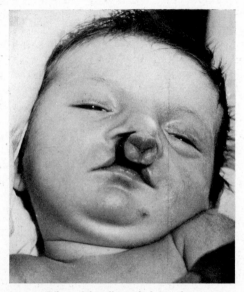

Bilateral harelip and cleft palate.

Macrocheilia has been referred to in the chapter on tumors as a congenital tumorlike enlargement of the lymphatic vessels, which may be progressive.

Pigmentations

The most important pigmentation is that which often occurs upon the lateral and inferior aspect of the tongue and in the buccal mucosa in Addison's disease. This has diagnostic significance, especially in negroes.

Inflammation

Stomatitis. ACUTE CATARRHAL STOMATITIS is more common in children than in adults. It may be due to mechanical, thermal or chemical irritants, may be the result of extension from inflammations of the pharynx and nose, may accompany acute infectious diseases such as scarlet fever, measles, typhoid fever, smallpox, etc., is common during the teething period and often accompanies gastric disturbances, particularly acute catarrhal gastritis. The mucous membrane is red, swollen, somewhat edematous and may show either excess or reduction of mucous secretion. Small white spots may appear due to necrosis or desquamation of the surface epithelium. Microscopically, there is, in addition to surface degeneration, hyperemia and edema, and a moderate infiltration of lymphoid cells and leukocytes.

ACUTE VESICULAR STOMATITIS may be caused by various irritants such as heat, or carious teeth, or may be an extension from vesicular or pustular processes about the lip, more particularly herpes, eczema and smallpox. The ordinary form is usually localized about the tip of the tongue, the lips and the buccal mucous membrane, where the vesicles are formed by a serous exudate under the squamous epithelium. There is usually a neighboring catarrhal inflammation and, if the vesicles rupture, small ulcers are formed. Early in the course of smallpox the hard, shot-like nodules may be found in the mucosa covering the hard and soft palate.

ACUTE FIBRINOUS STOMATITIS may be either an extension to the mucous membrane of the soft palate and lateral faucial walls, or to the base of the tongue, from diphtheria and other inflammations of the tonsils, or may be produced by the action of corrosive chemicals. Also fibrinous in character is the so-called APHTHOUS STOMATITIS which is more common in children during the period of teething but may accompany various acute infectious diseases. In adults it is more frequent in women during periods of pregnancy, the puerperium or during menstruation. The inflammation of the membranes is accompanied by the formation of slightly elevated yellowish-white plaques of irregular shape and size which, microscopically, show an exudate beneath the epithelium containing variable amounts of fibrin. Desquamation of the superficial epithelium may lead to ulceration.

ACUTE ULCERATIVE STOMATITIS may occur in young, ill-nourished children and is commonly associated with the presence of fusiform bacilli and spirochetes of Vincent. It also occurs in scurvy and in poisoning by mercury, lead, copper, and phosphorus. The lesions usually begin about the margins of the teeth, with hyperemia and swelling, and in scurvy there is a certain amount of hemorrhage. Ulceration rapidly proceeds along the gums and may involve the floor of the mouth and the teeth. Necrosis of the jaw bone may occur, particularly in cases of phosphorus poisoning. Infection may extend into the dental processes and is often followed by dropping out of teeth.

ACUTE GANGRENOUS STOMATITIS may be the result of saprophytic organisms invading wounds, may follow upon acute ulcerative stomatitis, or may occur as noma. The para-infectious disease called noma is a gangrenous process in the cheeks which may be primary there or may follow acute gangrenous stomatitis elsewhere. It is more common in young children, and is likely to be associated with scarlatina, measles, typhoid fever or other acute infectious diseases. The process rapidly extends through all the tissues of the cheek, appearing ultimately upon the cutaneous surface. It cannot be said that any special type of organism produces this condition but, as in other gangrenous inflammations of the mouth, the fusiform bacilli and spirochetes of Vincent are commonly found. The disease is usually fatal.

THRUSH is a form of stomatitis due to *Oïdium albicans,* occurring in ill-nourished children or in children and adults suffering from prolonged exhausting diseases. Slightly elevated, white or yellowish-white patches of irregular shape and size occur in various parts of the mouth, due to the growth in or upon the epithelium of the particular yeast concerned. This condition may extend to the pharynx, esophagus and even to the upper respiratory tract.

KOPLIK'S SPOTS are bluish-white, slightly elevated spots, a few millimeters in diameter, fairly numerous, which occur in the posterior buccal mucosa in the preëruptive stage of measles and constitute an important diagnostic sign. Similar spots may appear even earlier in the lachrymal caruncle. Microscopically, there is keratinization of the superficial epithelium under which is a collection of lymphocytes, large mononuclears and multinucleated giant cells.

TROPICAL SPRUE shows acute or chronic catarrh of the mouth often with aphthous spots. The catarrh may be present in the entire alimentary canal.

LUDWIG'S ANGINA is described by Ash-hurst as "a clinical entity consisting of septic cellulitis of the floor of the mouth and of the neck." It originates in inflammations of submaxillary glands and lymph nodes and may complicate dental infections. Suppuration is usual, constituting a phlegmon, and gangrene may supervene. Suppuration may extend into the mediastinum. Edema of the glottis may occur. Nearly one-third of the patients die.

CHRONIC STOMATITIS is characterized by a more or less diffuse thickening and keratinization of the superficial epithelium, with fibrosis of the underlying connective tissue and enlargement of the lymphoid nodules. The process when involving the filiform papillae of the tongue may give it an extremely shaggy appearance.

Leukoplakia oris, or *buccalis,* is more localized. Fox points out that it affects especially middle-aged men and is rare in women and in negroes. The direct cause seems to be local irritation particularly by tobacco, and syphilis is a predisposing cause in a large number of cases. The patches are of irregular shape and sometimes are referred to as geographic. They may appear upon lips, buccal mucous membranes, tongue, or other parts of the mouth, as slightly elevated, hard, clearly defined, yellowish or grayish-white plaques. Microscopically, the entire epithelial covering is thickened, and there is extensive keratinization of the epithelium between the papillae of the supporting connective tissue, and the latter frequently shows a low grade subacute or chronic inflammation. It may lead to carcinoma but may exist for years without malignant change.

Infectious Granulomata

Syphilis is the most frequent of these. Chancre may appear on lips, the buccal mucosa, particularly near the angles of the mouth, upon the tip of the tongue and even upon the tonsils. The secondary lesions may include an erythematous eruption or, more commonly, the so-called mucous patches. These are at first reddened areas, rapidly becoming slightly elevated plaques a few millimeters or a centimeter or more in diameter, fairly well defined, soft, and bluish-gray in color. Desquamation of the epithelium may leave shallow ulcers with a moist, smooth, only slightly reddened base. Gummata appear in the deeper tissues rather than upon the surface and finally produce projecting masses. These are more common in the soft palate than elsewhere. They may ulcerate and lead to severe hemorrhage.

Tuberculosis may occur as an extension from tuberculous lupus of the face, or as miliary or small conglomerate tubercles which are superficial and tend to ulcerate. It is not rare in the tongue, but is not often encountered elsewhere in the mouth; when it does occur it is most likely to affect gums and hard and soft palate. This type of lesion is practically always secondary to pulmonary tuberculosis, sometimes localizing in the mouth as the result of abrasions such as are produced by carious teeth, and indeed this may first call attention to the pulmonary disease.

Leprosy may appear in the mouth, particularly in the nodular lepromatous form. Actinomycosis and glanders also occur in the mouth.

Tumors

Benign Tumors. Fibroma and lipoma may occur in any part of the mouth, more commonly as somewhat pedunculated tumors of the mucous surface of the lips. Papillomata may occur in any part of the mouth, as is true also of the hemangioma. Macrocheilia has been referred to above; small lymphangiomas may occur in the buccal mucosa, especially near the lips. Dermoid cysts and other varieties of teratoma may occur, apparently as the result of faults in development of the branchial clefts. Presumably due to embryonal misplacement, are the so-called mixed tumors, like those of the parotid, occur (D'Aunoy).

The carcinomas of the mouth include the squamous cell carcinoma, likely to occur in association with jagged teeth, ill-fitting dentures, and on the lip especially of smokers. Transitional-cell carcinoma is also observed in various parts of the mouth. Lymphoepithelioma, made up of large cells often intermingled with lymphocytes, occurs principally in the posterior parts of the mouth where epithelium is in intimate contact with lymphoid tissue. Adenocarcinoma arises from glandular structures of the mouth and perhaps also from the so-called mixed tumors. Except for the adenocarcinomas, metastasis is not often widespread. Lympho-

sarcoma may arise in lymphoid structures, but other sarcomas are rare.

TONGUE

Congenital Malformations

The anterior portion or the entire tongue may be congenitally absent. The tip may be bifurcated or there may be actual lobulation of the tongue. Developmental

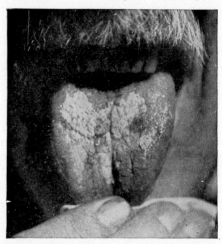

Leukoplakia of the tongue. From Hartzell, Diseases of the Skin.

fusion with the floor of the mouth or with the gums or even with the roof of the mouth are observed. Of most practical importance, however, is that condition known as "tongue-tie" in which the frenum is abnormally short, or extends out as far as the tip of the tongue. Remnants of the thyroglossal duct may produce cysts at the base of the tongue. These are usually lined by ciliated epithelium, and occasionally colloid may be produced in small acinic spaces.

Retrogressive Processes

The tongue is an important site of primary amyloidosis. Edema occasionally occurs, and the tongue is often affected in myxedema. Paralysis, such as may be due to lesion of the hypoglossal nerve in bulbar palsy, may lead to atrophy of the tongue.

Inflammations

Any of the inflammations discussed above as affecting the mouth may also affect the mucosa of the tongue. Glossitis occurs in connection with pellagra and other vitamin deficiencies, and in pernicious anemia. Abscess and other forms of interstitial inflammation as well as gangrene may occur from wounds of the tongue. A rare inflammation of subacute or chronic character is that known as *geographic tongue*. This occurs in infants and young children but rarely in adults. It sometimes shows a familial distribution. It usually begins near the tip of the tongue as a somewhat edematous yellowish-white spot, which spreads in all directions and very soon shows desquamation of

ulcerating lesion on the tongue margin, often in relation to carious teeth. It is usually secondary to pulmonary tuberculosis, but sometimes is said to be primary (see Feldman).

Syphilis may be present as chancre, secondary mucous patches or as gumma, the last being deep seated in the organ but occasionally appearing near the surface and ulcerating. Atrophy of the papillae of the base of the tongue is said to occur late in acquired syphilis.

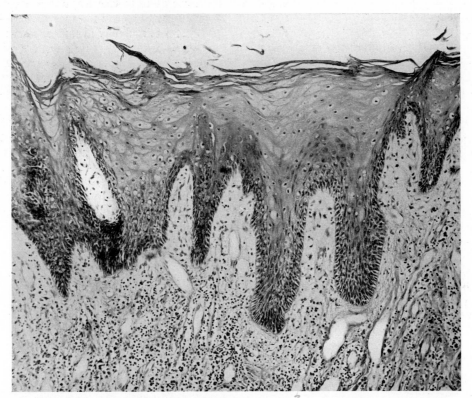

Leukoplakia of tongue. Note the keratosis and parakeratosis, the downward extension of the interpapillary epithelium and the lymphocytic infiltration of the underlying tissue.

the central part, leaving a smooth red surface lined by deeper epithelium. As it continues to spread, central healing occurs, the process usually running its course in about two weeks. Secondary areas may fuse with others, the whole process having an irregular outline suggesting a map-like contour. Recurrences are frequent and the disease may last over several years.

Infectious Granulomata

Tuberculosis is most frequent in males, appears usually as a conglomerate

Tumors

Benign tumors may occur in the substance of the tongue or as sessile or polypous tumors on the surface. Fibroma, lipoma, chondroma and hemangioma are reported. Congenital macroglossia is essentially a form of lymphangioma. Thyroid and parathyroid tumors have been observed which grow from embryonal displacements. Cysts may be derived from persistent thyroglossal ducts.

RANULA is a cystic condition in the lower surface of the tongue due to occlusion of salivary ducts.

Carcinoma of the tongue predominates in males, has an average age incidence of 58 years and is situated principally at the margin of the middle third of the tongue. There is often a history of carious teeth, ill-fitting dentures, use of tobacco, etc.; the coincidence of syphilis is fairly high. Most of the tumors are squamous cell carcinomas; transitional cell carcinoma and lymphoepithelioma are sometimes observed near the base. Adenocarcinoma is rare. The growth is slow and metastases occur principally in the sublingual and submaxillary lymph nodes. (Martin, et al.)

Sarcoma is extremely rare but may occur as a diffuse interstitial growth or sometimes as a projecting nodular growth. Even more infrequent is the occurrence of rhabdomyoma. The tongue is a site of predilection for the myoblastoma, referred to in the chapter on Tumors.

TEETH

Hypoplasia of the Teeth

Hypoplasia of the teeth may involve both the enamel and the dentin. Normal enamel is composed of characteristic rods united by interprismatic substance. Hypoplasia of the enamel is a deficiency of structure and calcification of the enamel occurring along the incremental lines. It is in reality a calcium deficiency of the enamel and is the result of a chronologic disturbance of amelogenic function during the time of enamelization. The result is imperfect calcification which involves both the rods and the interprismatic substance.

Such functional disturbances of the ameloblasts are caused by factors which interfere with calcium metabolism, such as dietary deficiencies, hyperthyroidism, fluorosis (due to fluorine in drinking water), and the acute exanthematous diseases. The deformity is manifested in that portion of the crown of the tooth which was in progress of calcification at the time the disturbance occurred. Calcification of the enamel of the tooth begins in the incisal portion of the tooth and progresses apically. Approximately five years elapse between the beginning and the completion of enamelization. Hypoplastic defects follow the growth lines (lines of

Retzius) and leave permanent records of the period at which the metabolic disturbance occurred.

These defects in enamelization are manifested grossly as pits, grooves of varying widths which encircle the tooth, or as microscopic defects in calcification. Upon eruption, the teeth are opaque, dull and chalky white in appearance. They soon become stained dark brown. It is doubtful that hypoplasia of the enamel, alone, is an important factor in the cause of dental caries, but gross defects of enamel contribute to the formation of bacterial plaques and may in this way contribute to the incidence of dental caries. Microscopically, the enamel rods are irregular in form and granular in character with an amorphous interprismatic substance. Corresponding defects in the dentin occur as irregular spaces with crescentic outlines of poor or uncalcified dentinal matrix. Such defects, while not contributing to the incidence of caries, are important factors in the rapidity of caries.

Syphilis

A specific deformity occurs with congenital syphilis, known as Hutchinson incisors and Fournier molars, in which there is a characteristic inhibition of growth and de-

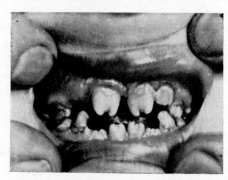

Hutchinson incisors in a 7-year-old boy.
(Courtesy of J. E. Rauschkolb, M.D.)

velopment of the enamel organ associated with severe hypoplastic defects of the enamel. There is no satisfactory evidence that direct invasion of *Treponema pallidum* into the enamel organs or tooth anlage is the cause of the hypoplasia (Hill). The teeth affected are the central and lateral incisors and first molars of the permanent dentition. These are the only teeth in the process of enamelization during the first and second year of life and their malformation is concurrent with other effects of syphilis in the newborn.

The deformity associated with Hutchinson incisors is lack of development of the central lobe. The mesial and distal lobes become inclined toward each other resulting in a tooth which is narrower at the incisal edge than at the gum line. Many times a cup-shaped depression exists between the mesial and distal lobes due to the lack of development of the central lobe. Crescent-shaped depressions may also occur in the incisal edge of the incisor teeth which are due to calcium disturbances. The Hutchinson tooth has normal width at the gum line with sides tapering to an incisal edge of diminished mesiodistal dimensions.

The enamel organs of the first molar teeth are also affected by congenital syphilis. They are undersized teeth and the first molar is usually smaller than the second molar. This lack of development results in teeth in which the cusps or mamelons are abnormally close together. The enamel formed during the first and second years is extremely hypoplastic and readily becomes involved by caries (Karnosh). Only about one-half of congenital syphilitics have this dental stigma, but its occurrence is more frequent than are the other members of Hutchinson's triad (Johnston et al.).

Dental Caries

Dental caries is a disintegration of the tooth structure which attacks both the enamel and the dentin. It begins on the surface of the tooth by the removal of the inorganic salts from the interprismatic substance, after which the enamel prisms are broken and washed away. Its progress in the enamel is comparatively slow but in the dentin it penetrates with great rapidity due to the presence of the dentinal tubules. Upon reaching the dentin, caries has a tendency to spread laterally following the dentino-enamel junction. This lateral destruction of dentin sometimes results in a rapid crumbling of the enamel due to the lack of support. Reactionary zones are demonstrable in the dentin of vital teeth beyond the region of active caries. This reaction manifests itself by partial or total obliteration of the dentinal tubules with a deposition of inorganic material either identical with or similar to the dentin itself.

Such zones are never seen in the dentin of nonvital teeth.

While causes of dental caries are not fully understood, many of its etiologic factors are known. Gross defects of the enamel, failure of the various embryonal tubes of the enamel to fuse properly, resulting in the formation of pits and fissures, and faults of form, position and occlusion of the teeth are contributing factors to dental caries. Miller believed caries to be due to the presence of

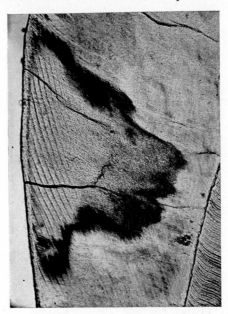

Ground section of tooth to show caries extending deeply into the enamel.

acids from bacterial growth held on the teeth by plaque formation. While this theory has been commonly accepted it is now known that accessory factors play a significant part in the etiology of dental caries. The organisms especially concerned are the oral lactobacilli. Although Clarke considers that the action of the *Streptococcus mutans* is necessary to break down the enamel before the oral lactobacilli can operate, McIntosh, James and Lazarus-Barlow find that the latter organism can produce sufficient acid to affect the enamel directly. Bunting and Palmerlee, and also Jay, believe these organisms are the chief acid-formers in the mouth. The presence of oral lactobacilli in expectorated saliva varies from none to one-half million per cubic centimeter. The numerical presence of these organisms in saliva is a reliable indicator of the activity of dental caries. Bunting, as well as Jay, further contends that adequate, well-balanced diets low in sugar definitely decrease oral lactobacilli in the mouth and markedly inhibit the activity of dental caries. Vitamin deficiencies are believed by several investigators to contribute to dental caries but results are not entirely uniform (see Boyd, et al.; Knowlton). Broderick claims that the amount of calcium in the blood and saliva determines the quality of the teeth and their susceptibility to caries.

The relation of the enamel to the individual has been the subject of much controversy. Fish and others claim that the enamel is the seat of certain metabolic activities such as recalcification, etc., through the agencies of fluids penetrating the substances from the dentin or from the oral secretions. Chase and others believe that the enamel after separation from the parent ameloblasts is a lifeless substance subject only to physicochemical changes. Since the enamel is a noncellular substance, reactions to injury cannot occur and neither regeneration nor repair is demonstrable. For many years attempts have been made to correlate variations in salivary secretions with the prevalence of dental caries but no such relationship has been shown to exist (see Marshall; Rosebury). The present evidence indicates that dental caries is the product of acids produced by sugar degradation through the medium of bacterial enzymes.

Peri-apical Diseases of the Teeth

Peri-apical diseases of the teeth are the result of degeneration and death of the tooth pulp. Traumatic injury may cause an occlusion of the blood vessels at the apex of the tooth and resultant infection of the pulp. Caries and the subsequent bacterial invasion may produce suppuration and necrosis of the pulp. Necrosis of the pulp followed by bacterial invasion either by direct extension through the dentin or by hematogenous infection, involves the peri-apical tissues and results in either an acute periodontitis or a dental granuloma. An acute periodontitis may suppurate to form an alveolar abscess. If a fistula form it usually discharges upon the oral mucosa on the buccal or labial side of the alveolar process but if in the lower jaw, may discharge upon the face.

A dental granuloma is a chronic proliferating periodontitis. It is not a specific infection but is called a granuloma because of its anatomic and histologic similarities to infectious granulomata. It is a nodule of connective tissue infiltrated with a variable number of lymphocytes, plasma cells and polymorphonuclear leukocytes. Epithelial cells which have their origin in the embryonal rests of Malassez are constantly present in dental granulomata. A proliferation of these epithelial cells forms islands which undergo necrosis because of the avascularity of the epithelium. This epithelial degeneration forms cystic areas. These are called dental or radicular cysts. Opinions differ concerning dental granulomata and their bacterial content. The organisms most commonly found in dental granulomata are streptococci of the nonhemolytic and viridans group. Staphylococci and pneumococci are also sometimes found (Rohdenburg and Franken). It is thought by some that all granulomata contain bacteria, but Hill's work indicates that the presence of bacteria is dependent upon the necrosis.

Pyorrhea Alveolaris

Pyorrhea alveolaris or periodontitis is a chronic suppurative inflammation of the periodontal membrane and gum margins surrounding the teeth. The early stages are evidenced by a gingival crevice of increased depth. This crevice is caused by a separation of the oral epithelium from the enamel epithelium and a downgrowth of oral epithelium to the bottom of the pocket. Bacteria accumulate within these crevices and inflammation, suppuration and necrosis follow. The gums surrounding the teeth are swollen, dark red in color, soft and bleed easily. The pockets vary in depth. The deeper ones, accompanied by severe destruction of the periodontal membrane, may cause the teeth to become loose.

Microscopically, there is a chronic inflammatory reaction of the soft tissues surrounding the teeth, accompanied by necrosis of the epithelium in the depths of the pocket. Local irritants such as calculus, faulty filling, loss of contact between the teeth which allows the packing of food, and traumatic occlusion are exciting causes of periodontitis. Factors other than local irritation are of importance in the etiology of this disease. Vitamin deficiencies and metabolic diseases, such as diabetes mellitus, are believed by various investigators to be primary causes. Bacteria, other than in the role of secondary invaders, probably are not an important etiologic factor, although this disease is especially frequent in unclean mouths (see Fisher). The presence of periodontitis favors phosphorus necrosis, mercurial stomatitis and the blue line of plumbism. Recession of the gums allowing the neck of the root of the tooth to become exposed but without pocket formation may result from local irritation.

Tumors and Cysts

Various connective tissue and epithelial tumors and cysts originate in the tissues of the maxilla and mandible. They may be associated with failure of the teeth to erupt and various malformations of the enamel, dentin and cementum. Odontomas are tumor-like growths derived from the special cells concerned in tooth development. Some odontomas are not true tumors but cystic cavities caused by degeneration of parts of the dental anlage.

Epithelial Odontomas. Radicular odontomas are cysts caused by degeneration of the epithelium of dental granulomas. They may be completely or partially lined with remnants of epithelium and are filled either with a clear or caseous fluid which is usually found to be infected. Follicular or dentigerous cysts arise around embedded or abnormally placed teeth which fail to erupt. They are believed to be caused by a degeneration of the stellate reticulum of the enamel organ. These cysts have the coronal portion of the tooth within the cystic cavity and the radicular portion protruding through the wall of the cyst. Microscopically, the wall of the cyst is of dense connective tissue, well vascularized in the external portion adjacent to the inner surface, which is lined with remnants of the external epithelium of the enamel organ. A thin bony shell of 1 to 3 mm. in thickness sometimes surrounds follicular cysts. Compound odontomas are composed of several or a large number of teeth included within the follicular wall. They are the result of supernumerary buds forming from the dental lamina. Most of the teeth formed are small and peg-shaped. They are frequently cystic.

ADAMANTINOMAS, as described in the chapter on Tumors, are tumors which arise from ameloblasts of the enamel organ or from remnants in the jaw of epithelium which has been displaced from the dental groove. They occur in solid and cystic forms, the latter usually multilocular. More common in the lower than in the upper jaw, they are locally invasive and may recur after removal, but rarely exhibit metastasis.

ENAMELOMAS are abnormal developments of enamel caused by disturbance of the enamel organs during the formation period of the enamel. They are irregular nodules of enamel and are not similar to the form or shape of teeth.

Connective Tissue Odontomas. These arise from the dental tissues of mesoblastic origin. Cementomas and dentinomas are irregular formations of cementum and dentin manifested either as an enlargement of the root of a tooth or as a nodular development on the sides of a root. Various composite forms of odontomas may occur.

A discussion of other tumors of the jaw is well presented by Geschickter.

SALIVARY GLANDS

Inflammations

These may occur in any of the salivary glands as the result of extension from the mouth or infection of the ducts, particularly when calculi are present, or, more especially in the parotid, may complicate septicemia or pyemia.

Parotitis. Of great importance is acute epidemic or infectious parotitis, or mumps, a highly contagious disease. This shows tender swelling of the parotid region, usually bilateral, with mild fever, but without leukocytosis. The disease lasts from one to two weeks. It may also involve the submaxillary glands. It is a catarrhal inflammation of the ducts and gland with hyperemia, edema, cloudy swelling and desquamation of epithelium and a mild infiltration of lymphocytes and a few leukocytes into the interstitial tissues. Upon recovery, the parotid is usually restored to normal. Commonly the disease may also affect the testis and sometimes the epididymis, especially at puberty. There may be complete recovery or residual fibrosis and atrophy. The disease may rarely show involvement of ovary, breast or pancreas.

Chronic inflammations, with fibrosis and glandular atrophy, may follow acute forms or be associated with calculi or plumbism. Mikulicz's disease, a symmetrical chronic inflammation which may also affect lacrimal glands, may be primary or symptomatic of other disease. Uveoparotid fever shows chronic inflammation in the parotid, sometimes nonspecific and sometimes with the lesions of Boeck's sarcoid.

Salivary Calculi

Salivary calculi are usually phosphatic but may be made of carbonates. Bacterial and mucous masses may constitute obstructive concrements. Calculi may attain great size and are more common in the submaxillary and sublingual ducts than in the ducts of Stensen. Obstruction by inflammation, by surrounding fibrosis or by calculi, leads to distention of the ducts and glands, sialocele, with subsequent atrophy of the glands. Obstruction of the sublingual duct may cause distention of the duct near its orifice under the tongue, producing the condition called ranula.

Infectious Granulomata

Tuberculosis may occur as the miliary or conglomerate form and the latter may constitute the so-called "cold abscess."

Syphilis may produce gumma.

Actinomycosis may also occur.

Tumors

Adenoma, fibroma, carcinoma, sarcoma and other tumors occur in the salivary glands. The most common is the so-called mixed tumor of the parotid, discussed in the chapter on Tumors. A high percentage are benign, but there is a notable potentiality toward malignant change; when this occurs the usual tumor is carcinoma. (See Stein and Geschickter.)

THROAT

Congenital Malformations

Defects in the final development and closure of the branchial clefts may result in the formation of cysts in the neighborhood of the fauces and pharynx. Either as the result of inflammation or of congenital malformation there may be stenosis or atresia of the fauces, of the soft palate and pharynx. Esophagopharyngeal diverticula are discussed under esophagus.

Inflammations

Acute catarrhal inflammations of the pharynx, tonsils, nasopharynx, and fauces are common in connection with colds, and various organisms may be isolated, including streptococcus, staphylococcus, pneumococcus, etc. These organisms, more particularly the streptococcus, may be the cause of epidemic sore throat. Similarly, catarrhal inflammation of varying severity may affect these parts in a variety of acute infectious diseases, notably scarlatina and diphtheria. The tonsils are likely to be the seat of an acute hyperplasia, not only in connection with the diseases mentioned above and accompanying catarrhal inflammations, but also in diseases where there is general lymphadenoid involvement, as for example, typhoid fever.

In acute follicular tonsillitis there is likely to be acute catarrhal inflammation of the fauces and pharynx. The tonsils are the seat of acute hyperplasia and the crypts are likely to be filled with leukocytic, fibrinous, necrotic or even suppurative material which appears upon the tonsillar surface as many foci of exudate 1 or 2 mm. in diameter. *Streptococcus haemolyticus,* as well as other organisms, may produce this condition.

Diphtheria, the general manifestations of which have been discussed in the chapter on Infectious Diseases, is likely to originate upon one or both tonsils. There is an associated catarrhal inflammation of fauces and pharynx as well as an acute hyperplasia on the tonsil itself. The surface shows the smooth white, or pale yellow, well defined, easily detached fibrinous exudate, which subsequently becomes yellow and rough on the outer surface, and more firmly attached. The diphtheritic inflammation may extend so as to involve fauces, nasopharynx, and larynx.

Vincent's angina, due to the spirochetes of Vincent and the associated fusiform bacilli, is commonly primary upon the tonsils but may appear anywhere else in the mouth.

There is at first a superficial destruction of the tissues which later produces a ragged, fairly well defined ulcer with gray, shaggy, necrotic base. The ulceration may extend widely both laterally and deeply.

Acute suppurative inflammation may involve any part of the throat, more especially as the result of invasion by streptococci or staphylococci. Beginning in the tonsils it may extend fairly widely in the peritonsillar tissues, constituting the condition commonly called quinsy or, more properly, acute suppurative peritonsillitis. Suppurative inflammations of the throat may also extend into the retropharyngeal tissues producing retropharyngeal abscess, which may cause serious obstruction to breathing. Tuberculosis may produce retropharyngeal "cold abscess."

Agranulocytic Angina. This occurs in connection with agranulocytosis or neutropenia, referred to in the chapter on Hematopoietic System. The throat may show only a few superficial ulcerations on the tonsils, or more extensive gangrenous destruction extending to esophagus and larynx. Microscopically, there is extensive necrosis, with bacterial masses, vascular thrombosis and a cellular reaction in which there are few or no polymorphonuclear leukocytes.

Chronic Inflammations. CHRONIC PHARYNGITIS is not uncommon in speakers and singers, particularly those with improper voice production. It is more especially a disease of adults and may appear as a granular form with hyperplasia of the small lymphadenoid foci in the pharynx. Chronic tonsillitis may appear at any time of life but is more common in childhood when it apparently is the result of repeated attacks of acute tonsillitis, or may be primarily chronic. It is essentially a subacute or chronic hyperplasia of the lymphadenoid tissues, often showing enlargement of the secondary nodules, increase in number of small lymphocytes and sometimes definite fibrosis. In association the crypts are often filled with desquamated cells and necrotic debris. This material is a favorable culture medium for various forms of bacteria and can be a source of absorption of bacterial products. Sometimes the bacteria and necrotic material are arranged in radial form, simulating the granules of actinomycosis. The enlargement of chronic hyperplasia

is often called, by clinicians, hypertrophy of the tonsils. The same condition in the pharyngeal tonsils is called adenoids. Enlargement of the tonsils may occur in lymphosarcoma, Hodgkin's disease, lymphoid leukemia and similar conditions. Leukoplakia, similar to that seen in other parts of the mouth, only rarely occurs upon the tonsils and pharynx.

Infectious Granulomata

Tuberculosis may be seen in these regions similar to that affecting other parts of the mouth. Tuberculous retropharyngeal abscess occasionally occurs. Of considerable importance is tuberculosis of the tonsil which occurs in from 2 to 3 per cent of all tonsils removed for pathologic examination. Weller divides tonsillar tuberculosis into three types, the focal crypt infection, the ulcerative lupus-like lesion, and diffuse miliary tuberculosis. How much significance tuberculosis of the tonsil has as a portal of entry of the organism into the body is unknown. It is often associated with other tuberculous lesions of the body and is especially frequent in connection with tuberculosis of the cervical lymph nodes; whether as a primary portal of entry or as secondary to the lymph node involvement, is not definitely known. (See Long, Seibert and Gonzales.)

Other Infections. Mucous patches of secondary syphilis are not uncommon in the throat. Gumma may form in the tonsils, fauces and pharynx and may ulcerate and occasionally produce severe hemorrhage. More rarely chancre occurs upon the tonsils. Rhinoscleroma not uncommonly extends so as to involve the tissues of the throat. According to Davis, actinomycosis does not occur in the human tonsil, and in suspected cases careful distinction must be made between this and actinomyces-like bodies found in chronic hyperplastic tonsillitis.

General Infection from Tonsils. Much discussion has arisen as to whether or not remote metastatic infections may be spread from the tonsils, especially such conditions as endocarditis, gallbladder disease, etc. The theory of elective localization has been discussed in the chapter on Principles of Infectious Disease. We consider it to be unproved. Nevertheless, the tonsils may provide a portal of entry in cases of septicemia and pyemia.

Tumors

Benign Tumors. Epignathus, a tumor-like embryonal mixture of tissues, appears in the pharyngeal wall. Fibroma, lipoma, chondroma, osteochondroma, angioma, and other benign tumors are occasionally found in the tissues of the throat. Papilloma covered by stratified squamous epithelium may appear in any part of the throat, but it is said to be most common about the uvula.

Carcinoma of the tonsil is not rare. It occurs principally in males, being most frequent in the sixth decade. It is usually a squamous-cell carcinoma, but transitional-cell forms and lymphoepithelioma also occur. Hemorrhage, pneumonia or asphyxia may be fatal. Metastasis occurs into lymph nodes of the neck; only rarely is it found below the level of the clavicle. (See Martin and Sugarbaker.)

Carcinoma of larynx, tongue or mouth may extend into the pharynx and tonsil.

Lymphosarcoma may be first observed in the tonsil, usually with involvement of the cervical lymph nodes, or may be secondary to the disease elsewhere. Other sarcomas are rare.

ESOPHAGUS

Ante Mortem Digestion — Lyell Brit. Med. J. 1935

Congenital Malformations

The commonest of these is an association of atresia with communication between esophagus and trachea, esophago-tracheal fistula. The esophagus itself may be simply narrowed or completely interrupted; in the latter case the upper part is blind and the lower part communicates with the trachea (Rosenthal). There may be congenital stenosis without tracheal fistula and there may be a congenital dilatation. Very rarely congenital aplasia, or agenesis of the esophagus, occurs in which both upper and lower parts terminate blindly, connected by a fibrotic muscular cord. This condition is usually associated with more general congenital malformations. A congenitally short esophagus may be associated with hiatus hernia, so that part of the stomach projects through the hiatus of the diaphragm into the thorax. This is referred to subsequently in the discussion of internal hernias.

15950

Retrogressive Processes

Postmortem softening is common at the lower end of the esophagus, due to the digestive action of gastric juice. Active hyperemia occurs in the early stage of inflammation. Edema of the lower end of the esophagus is said to occur after severe vomiting and sometimes accompanies acute diffuse peritonitis. Passive hyperemia is common in chronic heart and lung diseases, and is of importance because it may lead to the production of small submucous hemorrhages which break down to produce hemorrhagic erosions. Dilatation of the veins of the upper end of the esophagus sometimes occurs, in old people and also in others who, because of intrathoracic conditions, have obstruction to the superior vena cava. Varices of the lower end of the esophagus are frequent in cases of cirrhosis of the liver, may rupture and occasionally severe or fatal hemorrhage occurs. The cirrhosis is usually of the Laennec type, but other forms may be responsible. Hemorrhage from the esophagus may be due to abrasion from foreign bodies, ulcers, may occur in the various hemorrhagic diseases, and is often due to rupture of varices. Occasionally a thoracic aneurysm erodes into the esophagus with consequent fatal hemorrhage.

Corrosion of Esophagus

This results from the ingestion of corrosive poisons such as the strong acids, phenol, and strong alkalies. Included in the last group is commercial lye which, in this country, is frequently the cause of corrosion. The corrosive substances produce first an inflammation followed rapidly by more or less extensive necrosis. In the less severe cases the necrosis may be limited to the crests of the longitudinal folds and points of narrowness of the esophagus. In more severe cases necrosis may be extensive and deep throughout the esophagus. In the event of recovery cicatricial stenosis may cause partial or complete obstruction to swallowing. (See Clerf.)

Inflammations

Acute catarrhal inflammation sometimes occurs as the result of ingestion of too hot or irritant food or drink, or it may extend from a catarrhal inflammation of the pharynx. In the more severe cases of thrush of the upper alimentary canal the process may extend into the esophagus.

Acute fibrinous esophagitis, in which the exudate is usually deposited along the crests of the longitudinal folds, may complicate severe infectious diseases such as scarlatina, and typhoid fever, but true diphtheria of the organ is rare.

Superficial streptococcal infections are likely to show moderate degrees of necrosis of the mucous membrane. The pustules of smallpox may be encountered in the esophagus. More extensive suppurative inflammation of the esophagus may extend from the pharynx or throat and may follow abrasion by foreign bodies or corrosive poisoning, because of the entrance of pyogenic organisms. This may be superficial or may extend in a dissecting manner for considerable distances under the mucosa, and may ultimately lead to a suppurative peri-esophagitis. Acute esophagitis, sometimes ulcerative, is a frequent observation in autopsies on persons dead of infectious disease and prolonged exhausting diseases. Usually there are no symptoms clinically although the patient may complain of burning on swallowing. That it is due to the use of tubes, in diagnosis and treatment, is not certain.

Chronic catarrhal inflammation may be due to prolonged passive hyperemia and to repeated irritation such as occurs in alcoholism. It also accompanies paralysis of the esophagus and the various forms of dilatation. There is thickening of the mucosa, sometimes with the formation of small polypoid outgrowths, varying degrees of atrophy of the muscle, and fibrosis. Enlargement of glands from mucinous degeneration or obstruction produces the so-called chronic follicular esophagitis. Leukoplakia is common, but only rarely is it followed by carcinoma.

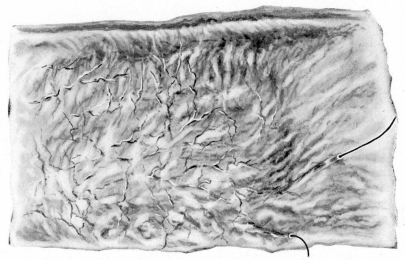

Varices of lower end of esophagus in a case of atrophic cirrhosis of liver. Horse hairs have been inserted at two points of rupture.

Infectious Granulomata

Tuberculosis may extend from the larynx or pharynx. Hematogenous miliary tuberculosis is more apparent in the musculature than in the mucosa. Tuberculous ulcers may occur perhaps as the result of swallowing infectious sputum or due to lymphogenous transport from neighboring foci of tuberculosis. Tuberculosis of mediastinal lymph nodes may extend to the esophagus and produce tuberculous ulceration (Clerf).

In syphilis there may be gummatous erosion of the esophagus. More significant, however, is the cicatricial stenosis or other alteration of form of the esophagus, due to contraction of scar tissue in the neighborhood of healed gummata.

Actinomycosis is rare.

Cysts

Congenital cysts usually are of relatively small size and occur in the lower third of the esophagus. They are often lined with ciliated columnar epithelium. They may be the result either of misplacement of lung anlage or failure of disappearance of embryonal esophageal tissue. Small retention cysts of the esophageal mucous glands may occur as the result of infection or may accompany chronic follicular esophagitis.

Ulcers

These are observed in tumors, following corrosion, occur in acute infectious diseases, especially typhoid fever, are seen in thrush, may be of decubitus type behind the cricoid, may be produced by foreign bodies and may occur in diverticula and dilatations. In the lower third, varicose veins may ulcerate. Peptic ulcers of aberrant gastric mucosa may also occur (Rector and Connerley).

Tumors

Benign Tumors. Papilloma, adenoma, fibroma, lipoma are not at all common and

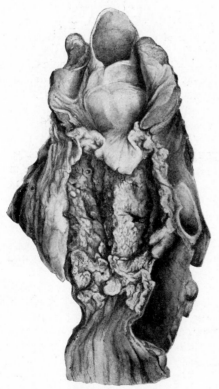

Eroding carcinoma of upper third of esophagus.

when they occur are likely to show somewhat elongated pedicles due to traction upon the

tumor by swallowing. Leiomyoma and rhabdomyoma are also said to occur.

Carcinoma of the esophagus affects males much more often than females and has its highest incidence in the sixth decade. The usual complaint is dysphagia due to obstruction. The tumor is usually in the form of a ring encircling the esophagus, but may occasionally be confined to one side of the wall. It may sometimes be a dense firm scirrhous type of tumor with constriction due to connective tissue growth and a relatively small amount of superficial necrosis; more commonly it is a fungating growth extending from 2 to 10 cm. along the esophageal wall, projecting into the lumen in massive form and showing extensive necrosis. It is especially likely to occur at the points of normal narrowness of the esophagus, namely, opposite the cricoid, the bifurcation of the trachea, and at the cardiac orifice of the stomach. Carcinoma is found in increasing order of frequency in the upper, middle and lower thirds of the esophagus. The most frequent microscopic form is squamous-cell carcinoma. Pearls are common, but may be necrotic. Basal cell types are rare. Adenocarcinoma and other forms of cylindrical-cell carcinoma are infrequent, usually occur in the lower third and may originate from the glands or undifferentiated rests of original epithelium.

The esophageal carcinoma usually appears as a single growth, and only rarely are there secondary smaller growths in the esophagus due to lymphatic dissemination. In rare instances a carcinoma involving one side of the esophagus may show what appears to be an implantation of tumor upon the opposite side. Metastasis occurs to the lymph nodes both above and below the lesion, but is more frequent and widespread in the latter situation, where it is especially likely to involve the nodes around the cardiac orifice of the stomach. Metastasis to the cervical lymph nodes is sometimes of importance in establishing a diagnosis. Metastasis to lungs and liver is not uncommon but more distant metastasis is unusual. The local extension of the tumor may result in perforation into the trachea, the bronchi or lungs, and occasionally into the pleural and pericardial sacs. Extension into the aorta may result in fatal hemorrhage. Involvement of the recurrent laryngeal nerve, either by direct extension or as the result of carcinomatous involvement of the mediastinal lymph nodes, may produce laryngeal paralysis.

Sarcoma is extremely rare, occurring especially in old age and the male sex, and usually found in the lower third of the esophagus. Grossly, it may be a submucous, nodular tumor or a flat diffuse tumor. The microscopic forms include spindle-cell sarcoma, lymphosarcoma and rare cases of leiomyosarcoma (French and Garland).

Secondary tumors of the esophagus are unusual. Carcinoma may spread from the stomach by direct extension, and similarly from the pharynx, the thyroid gland and the lung. Sometimes it may extend into the esophagus from neighboring lymph nodes such as those of the mediastinum. Secondary sarcoma is even more rare than secondary carcinoma.

Alterations of Lumen

Obstruction to the passage of food may be produced by the presence of foreign bodies, projecting tumors, or to a true stenosis of the wall, such as may be produced by scars following corrosion or such lesions as gumma. The lumen may also be narrowed by the presence of tumors within the wall and by various types of phlegmonous and other inflammations. Spasm of the esophagus may occur in any part of its wall but is most common at the cardiac end. Undoubtedly some of the cases of spasm are part of a psychoneurosis, but many cases have no such apparent origin, and except in rare instances where disease of the vagus nerve is found, the condition is without known cause. The lumen may also be narrowed by compression from without, such as may be produced for example by thoracic tumors, thoracic aneurysms, and thyroid enlargement. Above points of obstruction there is likely to be primarily a hypertrophy of the musculature of the esophagus followed by local dilatation.

Dilatation. This may affect the entire wall of the esophagus, either in a small part, or throughout the length of the tube, or it may be local in the form of diverticula. Local dilatation may occur above regions of constriction due to scars or tumors. Generalized dilatation, above the cardiac orifice of the stomach occurs rarely as a congenital lesion; it is usually due to a fault in passage of food from esophagus to stomach. This failure is

attributed by many to spasm of the cardiac sphincter, cardiospasm, and by others to failure of the sphincter to relax, achalasia. In either event, the basic trouble is with innervation. Increased vagal activity would cause

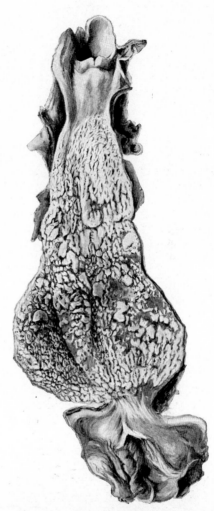

Dilatation of esophagus probably due to cardiospasm. Chronic catarrhal esophagitis and leukoplakia.

tonic esophagus and patent cardiac orifice; depression would lead to reduction of inhibition and the orifice would not open. Overactive sympathetics would cause contraction of sphincter; paralysis would cause unopposed vagal activity. Lesions of the vagus and also of Auerbach's plexus have been reported, but others have failed to find them. Evidently there is a fault of innervation, but the exact mechanism is not known. The esophagus may be moderately or so markedly dilated as to have a capacity of a liter or more. The longitudinal folds are more or less flattened and there is a chronic catarrhal inflammation. The muscle is hypertrophic but may be much attenuated. The sphincter muscle may be hypertrophic. (See Sodeman.)

Diverticula may be traction diverticula or pulsion (pressure) diverticula. Traction diverticula are small and occur in the anterior or lateral walls near the bifurcation of the trachea. They are usually funnel-shaped and rarely exceed a depth of 5 or 10 mm. The condition is commonly due to the contraction of scar tissue in the mediastinal lymph nodes or other tissues of the mediastinum, which when adherent to the esophageal wall lead to traction and diverticulum formation.

Pressure or pulsion diverticula, also sometimes called Zenker's diverticula, may occur in any part of the esophagus but are most common at the junction of esophagus and pharynx, and are therefore really esophagopharyngeal diverticula. The condition is commoner in advanced years and in the male sex. The dilatation is often saccular in character, may attain a diameter of several centimeters and may be so large that when filled with food it can compress the esophagus. The mucosa is usually thickened by a chronic catarrh and the muscle much attenuated or atrophic. The diverticulation is regarded as a sort of hernial projection of the lining of the esophageal wall between the fibers of the inferior constrictor of the pharynx. It is supposed that the increased effort in the first stage of deglutition, due to deformities of the mouth or swallowing of large pieces of food, may force the material upon this relatively weak part of the esophagus so as to produce local dilatation. The opening of the sac is in the posterior wall near the level of the cricoid cartilage, but when fairly large the sac itself is likely to project laterally and may be visible in the external surface of the neck.

STOMACH

Congenital Malformations

Sometimes the vertical fetal position of the stomach is retained in after life. The stomach may also occupy an abnormal position in connection with hernia through the diaphragm, and in situs inversus viscerum. Congenital closure of the cardiac or pyloric orifice is usually a part of more general malformation. Congenital diverticula, sometimes combined with inclusion of such glandular structures as pancreas, may occur in any part of the stomach. It is doubtful that hourglass stomach is of congenital origin.

Of great importance is congenital pyloric stenosis, sometimes called hypertrophic pyloric stenosis (see Sauer). There is little doubt that this is of congenital origin although symptoms usually are not observed until about two weeks after birth. The condition is more frequent in the male sex and sometimes shows familial distribution. The most striking feature is marked thickening or hypertrophy of the muscular walls of the stomach, beginning at the pyloric orifice and extending for 2 to 3 cm. along the pyloric canal. There is sometimes fibrosis of the submucosa and in many cases the mucosa is thrown into longitudinal folds. The pyloric orifice is much reduced and often will barely admit a probe. The exact cause is unknown. Some authors consider that it is primarily muscular and represents a tumor-like growth of the muscle in this situation. Others regard the hypertrophy of the muscle as secondary to spasm, which may be neurogenic, or due to faults of secretion leading to excessive contraction.

Postmortem Changes

Not infrequently rigor mortis of the gastric muscle will cause ring-like or complete contraction of the circular bundles. These deformities, however, can easily be removed by a moderate amount of traction. Postmortem digestion of the stomach is common and exhibits itself principally in the mucosa, at first along the cardiac end of the greater curvature and subsequently in other parts. The mucosa is soft and easily scraped off. Eventually the entire stomach wall may become involved and perforation may occur. The characteristic feature of these postmortem changes is that there is no reaction on the part of the tissues. Especially in connection with passive hyperemia of the stomach, postmortem digestion may lead to small extravasations of blood. The bacterial products of decomposition may act upon the blood pigment so as to produce a dark green, dark brown, or black discoloration referred to as pseudomelanosis.

Retrogressive Changes

Cloudy swelling is not at all uncommon in the glands of the gastric mucosa, occurring in connection with catarrhal inflammation, passive hyperemia and the other general conditions which produce cloudy swelling. Fatty degeneration occurs under similar conditions and is especially marked in the infectious diseases, high-grade anemias and phosphorus poisoning. Amyloid is likely to be found in the vessels, more particularly of the submucosa and the mucosa. Hematogenous pigmentation is not uncommon in cases of chronic passive hyperemia. Calcification occurs particularly as calcium "metastases" in the vessels and in the tunica propria near the acid glands. Atrophy is likely to attack the glands or the muscle or both. Atrophy of muscle is most apparent in the so-called chronic atrophic gastritis. Glandular atrophy occurs in the same condition and also appears in high grade anemias, especially pernicious anemia. The most significant functional change due to glandular atrophy is diminution or absence of gastric secretion, achylia gastrica.

Circulatory Disturbances

Active hyperemia occurs physiologically in the course of digestion. Pathologically, it may be a simple acute hyperemia due to the irritant character of foods and drinks. It may be a part of acute inflammations of various types and is likely to accompany various forms of enteric fevers. Passive hyperemia is extremely common and accompanies chronic diseases of heart or lungs, cirrhosis of the liver, thrombosis of the portal vein and similar conditions. There is a more or less diffuse reddening of the entire stomach, which after it has persisted for some time leads to a chronic catarrhal inflammation. Thus, the mucosa is likely to be thick, soft, red and covered with adherent viscid mucus.

Microscopically, there is cloudy swelling, fatty degeneration and mucinous degeneration of the glandular epithelium. The tunica propria is likely to be infiltrated with plasma cells, although this is difficult to determine positively, sometimes with polymorphonuclear leukocytes, and in more advanced stages there is fibrosis. Hematogenous pigmentation may be found in the tunica propria and in the submucosa; the latter also is fibrotic. Accompanying passive hyperemia there may be small petechiae in the submucosa and the mucosa, especially of the fundus, which may ultimately result in the production of multiple hemorrhagic erosions. Blood streaking and staining of vomitus secondary to the chronic catarrhs may be due apparently to leakage from overdistended capillaries.

In general anemias, the stomach is likely to be extremely pallid throughout and sometimes there is fatty degeneration of the epithelium in addition. The more severe chronic anemias, especially pernicious anemia, are frequently accompanied by atrophy of the mucous glands, sometimes in the form of chronic atrophic gastritis. Hemorrhage into the stomach may be the sequence of chronic passive hyperemia, hemorrhagic erosion, rupture of varices, erosion due to foreign bodies, and is of particular importance as an accompaniment of chronic ulcer and carcinoma of the stomach. It may also be of traumatic origin. In melena neonatorum, hematemesis may accompany the more common bloody diarrhea.

Inflammations

Acute catarrhal gastritis is believed to be extremely common although it is rarely observed at autopsy. It may apparently be caused by excess of food, food that is too hot or too cold, and irritant foods. The mucosa is the seat of active hyperemia, is swollen and covered with thick, sticky, glairy mucus. Microscopically, the principal changes are hyperemia associated with cloudy swelling and mucinous degeneration of the epithelium. The tunica propria is normally so rich in round cells that it is difficult to say whether or not there is an additional infiltration of lymphoid cells.

Acute fibrinous gastritis sometimes accompanies acute infectious diseases and may be the cause of the more severe gastric disturbances in the course of these diseases. It is only rarely that a true diphtheria of the stomach occurs, secondary to involvement of the throat.

Acute suppurative gastritis may occur in connection with pyemia and endocarditis, or as the result of infection of corrosive lesions. This is in the form of focalized abscesses in the wall of the stomach. Localized suppuration in the neighborhood of carcinomas and ulcers of the stomach may extend to produce an acute phlegmonous gastritis, as is true also of the erosions around foreign bodies. Suppurative lesions of the esophagus may extend into the stomach. Sometimes suppurations, as for example those in the lesser peritoneal cavity and in the pancreas or other neighboring organs, extend into the stomach.

ened, principally by proliferation of glandular epithelium. The enlarged glandular parts project between the ramifying connective-tissue septa of the tunica propria to present to the naked eye a mosaic-like marking of the mucous membrane.

Microscopically, the glands are elongated, and in the neighborhood of the muscularis mucosae, either coiled or sometimes bifurcated, resembling glands of Lieberkühn. Not infrequently goblet cells are encountered and sometimes the glandular lumen is filled

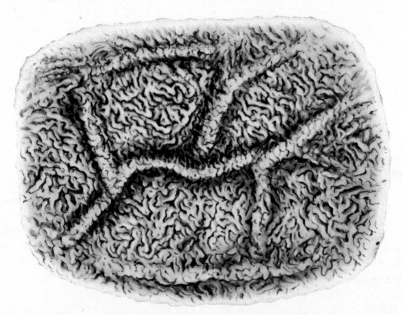

Chronic hypertrophic gastritis showing thick folded mucosa.

Chronic gastritis may affect principally the mucosa and submucosa or involve the entire thickness of the stomach. The forms involving the mucosa are referred to as chronic hypertrophic gastritis and chronic atrophic gastritis.

CHRONIC HYPERTROPHIC GASTRITIS may be due to chronic irritations similar to those which produce acute catarrhal gastritis; it may be due to retention of food in the stomach, such as may be caused by the scars of ulcers, obstructing influence of carcinoma, or constricting adhesions about the pyloric end of the stomach. The stomach may be of normal size or somewhat dilated. The rugae are likely to be somewhat more prominent than normal and less easily flattened by stretching. The mucosa is definitely thick-

with mucin. It is difficult to determine actual cell infiltration in the tunica propria, but in many cases a definite fibrosis can be made out, more particularly in the lines of depression of the mosaic-like marking. The muscularis mucosae is sometimes the seat of hypertrophy and the submucosa may be fibrotic. Occasionally a moderate hypertrophy of the muscularis is observed. Fibrosis of the muscularis and of the serosa also occurs. Sometimes proliferation of the epithelium appears to be of atypical character, but before such a diagnosis is made it is important to exclude the possibility of aberrant islands of intestinal glands, frequent in the stomach. Sometimes the hyperplasia of the glandular parts of the mucosa is excessive in various foci, so that there are projections of nodular character upon the mucous surface constituting the so-called verrucose catarrh or ÉTAT MAMELONNÉ.

CHRONIC ATROPHIC CATARRHAL GASTRITIS apparently may be due to the same causes as chronic hypertrophic, may be a later stage of chronic hypertrophic or may accompany prolonged high-grade anemias. In most cases the stomach is dilated. The mucosa is thin, pale, glossy and through it the vessels of the submucosa are clearly visible. The thinning affects all the coats and is accentuated by the variable degrees of dilatation of the stomach. Microscopically, the mucosa is found to be thin, and the glands short and well separated from one another. Cloudy swelling, fatty degeneration and mucinous degeneration occur in the glandular epithelium. The tunica propria is likely to be distinctly fibrotic. The muscularis mucosae is thin and attenuated and the submucosa fibrosed. There is atrophy and attenuation of the muscularis of the stomach associated with moderate fibrosis of this coat and also of the serosa. Alcoholism is often regarded as an important cause of both forms of chronic gastritis, but it is probable that gastric lesions are due to associated vitamin deficiencies rather than the alcohol. (See Berry.)

CHRONIC INTERSTITIAL GASTRITIS or chronic fibroplastic gastritis is not common, and is often difficult to distinguish from scirrhous carcinoma of the stomach. The causes of the condition are entirely unknown. It produces a form of stomach commonly referred to as "leather bottle" stomach. The organ is reduced in size and the wall considerably thickened, associated with marked increase in density. The character of the mucosa varies in different cases, sometimes being hypertrophic and sometimes atrophic. The outstanding feature is a marked increase in thickness of the submucosa, which in cross sections is prominent, pale, pearly and glistening.

Microscopically, there may be many fibroblasts or the connective tissue may be richly collagenous. It is generally thought that the thickening and increased density of the submucosa lead to the muscular atrophy which is commonly present. There is associated fibrosis of the musculature and the serosa. The term linitis plastica is often applied to this condition. In all cases, however, it is necessary to make careful examination in order to exclude scirrhous carcinoma of the stomach, which may be identical grossly. The possible fibrosis of syphilis is referred to below. Leukoplakia is rare.

Corrosion of the Stomach

The ingestion of corrosive poisons produces appearances in the stomach which vary with the character of the poison. Aschoff divides these into four different groups. The fixing corrosives include particularly phenol, mercuric chloride and formalin. These produce immediate death of the superficial parts of the stomach so that the cells are fixed in a solid, thick, firm but friable, pale or dark-brown mass. In the less severe cases this affects the ridges of the rugae but as a rule attacks the entire lining, fixing the rugae into conspicuous firm folds. Usually the patient dies almost immediately from shock. When death is not immediate, the tissue underneath the necrotic parts shows hyperemia, edema and inflammatory reaction.

Microscopically, the fixed cells show nuclear and cytoplasmic characters very much the same as with the ordinary types of fixation. The burning corrosives include especially sulfuric, hydrochloric and nitric acids. The superficial parts are discolored, soft, moist and necrotic, and can easily be scraped away. Sulfuric acid tends to char the tissue first yellow and then black, nitric acid stains yellow and dark brown, and hydrochloric acid pale yellow or white. Microscopically, this material is completely necrotic, and the degree of the reactionary hyperemia, edema and acute inflammation varies with the length of life following the poisoning. The softening corrosives include the strong alkalies, particularly sodium hydrate, potassium hydrate, lysol and lye. In these cases the discoloration is not so great as in the preceding group and the softening of the necrotic material much more pronounced. The weak corrosives, including oxalic acid, chromic acid, arsenous acid and phosphorus, produce lesser degrees of superficial necrosis, and since death does not ensue so quickly, the reactionary hyperemia and inflammation are likely to be marked.

Infectious Granulomata

Tuberculosis rarely affects the stomach. When it does, it is more common in males than females and occurs principally in early middle life. The most common lesion is tuberculous ulcer, but there may be a hyperplastic infiltrating lesion and disseminated miliary tubercles. The pyloric region is more often affected than the fundic. It is probably due to dissemination of organisms by the blood, but may extend through lymphatics; tuberculosis in the neighborhood may extend into the stomach. Swallowing bacilli is of little importance because they do not enter the intact mucosa. The idea that the acidity of the gastric juice prevents infection is not valid. (See Clagett and Walters.)

Syphilis. The only characteristic syphilitic lesion of the stomach is the formation of gumma, single or multiple and usually in the submucosa. The gumma may break down with ulceration. Cicatrization may lead to deformity including hourglass stomach and pyloric stenosis. Diffuse fibrosis is ascribed to syphilis. Furthermore local thickening and ulceration, with the microscopic picture of perivascular infiltration of lymphocytes and plasma cells, endarteritis, endophlebitis and "gummatoid" lesions are believed to be due to acquired syphilis (see Meyer and Singer; Williams and Kimmelstiel). We do not deny that this is true, but the lesion may readily be confused with chronic peptic ulcer and reticulum-cell sarcoma.

Congenital syphilis may affect the stomach in the form of gummata or in the form of diffuse round-cell infiltration of the various coats.

Other Infections. Actinomycosis and anthrax occasionally occur but usually are secondary to lesions elsewhere. Of importance is the fact that diseases of the lymphatic system such as typhoid fever, Hodgkin's disease, and lymphosarcoma may manifest themselves in the stomach. They may remain simply as lymphoid hyperplasias of the follicles or occasionally ulcerate to produce single or multiple ulcers which may be the source of hemorrhage.

Ulcer of the Stomach

Acute ulcers, which tend to heal, occur as the result of erosion of hyperplastic lymph follicles, may occur in infectious diseases without follicular hyperplasia, may be due to erosion of petechiae (hemorrhagic erosions) and may be due to erosion by foreign bodies.

Peptic ulcer, round ulcer or simple gastric ulcer, tends to persist and become chronic, heals slowly, if at all, and may exhibit several dangerous complications and sequels. Peptic ulcers of stomach and of duodenum are found in from 2 to 3 per cent of autopsies. They are encountered twice as often in males as in females. There is about an equal division between gastric and duodenal ulcers. The greatest incidence is in the fifth to the seventh decade, but many appear earlier. (See Gordon and Manning.) Chronic gastritis is a predisposing factor and there appears to be an "ulcer constitution" (Draper). Anemia has no demonstrable influence. Neither neurotic temperament nor enteroptosis appears to play a part. In animals, exhausting diseases and deficient diets favor the origin and persistence of ulcer (Ivy; Pappenheimer and Larimore).

The ulcer is usually a single, round or oval, sometimes elongated elliptic loss of continuity, situated in the posterior wall of the pyloric portion of the stomach near the lesser curvature. The pyloric part of the stomach is sometimes referred to as the ulcer-bearing area. Sometimes two or more ulcers occur. Only about 6 per cent are found in situations other than the ulcer-bearing area. The diameter varies from a few millimeters to 2 to 3 cm. or more. Within a few weeks of its origin, the ulcer extends into the muscular coats, but has little disposition to extend widely in a lateral diameter. In older ulcers the margins are indurated. The ulcer may be "punched out," or more commonly funnel shaped, often with "terraced" margins, the steps of the terrace representing smaller extent of destruction as the deeper coats are involved. The edges nearer the pyloric orifice are flatter or less steep than the other margins, presumably because of the rubbing of the food as it passes through the narrower part of the stomach. The ulcer is covered, and partly filled in, by a granular or slimy, pale, bloody or brown-tinged exudate, often digested or rubbed off in the autopsy specimen. Hyperemia is common around the margin and with the earlier ulcers may be widespread. Acute or chronic

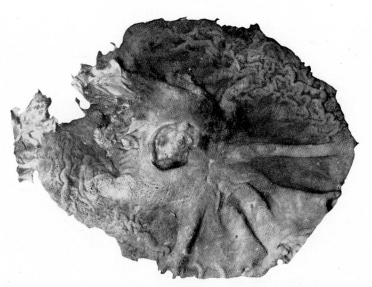

Chronic peptic ulcer showing radiating retraction lines. There is associated chronic hypertrophic gastritis.

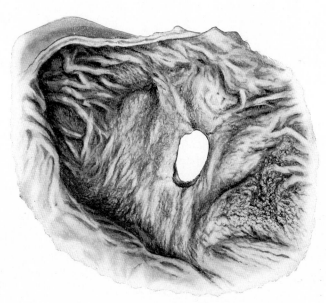

Perforated peptic ulcer of pylorus, showing terraced edge.

hypertrophic gastritis is common but not constant. In the early stages the underlying serosa often shows a deposit of fibrinous exudate, which later is represented by fibrous thickening or more often fibrous adhesions to surrounding structures.

Microscopically, as pointed out by Askanazy, four layers can usually be identified, namely, of exudation, of fibrinous necrosis, of granulation and of cicatrization. The exudate occupies the ulcer and extends for a variable distance into the tissues. It may be purulent, fibrinopurulent, or occasionally catarrhal, and not infrequently shows hemorrhage. Eosinophils are often present but in the later stages lymphoid and plasma cells may predominate. The zone of necrosis is usually definite but may be very thin in old ulcers. In addition to the ordinary nuclear and cytoplasmic changes of necrosis, there are often hyaline masses which stain as does fibrin, but show no network, no nodules, no asters, to characterize them as fibrin. They are probably derived from necrotic connective tissue. Granulation tissue, variable in extent and not different from granulation elsewhere, appears early in the course of the ulcer and is usually still present in old chronic ulcers. Scar tissue appears at the base of older ulcers and extends into the muscular and serous coats.

In addition to the destruction of the coats of the stomach there are often lesions of blood vessels and nerves. Acute periarteritis, with perivascular infiltration of leukocytes, lymphoid and plasma cells, and acute arteritis with penetration of these cells into the vascular wall, are common in and about the earlier ulcers. The inflammations become chronic in association with the older ulcers. Endarteritis deformans and obliterans are common. These may be due to involvement of the intima of the arteries, or much the same appearance may be due to thrombosis with organization and even canalization. Arteriosclerosis is frequently observed and may occur as a local process in young persons but Askanazy points out that ulcer patients 50 to 60 years of age or more may show no sclerosis of the gastric vessels. The nerves are interrupted with the destruction of the coats of the stomach and may show acute or chronic neuritis or perineuritis. The interrupted nerve bundles may elongate and become coiled to produce masses closely resembling the amputation neuroma.

In addition to the destructive and inflammatory changes in the mucosa, there may be a proliferation of epithelium upward to produce papilliform overhanging masses at the ulcer margin, or there may be growth downward along the edge and into the base of the ulcer. This downward proliferation must not be confused with carcinoma. Occasionally, the resistance of the ulcer base is so low that small dilatations or diverticula are formed.

When ulcers heal they do so by organization and consolidation of the defect with ingrowth and apposition of the mucosa and a complete or nearly complete regeneration of the mucosa (Ivy). The epithelial regeneration is complex, but the new cells are first mucus producing and then undergo differentiation to form the normal cells of the glands (see Popoff). The tunica propria participates in the formation of a new mucosa. The scar tissue may contract, so that there are radiating lines of retraction about the healed ulcer. Sometimes the cicatrization is more extensive, and if the ulcer be situated near the middle of the organ, contraction produces the "hour-glass stomach." If it be in the pyloric region the contraction may produce pyloric stenosis.

THE COMPLICATIONS of especial importance are hemorrhage, perforation and development of carcinoma. Hemorrhage is so common as to be regarded as a symptom. There may be occasional small hemorrhages, repeated small hemorrhages, with secondary anemia, or severe large hemorrhages which may be fatal. In the extension of the ulcer, large blood vessels may be eroded upon their lateral walls. Thrombi may be loosely formed or may be dislodged by peristalsis, gastric distention or by increase of blood pressure. Small hemorrhages may be due to hyperemia or to rupture of vessels in the granulation tissue. In the series of Gordon and Manning, hemorrhage occurred in 17.9 per cent and was more frequent in the acute than the chronic forms. If there be temporary renal insufficiency, as from anemia or chronic renal disease, there may be a marked rise of nonprotein nitrogen and urea in the blood, due to digestion of the blood, especially the erythrocytes, and the formation of urea. (See

Johnson; Chunn et al.) Many patients with gastric ulcer have a low level of ascorbic acid in the blood, probably because of low intake of vitamin C in the diet. Thus some of the bleeding from ulcers may be a manifestation of subclinical scurvy (Field et al.).

Ulcers may penetrate deeply and lead to perforation. In autopsy material this occurs in about 20 per cent of the cases, but may be less in the clinical cases. In the more acute ulcers this may lead to diffuse peritonitis, but frequently the slow progression of the penetration leads to inflammation of the serosa with development of fibrous adhesions, so that the effect of perforation remains localized. It may, however, expose surfaces of liver or pancreas and may produce gastrointestinal fistulae.

The possibility of transformation of gastric ulcer to carcinoma has practical importance, for if it were frequent, excision of ulcers would be indicated. Reports of the incidence of this change have varied widely, but successive studies have revised the figures downward. The ulceration of carcinomas is not rare, but usually these can be distinguished from chronic ulcers that have become carcinomatous. Only infrequently is the ulceration of a small carcinoma confusing. In the margins of chronic ulcers, the microscope often discloses alterations of regenerating epithelial cells that suggest carcinoma, but it is rare to find conclusive evidence. In a series of 141 cases of chronic gastric ulcer and 353 cases of gastric carcinoma, Klein found only 2 instances in which there were changes suggestive of development of carcinoma from ulcer. It is probable that the transformation is rare.

THE PATHOLOGIC PHYSIOLOGY of ulcer deals especially with gastric secretion and motility. It was long thought that hyperacidity is frequent in ulcer patients, but Carlson found that the acidity is not materially different from that of normal stomachs. Hyperperistalsis is frequent both clinically and experimentally, but this does not necessarily mean rapidity of emptying, and some cases have delayed emptying. Ivy found that hypermotility is due to an intrinsic nervous mechanism, augmented by the extrinsic system. Local spasm is extremely common as revealed by radioscopic examination, and is probably of the same nature. Palmer interprets the pain as due to the irritant effects of the acid gastric juice upon the inflammatory base of the ulcer, but Rabinovitch and associates attribute it to the perineuritis and perhaps the additional influence of edema and inflammation.

THE EXCITING CAUSE of gastric ulcer has been the subject of much clinical, anatomic and experimental study (see Karsner) and will be discussed in relation to faults of secretion, vascular lesions, parasites, neuromuscular influences, organs of internal secretion, cytolysins, and ferments.

Although no constant alteration of acidity is found in patients with peptic ulcer, it is possible that at the time of origin of the ulcer there may have been hyperacidity. By anastomosis of stomach and small intestine, so that unneutralized gastric juice impinges directly upon the intestinal mucosa, Mann observed the production of peptic ulcers of the intestine which tend to become chronic. If additional anastomosis provides access of alkaline duodenal contents near the junction of stomach and jejunum, the incidence of ulcer is reduced, thus indicating that acidity is of importance. Furthermore the experimental ulcer of cinchophen poisoning is associated with the production of large quantities of normally acid gastric juice and is prevented by administration of alkali (Bollman, Stalker and Mann). Of further probable significance is the fact that in man peptic ulcer of the duodenum is most frequent within 5 cm. from the pylorus. Kahn found that peptic ulcer is a great rarity in pernicious anemia, with its anacidity.

Stasis of gastric contents has been shown by Ivy and others to induce persistence of the ulcer. Bolton believes this to be due to irritation by the gastric contents. Sweet and his collaborators ascribe it to traction of the muscle, rendered hyperperistaltic by the obstruction, upon the margins of the ulcer. Kirsch and Stahnke state that penetration of the muscle of tunica propria is an important factor in chronicity. Ivy delayed healing by manipulation of an ulcer in an exposed pouch. Hyperperistalsis apparently favors the persistence of the ulcer.

The conical shape of gastric ulcer with the apex toward the serous surface suggests that it is due to infarction, but the same form could easily be due to destruction of such a nature that the mucous coat is more extensively involved than the submucosa and more resistant muscularis. As shown by Ivy, bland embolism does not produce infarction of the stomach. Although the vascular supply of the pyloric portion of the stomach is poorer than that of the fundus, infarction is rare in the human stomach, is usually massive, and occurs only when additional vascular lesions reduce the normally rich anastomosis. The extension of thrombosis into several arteries may account for the peptic ulcers in cases of polycythemia vera. The result of an infective embolus is to be regarded as an abscess. Those diseases, such as endocarditis and aortic thrombosis, in which bland embolism is common, rarely are complicated by gastric ulcer, and equally rare is gastric abscess in association with pyemia or septicemia. Acute and chronic arteritis and endarteritis are common in the neighborhood of gastric ulcer, but it is probable that they are secondary to the lesion rather than the cause of it. Arteriosclerosis is not usually severe in the earlier age periods of ulcer and is often absent (Askanazy).

Various micro-organisms have been found in gastric ulcer but interest centers about molds and bacteria. Molds are common but they are probably saprophytes that have nothing to do with the cause or persistence of the ulcer (Kirsch and Stahnke). Rosenau applies his theory of elective localization of streptococci to gastric ulcer. Although confirmed by some there is strong evidence against this view (see Holman). It cannot be said that any micro-organismal cause of gastric ulcer has been established.

It has been suggested that spasm of arteries or of muscularis mucosae might cause ischemia and consequent ulcer. The occurrence of acute and chronic neuritis might be thought to be responsible for the spasm, but these lesions are probably secondary rather than primary. Section of splanchnics (Ivy) and of vagi (Lasowsky and Ptschelina) is not followed by ulcer formation. Cushing noted the occurrence of acute peptic ulcers in patients with disease of the brain and Keller produced acute lesions in the stomach of the dog by operations on the brain. Boles and Riggs suggest that a generalized circulatory disturbance accompanying cerebral lesions may well be responsible for the ulceration,

but indicate that in some instances the ulcer may be neurogenic. The theory of neurovascular influence is attractive, may well apply to certain ulcers, but is not proved to be the origin in all or a majority. (See Haymaker and Anderson.) Dragstedt states that gastric juice can digest living gastric mucosa, but that this does not ordinarily take place because of protection by mucus and gastric contents. An excessive flow of gastric juice may overcome these protective factors and produce ulcer. It is possible that neurogenic factors may contribute to excessive flow of gastric juice. Local injection of many substances into the gastric wall of experimental animals leads to ulceration, but no special agent acting upon blood vessels has been demonstrated as a cause.

Anatomically, gastritis is frequently found in stomachs the seat of peptic ulcer; in our experience this is usually chronic hypertrophic gastritis. Which is cause, and which is effect, is difficult to say, but Konjetzny is of the opinion that inflammation, especially when acute, is a direct or indirect cause of the ulcer.

The work of Mann and others suggests the influence of ductless glands or their secretions, especially the adrenal and the thyroid. The studies of the relationship of disturbances of ductless glands, whether they are supposed to operate directly or through the intermediation of the autonomic nervous system, have not been sufficiently correlated to permit of satisfactory conclusions.

IN SUMMARY, it may be said that pathologically, peptic ulcer is an inflammatory lesion so situated that gastric juice probably augments the destruction of tissue. Various predisposing causes seem to be operative in the patients, but these are not conclusively established. The direct exciting cause of the ulcer has not been disclosed in such fashion as to be beyond doubt. The persistence or chronicity of the ulcer depends upon a variety of factors, none of which can be said to operate in all cases. Probably several of these factors act coincidentally. Thus, there must be considered especially, acidity and volume of gastric juice, stasis of neuromuscular or obstructive origin, the irritative and traumatic influence of gastric contents and the traction of muscle about the ulcer. (See Hurst and Stewart.)

Tumors

Benign tumors of clinical significance are not common but may be of importance and may produce marked obstruction to the pyloric outlet. The epithelial benign tumors include particularly the papilloma and the adenoma, which may be polypoid in character. The papilloma may be distinctly pedunculated or sessile, and is made up of a more or less intricate papillary outgrowth of connective tissue of the submucosa, sometimes also with cells from the muscularis mucosae, covered by cylindrical epithelium, occasionally with gland formation.

MUCOSAL POLYPS. Schindler and McGlone distinguish three varieties of mucosal polyps.

The inflammatory pseudopolyps occur in association with chronic gastritis, especially the atrophic form, as multiple relatively small nodules situated principally in the pyloric portion and sometimes with shallow ulcers between them. These nodules are composed principally of dense connective tissue infiltrated with plasma cells; irregular epithelial tubules are found on the surface.

Adenomatous polyps are the most common benign tumor of the stomach. They may be sessile or pedunculated, single or multiple, and are usually 1 or 2 centimeters in diameter but may be larger. Grossly, they are red and soft. Microscopically, they are composed of acinic and tubular epithelial structures, irregular as to size and outline and lined by columnar epithelium. The connective tissue stroma is usually moderate in amount.

Hyperplastic polyps are rare, moderate in size and usually multiple. They consist of lobulated masses of dense connective tissue on the surface of which are complex epithelial crypts lined by epithelium which is differentiated like that of the gastric mucosa. Mucosal polyps of the stomach may become carcinomatous.

FIBROMA of the stomach may appear in the submucosa or in the subserosa and more rarely in the muscularis. Occurring in the submucosa, the tumor may project into the stomach as a polypoid growth covered by cylindrical epithelium.

LIPOMA may be multiple but is usually small and of little significance.

MYOMA, FIBROMYOMA, NEUROFIBROMA, LYMPHANGIOMA and HEMANGIOMA of the stomach have also been described. (See Minnes and Geschickter.)

Malignant tumors of the stomach include sarcoma and carcinoma, the former being unusual and the latter very frequent.

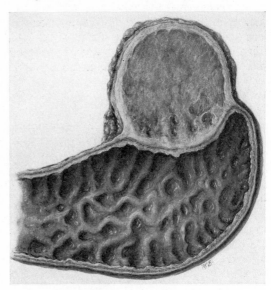

Fibroma in wall of stomach.

SARCOMA occurs principally in the fifth decade of life and about equally in the two sexes. It apparently originates more commonly from the submucosa than from other coats of the stomach. It may be a diffuse flat type of growth or a nodular projecting growth, sometimes pedunculated. The firm cross section is homogeneous, gray and fairly well vascularized. Sarcoma may appear in any part of the stomach but is more common in the pylorus and in the greater curvature. Goldstein found that of 592 sarcomas of the intestinal canal, 265 occurred in the stomach. Douglas estimates that sarcoma constitutes about 1 per cent of all tumors of the stomach. Lymphosarcoma is the most common form. Much more rare are fibrosarcoma, myxosarcoma and leiomyosarcoma. Reticulum-cell sarcoma may be localized and ulcerated, and may be confused with carcinoma. Metastasis, except in the case of lymphosarcoma, is likely to be limited to nearby lymph nodes and to liver (see D'Aunoy and Zoeller).

CARCINOMA. Carcinoma of the stomach is extremely common, constituting according to various statistics between 20 and 40 per cent of all malignant tumors of the body (Livingston and Pack). It is more frequent in men than in women and the majority of cases occur after 50 years of age, although its occurrence earlier in life is by no means rare. It runs its course in about two years although some cases terminate sooner and others last ten years or more. The digestive disturbances are due principally to obstruction of the passage of food through the pylorus. Pain is by no means a constant feature. Vomiting is

though it is possible that surface epithelium may rarely be the source. It may also be derived from mucosal polyps. Reference has been made above to the infrequent transformation of ulcer to carcinoma. Konjetzny is of the opinion that pre-existent chronic gastritis gives rise to the carcinoma, and that even if ulcer be present, the carcinoma is due to the associated gastritis rather than the ulcer. Extensive experimental work has been done, but has thrown little light on the human disease (see Klein and Palmer).

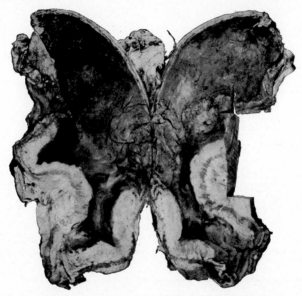

Cross section of carcinoma of pylorus, showing invasion through muscular coat. Army Medical Museum 17381.

likely to occur several hours after the ingestion of a meal and may be bloodstained or distinctly hemorrhagic. Occasionally, fragments of the tumor may be identified in the vomitus. Achlorhydria and increase of lactic acid are common but not constant. Anemia, of microcytic type, may result from repeated small hemorrhages, disturbances of metabolism of iron and perhaps some poisonous effect upon bone marrow. Macrocytic anemias may be due to metastases to bone marrow, failure of intrinsic factor in the diseased stomach or may rarely be part of an associated pernicious anemia (Goldhamer).

When the carcinoma is situated in the fundus, the symptoms are usually much less marked and may be absent, largely because there is little or no obstruction. Carcinoma originates in the glandular epithelium, al-

Forms of Carcinoma. Grossly, two forms are distinguished, the soft or medullary carcinoma and the hard or scirrhous carcinoma. All the forms are most frequent in the lesser curvature near the pylorus, but it is of interest to note that only rarely does cancer extend beyond the pyloric fold into the duodenum.

The soft cancers, which include particularly adenocarcinoma and carcinoma simplex, may be well localized and nodular in character, or more especially with the carcinoma simplex, may occasionally be diffuse. These soft cancers usually project into the stomach and show more or less marked ulceration. The tumor may be a cauliflower-like projecting mass, may be a more or less circumscribed ulcerating mass, may be distinctly focalized or extend in ring form completely around the pyloric end of the stomach. Beginning in the mucosa it rapidly extends into the submucosa and the muscularis, and involving the serosa may show localized extension along the serous surface or may be complicated by perforation. Not infrequently, owing to the slow course of the process, adhesions are formed around the margins of the point of perforation which limit the effects in the same way as is true of perforation of gastric ulcer. Rarely secondary small nodules, due to lymphatic transport rather than to implantation, appear in the submucosa in the immediate neighborhood of the primary tumor. Superficial ulceration is almost constant and there may be extensive necrosis of the tumor growth with the production of a large ulcer. Sometimes saprophytes gain entrance and the necrotic mass becomes gangrenous. Secondary changes in the stomach depend in large part upon the retention of food. There is usually primarily a hypertrophy of the stomach followed ultimately by dilatation. The mucosa shows chronic inflammation, sometimes hypertrophic and sometimes atrophic.

The scirrhous carcinoma of the stomach is almost invariably diffuse in type, beginning in the pyloric end of the stomach and extending in variable degrees toward the cardia. Here, there is thickening of all the coats, more especially the submucosa, due to the carcinoma, and of the muscularis in part because of tumor and in part because of hypertrophy. The stomach is small, of the "leather-bottle" type, and resembles very closely the stomach of chronic interstitial gastritis, or linitis plastica referred to above. Ulceration may occur in scirrhous carcinoma but is by no means a constant or necessary part of the picture. The final diagnosis usually rests upon microscopic examination.

Microscopically, three chief forms are distinguished, the adenocarcinoma, the carcinoma simplex and the scirrhous carcinoma. The adenocarcinoma is likely to show great variation in the number of lining cells. Infiltration of the tissue is likely to be extensive, but the degree of reactionary inflammation depends in part at least upon the degree of ulceration. If the latter be extensive, there is likely to be a considerable infiltration of polymorphonuclear leukocytes, and in the more long-standing cases granulation tissue

may constitute a considerable part of the tumor mass. Occasionally there is excessive production of mucin, with the formation of a mucinous or "colloid" carcinoma (see Stinson). Carcinoma simplex shows islands of relatively undifferentiated epithelium invading the tissues, and shows reactionary inflammation depending in large part upon the degree of ulceration. This type of growth is somewhat more commonly diffuse than is the adenocarcinoma. Here again, depending upon ulceration, there may be a considerable growth of granulation tissue.

Rarely there is observed the so-called "carcinoma in situ," a condition in which the mucosa may show a focus of pleomorphism of cells with loss of cellular polarity confined to the mucosa. Usually the surface is slightly ulcerated. (See Mallory.) This is probably a pre-invasive stage of carcinoma.

Squamous-cell carcinoma may originate in the cardia due to inclusions of esophageal epithelium. Squamous metaplasia of cylindrical cell carcinomas is rare.

Metastasis is more frequent from the medullary than from the scirrhous carcinoma. The lymph nodes surrounding the stomach are affected in a large percentage of cases, especially in the gastric-subpyloric and superior gastric groups of nodes (Coller, et al.). From these there may be more or less widespread extension into the peritoneum, which may be thickly studded with small or large metastases. In our own experience metastatic involvement of the omentum, apparently as a retrograde extension, has been more common from carcinoma of the cardia than from carcinoma of the pylorus. Metastasis to the liver is extremely common and it is probable that this is very largely due to lymphatic dissemination. Nevertheless, it is probable that in certain cases, if not in many, the tumor invades blood vessels and is transported to the liver through the portal veins. The nodules in the liver may be few and small or may be numerous and large, so that the liver is often markedly increased in size. It is unusual, however, for the liver to show marked alteration of function. Metastasis to bones is much more frequent than is commonly supposed. Widespread carcinomatosis is not frequent.

Secondary Tumors. Direct extension of carcinoma of the esophagus into the cardiac portion of the fundus is not rare. The presence of secondary nodules of such carcinoma in other parts of the stomach is probably due to lymphatic transport. Direct extension of carcinoma of the pancreas, biliary passages and liver is rare, as is also that from sarcomas of neighboring viscera. Metastastatic tumors are rare, but sometimes occur from carcinomas of breast, rectum and bronchi.

Alterations of Form and Position

Some of these have been mentioned, as for example, the reduction in size in chronic interstitial gastritis and the various stenoses or constrictions. Dilatation of the stomach may be acute or chronic. Acute dilatation may occur at any time as a result of pyloric stenosis, may be due to overloading of the stomach or to paralytic ileus of the duodenum. In addition, rare cases occur, in which the direct etiology is obscure, as for example, those which follow abdominal section or other operations, those which occur during the course of acute infectious diseases, particularly pneumonia, or during the course of chronic wasting and nervous diseases, and those which follow traumatic injury or occur in the midst of apparently perfect health. Clinically, there is vomiting, abdominal pain, distention and tenderness, marked thirst and scanty urine, followed by collapse and death.

Chronic dilatation is due to prolonged pyloric obstruction such as occurs in carcinoma, whether medullary or scirrhous. Sometimes polyps obstruct the pylorus. Pyloric hypertrophy of infants usually produces only moderate dilatation. A pyloric hypertrophy also occurs in adults, but this is probably secondary to chronic gastritis, both mucosal and interstitial (Konjetzny). Vomiting occurs usually two or more hours after eating. The vomitus shows reduced hydrochloric acid, sarcinae, yeasts, bacteria and undigested food. Fermentation or putrefaction produce variable quantities of lactic acid, butyric acid and even acetic acid. Gases such as hydrogen, carbon dioxide, and rarely marsh gas may lead to marked distention. Gas produced postmortem frequently causes moderate distention of stomach and intestines. The pathologic forms may show enormous distention, so that the greater curvature reaches the pubis.

Diverticula may form between the bands of scarring around old gastric ulcers or may be produced by traction of external adhesions.

Ptosis of the stomach is usually associated with ptosis of other organs, especially the transverse colon. It is probably acquired as the result of faulty posture. Roentgenograms may show the greater curvature nearly down to the pubis, but there is only moderate or no dilatation. Generally speaking, it has no special symptoms.

Foreign Bodies

Various foreign bodies are swallowed by accident or by design, and may accumulate in great quantity and variety in the stomach. They may be passed through the intestinal canal, may remain in the stomach or perforate. Hair balls, masses of swallowed hairs, are seen in the stomachs of cattle and cats, and in man occur occasionally in the stomachs of mental defectives. As they increase in size they conform to the outline of the stomach and produce abdominal swelling. Often symptomless, they may cause stasis, ulceration and even perforation. Other substances may accumulate in much the same fashion (Hart).

INTESTINES

Congenital Abnormalities

Absence. The intestines may be entirely or partly absent owing to congenital defects, more particularly when there is general malformation of the body. The intestine may be shorter than normal, more especially the large intestine. Occasionally, the appendix may be aplastic or completely absent. Heterotopias are not rare (Taylor).

Congenital atresias may occur in any part of the gut but are found especially in the duodenum, at the ileocecal junction and at the lower end of the large intestine. As a rule, the intestine above the point of constriction is dilated, filled with amniotic fluid or meconium and sometimes distinctly hypertrophic. The intestine below is usually collapsed and may be aplastic.

Of great importance are those atresias which occur in and about the rectum. Three chief forms are observed. In one the rectum reaches as far as the anus but does not communicate with it. In another, the point of atresia is slightly above the anal orifice so that there is a blind anal groove extending up a centimeter or more. In the more serious forms the rectum ends blindly a considerable distance from the anus and there is no anal groove. These atresias at the lower end of the gut may communicate by fistulous tracts either internally with the vagina in females or the bladder or urethra in males or externally in the midline of the perineum. Although these fistulae may be congenital in origin, it seems more likely that most of them are pathologic in nature and due to the pressure of the contents of the obstructed intestine.

elongation and with secondary hypertrophy of the muscular part of the wall. It is not incompatible with life and the patient may reach mature years, suffering only from retention of feces so that bowel movements are infrequent, sometimes separated by a week or more, and associated with considerable abdominal enlargement. It is possible that the disorder may be acquired. It is explained by overactivity of sympathetics with inhibition of colonic muscle and contraction of the sphincter, or underactivity of the parasympathetics with poor peristalsis and inadequate relaxation of sphincter. (See Turell.)

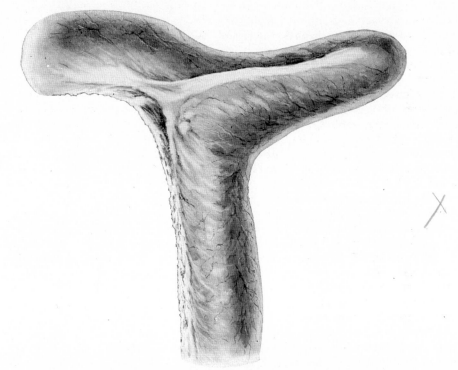

Meckel's diverticulum of small intestine.

structed intestine. There are in addition true congenital fistulae about the lower end of the abdomen due to failure of development of the cloaca.

Congenital Dilatation. Dilatation occurs above congenital atresias as has been noted. These are, however, in a sense acquired rather than strictly congenital. The most important congenital dilatation is that which is spoken of as *megacolon congenitum*, or HIRSCHSPRUNG'S DISEASE. In this condition the colon throughout its entire length is moderately or enormously dilated, usually with

DIVERTICULA. *Meckel's diverticulum* is common and is due to incomplete regression of the omphalomesenteric duct. Arising from the surface of the gut distal to the mesentery, it is usually but not always 80 to 100 cm. above the ileocecal junction and may be several centimeters long. It is subject to volvulus, to inflammation, to heterotopia of gastric or duodenal mucosa or pancreatic tissue, to peptic ulcer of gastric or duodenal tissues, and to benign and malignant tumor formation derived from the tube or heterotopic structures (Nygaard and Walters).

Acquired diverticula are referred to here for convenience. In the duodenum both congenital and acquired diverticula occur near the ampulla in the pancreatic part of the duodenum. In the small intestine, diverticula are found at the mesenteric attachment. In the large intestine they arise at or near the mesocolic attachment. In both parts of the intestine they are usually multiple. The diverticula of the large intestine occur in from about 25 to 30 per cent of all adults. They are usually symptomless but may be the seat of acute or chronic diverticulitis. Perforation may give rise to local or diffuse peritonitis. It is difficult to distinguish between acquired and congenital diverticula, and it is probable that most are acquired, perhaps as the result of local areas of deficiency of muscle. Most of the diverticula have a small amount of muscle in the wall but some, referred to as false diverticula, have no muscle whatever.

Congenital alterations of position of the intestine are exhibited principally in the form of transposition of the viscera and in the form of hernias.

A HERNIA is a protrusion of part of the intestine or of other abdominal organs, associated with exvagination of the peritoneum, through some part of the abdominal wall. This may be through some such orifice as the inguinal canal or an incomplete union of the abdominal wall at the position of the umbilicus, etc. Hernias may be classified as external when they project on the outer surface of the body, or internal when they project into other parts of the body cavity. Thus, the external hernias may be inguinal, crural or femoral, perineal, umbilical, or abdominal (projecting through the linea alba). These may be due to increase in size or inadequate closure of orifices, or may occur as the result of excess strain upon orifices, which although apparently properly closed exhibit congenital weakness. They may be truly acquired as the result of traumatic interruption of continuity of the abdominal wall. As the result of improper or incomplete repair of the abdominal wall in surgical operations, the scar may subsequently stretch, and hernia occur through the scar.

Internal hernias include those which occur through the diaphragm. These may be congenital or acquired; when acquired the usual cause is trauma. When occurring through the leaves of the diaphragm the left side is usually involved so that stomach and portions of the intestine are found in the thorax. Hiatus hernias may be due to congenitally short esophagus or to deficiency of formation of the diaphragm at the hiatus. There is herniation of part of the cardia of the stomach. (Polley.) Internal hernia may also occur into retroperitoneal spaces, more particularly that which exists at the point where the duodenum joins the jejunum. Covering the abdominal contents in the case of external hernias are the peritoneum, various fascias, muscle remnants, skin, etc., completely described in the textbooks on surgery.

Ordinarily, the contents of external hernia may be pressed back into the abdomen and the hernia is said to be reducible. Adhesion to the wall of the sac or the hernial ring may render the hernia irreducible. Adhesions between coils of gut or folds of omentum may result in the formation of a tumor-like mass reducible or not, depending upon adhesions to the sac wall. The accumulation of intestinal contents in coils of gut in the hernia may obstruct the intestine and the hernia is said to be incarcerated. The hernia is strangulated when, either as the result of incarceration or otherwise, the circulation of blood is obstructed, with consequent blood stasis, edema, hemorrhage, or necrosis and gangrene. Even without gangrene mild degrees of acute fibrinous peritonitis occur. Gangrene leads to local acute peritonitis, which, especially when perforation occurs, may become widespread.

Organic Obstruction

This term indicates the invagination of an upper segment of gut within a lower segment. This may be of small intestine into small intestine, small intestine usually with cecum into large intestine, large intestine into large intestine, or rectum externally through the anus as "prolapsus recti." The outer sheath of the lower part of gut, the ensheathing layer, is called the intussuscipiens. The two layers of upper segment which are folded upon each other within the sheath constitute the intussusceptum. Except in prolapsus recti, intussusception usually gives rise to intestinal obstruction. The peristaltic action of the intussuscipiens exerts a pull upon the intussusceptum which is finally halted in its downward passage by the mesenteric attachment. Since the vascular supply and drainage of the intussusceptum are within the mesentery, there is interruption first of venous drainage and then of arterial supply. There follows blood stasis and edema of the intussusceptum which further interferes with circulation. Infection of the enclosed wall is followed by local peritonitis and consequent fixation of the intussusceptum. Finally, necrosis and gangrene, with all the dangers and sequences of perforation, occur. Intussusception is more common in children than adults. Postmortem or agonal intussusception is distinguished by lack of local peritonitis and ready reducibility. This is also more common in children than in adults. It is common in laboratory animals, especially guinea-pigs and rabbits. In children there is usually no discernible cause, but in adults peristaltic action upon tumor masses in the small intestine may pull the segment down to form the intussusceptum.

Volvulus. This term indicates a twisting of a coil of gut upon itself or a twisting in the long axis. The former is more common and is especially likely to occur in the sigmoid flexure. The mesosigmoid may be congenitally long or elongated by traction of adhesions, so that the sigmoid is a long, more or less angulated loop. Twisting of the mesosigmoid may bring the basal segments in contact so that they mutually press upon one another, become obstructed and strangulated. Similar volvulus may occur at the ileocecal junction due to long mesocecum. Volvulus of the small intestine is less common. Spiral twisting upon the long axis of the gut is unusual and is more often observed in the small intestine. Torsion, with secondary hyperemia, hemorrhage, edema, necrosis and sometimes infection may affect the omentum or epiploic appendages.

Intestinal Obstruction. This is usually classified as mechanical and dynamic, or paralytic. The former is due to conditions which physically obstruct the lumen such as hernial incarceration and strangulation, obstruction by fibrous adhesions, intussusception, volvulus, obstructing bodies such as swallowed foreign bodies, gallstones, inspissated masses of feces, tumors of the gut, tumors or similar masses compressing the gut, strictures of congenital or acquired origin,

the latter usually inflammatory in character. Paralytic obstruction is due to acute peritonitis or to infarction of the gut. It may also be due to abdominal operations, extra-abdominal colics such as that due to renal calculus, infectious diseases such as pneumonia which probably operate through toxic products of the disease, and nervous diseases affecting spinal cord and sympathetic system.

Symptoms and signs such as abdominal distention and pain, hyperperistalsis above the point of mechanical obstruction, diminishing as distention of the gut increases, retention of intestinal contents and vomiting which ultimately becomes fecal, vary with the type, location and completeness of the obstruction. Finally a shock-like condition develops and death supervenes. The symptoms are more severe when the obstruction is high in the small intestine than when it affects the large intestine. The obstruction and associated symptoms are referred to as ileus.

The abdominal distention is due to filling of the intestine with solid, liquid and gaseous contents. The accumulation of gas may produce marked meteorism. This is primarily due either to accumulation above obstruction or in the paralyzed gut, and is augmented by secondary circulatory effects due to the distention. The abdominal distention may be so great as to interfere with heart action, especially it seems by reducing flow through the abdominal veins and into the atria. Vomiting is due in part to accumulation of intestinal and gastric contents, in part to reverse peristalsis and is contributed to by reflex irritation from the distended intestine (see Crowley). Pain is due principally to colicky contractions of gut segments and perhaps to other factors.

The most frequent cause of acute intestinal obstruction is strangulation of the gut in external hernias. McIver found this to be the cause in 44 per cent of 335 patients. About 10 per cent were due to tumors. Fairly frequent were cases of obstruction due to bands and adhesions. Next were cases of intussusception. Obstruction is said to be simple, when there is no apparent damage to the gut wall, as may be true in obstruction by adhesions and foreign bodies, and is said to be strangulated when the wall is injured. Usually the onset of symptoms is abrupt and the course stormy.

Experimental and clinical studies have been numerous and have thrown much light on the subject. Vomiting is severe in high intestinal obstruction. The loss of water and salt is marked and may be fatal. The dehydration may be accompanied by retention of nitrogenous products in the blood and moderate renal insufficiency, but this probably is not a cause of death. Loss of water and salt may be marked in low intestinal obstruction, but it is likely that death is due to absorption of poisonous material from the gut. Whether such materials are produced in the intestine independently of disease of its wall is controversial. The same is true of the question as to whether the normal contents of the bowel are poisonous or whether there must be some action by secretions or bacteria to render the contents poisonous. The evidence favors the view that the poisonous material is the result of bacterial action upon the injured wall. The substance, however, is not a true toxin. In low obstruction there is often a fall of blood pressure together with hemoconcentration; all the manifestations of shock occur, as described in the chapter on Disturbances of Circulation. The significance of distention of the intestine is great, as indicated by the favorable results of decompression by the Miller-Abbott tube. This reduces distention and washes out intestinal contents and gas. The compression of the gut wall may reduce absorption of poisonous materials but this is not finally proven. As mentioned above, reflex stimulation is probably important in reference to vomiting. Starvation is an item of only secondary importance. (See Besser.)

Retrogressive Processes

Chronic passive hyperemia may lead to hemosiderosis of the intestinal wall. The pigment of hemosiderosis may be in sufficiently large amounts to give a distinct light brown color to the mucosa. Melanosis is a dark brown or black pigmentation of the mucosa, which may affect the entire gut but is usually more prominent in or limited to the large intestine (Stewart and Hickman). It usually does not affect the lymphoid structures or the glands. It appears as an amorphous granular pigment in the connective tissue of the mucosa and does not respond to the tests for iron. Its chemical composition is not definitely known. It occurs under a variety of circumstances of which constipation and wasting diseases seem to be important.

Chronic inflammations may produce pigmentation, probably hematogenous, of the tips of the villi and in the neighborhood of the lymph follicles. Not infrequently dark brown pigmentation affects the lymph follicles, particularly those of the large intestine, where the pigmented points are so close together as to produce the so-called "shaven beard" appearance. This is believed to be the late result of inflammation of a hemorrhagic character. Pseudomelanosis, such as affects the stomach, may also occur in the intestine as the result of action of hydrogen sulfide upon blood. The muscle of the gut may undergo atrophy, usually simple, but occasionally a brown atrophy with relative or absolute increase in the muscle pigment. The glands may show cloudy swelling, mucinous degeneration, fatty degeneration, atrophy, etc., in connection with inflammations; and soon after death they show postmortem decomposition. In secondary amyloidosis, the vessels of the intestines may be affected; in some cases of primary amyloidosis, tumorlike nodules of amyloid may occur in the muscle.

Disturbances of Circulation

Active hyperemia occurs physiologically during digestion and pathologically as the result of local irritation and acute inflammation. The redness of active hyperemia usually disappears soon after death. Passive hyperemia is common especially as the result of cardiac disease, disease of the liver, particularly cirrhosis, chronic disease of the lungs, thrombosis of the portal vein or vena cava, and may be observed locally in such conditions as intussusception, volvulus and incarcerated or strangulated hernia. Grossly, the intestine is likely to be somewhat thickened, of dark red or purple color, in the prolonged cases pigmented as noted above, and is likely to show catarrhal inflammation of the mucous membrane. Associated edema may be slight or marked and usually is most apparent in the submucosa. Submucosal hemorrhages are occasionally observed.

Varicose veins are rare in the intestinal canal. Hemorrhoids or anal hemorrhoids are varicose dilatations of the hemorrhoidal plexus in and about the anus. They may be internal to the orifice, or external with projection on the cutaneous surface, or both. The cause is not known, but there is probably some inherent constitutional weakness of the venous walls that favors varicosity. Constipation favors their development and they may be enlarged as the result of passive hyperemia of the portal system. They are nodular masses, a few millimeters or more in diameter, clustered together and compressible. Thrombosis may take place, especially when there is local infection. This renders them firm; organization of the thrombus may cause shrinkage and increased firmness. Minor degrees of hemorrhage are common, especially where infection is present, and occasionally frequently repeated hemorrhages may lead to slight anemia. Large hemorrhages rarely occur.

Embolism in the arteries of the intestinal canal is not uncommon. The emboli arise from endocarditis, thrombi within the heart, thrombi upon diseased aorta or in other situations. Occasionally thrombosis appears to be primary in these vessels. The anastomosis of vessels in the rectum makes it improbable that minor occlusion is of any significance unless the embolus be infected. In the small intestines, and to a certain degree in the large intestines, in spite of fairly free anastomosis, occlusion of arteries usually leads to hemorrhagic infarct of the area supplied. If this be limited to the small area over the convexity of the gut, adhesion may prevent rupture into the general peritoneal cavity. If the embolus be infected, local suppuration may ensue rapidly. Obstruction of a larger branch means necrosis of a larger or smaller segment of the entire intestinal wall, which primarily interrupts the continuous flow of peristaltic movement producing ileus and secondarily leads to gangrene, rupture of the intestine and widespread peritonitis.

Hemorrhage from the intestinal canal may be small, large or even sufficient to be fatal. It may be due to hyperemia principally of the passive type, to infarction as indicated above, to acute inflammations, more particularly those which lead to necrosis of the mucosa, to ulcers such as gastric and duodenal ulcers and those of tuberculosis, syphilis, typhoid fever and to tumors. Blood diseases, especially those with a hemorrhagic

disposition, melena neonatorum, those infectious diseases which lead to hemorrhage elsewhere, foreign bodies and wounds from the outside, hemorrhoids, all may lead to hemorrhage. If hemorrhage originate low in the colon, in the rectum or in the anus, the blood in the stools is bright red. If the hemorrhage originate in stomach or small intestine, it is digested and disintegrated by the time it appears in the stools; this gives rise to "tarry" stools.

Inflammations

Inflammations of the intestinal canal may be particularly prominent in one part or another, and are usually named more or less specifically as duodenitis, enteritis, appendicitis, typhlitis, colitis, sigmoiditis and proctitis. As a rule, it is usual to find some extension beyond the situation principally indicated by the name. Thus, an inflammation of the colon is likely to show simultaneous involvement of the lower portion of the small intestine, and conversely any enteritis is likely to show a more or less extensive associated colitis.

Acute catarrhal inflammation may be due to any of those causes indicated in discussing the catarrhs of the stomach, including various irritant foods and drink, as well as the irritation of decomposing or stagnant foods, irritant and escharotic poisons and those poisons generally grouped under the term "food poisoning" including products of the botulinus, enteritidis and paratyphosus groups. Grossly, the affected part of the intestine shows a soft, thick, red mucosa covered by viscid adherent mucus. The submucosa may be edematous. The muscularis shows little or no change.

Microscopically, there is mucinous degeneration of the epithelium and infiltration of lymphoid and plasma cells into the mucosa. More severe cases may show infiltration of polymorphonuclear leukocytes. Desquamation of epithelium is a common feature both grossly and microscopically, and more particularly with catarrhal inflammation of the rectum and lower large intestine, the desquamation may be so active as to constitute tubular casts of the intestinal lining. In the more severe cases this is referred to as desquamative enteritis, colitis, or proctitis, as the case may be.

Acute follicular enteritis is more common in children than adults and may be the morphologic basis of some forms of "summer complaint" of children. In some cases dysentery bacilli or large numbers of anaerobic gas bacilli may be recovered, but in many no definite pathogenic bacteria are found. The enteritis or enterocolitis is catarrhal in type, associated with hyperplasia of the solitary lymphoid follicles; which project as fairly firm, pallid or hyperemic nodules. These may undergo necrosis and ulcerate to produce acute follicular ulcerative enteritis.

Acute fibrinous inflammations of the intestine are well represented in bacillary dysentery, to be discussed subsequently. Acute fibrinous inflammation may also accompany acute infectious diseases, more particularly pyemia. Mercurial poisoning often shows an ulcerative and fibrinous inflammation of the lower ileum and upper part of the large intestine. A somewhat similar condition is sometimes observed in uremia. In fibrinous inflammation there is usually a profound catarrhal inflammation associated with considerable desquamation and deposit of fibrin upon the surface. The mucosa and submucosa are edematous and there is usually a rich infiltration of polymorphonuclear leukocytes.

Acute phlegmonous inflammation may follow acute fibrinous forms, especially when ulceration occurs; or a more localized suppuration may be introduced through ulcers such as those of tuberculosis or carcinoma; and occasionally the intestine may be involved in cases of pyemia.

Chronic catarrhal inflammation of the intestine is usually due to the passive hyperemia of chronic heart, lung or liver diseases. The thickened mucosa is often covered by mucus, and may be pigmented. In cases of long duration, atrophy may be found in mucosa and even in the muscularis. Rarely the glands may be dilated to produce a cystic form of the lesion. Polyp formation is less frequent than in similar disease of the stomach. Any of these forms may be accompanied by slight or marked ulceration. A chronic ulcerative enteritis has been described as due to histoplasmosis (Henderson and Pinkerton).

Ulcerative colitis is usually chronic in nature and course. The lesions, both grossly and microscopically, resemble those to be described in the chronic forms of bacillary dysentery. Thought to be due to specific streptococci, and also to be influenced by constitutional factors, the cause has not been conclusively identified (see Paulson).

Regional ileitis affects males and females about equally, occurs at all age periods but is most frequent in the third decade. The symptoms may be those of acute inflammation in the abdomen or those of chronic partial intestinal obstruction. The roentgenogram shows fairly characteristic filling defects. Various causes including bacteria, animal parasites, allergy, etc., have been considered but none has been proved. In most cases the terminal ileum is affected, but the lesion may extend into the cecum and may occur in various regions of the small intestine.

In the acute stages, the intestinal wall is swollen by edema and hyperemia and the serosa may be slightly dull. The mucosa is also edematous and may show mucosal ulcers sometimes covered by fibrinous exudate. In the chronic stages, the wall is thick, firm, "like a garden hose," and fibrous peritoneal adhesions may be extensive. Microscopically, the acute stage shows principally edema with relatively few exudative cells. In the chronic stage there is fibrosis of all coats and often a hypertrophy of muscle. Ulceration is deeper in the chronic lesions and may perforate, but peritoneal inflammation is usually limited by the adhesions. (See Shapiro.)

Gas Cysts

Gas cysts of the intestines, or intestinal pneumatosis, are uncommon. The lesion is due to the presence of gas or air in the lymphatics of the intestine and mesentery, appearing as numerous bubbles in cysts whose walls are thin and transparent, tending to become thicker and more opaque as the result of granulation and organization. In most cases there is ulceration in the stomach or some other part of the intestinal canal, affording a portal of entry for air or intestinal gas, which if introduced under pressure such as may be produced by vomiting could infiltrate widely in the lymphatics. We support this mechanical theory, but others have proposed that the gas is due to bacterial action in the lymphatics or that the disease is neoplastic. (See Mills.)

Special Infections

Several infectious diseases have their most prominent pathologic and clinical manifestations in connection with the intestinal canal. Although general manifestations are variable in the acute and chronic inflammations, they are of great significance in these special infections. These include particularly typhoid fever, bacillary dysentery, amebic dysentery and cholera. Infectious granulomata as they affect the intestines will be referred to in a separate section.

Typhoid Fever. The general aspects of typhoid fever have been considered in the chapter on Principles of Infectious Disease. The discussion here will be directed toward the lesions in the intestine. The chief manifestations are in the ileum with involvement of the lymphoid aggregates, especially the Peyer's patches.

The degree of involvement of the large intestine varies in individual cases. In occasional cases the lymphoid follicles of the stomach are involved. The small intestine is likely to show acute catarrhal inflammation in association with the changes in the Peyer's patches. In the Peyer's patches and to variable degrees in the solitary follicles, the first change is hyperemia. Following this there is acute hyperplasia of the lymphoid nodules. Thus, the patches are enlarged in all diameters and project into the intestine. The surface is likely to be convoluted so as to resemble the brain of a small animal. In the later periods of this stage hyperemia is likely to be only slight. Next comes necrosis of the lymphoid apparatus with desquamation of the necrotic material into the intestinal lumen, and the formation of an ulcer coextensive with the Peyer's patch. The ulcer shows elevated ragged margins and a somewhat roughened, necrotic, usually pallid base, not extending beneath the submucosa. Without secondary infection the further progress includes healing of this true typhoid ulcer by organization of the base and growth of surface epithelium. Glandular epithelium does not regenerate to any considerable degree, and it is probable that regeneration of lymphoid tissue is not extensive.

Microscopically, the stage of hyperplasia shows multiplication of lymphoid and endothelial cells, sometimes associated with slight infiltration of polymorphonuclear leukocytes. Early in the course, hyperemia is prominent but subsequently decreases. An important feature of the stage of hyperplasia is the phagocytic activity of the large mononuclear cells, which contain not only typhoid bacilli but also cell fragments, nuclear fragments and erythrocytes. In the stage of ul-

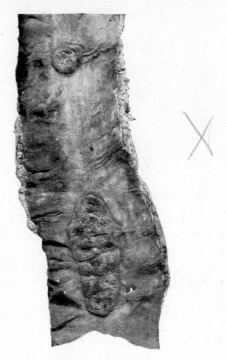

Swelling of Peyer's patches in typhoid fever. Army Medical Museum 30456.

ceration the remnants of hyperplastic lymphadenoid tissues are easily observed in the margins and the base, but, even without severe secondary infection, there is likely to be a moderate or marked infiltration of polymorphonuclear leukocytes under the necrotic material remaining in the ulcer. Granulation and epithelial regeneration are not markedly different from that occurring under other conditions.

The surface of the typhoid ulcer may become secondarily infected and hence extend deeply into the muscularis and even the serosa. Hemorrhage from vessels incompletely filled by thrombosis or those from which thrombi may be dislodged by gaseous distention of the gut may be severe or even fatal. Perforation into a space protected by adhesions may produce local abscess, and perforation into the peritoneal cavity a widespread acute suppurative peritonitis.

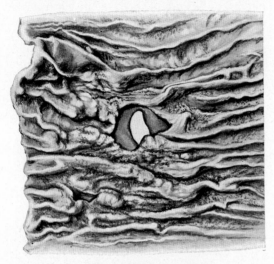

Perforated typhoid ulcer of ileum.

Infections by the paratyphoid bacilli are in general less severe as regards both general symptoms and local lesions.

Bacillary Dysentery. The term dysentery has been employed clinically to signify bloody and mucous diarrhea accompanied by straining and tenesmus, the stools as a rule being small and frequent. Pathologically, the term is restricted to two conditions with definite causes, the one, bacillary or epidemic dysentery and the other, amebic dysentery. Detailed references are not given here because they are covered by Callender. The disease occurs in epidemic and in endemic form. It is observed particularly under conditions of crowding such as occur in asylums and in army camps. It constitutes one of the forms of summer diarrhea in children.

It is a specific acute infectious disease, with fever, prostration and the special disorders of dysentery. The course is usually a few weeks but occasionally the disease may be of longer duration. It may be caused by *Shigella dysenteriae,* or by separate forms morphologically similar but differing as to fermentation and immunologic characters. The latter include particularly the Hiss, the Flexner, the Strong and the Sonne forms, usually grouped as varieties of *Shigella parady-*

senteriae. The first form produces the most severe disease. In the second group are those

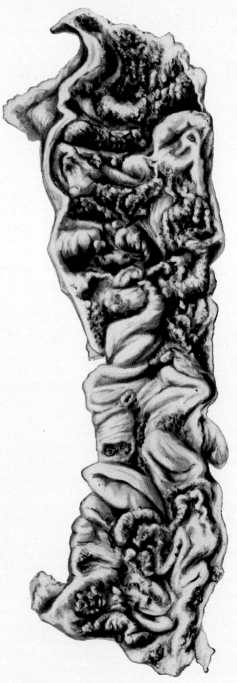

Fibrinous exudate and ulceration in bacillary dysentery.

which produce dysentery in adults and summer diarrhea in children.

The organisms enter by the mouth and

produce lesions in the large intestines associated with secondary toxic manifestations. They can be recovered from stools in early stages of the disease, particularly when cultures are made from small masses of bloody mucus, and can also be recovered after death directly from the mucous membrane. It is only rarely that they are found in the blood.

The intestinal lesions are confined almost entirely to the large intestine, although occasionally there is slight extension upward into the lower ileum, and sometimes the appendix is involved. In the large intestine, the lower part and the rectum are likely to show the most severe inflammation. In the earlier stages the inflammation may apparently be simply a catarrhal inflammation, or pseudo-membranous or even suppurative in character, but ulceration rapidly ensues. The ulcers are primarily in small foci but rapidly extend to involve a large part of the wall. They may be so extensive that only small islands of mucosa remain as red, swollen patches, sometimes covered with fibrin or with pus. The ulcers may penetrate only into the submucosa but not infrequently involve the muscularis. The edges may be sharp or may be markedly undermined. The base is usually of brown color due to hematogenous pigmentation.

Microscopically, the epithelium of the mucosa undergoes considerable necrosis early in the process, and may be surmounted by a network of fibrin enmeshing leukocytes and other inflammatory cells. The margins of the ulcer show an infiltration of polymorphonuclear leukocytes associated with lymphoid cells, large mononuclear cells and sometimes eosinophils. This inflammatory process also appears in lesser degrees throughout the intestinal coat and is commonly associated with inflammatory edema. As the disease progresses, reaction of the fixed connective tissue becomes apparent, with the production of granulation tissue, followed by greater or lesser degree of cicatrization. Epithelialization of the surface occurs from the remaining islands of living tissue. Secondary infection may play a prominent part, so that suppuration or phlegmonous inflammation of the gut wall occurs and, in occasional cases, a gangrenous type of inflammation is observed.

In severe cases the inflammation is so marked that the peritoneal coat is involved

in a slight fibrinous exudate, which tends to produce fibrous adhesions. Perforation of the gut with general peritonitis is not common, since as a rule adhesions precede the perforation. Therefore, in case of perforation there is likely to be produced localized pericolic or perirectal abscess. The progress of the inflammation is such that massive hemorrhage from the ulcers is not common, because thrombosis is usually well established.

In contrast to amebic dysentery, which may produce large solitary abscess of the liver, bacillary dysentery only rarely produces abscess of the liver, and when observed, they are usually multiple. Acute inflamma-

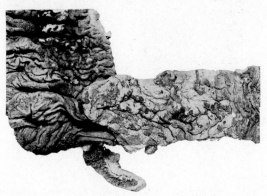

Superficial necrosis of mucosa of lower ileum and cecum in bacillary dysentery. Army Medical Museum 6301.

tion, sometimes leading to abscess formation, may be observed in situations other than the liver, as for example, in the skeletal muscle and in the parotid gland. Acute endocarditis, myocarditis or pericarditis occur but are infrequent. The exotoxic manifestations in the nervous system are by no means constant and are principally in the form of peripheral neuritis. Nonsuppurative inflammations of the joints are not uncommon and are believed to be due to the endotoxin absorbed from the intestines. After recovery, cicatrization takes place but only rarely does this go on to contraction of such degree as to produce stricture.

Although relapses occur, reinfections are unusual. During the course of the disease the patient develops specific agglutinins but usually not in titres higher than one to fifty. More especially in Shiga dysentery the use of therapeutic immune serum is of value. This is usually a polyvalent antitoxic serum.

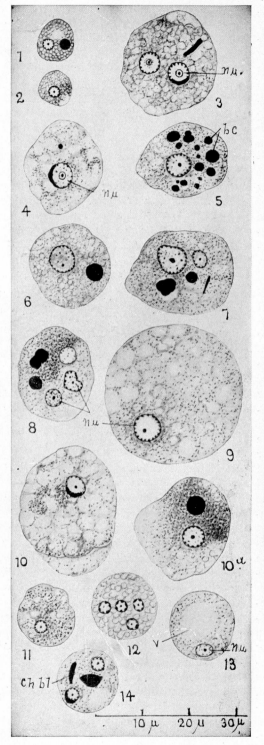

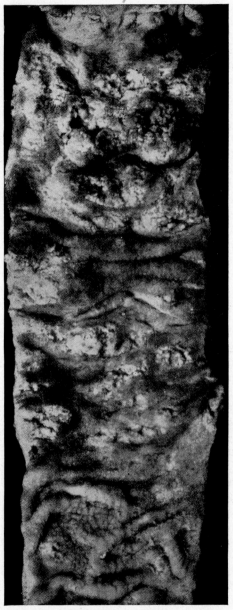

Figs. 1-8—*E. histolytica*, ameba from the cultures. (1, 2) Small forms; (3, 7) Amebae, with two nuclei, one of which is smaller than the other; (5) amebae full of ingested blood corpuscles; (4) ameba with large vacuoles; (8) three-nucleate amebae.

Nu., Nucleus; *b.c.*, blood corpuscles.

Figs. 9-11—*E. histolytica* from the ulcers of the large intestine of cats. (9, 10) Large vacuolate amebae; (10*a*) amebae showing pseudopodia. (11) Smaller, less vacuolated ameba.

Figs. 12, 13, 14—Cysts from the cultures.

Nu., nucleus; *v.* vacuoles; *ch. bl.*, chromatin block.

Fig. 114—Portion of large intestine of cat 1. Note the ulcerated areas. (Magnification, 3 diameters). From D. W. Cutler, Jour. Pathology.

Endamoeba histolytica and lesions in the colon.

Prophylactic vaccination has not been widely employed because of the severity of local and general reaction due to the injection. It is likely that with the production of vaccines which do not produce such severe reactions, vaccination may be widely practiced. (See Macumber.)

Amebic Dysentery. This is due to *Endamoeba histolytica*, but since the presence of these organisms does not necessarily lead to dysenteric manifestations, the name amebiasis is preferred. It is sometimes called tropical dysentery, but is not confined to tropical or subtropical countries. It is endemic in many parts of the world, and in the United States it is said that amebae or their cysts can be recovered in the stools of from 5 to 10 per cent of the population. The carrier state, then, is not uncommon. It is more frequent in adults than in children and may spread in institutions and armies. The organisms are transferred in water and food.

The *E. histolytica* is an actively motile ameba usually 20 to 30 micra in diameter, but sometimes measuring from 18 to 40 micra. In the fresh actively motile state the ectoplasm and endoplasm are not clearly defined, but as motility is reduced there still remains an active thrusting out of pseudopodia of almost entirely clear ectoplasm. The nucleus is vesicular and contains less chromatin than other intestinal amebae. The cytoplasm may contain many erythrocytes or a few leukocytes or other cells, but only rarely contains bacteria and intestinal debris, in contrast to the nonpathogenic *E. coli*. The organisms are recoverable in smears of the feces, especially from masses of mucus, and may be cultivated with difficulty. Tissue sections and inference from the observation of liver and brain abscesses indicate that they may gain access to the blood stream. The cysts are encountered in the feces during the disease, in carriers who have recovered from the disease and in those carriers who ingest, harbor and discharge the parasites without suffering from the disease. The cysts are thick-walled spheroids with a maximum diameter of 20 micra, with clear cytoplasm and one, two, or four fairly dense nuclei; sometimes there is a glycogen globule but no other material in the cytoplasm. Lesions have been produced experimentally in kittens, monkeys, mice and rats; from the study of these, information has been collected as to the course of the disease.

The lesions of amebic dysentery are confined almost entirely to the large intestine. Although the disease is chronic in nature there may be clinically acute cases or exacerbations of the chronic cases. These, however, show no distinguishing features pathologically. In the early stages, there is an acute catarrh of the mucosa associated somewhat

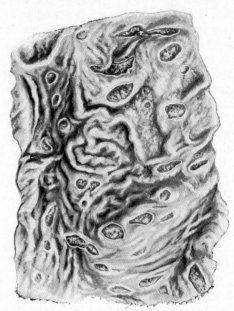

Thickening of gut and chronic ulcers in amebic dysentery.

later with the appearance of small nodules with minute central ulcers. The ulcers tend to coalesce laterally along the valvulae conniventes, may grow to considerable size and are usually disposed laterally in the gut. The outline is irregular and the edges are usually thick and elevated. Although not always the case, there is usually marked undermining of the edges with extension of numerous small fistulae under the mucosa. Deep extension of the ulcers is usually the result of secondary infection. The intervening mucosa may continue to be edematous, but only when secondarily infected shows fibrin formation or suppuration. The inflammation of the intestinal wall is of chronic character and as a consequence there is little or no localized fibrinous peritonitis or subsequent adhesion. The older cases usually show marked thickening of the intestinal wall due to fibrosis, but this is not invariably the case since in some instances there is actual thinning of the wall.

Microscopically, the earlier lesions show catarrhal inflammation with production of mucus. Penetration of the amebae into the mucosa and thence into the submucosa, is accompanied by coagulation necrosis of the mucosa and submucosa, followed by liquefaction and ulceration. Cells which infiltrate in the neighborhood are principally lymphocytes, large mononuclear cells and a relatively small number of leukocytes. In these areas the amebae can be identified as large cells whose nuclei are small, fairly dense and often polychromatic. The cytoplasm is not vacuolated but may contain red blood corpuscles, and an occasional leukocyte. Secondary infection and gangrene may occur. Perforation, with acute widespread peritonitis and death, is more common in amebic than in bacillary dysentery, probably because of the failure of formation of adhesions in the former. Hemorrhage from the ulcers may be slight or severe.

The prominent sequel of amebic dysentery is the so-called abscess of the liver, usually fairly large and solitary, and occasionally multiple. The organisms are carried by the portal vein into the liver and set up there a coagulation necrosis followed by liquefaction, similar to that in the gut. Sometimes bacteria gain entrance with the amebae and produce a true abscess. Without such infection the margin of the necrotic area shows an infiltration of lymphoid, plasma cells and monocytes and in the earlier stages a considerable number of amebae. As time goes on, the connective tissue proliferates and encapsulates the area, or the process may extend to the surface of the liver and rupture. With extension of the necrotic mass upward, adhesions form between liver, diaphragm and lungs, so that perforation may occur into the lung followed by expectoration of brownish-red pus containing amebae. Occasionally healing occurs, the contents become semisolid or gelatinous and may ultimately become completely cicatrized. Abscesses may occur also in spleen and brain; abscesses in the skin may lead to ulceration. The disease may ultimately lead to polyps of the colon and Reed and Anderson report that carcinoma may occur. (See Callender; Meleney.)

Asiatic cholera is due to *Vibrio comma* or Komma bacillus of Koch, and is transmitted particularly by water and food, occurring often as epidemic and in certain countries apparently endemic forms. The incubation period is approximately 24 to 48 hours and the disease is characterized in the milder cases simply by diarrhea. In more severe cases there are diarrhea, vomiting and prostration, and in the most severe cases these symptoms are accompanied by collapse, delirium, coma and death. The diarrhea is in the form of a large discharge of watery stools, the so-called "rice water" stools, the granules being principally bacterial masses, mucus and desquamated epithelium. The loss of water in the stools leads to dehydration and to the various sequels of hemoconcentration going on to anuria and acidosis. At autopsy, there is marked rigor mortis, thick blood, dryness of the serous cavities, cloudy swelling of kidneys and of other viscera, but the spleen is not usually enlarged. Bronchopneumonia, cholangitis and cholecystitis are frequent.

The intestinal lesions usually affect the entire small intestine, may extend into the colon and rarely into the stomach. The intestinal content may be thin and watery or rather thick, turbid, and viscid. The intestinal mucosa may be smooth, somewhat pallid and translucent, or of pink color, covered with adherent mucus. There is moderate enlargement of the lymphoid apparatus of the intestinal canal, often showing in the center of the follicles a small opaque area of necrosis. In the lower part of the intestines there may be petechiae. Hyperemia is present in the various coats of the intestine, involving not only the peritoneal coat but also the mesentery. Sometimes the peritoneum contains a thick cloudy fluid which shows numerous desquamated mesothelial cells. Microscopically, in addition to general hyperemia, usually without any edema, there is necrosis and desquamation of the surface epithelium, acute hyperplasia of the lymphoid apparatus with necrosis in the centers of the follicles. Properly stained, the vibrios may be found in the mucus adherent to the surface, on the surface and in the intestinal crypts. The kidneys may show advanced cloudy swelling and even necrosis of the epithelium, and sometimes hyaline droplet formation in the tubular epithelial cells. The mesenteric lymph nodes are likely to be enlarged and soft, and microscopically show acute hyperplasia with necrosis.

The diagnosis depends upon identification of organisms in the stools. Blood cultures are rarely if ever positive. Nevertheless at autopsy, organisms can be recovered from intestine, spleen, mesenteric lymph nodes, biliary passages and pneumonic foci. The systemic manifestations are due in part to dehydration and in part to intoxication. In nonfatal cases, organisms persist in the stools for a few weeks. The carrier state sometimes occurs, presumably because of infection of the gallbladder. Immunity develops and can be induced by vaccination.

Infectious Granulomata

Tuberculosis. Tuberculosis is the most frequent of the infectious granulomata in the intestinal canal. It may be primary or secondary. Primary infection by way of the intestine is infrequent in the United States and is usually attributable to milk from tuberculous cows. Thus, the organism is commonly the bovine form. The lesions in the intestine are like those of secondary tuberculosis, but may be more localized; the mesenteric lymph nodes are often extensively involved. (See Reichle.)

Secondary tuberculosis of the intestine is found in about 70 per cent of fatal cases of tuberculosis. It is usually secondary to chronic pulmonary tuberculosis but also occurs in disseminated miliary tuberculosis. It is more frequent and more extensive in females and negroes than in males and whites. It may be due to swallowing of infected sputum or to dissemination by blood and lymphatics. The lesions are found principally in Peyer's patches and solitary lymphoid follicles, especially in the lower ileum. The disease may extend higher in the ileum and rarely into jejunum or even duodenum; extension into the cecum and colon is not infrequent.

The earliest change is the development of miliary or conglomerate tubercles in the follicles of the solitary nodes and of Peyer's patches. Following enlargement and fusion, caseation occurs with subsequent ulceration of the surface. By the time ulceration occurs, there is usually a chronic catarrhal inflammation of the neighboring parts of the intestine. The ulcers tend to enlarge laterally because of the fact that the tuberculous process follows the intestinal lymphatics. It is not common for secondary infection to occur, but in some instances fusion of neighboring ulcers may produce an extensive area of ulceration extending for 20 cm. or more along the intestine, and in such cases an acute pseudomembranous inflammation or even gangrene may be observed over the surface of the ulcer.

Microscopically, the ulcer in the earlier stages is surrounded simply by a caseous mass with the usual marginal arrangement of epithelioid and lymphoid cells. Outside this zone there is likely to be a subacute inflammatory reaction with infiltration of lymphoid, plasma and large mononuclear cells. In the neighborhood of the ulcer, more particularly in the submucosa and under the peritoneum, but sometimes also in the muscularis, miliary tubercles with small foci of central necrosis and with or without giant cells are often found. When secondary infection becomes marked, the acute inflammatory reaction may entirely obliterate the characteristic features of tuberculosis. Tubercle bacilli are usually demonstrable microscopically unless the secondary infection is severe.

Characteristically, the ulcers are elliptical and so situated that their long axis is transverse to the long axis of the gut, but sometimes, more especially in the early lesions, they are circular or may even be coextensive with Peyer's patches. The ulcer has an irregular margin and thick, elevated, undermined edges in which small tubercles may be found. The base is often cheesy, with small nodules representing tubercles, but when secondarily infected it may be stained brown by blood or show a moderate degree of suppuration. The most important diagnostic feature is the demonstration of tubercles in the peritoneal surface immediately underlying the ulcer. Often the tubercles occur in bead-like chains in the neighboring lymphatics. Depending in part upon the rapidity of the tuberculous process and in part upon the beginning of secondary infection, the peritoneum may show a deposit of fibrin, which in later stages may become organized and produce fibrous adhesions.

Under favorable conditions the ulcer may heal by cicatrization and epithelialization. If the original ulcer were fairly extensive, cicatricial contraction may occur with the production of stenosis of the gut. Perforation of the intestine may occur, but the slow course usually leads to a preceding fibrous adhesion so that only local peritonitis or abscess formation results. Small hemorrhages, sufficient to be demonstrable microscopically in the stools or even to stain the stools grossly, are not infrequent, but large fatal hemorrhages are distinctly unusual. Extension and perforation of ulcers near the anus in the lower part of the rectum produce perirectal "cold abscesses" which may rupture through the perineum and produce fistulae. The extension of the tuberculous process into the peritoneum may produce a widespread acute or chronic tuberculous peritonitis. In various parts of the intestinal tract, from duodenum to rectum, more especially in colon and rectum, tuberculous granulation tissue may produce large, dense, obstructive masses, which both clinically and upon gross examination may be confused with carcinoma. (See Stewart.)

Syphilis. Syphilis of the intestines may be either congenital or acquired. The congenital lesions are usually in association with lesions of the other viscera such as lung, liver, etc. The most definite lesions in the intestine, namely, small, flat, single or multiple gumma-like processes, occur in the ileum although they may be found elsewhere. These may undergo ulceration as is true of the acquired lesions. In even more rare instances miliary gummata may be found in the gut (see D'Aunoy and Pearson). Lesions of the intestinal tract in acquired syphilis occur as gummata late in the disease. They affect particularly the rectum, the sigmoid and other flexures as well as other parts of the colon, but are rarely observed in the small intestine. The primary condition is apparently single or, more rarely, multiple gumma formation of the mucosa or submucosa, producing an elevated nodular tumor-like growth. The gumma breaks down to form an ulcer, chronic in type, and often extending transversely in the intestine. The microscopic picture of gumma, together with perivascular infiltrations of lymphoid and plasma cells, chronic obliterative arteritis and phlebitis, is often obscured by the acute inflammation of secondary infection. Perforation is rare and the

resultant peritonitis localized by the preexistent fibrous adhesions. Cicatricial contraction may lead to stenosis of the gut.

Lymphogranuloma Venereum. Stricture of the rectum, situated a few centimeters above the anus, is more frequently due to this disease than any other. Tuberculosis, syphilis and amebiasis are only rare causes of fibrous stricture in this situation and the same is true of carcinoma. Occasional cases of more diffuse fibrous thickening of the colon may perhaps be due to extension of lymphogranuloma venereum. (See Martin.)

Actinomycosis most often affects the colon, in or near the cecum. There is found a more or less extensive deep ulcer with the small yellow actinomyces granules in the pus. Chronic adhesions of the neighborhood are common and the process extends through these to form fistulae with neighboring coils of intestine, or other viscera, may produce acute diffuse peritonitis, may invade the liver and other solid organs, or may penetrate through the diaphragm into the pleura and lung.

Lesions of the Lymph Nodes

The lymph nodes, including both solitary follicles and Peyer's patches, may be involved as part of the general enlargement of the lymph nodes of the body incident to such diseases as lymphoid leukemia or its aleukemic form, and lymphosarcoma. Hodgkin's disease may similarly affect the intestines.

Ulcers

These include ulcers due to various inflammatory diseases mentioned above, scybalous or stercoral ulcers and ulcers due to tumors benign and malignant. The peptic ulcer, described above as it affects the stomach, also occurs in the duodenum.

DUODENAL ULCERS of this type are usually solitary but may be multiple. They are found as a rule in the first part of the duodenum upon the posterior wall. The ulcer is generally round, slightly terraced and of essentially the same general and microscopic character as that of the stomach. Clinically, it seems to be more common than ulcer of the stomach but postmortem statistics usually show it to be less so. Its cause is not known but perhaps the action of gastric juice has some important influence. It has a distinct tendency to heal and the scar may produce slight deformity; occasionally small diverticula occur. Ulceration of the intestine may occur in from about 2 to 4 per cent of cases of severe burns, but the mechanism of ulceration is not known. These "Curling's ulcers" occur more often in duodenum than stomach, and may be single or multiple. As with other duodenal ulcers, hemorrhage is common and may be fatal; perforation also occurs. (See Harkins.) Peptic ulcers of the jejunum are rare except as a sequel of gastro-jejunostomy. There is doubt as to whether the gastric juice causes this lesion, or whether it is due to trauma at the time of operation, or to other cause.

Tumors

Congenital tumors are unusual. Dermoid cysts occur especially in the small intestine, and we have observed one case of hemangio-endothelioma of the small intestine, probably of congenital origin.

Benign tumors are not uncommon, especially lipoma and adenoma. Such tumors originate in the mucosa or submucosa and, projecting into the lumen of the gut, may be exposed to the peristaltic action so as to become pedunculated, the pedicles sometimes being extremely long.

LIPOMA is particularly common in the colon but may be observed in other situations. It apparently arises in the submucosa and projects first as a lobulated nodule which subsequently becomes polypoid. Solitary tumors of this sort occur in the peritoneal coat, more especially in obese individuals. This must not be confused with the fat increase in the epiploic appendages which sometimes may be almost tumor-like in character.

ADENOMA of the intestine is much more common in the colon than in the small intestine. The glands proliferate to form first a sessile, slightly projecting mass which increases in size and becomes pedunculated. The movement of intestinal contents or peristaltic action may lead to considerable elongation of the pedicle. Sometimes adenomas seem to be traced to previous inflammation, but for the most part they are true neoplasms.

MULTIPLE POLYPOSIS is usually confined to the large intestine. The number varies from a few to a hundred or more. The polyps are adenomatous. This disease may be observed at any time of life and occurs about equally in males and females. As was noted in the chapter on Tumors, it is a hereditary condition. Malignant change may be found in one or several of the adenomas, and adenomatous polyps are often the forerunners of carcinoma. (See McKenney.)

FIBROMA may occur as a polypoid tumor in the lumen, especially in the rectum.

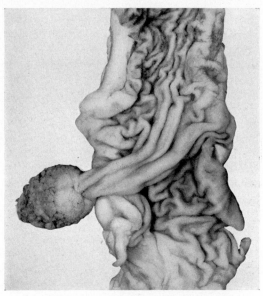

Pedunculated adenomatous polyp of colon.

This and other polypoid tumors of the rectum may project through the anus. Fibroma, myoma, fibromyoma and adenomyoma grow in the wall of the intestine and may project outward or inward. Neurofibromas may be single or, in cases of neurofibromatosis, multiple.

The hemangioma and lymphangioma are rare, and probably congenital. They grow as flat, bulky masses, infiltrating the wall and obstructing by their bulk rather than by polypoid growth into the lumen. Bleeding is a frequent result of benign tumors, whether they be intramural or polypoid. Obstruction may be due to bulk of the tumor, or, especially in the small intestine, a nodule may be drawn down by peristalsis so as to produce intussusception.

Many carcinomas of the large intestine originate in adenomatous polyps. Swinton and Warren found this to be true of

14 per cent of their 827 cases, but admit that the actual figure is probably distinctly higher. Squamous-cell carcinoma occurs in the anus and neighboring rectum; metastasis is usually first to the inguinal lymph nodes.

The symptoms include constipation or intermittent diarrhea, bleeding, and partial or complete obstruction. Disturbances of hepatic function occur, and may be responsi-

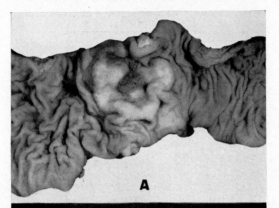

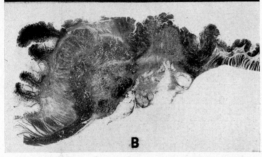

A. Polypoid ulcerative carcinoma of sigmoid flexure of colon. B. Low power photomicrograph of ulcerating-infiltrating carcinoma of sigmoid flexure. Note hypertrophy of muscle at left (proximal portion), ulceration in middle and massive tumor below replacing muscle and extending to mesocolic attachment.

ble for delayed healing of wounds, refractory character of anemia, hemolytic reactions to transfusion, reduction of plasma proteins and of prothrombin (see Abels, et al.).

CARCINOID. Sometimes called argentaffin tumor, this is usually a nodule originating in the submucosa. It often projects into the lumen as a rounded smooth nodule, a few millimeters or a centimeter or more in diameter, sessile and firm. Microscopically, there are nests of small polyhedral cells, sometimes producing small acini; silver stains show many of the cells to be argentophilic. The Kulschitsky argentophile cells, from which the lesion is probably derived, are situated in all parts of the gastro-intestinal tract, but carcinoids are about twice as frequent in the appendix and the distal ileum as elsewhere; only a few have been reported in the duodenum, and still fewer in duodenum, stomach and Meckel's diverticulum. Malignancy, with metastasis usually limited to the regional lymph nodes, is infrequent and in our experience rare. It accompanies tumors of the ileum rather than those of the appendix. (See Ariel; Porter and Whelan.)

Malignant Tumors. Of these, carcinoma is the most common. The small intestine is involved in about 2.5 per cent of all intestinal carcinomas, and of these nearly half are in the duodenum (Eger). Since carcinomas of the duodenum are most frequent in the second portion and ulcers in the first portion, and since there is a wide disproportion in incidence of the two, it is unlikely that duodenal ulcer has any practical bearing on duodenal carcinoma. The carcinomas in the duodenum are usually adenocarcinomas, whereas in the jejunum and ileum they are likely to be undifferentiated. Metastasis is local and late.

CARCINOMA OF THE LARGE INTESTINE occurs more often in males than females. The incidence is highest in the sixth decade, but a little earlier for women than men. More than half are situated in the rectum. Of those in the other parts of the large intestine, about one-third are in the sigmoid, about one-third in the proximal colon up to and including the hepatic flexure, and the other third in the transverse colon, splenic flexure and descending colon. Karsner and Clark distinguish grossly (1) projecting or polypoid, (2) infiltrating or ulcerative, and (3) stenosing forms. Microscopically, the picture varies from well-differentiated adenocarcinoma to undifferentiated carcinoma simplex. Mucin production is observed, and in from 5 to 10 per cent of the cases the tumor is a mucinous adenocarcinoma. Stenosis may be due to scirrhous cancer, to cicatricial constriction and to bulk of the tumor. Ulceration is frequent and may lead to lymph-node hyperplasia which resembles metastasis grossly. Direct extension to surrounding structures occurs more especially with the rectal carcinomas. The peritoneum may be directly involved and become the seat of widespread

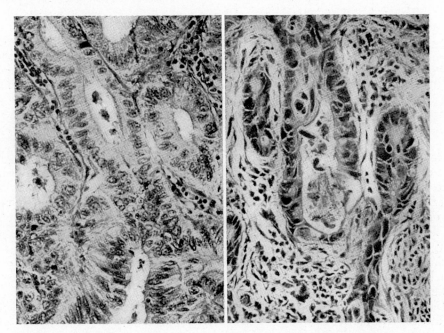

Malignant adenoma of colon. Carcinoma grade I.

Adenocarcinoma of colon. Carcinoma grade II.

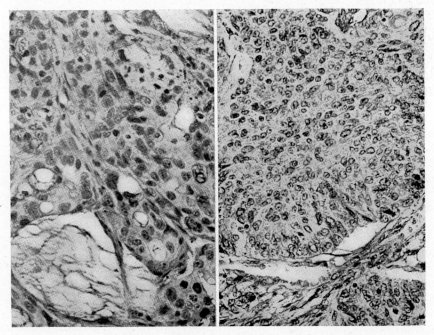

Adenocarcinoma of colon. Carcinoma grade III. Also shows mucin production.

Carcinoma simplex of colon. Carcinoma grade IV.

tumor. Metastasis to regional lymph nodes is common. Usually metastasis to viscera is confined to organs below the diaphragm, especially liver, but not infrequently is found in lungs and other organs. Probably because of lymphatic drainage, carcinomas of the rectum and sigmoid are more likely to metastasize than those of the upper colon.

SARCOMA of the intestines may be of various types, but most common is the lymphosarcoma. This may or may not arise primarily in the gut. The ileum is the usual site; the colon may be involved but the duodenum only rarely. The multiple, spherical, soft, reddish-gray nodules, several millimeters or more in diameter, involve submucosa first and then project into the lumen. Microscopically, they show the usual features of lymphosarcoma. Involvement of the intestines in leukemia may be almost identical. The nodules may ulcerate and suppurate; When they cause obstruction it is usually due to intussusception. Other forms of sarcoma are rare, occur more often in males than females, are usually nodular, may occasionally circumscribe the gut sometimes with narrowing of the lumen, but are only rarely polypoid. We have observed a case of spindle-cell sarcoma primary in a Meckel diverticulum.

MELANOMA occurs at or near the anus, but has been reported as a rare occurrence in small intestine. In the lower rectum it probably arises in embryonally misplaced skin. It may be highly malignant.

SECONDARY CARCINOMA of the intestine may be solitary but is more usually multiple. It may be a retrograde involvement through the lymphatics as the result of metastases in lymph nodes; it may be an implantation in the abdominal cavity, or may be secondary in close proximity to a primary carcinoma of the gut itself. Melanotic tumors, whether they be of the skin or of the choroid, more especially the former, are likely to show metastases in the intestinal canal. The wide dissemination of the various forms of sarcoma includes involvement of the intestines.

Parasites

A wide variety of animal parasites may infest the intestine. These are discussed in the text books of protozoology. The tape worms do not produce significant pathologic alterations of the intestine, but as has been

indicated, the *Diphyllobothrium latum* may lead to profound anemia. Of the round worms, the larva of *Trichinella spiralis* may be found in intestinal muscle. *Ascaris lumbricoides* may apparently cause ulcers of the lower gut, may constitute the nidus of intestinal concrements, or may accumulate in balls to obstruct the lumen. *Oxyuris vermicularis* and *Tricocephalus dispar* are of little importance pathologically. *Ankylostoma duodenale* and *Necator americanus* attach themselves to the mucosa of jejunum and upper ileum, and by their injury produce multiple small hemorrhages. The secondary anemia, as the result of the hemorrhages and possibly also of products of the worms, may be prolonged and severe and is usually accompanied by eosinophilia.

The flat worms may gain entrance to the body through the alimentary tract but do not lead to disease there. *Distomum hematobium* probably gains entrance through the skin. The worms may gain access to the veins of the rectum from those of the pelvis.

The most important pathogenic rhizopod is the *Endamoeba histolytica*, the cause of amebic dysentery. The flagellates, such as *Lamblia intestinalis*, *Trichomonas intestinalis* and subgroups, *Tetramitus mesnili*, are found in the stools of patients with and without diarrhea, but their pathogenicity is not established. The same is true of *Blastocystis hominis*. On the other hand, it is now found that *Balantidium coli* may invade the mucosa of the intestine, principally the colon, and produce chronic inflammation and ulceration (see Hegner; Young).

Foreign Bodies

Swallowed foreign bodies of all characters may enter the intestine. Shellac, and various minerals administered as drugs, may form intestinal concrements. Parasites, gallstones, hair and other swallowed foreign bodies, may be the nidus for calcified, sometimes laminated, hard or friable enteroliths. Masses of feces may by inspissation, sometimes associated with calcareous deposit, form concrements. All these are of importance as possible causes of obstruction, ulceration or perforation. Ordinary inspissated fecal masses called scybala, stagnant in cecum, flexures or diverticula of the colon, may produce chronic ulcers with more or less extensive non-specific granulation tissue, the so-called scybalous or stercoral ulcers.

Appendix

Although in consideration of the intestinal canal there has been no sharp division of diseases of the different segments, the great clinical significance of the diseases of the appendix, more especially of inflammatory nature, justifies a brief separate discussion.

Acute Appendicitis. The milder manifestations of acute appendicitis affect principally the mucous membranes, and the more severe forms extend through the width of the wall of the appendix. Secondary inflammation may be due to extension of inflammation from the cecum as in typhoid fever, tuberculosis and dysentery. Inflammation may also extend from the female internal genitalia, particularly the fallopian tubes, to the appendix. Infection may also be carried by the blood stream as in cases of septicemia and pyemia. Although we speak of primary inflammations of the appendix, it is not clearly established that they do not originate in the cecum and thus invade the appendix, but, since the manifestations are so strikingly within the appendix and are cured by removal of that organ, this conception is practically acceptable.

FOREIGN BODIES are frequent in the appendix, including fecal concrements and

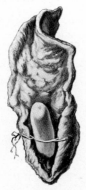

F e c a l concrement in appendix.

fecaliths, vegetable seeds, metallic objects and parasites, especially *Oxyuris vermicularis*. The presence of foreign bodies has led to the thought that obstruction to the lumen of the appendix may cause inflammation. This view has been championed by Wangensteen and his associates (see Dennis, et al.) but the observations of Bowers show that no obstruction is demonstrable in 80 per cent of cases of appendicitis. If obstruction incites the disease, it does so infrequently, although it may play a part in determining perforation. Ashburn reports the presence of oxyurids in 7.9 per cent of surgically removed appendices, but concludes that they do not cause inflammation. As with other parts of the intestinal tract, the identification of pathogenic organisms is somewhat difficult. The vast majority of cases shows the presence of colon bacillus (Warren). A moderate number shows the presence of streptococci of various types and a small number shows the presence of a wide variety of other organisms. Admitting the possible fallibility of bacteriologic methods in these circumstances, nevertheless, it seems apparent that from the bacteriologic point of view, appendicitis is not a specific disease.

IN ACUTE CATARRHAL APPENDICITIS, although the symptoms may be severe clinically, the appendix is likely to show relatively little gross morbid anatomic change other than slight swelling, moderate hyperemia, and thickening of the mucosa with accumulation of mucus upon its surface. Microscopically, there is found cloudy swelling of the appendical epithelium, marked accumulation of mucus, infiltration of lymphoid cells and polymorphonuclear leukocytes into the tunica propria and between the gland cells. Sometimes ulceration is present. In the submucosa the lymphoid tissue generally shows a slight infiltration of polymorphonuclear leukocytes. Except for the possibility of edema, the other coats are likely to show little change. As with catarrhal inflammation elsewhere, the mucous exudate may become purulent in character and may, either with or without ulceration, pass over into the diffuse form.

ACUTE DIFFUSE APPENDICITIS is definitely exudative in character and is disposed to become suppurative in type. Grossly, the appendix is usually swollen, markedly hyperemic and soft. The lumen may be filled with mucopurulent or purulent material. Ulceration is distinctly more common than in the catarrhal form. The peritoneal surface may be covered with a thin film of fibrinous or fibrinopurulent exudate. Microscopically, the milder cases show, in addition to those features described in catarrhal appendicitis, considerable edema and exudation of polymorphonuclear leukocytes. The leukocytes

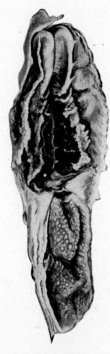

Appendix showing at one end acute catarrhal appendicitis with follicular hyperplasia, and at other end acute diffuse appendicitis with ulceration.

may accumulate in masses to constitute small pockets of pus. The associated necrosis of tissue may lead to perforation of the appendix. When suppuration is pronounced the condition is often called acute suppurative appendicitis.

ACUTE GANGRENOUS APPENDICITIS may be due to invasion of saprophytic organisms through ulceration in some other form of appendicitis, or may be accounted for by vascular occlusion resulting from thrombosis infective in character, or from malposition of the organ. Grossly, the appendix is swollen, hyperemic, covered with fibrinous or fibrinopurulent exudate and shows brown or green discoloration in the foci of gangrene. These may be focalized near the tip, or in any other

part of the organ, or may be diffuse. Microscopically, the picture is much the same as in acute diffuse or suppurative appendicitis with foci of gangrenous necrosis.

THE COMPLICATIONS of acute appendicitis depend in certain measure upon the severity of the disease. With only moderate peritoneal involvement, as in the catarrhal and milder diffuse disease, the process may heal and the fibrinous peritonitis lead to more or less dense fibrous adhesions. Adhesions sufficiently extensive may produce partial or complete intestinal obstruction. If perfora-

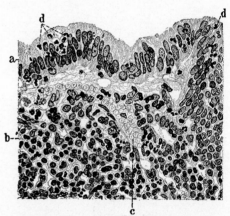

Acute catarrhal appendicitis. The section shows a small portion of the surface epithelium (a) with part of a gland on the right-hand side, and the membrana propria (b) containing a dilated capillary (c). The epithelium and membrana propria are moderately infiltrated with polymorphonuclear leukocytes (d). From Kelly and Hurdon, The Vermiform Appendix and Its Diseases.

tion occur after fibrinous or fibrous adhesions bind the organ to neighboring structures, there may be an inflammation limited to the region. If, however, these adhesions be broken through or have not been established, perforation produces an acute diffuse peritonitis. Infective thrombosis of the appendical veins may extend to the portal vein and ascend to the liver, ultimately producing multiple abscesses. Occasional cases of septicemia or pyemia occur without extensive thrombosis. The drainage of the peritoneum toward the diaphragm probably accounts for the occurrence of subdiaphragmatic abscess and its sequels.

Chronic Appendicitis. Chronic catarrhal appendicitis differs from the acute form in that there is relatively less swelling or hyperemia. Microscopically, fibrosis may be present in the tunica propria and submucosa, and in these areas local histo-eosinophilia is likely to be more pronounced than in the acute form. Mucinous degeneration is prominent. There is much discussion as to

consistency. The lumen may be narrowed or completely obliterated. Microscopically, fibrosis is found in all the coats, sometimes associated with atrophy of the muscularis. Between muscularis and submucosa there is often a considerable accumulation of fat. Associated with the fibrosis of submucosa,

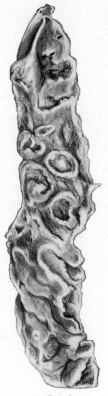

Involvement of appendix in typhoid fever showing typhoid ulcers.

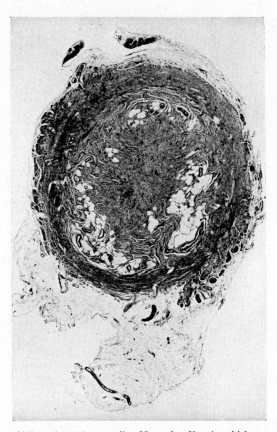

Obliteration of appendix. Note the fibrosis which replaces mucosa, and fibrosis and fat in submucosa.

whether or not chronic interstitial appendicitis exists, that is as a chronic progressive inflammation. Fibrosis may represent the cicatrization of a previous acute appendicitis (see Hellwig). The continuance of slight symptoms may be due to cicatricial involvement of sympathic nerves rather than to progressive inflammation (see Rohdenburg).

Involutionary changes of the appendix occur in advanced life, but exactly comparable changes may be seen in early life. Sometimes this is called chronic obliterative appendicitis, but there are no microscopic features of inflammation. The appendix is likely to be reduced in diameter and of firm

there is usually atrophy or partial disappearance of glands and of the lining epithelium. The lymphoid follicles and lymphoid tissue generally, are usually atrophic. The lumen is partially obliterated. The condition may progress so that the mucosa disappears and the lumen is completely obliterated. There is found a central mass of connective tissue surrounded by fat and then by fibrotic muscularis with or without atrophy.

Infectious Granulomata. Tubercles may be found in the peritoneum of the appendix as a part of widespread tuberculous peritonitis. Tuberculous involvement of the mucosa with ulceration is usually an extension from the same process in the intestine. Actinomycosis occurs in the appendix and suggests the possibility that the organisms may have been carried upon grains which lodge in the appendix.

Tumors of Appendix. The carcinoid, described among tumors of the intestine, is fairly common in the appendix. True carcinoma is rare. Microscopically the latter shows greater invasiveness, reaction in the margins, often acinus formation and is much more likely to exhibit mitotic figures. The cells may be definitely cylindrical in shape

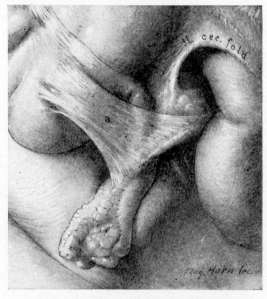

Peritoneal adhesions about a previously inflamed appendix. From Kelly and Hurdon, The Vermiform Appendix.

as compared with the cuboidal or polygonal cells of the carcinoid. Benign tumors are also rare. Malignant tumors elsewhere may metastasize to the appendix but the usual involvement is by direct extension, as for example from the cecum.

Foreign Bodies. Various foreign bodies which may be swallowed may ultimately lodge in the appendix. It is probable that many foreign bodies considered to be vegetable seeds, are merely concentrically laminated fecal concrements. The stagnant current of material in the appendix predisposes to the formation of small scybalous masses of feces which remain in situ. Except

for *Oxyuris vermicularis*, intestinal parasites are not likely to occur in the appendix.

Epiploic Appendages

In obese subjects, the epiploic appendages may attain considerable size and may be mistaken for lipomas. There are infrequent instances of torsion and infarction with symptoms of acute abdominal inflammation which may resemble those of acute appendicitis; rarely this is followed by abscess formation and diffuse peritonitis (see Pines, et al.). It is also possible that this may occur without symptoms and the appendices may become detached as free fibrous bodies.

PERITONEUM

Congenital Deformities

Congenital deformities are of little significance in the peritoneum, except where the folds which normally appear are accentuated or improperly formed so as to constitute fairly large bands in the peritoneal cavity. These are sometimes referred to as congenital adhesions but are simply faults of development. Their particular significance is that they may lead to intestinal obstruction.

Circulatory Disturbances

Active hyperemia occurs in the early stages of acute peritonitis and may accompany inflammation of organs within the peritoneum. It is also likely to occur when there is sudden removal of pressure from within the peritoneum by withdrawal of large quantities of fluid.

Passive hyperemia occurs as the result of chronic diseases of liver, lungs and heart, and as the result of the obstruction of outflow from the veins by thrombosis or from compression. Such passive hyperemia occasionally leads to hemorrhage, but its greatest importance is that it disturbs the drainage from the peritoneal cavity and results in accumulation of fluid, or ascites.

Laennec cirrhosis of the liver produces passive hyperemia in the portal circulation. The formation of peritoneal fluid is not seriously interfered with but its drainage is obstructed so that it may accumulate in extremely large quantities. Passive hyperemia as the result of heart disease is an important cause of ascites, but as a rule does not lead to such large accumulation of fluid as is true of Laennec cirrhosis of the liver. Chronic fibrosis of the lung and emphysema may also produce ascites. Compression of the portal veins or of the inferior vena cava by tumor masses, large lymph nodes and fibrous adhesions as well as thrombosis within the vessels, either the result of infectious thrombosis or of tumor thrombosis, may also produce ascites. These conditions are discussed in the chapter on Liver and Pancreas.

Ascites must be regarded as an edema of the peritoneal cavity. The fluid is therefore thin, watery, pale yellow, of low specific gravity ranging between 1004 and 1015, with a low content of protein which rarely exceeds 3 per cent. Microscopically, there are found a few cells, usually of endothelial character, showing cloudy swelling or fatty degeneration, and a few leukocytes similarly degenerated. Ascites may also be observed under conditions where the edema may be more or less general, such as in chronic Bright's disease and nutritional edema. The serous exudate of tuberculous peritonitis and of involvement of the peritoneum by malignant tumors may closely resemble ascites. It is often difficult to distinguish an exudate of this sort and a true transudate such as characterizes ascites. Chronic fibrous peritonitis may produce ascites either generalized, or as localized saccules within the adhesions. Chylous ascites is usually the result of obstruction to the thoracic duct such as occurs from malignant tumor invasion, tuberculosis and other diseases. Chronic peritonitis may also so obstruct the drainage from the lymphatics of the intestines as to lead to chylous ascites. The fluid of ascites may sometimes be slightly milky because of degeneration of the cells which it contains, so-called chyliform ascites. Ascites leads to discomfort because of the pressure of fluid and because of the limitation of expansion of the thorax. If long continued it may lead to a chronic fibrous peritonitis.

Hemorrhage of the peritoneum may be due to direct trauma, such as by stab wounds and surgical operations, or may be due to indirect trauma, such as injury to the abdomen with rupture of the internal viscera or vessels. Hemoperitoneum is not uncommonly caused by hemorrhage from the genital canal, particularly in females where it may be due to rupture of graafian follicles, corpus luteum, or hemorrhage from extra-uterine pregnancy. Hemorrhage may also be due to infarction, particularly of the intestine, rupture of aneurysms in the abdominal cavity, chronic passive hyperemia, tuberculosis of the peritoneum, hemorrhagic diseases, tumors of neighboring viscera and of the peritoneum.

Peritonitis

Both acute and chronic forms may either be local or diffuse. The localization of acute forms may be due to origin within a viscus, as the appendix, or to the presence of pre-existing limiting adhesions. Acute peritonitis may be due to chemical irritation such as the presence of bile, the fluid of ruptured cysts, prolonged ascites, and in the days of antiseptic surgery, was sometimes due to chemicals employed for antisepsis. This as a rule is an acute fibrinoserous peritonitis, but may become suppurative. Bacterial causes include streptococcus, staphylococcus, colon bacillus, pneumococcus, anaerobes, and particularly in local form around the female genitalia, the gonococcus. As the result of perforation of the gut, saprophytes may gain entrance and produce a gangrenous type of peritonitis.

The acute inflammations of the peritoneum may arise as the result of extension by contiguity from inflammation within the intestines, within the uterus, particularly in puerperal sepsis, within the gallbladder, the urinary bladder, the pleura and other neighboring locations. In some instances the bacteria may precede or follow the extension of the inflammatory process. Extension of inflammation by continuity is best exemplified in extension of inflammation from the fallopian tubes. Thus, gonococcal inflammation may extend directly through the fimbriated end into the peritoneum, but as a rule, leads only to a local peritonitis. If the primary tubal inflammation be streptococcal in type, a diffuse peritonitis may occur. Of great importance are those forms of peritonitis due to perforation of viscera within or neighboring upon the peritoneum. The pneumococcal peritonitis of nephrosis in childhood and streptococcal peritonitis without local cause, ap-

Phrenic peritonitis see Stanley Arch Int M 78:1 '46

pear to be derived from throat infections, but whether the peritoneal involvement is due to hematogenous transfer or to swallowing and extension through the intestinal wall is not established. The acute inflammations of the peritoneum do not differ essentially from those of other serous membranes and may therefore be acute fibrinous, acute fibrino-purulent, acute suppurative, acute hemor-rhagic and acute gangrenous.

Adhesions. Adhesions are due to the organization of acute exudate upon neighbor-ing surfaces of the peritoneum. Even with the most careful aseptic technic in surgery, the interruption of surface continuity results in a slight degree of fibrinous exudation, and as a consequence more or less extensive ad-hesions are almost constant following surgical operation in the peritoneum. Of course, the smaller the amount of trauma, the less exten-sive the adhesions. Inflammations of appen-dix and gallbladder, inflammatory and ulcera-tive processes of stomach and intestines may show peritoneal involvement and lead to sub-sequent adhesions. Extensive adhesions in the pelvic peritoneum are extremely common as the result of gonorrhea in the female. Unless the causative inflammation be more or less continuous, as may be true of gonorrhea, the adhesion is simply a cicatrizing process and has a subsequent history similar to that of scars anywhere. The primary event is con-traction of the scar so that viscera may be tightly bound together. In some instances the movement of the abdominal viscera may pro-duce traction upon the scar and elongate it to form a fibrous band. As with congenital de-formities of the peritoneum these adhesions of inflammatory origin may alter the position of viscera, and more especially where they are elongated to form bands or cords, may lead to strangulation of sections of intestine or produce obstruction by torsion.

Chronic peritonitis, in order to be so classified, must be a progressive chronic inflammation. Occasionally, a fairly wide-spread organizing fibrinous or chronic fibrous peritonitis may be observed, particularly as the result of chronic passive hyperemia and long standing ascites. Occasionally, a chronic peritonitis may in itself so dam back lym-phatic outflow as to produce ascites. The involvement of the peritoneum in the pro-gressive fibrosing inflammations of serous membranes, called multiple serositis, is usu-ally restricted to the subdiaphragmatic and upper part of the peritoneum. Chronic peri-tonitis may also appear in local forms upon the surfaces of organs, more particularly the spleen and the liver. There is a progressive deposit of fibrous connective tissue with thickening and stiffening of the capsule of the organ, and subsequent hyalinization to constitute the "zuckerguss" splenic or hepatic capsulitis.

Infectious Granulomata

Tuberculosis of the peritoneum is most commonly the result of direct extension such as from tuberculous enteritis and mesenteric lymphadenitis. It may also extend from the

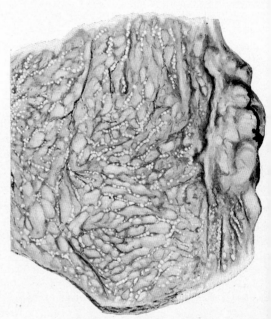

Miliary tuberculosis of omentum.

pleura, the female internal genitalia, bones, adrenals, kidneys and other viscera. Although it may occur as a part of a disseminated mili-ary tuberculosis, it is not likely in this form to lead to such extensive lesions as when due to direct extension. Laennec cirrhosis of the liver with its consequent disturbance of peri-toneal circulation, apparently serves some-times as a predisposing cause for peritoneal tuberculosis. In the acute form, miliary tu-bercles are found widely distributed over the surface of the peritoneum, in some cases as-sociated with a mild acute fibrinous peritonitis, and even with an acute fibrinoserous peritonitis.

In the more chronic forms the tubercles are larger and often fibrotic. Even in man, although the process is more characteristic in cattle, the tubercles may enlarge and show progressive fibrosis so as to constitute fairly large pearl-like masses, either sessile or pedunculated, constituting the so-called "perlsucht" disease. In the chronic forms of peritoneal tuberculosis, the fibrosis is not limited entirely to the tubercles and extensive adhesions are likely to be produced, sometimes to such an extent that it is difficult to separate one coil of gut from another. These adhesions may be the result of an early acute fibrinous process or apparently may be entirely chronic in nature. Either with or without these adhesions, fluid may accumulate in large quantities. This varies in character from a fluid of low specific gravity with the characters of transudate, to that of higher specific gravity more nearly resembling serous exudate. It would appear that fluid accumulation may be due to faults in lymphatic drainage resulting from the tuberculosis, or may be due to the subacute or chronic inflammation with serous exudation. Hemorrhage into the fluid is not uncommon.

Tumors

After a tumor of the peritoneum has developed, it is often difficult to say whether it originated in the mesothelium, in the peritoneal connective tissue or in the underlying tissues. It is therefore advisable to discuss the tumors that affect the peritoneum without further reference to the exact site of origin.

Benign tumors include lipoma, fibroma, myxoma, leiomyoma usually originating in the omentum, neurofibroma, ganglioneuroma, angioma both of lymphatic and blood vascular type, sometimes combined with endothelial proliferation to constitute angio-endothelioma. Various types of sarcoma are observed and there is also found a tumor called the endothelioma or mesothelioma, originating presumably from the mesothelium, growing as a more or less diffuse nodular mass and showing histologically sheets of cells of mesothelial or endothelial character. We have observed one such case in the omentum. It is always difficult, however, to distinguish between this type of tumor and an epithelial tumor which may have originated in misplaced epithelium. Cyst formation may occur in the lymphatics, more particularly in the mesentery, and sometimes contain chylous material. Dermoid cysts, echinococcus cysts, and cysts formed by encapsulation of foreign material such as blood, are sometimes observed, and in intestinal pneumatosis the gas cysts may be observed in peritoneum and mesentery. Tumors of cystic character may show the same character in peritoneal metastases.

Secondary carcinoma of the peritoneum is common, originating particularly from carcinoma of the various organs partially or completely covered by peritoneum. Metastasis may also occur from more remote situations such as the breast. The nodules may be multiple and minute, somewhat resembling tuberculosis, or may be larger and more diffuse. The irritation of the tumor sometimes produces a low grade of inflammation leading subsequently to more or less extensive adhesions. According to extent or situation, ascites may appear or there may be a serous type of exudation. In either case, the fluid is likely to be somewhat bloody. An important source of secondary carcinoma of the peritoneum is the papilliferous cystadenoma of the ovary. Either infiltrating the omentum, mesentery, or extending diffusely over the surface of the peritoneum, the papilliferous structure is more or less reduplicated and there is poured out either into cysts or free into the abdominal cavity a large quantity of gelatinous mucous material. This constitutes one of the forms of pseudomyxoma peritonei, but a closely similar condition grossly may be produced by secondary invasion of mucinous carcinomas from other points of origin. The rupture of cysts containing mucin or mucoid may determine the presence of considerable amounts of these substances within the peritoneum, usually leading to a variable degree of chronic fibrous peritonitis.

Foreign Bodies

Foreign bodies include needles and similar metallic substances which may erode through the gut, and gallstones and other foreign bodies of the intestines entering the peritoneum because of perforation. Sometimes epiploic appendages become strangulated and detached and constitute foreign bodies. There are also found the so-called corpora libera, small firm pearly connective-tissue masses, probably made up of organized cicatrized fibrin and resembling similar foreign bodies found in the joint cavities.

The encapsulation of small foreign particles, such as pieces of surgical sponges, small vegetable or other granules which may penetrate through ulcers or gain access to the deep lymphatics of the gut, may produce nodules, usually localized, which resemble tubercles grossly and show foreign body giant cells microscopically, the so-called foreign body tubercles or pseudotubercles.

REFERENCES

Abels, J. C., P. E. Rekers, G. E. Binkley, G. T. Pack, and C. P. Rhoads: Metabolic Studies in Patients with Cancer of the Gastrointestinal Tract. II. Hepatic Dysfunction, Ann. Int. Med., 16: 221, 1942.

Ariel, I. M.: Argentaffin (Carcinoid) Tumors of the Small Intestine: Report of Eleven Cases and Review of the Literature, Arch. Path., 27: 25, 1939.

Aschoff, L.: Pathologische Anatomie, 5th ed., Jena, 1921.

——: The Relation of Mucosal Erosions to the Development of Ulcer of the Stomach, Lectures on Pathology, New York, 1924, p. 279.

——: Appendicitis, translated by G. C. Pether, London, 1932.

Ashburn, L. L.: Appendiceal Oxyuriasis. Its Incidence and Relationship to Appendicitis, Amer. Jour. Path., 17: 841, 1941.

Ashhurst, A. P. C.: Ludwig's Angina, Arch. Surg., 18: 2047, 1929.

Askanazy, M.: Ueber Bau und Entstehung des chronischen Magengeschwürs, sowie Soorpilzenbefunde in ihm, Virchow's Arch. Path. Anat., 234: 111, 1921; 250: 370, 1924.

Bell, J. R.: Gastric Ulcer and Achlorhydria, Arch. Int. Med., 32: 663, 1923.

Berry, L. H.: Chronic Alcoholic Gastritis. Evaluation of the Concept in One Hundred Cases, Jour. Amer. Med. Asso., 117: 2233, 1941.

Besser, E. L.: Cause of Death in Cases of Mechanical Intestinal Obstruction: Consideration of Certain Confused Issues and Review of Recent Literature, Arch. Surg., 41: 970, 1940.

Blessing, G.: Allgemeine Pathologie und pathologische Anatomie der Zähne und der Mundhöhle, Ergeb. Allg. Path. u. Path. Anat., 17¹: 859, 1914.

Boles, R. S., and H. E. Riggs: Neurogenic Factors in the Production of Acute Gastric Ulcer, Jour. Amer. Med. Asso., 115: 1771, 1940.

Bollman, J. L., L. K. Stalker, and F. C. Mann: Experimental Peptic Ulcer Produced by Cinchophen, Arch. Int. Med., 61: 119, 1938.

Bowers, W. F.: Appendicitis, with Especial Reference to Pathogenesis, Bacteriology and Healing, Arch. Surg., 39: 362, 1939.

Boyd, J. D., C. L. Drain, and M. V. Nelson: Dietary Control of Dental Caries, Amer. Jour. Dis. Child., 38: 721, 1929.

Broderick, F. W.: The Effect of Endocrine Derangement on the Teeth, Dental Cosmos, 63: 135, 1921.

Bunting, R. W., E. Delves, and D. G. Hard: Report of Recent Experiments in the Control of Dental Caries, Jour. Dent. Res., 10: 374, 1930.

Bunting, R. W., and F. Palmerlee: The Role of B. Acidophilus in Dental Caries, Proc. Soc. Exper. Biol. and Med., 22: 296, 1924-25.

Callender, G. R.: Dysentery, Arch. Path. and Lab. Med., 3: 665, 1927.

Carlson, A. J.: The Secretion of Gastric Juice in Health and Disease, Physiol. Rev., 3: 1, 1923.

——, T. E. Boyd, and J. F. Pearcy: The Reflex Control of the Cardia and Lower Esophagus in Mammals, Arch. Int. Med., 30: 409, 1922.

Chase, S. W.: A Critical Review of the Controversy Concerning Metabolism in the Enamel, Jour. Amer. Dent. Asso., 18: 697, 1931.

Chunn, C. F., and H. N. Harkins: Experimental Alimentary Azotemia: Comparative Effects of Red Cells and Plasma, Proc. Soc. Exper. Biol. and Med., 47: 7, 1941.

——, ——, and R. T. Boals: Alimentary Azotemia and the Bleeding Peptic Ulcer Syndrome, Arch. Surg., 43: 773, 1941.

Clagett, O. T., and W. Walters: Tuberculosis of the Stomach, Arch. Surg., 37: 505, 1938.

Clarke, J. K.: On the Bacterial Factor in the Aetiology of Dental Caries, Brit. Jour. Exper. Path., 5: 141, 1924.

Clerf, L. H.: Cicatricial Stenosis of the Esophagus Caused by Commercial Lye Preparations, Jour. Amer. Med. Asso., 80: 1600, 1923.

——: Tuberculous Periesophageal Abscess Producing Stenosis; Report of One Case, Ann. Otol. Rhin. and Laryng., 49: 793, 1940.

——: Diseases of the Esophagus. Esophagoscopic Considerations, Arch. Surg., 41: 1043, 1940.

Coller, F. A., E. B. Kay, and R. S. McIntyre: Regional Lymphatic Metastases of Carcinoma of the Stomach, Arch. Surg., 43: 748, 1941.

Cooke, H. H.: Carcinoid Tumors of the Small Intestine, Arch. Surg., 22: 568, 1931.

Crowley, R. T.: Reflex Changes in Respiration Induced by Distention of the Small Intestine, Arch. Surg., 44: 707, 1942.

Cushing, H.: Peptic Ulcers and the Interbrain, Surg., Gynec. and Obst., 55: 1, 1932.

Dameshek, W., and M. Ingall: Agranulocytosis (Malignant Neutropenia). Report of Nine Cases, Two with Recovery, Amer. Jour. Med. Sci, 181: 502, 1931.

D'Aunoy, R.: Mixed Tumors of the Palate, Amer. Jour. Path., 6: 137, 1930.

——, and B. Pearson: Intestinal Lesions in Congenital Syphilis: A Histologic Study, with a Report of Three Additional Cases, in all of Which Spirochetes Were Identified, Arch. Path., 27: 239, 1939.

——, and A. Zoeller: Sarcoma of the Stomach, Report of Four Cases and Review of the Literature, Amer. Jour. Surg., 9: 444, 1930.

Dennis, C., R. E. Buirge, R. L. Varco, and O. H. Wangensteen: Studies in the Etiology of Acute Appendicitis: An Inquiry into the Factors Involved in the Development of Acute Appendicitis Following Experimental Obstruction of the Appendical Lumen of the Rabbit, Arch. Surg., 40: 929, 1940.

Douglas, J.: Benign Tumors of the Stomach, Ann. Surg., 77: 580, 1923.

——: Sarcoma of the Stomach with Report of Three Cases, Ann. Surg., 71: 628, 1920.

Dragstedt, L. R.: Pathogenesis of Gastroduodenal Ulcer, Arch. Surg., 44: 438, 1942.

Draper, G.: Human Constitution, Philadelphia, 1924.

Eger, S. A.: Primary Malignant Disease of the Duodenum, Arch. Surg., 27: 1087, 1933.

Eusterman, G. B.: Gastric Syphilis: Observations Based on Ninety-three Cases, Jour. Amer. Med. Asso., 96: 173, 1931.

Ewing, J.: Neoplastic Diseases, 4th ed., Philadelphia and London, 1940.

Feldman, W. H.: Tuberculosis of the Tongue with a Case Report, Amer. Jour. Path., 3: 241, 1927.

Field, H., Jr., W. D. Robinson, and D. Melnick: Vitamins in Peptic Ulcer, Ann. Int. Med., 14: 588, 1940.

Fischer, W.: Speiseröhre, in F. Henke and O. Lubarsch: Handbuch der speziellen pathologischen Anatomie und Histologie, Berlin, 4¹: 74, 1926.

Fish, E. W.: The Circulation of Lymph in Dentin and Enamel, Jour. Amer. Dent. Asso., 14: 804, 1927.

Fisher, J. H.: Pyorrhea Alveolaris: The Role of Certain Microörganisms Found in the Lesions, Amer. Jour. Path., 3: 169, 1927.

Foster, W. C.: Acute Intestinal Obstruction. The Correlation of Recent Experimental Studies and Clinical Application, Jour. Amer. Med. Asso., 91: 1523, 1928.

Fox, H.: Leukoplakia Buccalis, Jour. Amer. Med. Asso., 85: 1523, 1925.

French, L. R., and L. H. Garland: Leiomyosarcoma of the Esophagus, Amer. Jour. Roentgenol., 45: 27, 1941.

Friedman, J. C., and W. W. Hamburger: Experimental Chronic Gastric Ulcer, Jour. Amer. Med. Asso., 63: 380, 1914.

Gatch, W. D., H. M. Trusler, and K. D. Ayres: Causes of Death in Acute Intestinal Obstruction, Surg., Gynec., and Obst., 46: 332, 1928.

Geschickter, C. F.: Tumors of the Jaws, Amer. Jour. Cancer, 24: 90, 1935.

Goldhamer, S. M.: Macrocytic Anemia in Cancer of the Stomach Apparently Due to Lack of Intrinsic Factor, Amer. Jour. Med. Sci., 195: 17, 1938.

Goldstein, H. I.: Primary Sarcoma of the Intestines. A Review of Recorded Cases, Amer. Jour. Surg., 35: 240, 1921.

Gordon, J. S., and J. J. Manning: An Autopsy Survey of Gastroduodenal Ulcers in the Philadelphia General Hospital 1920-1937, Amer. Jour. Med. Sci., 202: 423, 1941.

Hardt, L. L. J.: Studies of the Cause of Pain in Gastric and Duodenal Ulcers, Arch. Int. Med., 29: 684, 1922.

Harkins, H. N.: Acute Ulcer of the Duodenum (Curling's Ulcer) as a Complication of Burns; Relation to Sepsis, Surgery, 3: 608, 1938.

Hart, W. E.: Phytobezoars, Jour. Amer. Med. Asso., 81: 1870, 1923.

Haymaker, W., and E. Anderson: Functions and Clinical Syndromes of the Hypothalamus, Internatl. Clin., 2: 253, 1940.

Hegner, R.: Pathogenicity of Human Intestinal Protozoa, Arch. Path. and Lab. Med., 3: 1009, 1927.

Hellwig, C. A.: Obliteration of the Vermiform Appendix, Amer. Jour. Obst. and Gynec., 18: 332, 1929.

Henderson, R. G., H. Pinkerton, and L. T. Moore: Histoplasma Capsulatum as a Cause of Chronic Ulcerative Enteritis, Jour. Amer. Med. Asso., 118: 885, 1942.

Hill, T. J.: The Epithelium in Dental Granulomata, Jour. Dent. Res., 10: 323, 1930.

——: An Investigation of Spirochetosis of the Dental Anlage in Congenital Syphilis, Amer. Jour. Path., 7: 515, 1931; see also Bunting, R. W., and T. J. Hill: A Text Book of Oral Pathology, 2d ed., Philadelphia, Lea and Febiger, 1940.

Hirsch, E. F.: The Gastric Mucosa in Delirium Tremens, Arch. Int. Med., 17: 354, 1916.

Holman, W. L.: The Relative Longevity of Different Streptococci and Possible Errors in the Isolation and Differentiation of Streptococci, Jour. Infect. Dis., 15: 293, 1914.

——: Spontaneous Infection in the Guinea-Pig, Jour. Med. Res., 35: 151, 1916.

——: Focal Infection and "Elective Localization." A Critical Review, Arch. Path., 5: 68, 1928.

Hurst, A. F., and M. J. Stewart: Gastric and Duodenal Ulcer, Oxford Univ. Press, 1929.

Ivy, A. C.: Contributions to the Physiology of the Stomach, Arch. Int. Med., 25: 6, 1920.

——: Studies on Gastric and Duodenal Ulcer, Jour. Amer. Med. Asso., 75: 1540, 1920.

——, J. E. McCarthy, and B. H. Orndoff: Studies on the Effect of Roentgen Rays on Glandular Activity, IV, Effect of Exposure of Abdominal and Thoracic Areas to Roentgen Rays on Gastric Secretion: Note on Roentgen Cachexia, Jour. Amer. Med. Asso., 83: 1977, 1924.

Jay, P.: The Bacteriology and Immunology of Dental Caries, in Dental Science and Dental Art, edited by Samuel H. Gordon, Philadelphia, Lea and Febiger, 1938, p. 348.

Johnson, J. B.: The Pathogenesis of Azotemia in Hemorrhage from the Upper Gastro-intestinal Tract, Jour. Clin. Investi., 20: 161, 1941.

Johnston, W. D., B. G. Anderson, and P. F. McAlenney: Effects of Congenital Syphilis on the Teeth and Associated Structures in Children, Amer. Jour. Orthodont. and Oral Surg., 27: 667, 1941.

Kahn, J. R.: Absence of Peptic Ulcer in Pernicious Anemia, Amer. Jour. Med. Sci., 194: 463, 1937.

Karnosh, L. J.: Histopathology of Syphilitic Hypoplasia of the Teeth, Arch. Dermat. and Syph., 13: 25, 1926.

Karsner, H. T.: The Pathology of Peptic Ulcer of the Stomach, Jour. Amer. Med. Asso., 85: 1376, 1925.

——, and B. Clark, Jr.: Analysis of 104 Cases of Carcinoma of the Large Intestine, Amer. Jour. Cancer, 16: 933, 1932.

Keller, A. D.: Ulceration in the Digestive Tract of the Dog following Intracranial Procedures: Preliminary Study, Arch. Path., 21: 127, 1936.

Kirsch, E., and E. Stahnke: Die heilungsverzögernde Wirkung des Muskelzerstörung im chronischen Magengeschwür, Frankfurt. Zeitschr. Path., 33: 269, 1926.

——: Pathologisch-anatomische, klinische und tierexperimentelle Untersuchungen über die Bedeutung des Soorpilzes für das chronische Magengeschwur, Mitt. Grenzgeb. Med. u. Chir., **36**: 174, 1923.

Klein, A. J., and W. L. Palmer: Experimental Gastric Carcinoma: A Critical Review with Comments on the Criteria of Induced Malignancy, Arch. Path., **29**: 814, 1940; *see also* Jour. Nat. Cancer Inst., **1**: 559, 1941.

Klein, S. H.: Origin of Carcinoma in Chronic Gastric Ulcer, Arch. Surg., **37**: 155, 1938.

Knowlton, G. C.: Relation of Diet to the Production of Dental Caries in Young Rats, Proc. Soc. Exper. Biol. and Med., **27**: 757, 1929-30.

Kocher, Th.: Die Lehr von der Brucheinklemmung, Deutsch. Zeitschr. Chir., **8**: 331, 1877.

Konjetzny, G. E.: Der Magenkrebs, Stuttgart, Enke, 1938.

Lasowsky, J. M., and A. N. Ptschelina: Ueber trophische Magenstörungen unter der Einwirkung beiderseitiger Vagotomie, Virchow's Arch. Path Anat., **285**: 755, 1932.

Lignac, G. O.: Ueber sogenannte "Melanosis" coli, Krankheitsforschung, **2**: 162, 1925.

Livingston, E. M., and G. T. Pack: End Results in the Treatment of Gastric Carcinoma, in Treatment of Cancer and Allied Diseases, New York, Hoeber, 1940, vol. 2, p. 1110.

Long, E. R., M. V. Seibert, and L. M. Gonzalez: Tuberculosis of the Tonsils: Its Incidence and Origin, Arch. Int. Med., **63**: 609, 1939.

Lynch, J. M., and J. Felsen: Tumors of the Colon and Rectum, New York, 1925.

Macumber, H. H.: Acute Bacillary Dysentery: A Clinicopathologic Study of Two Hundred and Sixty-Three Consecutive Cases, Arch. Int. Med., **69**: 624, 1942.

Mallory, T. B.: Carcinoma in Situ of the Stomach and Its Bearing on the Histogenesis of Malignant Ulcers, Arch. Path., **30**: 348, 1940.

Malone, R. H.: A Contribution to the Pathology of Amoebic and Bacillary Dysentery, Bull. Internatl. Asso. Med. Museums, **8**: 144, 1922.

Mann, F. C.: A Study of the Gastric Ulcers Following Removal of the Adrenals, Jour. Exper. Med., **23**: 203, 1916.

——, and C. S. Williamson: The Experimental Production of Peptic Ulcer, Ann. Surg., **77**: 409, 1923.

Marshall, J. A.: The Etiology of Dental Caries, Physiol. Rev., **4**: 564, 1924.

Martin, C. F.: Stricture of the Rectum, Jour. Amer. Med. Asso., **101**: 1550, 1933.

Martin, H. E., H. Munster, and E. D. Sugarbaker: Cancer of the Tongue, Arch. Surg., **41**: 888, 1940.

——, and E. L. Sugarbaker: Cancer of the Tonsil, Amer. Jour. Surg., **52**: 158, 1941.

McIntosh, J., W. W. James, and P. Lazarus-Barlow: An Investigation into the Etiology of Dental Caries, Brit. Jour. Exper. Path., **3**: 138, 1922-23; **5**: 175, 1924; **6**: 260, 1925.

McIver, M. A.: Acute Intestinal Obstruction, I, II, III, Arch. Surg., **25**: 1098, 1106, 1125, 1932.

McKenney, D. C.: Multiple Polyposis: Congenital, Heredofamilial, Malignant, Amer. Jour. Surg., **46**: 204, 1939.

Meleney, H. E.: The Pathology of Amebiasis: Clinical Lecture at the Cleveland Session, Jour. Amer. Med. Asso., **103**: 1213, 1934.

Meyer, K. A., and H. A. Singer: Syphilis of the Stomach with Special Reference to Its Recognition at Operation, Arch. Surg., **26**: 443, 1933.

Miller, W. D.: The Agency of Acids in the Production of Caries of Human Teeth, etc., Dental Cosmos, **25**: 337, 1883.

Mills, H. W.: Gas Cysts of the Intestine, with Report of Three Cases, Surg., Gynec. and Obst., **40**: 387, 1925.

Minnes, J. F., and C. F. Geschickter: Benign Tumors of the Stomach, Amer. Jour. Cancer, **28**: 136, 1936.

Nygaard, K. K., and W. Walters: Malignant Tumors of Meckel's Diverticulum. Report of a Case of Leiomyosarcoma, Arch. Surg., **35**: 1159, 1937.

Olitsky, P. K., and Kligler, I. J.: Toxins and Antitoxins of Bacillus Dysenteriae Shiga, Jour. Exper. Med., **31**: 19, 1920.

Palmer, W. L.: Peptic Ulcer and Gastric Secretion, Arch. Surg., **44**: 452, 1942.

Pappenheimer, A. M., and L. D. Larimore: The Occurrence of Gastric Lesions in Rats and Their Possible Relation to Dietary Deficiency, Proc. Soc. Exper. Biol. and Med., **21**: 141, 1923; *see also* Jour. Exper. Med., **40**: 719, 1924.

Paulson, M.: The Present Status of Idiopathic Ulcerative Colitis, with Especial Reference to Etiology, Jour. Amer. Med. Asso., **101**: 1687, 1933.

Pessin, S. B.: The Enterochromo-Argentaffin Cells, Arch. Path., **11**: 171, 1931.

Pines, B., J. Rabinovitch, and S. B. Biller: Primary Torsion and Infarction of the Appendices Epiploicae, Arch. Surg., **42**: 775, 1941.

Polley, H. F.: Congenital Short Esophagus with Thoracic Stomach and Esophageal Hiatus Hernias, Jour. Amer. Med. Asso., **116**: 821, 1941.

Popoff, N. W.: Pathology of the Stomach, Arch. Path., **31**: 220, 1941.

Porter, J. E., and C. S. Whelan: Argentaffine Tumors. Report of 84 Cases; 3 with Metastases, Amer. Jour. Cancer, **36**: 343, 1939.

Portis, S. A., and R. H. Jaffe: A Study of Peptic Ulcer Based on Necropsy Records, Jour. Amer. Med. Asso., **110**: 6, 1938.

Rabinovitch, J., B. Pines, and I. Teicher: Pathogenesis and Pathologic Changes in Peptic Ulcer, and Production of Pain, Arch. Int. Med., **67**: 620, 1941.

Rector, L. E., and M. L. Connerley: Aberrant Mucosa in the Esophagus in Infants and in Children, Arch. Path., **31**: 285, 1941.

Reed, A. C., and H. H. Anderson: Amebiasis and Cancer of Colon, Amer. Jour. Med. Sci., **191**: 237, 1936.

Reichle, H. S.: Primary Tuberculous Infection of the Intestine, Arch. Path., **21**: 79, 1936.

Reynolds, L., and C. W. McClure: Motor Phenomena Occurring in Normal Stomachs, in the Presence of Peptic Ulcer and Its Pain, as Observed Fluoroscopically, Arch. Int. Med., **29**: 1, 1922.

Ritchie, G.: Argentaffin Tumors of the Small Intestine: A Report of Four Cases, One with Metastases, Arch. Path., **10**: 853, 1930.

Rohdenburg, G. L.: So-called Chronic Appendicitis, Arch. Path. and Lab. Med., **3**: 947, 1927.

——, and S. W. A. Franken: Dental Granulomas, Jour. Amer. Med. Asso., **93**: 191, 1929.

Rosebury, T.: The Problem of Dental Caries, Arch. Path., **15**: 260, 1933.

Rosenthal, A. H.: Congenital Atresia of the Esophagus with Tracheo-esophageal Fistula: Report of Eight Cases, Arch. Path., **12**: 756, 1931.

Rost, F.: The Pathological Physiology of Surgical Diseases, Trans. by S. P. Reimann, Philadelphia, 1923.

Sauer, L. W.: Hypertrophic Pyloric Stenosis (A Monographic Review), Arch. Pediat., **41**: 145, 1924.

——: Pyloric Hypertrophy in Hypertrophic Pyloric Stenosis, Amer. Jour. Dis. Child., **27**: 608, 1924

Schaffer, A. J., and A. W. Jacobsen: Mikulicz's Syndrome, Amer. Jour. Dis. Child., **34**: 327, 1927.

Schindler, R., and F. B. McGlone: Familial Occurrence of Hyperplastic Gastric Polyps, Arch. Surg., **41**: 1483, 1940.

Shapiro, R.: Regional Ileitis. A Summary of the Literature, Amer. Jour. Med. Sci., **198**: 269, 1939.

Singer, H. A.: Leukoplakia of the Stomach: Report of a Case, Arch. Path., **9**: 676, 1930.

——: Syphilis of the Stomach, with Special Reference to the Significance of Spirochetes, Arch. Int. Med., **51**: 754, 1933.

Sodeman, W. A.: Cardiospasm or Achalasia of the Esophagus, Ibid., **199**: 132, 1940.

Stein, I., and C. F. Geschickter: Tumors of the Parotid Gland, Arch. Surg., **28**: 492, 1934.

Stewart, M. J.: Pathology of Intestinal Tuberculosis, Tubercle, **9**: 409, 1927-28.

——, and E. M. Hickman: Observations on Melanosis Coli, Jour. Path. and Bact., **34**: 61, 1931.

Stinson, J. W.: Colloid Carcinoma of the Stomach, Surg., Gynec. and Obst., **46**: 180, 1928.

Sweet, J. E., L. T. Buckman, A. Thomas, and E. M. Bell: The Pathogenesis of Peptic Ulcer, Arch. Surg., **6**: 837, 1923.

——, M. M. Peet, and B. M. Hendrix: High Intestinal Stasis, Ann. Surg., **63**: 720, 1916.

Swinton, N. W., and S. Warren: Polyps of the Colon and Rectum and Their Relation to Malignancy, Jour. Amer. Med. Asso., **113**: 1927, 1939.

Taylor, A. L.: The Epithelial Heterotopias of the Alimentary Tract, Jour. Path. and Bact., **30**: 415, 1927.

Turell, R.: Diseases of Colon and Rectum, Amer. Jour. Med. Sci., **202**: 282, 1941.

Warren, S.: The Etiology of Acute Appendicitis, Amer. Jour. Path., **1**: 241, 1925.

Weller, C. V.: The Incidence and Histopathology of Tuberculosis of the Tonsils, Arch. Int. Med., **27**: 631, 1921.

——: Tonsillar Tubercles Containing Intracellular Concretions Simulating Foreign Body Pseudotubercles, Ann. Otol., Rhinol. and Laryng., **31**: 110, 1922.

Wilensky, A. O., and W. Thalhimer: The Etiological Relationship of Benign Ulcer to Carcinoma of the Stomach, Ann. Surg., **67**: 215, 1918.

Williams, C., and P. Kimmelstiel: Syphilis of the Stomach, Jour. Amer. Med. Asso., **115**: 578, 1940.

Windholz, F.: Ueber erworbene Syphilis des Magens, Virchow's Arch. Path. Anat., **269**: 384, 1928.

Young, M. D.: Balantidiasis, Jour. Amer. Med. Asso., **113**: 580, 1939.

Zironi, G.: Experimenteller Beitrag zur Pathogenese des Ulcus rotundum des Magens, Arch. f. Klin. Chir., **91**: 662, 1910.

17

Liver and Pancreas

LIVER

Congenital Anomalies

The right or left lobes may be small or absent, and in severe general anomalies the liver may be absent. The lobes may show divergence from relative size and shape, may be more or less numerous than normal. If the left lobe be unusually large the organ is sometimes called the "beaver tail" liver. A tongue-like downward projection of the right lobe, the so-called Riedel's lobe may be confused with malposition of the kidney. The liver is on the left side in situs viscerum inversus. It may be much altered in position in cases of diaphragmatic and umbilical hernia.

Acquired Abnormalities of Form and Position

The contraction of scars, of wounds, ruptures, abscesses, etc., may produce deformities; and in syphilis the cicatricial contraction about gummata may produce a pseudolobation of the liver, the so-called hepar lobatum. The "corset" liver, due to pressure of corset, belt, etc., usually shows one or more folds in the upper surface of the liver, extending transversely (coronal) or obliquely, variable in depth, and in the depths of the fold sometimes showing fibrosis of the capsule. Pressure of a fixed costal margin in the aged, or in a kyphoscoliosis may produce much the same picture. Parallel sagittal folds in the upper surface, usually two or more in number, may be of congenital origin, or may accompany chronic disease of the lungs such as chronic emphysema. Abnormal folds of gut may leave their imprint upon the surface of the liver. As a result of cloudy swelling, passive hyperemia or other changes which produce a large soft liver, the impression of ribs may be seen on the upper surface.

Postmortem Changes

In addition to the general softening and autolysis which may affect the liver, the most important postmortem change anatomically is the so-called foamy liver. This is due to the presence of anaerobic gas-forming bacilli from the intestinal canal or from infected wounds. These multiply after death, especially if the body be kept warm, and produce numerous bubbles of gas. Decomposition proceeds rapidly and the liver becomes soft and spongy. Microscopic examination shows gas bubbles, dead cells, and numerous bacilli in the blood vessels.

Pigmentation

Brown Atrophy. In advanced life and also as the result of prolonged wasting

546

diseases such as tuberculosis and carcinoma, the liver is sometimes the seat of brown atrophy. It is reduced in size and increased in consistency. It shows a deep brown color externally and in the cross section. The color is due to a relative and probably absolute increase in a noniron-bearing pigment normally present in the cells. Hemosiderosis in the liver is extremely common, particularly as the result of chronic passive hyperemia.

The liver grossly may not show definite pigmentation, but microscopically the cells of the liver cords in the central zone of the lobules contain quantities of iron bearing golden brown granular pigment. This may also be observed in small amounts in the endothelial cells of the sinusoids. In pernicious anemia and sometimes in profound secondary anemias the liver may be extensively pigmented with hemosiderin so as to be of light brown color to the naked eye. Microscopically, the iron-bearing golden-brown granules of pigment are found distributed in the parenchymatous cells throughout the lobules and not especially confined to the central zone.

Hemochromatosis probably affects the liver before the other organs. As indicated in the chapter on pigmentations, the pigment is in part hemosiderin and in part hemofuscin. It is deposited first in the sinusoidal endothelium, then in the lining epithelium of the small bile ducts and cells of the connective tissue stroma and ultimately in muscle cells of the blood vessels. It appears first in the periphery of the lobule and later in the center. Fibrosis with distortion of architecture is usually present to produce "pigment cirrhosis."

In malaria the liver may be the seat of pigmentation visible to the naked eye. Upon microscopic examination pigment is found as dark-brown granules, which do not respond to the iron test, situated principally in the Kupffer cells of the sinusoids. In argyria the silver pigment may be found under the endothelial cells of the sinusoids. Carbon is sometimes found in the form of opaque granules and spicules in the connective tissue due to transfer from anthracotic lung or mediastinal lymph nodes.

Bile pigmentation may be observed as a diffuse pigmentation of the liver in any variety of jaundice. The color of the fresh specimen is usually yellow but after oxidation of the bilirubin to biliverdin it becomes green. As the result of stasis of bile following obstruction either to the larger or smaller ducts, the pigment accumulates in small solid masses in the bile canaliculi within the cells and in the bile capillaries which course between the cells. This accumulation is more often observed in the center of the lobules than in the periphery but may be observed in either situation. The pigment masses may be phagocytosed by Kupffer cells of the sinusoids and by migratory macrophages.

Degenerations and Infiltrations

Cloudy swelling is common in the liver, particularly as the result of acute infectious diseases. Among other causes are passive hyperemia, general anemias, leukemias, poisoning by metals such as arsenic, antimony and lead, and other agents such as carbon monoxide, alcohol, chloroform, iodoform and ether. The gross picture is usually altered by passive hyperemia, because the various causes of cloudy swelling of the liver affect the heart also, with consequent congestive failure. In a general way, however, the liver is somewhat enlarged, with a tense capsule. It is of reduced consistence, pallid in color, cuts with decreased resistance and shows a pallid, moist, bulging, friable cross section.

Microscopically, practically all the cells are affected, although as the result of passive hyperemia the lesion may be most marked in the central zone. The cells are swollen but their outline may be more distinct than usual, because the tension of the capsule leads to compression of the margins of the swollen cells. The cytoplasm is pale and distinctly granular. The nuclei are not affected. In passive hyperemia, where the lesion is most pronounced in the central zone, the dilated capillaries may prevent marked swelling of the cells. Hydropic degeneration or infiltration is probably simply an advanced stage of cloudy swelling, where the water imbibition is so marked as to lead to the presence of microscopically visible droplets. The center of the droplets of water may show a minute acidophilic mass which stains as does fibrin.

Fatty Degeneration. Provided the cause be removed, cloudy swelling may progress to complete recovery, but with continuance or unusual severity of the same causes as those of cloudy swelling, the condition progresses to fatty degeneration. Prolonged passive hyperemia is especially likely to produce fatty degeneration in the central zones. The condition may also be observed around abscesses, infarcts, and foci of necrosis. In addition to the general conditions enumerated above, there are poisons that are particularly prone to produce fatty degeneration, notably phosphorus, carbon tetrachloride, phloridzin, etc. As is true of cloudy swelling, the disease underlying the fatty degeneration also leads to passive hyperemia so that the condition is not often observed in uncomplicated form.

Grossly, however, the liver is likely to be reduced in size with a flaccid capsule and sharp rather than rounded edges. The organ is soft, cuts with diminished resistance and shows a nonbulging or retracted cross section. Both outer surface and cross section are of yellow color. Microscopically, the lesion affects the central zone more strikingly than the peripheral zone. The cells may be enlarged but usually are reduced in size. The cytoplasm is granular, as a part of the cloudy swelling, and contains a variable number of minute fat droplets. The nucleus is usually normal but sometimes slightly pyknotic. The gross features may resemble more closely those of cloudy swelling when the fatty degeneration is of only slight degree, and the microscopic findings show only slight fatty degeneration. In most cases the two conditions are intermingled and one or the other may predominate.

Fat Infiltration. The causes, mechanism of development and effects of fat infiltration of the liver have been discussed in the chapter on Degenerations and Infiltrations. Here, only the pathologic anatomy will be reviewed. The organ is increased in weight but not in specific gravity. The size is increased in all dimensions, the inferior border is rounded and the organ is yellow. The capsule is smooth, glistening and tense. The organ cuts with normal resistance and the knife becomes greasy. The cross section bulges slightly, is yellow, slightly moist, somewhat fragile, and the lobular markings are somewhat obscured.

Microscopically, the principal change is in the parenchymal cells. The cell contains a large droplet of fat and has a narrow surrounding zone of cytoplasm; the nucleus is in the periphery of the cell and often elongated. This is the so-called signet-ring cell. In milder degrees of involvement, the peripheral cells of the lobule are affected, but in the marked cases all the cells show the change.

Amyloid. The liver, spleen and kidneys are the principal organs affected in secondary amyloidosis, the causes of which have been discussed in the chapter on Degenerations and Infiltrations. The organ is enlarged, firm, pale, shows rounded edges and a tense capsule. It cuts with normal resistance and shows a slightly bulging or nonbulging, pale, moist, slightly bleeding, more or less smooth glassy surface. Depending upon the degree of involvement the glassy character may be in numerous foci or diffusely distributed. The usual tests for amyloid, such as iodine and sulphuric acid, are diagnostic. Microscopically, the amyloid is found as a homogeneous hyaline mass, situated primarily between the endothelial cells of the sinusoids and the liver cords. This increases in size so as to compress and produce atrophy and complete disappearance of liver cords. As the disease progresses the larger masses may become more or less confluent, and amyloid is also observed in the arteries of the portal spaces. Primary amyloidosis is not likely to affect the liver.

Hyalin is observed grossly in cases of extensive thickening by fibrosis of the liver capsule, producing the so-called "zuckerguss" or sugary liver. Microscopically, it may be observed in the connective-tissue masses in cirrhosis of the liver and in the blood vessels of the liver. Hyaline droplets may be found in the epithelial cells in cirrhosis and other lesions.

Glycogen is normally present in the liver and may be increased by feeding with carbohydrates. The amount is reduced in untreated diabetes mellitus, but increases on administration of insulin especially when glucose is also given (Wirtschafter and Korenberg).

Hepatic Necroses. Necrosis of the liver may be incident to traumatic injury, to abscesses and to infarction. There is, however, a group of necroses which, because of their situation and nature require special comment. These affect special parts of the obule and may be central, midzonal, periph-ral or focal. The liver is usually the seat of degenerations and passive hyperemia, but the foci of necrosis are only rarely large enough to be visible grossly.

CENTRAL NECROSIS is a common accompaniment of passive hyperemia. The central veins and neighboring sinusoids are enlarged and engorged with erythrocytes. The intervening parenchymal cells show hyaline or granular necrosis and often disappear completely. This occurs in prolonged passive hyperemia whether there be associated infection or not. Prolonged chloroform anesthesia may produce central or more extensive necrosis, more often hyaline than granular. This is probably due to combination of the chloroform with sulfhydryl groups with consequent inactivation of intracellular enzymes (Miller, et al.). Sometimes the necrosis in so-called acute yellow atrophy is central. Various poisons, some of which are industrial hazards, may produce central necrosis, including carbon tetrachloride, trinitrotoluene, dinitrotoluene and certain naphthalines. Although the experimental injection of diphtheria toxin produces central necrosis, the necrosis in diphtheria of man is usually focal.

MIDZONAL NECROSIS (of the middle zone) may occur around the central necrosis of passive hyperemia and may accompany a variety of acute infectious diseases. In fatal cases of yellow fever there is marked fatty degeneration and necrosis, midzonal in distribution. In addition to nuclear inclusion bodies there are cytoplasmic acidophilic hyaline masses, called Councilman bodies, probably necrotic cells. Comparable midzonal necrosis is found in the liver following fatal burns of the body (Belt). Buis and Hartman report that it is central, but this may well be due to the effects of tannic acid used in treatment (see Wells, et al.).

NECROSIS OF THE PERIPHERAL ZONE, either focal or more extensive, is seen in eclampsia, phosphorus poisoning, which may however be central, and experimentally following intravenous injection of chloroform (Schultz et al.). More diffuse necrosis involving two or more zones may result from extension of any of the conditions noted above, and also results from poisoning by mercury and arsenic.

BY FOCAL NECROSIS is meant the death of a small group of cells, which may appear in any of the zones, but is probably more common in the middle zone than elsewhere. Focal necrosis is due to acute infectious diseases, outstanding among which is typhoid fever. Nevertheless, it may be observed in diphtheria, scarlatina, measles, septicemia and other types of infection. Experimentally, the injection of ether or of specific hemagglutinative and hemolytic immune sera also produces focal necrosis which is likely to be hyaline in character.

The degree of reaction to the necrosis depends in part upon the extent of the lesion and the length of time the patient or animal survives the injury. Infiltrations of polymorphonuclear leukocytes, lymphocytes and mononuclear cells, particularly the endothelial type of cell, is variable. In some instances the polymorphonuclear leukocytes predominate, especially in the earlier stages. In others, notably the focal necrosis of infectious disease, although the polymorphonuclear leukocytes predominate early in the lesion, in the later stages the infiltration is principally by large mononuclear cells which are actively phagocytic.

In rare instances, reflux of pancreatic juice into the liver because of obstruction of the common duct, may lead to small regions of necrosis in the liver with the general features of fat necrosis. These foci are not confined to any particular zone of the lobule. (See Schiller.)

Numerous observers have noted the presence of thrombi in the capillaries. The studies of Mallory and of Opie indicate that occlusion of the sinusoids by small foreign bodies may produce necrosis. This, however, is not so extensive as is observed in other conditions. Our own studies show that the circulation in the sinusoids is not entirely obliterated by the presence of the hyaline thrombi of immune serum necrosis. Mallory has indicated further that occlusion of the sinusoids by endothelial cells transferred from the spleen is associated with the focal necrosis seen in typhoid fever. It seems probable, however, as the result of our investigations and of those of others, that in addition to the partial or complete occlusion of the circulation of the sinusoids, there must be some cytolytic or cytotoxic action.

Functionally, there may or may not be

severe disturbance attributable to the liver. In the more extensive necroses, jaundice is not uncommon, but it is at least probable that the jaundice is not only obstructive due to interruption of the bile canaliculi but also of hemolytic origin due to the same cause which leads to necrosis. Whipple finds that the amount of fibrinogen in the blood is reduced, probably accounting for decreased coagulability of the blood, and that the amount of lipase is increased. The ammonia of the urine may be increased in certain conditions of this kind, indicating a reduced detoxifying action on the part of the liver. In experimental liver necroses, an accumulation of non-protein nitrogen in the blood, a reduced tolerance to sugars and usually a terminal acidosis is found in addition to the alterations in fibrinogen and lipase.

Eclampsia. This is one of the toxic complications of pregnancy and usually ap-

tion, hyperemia, hemorrhage and small foci of necrosis.

Microscopically, the foci of necrosis are small or extensive and are in the periphery of the lobule. The cell cords are disorganized, the cells are the seat of cloudy swelling and necrosis and often contain vacuoles (not fat) in the cytoplasm. The sinusoids often contain hyaline thrombi and sometimes syncytial masses, apparently from the chorionic villi. The process may merge into an acute yellow atrophy. Various lesions are found in the kidney, including glomerulonephritis, acute necrotizing arteriolitis, mild or severe nephrosis, pyelitis, and in some instances it escapes. The myocardium may be degenerated. The central nervous system may show focal hemorrhages, necrosis and thrombosis.

The cause of eclampsia is unknown. Various theories have implicated hypotheti-

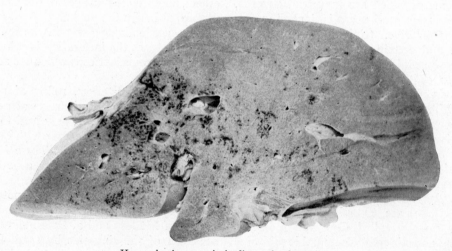

Hemorrhagic necrosis in liver of eclampsia.

pears in the later months or in the early puerperium, but is occasionally observed early in pregnancy. Clinically, in addition to decreased urinary output and subcutaneous edema, the outstanding features are convulsions, often associated with persistent vomiting. The anatomic lesions are most striking in the liver but these do not correspond in severity with the clinical manifestations. There may be merely hyperemia, fatty degeneration, small foci of necrosis and slight leukocyte infiltration or there may be massive infarcts, necroses and hemorrhages. More characteristic are extensive fatty degenera-

cal poisons originating in the breast, placenta, and the fetus itself. In cattle, removal of the breast is said to be beneficial, but this has not been shown to be true in women. Emptying the uterus of women often leads to recovery, but the fetus may be quite normal. The placenta also is usually normal anatomically and no poison has been consistently identified in it. Kappeler-Adler suggests that the disease may be due to histamine, but even so the origin of the histamine is not indicated. Integrity of the ovary and hypophysis is essential to normal pregnancy, but there are no clear indications of functional alterations in eclampsia. It has been thought that the hepatic lesion is due either to emboli from the placenta, or to the production of thrombi by incompletely transformed proteins derived from placenta or intestine, but neither of these theories is established. There are disturbances of salt and water metabolism and reduction of plasma albumin, but these are probably secondary rather than causative. (See Stander.)

ACUTE DIFFUSE NECROSIS. In addition to the localized necroses noted above, the lobules may be the seat of more widespread or diffuse necrosis. This may occur in acute infectious diseases, such as scarlatina and measles, infectious jaundice, and poisoning by phosphorus, arsenic, mercury, chloroform, cinchophen, carbon tetrachloride and other agents. Some of these start in one part of the lobule and extend throughout, as for example, phosphorus poisoning with its primary peripheral zonal necrosis and chloroform with its central necrosis. Indeed, the peripheral zonal necrosis of eclampsia may become diffuse.

In addition, there is a diffuse necrosis of unknown cause often called acute yellow atrophy. The symptoms and signs of the former group may closely resemble those of acute yellow atrophy or may be much milder and end in recovery. The outcome of all these forms of necrosis may be toxic cirrhosis, discussed subsequently.

ACUTE YELLOW ATROPHY. Although the liver may be much reduced in size, this is not due to atrophy in the ordinary sense but to destruction of hepatic parenchyma. A preferable term would be diffuse toxic necrosis. The disease sometimes complicates infections and may occur in pregnancy, but the typical cases are without identifiable cause. It is suggested that poisons generated in the intestinal canal may be the cause, but this is not proved. In experimental animals, dietary deficiencies of certain types of fats, dietary substitutions, deficiencies of members of the vitamin B complex, feeding of butter yellow, etc., have led to necrosis resembling that of diffuse toxic necrosis, but the application of these to man is not clear. The disease is most common in early adult life and attacks females much more often than males. It runs a course varying from a few days to a few weeks, usually initiated with gastro-intestinal symptoms followed by reduction in size of liver, jaundice, coma, and sometimes multiple hemorrhages in various organs. The urine characteristically contains leucine and tyrosine as well as other amino-acids and purines. Analysis of the liver shows the presence of essentially the same products. The blood is much the same as in many other liver necroses except for the large amount of leucine, tyrosine, other amino-acids, and bile pigments and salts. Whereas in chloroform, phosphorus and *Amanita phalloides* poisoning, the early change affects the cytoplasm principally in the form of fatty degeneration with necrosis apparently secondary, in acute yellow atrophy the necrosis is primary, the nuclei being destroyed early in the course of the condition, the cytoplasm undergoing autolysis subsequently.

At autopsy the liver is found to be much reduced in size, sometimes as small as 750 grams, and is situated well toward the spinal column. The organ is extremely soft, somewhat elastic, shows sharp edges, a wrinkled capsule and flattens remarkably when laid on the table. Through the capsule numerous yellow or grayish-red, often slightly depressed, patches are observed. The organ cuts easily and the cross section usually shows retraction. It is soft, distinctly friable and of a diffuse yellow color. In somewhat later stages, however, the yellow may be mottled with red and in still later stages the color may be a diffuse yellowish-red. In the red areas the consistence is less "mushy" than elsewhere. Upon exposure to the air the color may become green, since it is largely due to bile pigment. In later stages, when connective tissue growth has partly replaced the necrotic liver substance and regeneration is in progress, the consistence is greater than in the early stage and ultimately toxic cirrhosis may develop.

Microscopically, the degenerative and necrotic processes are almost coextensive with the lobules, and in our experience the most severe lesion has been in the central part of the lobule. In the necrotic areas the nuclei are completely absent and the cytoplasm may be granular, the seat of fatty degeneration, or has completely disappeared. In areas of complete disorganization, albuminous granules, small globules of fat, small solid masses of bile pigment and crystals which are probably crystallized bile pigment are found. The sinusoids are often widely distended and in the disorganized area small foci of hemorrhage are observed. When the liver is red these areas of hyperemia and of hemorrhage are more pronounced. If the patient survive, fibrosis and regeneration make their appearance. The connective tissue grows principally from the pre-existing connective tissue of the portal space. In his exhaustive review of the whole topic of acute yellow atrophy, Roman discusses the part played by bile ducts and liver cells in regeneration. There is little doubt that there is genuine proliferation of bile ducts, but this contributes little or nothing to the formation of new pseudolobules. The bulk of new formation of liver cells is

sular rupture or may be divided into bleeding fragments which undergo necrosis. Hemorrhage and shock may be fatal within a short time or two or three days after the injury. Sterile peritonitis may occur from leakage of bile. Penetrating wounds or ruptured stomach or intestine may be followed by bacterial peritonitis. (See Krieg.)

Circulatory Disturbances

Passive hyperemia of the liver is due principally to chronic disease of the heart or congestive failure. It may also be the result of chronic diseases of the lung with stasis in the right side of the heart, to tumors or fluid in the thorax compressing the inferior vena cava, or to disease within the inferior vena

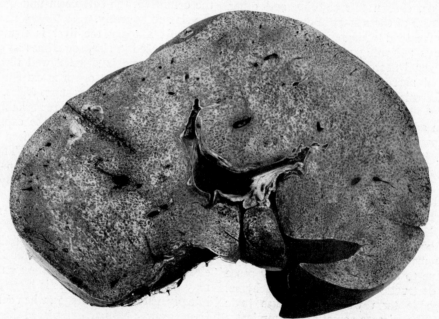

Passive hyperemia of liver, showing enlarged central zones. Army Medical Museum 13354.

from pre-existing surviving cord cells, and a functional communication with bile ducts may occur.

Trauma

Traumatic injury of the liver may be due to penetrating wounds or caused by crushing of the abdomen, such as occurs in automobile accidents. In the former the missile or knife may penetrate other viscera as well and in the latter other organs, both solid and hollow, may be ruptured. In the crushing injuries, the liver may show a cap-

cava itself. The distance between the entry of the hepatic vein into the inferior vena cava and of the latter into the right atrium is so short, that effects are quickly evident in the central veins and the sinusoids.

The appearance of the liver varies considerably, depending upon the duration and degree of the hyperemia. In the earlier stage the liver is large, with tense capsule, rounded edges, fairly firm and of dark red or purple color. It cuts with normal resistance and shows a soft, bulging, freely bleeding cross section in which the central zones are found to be dark red or purple, enlarged and some-what depressed below the slightly bulging, yellow or brown peripheral zone. In a later stage the liver may be of normal or reduced size and the color altered by the presence of cloudy swelling or fatty degeneration. Be-cause the liver loses much blood by draining into other tissues after death, the organ may be much larger in life than at autopsy. Owing to the peculiar lobular construction of the human liver, the distention of the central zones may become so great as to establish what appears grossly to be an interlacing network of communicating, red, slightly de-pressed lines about a millimeter wide which are fused central zones of neighboring lob-ules. At this stage there is usually well-marked fatty degeneration of the surrounding liver cells. This constitutes the so-called nut-meg liver of chronic passive hyperemia. Still later the liver is considerably reduced in size and is said to be the seat of red atrophy. This may represent either an advance of the nutmeg liver or may not have been preceded by any such condition. Ultimately fibrosis may be sufficiently advanced to form cardiac cirrhosis, which is discussed below.

Microscopically it is possible to dis-tinguish several grades or degrees of passive

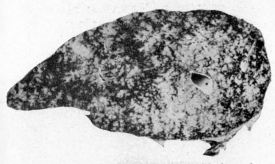

Chronic passive hyperemia of the liver with fatty de-generation ("nutmeg" liver).

hyperemia. The mildest is that in which there is distention of the central vein and the neigh-boring parts of the sinusoids. The cells of the central zone appear to be reduced in size, which is generally thought to be atrophy, although Mallory states that it may also rep-resent elongation of the cells. There may be cloudy swelling, a deposit of hemosiderin in the cells, and edema. In another type of lesion there may be fatty or vacuolar degen-eration, with only little distention of the vein

and sinusoids. In some instances, these cells may be so swollen by degeneration that the sinusoids appear to be compressed and the hyperemia is most marked in the immediately neighboring middle zone of the lobule. Cen-tral necrosis also occurs, as indicated above. In the nutmeg liver, the degenerations are marked and the hyperemic regions of neigh-boring lobules fuse. After death, the blood drains out of the liver in considerable quan-tity. This causes a certain amount of firm-ness and the collapse of the central zones may produce a slight nodularity. Zimmerman and Hillsman report that there is little dis-turbance of function even in most severe passive hyperemia, except when necrosis su-pervenes.

Edema. This may be local in regions of the liver or widespread. It is characterized by widening of the spaces between the cells of the cords and the lining cells of the si-nusoids. Precipitation of protein by fixa-tion causes the presence of finely granular protein aggregates in the spaces. It may be due to physical causes, as in passive hyper-emia, or to relatively increased vascular per-meability in a variety of general diseases (Keschner and Klemperer).

Embolism. As with embolism of other organs, the primary cause may be found in the arterial system with transport to the liver through the hepatic artery or, in the tribu-taries of the portal system with transport through the portal vein. Thus, endocarditis, arteritis, thrombophlebitis, sclerosis, throm-bosis and other similar lesions may produce embolism in the liver. Rarely, retrograde embolism from the inferior vena cava or the right heart may occur into the hepatic vein.

Thrombosis. Thrombosis in the portal vein may be due to tumors in the liver either primary or secondary, compression of veins by tumors, gallstones, and other lesions out-side the liver, cirrhosis of the liver, thrombo-phlebitis, cholangitis. It may complicate sclerosis of the veins, as discussed later. Thrombophlebitis in any part of the portal tributaries may progress to involve the chief vein. The same conditions may cause throm-bosis in the hepatic veins. Thrombosis of the hepatic artery is usually due to arteriosclero-sis but may be of other thrombotic or embolic origin (see Morgan, Lieber and Stewart). Oc-casional cases of aneurysm of the hepatic

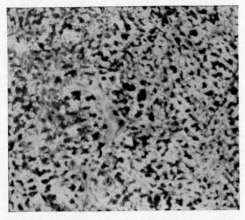

Moderate passive hyperemia limited to central zones.

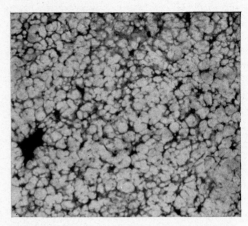

Laennec cirrhosis, to show fibrosis and distortion of architecture.

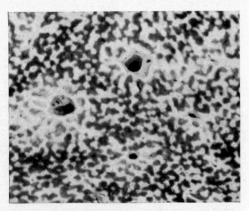

Advanced passive hyperemia with fusion of adjacent central zones.

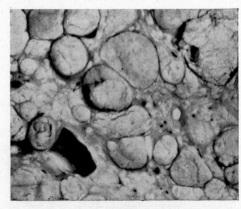

Laennec cirrhosis with large nodules of "regeneration."

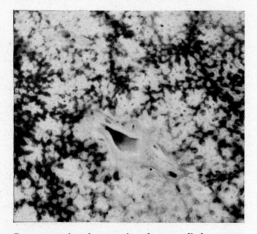

Severe passive hyperemia, the so-called nutmeg liver.

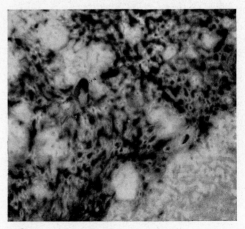

Primary carcinoma. Invasion without compression of hepatic substance.

Macrophotographs of gross sections of liver, magnified about 2 diameters.

artery are observed and these may be complicated by thrombosis.

The extensive anastomoses within the liver of branches of the hepatic artery and of the portal vein, both within their own circulation and between each other, are such that the occlusion of the intrahepatic branches often has no observable effect, as pointed out by Winternitz. Occlusion of the main branch of the portal vein may lead to no change in the liver other than a moderate hyperemia. There may, however, be some atrophy of the liver cells. Similarly, occlusion of the hepatic vein may produce a distinct hyperemia or no effect. Either of these conditions may produce passive hyperemia of the vessels of the abdominal cavity, with hyperemia of the intestines, enlargement of the spleen and sometimes ascites. The establishment of collateral circulation through the hepatoduodenal ligament may relieve the passive hyperemia in the abdomen. Occlusion of the entire hepatic arterial supply leads to infarction, unless collateral circulation is established. Occlusion of small branches is without effect. It is usually due to occlusion of intrahepatic branches of the portal vein, but occlusion of the main portal vein does not cause infarction because of the supply of blood from the arteries (see Zimmerman).

Infarction. This lesion in the liver is distinctly unusual. Pale yellow areas near the surface, somewhat resembling infarction, are frequently observed, but there is no necrosis. The so-called atrophic red infarct of Zahn cannot be regarded as a true infarct since there is only hyperemia and atrophy of the parenchymatous cells. As observed at autopsy most infarcts of the liver are hemorrhagic although some may be white or anemic. They may be of conical or of cylindrical form, usually sharply defined, and either swollen or retracted, depending upon duration. Collateral hyperemia is not marked and reactionary fibrosis is usually slight in degree. Occlusion of hepatic veins leads to necrosis, which may or may not be regarded as infarction depending upon definition of the term. "Complete block of the arterial blood supply always leads to infarction, even in the presence of full venous circulation." It cannot be said that direct trauma causes infarction because of the uncertainty as to whether necrosis or vascular thrombosis occurs first.

Hemorrhage in the liver occurs as the result of vascular occlusion, chronic passive hyperemia, especially with necrosis, eclampsia, phosphorus poisoning, various infectious diseases, hemorrhagic diseases, infarction, and traumatism. It may be observed as subcapsular hematoma in infants born of mothers suffering from infectious or toxic diseases.

Portal Phlebosclerosis. As a sequel of prolonged passive hyperemia, such as may accompany hepatic cirrhosis, the veins of the portal system may show fibrosis, sometimes marked in the intima. Comparable changes may occur in the veins in the liver. As a rule this is only slight. Portal phlebosclerosis may also be primary, with onset at comparatively early age and enlargement of the spleen; but anemia and ascites do not occur (see Reich). Slight fibrosis of the portal vein may occur in connection with the Cruveilhier-Baumgarten syndrome, in which associated with persistence of the umbilical vein there is distention of veins of abdominal wall especially around the umbilicus (caput medusae) venous murmur in these veins, ascites, fibrosis of liver and slight or marked splenic enlargement (Armstrong, et al.).

Inflammation

Acute Suppurative Inflammation. The infectious agent producing suppurative inflammation of the liver, or abscess formation, may be introduced through the portal vein, the hepatic artery, the hepatic vein, the biliary passages or by direct extension. With few exceptions, such as amebic abscess and those forms which occur as the result of direct extension, abscess of the liver is usually multiple. The most common mode of entry is through the portal vein as the result of ulcerative or suppurative lesions connecting with its tributaries. Suppurative or ulcerative appendicitis with peri-appendical abscess constitutes the most common point of origin. Ulcers and suppurative lesions of the stomach, small and large intestines are of importance. Among these is bacillary dysentery, which has been discussed in the preceding chapter. Abscesses in such organs as pancreas, spleen and especially abdominal lymph nodes may cause abscess in the liver. However, multiple abscesses of the liver are occasionally found without any demonstrable portal of entry. In this group of cases, however, it is important always to examine for actinomyces which may gain access to the liver without gross lesion of the intestine.

The infection in the liver starts, as a rule, as a suppurative thrombophlebitis of the smaller tributaries of the portal veins. From this lesion emboli are detached and lodge in the intrahepatic branches of the portal vein, pylephlebitis. Occasionally, the extension is by a progressive thrombophlebitis extending along tributaries to the main stem of the portal. Grossly, the liver is usually somewhat enlarged, dark and either gray or yellow, depending upon the degree of associated cloudy swelling or fatty degeneration, or green in color due to the escape of bile. The capsule is tense and smooth, except when abscesses near the surface involve the capsule in an acute fibrinous or fibrinopurulent perihepatitis. Upon cross section, the abscesses are found distributed more or less uniformly throughout the liver, but as a rule are much more numerous in the right than in the left lobe. They may vary in size from 3 mm. to several centimeters. The outline is often irregular, giving the impression that several small abscesses have coalesced. The degree of destruction of hepatic tissue varies. Trabeculae of connective tissue may course through the abscess and sometimes fairly solid masses of necrotic parenchymal cells are observed. The pus may be yellow, green, nonodorous, or foul, depending upon the type of organism involved. The origin is such that colon bacilli frequently contaminate the abscess and other gas formers may gain entrance. There is usually a marginal zone of hyperemia. The liver shows variable degrees of hyperemia, cloudy swelling, fatty degeneration and sometimes bile stagnation.

Microscopically, it appears that the organisms in the emboli multiply rapidly to fill a branch of the vein, around which there is a zone of leukocytes, further surrounded by a zone of necrotic liver cells. This primarily portal situation of the abscess may rarely be noted grossly. As the area of suppuration increases in size it is often preceded by the necrosis of hepatic cells and a small zone of hyperemia. Fatty degeneration is often more pronounced in the neighborhood of the abscess than elsewhere in the liver.

AMEBIC ABSCESS is found in the right lobe of the liver in about half the cases and is solitary in about 55 per cent of the cases. The organism enters through the portal vein, lodges in the portal space, and produces necrosis of surrounding regions with little inflammatory reaction (Palmer). Neighboring necrotic masses fuse to form larger abscesses. Although at first fibrin and an occasional polymorphonuclear leukocyte are seen, the principal response is an infiltration of small and large mononuclear cells, and stimulation of fibrosis. In spite of the development of a connective-tissue reaction in the margin, the abscess slowly extends and may reach large proportions. Rupture may lead to a widespread peritonitis and death, although surgical puncture of the abscess by a trocar is frequently practiced without danger, because of the presence of fibrous adhesions on the hepatic surface. Although the abscess content may be purulent it is more commonly soft, granular and cheesy. Occasionally, jaundice may accompany the lesion. It is only rarely that amebic abscess is multiple. The solitary abscess is usually in the right lobe, may grow to enormous size. As much as 8 liters of necrotic material have been removed.

Other Portals of Entry. The hepatic artery and the hepatic vein only occasionally furnish a portal of entry for hepatic abscess. In cases of endocarditis or of pyemia, emboli may enter through the hepatic artery. When abscesses occur in this way they are usually multiple but small, and often appear to follow the distribution of one of the smaller branches of the artery. A suppurative thrombophlebitis of the inferior or superior vena cava may extend by retrograde thrombosis or embolism into the liver. Such an occurrence is rare.

Suppuration in the gallbladder and biliary passages may extend along the intrahepatic biliary passages and produce multiple abscesses of the liver. Generalized jaundice is common in this condition and the contents of the abscess are usually bile stained. Although at autopsy the exact origin of such abscesses may not be apparent, yet the presence of jaundice and more particularly the presence of a more or less generalized suppurative cholangitis indicates the derivation.

Abscesses in the liver arising by direct extension are usually superficial. Such a process may extend from suppurative disease of the gallbladder or bile passages, sub-

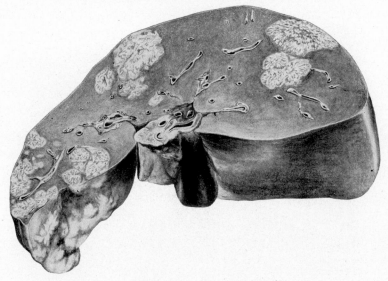

Multiple abscesses of liver.

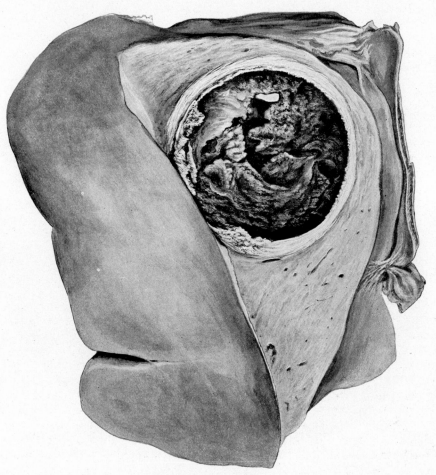

Amebic abscess of liver.

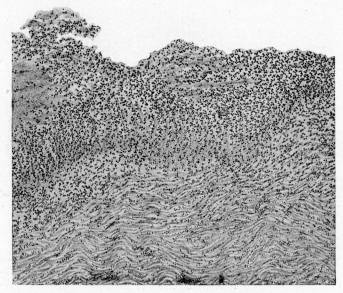

Marked fibrosis in wall of amebic abscess of liver.

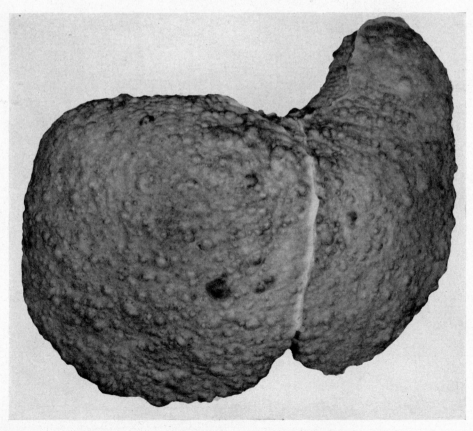

Outer surface of Laennec cirrhosis of the liver.

diaphragmatic abscesses, abscesses of kidney and perirenal tissue, pancreas and other neighboring positions, and may result from perforation of ulcers of stomach and duodenum. Sharp foreign bodies may penetrate through stomach or intestine and lodge in the liver to produce abscess formation.

Acute Nonsuppurative Inflammations. Acute hepatitis of this variety is essentially an alterative (degenerative) inflammation. The parenchymal component varies from cloudy swelling to necrosis. The interstitial or mesenchymal component is found in the form of infiltration of polymorphonuclear leukocytes or lymphoid and large mononuclear cells, or mixtures. In addition certain authorities accept Roessle's view that the accumulation of fluid between capillaries and cord cells is an inflammatory component and represents a serous hepatitis. This, however, is not fully established. Mild forms of acute hepatitis may occur in association with acute infectious diseases. They may be without known cause and constitute the underlying lesion of so-called catarrhal jaundice. Some of the infectious diseases and certain intoxications, such, for example, as poisoning by cinchophen or carbon tetrachloride, etc., may produce extensive necrosis, and because of the associated injury and reaction of the mesenchymal tissues are often regarded as acute hepatitis. The acute inflammatory reaction in these conditions is slight, but may be followed by extensive fibrosis. The milder forms of acute hepatitis may heal completely. Patients with cirrhosis of the liver may occasionally give a history of having had previous attacks of what clinically appears to have been acute hepatitis (Bloomfield).

Chronic Hepatitis. Cirrhosis. As with other parenchymatous viscera, it is often difficult to distinguish in the liver between fibrous overgrowth representing cicatrization and that which is progressive in character and regarded as chronic inflammation. In certain cases it is easily possible to recognize scar formation. In most instances, however, it is plainly evident clinically that the more diffuse forms of connective-tissue overgrowth are progressive in character, microscopically show lymphoid and other mononuclear cells in the masses of connective tissue, and therefore are regarded as chronic inflammations.

This progressive overgrowth of connective tissue, with the associated changes in the parenchyma, is usually referred to as cirrhosis of the liver. The most common form is that called atrophic or Laennec cirrhosis. Other forms include obstructive biliary cirrhosis, capsular cirrhosis, syphilitic cirrhosis, the cardiac cirrhosis of passive hyperemia, and hypertrophic biliary cirrhosis. Somewhat different classifications are offered by other authors. It is not clearly apparent, however, that in these various diseases there is sufficient uniformity of cause or effect to justify classification of them all as a part of one great unit. Our consideration will attempt to group them in as far as possible. That form due to syphilis will be considered with the subject of syphilis rather than under cirrhosis. The term cirrhosis, indicating a yellow color, is a misnomer, since many of the livers are not of yellow color. A comprehensive discussion is found in the book of Eppinger and in Askanazy's account of the first conference of the International Society for Geographic Pathology.

Laennec Cirrhosis. This is often called atrophic cirrhosis, but this term is misleading in that the liver is by no means always reduced in size. The name "portal cirrhosis" is anatomically correct because the fibrosis is in the portal spaces, but incorrectly implies origin of the disease in the portal vein. The old names gin-drinker's liver and hobnail liver are being abandoned. Laennec cirrhosis is a disease principally of the male sex and middle life, sometimes appears to be familial, usually is accompanied by ascites and exhibits jaundice for short periods or as a terminal event in about one-third of the cases. Fibrosis of the liver and destruction of parenchyma are prominent, but the term cirrhosis definitely connotes distortion of the architecture.

The cause of Laennec cirrhosis has been extensively studied both in man and experimentally. Consideration has been directed especially to two factors, namely infections and dietary influences. Infectious diseases may be responsible for hepatic necrosis but the later lesions are usually like those of toxic cirrhosis. Infectious disease often precedes the development of juvenile cirrhosis (Moon), but this is not typical Laennec cirrhosis. Bacteria, especially streptococci, are observed in certain cirrhotic livers. These items are suggestive but not conclusive. Sometimes tuberculosis or syphilis may be associated but there is no real indication that they are causative.

A history of alcoholism, especially the use of spirituous liquors, is given by many patients with Laennec's cirrhosis, but others have no such record and many alcoholics have no cirrhosis. Experimentally, alcohol, if given with an adequate diet, does not produce

there be a high fat diet with the low protein diet. The nature of the fat has some influence, because some fats appear to be more firmly fixed in the liver than others. The ultimate production of cirrhosis in depancreatized animals with fatty livers has been referred to in the chapter on Degenerations and Infiltrations. There is evidently importance to be attached to the amino-acids. The hepatic injury and cirrhosis of low protein

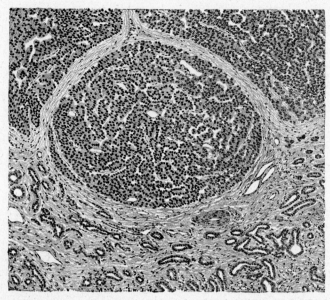

Laennec cirrhosis of liver showing multiplication of interlobular bile ducts.

cirrhosis. Alcoholics may have dietary deficiencies because they often eat very little. Intake of fats, proteins or carbohydrates, or all three, and of vitamins, especially vitamin B, may be much reduced. Whether the deficiencies of themselves lead to cirrhosis, whether they render the organ more susceptible to alcohol or injurious substances from the intestinal canal, or whether they permit the direct action of some other dietary factor, is not settled.

Extensive experimental work has been done, especially with rats and rabbits. It is probable that the caloric value of the diet is of no importance. Of the various constituents of the diet, study has been directed especially to proteins, fats and vitamin B. Prolonged deficiency of protein will lead to cirrhosis, but this is more striking if the protein is poor in methionine. The same is true if

diets is emphasized by low methionine content, but this is prevented by use of cystine or choline. What the influence of the sulfur content of these amino-acids is has not yet been clarified.

Prolonged feeding of excess l-cystine also leads to cirrhosis; the effect is diminished by lard and by cod-liver oil but not by butter fat. When dietary alterations are made, feeding of butter yellow causes cirrhosis (later carcinoma). If in addition to dietary alterations, yeast be withheld, the cirrhosis is augmented. That this is due to vitamin deficiency due to absence of yeast from the diet is not certain. Neither thiamin nor any component of the B_2 complex can be held responsible. Perhaps, however, the presence of sulfur-containing amino-acids is of importance. The effects of low protein diets are increased by addition of alcohol.

PLATE XIV

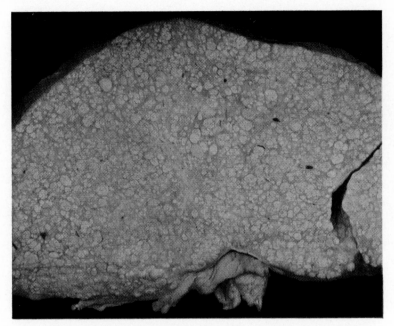

Cross section of liver the seat of Laennec cirrhosis. Note color of parenchymal nodules and disruption of lobular architecture.

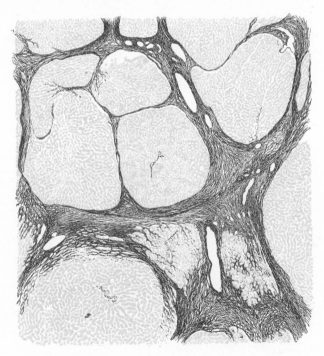

Laennec cirrhosis of liver stained by Mallory connective-tissue stain. The connective tissue is stained blue and the parenchyma pale yellow.

The application of the experimental results to man is not altogether clear, but the reduced protein stores of cirrhotics, the marked alterations of diet, the occasional demonstration of vitamin deficiencies, all point toward dietary factors as of great importance, either directly or by an influence on the hepatic cells making them susceptible to the effects of alcohol or some other poison. (See Rich and Hamilton; György and Goldblatt; Earle and Victor; Lillie, Daft and Sebrell.)

In addition to the methods indicated above, cirrhosis has been produced experi-

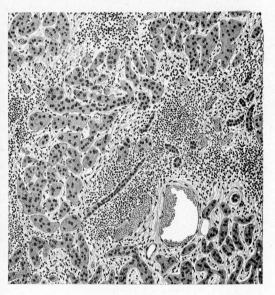

An area of cirrhosis in which perilobular infiltration of lymphoid cells is marked.

mentally by a variety of inorganic and organic agents. Only a few of these produce such distortion of lobular pattern as to justify the diagnosis of cirrhosis; these include phosphorus, especially in combination with alcohol, manganese chloride when combined with phenylhydrazine, carbon tetrachloride and tar. (See Moon.) Certain other agents, including buckwheat, seeds of *Amsinckra intermedia*, and various metals, including copper, salts of arsenic, selenium and others, will produce a fibrosis closely resembling but not usually identical with the human disease.

The pathogenesis of the lesion is in dispute. Whether the fibrosis is a reparative process secondary to liver cell destruction or is primary with secondary compression and destruction of cells is not positively known. Pearce's work indicates that cell destruction is primary, and this view is widely accepted. It does not explain the progressive character of the fibrosis, which we believe to be chronic inflammation probably induced by the same agent that led to cell destruction. (See Moon; Bloomfield.)

Grossly, the liver varies in size. It may be enlarged even in fatal cases, although clinically it may be at first enlarged and subsequently much smaller. Reduction in size may be extreme, down to weights of 600 or 700 grams. The smaller livers are increased in specific gravity because of the relative increase in amount of connective tissue. The shape is usually about normal since the process involves the entire liver fairly equally. The edges are usually sharp, although in those cases where there is associated fat infiltration they may be rounded. The color is ordinarily a reddish-brown but may be yellow due to fat infiltration, or yellowish-green due to bile stagnation. The outer surface is uniformly nodular, sometimes more strikingly so in the lower surface. In different cases nodules may be small, varying between 2 and 3 mm. in diameter, or larger, ranging in the neighborhood of 5 mm. in diameter. They are generally spherical, well defined, project above the outer surface, are relatively soft, and are of reddish-brown or brownish-yellow color, separated from one another by a dense gray, retracted, connective tissue network.

The organ is firm in consistence and cuts with increased resistance. The cross section is firm, more or less retracted, and shows an interlacing network of dense gray fibrous connective tissue, with intervening, slightly bulging parenchymatous tissue similar to that seen in the nodules on the outer surface. The size of the nodules depends in part upon the number of lobules included in the connective-tissue network. In cases where the nodules are small the condition is referred to as a monolobular cirrhosis; where larger it is referred to as multilobular cirrhosis. This distinction is not strictly accurate since in the smaller nodules several lobules are likely to be included. Often nodules of light yellow color and of soft consistence which represent foci of so-called nodular regeneration are found not only on the outer surface but also in the cross section. When the cirrhosis is a part of hemochromatosis, the brown color of the liver is obvious and the organ responds even grossly to the potassium ferrocyanide-hydrochloric acid test for iron.

Microscopically, if the section be taken near the surface, the irregular surface outline is observed. The capsule is normal or only slightly thickened over the nodules but usually dense and fibrotic in the interspaces. Instead of the normal arrangement of perilobular connective tissue, only partly dividing lobules from one another, there is a complete lobulation by the thick fibrosis. Within the oval or circular spaces of this network one or more lobules may be identified. As a rule, the connective tissue is of adult type, rich in fibrils and with dense nuclei, but occasionally, younger types of fibroblastic connective-tissue cells are observed. There is a variable infiltration of lymphoid cells sometimes associated with large mononuclear and plasma cells and even a few leukocytes.

A definite increase in the number of small bile ducts is found within the dense masses of connective tissue. These appear to ramify through the connective tissue and often show clubbed ends suggesting an abortive new formation of lobules. Indeed, the extension of the bile duct with the clubbing of the ends may go on to the formation of large masses of irregularly distributed and arranged cells, morphologically similar to those of the liver cords. These do not show definite cord-like arrangement, show little in the way of bile canaliculi and are not regularly vascularized. This is the microscopic picture of the nodules spoken of grossly as so-called regenerative. There is no indication, however, that any true regeneration of hepatic structure takes place.

As a rule the connective-tissue overgrowth is sharply defined, but occasionally branching processes of connective tissue penetrate a short distance between the cords of the lobules. The parenchymatous cells are definitely reduced in number and are usually the seat of variable degrees of cloudy swelling, sometimes with slight fatty degeneration in the central zones. As a rule, the central cells are small and appear to be atrophic but the peripheral cells may be larger than normal and are presumably hypertrophic. The nuclei vary in size and in staining capacity and sometimes show budding forms within

the cells suggesting amitotic division. Not infrequently moderate hemosiderosis of the central zone is observed. In the cases with prolonged jaundice, bile pigment may be found in the canaliculi and bile capillaries.

Laennec cirrhosis may progress far anatomically before functional changes are demonstrable. The numerous functions of the liver are more and more disturbed, including carbohydrate and protein metabolism and the so-called detoxifying mechanisms. Macrocytic hyperchromic anemia develops independently of hemorrhage. Deficiency of prothrombin, with hemorrhagic tendency, is apparently due to interference with synthesis of vitamin K. Jaundice is probably due in part to destruction of parenchyma and in part to compression of the finer biliary passages by fibrous tissue. The patient ultimately may go into coma and end in "liver death." (See Snell and Butt.) Renal insufficiency develops as a part of the "hepato-renal syndrome." The principal associated renal lesion is a nephrosis; in cases with jaundice the renal cells are stained by bile, so-called bile nephrosis.

Of especial interest are passive hyperemia in the portal venous system, portal hypertension, and ascites. The reason for the evident obstruction to circulation in the liver has been widely discussed. In our opinion the view expressed by McIndoe is probably correct and the disturbance is due to reduction of the vascular bed of the cirrhotic liver; the communications between the portal venous and the hepatic venous and the arterial systems become irregular in distribution and quantitatively reduced. It is possible, however, that disturbance of relation between blood flow in hepatic arteries and portal veins may interfere with passage of blood through the latter (Dock).

Ascites is the excessive accumulation of a transudate in the peritoneal cavity. It is one of the frequent signs of hepatic cirrhosis. As a rule the fluid is pale yellow, limpid, of low specific gravity and contains but few cells. It may at times be of darker color and higher specific gravity, probably because of partial resorption of water. In time, especially after repeated paracenteses, the peritoneum may show fibrous thickening and adhesions. Accumulation of fluid may vary from time to time and in some cases may be slight or absent. This indicates that the portal hypertension of passive hyperemia is not the sole cause of ascites. The reduction of plasma proteins in the blood of cirrhotics with ascites indicates that reduced osmotic pressure is an important factor (Post and Patek). This reduction may not be sufficient to cause general edema, but when associated with portal hypertension, the combination of the two factors determines the local edema called ascites. Occasionally anal hemorrhoids may be augmented in size.

More frequent is the dilatation of veins at the lower end of the esophagus, esophageal varices, rupture of which may lead to severe or fatal hemorrhage. If adhesions form between the liver and abdominal walls the drainage of the portal circulation may be improved. Commonly, however, collateral circulation is provided by enlargement of veins which can carry the blood from the portal area directly to the thorax without passing through the liver, communicating ultimately with either the inferior or superior vena cava. The superficial abdominal veins may partake in this process and show lines from the groin toward the umbilicus and thence up toward the chest. Marked venous enlargement around the umbilicus is referred to as the caput Medusae. The evidence of obstruction to portal circulation is found in increased portal pressure. The flow into the various collaterals probably begins early in the course of the disease.

FATTY CIRRHOSIS. Although grossly and microscopically this condition appears to be merely a combination of fat infiltration and Laennec cirrhosis, there is probably an intimate relation between the two. In the chapter on Degenerations and Infiltrations, there is a discussion of the mechanisms of fat infiltration and the fact that in experimental animals this may proceed to cirrhosis. Furthermore, it may be that there is an alteration of metabolism of fats so that the liver anchors certain types of fat with consequent injury to the cells (Spellberg et al.). In man there is often a history of alcoholism or the coexistence of diabetes mellitus. The lesion is probably a sequel of alcoholism, inadequate diet and vitamin-B deficiency. Fat infiltration is followed by perilobular fibrosis. Later the fibrosis alters the architecture of the liver

with the production of nodules. (See Connor.)

OBSTRUCTIVE BILIARY CIRRHOSIS. The result of prolonged stagnation of secretion of a gland is usually atrophy of the secreting substance and overgrowth of supporting connective tissue. Experimentally this occurs in the liver as the result of prolonged obstruction to the hepatic duct. After several weeks, rabbits show an obstructive biliary cirrhosis which resembles very closely Laennec cirrhosis with extreme jaundice. It is probable that this process conforms closely to that in other glands.

In man, obstructive biliary cirrhosis is uncommon, partly because modern surgery relieves the obstruction, and partly because the various changes incident to prolonged stagnation of bile lead to death before cirrhosis appears. Nevertheless, occasional cases are observed in which there is partial or almost complete obstruction to the outflow of bile as the result of concretions, tumors or inflammatory strictures in adults and congenital anomalies of the bile ducts in infants, in which the liver is icteric and the seat of a nodular type of cirrhosis. The microscopic picture of perilobular fibrosis is combined with bile pigmentation and often an infiltration of lymphocytes, plasma cells and sometimes polymorphonuclear leukocytes in and about the bile ducts. This inflammation may indicate infection, but this is not necessarily true, and the cirrhosis may progress without infection. (See Judd and Counseller; MacMahon and Mallory.)

TOXIC CIRRHOSIS. Recovery from any of the acute diffuse necroses described above may result in extensive fibrosis of the liver. Clinically this condition appears to be progressive, but there is uncertainty as to whether shrinkage in the size of the liver is due to contraction of scar tissue or to progressive chronic inflammation; our opinion favors the latter. The condition may closely resemble Laennec cirrhosis, but more often the liver is of normal or only moderately reduced size, slightly if at all nodular, with widespread diffuse fibrosis. Microscopically, the lobules vary in size and form. There may be remnants of the earlier necrosis. Fibrosis is diffuse and of irregular distribution. Proliferation of bile ducts and cellular infiltration may be marked or slight and are more

✗ In congenital atresia see
Ladd   Annals Surgery   102 : 742   1935
            "   "   112   1940
Donovan   SGO   1940

variable than in Laennec cirrhosis. A somewhat similar picture is presented by so-called INFECTIOUS CIRRHOSIS, except that inflammation may be notable in the finer biliary passages and even in the parenchyma (MacMahon).

PERILOBULAR FIBROSIS. In advanced life, also in connection with chronic intoxications such as lead poisoning, chronic infectious disease such as tuberculosis and syphilis, the connective tissue of the portal spaces may be increased in amount and even show slight multiplication of bile ducts and infiltration of lymphocytes. It may lead to slight roughening of the liver surface. Only when the fibrosis is accompanied by actual distortion of the lobular architecture is a diagnosis of cirrhosis justified.

CAPSULAR PSEUDOCIRRHOSIS. Fibrosis of the capsule of the liver may extend for 1 or 2 cm. into the substance of the organ especially along the lines of the perilobular connective tissue, but the process is not widespread and hence is not regarded as a true cirrhosis. The involved regions may show reduction in amount of parenchyma but the organ is not likely to be nodular. The lesion occurs in syphilis and other chronic infections, and as a part of multiple serositis together with fibrosis of pleura and pericardium, the so-called Pick's disease.

CENTRAL OR CARDIAC CIRRHOSIS. In the discussion of passive hyperemia of the liver, attention was drawn to the ultimate fibrosis that may develop in the central zone. This may increase considerably so that the liver at autopsy is firm, red and reduced in size. Fibrosis in fused central zones, together with collapse of the hyperemic zones after death may produce slight or moderate nodularity of the organ. The relative anoxia of the liver may render the tissues more susceptible to injurious agents and consequently there may be perilobular fibrosis. (See Katzin et al.)

HYPERTROPHIC BILIARY CIRRHOSIS. Often called Hanot cirrhosis, the liver in this disease is enlarged, but differs in appearance from the large livers of Laennec cirrhosis. Many pathologists of extensive experience have never seen a case and doubt that it exists as an entity. List, however, using modern methods, has described two cases that appear to be characteristic. The disease is thought to be more frequent in France than

elsewhere, is of insidious onset and is accompanied by great enlargement of the liver and spleen and marked jaundice. Jaundice is apparently due, as suggested by Eppinger, to obstruction in the finest biliary passages. It is not complete and the stools are not acholic. The formation and destruction of bile are probably not interfered with since there is usually no urobilin in the urine. Intermittent fever is commonly observed. The cause of this variety of cirrhosis is even more obscure than that of Laennec cirrhosis. Various acute infectious diseases, alcohol, and syphilis have been incriminated, but without proof.

Grossly, the liver is considerably enlarged, attaining a weight of as much as 5

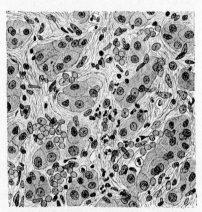

Intra-lobular fibrosis in hypertrophic cirrhosis of liver, separating the liver cords.

kg. The capsule is tense, the edges rounded, the organ firm and of yellow or greenish-yellow color. It cuts with increased resistance and shows a more or less retracting, firm, uniformly fibrotic cross section with little or no lobular distinction. Microscopically, the jaundice may or may not be apparent in the form of solid masses of pigment. Fibrosis is moderate in the perilobular connective tissue, but reaches extensively between the liver cords, a feature which distinguishes this disease from the perilobular fibrosis of the other forms of cirrhosis. This conception of hypertrophic cirrhosis is that originally given by Hanot, but subsequently he and others confused the lesion with the early stages of Laennec cirrhosis. Diffuse capillary cholangitis, such as may accompany obstructive lesions of the hepatic duct, is sometimes but not invariably present. Hence it is not likely that this disturbance is primary in the disease.

Infectious Granulomata

Syphilis. CONGENITAL SYPHILIS may or may not lead to anatomic lesions, but if fatal in early life, is likely to show large numbers of spirochetes. Definite lesions are likely to be of one or two forms, probably essentially dependent upon failure of the parenchyma to develop completely. Thus, there may be a mass of round cells in the perilobular spaces presumably representing mesoblast, or there may be a mass of mature connective tissue, associated with lymphoid and plasma cells, an increased number of the bile ducts and distortion of lobules. In the other important form there is a more diffuse growth of fibrous tissue within the lobules, surrounding capillaries and sinusoids, separating and distorting the liver cords. Grossly, the liver may be large, normal in size or small, is usually firm and sometimes shows slight nodularity of the outer surface and cross section, especially when the fibrosis is marked in the perilobular spaces. In either form of fibrosis, small areas of focal necrosis may be frequent or there may be multiple miliary gummata. It is at least possible that the focal necroses represent the early stage of miliary gumma formation. Large gummata are infrequent.

ACQUIRED SYPHILIS affects the liver in a variety of ways. Jaundice may occur in the secondary or even tertiary stage of syphilis, presumably due to degenerative lesions of the liver cells or perhaps acute parenchymatous inflammation. Chronic perihepatitis may occur in the form of thick fibrosis of the capsule of the liver, often hyalinized, occasionally calcified, and is usually associated with adhesions. This may result in the so-called capsular cirrhosis. Many observers are of the opinion that a perilobular fibrosis diffuse in extent, and often progressing to more or less marked nodularity, occurs in syphilis. This is of the nature of the generalized fibrosis in late syphilis. Gummata may occur in the substance of the liver or project as nodular masses above the surface of the organ. They may be single or multiple and may attain a diameter of 5 cm. or more. They are distinguished by a fairly solid necrotic content and dense fibrosis in the margin.

Great distortion of the liver may occur as the result of contraction of scar tissue in radiating lines around gummata in the substance of the organ. Thus, the outer surface is broken up into many smaller lobes, producing the so-called hepar lobatum. The intervening substance may be apparently normal, or the seat of a perilobular fibrosis. Section of the liver shows the radiating lines of connective tissue communicating centrally with the remains of a gumma, or sometimes a nodule definitely distinguishable as a gumma, and peripherally with the retracted parts of the liver surface. Microscopically, the small arteries in the neighborhood of the dense areas of connective tissue may show chronic obliterating or deforming endarteritis. The masses of connective tissue are often infiltrated with lymphoid or plasma cells, and may occasionally show multiplication of bile ducts. Amyloidosis of the liver may be caused by syphilis. The subject of congenital and acquired syphilis of the liver is admirably reviewed by Herxheimer.

Tuberculosis. There are three important forms of tuberculosis of the liver. Miliary tuberculosis of the liver is common in disseminated miliary tuberculosis. Often the miliary tubercles are not visible to the naked eye but are found upon histologic examination, occupying principally the perilobular connective tissue. In these circumstances they are usually extremely small and composed only of epithelioid and lymphoid cells with relatively few giant cells and little or no necrosis. Such grossly invisible tubercles may be assumed to be present in most cases where there is hematogenous miliary tuberculosis involving lungs, spleen and kidneys. Small conglomerate tubercles may be visible grossly as minute gray points or larger miliary tubercles, one or two millimeters in diameter. Microscopically, these are found to be either large miliary tubercles with central necrosis or small conglomerate tubercles.

Conglomerate tuberculosis of the liver may be secondary to pulmonary tuberculosis or to abdominal or even genito-urinary tuberculosis. There may be several foci attaining a diameter of about 7 mm. or more, or rarely there are large solitary tubercles with a diameter of several centimeters. The latter may show a fibrous wall and must be differ-

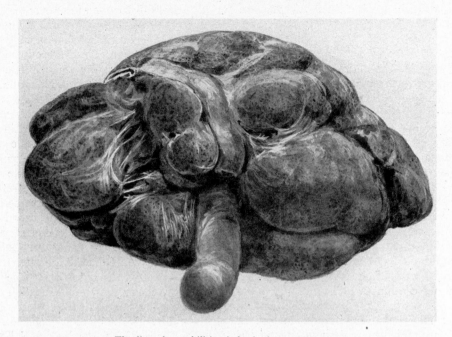

The liver in syphilitic cirrhosis, hepar lobatum.

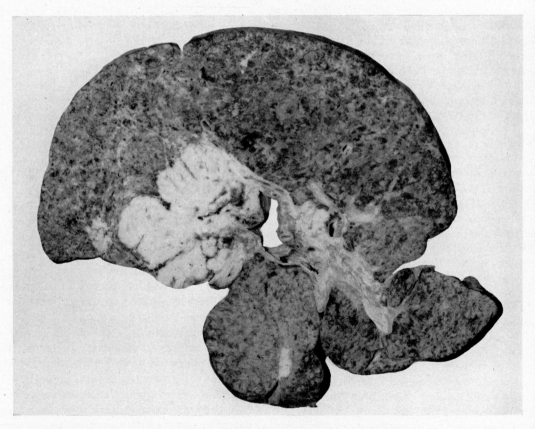

Cross section of liver, the seat of multiple gummas and hepar lobatum. The smallest gumma in the quadrate lobe is partly cicatrized and accompanied by retraction of the outer surface.

entiated from gumma, usually by means of staining for the tubercle bacilli.

The third form which is uncommon, is characterized by involvement of the biliary passages, and bile staining of the content of the tubercles. It is sometimes named tuberculous cholangitis or pericholangitis. The liver shows tuberculous masses varying from a few millimeters to a centimeter or more in size, usually clearly defined and containing bile stained, cheesy material. Occasionally, secondary infection occurs producing abscesses. According to the studies of Winternitz, such a process may arise by invasion of the intrahepatic bile ducts by caseous tubercles in the perilobular connective tissue, or may be due more rarely to an ascending tuberculous infection of the biliary passages. Certain authorities regard tuberculosis as a possible cause of Laennec cirrhosis of the liver, but this cannot be accepted as final, and it is at least possible that some other associated condition is more directly the cause than is the tuberculosis. Amyloidosis of the liver may occur in connection with direct tuberculous infection of the organ.

Actinomycosis is not rare in the liver and may be observed secondary to intestinal actinomycosis and due to extension either directly or through the retroperitoneal tissue. It may also be metastatic from actinomycosis in more distant parts of the body.

Lymphomatous Nodules

Since small lymphoid aggregates occur in the liver normally, it is to be expected that diffuse disease of the lymphoid apparatus will be observed also in the liver. Thus, in lymphoid leukemia it is not uncommon to find grossly visible, pale gray nodules representing the rich infiltration of lymphoid cells in the perilobular spaces. The same is true sometimes in lymphosarcoma. Hodgkin's disease can also affect the liver in this fashion. These conditions have been discussed in the chapter on Hematopoietic System.

Tumors

Benign Tumors. CAVERNOUS HEMANGIOMA. The commonest tumorous condition of the liver is the cavernous hemangioma, sometimes called cavernoma. This is a very common incidental finding at autopsy, especially in adults. The cavernoma may be single or multiple, usually situated immediately under the surface of the liver and varying in size from a few millimeters to several centimeters. It is a well-defined purple or dark-blue mass, which bleeds freely and retracts somewhat below the cross section of the organ. When the blood is washed out, the mass has a somewhat spongy appearance. Microscopically, it is made up of an inter-

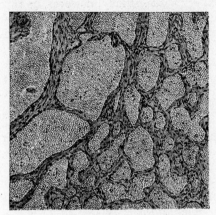

Cavernous hemangioma of the liver.

lacing network of dense connective tissue enclosing fairly large spaces lined with endothelium and filled with blood. It may or may not be definitely encapsulated and sometimes shows connection between the blood spaces and the sinusoids of the liver.

Characteristically, the cavernous hemangioma is benign both pathologically and clinically, but rare cases occur in which the tumor becomes locally invasive. We have observed one case in which the liver weighed more than 16 kg., due to extensive invasion of a cavernous hemangioma. Since the condition occurs more frequently in adults than in children, it is assumed by some that the spaces represent dilatation of sinusoids with disappearance of parenchyma. On the other hand, the condition has so much in common with the hemangiomata of the skin that it is regarded as of congenital origin. In this sense it is looked upon as a hamartoma which, when it undergoes true tumor formation, becomes a hamartoblastoma. It may rarely be associated with similar lesions in other organs.

ADENOMA of the liver is relatively uncommon. The growth may be single or multiple. The size varies from a few millimeters to several centimeters. The tumor may bulge slightly above the capsule, and in cross section is soft, bulging, light yellow, or brown in color and distinctly friable. It is well defined, compresses the surrounding substance and is sometimes encapsulated.

Microscopically, the tumor cells resemble liver cells, irregularly arranged but sometimes with interlacing capillaries between cell cords. It may, however, be tubular or acinic in character probably representing a multiplication of bile ducts. Both the liver-cell adenoma and the tubular biliary adenoma may secrete bile. In the former it appears as masses of pigment within or near the cells and in the latter may so distend the spaces as to produce a cystadenoma.

ADRENAL INCLUSIONS are sometimes observed and may give rise to growth of tumor. FIBROMA, LIPOMA AND NEUROFIBROMA have been observed.

Malignant Tumors. CARCINOMA may be primary or secondary in the liver. Counseller and McIndoe report an incidence of primary carcinoma of 0.14 per cent in 42,276 autopsies. It affects males more often than females and is most common in the fourth and fifth decades of life, although it may occur in infancy and childhood. In adults, Laennec cirrhosis is a common accompaniment (Winternitz; Jaffe; Karsner; McIndoe and Counseller) and the history commonly shows presumptive etiologic factors of cirrhosis together with its symptoms.

Eggel differentiates three forms grossly. In the nodular form there are numerous nodules variable in number and size, usually clearly separated from the liver tissue. In the massive form the tumor constitutes a large mass occupying either an entire lobe or the greater part of it. It is poorly defined and shows neighboring small secondary nodules. In the diffuse form the whole liver is infiltrated with numerous small tumor nodules often no larger than a lobule, each enclosed in a connective tissue band so that the lesion is only differentiated from cirrhosis by the aid of a microscope. It is important to note that in all of these forms the tumor appears as a distinctly invasive and not compressive growth. Icterus is common and the liver may be deeply pigmented.

Microscopically, the carcinoma may be undifferentiated or may resemble an adenocarcinoma. The cells of the former are supposed to originate from hepatic cord cells and the latter from bile ducts, but there is no proof for this assumption. What seem to be acini are often short tubular structures and this form of tumor is really a tubulo-acinic carcinoma. Moderate pleomorphism of cells is found in both forms but mitotic figures are infrequent; invasion is well marked. Bile pigment may be found in tumor and in surrounding liver. The association with cirrhosis suggests that the carcinoma may be the outcome of epithelial proliferation of cirrhosis, but carcinoma occurs without cirrhosis and may even occur in early life (Rosenbusch). Intrahepatic metastasis appears to be common, but what seem to be metastatic nodules may be additional foci of primary carcinoma, i.e., the tumor may be multicentric (McIndoe and Counseller). Invasion of blood vessels is often seen, and metastasis to the lungs is common. Occasionally metastasis is widely distributed.

Secondary carcinoma of the liver is most frequently metastatic from the stomach, but may invade the liver from other parts of the alimentary canal, the organs of the abdominal and pelvic cavities, the respiratory tract, the skin, the breast and other situations. Grossly, the nodules may be multiple or single, usually the former. When multiple, they present a greater degree of uniformity in size than is true of the multiple nodules of primary carcinoma. They grow rather by a combination of invasion and compression and are accordingly more sharply defined than is true of primary carcinoma. Jaundice is less frequent in secondary than in primary carcinoma; cirrhosis is much less frequent and is to be regarded as an incidental finding. The nodules are often pale gray or pale yellow in color, soft, bulge in the cross section and show early necrosis. Nodules in the outer surface, after they have undergone central necrosis, often show a central depression, the so-called umbilication.

SARCOMA. Primary sarcoma is rare and may occur as single or multiple nodules. Spindle-cell sarcoma, round-cell sarcoma and various subvarieties are described. The hemangio-endothelioma is probably also to be included in the group of malignant connective-tissue tumors. Sarcoma appears also to be associated with cirrhosis of the liver

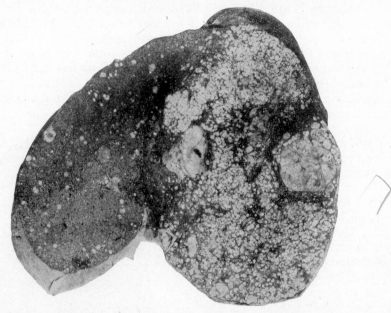

Extensive primary carcinoma of liver. Army Medical Museum No. 39163.

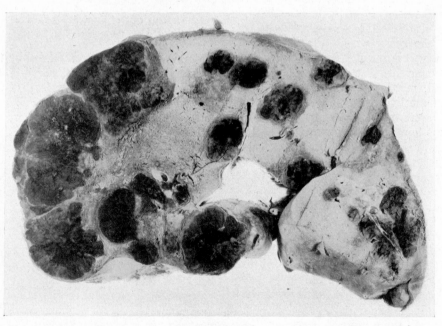

Multiple nodules of metastatic melanoblastoma in liver.

(Jaffe). Experimentally it has been produced by infection with cysticercus fasciolaris (Bullock and Curtis).

The round-cell forms represent some variety of lymphosarcoma. The spindle-cell forms may possibly be confused with spindle-cell formation in carcinoma, in which, as in the thyroid, the reactionary connective-tissue growth may lead to elongation of the epithelial cells. Any form of sarcoma, primary in other situations, may show metastases in the liver. Outstanding among these is the melanoblastoma of the choroid coat of the eye, which apparently produces metastasis in the liver more often and to a greater extent than in other organs. Extensive infiltration of the liver may also occur as secondary to malignant transformation of pigmented moles of the skin.

Cysts

Experimentally, McMaster and Rous have shown that obstruction to the bile passages may lead to wide distention of the ducts, without ballooning of the organ itself, a hydrohepatosis. The failure of marked enlargement of the liver is attributed to the low secretory pressure. In man, local distention may become cystic in character, particularly as the result of cicatricial obstruction to pre-existing bile ducts within the liver, or to secretion within newly formed bile ducts without sufficient outlet. Such cysts are usually small, multiple, occur within the substance of the liver and may contain bile or colorless secretion. More common are multiple cysts immediately under the capsule of the liver, variable in size, projecting above the surface, thin-walled, and usually containing clear limpid fluid. Occasionally a thicker viscid fluid or even bile may be observed. The cysts are usually lined with cylindrical epithelium but occasionally ciliated epithelium or flat epithelium is seen. This appearance is commonly associated with congenital cyst-adenoma of the kidney, and is believed to be due to a congenital fault in the development of the bile passages. Lymphatic cysts have been described. The important parasitic cyst in the liver is the echinococcus cyst.

Parasites

Echinococcus Cysts. Infestation of man by this parasite occurs more frequently in central and northern Europe than elsewhere, and sporadic cases in this country are almost invariably in individuals who have migrated from those parts of the world. The *Taenia echinococcus* occurs in large numbers in the gut of the dog. The worm measures about 6 mm., the head and neck being about

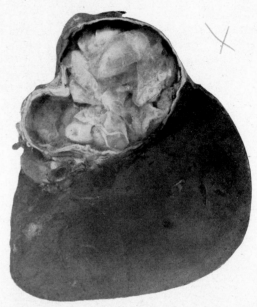

Echinococcus cyst of liver. Army Medical Museum 39163.

3 mm. in length and accompanied by three or four small segments or links. The ova (embryophore) contained in the feces of the dog, may be taken into the intestinal canal of man and a wide variety of other animals. The hexacanthus embryo hatches in the stomach or intestine, bores through the gut wall and is conveyed by either blood or lymph stream to almost any part of the body. This mode of entry predisposes the liver to infestation.

In the liver, as in other organs, there is subsequently formed a slowly growing cysticercus or larval stage. The fully developed cyst shows a wall made up microscopically of concentric laminae of hyaline chitinous-like material, and is lined by the "germinal cells" from which grow "daughter" cysts and in turn "granddaughter" cysts and so on in the same fashion. The parent cyst may grow to great size. The daughter cysts vary in size from a few millimeters to a centimeter or more and often are free in the larger cyst. Their walls are thin and translucent. A low-grade chronic inflammatory reaction about the parent cyst leads to the formation of a fibrous capsule. The cyst content is usually a thin, limpid, colorless fluid, of low specific gravity, containing salt, very little protein, cholesterol, creatin, sometimes sugars presumably derived from glycogen, and other substances. It is irritant to the skin and is said to be toxic for animals. Rupture into the peritoneum may be followed by inflammation, intoxication and even death (Wells). Used as an antigen, the fluid shows precipitin reactions and complement fixation with the patient's serum. The fluid contains scolices, or more often free hooklets, and may

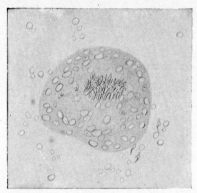

Scolex and hooklets recovered from fluid of echinococcus cyst.

be the source of secondary cysts. In old cysts the fluid may become inspissated and of putty-like character, in which stage daughter cysts, scolices and hooklets are often absent. Rarely, instead of this endogenous formation of daughter cysts, exogenous formation may lead to a more or less focal collection of cysts. (See Loucks; Arce.)

The so-called multilocular echinococcus cyst is rare as a primary condition. It invades the liver widely, producing cysts of variable size, the larger ones of which show a rough, shaggy wall. The contents are often gelatinous in character, the whole condition sometimes resembling mucinous carcinoma. The intervening liver is fibrotic and may show extensive bile duct multiplication. It is believed that this is due to a slightly different worm, the *Taenia multilocularis*, peculiar in larger scolex, larger number of segments, arrangement of uterus and most especially in its

disposition to produce the multilocular cyst in its larval stage.

In Africa and Asia, bilharziasis or schistosomiasis may be accompanied by marked enlargement of liver and spleen. The former may subsequently be much reduced in size because of irregular fibrosis due to the presence of ova of *Bilharzia mansoni* (in Africa) or *Bilharzia japonica* (in Asia). The enlargement of the spleen is due in part to passive hyperemia and in part to the irritation of the ova.

Pentastomum denticulatum, the larval stage of *Pentastomum tenioides*, occurring in the nose of dogs, forms multiple minute nodules in the human liver, sometimes fibrous and more often calcified. Invading more especially the biliary tracts and exciting inflammation in the perilobular connective tissue, occasionally with abscess formation, are rare infestations by *Fasciola hepatica*, *Dicrocelium lanceolatum*, *Opisthorchis felinus*, *Clonorchis sinensis*. *Ascaris lumbricoides* may occur in the larger bile passages and produce icterus (Motta). *Coccidium oviforme* produces papillary proliferation of the biliary passages very commonly in the rabbit and is said to occur in man.

Foreign bodies may be encountered in the liver as the result of wounds or from penetration through some part of the intestinal canal.

GALLBLADDER AND BILE DUCTS

Congenital Anomalies

Absence. The gallbladder may be congenitally absent. It may show a longitudinal fissure sometimes deep enough to divide it into two bladders, even with separate ducts. It may show an hourglass form due to transverse fissure. It may lie under the left lobe. It may be embedded in the substance of the liver or may more rarely be separate as a "floating" gallbladder.

Malformations. Various abnormalities are found in the union of the two main hepatic ducts with each other and with the cystic duct. The common duct may be very short and is sometimes double. It may show abnormalities of union with the pancreatic ducts. The papilla may be double or may be situated high in the duodenum. In congenital

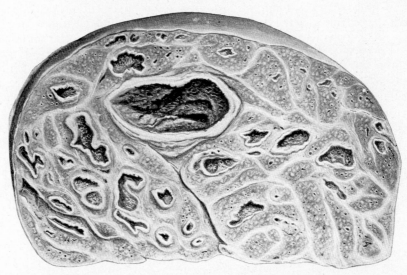

Multilocular echinococcus cysts of liver, showing the usual extensive fibrosis of the
organ and the shaggy lining of the cyst walls.

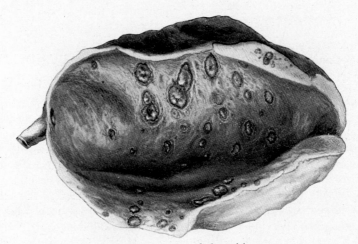

Acute ulcerative cholecystitis.

Lysated ducts 15902

absence of the gallbladder, the common duct may be dilated.

CONGENITAL ATRESIA of the bile ducts is of considerable clinical importance. It may affect any part of the hepatic, cystic or common ducts. The affected parts may be solid cords or entirely absent. The gallbladder may be absent, rudimentary or dilated.

Retrogressive Changes

Passive hyperemia and edema may result from general passive hyperemia or that of hepatic cirrhosis. Minute hemorrhages may occur in these circumstances or may accompany inflammations. Necrosis and gangrene may occur in the rare cases of "floating" gallbladder, when it twists upon the duct. Atrophy may follow chronic inflammations.

Inflammation

The causative agent of inflammation may enter the gallbladder either from the duodenum or by way of the portal circulation, occasionally through the general circulation as in pyemia, sometimes through lymphatics from neighboring inflammation, and rarely as a direct invasion from inflammation of the peritoneum. Various bacteria may be associated, especially colon bacilli, typhoid bacilli, streptococci, staphylococci and others. Transfer of organisms from the intestinal canal may be by inflammation of the ducts or through the blood stream. The acute inflammations may be catarrhal, suppurative, or fibrinous. The chronic inflammations may be catarrhal, suppurative or pseudomembranous forms, and may be a chronic ulcerative type.

Acute Catarrhal Inflammation. It is thought that inflammations of the duodenum may extend into the common duct to produce a catarrhal choledochitis. Formerly it was assumed that painless jaundice of short duration, so-called catarrhal jaundice, is due to obstruction by swelling of the duct or plugging by mucus. It is now generally considered that "catarrhal jaundice" is the result of a mild acute hepatitis, and thus of intrahepatic rather than extrahepatic origin. (Gaskell.) More severe catarrhal inflammation may result from obstruction to the outlet of bile, and infection with organisms such as colon bacillus. Poisons such as phosphorus and arsenic may produce catarrhal inflammations of the intrahepatic ducts. Catarrhs also accompany various infectious diseases, particularly typhoid fever, cholera and smallpox.

When seen at autopsy, catarrhal inflammation is usually an incidental finding. The mucosa is red, swollen, and covered with gray, viscid mucus. Microscopically, there is cloudy swelling and sometimes mucinous degeneration of the epithelium, hyperemia, edema and infiltration of mononuclear cells and a few polymorphonuclears. (See Klemperer, et al.)

Acute Suppurative and Fibrinous Inflammations. The acute suppurative form usually originates in ulcers, which may be secondary to fibrinous inflammation, to chronic ulcerative forms, or to the erosion by gallstones. The suppuration may become extensive, producing a phlegmonous type of cholecystitis or cholangitis. Local inflammation of the surrounding peritoneum may occur; sometimes there is direct invasion of the liver by the abscess; or there may be extension along the intrahepatic bile ducts with the production of multiple abscesses. If the outlet of the gallbladder be obstructed, pus may accumulate within the gallbladder, producing the so-called empyema of the gallbladder. The acute fibrinous forms are often combined with ulcer formation. The ulcer may erode into blood vessels with subsequent hemorrhage, or may perforate through the gallbladder to produce local or general suppurative peritonitis.

Chronic inflammations may follow any of the acute forms. In the usual chronic catarrhal inflammations of the gallbladder there is considerable distention of the bladder with thinning of the walls. Often the content is a thin, only slightly viscid, clear, brown or colorless fluid. More especially in older persons the chronic catarrh may be accompanied by papillary outgrowth from the lining mucosa. On the other hand, the chronic catarrh as well as the acute suppurative and fibrinous inflammations, may lead to a chronic productive or fibroplastic type of inflammation in the entire wall of the gallbladder and ducts, which become considerably thickened due to fibrosis of all the coats. The contraction of the fibrosis tissue may produce interlacing trabeculation of the lining of the gallbladder.

As the process continues the gallbladder is reduced in size and finally may have an extremely small cavity. Sometimes the fibrosis is followed by calcification and even ossification. Accompanying the condition there is likely to be a productive pericholecystitis and pericholangitis with adhesions to the surrounding structures. Chronic ulcerative cholecystitis differs from the other forms principally in the presence of multiple ulcers. It is usually accompanied by cholelithiasis, may perforate, or may lead to suppurative cholangitis. Cholesterol may be deposited in the mucosa of the chronic cholecystitis as multiple miliary nodules, producing the so-called strawberry gallbladder. (See Graham et al.)

Infectious Granulomata

These are rare. Gumma may occur in the gallbladder in either congenital or acquired syphilis, and lead to stenosis or obliteration. Tuberculosis may enter the gallbladder from neighboring tuberculous lymph nodes or the organ may be involved in a generalized miliary tuberculosis. In the more extensive cases, tuberculous ulcers are found in the mucosa. Actinomycosis occasionally involves the gallbladder from intestinal canal or liver.

Cholelithiasis

The composition of biliary concrements and the mechanism of their formation have been discussed in the chapter on Mineral Infiltrates and Concrements. As judged by clinical manifestations, cholelithiasis occurs most commonly between the ages of 30 and 55 years, although it may occur at almost any period of life. It is much more frequent in women than in men and occurs especially during and after pregnancy. There appears to be a familial disposition to the disease, but it is not conclusively demonstrated as hereditary. The most characteristic sign of the presence of concrements is biliary colic, but some cases give only manifestations of irritation or inflammation of the gallbladder and others are entirely symptomless.

From observation of gallbladders obtained at operation and at autopsy, it may be said that concrements may produce no significant lesion of the gallbladder. This appears to be especially true of the multiple-faceted concrements. There may be merely a

slight catarrhal inflammation of bladder and ducts. The sphincter of Oddi does not prevent entry of bacteria from the intestinal canal, and such an irritative catarrh may predispose to inflammations of greater severity, as have been described above. When stones are lodged near the neck of the gallbladder for a con-

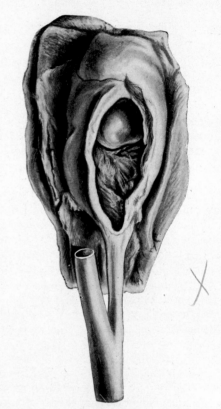

Cholelithiasis.

siderable period, local atrophy with fibrosis and possibly constriction, may occur. Ulceration may take place and this may perforate; if fibrous adhesions have formed, there may be a localized abscess or occasionally perforation into the stomach or duodenum with establishment of fistula; sometimes perforation extends into the peritoneal cavity with development of widespread peritonitis. Lodgment of the concrement in the cystic duct may produce distention of the gallbladder. Lodgment in the common duct may produce jaundice, in prolonged cases obstructive biliary cirrhosis, and if associated with infection, extensive intrahepatic cholangitic multiple abscesses. The prolonged irritation of gallstones may result in carcinoma. Concrements entering the intestinal canal usually pass out in the feces, but rarely may produce intestinal obstruction.

Obstruction of Bile Ducts

This may occur within the liver by tumor invasion or by contraction of fibrous tissue. Obstruction of the extrahepatic ducts may be due to acute inflammations, concrements, foreign bodies or parasites, tumors within or outside the ducts, enlarged lymph nodes and by the contraction of scars in the duodenum or of peritoneal adhesions. The icterus of biliary obstruction is not due to extrahepatic bile formation nor to tearing of bile capillaries but probably to resorption (Scheunert).

Prolonged obstruction may cause extensive dilatation of the ducts (hydrohepatosis), and even though icterus persist, the bile is replaced by a thin colorless fluid secreted by the ducts. Rous and McMaster showed that this fluid is secreted with moderate pressure, is alkaline and practically devoid of cholesterol and cholates. Obstruction of the cystic duct may lead to reduction in size of the gallbladder because of resorption of bile but later the size is increased by secretion from the mucosa. The fluid is like that seen in obstructed ducts except that it is often more viscid because of a richer content of mucus. This is called hydrops of the gallbladder or *hydrops cystidis felleae*. The wall is usually thin and the muscle atrophic, or there may be chronic inflammation. Rupture is rare. Obstruction of the common duct may produce changes like those due to hepatic duct obstruction, but the gallbladder distention is of lesser degree than that seen with cystic duct obstruction.

Tumors

Benign tumors of gallbladder and bile ducts are uncommon, and include papilloma, which may be diffuse, adenoma, which may be cystic, fibroma, neurofibroma, amputation neuroma, myxoma and various mixtures.

Malignant Tumors. Sarcoma occurs, but is rare.

CARCINOMA of the gallbladder is fairly frequent and is much more common in women than in men. Cholelithiasis often accompanies the carcinoma. It may be primary and lead to carcinoma by irritation, or the functional disturbances of the carcinoma may induce the formation of concrements. Sometimes the carcinoma is a localized cauliflower-like mass projecting into the lumen, but usually it is a diffuse infiltrating tumor with direct extension into neighboring structures, especially the liver; it may also produce metastases in the liver. Depending upon the site of the tumor and the degree of fibrosis, the gall-

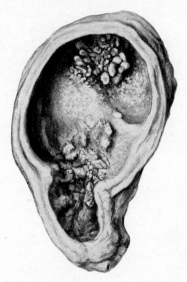

Multiple papillomata of gallbladder.

bladder may be distended or shrunken. The common microscopic form is an undifferentiated cylindrical-cell carcinoma simplex, but adenocarcinoma is frequent and mucinous carcinoma is not rare. Squamous-cell carcinoma occasionally occurs, probably due to epithelial metaplasia in chronically inflamed gallbladders, although metaplasia may occur in cylindrical-cell carcinomas.

Primary carcinoma of the extrahepatic bile ducts is infrequent, occurs more often in men than in women, and is a disease of old age (Shapiro and Lifvendahl). It may be scirrhous or medullary, and usually extends along the ducts. It is usually some variety of adenocarcinoma and is found most often in the common duct, but it may occur in hepatic or cystic duct or at the ampulla. It is not likely to metastasize widely. As a rule there is stenosis of the common duct, sometimes with stenosis of the pancreatic duct and secondary atrophy of the pancreas. As has been mentioned when discussing tumors of the liver, the tubular variety of primary carcinoma of the liver is presumed to originate from intrahepatic bile ducts. Secondary tumors of the gallbladder and of the extrahepatic bile ducts usually invade by direct extension from other situations, but rarely true metastases may be encountered. (See Kirschbaum and Kozoll.)

PANCREAS

Congenital Anomalies

Absence of the pancreas is confined to severe monster formation. The head of the pancreas may be large, may partly or completely encircle the duodenum, or may be almost completely separated from the tail by a small midportion. Accessory pancreas, usually multiple, may be found in jejunum, duodenum, stomach, mesentery and other situations. Accessory spleens may be found in the tail of the pancreas. Transposition occurs in situs viscerum inversus. The duct may be double (persistence of duct of Santorini) and may enter the duodenum or even the stomach independently of the common bile duct. Obliteration of the pancreatic duct may accompany congenital obliteration of the bile ducts.

Retrogressive Changes

The most important pigmentation is that in hemochromatosis. This has been discussed in the chapter on Pathologic Pigmentation. The lesion is usually associated with that type of diabetes known as *diabete bronzé*. The pigments, hemosiderin and hemofuscin, are found in the connective tissue, which is usually increased in amount (fibrosis) and also in cells of the acini and the islets. The organ may be grossly brown in color and is usually firm.

Cloudy swelling and fatty degeneration occur under the usual conditions, such as infectious diseases and various kinds of poisoning. Fat infiltration is often referred to as lipomatosis of the pancreas. It occurs especially in obesity. The fat is found in the interlobular connective tissue, and a variable degree of atrophy of the parenchyma is commonly associated. In extreme cases the organ is a fatty mass with little pancreatic substance visible. Amyloid occurs in the smaller vessels and sometimes in the islets, in cases of extensive amyloidosis. Arterioles are often involved in widespread arteriolar sclerosis and may exhibit hyaline necrosis. Moderate degrees of atrophy are frequent, but rarely atrophy may be so marked that the stools are fatty and the liver may show marked fatty change (Norris, et al.).

Fat necrosis is more truly a fat tissue necrosis involving the cytoplasm and nucleus as well as the fat, and has been discussed in the chapter on Necrosis and Somatic Death. It occurs in acute necrosis, in hemorrhage in the pancreas, in obstruction of the ducts, especially by gallstones, following trauma of the pancreas and any condition which destroys pancreatic tissue and liberates the enzymes. Rare cases are found without identified cause. It affects the fat of the pancreas, omentum, mesentery, abdominal wall and may rarely occur more remotely, as in the liver and subcutaneous fat. The foci rarely exceed a few millimeters in diameter and appear as well-defined, firm, yellow or gray, dry soapy nodules, sometimes surrounded by small zones of hyperemia. The necrosis is apparently due to liberation from the pancreas of lipase and trypsin, the latter destroying cellular tissue and the former splitting the fat. Herbert finds that the necrotic tissue contains neutral fat, fatty acids and soaps, part of which may be crystalline. There is a marked increase of calcium, little of which exists as soap. The product of hydrolysis is acid, with very little soap formation.

Microscopically, many of the fat cells show the cytoplasmic and nuclear change of necrosis. The fat globules are largely replaced by a finely granular basophilic substance, probably calcium and soaps. If crystallization has occurred, acicular spaces are observed due to solution of the crystals in the process of embedding and staining. There may be reactionary marginal hyperemia, usually with hemorrhage, or there may be reactionary inflammation, sometimes suppurative. The glycerol liberated, the amount of fatty acids formed, the amount of soap formed, even though it be slightly soluble, is not sufficient to account for the intoxication which may accompany the condition, so that it is assumed that the causative disease rather than the fat necrosis leads to severe symptoms when they are present.

Circulatory Disturbances

Passive hyperemia occurs with general passive hyperemia. The pancreas may be large, dark red or purple, and firm. Minute hemorrhages are not infrequent in passive hyperemia and in the hemorrhagic diseases. Large hemorrhages are sometimes observed, formerly called pancreatic apoplexy, associated with the signs and symptoms of acute pancreatic necrosis. These hemorrhages are due to acute necrosis, but may be so large as to obscure the necrosis. Rare cases of sudden death may show this hemorrhagic lesion as the only significant observation at autopsy. The mechanism of "pancreatic death" is not known, but there is usually necrosis, hemorrhage or peritonitis.

Acute Pancreatic Necrosis

Much attention has been given to so-called acute hemorrhage and gangrenous pan-

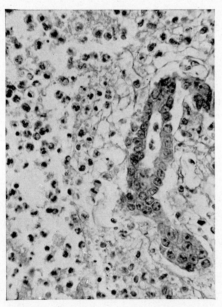

Cellular exudation in acute pancreatic necrosis.

creatitis, but as the lesion is studied it becomes apparent that hemorrhage is secondary to necrosis and that what appears to be gangrene is agonal or postmortem. Thus it is desirable to regard the condition as primarily necrotic in character. The destruction of tissue, however, is likely to be accompanied by hemorrhage, variable in degree, and by exudation. This interpretation differs from that of Fitz in his original communication, but newer methods of study and more extensive material justify it.

Acute hemorrhagic necrosis occurs most frequently in obese individuals in middle life. According to Gruber, 65 per cent of the cases are in females and 35 per cent in males. About 53 per cent of the patients are obese. A history of previous gastro-intestinal disturbance is obtained in from 60 to 70 per cent of the cases. The disease is marked by sudden onset with pain and collapse, and usually runs a rapid course with death in a few days. Surgical operation in early cases shows a swollen and edematous but firm pancreas without discoloration.

Later and at autopsy, when the disease has run its course, the organ is large, firm except for soft areas of necrosis, and discolored by hyperemia and hemorrhage. As indicated above, hemorrhage may be massive. Especially if the autopsy be deferred, postmortem changes advance rapidly so that the color becomes gray or black and the odor foul. It may be that gangrene can occur in life from extension of saprophytes from the intestine, but it is practically never observed at surgical operations.

Microscopically, foci of necrosis of the pancreatic tissue, variable in size, are found. Surrounding and extending into these is inflammatory exudation, with many polymorphonuclear leukocytes, variable numbers of lymphocytes and large mononuclears, not infrequently enmeshed in fibrin. The degree of hemorrhage may be slight, moderate or massive. Blood vessels may show destruction, complete or partial, in the necrotic masses. Arteritis and phlebitis, with or without thrombosis, are sometimes found, but they are usually remote from rather than near the regions of necrosis. Arteriolitis may also be found. Fat necrosis, as described above, is practically constant.

The abdominal cavity often contains a serous or serohemorrhagic exudate, which was thought to be responsible for the shock-like or toxic manifestations, but Whipple and also Ireneus found that this material is not poisonous. Dragstedt believes that the poisonous material, supposed to operate in the disease, is made up of proteinogenous amines from bacterial decomposition of proteins or their split products.

In prolonged cases, or occasionally in those of short duration, inflammatory reactions, often with suppuration, may extend widely in the greater and lesser abdominal cavities, into retroperitoneal tissues and ultimately around the kidneys or into the thorax. In the widely extensive disease, dead pancreatic tissue may lie free as a sphacelus. Thrombosis in the splenic veins may be severe

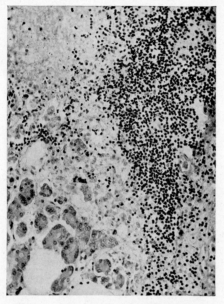

Hemorrhage in acute pancreatic necrosis.

and extensive. Gruber reports the occurrence of diabetes in some of a small number of patients who have recovered from the necrosis.

The pathogenesis of the disease has been extensively studied. The problems concern anatomic relations of the biliary and pancreatic ducts, disease within or around the pancreatic ducts, the possible action of bile or of pancreatic juice, vascular injury and infection. In a small number of cases, it is found that a stone is lodged in the ampulla of Vater and that the entrance of the pancreatic duct is in such a position that bile could flow into it (Opie). It is thought that inflammation of the common duct and perhaps spasm of the sphincter of Oddi may have the same effect.

Dragstedt and his associates believe

that the bile salts destroy the walls of small ducts so as to permit destructive action upon the gland. Experiments indicate that other irritative substances may have the same effect. In their opinion it is not necessary to assume that differential pressure between the biliary and pancreatic systems is necessarily of significance, because anastomosis of the ductal systems of Wirsung and Santorini may provide for a common channel with outflow from the latter duct. Rich and Duff believe that there must be pressure within the ductules sufficient to produce rupture and that inactivated or activated pancreatic trypsin injures blood vessels with consequent hemorrhage and necrosis. Whether activation is necessary or not is a disputed point. Conclusive evidence that vascular injury is primary is still wanting. Experimental infarction produces localized necrosis but this does not go on to widespread disease (Smyth).

Both clinically and at autopsy there is a high incidence of disease of the biliary passages in cases of pancreatic necrosis, but from the other point of view pancreatic necrosis is not a frequent complication of disease of biliary passages (Weiner and Tennant). Bacteria are secondary invaders rather than causative. Rich and Duff emphasize the frequently observed metaplastic proliferation of lining epithelium of small ducts as a cause of obstruction with resultant increased pressure, rupture and vascular injury. Ligation of the main duct, however, leads to atrophy rather than necrosis. The onset of the disease often follows a heavy meal or consumption of alcohol, but neither experimentally nor in man can the disease be related definitely to secretory activity of the pancreas. It cannot be said that any of the conditions outlined above is constantly present.

Inflammation

Acute Inflammations. The term acute pancreatitis can well be limited to those conditions in which the inflammation is considered to be the primary event, even although necrosis and hemorrhage may supervene. Suppuration in the pancreas may be due to direct extension of a peptic ulcer into the organ, involvement of the pancreas as the result of purulent peritonitis of the lesser peritoneal cavity, or similar inflammation in other nearby organs, and rarely occurs as a part of pyemia.

Conversely abscess of the pancreas may rupture into the greater or lesser peritoneal cavity or into neighboring organs such as the stomach. Abscess of the pancreas shows the usual gross and microscopic features of abscess in any situation, except that there is usually an associated fat necrosis. Only rarely is acute pancreatic necrosis or hemorrhage severe. Diffuse nonsuppurative inflammations may be observed as an uncommon complication of mumps.

Chronic Inflammations. As age advances, the amount of supporting connective tissue of the pancreas gradually increases,

nal perisialodochitis." In the interacinar forms, the connective-tissue growth is principally between the acini separating them, thus rendering them more distinct. Rarely, the connective tissue may extend into the acini and isolate individual cells. This interacinar form of pancreatitis is more frequently associated with diabetes mellitus, than is the interlobular form.

The causes of chronic interstitial pancreatitis include all those causes which may produce fibrosis in various internal viscera, such as chronic poisoning either of internal origin including gout, rheumatism, etc., or of external origin, such as alcohol, lead and other ingested poisons. Of especial impor-

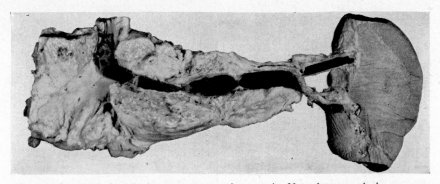

Thrombosis of splenic vein in acute pancreatic necrosis. Note fat necrosis in pancreas.

and it is sometimes difficult to distinguish in adult life between minor degrees of chronic pancreatitis and the ordinary increase in connective tissue. As a rule, however, foci of lymphoid and other mononuclear cells, or wide distribution of these cells, indicate the inflammatory nature of the condition. Opie recognizes two varieties of chronic interstitial pancreatitis, namely, the interlobular and the interacinic. In either case the organ is distinctly firmer than normal, and when the connective tissue is interlobular the broad bands of connective tissue separating the parenchyma may be visible in the cross section of the organ.

Microscopically, the interlobular forms show definite overgrowth of connective tissue, which separates more distinctly the pancreatic lobules. In this condition, overgrowth of connective tissue separating the acini is not likely to be at all marked. Rarely, the overgrowth of connective tissue may be so definitely distributed about the pancreatic duct as to justify the term "chronic abdomi-

tance is the fact that obstruction to the pancreatic duct by calculi, either within the pancreatic duct or in the ampulla of Vater, obstruction by the presence of tumors or chronic inflammatory masses, is followed by atrophy, or disappearance of the acini, overgrowth of connective tissue, and persistence of the islands of Langerhans. Chronic interstitial pancreatitis is sometimes associated with cirrhosis of the liver and it seems probable that the cause of the latter operates to produce the former. Some cases are entirely obscure as to origin.

Infectious Granulomata

Tuberculosis rarely affects the pancreas. Even in most advanced cases of generalized miliary tuberculosis, the pancreas often escapes, and when miliary tubercles are reported they are usually in the interstitial tissue rather than in the parenchyma. Tuberculous involvement may extend from tuberculosis of neighboring lymph nodes and other organs.

In congenital syphilis, the pancreas is often found to be large and firm. Microscopically, it shows what may be signified as a more or less specific form of chronic interstitial pancreatitis. As with other organs in congenital syphilis, the parenchyma is poorly developed and the acini are likely to show fewer cells than in normally developed organs. The mesoblastic tissue remains in excess and shows greater or lesser differentiation toward the adult type of interstitial connective tissue. Perivascular and adventitial infiltration of lymphoid cells is likely to be prominent. Special stains show large numbers of spirochetes. The relative increase of connective tissue affects the intralobular and interacinar connective tissue, and there may be intra-acinar fibrosis. Acquired syphilis may show diffuse interlobular or interacinar fibrosis, with infiltration of small and large mononuclear and plasma cells. Gumma of the pancreas is rare.

Tumors

The benign tumors are relatively infrequent and include lipoma, myxoma, chondroma and fibroma. Adenomas of the duct-acinar system may be solid or cystic, the latter being sometimes papilliferous.

ISLET CELL ADENOMAS are infrequent but are of importance because some are associated with the syndrome of hypoglycemia. Surgical removal usually results in cure. Neither grossly nor microscopically are there criteria by which those associated with hypoglycemia can be distinguished from those which are not. It is probable that there are no differences in number or character of the beta cells. Hypoglycemia is not likely to be associated with these tumors in older age groups. Although the adenoma may be found in any part of the pancreas, it is most frequent in the tail; only rarely is there more than one.

Grossly, the tumor is generally spherical, 1 or 2 cm. in diameter or larger, darker in color than the surrounding pancreas, well defined with compression of neighboring pancreas and sometimes encapsulated. Microscopically, the cells are like the cuboidal or polygonal cells of the normal islet, arranged in cords which are separated from each other by numerous capillaries; the appearance closely resembles that of a greatly enlarged islet. Occasionally small tubules or acini are seen. The tumor is probably derived from ductules rather than from pre-existent islets. (See Duff.)

Malignant Tumors. PRIMARY CARCINOMA of the pancreas may be of islet cell type or of acinus-duct type. The former is rare and may be accompanied by hypoglycemia. The carcinoma derived from ducts or acini is the

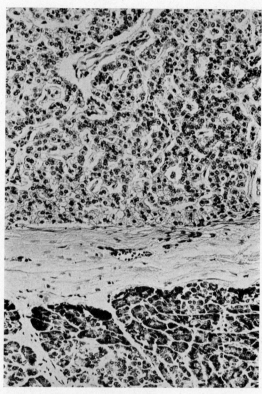

Adenoma of pancreas. Above are the cellular cords of the adenoma. Below the capsule of the tumor is pancreatic tissue.

most frequent tumor of the pancreas. It affects males much more often than females, occurs principally in later middle life and runs a rapid course. It originates in the head of the pancreas far more often than in the tail; it may spread widely in the organ.

Grossly, the tumor is more frequently a scirrhous than a medullary carcinoma. It may be a large projecting mass of several centimeters in diameter or may be so small as to be found with difficulty. Microscopically, it is possible to distinguish the carcinoma simplex and the adenocarcinoma. True mucinous carcinoma is infrequent. Very rarely the carcinoma may show metaplasia with the formation of squamous epithelial cells. The size and shape of the cells varies in different carcinomas and it is suggested that if the type of cell be of large round form, the origin is from the acinic cells; if the cells be cylindrical in character it is supposed that the tumor originates in the pancreatic ducts. The determination of derivation purely on the

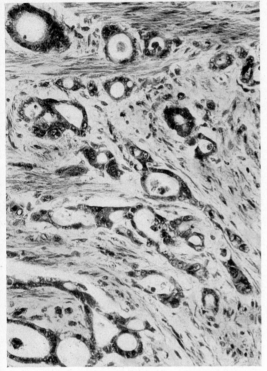

Scirrhous adenocarcinoma of pancreas.

basis of cells found is often fallacious. The tumor may extend directly into the duodenum and into the neighboring peritoneum.

Metastases occur principally to the regional lymph nodes and in a large percentage of cases to the liver. Occasionally they may be widespread. The presence of the tumor may cause obstruction to the pancreatic duct and resultant fatty stools. Involvement and compression of the common duct may produce icterus. Tumor thrombi may occur in the portal veins with all the sequences of stagnation of circulation in the portal area. Rarely intestinal obstruction is caused by the carcinoma. Destruction of the pancreas may be so extensive as to produce diabetes mellitus, but this is rare.

THE SARCOMA is a rare primary tumor in the pancreas and is said to occur most frequently in the head of the organ. It is usually a lymphosarcoma but may be a spindle-cell sarcoma or other type.

SECONDARY TUMORS in the pancreas are not especially common. Secondary carcinoma sometimes occurs. Of the sarcomas which may be secondary in the pancreas, the melanoblastoma is distinctly the most frequent.

Cysts

There are three forms of true cysts of the pancreas which show a lining of epithelial cells, and in addition a fourth form which is referred to as pseudocyst or cystoid.

The so-called proliferation cysts such as occur in adenoma and adenocarcinoma are among the true cysts.

Cystic fibrosis of the pancreas is of great importance in young children. It is probably congenital and due to dysontogenetic and unbalanced growth of ducts and mesoblast. The organ is small, firm and contains numerous thick walled cysts, a few millimeters to a centimeter in diameter. Microscopically, there is marked fibrosis, dilatation of the ducts, and cysts with a single layer of lining epithelium and containing acidophilic homogeneous or laminated concrementous material. Its occurs in infancy and childhood, is about twice as frequent in girls as in boys and is the basis of one of the forms of celiac disease, fatty diarrhea, pulmonary disease (including bronchopneumonia, bronchiectasis and abscess) and often is accompanied by deficiency of vitamin A. (See Anderson.)

Retention cysts may involve the larger ducts of the pancreas either in a diffuse general dilatation or a more nodular type of dilatation. This is usually due to calculi in the ducts, to pressure or invasion by tumor, or compression by inflammatory masses. Multiple retention cysts are observed occasionally in the smaller ducts, due apparently to fibrosis of the organ leading to compression of the smaller divisions of the duct system.

Pseudocysts or cystoids are believed to originate principally from hemorrhage or trauma and represent subsequent encystment of a hematoma. These are usually solitary, large, occur in the tail of the pancreas, and project outside the organ, sometimes ultimately becoming more or less separated from it. The contents may be serous, serosanguinous or bloody.

Pancreatic Calculi

These are probably entirely the result of inflammatory disease in the duct, since experimental ligation of the duct does not lead to their formation. As with the salivary glands, the calculi are usually made up of calcium phosphate or in some instances of calcium carbonate, and in the pancreas there is usually a mixture of other salts. The calculi may be single or multiple and often attain considerable size. They are granular on the outer surface, pale yellow or grayish-white in color, soft and easily broken up. They may lead to obstruction of the duct, with consequent atrophy of the parenchymatous substance, other than the islets of Langerhans, and considerable fibrosis. There may be moderate or cystic dilatation of the larger ducts, usually associated with a chronic catarrh. Occasionally fat necrosis takes place. In some instances secondary infection occurs and suppuration ensues.

Foreign Bodies and Parasites

The most important foreign body is the gallstone. This, situated in the pancreatic duct, may show additional deposits of calcium salts, and depending upon the degree of obstruction, leads to the sequences enumerated above under pancreatic calculi. The animal parasites include the echinococcus cyst, occasionally ascarids and rarely some of the forms of distoma.

Pancreatic Disease in Diabetes Mellitus

The functional relation of the islets of the pancreas to sugar metabolism is well established, although there is an interrelation of the islet function with that of other endocrines, notably the pituitary and adrenal. Nevertheless, anatomic lesions of the pancreas are not constantly present in diabetes mellitus. These may be considered as they bear on disease of the pancreas as a whole or on lesions of the islets. Among the former are included fibrosis, fat infiltration, arteriosclerosis, acute pancreatic necrosis, abscess, carcinoma and others. Diabetes occurs in connection with these lesions, but destruction of the organ must be extensive, involving ap-

proximately seven-eighths of the gland in order to be significant. Hydropic degeneration of the islet cells may occur but it is by no means frequent.

Other changes in the islets include fibrosis which ultimately replaces the islets and becomes hyalinized, lymphocytic infiltration, fat infiltration, and hemorrhage. Fibrosis and hyalinization seem to be more frequent

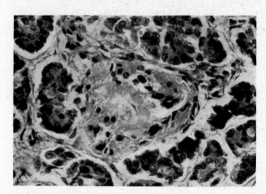

Fibrosis of an islet of Langerhans in a case of diabetes.

in the islets of diabetics than of others, but many cases do not show these changes and the changes are not uncommon in nondiabetics. There are, then, no regular or diagnostic lesions in the pancreas. (See Warren.) Infants born of diabetic mothers may show more or less marked increase in size of the islets, but this is not constant and may occur in infants of nondiabetic mothers (see Potter, et al.).

The lesions in the islets may vary markedly in the same pancreas and a considerable number may be normal. Glycogen infiltration of the cells of Henle's loops in the kidneys, ordinarily common, is often absent in insulin-treated cases. There is likely to be fibrosis of myocardium, arteriosclerosis and vascular disease of the kidneys. The vascular lesions probably are the important feature in causing infarction of extremities (gangrene) frequent in diabetics, especially those who are obese. (See Warren.)

REFERENCES

Albrecht, F.: Pathologie der Bauchspeicheldrüse, Ergebn. d. allg. Path. u. path. Anat., 15(2): 783, 1911.

Allen, F. M., E. Stillman, and R. Fitz: Total Dietary Regulation in the Treatment of Diabetes,

Monograph No. 11, Rock. Inst. for Med. Res., New York, 1919.

Anderson, D.: Cystic Fibrosis of the Pancreas and Its Relation to Celiac Disease, Amer. Jour. Dis. Child., 56: 344, 1938.

Arce, J.: Hydatid Disease (Hydatidosis): Pathology and Treatment, Arch. Surg., 42: 1, 1941.

Armstrong, E. L., W. L. Adams, L. J. Tragerman, and W. E. Townsend: The Cruveilhier-Baumgarten Syndrome; Review of the Literature and Report of Two Additional Cases, Ann. Int. Med., 16: 113, 1942.

Askanazy, M.: Comptes Rendus de la Premiere Conference Internationale de Pathologie Geographique, Geneva, Kundig, 1932.

Belt, T. H.: Liver Necrosis Following Burns, Simulating the Lesions of Yellow Fever, Jour. Path. and Bact., 48: 493, 1939.

Bloomfield, A. L.: The Natural History of Chronic Hepatitis (Cirrhosis of the Liver), Amer. Jour. Med. Sci., 195: 429, 1938.

Buis, L. J., and F. W. Hartman: Histopathology of the Liver Following Superficial Burns, Amer. Jour. Clin. Path., 11: 275, 1941.

Bullock, F. D., and M. R. Curtis: Further Studies on the Transplantation of the Larvae of Taenia Crassicollis, etc., J. Cancer Res., 10: 393, 1926.

Connor, C. L.: Fatty Infiltration of the Liver in the Development of Cirrhosis in Diabetes and Chronic Alcoholism, Amer. Jour. Path., 14: 347, 1938.

———: The Etiology and Pathogenesis of Alcoholic Cirrhosis of the Liver, Jour. Amer. Med. Asso., 112: 387, 1939.

Counseller, V. S., and A. H. McIndoe: Primary Carcinoma of the Liver, Arch. Int. Med., 37: 363. 1926.

Dock, W.: The Role of Increased Hepatic Arterial Flow in the Portal Hypertension of Cirrhosis, Trans. Asso. Amer. Phys., Vol. 57, 1942, in press.

Dragstedt, L. R., H. E. Haymond, and J. C. Ellis: Pathogenesis of Acute Pancreatitis (Acute Pancreatic Necrosis), Arch. Surg., 28: 232, 1934.

Duff, G. L.: The Pathology of Islet Cell Tumors of the Pancreas, Amer. Jour. Med. Sci., 203: 437, 1942.

Earle, D. P., Jr., and J. Victor: The Effect of Various Diets on the Liver Damage Caused by Excess Cystine, Jour. Exper. Med., 75: 179, 1942.

Eggel, H.: Ueber das primäre Carcinom der Leber, Beiträge z. path. Anat. u. z. allg. Path., 30: 506, 1901.

Eppinger, H.: Die Leberkrankheiten, Vienna, Springer, 1937.

Ewing, J.: Neoplastic Diseases, Ed. 4, Philadelphia and London, 1940.

Fitz, R. H.: Acute Pancreatitis, Med. Record, 35: 197, 225, 253, 1889.

Gaskell, J. F.: The Changes in the Liver in a Fatal Case of Epidemic "Catarrhal" Jaundice, Jour. Path. and Bact., 36: 257, 1933.

Graham, E. A., W. H. Cole, G. H. Copher, and S. Moore: Diseases of the Gall Bladder and Bile Ducts, London, 1923; Elman, R., and E. A. Graham: The Pathogenesis of the "Strawberry" Gallbladder (Cholesterosis of the Gallbladder), Arch. Surg., 24: 14, 1932.

Gruber, G. B.: Pathologie der Bauchspeicheldruse, Henke-Lubarsch Handbuch d. spez. path. Anat. u. Hist., Berlin, Springer, 5², p. 211, 1929.

György, P., and H. Goldblatt: Observations on the Conditions of Dietary Hepatic Injury (Necrosis, Cirrhosis) in Rats, Jour. Exper. Med., 75: 355, 1942.

Hall, E. M., and W. Ophüls: Progressive Alcoholic Cirrhosis, Amer. Jour. Path., 1: 477, 1925.

Herbert, F. K.: Pancreatic Fat Necrosis, a Chemical Study, Brit. Jour. Exper. Path., 9: 57, 1928.

Herxheimer, G.: Zur Aetiologie und pathologischen Anatomie der Syphilis, Ergeb. d. allg. Path. u. path. Anat., 11¹: 1, 1906; Zur pathologischen Anatomie der kongenitalen Syphilis, ibid., 12: 499, 1908.

Ireneus, C., Jr.: Experimental Bile Pancreatitis with Special Reference to Recovery and to the Toxicity of the Hemorrhagic Exudate, Arch. Surg., 42: 126, 1941.

Jaffe, R. H.: Sarcoma and Carcinoma of the Liver Following Cirrhosis, Arch. Int. Med., 33: 330, 1924.

Judd, E. S., and V. S. Counsellor: The Effects of Obstructive Lesions of the Common Duct of the Liver, Jour. Amer. Med. Asso., 89: 1751, 1927; see also Counsellor, V. S.: Ann. Surg., 87: 210, 1928.

Kapeller-Adler, R.: Significance of Isolation of Histamine from the Urine in the Toxaemia of Pregnancy, Jour. Obst. and Gynec., Brit. Emp., 48: 155, 1941.

Karsner, H. T.: A Clinicopathological Study of Primary Carcinoma of the Liver, Arch. Int. Med., 8: 238, 1911.

——— and J. C. Aub: An Investigation of the Origin of Immune Serum Necrosis of the Liver, Jour. Med. Research, 28: 377, 1913.

Katzin, H. M., J. V. Waller, and H. L. Blumgart: "Cardiac Cirrhosis" of the Liver: A Clinical and Pathologic Study, Arch. Int. Med., 64: 457, 1939.

Keschner, H. W., and Klemperer, P.: Frequency and Significance of Hepatic Edema, Arch. Path., 22: 583, 1936.

Kirschbaum, J. D., and D. D. Kozoll: Carcinoma of the Gall Bladder and Extrahepatic Bile Ducts. A Clinical and Pathological Study of 117 Cases in 13,330 Necropsies, Surg., Gynec. and Obst., 73: 740, 1941.

Klemperer, P., J. A. Killian, and C. G. Heyd: The Pathology of "Icterus Catarrhalis," Arch. Path. and Lab. Med., 2: 631, 1926.

Krieg, E. G.: Hepatic Trauma. Analysis of Sixty Cases, Arch. Surg., 32: 907, 1936.

Lillie, R. D., F. S. Daft, and W. H. Sebrell, Jr.: Cirrhosis of the Liver in Rats on a Deficient Diet and the Effect of Alcohol, Publ. Health Rep., 56: 1255, 1941.

List, C. F.: Ueber das Problem der hypertrophischen Leberzirrhose an Hand von zwei sezierten Fällen, Frank. Zeitschr. f. Path., 34: 242, 1926.

Loucks, H. H.: Hydatid Cyst. A Review and a Report of Cases from North China, Nat. Med. Jour. China, 16: 402, 1930.

MacMahon, H. E., and F. B. Mallory: Obstructive Cirrhosis, Amer. Jour. Path., 5: 645, 1929.

———: Infectious Cirrhosis, Amer. Jour. Path., 7: 77, 1931.

Mallory, F. B.: A Histological Study of Typhoid Fever, Jour. Exper. Med., 3: 611, 1898; Necroses of the Liver, Jour. Med. Research, 6: 264, 1901; Chronic Passive Congestion of the Liver, ibid., 24: 455, 1911; Cirrhosis of the Liver, Five Different Types of Lesions from Which It May Arise, Johns Hopk. Hosp. Bull., 22: 69, 1911.

Mann, F. C.: The Effects of Complete and Partial Removal of the Liver, Medicine, 6: 419, 1927.

McIndoe, A. H.: Vascular Lesions of Portal Cirrhosis, Arch. Path. & Lab. Med., 5: 23, 1928.

McIndoe, A. H., and V. S. Counseller: Primary Carcinoma of the Liver of Possible Multicentric Origin Occurring in a Case of Portal Cirrhosis, Amer. Jour. Path., 2: 557, 1926.

McMaster, P. D., and P. Rous: Hydrohepatosis, a Condition Analogous to Hydronephrosis, Proc. Nat. Acad. Sci., 9: 19, 1923.

Miller, L. L., J. F. Ross, and G. H. Whipple: Methionine and Cystine, Specific Protein Factors Preventing Chloroform Liver Injury in Protein-depleted Dogs, Amer. Jour. Med. Sci., 200: 739, 1940.

Moon, V. H.: Infection as a Cause of Juvenile Cirrhosis, Amer. Jour. Med. Sci., 177: 681, 1929; Histogenesis of Atrophic Cirrhosis, Arch. Path., 13: 691, 1932; Experimental Cirrhosis in Relation to Human Cirrhosis, Arch. Path., 18: 381, 1934.

Morgan, D. R., M. M. Lieber, and H. L. Stewart: Hepatic Infarction in Myelogenous Leukemia and Periarteritis Nodosa, Amer. Jour. Med. Sci., 192: 540, 1936.

Motta, L. C.: Ascariasis of Intrahepatic Bile Ducts, Jour. Amer. Med. Asso., 82: 85, 1924.

Norris, E. H., A. H. Beard, and L. S. Gerber: Atrophy of the Pancreas with Extreme Fatty Metamorphosis of the Liver and Steatorrhea, Arch. Path., 26: 1234, 1938.

Opie, E. L.: Zonal Necrosis of the Liver, Jour. Med. Research, 12: 147, 1904; Diseases of the Pancreas, Philadelphia, Lippincott, 1903.

Palmer, R. B.: Changes in the Liver in Amebic Dysentery with Special Reference to the Origin of Amebic Abscess, Arch. Path., 25: 327, 1938.

Pearce, R. M.: The Experimental Production of Liver Necroses by the Intravenous Injection of Hemagglutinins, Jour. Med. Research, 12: 329, 1904; Regenerative Changes in the Liver, ibid., 15: 99, 1906.

Post, J., and A. J. Patek, Jr.: Serum Proteins in Cirrhosis of the Liver. I. Relation to Prognosis and to Formation of Ascites, Arch. Int. Med., 69: 67, 1942.

Potter, E. L., H. P. G. Seckel, and W. A. Stryker: Hypertrophy and Hyperplasia of the Islets of Langerhans of the Fetus and of the Newborn Infant, Arch. Path., 31: 467, 1941.

Reich, N. E.: Primary Portal Phlebosclerosis, Arch. Int. Med., 69: 117, 1942.

Reichle, H. S.: Toxic Cirrhosis of Liver due to Cinchophen, Arch. Int. Med., 44: 281, 1929.

Rich, A. R., and G. L. Duff: Experimental and Pathological Studies on the Pathogenesis of Acute Hemorrhagic Pancreatitis, Bull. Johns Hopkins Hosp., 58: 212, 1936.

Rich, A. R., and J. D. Hamilton: The Experimental Production of Cirrhosis of the Liver by Means of a Deficient Diet, Bull. Johns Hopkins Hosp., 66: 185, 1940.

——: Further Studies on Cirrhosis of the Liver Produced by a Dietary Deficiency, Trans. Asso. Amer. Phys., 55: 133, 1940.

Roger, G. H.: Physiologie Normale et Pathologique du Foie, Paris, 1922.

Roman, B.: Acute Yellow Atrophy of the Liver, Arch. Path. & Lab. Med., 4: 399, 1927.

Rosenbusch, H.: Zur Enstehung des primären Lebercarcinoms, Virchow's Arch. f. path. Anat., 261: 326, 1926.

Rous, P., and P. D. McMaster: The Concentrating Activity of the Gall Bladder, Jour. Exper. Med., 34: 47, 1921; Physiological Causes for the Varied Character of Stasis Bile, ibid., 34: 75, 1921; Rous, P.: The Biliary Aspects of Liver Disease, Amer. Jour. Med. Sci., 170: 625, 1925.

Scheunert, G.: Die Morphologie des experimentellen Stauungsikterus, Beitr. z. path. Anat. u. z. allg. Path., 86: 455, 1931.

Schiller, W.: Liver Cell Fat Necrosis Caused by Pancreatic Reflux, Surg., Gynec. and Obst., 72: 70, 1941.

Schultz, E. W., E. M. Hall, and H. V. Baker: Repair of the Liver Following Injection of Chloroform into the Portal System, Jour. Med. Research, 44: 207, 1923-24.

Shapiro, P. F., and R. A. Lifvendahl: Tumors of the Extrahepatic Bile-Ducts, Ann. Surg., 94: 61, 1931.

Smyth, C. J.: Etiology of Acute Hemorrhagic Pancreatitis with Special Reference to the Vascular Factors. An Analysis of Autopsies and an Experimental Investigation, Arch. Path., 30: 651, 1940.

Snell, A. M., and H. R. Butt: Hepatic Coma: Observations Bearing on Its Nature and Treatment, Trans. Asso. Amer. Phys., 51: 321, 1941.

Spellberg, M. A., R. W. Keeton, and R. Ginsberg: Dietary Production of Hepatic Cirrhosis in Rabbits, with an Analysis of the Factors Involved, Arch. Path., 33: 204, 1942.

Stander, H. J.: The Toxemias of Pregnancy, Medicine, 8: 1, 1929.

Warren, S.: The Pathology of Diabetes Mellitus, Philadelphia, Lea & Febiger, Ed. 2, 1938.

Warthin, A. S.: The New Pathology of Syphilis, Harvey Lectures, Philadelphia, 1917-19, p. 67; Syphilis of the Pancreas with Reference to the Coincidence of Syphilitic Pancreatitis and Diabetes, Trans. Asso. Amer. Physicians, 31: 387, 1916.

Weiner, H. A., and R. Tennant: A Statistical Study of Acute Hemorrhagic Pancreatitis (Hemorrhagic Necrosis of Pancreas), Amer. Jour. Med. Sci., 196: 167, 1938.

Wells, D. B., H. D. Humphrey, and J. J. Coll: The Relation of Tannic Acid to Liver Necrosis Occurring in Burns, New England Jour. Med., 226: 629, 1942.

Wells, H. G.: Chemical Pathology, 4th ed., Philadelphia, 1920.

Whipple, G. H.: A Test for Hepatic Injury: Blood Lipase, Johns Hopkins Hosp. Bull., 24: 357, 1913; Pregnancy and Chloroform Anaesthesia, Jour. Exper. Med., 15: 246, 1912; Insusceptibility of Pups to Chloroform Poisoning During the First Three Weeks of Life, ibid., 15: 259, 1912; Acute Hemorrhagic Pancreatitis, etc., Surg., Gynec. and Obst., 17: 541, 1913.

Whipple, G. H., and J. A. Sperry: Chloroform Poisoning, Liver Necrosis and Repair, Johns Hopkins Hosp. Bull., 20: 278, 1909.

Wilder, R. M.: Clinical Diabetes and Hyperinsulinism, Philadelphia, Saunders, 1940.

Winternitz, M. C.: Tuberculosis of the Stomach: Tuberculous Cavities of the Liver; with Report of a Case, Johns Hopkins Hosp. Bull., 19: 223, 1908; The Effect of Occlusion of the Various Hepatic Vessels upon the Liver, ibid., 22: 396, 1911; Primary Carcinoma of the Liver, Johns Hopkins Hosp. Reports, **17**: 143, 1916.

Wirtschafter, Z. T., and M. Korenberg: Diabetes Mellitus, Baltimore, Williams & Wilkins, 1942.

Zimmerman, H. M.: Infarcts of the Liver and the Mechanism of their Production: Report of a Case, Arch. Path., **10**: 66, 1930.

Zimmerman, H. M., and J. A. Hillsman: Chronic Passive Congestion of the Liver: An Experimental Study, Arch. Path., **9**: 1154, 1930.

18

The Urinary System

THE KIDNEYS

Congenital Anomalies

Agenesis and Hypoplasia. Bilateral absence, agenesis or aplasia, of the kidneys is rare, is incompatible with life and is associated with monster formation. Unilateral agenesis is not uncommon and is observed especially on the right side and in males (Huffman). The opposite kidney is usually hypertrophic and attains a weight equal to that of two normal kidneys. Bilateral hypoplasia is rare and incompatible with life.

Unilateral hypoplasia is infrequent and the opposite kidney shows a corresponding hypertrophy.

The fused or horseshoe kidney is unusual but not rare, having been found according to Keyes in 30 cases in 21,218 autopsies. The lower poles of the two kidneys are connected either by an isthmus of renal substance or by a connective tissue band. Fusion at other parts is extremely rare. The renal pelves may be fused, or separate, or may be anomalous. The ureters pass anterior to the isthmus and they, as well as the arteries, may be anomalous.

Dystopia, congenital misplacement of the kidney, indicates an anomaly dependent upon a failure of the kidney to ascend to the normal position. The kidney may therefore be found in the lower abdomen or pelvis. This anomaly usually affects the left kidney but may affect both. Such a position of the kidney may lead to erroneous clinical diagnoses of tumor or inflammatory mass. More or less complex anomalies of arteries and veins and malformations of parts of the genital tract are frequently associated with dystopia of the kidney (Huffman).

Fetal lobulation of the kidneys is a persistence into adult life of the fetal lobes and is so common as to be regarded as normal. Frequently in adult life the two poles of the kidneys are found to be separated by an ingrowth of cortex, often with more or less complete division of the renal pelvis into two parts, called bipolar kidney. Accessory kidneys are rare.

The congenital anomalies of the types mentioned are usually ascribed to misplacement or other alteration of the renal buds (Huntington). The congenital cystic kidney will be considered with cysts.

Acquired Alterations of Position

Nephroptosis, or floating or movable kidney, is an acquired downward displace-

586

ment of the organ which is more common in women, especially those of advanced years, and affects the right more often than the left kidney. Although it may occasionally be congenital, it occurs usually in connection with general ptosis of the abdominal viscera such as may be observed in old age with wasting of the belly fat, or as a sequel of pregnancy. Downward displacement of the liver from tight lacing or the weight of tumors, atrophy of fat in wasting diseases, and even trauma,

of prolonged passive hyperemia. The iron-bearing pigment is found in the cells of the convoluted tubules and sometimes in other parts of the tubules. Rarely it is found in the interstitial connective tissue. Hemoglobinemia, after passing the threshold of excretion by the kidney, leads to hemoglobinuria. This occurs especially in the so-called blackwater fever of malaria, poisoning by potassium chlorate, extensive burns of the body surface; it is occasionally observed in the

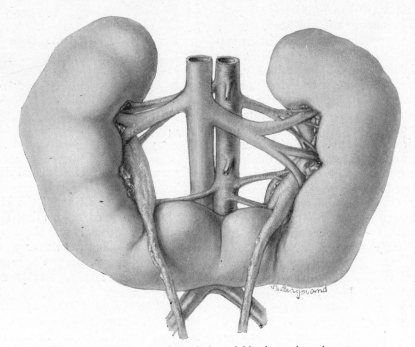

Horseshoe kidney, showing relation of blood vessels and ureters.

may cause nephroptosis. The kidney is in a lower and more horizontal position than normal; in extreme cases it may move downward and forward to the iliac fossa. Ptosis may interfere with renal blood flow and thus cause orthostatic hypertension (McCann and Romanowsky). Kinking of the ureter may produce hydronephrosis, a distention of the renal pelvis with subsequent atrophy and fibrosis of the kidney. In rare cases the organ may undergo necrosis as a result of torsion of the blood vessels.

Pigmentation and Mineral Deposits

The deposition of hemosiderin in the kidney is uncommon and perhaps occurs more often as the result of pernicious anemia than

course of pregnancy and may result from prolonged muscular exercise as in long marches. The cortex and peripheral parts of the medulla are of a dark brown color. Much the same color is observed in cases of methemoglobinemia and methemoglobinuria.

Transfusion reactions may be accompanied by hemoglobinuria and renal insufficiency. The latter has been thought to be due to blocking of tubules by hemoglobin casts, but de Navasquez points out that the number of nephrons blocked is relatively small and thinks the renal insufficiency due in large part to low blood pressure and inadequate glomerular flow. A further factor is degeneration of tubular epithelium (see Ayer and Gauld).

In cases of icterus of any origin the kidney may be deeply pigmented. In infants bilirubin may be deposited as needle-like crystals or rhomboid plates in the lumina of the tubules, or sometimes in the epithelium and even in the connective tissue. Hemoglobin and bilirubin may pigment tubular casts and also necrotic epithelium. The pigment of ochronosis may be found in convoluted tubules and glomeruli, and may stain casts.

Deposition of urates occurs in the so-called uric acid infarcts of infants and in the gouty kidney. Uric-acid infarcts are common in the kidneys of the new-born. Grossly the tips of the pyramids show radiating yellow, glossy streaks, and sandy material may be found in the pelvis. Microscopically, the tubules contain minute, laminated, radially striated spheres of crystalline material. These are made up principally of sodium urate, but contain also calcium, phosphates and oxalates. At birth, the destruction of leukocytes produces an excess of uric acid in the blood. As the strongly acid urine is secreted, sodium urate is formed. This is precipitated probably as the result of a colloidal reaction induced by small amounts of protein contributed by the renal epithelium. The lesion is not a true infarct and clears up in a few days.

The gouty kidney also shows precipitation of urates, the result of rich uric-acid content of the blood, but deposited in the kidney over the course of years rather than of a few days. Grossly, small nodular or diffuse, pale yellow, chalky deposits are found in the pyramids and sometimes in the neighboring cortex. Microscopically the crystals of sodium urate are principally in the interstitial tissues but may be found in tubules and vascular walls (Fahr). There may be destruction of tubular epithelium and supporting tissues, and the chronic inflammatory reaction may be accompanied by foreign body giant cells.

In the aged, and in chronic nephritis, the tips of the pyramids may show small nodules of calcium. CALCIUM DEPOSITION in the arteries, interstitium of cortex and occasionally glomerular capillaries, occurs in metastatic calcification and after experimental administration of excessive doses of irradiated ergosterol. Calcification of necrotic tubular epithelium is common in mercuric chloride poisoning. In ARGYRIA, the minute black granules of pigment are found in the membrana propria of the glomerular loops.

Retrogressive Changes

Cloudy swelling, fatty degeneration and amyloidosis are of especial significance because they may produce signs and symptoms similar to those of Bright's disease. In the discussion of that topic these lesions will

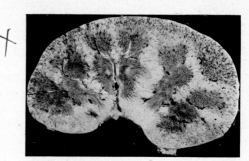

Advanced cloudy swelling of kidney. Army Medical Museum, No. 13331.

be grouped under the general heading of nephrosis.

Cloudy swelling of the kidneys occurs in all those conditions described in discussing the general pathology of cloudy swelling, including particularly the acute infectious diseases, passive hyperemia, profound anemias and various forms of poisoning.

The kidney is soft, swollen, increased in weight, but as a rule does not attain the size and weight observed in acute nephritis. The capsule strips readily, the organ cuts with normal resistance and shows a thick, bulging, pallid, "parboiled" cortical substance in which the glomeruli are usually visible as small red points. The lighter cortical striations are wider than are the darker. The change affects the cells of the convoluted tubules more strikingly than others, as is shown microscopically by the increase in size and increased granularity of the cells. The increase in size may lead to almost complete obliteration of the tubular lumina, but in the later stages the parts of the cell next to the lumen apparently drop away and the thickness of the cell ultimately is reduced. Where the lumen is open there is usually a deposit of albuminous granular material. In uncomplicated cloudy swelling the glomeruli are normal.

In cases where there is excessive imbibition of water, the microscopic picture is that of hydropic infiltration with large droplets in the tubular cells. The tubular epithelium may also show hyaline droplets. It seems at least possible that the milder renal disturbances, such as albuminuria, oliguria and cylindruria, occurring in acute infectious diseases are due to cloudy swelling, a condition found almost constantly at autopsy in such cases.

Fatty degeneration occurs under much the same conditions as cloudy swelling, except that the causes persist longer or operate with greater intensity. It is especially likely to be prominent in severe anemias and is common in various forms of chronic renal disease. Fatty degeneration is also found in diabetes, exophthalmic goiter, in pregnancy if complicated by eclampsia or nephritis and in poisoning by fungi, by phosphorus and other agents. The condition in itself has no particular influence upon the size of the kidney but may be the cause of considerable reduction of consistency. Grossly, there may be irregularly defined yellow patches several millimeters in diameter on the outer surface, but as a rule this change is more prominent in the cross section, especially in the interpyramidal cortical substance. Less commonly the entire cortex is of a diffuse yellow color.

Demonstrated by special methods, the fat appears in the early stages as small globules within the cell near the basement membrane, and in later stages may involve the entire cell. The epithelium of the loops of Henle and the distal convoluted tubules may contain fat normally (Fuller), but fat in the proximal convoluted tubules always means pathologic alteration. This is usually neutral fat, but cholesterol and its esters and other lipids may be found. Degenerate epithelium may also show anisotropic lipoid droplets, especially numerous in chronic lipoid nephrosis. Most investigators believe that severe fatty change reduces the functional capacity of the kidney, a view with which Fahr disagrees. Fatty degeneration of the glomeruli is common in certain forms of chronic renal disease, especially in chronic glomerulonephritis. (See Dible and Hay.)

Glycogen. The deposit of microscopically demonstrable glycogen occurs practically only in connection with diabetes mellitus. With special stains it is seen as droplets, especially in the ascending limb of Henle's loop. In ordinary preparations the glycogen is dissolved out and the cells are vacuolated. Insulin treatment reduces the amount of glycogen.

Hyalin occurs in various chronic diseases of the kidney, affecting particularly the interstitial connective tissue, the blood vessel walls, the capsule of the glomeruli, and the capillaries of the loops. Hyalin in the form of droplets may also be observed in the capillary loops in connection with acute infectious diseases, especially diphtheria. Epithelial hyalin, in the form of hyaline droplets in the tubular cells, occurs in various acute and chronic renal diseases.

Amyloidosis of the kidneys is practically always of a secondary type and is

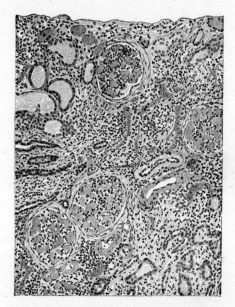

Amyloid in the loops of the glomerular tufts and in the walls of small arteries.

usually associated with amyloidosis elsewhere, particularly in the liver and the spleen. The lesion is most frequently secondary to tuberculosis, but other diseases may be responsible. The nature of amyloid and its distribution in the kidneys is discussed in the chapter on Degenerations and Infiltrations.

Characteristically, the kidney of amyloidosis is the large white kidney. It is large and firm, the capsule strips readily and leaves a pale, smooth outer surface. The organ cuts with slightly increased resistance, showing a pale, glassy cross section with increase in width of both cortex and medulla; the use of Lugol's solution and dilute sulfuric acid demonstrates the presence of amyloid. In rare instances, the kidney ultimately becomes fibrous and shrunken. Microscopically, the homogeneous amyloid is found in glomerular tufts, arteriae rectae and basement membrane of tubules; metachromatic aniline stains demonstrate the amyloid nature of the homogeneous material. Bell and Hartzell maintain that fibrosis of the glomerular tufts appears even in the large kidney and that the disease is a nephritis rather than a nephrosis. In our opinion, it is a nephrosis.

Clinically, there is likely to be albuminuria together with the presence of casts in the urine, some of which appear to be made of amyloid. The studies of Berg show

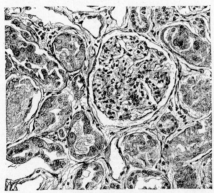

Necrosis and desquamation of tubular epithelium as the result of poisoning by male fern.

that in the later stages of amyloidosis, proteins of large molecular size such as globulins and fibrinogen pass through the glomerular filter. Ultimately the interference with renal function may go on to the development of uremia and death. Only occasionally is hypertension observed and then it appears in connection with the small contracted amyloid kidney rather than with the large white kidney (See Mark and Mosenthal). In the classification of Bright's disease, given further on, amyloidosis is included as one of the forms of chronic nephrosis.

Atrophy of the kidney may affect the whole organ or only part of it. A general atrophy may be due to reduction in the size of the lumen of the renal artery, to general wasting diseases, and may be seen as part of the wasting of the body in advanced age. Another cause of general atrophy is hydronephrosis, referred to subsequently. Chronic disease of arteries and of arterioles in the kidney leads to localized foci of atrophy, described below.

Necrosis of the kidney is observed in infarction and in bilateral cortical necrosis, described below. Necrosis of tubular epithelium occurs in different kinds of poisoning, as for example poisoning by mercuric chloride, arsenic, diethylene glycol and male fern. Foci of necrosis with desquamation of the epithelial cells is common in the inflammations of the kidney.

Circulatory Disturbances

Active hyperemia is observed especially in the various types of acute inflammation of the kidney.

Passive hyperemia is common, and clinically is often accompanied by changes in the urine. At postmortems, variable degrees of hyperemia are observed as a result of death from almost any cause, and the condition becomes more prominent by the settling of blood back into the kidneys. The most important cause of prolonged passive hyperemia is disease of the heart. It also occurs in chronic diseases of the lungs and pleura. Involvement of the renal veins or the inferior vena cava by tumors or thrombosis, pressure by tumors and inflammatory swelling, and probably also the accumulation of large quantities of fluid in the peritoneal cavity such as occurs in the ascites of hepatic cirrhosis, may cause passive hyperemia of the kidneys.

In the earlier stages the kidney is large, dark red in color, with a tense capsule which strips with ease. The outer surface is smooth and moderately firm. The organ cuts with normal resistance and shows a moderate thickening of the entire substance and in the cross section is dark red and bleeds freely. The color of the pyramids is purple in contrast to the dark red of the cortex. The glomeruli may be seen as prominent dark red points. The stellate veins of the outer surface as well as those of the pelvis are usually prominent.

As time goes on, interstitial connective

tissue increases in amount and the kidney is reduced in size and increased in consistency, usually smooth, however, and only rarely granular on the outer surface. The greater the amount of connective tissue the more adherent is the capsule and the more resistant is the organ to cutting. Correspondingly, as the fibrous overgrowth continues, the cortex is reduced in thickness and the pyramids are likely to show the gray color of fibrosis near their tips. The glomeruli continue to be visible grossly as red points.

Microscopically, practically all the vessels of the kidney are distended with blood, more especially those of the venous circulation. The glomerular tufts are filled with blood and may occupy the entire capsular space. The tubular epithelium is the seat of cloudy swelling. In the tubular lumina, and also in the subcapsular space where it is patent, there is a granular albuminous precipitate. Small interstitial hemorrhages are sometimes observed and red blood corpuscles may be seen within the tubular lumina. Although hyaline and granular casts may be found in the urine, it is unusual to observe them in the kidney section. In later stages there may be slight or moderate diffuse fibrosis. At this stage the capsule of Bowman and occasionally the tuft may show fibrosis. As has been mentioned above, hemosiderosis is not common in passive hyperemia.

Clinically, the urine is often reduced in amount and of high specific gravity, presumably due to slowing and reduced pressure of the blood current through the glomeruli. There may be considerable amounts of albumin, frequently hyaline and sometimes granular casts, and also red blood corpuscles. The renal excretory function is not materially altered. Dyes used to test function are readily excreted and there is no significant retention of nitrogenous metabolites.

Edema is observed in the kidney in the course of inflammations but is apparently more prominent when the glomeruli are seriously injured. It may also be seen in cases of suppression of urine.

Solid emboli usually originate from vegetations on the cardiac valves and from thrombi in the chambers of the heart or on sclerotic patches in aorta and arteries. Solid emboli may be bland or infected; the former lead to bland infarction and the latter to

hematogenous abscesses. In fat embolism, globules of fat are frequently found in the capillaries of the glomerular tufts. Bacterial embolism may also occur in the glomerular capillary loops. Cells from the placenta and also giant cells of bone marrow are occasionally found in the capillaries of the kidney. In cases of embolism of amniotic fluid, squames may be found in the glomerular capillaries.

Infarction. Septic or infected emboli produce abscesses of the kidney, which will be discussed subsequently. Bland infarction

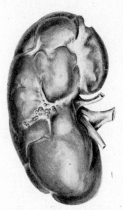

A kidney, the seat of numerous healed infarcts and fetal lobulation.

of the kidney is due to solid emboli, such as has been mentioned above. Clinically, the lodgment of an embolus in the kidney may cause pain in the flank and subsequently there may be blood in the urine, but generally speaking, infarcts in the kidney are never sufficient in number or size to produce any serious disturbance of renal function. Infarcts of the left kidney are slightly more frequent than those of the right, probably because the left renal artery comes off from the aorta somewhat obliquely instead of at a right angle as is true of the right renal artery.

Both experimentally and in man, the earliest stage of infarction is in the form of the red infarct. This is slightly swollen, conical in form, deep red in color and relatively dry in the cross section. Microscopically, there is cloudy swelling in the early stages, then fatty degeneration and finally necrosis of the tubular epithelium. There is marked hyperemia, conglutination of the red corpuscles, and slight hemorrhage into the interstitial substance, the glomerular spaces and the tubular lumina.

Owing to the fact that decolorization appears early in the kidney, the white or anemic infarct is far more common than is the red infarct. In the earlier stages the white infarct is distinctly swollen, bulges upon the outer surface, is pale yellow in color, soft in consistency, friable and surrounded by a narrow zone of reactive hyperemia. The cross section is irregularly triangular in shape, extending through cortex and sometimes involving medulla, soft, relatively dry and friable. Microscopically, there is cloudy swelling in the early stages, and in the later stages necrosis of the tubular epithelium. The architecture of the kidney is preserved and the blood in the glomerular loops is more or less conglutinated. Later, the cells of the glomerular tufts and of the interstitial connective tissue show nuclear degeneration and solution and finally complete disappearance of the fibrillar substance. The margins show reactive hyperemia, infiltration of large and small mononuclear cells and leukocytes, small globules of fat, apparently transported from the necrotic central part, and sometimes small amounts of blood pigment.

Essentially the same changes occur in the kidney substance when the entire renal artery is occluded. The presence of passive hyperemia has apparently no effect upon the course of the infarct. In still later stages the necrotic mass is reduced in size and surrounded by a zone of organization and then of cicatrization. If the infarct be small it may become completely cicatrized, but it is only rarely that small areas of necrosis are not visible in the center of the healed infarct. The shrinkage of the conical mass of fibrosis, with a central necrotic mass of varying size, produces an irregular retraction of the outer surface of the organ, which may involve the entire thickness of the cortex and sometimes the medulla.

Bilateral Cortical Necrosis. This disease occurs principally in women during the fourth decade but may occur earlier and later. Frequently the onset is during the course of pregnancy or in the puerperium. Nevertheless, women who have never borne children may be affected and the disease occurs in men and children. The onset is usually with pain in the flanks followed by oliguria or complete anuria that may last from two to several days. Grossly the kidneys are enlarged and in the cross section show extensive pale yellow necrosis of the cortex, involving both outer and interpyramidal cortex. Occasionally minute points of hemorrhage are observed.

Microscopically there is complete necrosis of the tubules in the cortex associated sometimes with fibrinous thrombi in small arteries and in the capillaries of the glomeruli. Ultimately the glomeruli are destroyed. The necrosis is evidently due to ischemia brought about by obstruction of the small cortical arteries and the arterioles. The reason for this obstruction is not known and discussion varies as to whether it is neurogenic or due to inflammatory disease of these blood vessels. (See Duff and More.)

Hemorrhage. Hemorrhage into the kidney may give no sign clinically, but if there be extension into the surrounding tissue there may be general symptoms and signs of severe hemorrhage. One of the causes of blood in the urine (hematuria) is renal hemorrhage. Hemorrhage occurring in the kidney itself may be due to active or passive hyperemia, to the presence of malignant tumors, to infarction, to inflammations of various kinds, to specific inflammations particularly tuberculosis, and to direct or indirect trauma. Hemorrhage in the perirenal tissue may be extensive and is usually due to trauma, but cases are observed occasionally in which no cause can be discovered. Such a perirenal hematoma may be entirely absorbed. In other cases a capsule of fibrous tissue may form and the sac may contain pigmented fluid. Of much clinical importance is the so-called idiopathic or essential hematuria. Keyes includes under essential hematuria that due to a variety of definite causes such as hemophilia, scurvy, purpura, poisoning by drugs such as turpentine and cantharides, parasites, especially the *Distoma hematobium*, acute infectious diseases, hydronephrosis, movable kidney, calculi, chronic nephritis, inflammation of the renal papillae, and the so-called angioneurosis.

Of much clinical importance is the so-called idiopathic or essential hematuria, in which none of these special conditions is found. Sometimes the cystoscopic examination will show that the blood comes from only one kidney. Often in such cases the kidney is excised and submitted for pathologic examination. In some of these cases there are only slight cloudy swelling and sometimes the most minor degrees of inflammation. In others there may be small patches of fibrosis throughout the kidney and it is possible that the inflammation originally producing this fibrosis may so weaken capillary walls that they rupture when pressure is slightly increased.

Vascular Disease of the Kidneys. Disease of the arteries and the arterioles is of especial significance because of the likelihood of secondary effects upon the excretory and other functions of the kidneys. The acute arterial and arteriolar inflammations lead to acute localized or widespread inflammation in the renal substance. Arteriosclerosis of the large and small arteries leads to atrophy of segments of the cortex, associated with growth of connective tissue. Comparable disease of the arterioles may bring about essentially the same changes in smaller foci. The arterial disease is irregularly distributed and consequently the atrophic segments vary in size and distribution. Arteriolar disease is more uniformly distributed and so are the foci of atrophy. These states are included in the general category of nephrosclerosis. The condition is called arterial nephrosclerosis when the disease affects large and smaller branches of renal artery, or arteriolar nephrosclerosis when the arterioles are involved. In the later discussion of Bright's disease, it will be found that nephrosclerosis is one of the conditions included. This is principally because arteriolar nephrosclerosis may be accompanied by various clinical manifestations similar to those of Bright's disease.

These conditions will be discussed under the headings, acute arteritis, arterial nephrosclerosis, acute arteriolitis and arteriolar disease including arteriolar nephrosclerosis.

ACUTE ARTERITIS. Acute inflammations of arteries occur as the result of infective embolism and secondary to suppurative disease in the kidney. In addition there are rare cases in which acute arteritis of various forms, especially proliferative and exudative, occurs without demonstrable cause. These may produce slight or marked functional changes. As part of the general manifestations of periarteritis nodosa, the kidneys may be affected. There may be albuminuria, hematuria and ultimately severe and even fatal renal insufficiency.

Grossly the kidneys are usually swollen, hyperemic, soft and the seat of multiple infarcts and foci of hemorrhage. Microscopically, the arteries are characteristically inflamed as described in the chapter on Cardiovascular System, and the disease may extend as an exudative arteriolitis and glomerulitis. The tubules show cloudy swelling and the lumina may contain casts, red blood cells and leukocytes. The infarcts are like those usually seen.

ARTERIAL NEPHROSCLEROSIS. The functional changes are minimal or absent. The disease occurs principally in late middle and advanced life. The simple intimal arteriosclerosis of large and medium sized arteries is not uniformly distributed. In a variable number of vessels, the lumen is gradually reduced in size and finally practically occluded. This gradual reduction of blood supply to the given part of the kidney results in atrophy of the parenchyma, either as the result of faulty nutrition, inactivity, or both, and substitution by connective tissue. Because of the loss of renal substance and retraction of the connective tissue, the outer surface of the kidney shows irregularly stellate areas of retraction, varying from a few millimeters to a centimeter or more in diameter, in the base of which the organ is firm and gray due to the fibrosis. In cross section the triangular areas of fibrosis below the surface depressions may extend entirely through the cortex and sometimes into the medulla. The visible arteries are usually the seat of considerable sclerosis. The larger vessels, however, may be distinctly sclerotic without producing nephrosclerosis.

Microscopically, the atrophic areas show definite atrophy of the tubules and their cells, sometimes with complete disappearance. The intervening connective tissue is fibrotic, sometimes moderately infiltrated with lymphoid cells. The glomeruli show variable changes. In the areas less markedly involved, fibrosis of the capsule of Bowman, moderate in extent, may be found. There may be slight fibrosis of the tufts, but

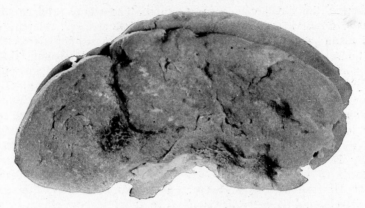

Arterial nephrosclerosis. Kidney about normal size with coarse foci of retraction, not uniform in size.

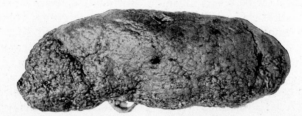

Arteriolar nephrosclerosis. Kidney is somewhat reduced in size. Fine lines of retraction result in projecting nodules fairly uniform as to size.

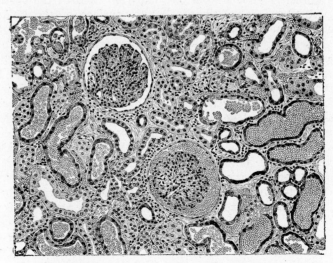

Acute degenerative glomerulonephritis with hemorrhage into subcapsular space and thence into tubules.

more characteristic is a certain degree of lobulation of the tufts with minor thickening of the walls of the individual capillaries. Subsequently, the fibrosis of both capsule and tufts becomes more marked, and ultimately the glomerulus may be converted into a small ball of fibrous tissue. The medium-sized and smaller arteries show extensive endarteritis deformans or obliterans. Tubules adjacent to the atrophic areas often show dilatation and this may become sufficiently marked to produce grossly visible retention cysts.

ACUTE ARTERIOLITIS may occur as a primary disease or may be superimposed on arteriolar sclerosis. The primary disease affects children more often than those who are older. The onset is usually abrupt and the disease fatal within about two weeks. Although much like acute glomerulonephritis clinically, it differs in that there is no history of preceding acute infection and the hypertension may be marked. There is widespread arteriolar inflammation, especially pronounced in the kidneys. Grossly, the kidneys resemble those of acute glomerulonephritis save for the presence of numerous petechiae. Microscopically many of the arterioles are thick, show extensive hyaline necrosis of their walls and exudation especially of polymorphonuclear leukocytes. The inflammation may extend in a fairly wide zone around the arterioles and is likely to progress into associated glomeruli. The tubules show cloudy swelling and foci of necrosis of their cells; hyaline casts, erythrocytes and leukocytes may be found in the tubular lumina. There is no reason for assuming that this acute disease may be transformed into a chronic arteriolar sclerosis.

As will be indicated later, an acute necrotizing arteriolitis may be superimposed on arteriolar sclerosis, but although the hyaline necrosis is conspicuous, there is little or no exudation. This lesion, however, probably occurs only when renal insufficiency is present (Goldblatt). Thus it differs from the primary acute arteriolitis in its microscopic appearance and in that it is caused by renal insufficiency or uremia. (See Schürmann and MacMahon; MacMahon and Pratt.)

CHRONIC ARTERIOLAR DISEASE may or may not be associated with a grossly observable lesion of the kidney. In either form, however, there may be associated persistent hypertension. If there be no alteration of the renal structure visible to the naked eye we refer to the disease as arteriolar sclerosis of the kidney. If there be gross distortion of the architecture of the organ by fibrosis, the lesion is referred to as arteriolar nephrosclerosis. In either event arteriolar disease is usually present in organs of other parts of the body. In the case of arteriolar disease of the kidney, the organ may be of normal size or slightly increased in size, not especially firm and show no distinctive features. Nevertheless, microscopically there is pronounced sclerosis of the arterioles throughout the kidney but as a rule this is manifest particularly in the preglomerular arterioles. Associated with this there may be glomerular lesions comparable to those described below in connection with arteriolar nephrosclerosis.

ARTERIOLAR NEPHROSCLEROSIS. Although arteriolar disease may be present elsewhere in the body, the kidney is the only organ that is likely to show distinctive anatomic alterations grossly. The kidney may be of normal size; it may be slightly or occasionally much reduced in size. It is red, pale or mottled. The capsule strips with increased resistance. The outer surface is finely and uniformly granular in character. Small nodules of parenchyma, usually less than a millimeter in size, project slightly above a reddish-gray network of retracted connective tissue. The organ is firm and cuts with increased resistance. The cross section, usually somewhat retracted, shows a narrowed cortex with irregular striae, and pyramids reduced in size with pale fibrous tips. The pelvis is normal, but the peripelvic fat increased in amount. The visible renal arteries may or may not be sclerotic.

Microscopically, there is diffuse fibrosis, augmented near the areas of retraction of the outer surface and in these regions often accompanied by infiltration of lymphoid cells. The arterioles, especially those afferent in the region of the glomeruli, are thickened, fibrous and often hyalinized. The glomeruli vary from normal to conversion into fibrous balls. Many show fibrosis of the capsule of Bowman and of the glomerular tufts. Special stains show that the tuft basement membrane is thickened and wrinkled (McGregor). Occasionally adhesions between tuft and capsule occur. More definitely inflammatory lesions are not common, except as a superimposed condition. The tubular epithelium usually shows cloudy swelling and often fatty degeneration. The tubular units are atrophic in many areas and hypertrophic in others. The atrophy is probably due to the arteriolar disease, but not necessarily the result of occlusion of glomerular circulation (Oliver). Cystic dilatation may be observed. The larger arteries are usually the seat of intimal arteriosclerosis.

The association of persistent hypertension is referred to in the chapter on the Cardiovascular System. Clinically a distinction is made between so-called benign and malignant hypertension. Benign hypertension progresses slowly with little or no clinical evidence of renal incompetency. Except for intercurrent disease, the patients die of failure of the hypertrophic heart or cerebral hemorrhage. If they develop renal disturbance, it appears insidiously and progresses slowly, evidently because of gradual destruction of glomeruli. For a long time there may be only slight albuminuria, cylindruria and slight decrease in output of test dyes, with little or no retention of nitrogenous products.

The term malignant hypertension is sometimes applied to the later stages just described or to a more rapidly progressive renal disease with marked interference with renal function and hematuria. Anatomically this is associated with a rapid progress of arteriolar sclerosis, or to acute hyaline necrosis of the sclerotic arterioles or to the superimposition of acute exudative arteriolitis (Klemperer and Otani). Death from renal insufficiency is more common in patients under than over 50 years of age (Moritz and Oldt). In such cases the number of patent glomeruli may be reduced 75 per cent or more (Moritz and Hayman). Changes in the eye grounds are like those in chronic glomerulonephritis as described below.

Inflammations

These may be exudative or alterative (parenchymatous). The exudative forms of inflammation include those due to pyogenic bacteria and to other organisms such as the tubercle bacillus; these will be considered after the discussion of the alterative inflammations. The alterative forms include lesions in which degenerations of the tubular epithelium are conspicuous, but associated with them are either proliferative or nonsuppurative exudative changes. The term Bright's disease is employed clinically to indicate the presence of disease of the kidneys, associated in variable degrees with hypertension, albuminuria, cylindruria, hematuria and decrease in renal excretory function. Among the anatomic lesions of Bright's disease are included different types of nephrosis, glomerulonephritis (hemorrhagic Bright's disease), vascular disease of the kidney and pyelonephritis.

Classifications of Bright's disease have been based upon etiologic, pathogenetic, functional, clinical, and morphologic viewpoints. Etiologic classification is unsatisfactory because the causes are often unknown, pathogenetic because the primary lesion is often obscured by advanced changes, clinical and functional because of the great difficulty in setting up groups that are sufficiently distinctive, purely morphologic because of the frequent lack of correlation between anatomic and functional alterations. The most widely accepted classification, namely that of Volhard and Fahr, into nephrosis, nephritis and nephrosclerosis is largely morphologic, but the lesions can be more closely correlated with the clinical features than is true of other classifications. There is no necessary interrelationship of the three forms of disease.

Nephrosis. This term refers to degenerations of the kidney, without features of genuine inflammation and has gained wider usage than nephropathy and nephrodystrophy.

ACUTE NEPHROSIS represents the effects upon the kidneys of various diseases, especially the acute infectious diseases; of intoxications, such as the toxemias of pregnancy; of ingested poisons, such as mercuric chloride; and of injurious substances originating in the body, such as hemoglobin and bile acids. Ordinarily the functional disturbances are not severe. Occasionally, however, the degenerations are so marked and the functional manifestations so great that even without signs of inflammation the condition is called acute tubular nephritis (Wolbach and Blackfan).

CHRONIC NEPHROSIS. Prolonged but relatively slight degeneration together with moderate diffuse fibrosis may accompany metabolic diseases such as gout, chronic arthritis, diabetes, etc., and the condition is often called chronic nephrosis. There are, however, two special conditions that are classified as chronic nephrosis, namely amyloidosis and lipoid nephrosis. Amyloidosis has been discussed above and reference was made to the fact that some believe there is an inflammatory component.

Chronic lipoid nephrosis is a term applied to a group of cases including more children than adults, in which there is albuminuria, usually pronounced, cylindruria and anisotropic lipoid droplets (cholesteryl esters) in the urine, with edema, reduction of plasma proteins and reversal of albumin: globulin ratio, and hypercholesterolemia (Leiter). Hypertension, hematuria and renal insufficiency are not part of the disease. Death may be due to the disease, but is often due to intercurrent infections, especially peritonitis usually pneumococcal. The kidneys are usually large, only occasionally reduced in size, are firm and pale, without petechiae. Microscopically, the connective tissue is somewhat increased and may be edematous. The tubules show profound cloudy swelling, are often vacuolated and sometimes necrotic, contain fat and with the Nicoll prisms show doubly refractile droplets of cholesteryl esters in considerable quantity. The glomerular tufts are anatomically normal in early stages, even though highly permeable for proteins. In later stages there may be slight thickening of the basement membranes. The patient may recover or the disease may be much prolonged with the possibility of transformation to chronic glomerulonephritis. Clinically there are cases of nephritis in which the albuminuria and edema dominate the picture; the nephritis is said to have a "nephrotische Einschlag," probably best translated as nephrotic component. The cause of lipoid nephrosis is not known, but it has been suggested that it may be due to infection, especially pneumococcal (Blackman). At any rate, the renal disturbance is but one part of a widespread disturbance of protein metabolism. (See Murphy, et al.)

Nephritis. DIFFUSE GLOMERULONEPHRITIS. This occurs in acute, subacute and chronic forms. The kidneys show marked tubular degeneration. The inflammatory component is usually found especially in the glomeruli. In the acute disease, this component is proliferative, affecting endothelium of the capillaries and sometimes the epithelium of the tuft and capsule; occasionally the glomerular lesions are degenerative or exudative without suppuration. In the subacute and chronic forms, the reaction is principally proliferation of connective tissue in the glomeruli and interstitial tissues. The patient with acute nephritis frequently recovers (about 60 per cent). He may die in the acute phase, but this happens in only from 5 to 15 per cent of the cases. The disease may become latent, with only slight manifestations, and, either after this stage or without it, may become chronic, but figures of the incidence of this latter sequel vary widely, from 6 to 35 per cent. (See Addis and Oliver; Matthews.)

ACUTE DIFFUSE GLOMERULONEPHRITIS. This disease affects children and young adults especially, but may occur in later life. It is characterized by malaise, occasionally slight fever, albuminuria, hematuria, edema, convulsions, and indications of decreased excretory function of the kidneys; in later stages moderate hypertension occurs.

CLASSIFICATION
OF BRIGHT'S DISEASE

Nephrosis
  Acute (Degenerations and necroses)
  Chronic
    Amyloid
    Lipoid

Nephritis
  Diffuse Glomerulonephritis (Hemorrhagic Bright's disease)
  Acute (Varieties of glomerular lesion)
    Degenerative
    Proliferative
      Intracapillary
      Extracapillary (Subcapsular)
    Exudative
  Subacute
  Chronic
  Focal glomerulonephritis
  Other special forms
  Pyelonephritis

Nephrosclerosis
  Arterial
  Arteriolar (Hypertensive)

The most common precursor is acute infection of the upper respiratory tract, especially sore throat and tonsillitis. Other infections include otitis and sinusitis, scarlet fever, infections of the skin, pneumonia, rheumatic fever and in a few cases a variety of other infections such as erysipelas, diphtheria, typhoid fever and various forms of surgical infections. Pregnancy may excite pre-existent renal disease to activity, or toxemias of pregnancy may be associated with nephrosis, glomerulonephritis or acute arteriolar disease (Zimmerman and Peters). The occurrence of "trench nephritis" in World War I and certain instances in civil life suggest that exposure to cold may predispose to or excite the disease, but experimentally lesions of the kidney following prolonged exposure to cold do not resemble human nephritis (Mackay et al.). Prolonged physical exertion, as in long marches, may produce temporary albuminuria, but there is no indication that this is due to nephritis. This discussion should not convey the impression that nephritis is a frequent complication of the common acute infectious diseases. It is not, and it complicates only a small percentage of cases of scarlet fever (Kannerstein).

The bacteria associated with the primary disease are especially *Streptococcus haemolyticus* and to a lesser degree *S. viridans*. Pneumococci are also frequently recovered, but staphylococci only occasionally. (See Hayman and Martin; Matthews.) There is usually a latent period between the primary infection and the development of nephritis, which in the case of scarlet fever is often about three weeks. This latent period becomes shorter in recurrences.

Various manifestations suggest three possibilities as to pathogenesis, namely (a) direct action of bacterial toxins on the kidneys, (b) transfer of infection to the kidneys and (c) antigen-antibody reactions. Certain products of bacteria, such as toxins and autolysates, pneumococci, streptococci and staphylococci, produce renal lesions in experimental animals but these are not exactly like the human disease. Furthermore they often do not show the latent period. Living bacteria may produce comparable experimental lesions, but in man bacteria are not often found in the urine of the patient nor in the kidneys at autopsy.

Many investigations have been made of possible immune or allergic reactions. The bacterial products, referred to above, are more active if the kidney has previously been sensitized. Schwentker and Comploier report that by injecting rabbits repeatedly with a mixture of rabbit kidney substance and staphylococcal or streptococcal toxin, complement-fixing antibodies are produced by the animals. One of these antibodies was fixed by the serum of a large percentage of scarlet-fever patients and only a few of the normal controls. They proposed the hypothesis that the bacterial toxin of scarlet fever alters the proteins of the renal cells in the early stage of the disease. The altered protein is liberated as the cells are repaired and in the course of the latent period new antibodies are produced which are specific for and react with the renal cells. Kay and associates repeated this experiment except that they used human kidney instead of rabbit kidney. They found no reacting substance in the blood of 78 patients with scarlet fever. Although this fails to support the hypothesis, they are not ready to deny it. Nevertheless, the whole idea of auto-immune bodies has little as yet to support it. Perhaps in time more definite information will accrue.

It has also been found that immunization of animals of one species by suspensions of perfused kidney tissue from another species produces a nephrotoxic serum against the first species. Most of the experiments have been done with a nephrotoxic serum for rabbits prepared in ducks, and a nephrotoxin for rats prepared in rabbits. This produces a nephritis more closely resembling that of man than any other experimental form. Nevertheless there are certain minor differences. The latent period is short, a few hours in rats and about a week in rabbits. Whether the nephrotoxic serum acts directly or through the elaboration of a new auto-nephrotoxin (Kay) is uncertain, but the former seems more probable. Certain physiologic observations with this form of nephritis are valuable, but that the mechanism of its production throws light on the human disease is uncertain. (See Smadel.)

Renal lesions, usually nephrosis rather than nephritis, have been produced by parenteral infections or feeding of a wide variety of agents, especially uranyl nitrate, cantharadin, arsenous acid, mercuric chloride, sodium tartrate, as well as numerous other substances, but the information obtained has only little bearing on human nephritis. (See Horn.)

The histogenesis of glomerulonephritis is pieced together by observations in man due to direct or indirect action of the injurious agents that excite the glomerular lesions.

GROSS MORBID ANATOMY OF ACUTE GLOMERULONEPHRITIS. Although acute glomerulonephritis is divided into different forms on microscopic examination, as indicated in the boxed chart, the gross changes are practically the same for all. Occasional instances of acute nephritis occur in which the kidney, grossly, appears to be practically normal. Usually, however, the organ is en-

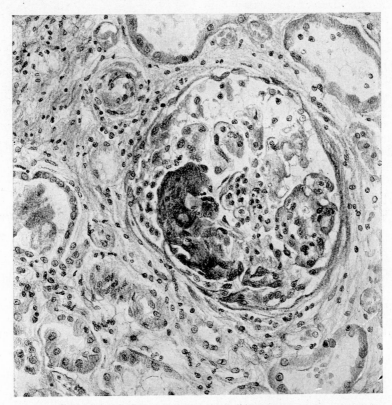

Acute exudative nephritis, showing extensive fibrin formation in the subcapsular space, as well as swelling and proliferation of the capsular epithelium.

and experimental animals, attention being directed to the glomerular lesion. Probably the first change is wide dilatation of the capillaries of the tuft (Dunn). Following this there may be degeneration with hemorrhage from the tuft, nonsuppurative exudation in and around the tuft, or proliferation of the endothelium of the capillaries or the epithelium of tuft and capsule. Special stains may sometimes disclose swelling and beading of the basement membrane of the tuft. The degenerations of tubular epithelium, common to all forms of nephritis, are probably larged, sometimes considerably, the consistency is reduced and the capsule is tense and strips with ease. The outer surface is smooth and may be pale gray, red or mottled in color. The organ cuts with reduced resistance and shows a soft, bulging, moist cross section, which may or may not bleed freely, depending upon the accompanying hyperemia. The cortex is moderately or considerably thickened, the striations are obscured or broken, and the glomeruli instead of appearing as red points appear as grayish-white points, giving the cortex a sanded appearance. The pyramids may be slightly swollen but as a rule are practically normal. The peripelvic fat and pelvis are normal.

MICROSCOPIC CHARACTERS. These vary in accordance with the different forms. In all varieties of acute diffuse glomerulonephritis there are various retrogressive changes in the tubular epithelium, affecting particularly that of the proximal convoluted tubules. These include cloudy swelling, fatty degeneration, usually minor in degree, hydropic infiltration, hyaline-droplet formation and necrosis. In some cases the desquamation of degenerated and necrotic epithelium is so great that the term desquamative nephritis is applied. Granular albuminous detritus is found in the tubules and also in the subcapsular space of the glomerulus. The casts found in the tubules are usually hyaline, which may show adherence of epithelium, of leukocytes, or of red blood corpuscles. In addition, finely and coarsely granular casts, epithelial, leukocytic, blood and fibrin casts may be observed. There may or may not be extensive hyperemia. Edema of the interstitial connective tissue is fairly common and occasionally there is slight infiltration of lymphoid and plasma cells.

The lesions in the glomeruli, referred to as glomerulitis, distinguish the various microscopic forms of acute glomerulonephritis, the other lesions being essentially the same in all three forms.

Degenerative glomerulitis may show severe degeneration or necrosis of the cells of the glomerular loops, which permit of rupture of the capillaries and hemorrhage into the subcapsular spaces and thence into the tubules. Often the actual demonstration of degenerative lesions of the cells is difficult or impossible and is inferred by the presence of the hemorrhage.

Exudative Glomerulitis. Capillaries show many polymorphonuclear leukocytes, and they may pass through the capillary walls and appear in the tubules and in the urine. Rarely the glomerular tufts may be converted into small abscesses. It seems probable that the accumulation of leukocytes is so great that circulation is impeded or completely stopped in the capillary loops, and it is stated that the leukocytes may remain in this situation after the process becomes chronic in character.

Proliferative glomerulitis is divided into two forms, the intracapillary form and the extracapillary or subcapsular form. In the intracapillary form the entire tuft is considerably enlarged and often occupies the entire capsular space. The capillary loops are free of blood, due to swelling and proliferation of the capillary endothelium. Oc-

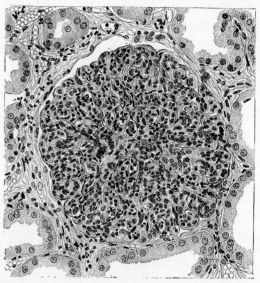

Acute glomerulonephritis. The glomerular tuft is much enlarged by proliferation and swelling of its constituent cells. No blood is found in the capillary loops.

casionally, a few polymorphonuclear leukocytes may be observed in the capillary loops and in the interstitial connective tissue. In the extracapillary or subcapsular form there is swelling and proliferation of the epithelium underlying the capsule of Bowman. The mass of cells may form a circular rim around the glomerulus or a crescentic mass. The tuft itself may be somewhat compressed by this proliferation. As a general rule, these forms of acute glomerular nephritis can be well distinguished from one another, but there are occasional cases in which confusion is likely and in which usually the final diagnosis is made upon the predominance of one change over the other.

SUBACUTE AND CHRONIC DIFFUSE GLOMERULONEPHRITIS. According to the views of Löhlein, nephritis or glomerulonephritis can be divided into three varieties or stages; namely, acute glomerulonephritis with a duration of days or weeks, subacute glomerulonephritis with a duration of one or several months, and chronic glomerulonephritis with a duration of a year or more. Many authorities have accepted this classification, but some prefer to regard the subacute form as an early stage of a chronic glomerulonephritis. In most, if not all, instances chronic glomerulonephritis is the sequel of an acute nephritis. Acute nephritis may heal, may lead to death, or may become chronic either directly or after a period of latency. Cases are described in which it is supposed that the disease is primarily chronic with insidious onset, but probably there was, in these instances, an unnoticed acute nephritis as the original disorder. It has been suggested that gout, syphilis, lead poisoning, chronic rheumatism and prolonged intestinal disturbance may lead to chronic glomerulonephritis, but the lesion is usually a nephrosclerosis, as has been shown in lead poisoning (Nye).

IN THE SUBACUTE STAGE of glomerulonephritis, the kidney is still considerably enlarged. The consistency may be soft, as in acute nephritis, or there may be some firmness, depending in large part upon the overgrowth of connective tissue. The capsule usually strips with ease but may be slightly adherent. The outer surface is usually pale but may be red or mottled red and gray. The organ cuts with normal or very slightly increased resistance and shows a thick, bulging cortex, colored like the outer surface, with obscured striations and pale bloodless glomeruli. The pyramids may be somewhat swollen but usually only slightly so. The peripelvic fat and pelvic mucosa are normal.

Microscopically, the tubular epithelium shows cloudy swelling and fatty degeneration, hydropic infiltration, hyaline droplet formation, necrosis and sometimes doubly refractile lipoid globules. The tubules may show all the varieties of lesion noted in discussing acute glomerulonephritis, and sometimes contain blood. The interstitial tissue may show edema, and infiltration of polymorphonuclear leukocytes and eosinophils. It is likely to show marked and sometimes massive increase of connective tissue, especially in the cortex; the cells are often fibroblastic in appearance. The blood vessels may be engorged; arteriosclerosis is common. Hemor-

rhage may be observed in cases of mottled kidney. The glomeruli may resemble very closely those of acute glomerulonephritis. Following acute exudative glomerulonephritis there is likely to be some proliferation of connective tissue within the capillary loops, definitely enclosing the leukocytes. In the intracapillary forms the earliest change seen in the nature of chronicity is an increase in the amount of collagenous material between the endothelial cells, subsequently going on to definite fibrosis. The glomerular tuft may be distinctly lobulated and there may be adhesions between the tuft and the capsule of Bowman. In a general way, the subacute extracapillary glomerulonephritis is more severe clinically than the intracapillary variety. In the microscopic picture, the circles or crescents of proliferated subcapsular cells persist and show fusion, fibrosis and hyalinization. Some of the glomeruli may show more advanced fibrosis and hyalinization, and conversion into small balls of fibrous tissue with ultimate hyalinization.

IN CHRONIC GLOMERULONEPHRITIS the kidney is usually but not invariably reduced

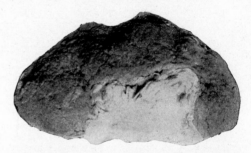

Chronic diffuse glomerulonephritis. Kidney is much reduced in size with irregular retractions of outer surface. Comparable changes may be observed in marked arteriolar nephrosclerosis and microscopic diagnosis is required.

in size and weight. For descriptive purposes it is possible to divide this condition into two forms, the nongranular and the granular form of chronic glomerulonephritis. This does not mean that these are separate and distinct forms, or that the nongranular form may not change subsequently into a granular form. Nevertheless, the nongranular form may show considerable reduction in size of the kidney without granulation of the surface. As a rule, the reduction in size is slight or moderate in the nongranular form.

The organ is of increased firmness, the capsule strips with slight difficulty and discloses a generally smooth outer surface. The color may be pale gray or grayish-yellow, or may be spotted with areas of yellow several millimeters in diameter. In other cases the outer surface is red or mottled. The organ cuts with very slightly increased resistance and shows a slightly bulging or non-bulging, moist, slightly bleeding cross section. The cortex is usually slightly reduced in thickness and shows color similar to that kidneys is closely similar to that to be described in the granular variety.

The granular form of chronic glomerulonephritis may show slight, moderate or marked reduction in the size of the kidney. In one of our cases, a man twenty-two years old, the kidneys weighed together 60 grams. The consistency and granularity of the kidney are in a general way in keeping with the reduction of size. The smaller kidneys are of leathery consistency. The capsule strips with difficulty, also depending upon the degree of

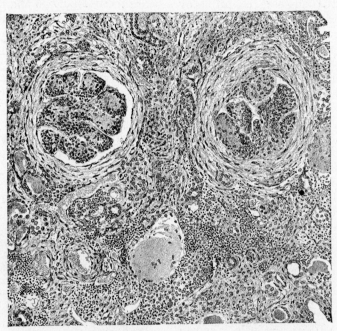

Chronic glomerulonephritis, showing extensive fibrosis of interstitial tissue with associated infiltration of lymphoid cells. The glomerular capsules are markedly fibrotic. The tufts are the seat of extensive fibrosis and also focal fibroid areas, probably the scars of a focal glomerulitis.

on the outer surface. The striations are blurred, broken and the tissue may be spotted or flecked with yellow. The glomeruli are generally pale and bloodless. The pyramids show no important change save for slight fibrosis near their tips. The peripelvic fat is often moderately increased in amount. The pelvic mucosa is normal. Microscopically, it may be possible to observe a waviness of outline of the outer surface of the organ. The connective tissue shows a diffuse overgrowth, often with a slight infiltration of lymphoid and plasma cells. In other respects the microscopic appearance of these fibrosis, and tears with it small pieces of renal substance. The outer surface shows fairly uniformly sized projecting granules, although there is less uniformity than is observed in nephrosclerosis of arteriolar variety. The projections are composed of parenchyma and may be pale gray or yellow in color. In some instances, however, they are red. The retracted part is made up of connective tissue, usually of pale gray but sometimes of red color. In occasional instances the connective tissue network shows minute, glossy, yellow points made up of the fatty or lipoidal detritus of destroyed parenchyma. The organ cuts with increased resistance and in many cases retracts below the line of section. The cross section is firm and moist and of the same general color as the outer surface. The cortex is irregularly reduced in thickness, often shows lack of distinction from the pyramids, and shows irregularity and blurring of the striations. The glomeruli are in large part pale and bloodless but some may be red. The markings of the pyramids are usually well preserved, but the entire substance of the pyramid is reduced in amount and the tips are almost always gray and fibrous. The peripelvic fat is usually considerably increased in amount. The pelvic mucosa is normal.

Microscopically, the renal capsule shows considerable fibrous thickening. The interstitial connective tissue is diffusely overgrown, more especially in irregular focalized areas and in bands at right angles to the outer surface. As a rule the glomeruli are not uniformly affected, presumably due to the recovery from acute disease on the part of a certain number of them. In the affected glomeruli there is usually fibrosis of the capsule and fibrosis of the glomerular tufts, more particularly near the center of the loops. There may be fibrous adhesions between lobules of tuft and capsule. Sometimes small spaces are thus formed, which when lined by epithelium give a pseudoacinic appearance. Depending upon the lesion in the acute stage, it may be possible to find a few leukocytes within the glomerular tufts or remnants of subcapsular epithelial proliferation. Some glomeruli are converted into balls of fibrous tissue and others show partial or complete hyalinization. A number of glomeruli may show only thickening of the capsule with preservation of the circulation in the tufts, others show general enlargement, and still others are essentially normal.

The changes in the tubules vary greatly in degree and in situation. In the usual sections, tubules near and in the region of fibrosis may be slightly or markedly atrophic. In less fibrotic regions there are large tubules sometimes with large cells and sometimes with flattened cells. Dilatation may result in the formation of cystic spaces, some of which are visible grossly and may attain great size. The tubular epithelium shows cloudy swelling, hydropic degenera-

tion, fatty degeneration and hyaline droplets; necrosis and desquamation may affect small groups of cells. The tubular lumina often contain casts of different varieties, the hyaline casts predominating. Mitotic figures

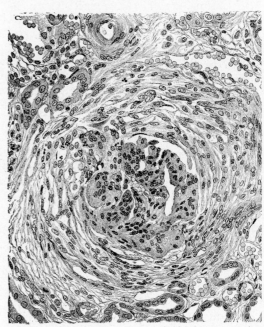

Detail of subacute or subchronic capsular glomerulonephritis. Note the great proliferation of subcapsular cells and compression of the capillary tuft.

may be found in glomeruli and tubules (Hartz et al.). There may be regeneration of tubular epithelium and sometimes the formation of small nodules of adenoma-like hyperplasia.

The extensive studies of Oliver, by serial section and reconstruction, show that there are atrophic and hypertrophic changes in the tubules and that the same tubule may show both in different portions. Even though the glomeruli may be shrunken or absent, the tubular cells retain the microscopic character of functioning cells. Constriction of tubules at different levels may detach tubules from glomeruli so that there are aglomerular tubules and atubular glomeruli. Indeed a segment of tubule may be separated both from its distal part and also from its glomerulus. The nutrition of the tubular part of a nephron whose glomerulus is destroyed is by means of a communication between afferent and efferent arteriole through the vessel of Ludwig. The arteries of the kidney may be essentially normal or they may show slight or marked arteriosclerosis; sometimes there is duplication of elastica, fibrosis of media and fatty degeneration of media and intima.

Chronic glomerulonephritis may be complicated by a superimposed acute glomerulonephritis. In some instances arteriolar sclerosis may be present and it may be difficult to determine whether the glomerular lesions are due to the arteriolar disease or whether there is the so-called combination form of glomerulonephritis and arteriolar disease.

FOCAL GLOMERULONEPHRITIS. This occurs in an acute form and in a healed stage. It is most frequently a complication of endocarditis lenta but may occasionally be observed in other infectious diseases. Many believe that the lesion in the glomeruli is due to embolism of bacteria into the capillaries but others suggest the possibility of action by injurious products of bacteria. Clinically there may be albuminuria and hematuria but generally there is little or no reduction of renal excretory function. Occasionally the kidney may show no significant gross lesion but as a rule it is swollen, soft, hyperemic, cuts with reduced resistance and shows a bulging thickened cortex. On the outer surface and in the cross section there are likely to be numerous minute petechiae, which give the kidney the so-called "flea bitten" appearance.

Microscopically the disease is found to be focal in that only about 15 to 40 per cent of the glomeruli are diseased, and in that the involvement in the individual glomeruli usually does not affect the entire tuft. The lesion may affect any part of the tuft and rarely the entire tuft. There is swelling of the epithelium of the tuft with compression and obliteration of the capillaries, followed by necrosis of the swollen cells and fusion to form a mass of finely granular acidophilic material, sometimes containing a small amount of fibrin. It is reported that some of the cases which complicate endocarditis lenta may show streptococci in the affected portions of the glomeruli. Instead of proceeding to a chronic stage, the necrotic focus undergoes cicatrization to produce the healed stage of this disease. In the same kidney there may be various stages between the

acute and the healed lesion. In the acute stage there are degenerations of the tubular epithelium; in the healed stage there may be atrophy of the tubules which come off from diseased glomeruli. In either stage the unaffected glomeruli appear to be entirely normal morphologically.

OTHER SPECIAL FORMS. *Acute Tubular Nephritis.* Reference was made above to the fact that there are occasional instances, especially in children, where the clinical manifestations are severe enough to justify a diagnosis of nephritis, whereas the anatomic manifestations are principally those of degeneration of the tubular epithelium, sometimes with a moderate degree of interstitial edema. Wolbach and Blackfan and others call this acute tubular nephritis. The name acute tubular nephritis may be applied also when marked tubular disease is associated with only slight glomerular disease.

Acute Nonsuppurative Interstitial Nephritis. This may be merely an incidental finding at autopsy, or the patient may show indications of renal insufficiency, and die in uremia. Councilman originally described this

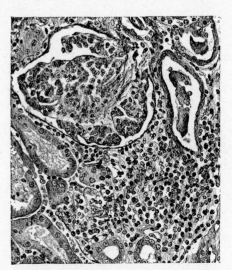

Acute interstitial nephritis, showing extensive infiltration of mononuclear cells into the interstitial substance. The glomerular tuft shows acute glomerulitis.

as a complication of various acute infectious diseases. Since then it has been observed in connection with the hemolytic reactions of transfusion, in food poisoning, and in the hepatorenal syndrome. Nevertheless, the disease is rare and cannot be ascribed to any one particular condition. Grossly, the kidney is large, soft, and cuts with decreased resistance. In the cross section the swollen parenchyma is somewhat glossy and shows irregularly disposed gray streaks in the cortex. Occasionally a few petechiae are found.

Microscopically, exudation is observed in a few or many foci distributed in the interstitial connective tissue. In some instances this exudate is largely serous, in others it is made up of a collection of cells including polymorphonuclear leukocytes, lymphocytes, large mononuclears, plasma cells and eosinophils. The glomeruli may be unaffected or there may be a precipitate of protein material in the subcapsular space. Occasionally there is acute diffuse intracapillary glomerulonephritis and rarely acute focal glomerulonephritis. The tubules show various changes from cloudy swelling on through to necrosis. There are likely to be many casts in the tubular lumina, some of which are found to be leukocytic. In establishing a diagnosis, care must always be taken to exclude the early effects of acute ascending pyelonephritis. (See Kimmelstiel.)

Other Glomerular and Associated Lesions. Owing especially to the work of Goormaghtigh, attention has been directed to what is spoken of as the "juxtaglomerular apparatus." This consists of a group of cells situated at the angle of the afferent and efferent arterioles of the kidney, called "polkissen." The cells in part resemble fibrous tissue cells and in part are supposed to be afibrillar smooth muscle cells. That part of the distal convoluted tubule near the glomerulus may show enlargement of the epithelial cells proximal to the glomerulus. Hyperplasia, as well as various degenerative changes and fibrosis, are said to occur in the polkissen. That these are regularly associated with lesions of the kidney and with hypertension has not been established in the case of man. The suggestion that the juxtaglomerular apparatus is an endocrine organ has not been established (Goormaghtigh; Edwards).

Intercapillary glomerulosclerosis has been described as occurring especially in diabetics. Grossly the kidney may show no alteration but microscopically the glomeruli show a considerable increase in the intercapillary connective tissue which often forms in fairly large globular masses and is often hyalinized. The capsule of Bowman may show slight fibrous thickening. It has not been established that there is any definite functional disturbance associated with this lesion. As a matter of fact, Horn and Smetana have found, in a series of cases, that it was observed about as frequently among those who were the victims of hypertension and vascular disease of the kidneys without diabetes, as among diabetics.

FUNCTIONAL DISTURBANCES. The clinical manifestations of glomerulonephritis are due to alteration of excretory function of the kidney, associated metabolic disturbances and other changes. The principal alterations include decrease or increase in the volume of urine, changes in specific gravity, "fixation" of specific gravity, albuminuria, casts in the urine, hematuria, retention of electrolytes and water, edema, retention of protein metabolites, anemia, hypertension, retinal lesions and uremia. These phenomena may occur in other diseases and in other lesions of the urogenital system but will be discussed here principally as they are observed in Bright's disease.

Oliguria means a reduction in the total amount of urine excreted. Ordinarily the urine is dark, rich in solids and has a high specific gravity. This change may occur in acute nephritis, in the acute nephroses, particularly that due to mercuric chloride and as a late stage of any renal disease. The mechanism is by no means clear. It has been thought that swelling of the tubular cells and edema of the interstitial tissues reduces circulation through the tissues, but experimentally this has been shown not to be the case (Hayman; Moore and Hellman). Glomerular filtration is probably reduced in acute diffuse glomerulonephritis, but while this would reduce urinary volume it does not explain increased concentration of solids. The nephroses show no morphologic changes in the glomeruli, but this does not exclude the possibility of functional alteration. It may be that with marked disease of the tubular epithelium the osmotic pressure of the blood in surrounding capillaries is operative on the tubular urine. Thus water would be resorbed and the urine reduced in volume and increased in specific gravity; this, however, is only speculation. Oliguria may progress to complete suppression of urinary output, called anuria.

Polyuria means an increase in output of urine. Usually the urine is pale, poor in solids and of low specific gravity. This may be observed in the early stages of acute nephritis in both man and experimental animals, probably because of the dilatation of capillaries in practically all the glomeruli. It is also observed in patients who are losing the fluid of edema. In chronic glomerulonephritis and in chronic arteriolar disease, this disturbance is common, and occurs in spite of a reduction of vascular bed and markedly decreased perfusion rate (Hayman). In these diseases, however, hypertension is often present and it is possible that this may increase the rate of filtration in those glomeruli not destroyed by the disease. The disease of the tubular epithelium may be such that resorption is decreased (Richards). Thus the urine would approximate the glomerular filtrate. This presupposes a different order of tubular disease from that which permits direct oncotic action of the blood in the production of oliguria.

This failure of the kidney to concentrate urine is called hyposthenuria. There are various theories to explain this but the evidence is strongly in favor of the view that it is due to reduced resorption by the tubular epithelium (Hayman, Shumway, Dumke and Miller). Even when water is withheld from the patient, the urine still remains dilute. Clinically, advantage is taken of this fact in a simple test of renal function. If the urine remains dilute, the condition is said to represent "fixation" of specific gravity.

Albuminuria, or more correctly proteinuria, is due to the filtration of protein through the glomerular capillary membranes. It may be produced by a wide variety of local lesions in the urogenital tract, inflammations, may be reflex, orthostatic, due to exercise, occurs in passive hyperemia and in the nephroses. Thus it cannot be looked upon as a certain sign of Bright's disease. The suggestion has been made that the protein is derived from renal epithelium and other organs but the investigations of Widdowson, by a variety of tests, indicate plainly that the protein in the urine is identical with serum protein. It has also been suggested that this is an altered or toxic form of protein, but Hayman and Bender injected plasma from nephritic patients intravenously into normal subjects and could not demonstrate the production of albuminuria. Certainly, most of the protein is the smaller molecular albumin, but with more and more marked disease of the glomeruli, larger molecular substances may pass through so that ultimately globulin and even fibrinogen may appear in the urine.

Cylindruria means the presence of casts in the urine. These originate in the tubules of the kidney by condensation or agglomeration of various constituents. The

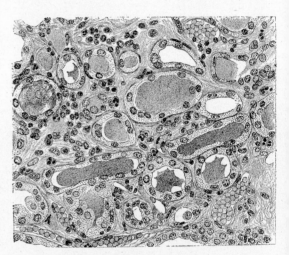

Casts in the renal tubules.

commonest are the hyaline casts. Although some of these may be agglomerates of epithelial hyaline droplets, it is probable that buds of vacuolated cytoplasm of the tubular cells become constricted and drop into the lumen to form a reticulum of circles often seen in sections, then fuse to form granular casts and condense into hyaline casts (Jackson). As these pass down the tubules, cellular and other debris may become adherent. Thus granular casts may be due to adherence of granular material to hyaline casts or may be made up entirely of protein granules. Casts may also be made up of desquamated epithelial cells, leukocytes, or erythrocytes, or mixtures of these and occasionally are masses of fibrin. The Addis count of casts, erythrocytes and leukocytes is used clinically for diagnostic and prognostic purposes.

Hematuria means the presence of blood in the urine. This may be due to a wide variety of inflammatory and neoplastic lesions of the urogenital tract or the presence of calculi and foreign bodies. It is in these states that the blood may be present in great amounts. In Bright's disease the amount of blood is relatively small, but numerous erythrocytes are observed in the urine and the urine will respond to the various tests for the presence of blood. It occurs in any of the forms of acute Bright's disease and theoretically should be more marked in degenerative glomerulonephritis than in other forms, but in practice there is no close correlation. It also occurs in chronic glomerulonephritis and may be observed occasionally in the latent stages of glomerulonephritis. It occurs in both the acute and chronic forms of arteriolar disease of the kidney. The microscopic examination of the kidneys strongly suggests that most of the hematuria is due to leakage of erythrocytes through the capillaries of the tufts.

Electrolyte Balance. The principal disturbance of electrolyte balance is found in retention of sodium chloride, phosphates and sulfates. Indeed, inorganic sulfates may be retained much earlier than is true of any of the products of nitrogen breakdown. The evidence concerning magnesium, potassium and calcium does not indicate any consistent failure of the kidney to excrete these substances. The bearing of retention of salts on edema will be referred to later.

The retention of phosphates determines a fall in the serum calcium. The consequent disturbance of calcium and phosphorus metabolism probably accounts for the occurrence of renal rickets and renal dwarfism. These may be associated with any chronic renal disease but are observed more especially in connection with chronic arteriolar disease of the kidneys and sometimes associated with hydronephrosis due to congenital faults in bladder and urethra. (See Mitchell and Guest.) In adults, the low calcium may stimulate the parathyroid glands to hyperplasia. Hyperfunction of the parathyroids may cause an increase in amount of calcium in the blood together with the retained phosphorus. Furthermore the activity of the parathyroid may cause osteoporosis and fibrosis of the marrow of the bones.

Thus, the fault in the bones, together with the oversaturation of the blood with phosphate and calcium, may result in metastatic calcification (see Herbert, et al.).

Edema is due to retention of water in the tissues of the body. That which is associated with renal disease is less dependent upon hydrostatic factors of posture than is cardiac edema. Thus it is likely to be widespread rather than limited to dependent parts, although it may be more pronounced in dependent parts than elsewhere. It often appears in the lower eyelids before other situations, probably because of the distensibility of the soft tissues of the lids, which is not restricted by local tissue pressure, or by restraining skin. It is likely to develop in sleep because of the relatively sluggish lymph flow and become less marked during the day (Burch). The accumulation of water is accompanied by a retention of salt in the body. It is unlikely that water retention is a cause of the salt retention, but salt retention may determine water retention in the maintenance of isotonicity.

As mentioned earlier, there is a loss of protein through the kidney, and protein metabolism may be disturbed in other ways. Most cases of renal edema show a reduction in total plasma proteins but the occurrence, disappearance or degree of edema cannot be closely correlated with the amount of reduction of plasma proteins. Nevertheless, much of the edema must be due to a decrease of the osmotic pressure of the blood. The reduction in amount of plasma proteins brings about decreased osmotic pressure of the blood to a degree that even in the presence of normal or subnormal hydrostatic pressure, edema occurs. It is suspected that there is also an increase of capillary permeability, but this is not proved.

Protein Metabolites. Accumulation of the products of protein metabolism in the blood and body fluids may be absent, slight or marked. This is due to a reduction in the permeability of the kidney for the various substances, including especially urea, uric acid and creatinine (Myers and Muntwyler). The reduction in permeability is effective first for uric acid, then urea and then creatinine, but this does not mean that in the advanced case these bodies are retained proportionately. Since the amount present in the blood is due to accumulation over a period of time, there is no clear indication of the actual functional capacity of the kidney at the moment of analysis. More exact and more delicate is determination of the capacity of the kidneys to clear the blood of products of protein metabolism, especially urea and creatinine. Although the measure of accumulation is valuable clinically, the clearance tests are more dependable. (See Smith.) Various other simpler tests of renal excretory capacity depend upon the rate of excretion of dyes, such as phenolsulfonephthalein and indigo carmine, and of certain substances such as lactose and amylase. Simplest of all is the determination of fixation of specific gravity, referred to above. Withholding of water from the diet is followed by increased concentration of urine and increased specific gravity. In renal insufficiency the urine remains dilute, the specific gravity increases only slightly and is said to be fixed in the vicinity of the so-called isosthenuric level of 1.010.

Anemia of normocytic normochromic type is a common accompaniment of diffuse glomerulonephritis, both in the acute and more particularly in the chronic forms. The amount of blood lost in the urine is not sufficient to account for the anemia and there is no reason for assuming that the loss of protein is of significance. There is no adequate proof for the view that it is due to poor absorption of food and of iron. Brown and Roth suggest, from their studies, that neither hemolysis due to retained products of metabolism or to toxic agents, dietary deficiency nor loss of protein in the urine is the cause. They ascribe the anemia to decreased functional activity of the bone marrow as a part of the general and widespread injury in the disease.

Hypertension of moderate degree may occur in acute diffuse glomerulonephritis and disappears if the nephritis heals. Persistent hypertension with associated cardiac hypertrophy is common in chronic diffuse glomerulonephritis and other forms of chronic renal disease. The clinical manifestations are similar to those that accompany any type of persistent hypertension. In the chapter on Cardiovascular System there is a discussion of hypertension, in which it is pointed out that the so-called essential form is due to reduced blood flow in the kidney,

and the formation of a pressor substance. In chronic diffuse glomerulonephritis it is probable that the disease of the glomeruli brings about sufficient alteration of circulation to have the same functional effects. We are of the opinion that the hypertension of renal disease is of essentially the same nature as the so-called essential hypertension. Nevertheless, as was pointed out in the earlier discussion, this view is disputed by some investigators.

Albuminuric Retinitis. Examination of the eye grounds often discloses what is spoken of as albuminuric retinitis. The retina shows narrowed, beaded and sometimes tortuous arteries and arterioles which may compress veins at cross-overs, often hemorrhages and white or yellow spots around a swollen nerve head and around a hyperemic macula. These spots are spoken of as exudate but microscopic examination of such eyes shows that they are due simply to fatty degeneration of the retina. The fatty degeneration is probably due in part to reduction of lumen of arterioles and in part to prolonged spasm. There is no demonstrable inflammation. The arterial and venous changes accompany hypertension rather than albuminuria. Thus, albuminuric retinitis is neither albuminuric nor is it a retinitis.

Acid intoxication is not frequent in the milder stages of nephritis, but when renal insufficiency becomes marked, acidosis may reach high degrees. It is uncommon for the acidosis of Bright's disease to show an associated ketosis. There are various symptoms including dyspnea and hyperpnea. Atchley and Benedict attribute the acidosis to retention of phosphate and sulfate ions, the base being supplied by carbonate and chloride. Nevertheless, the actual mechanism of development of acid intoxication is not altogether clear. Statements to the effect that acidosis is a cause of nephritis are contradicted by the work of various investigators, including Karsner, Reimann and Brooks, as well as Seegal.

Uremia. Patients who die of renal insufficiency are said to die of uremia. Exactly what is meant by uremia is not clearly established. Nevertheless, there is an association of headache, drowsiness, vomiting, convulsions and coma, together with twitchings of the extremities and other symptoms, which appear to be associated directly with the renal insufficiency. It cannot be said that any single cause has been determined for this condition. Harrison and Mason point out that these various disturbances are the result of alterations of the internal environment of the body, as indicated by the changes referred to above. The retention of phenol derivatives may be related to the onset of stupor and coma (Dickes).

The acidosis together with the loss of base may be of importance in the production of disturbances of respiration. The depletion of chloride and of water probably accounts for an increase in the catabolism of protein and may impair the excretion of the end products by the kidney. The deficiency of calcium is probably concerned with the motor irritative phenomena such as twitching and convulsions. This may be contributed to further by the accumulation of compounds of guanidine. It is suggested that the accumulation of urea may initiate ammoniacal fermentation in the alimentary canal and may interfere with processes of detoxification by the liver and other bodily mechanisms. They picture the whole process as death of the organism due to an environment poisoned by products of its own metabolism.

Suppurative or Purulent Inflammation. Infection gains access to the kidney by three pathways, through the blood stream, by ascent from the lower urinary tract and by direct extension from surrounding structures.

Transfer of bacteria through the blood stream occurs in cases of pyemia or septicemia and infectious processes in the cardiovascular system, especially bacterial endocarditis. The bacteria most frequently encountered are staphylococci or streptococci, but other organisms occasionally are found. The organisms usually lodge in the capillary loops of the glomeruli and occasionally in other capillaries and produce multiple abscesses. The consequence is hematogenous or metastatic suppurative nephritis.

Grossly, such a kidney is usually swollen, hyperemic and soft. The capsule strips easily but may tear with it the outer wall of superficial abscesses. The outer surface shows numerous small abscesses, usually about a millimeter in diameter but some-

times larger, scattered diffusely over the surface or sometimes arranged in small groups. The abscess itself is white or pale yellow and soft, and pus can be expressed from it. There is usually a surrounding zone of marked hyperemia. The organ cuts with normal resistance and shows a slightly bulging, soft, swollen, hyperemic, bleeding cross section. Usually the abscesses are found principally in the somewhat thickened bulging cortex, but occasionally they are found also in the medulla and in rare instances they are confined to the pyramids.

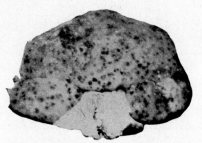

Child's kidney, the seat of pyemic abscesses and petechiae (staphylococcus aureus).

Microscopically, it is not uncommon to find a clump of bacteria in the center of the abscess, and if the condition be sufficiently early the organisms may be found in the glomerular loops or sometimes in the intertubular capillaries. Around the bacteria there is an area of necrosis, surrounded immediately by a rich infiltration of polymorphonuclear leukocytes, grading off into a zone of intense active hyperemia. The tubules are usually the seat of advanced cloudy swelling, sometimes with fatty degeneration and with necrosis. Hemorrhage into the interstitial tissues, as well as into the tubular lumina, is not uncommon. The glomeruli not affected by the bacteria may be the seat merely of a hyperemia or may show any of the forms of acute glomerulitis.

There are two other varieties of hematogenous suppurative nephritis. One is in the form of infected infarcts caused by emboli which contain infective bacteria. The other, not very common, is that form in which, whether abscesses form in the glomeruli or not, the destruction of the glomeruli may permit the bacteria to gain access to the urinary stream, subsequently to lodge in the collecting tubules in the pyramids. In this form, without definite lesion in the renal pelvis, streaks of suppuration are found radially disposed in the cross section of the pyramids. These streaks show a central collection of pus and necrotic material surrounded by reactionary hyperemia. This form is often referred to as the excretion form of hematogenous suppurative nephritis.

In contrast to the hematogenous or metastatic variety of nephritis there is the so-called ascending or urinogenous form of suppurative nephritis, or ACUTE PYELONEPHRITIS. Grossly, the kidney shows all the signs of advanced cloudy swelling and may be markedly enlarged. In cross section the renal pelvis is the seat of suppurative inflammation, with or without distention of the cavity. Radiating from the tips into the substance of the pyramids, there are streaks of pus with a surrounding area of hyperemia. Sometimes these extend outward into the cortex and may even pass through the cortex to produce perinephric abscesses. Microscopically, the changes are found principally in the pyramids. The central mass of necrosis is surrounded by infiltration of polymorphonuclear leukocytes and mononuclear cells and then by a zone of hyperemia. The tubules may contain masses of leukocytes sometimes sufficiently solidified to form casts, and in some instances bacteria can be identified in the tubular lumina and in the lining cells.

Most such cases have their origin in a suppurative cystitis which ascends through the ureter, involves the renal pelvis and then the kidney. The organism particularly associated with this condition is the colon bacillus but others are occasionally found. The possible modes of transport of infection from the bladder are by way of the ureteral lumen, by way of its lymphatics, or by means of the general blood circulation. Since the flow of urine is downward, it has been supposed that bacteria cannot ascend through the ureteral lumen, but experimentally, at least in the guinea pig, obstruction of ureters and disturbances of innervation are followed by ascent of bacteria into the pelvis (Kellaway et al.). In other animals and in man, obstruction to the neck of the bladder permits of urinary reflux into the ureters when positive pressure is applied to the bladder,

thus providing for upward dissemination of bacteria (see Eisendrath, Katz and Glasser). Paralysis of the bladder and section of ureteral valves permits an ascending infection through the ureteral lumen (Barber and Draper). If inflammation extend from the bladder into the ureteral lumen, ureteral movement is diminished, and inflammation and infection may proceed upward.

It has also been shown that infection may extend from the bladder into the pericystic and ureteral lymphatics. The latter drain toward the renal pelvis and it is possible that bacteria so transferred may enter the kidney (Eisendrath and Schultz). Nevertheless cases are observed without inflammation in the ureteral lymphatics and it is difficult to believe this is the sole or chief route of ascent. The assumption that bacteria enter the blood stream from lower urogenital infections and are selectively deposited in the kidneys without involvement of other organs has no real support. Our view is that although other factors may operate, the principal mode of ascent is by extension of the inflammation into the mucosa of the ureters and pelvis and thence into the kidney.

CHRONIC PYELONEPHRITIS. Patients with hematogenous abscesses usually die of the underlying pyemia. Acute pyelonephritis may heal or may become subacute and later chronic; healing may occur in any of these stages. In the chronic or healed chronic stage, the kidney may be of normal size, slightly or markedly reduced in size. Often the effects differ markedly in the two kidneys. The organ is firm and the capsule strips with increased resistance. The outer surface may be red, gray or mottled but is usually characterized by foci of retraction. These vary greatly as to size but, regardless of the size, the base of the retraction is flat, finely granular and densely fibrous. This is true scarring of old inflammatory foci and has not the conical form of healed infarcts or of arterial nephrosclerosis. The kidney cuts with increased resistance and shows a nonbulging or retracted cross section, in which the cortex is irregularly reduced in thickness, the striations and distinction from medulla obscured and the pyramids fibrotic, especially toward the tips. The pelvic mucosa is usually thick and dense, with a finely granular surface.

Microscopically, changes are observed particularly under the depressions of the outer surface. The interstitial tissue is richly collagenous and contains foci of lymphocytes, plasma cells, large mononuclear cells, sometimes eosinophils and an occasional polymorphonuclear leukocyte. The tubules are usually atrophic except that toward the border of the fibrotic region and between

toward the squamous form. The underlying connective tissue is infiltrated by cells like those which occur in the interstitial tissue of the cortex. Subacute pyelonephritis shows somewhat more marked inflammatory change and if healing has occurred the inflammatory lesions are practically absent.

Subacute and chronic pyelonephritis is more frequent in females than males; the sex difference is more striking in negroes. It affects principally those in early middle life.

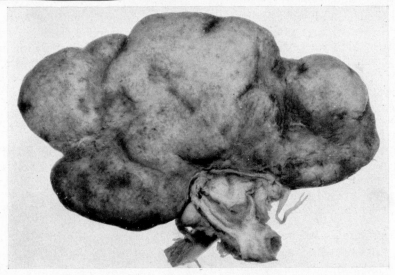

Outer surface of kidney in chronic pyelonephritis. Note depressions of irregular size and distribution with relatively flat base. Kidney about normal size.

such regions there may be marked dilatation of tubules which often contain large hyaline casts (incorrectly called colloid casts). If the disease be active, polymorphonuclear leukocytes, free or as casts, appear in the tubules, but if the condition be healed this is not true. The glomeruli show variable degrees of fibrosis of capsule and tuft, on to complete fibrosis, but many are morphologically normal. Sometimes the preglomerular and other arterioles are thickened and when death occurs in uremia show acute hyaline necrosis. Nevertheless, these changes do not necessarily occur. The larger arteries often show intimal sclerosis. The intermediate and smaller arteries often show a proliferation of connective-tissue cells of the intima, a proliferative endarteritis. The epithelium of the pelvic mucosa may be desquamated, hyperplastic or may show prosoplastic metaplasia

This disease is one of the frequent causes of hypertension and the kidneys usually show well-marked arteriolar disease. Hypertension may be due to unilateral renal involvement; if this can be reasonably established clinically, surgical removal of the kidney results in cure of the hypertension. Renal insufficiency in the later stages of the disease is practically indistinguishable clinically from the terminal stages of chronic glomerulonephritis and of arteriolar renal disease. Uremia, with all its manifestations, leads to death. (See Weiss and Parker.)

Suppurative nephritis resulting from direct extension is rare. It is due to penetration of perinephric abscesses into the renal substance, as indicated later.

Perinephric Inflammations. The most important inflammations in this region are abscesses, referred to usually as perinephric abscess, or tautologically as perinephritic abscess. Probably the most frequent point of origin is renal abscess, which may extend directly or by way of lymphatics into the perirenal fat. In cases of pyemia, abscesses may develop in the perinephric area, independently of any preceding renal infection. Direct extension may occur from neighboring structures as suppurative inflammations of appendix, intestines, vertebrae, internal genitalia, and pleura. Infection of the lower urogenital tract may extend through the peri-ureteral tissues and lymphatics into the perinephric tissues without preliminary involvement of the kidney (see Rolnick). Any of these inflammations may then involve the kidney.

Fibrosis of the capsule and perinephric tissues may occur as the result of acute inflammations in that region, or probably also as secondary to renal suppuration. Contraction may compress the kidney and depress its function. O'Connor regards it as a chronic inflammation, chronic cicatrizing perinephritis, but it may be merely a scarring of the acute lesion, or perirenal sclerosis.

Infectious Granulomata

Tuberculosis. Infections of the kidney by tubercle bacilli may follow the same routes as those indicated for pyogenic organisms. Tuberculosis of the kidney in massive form may be rarely the result of direct extension of tuberculosis of neighboring structures, particularly of the spinal column. The hematogenous variety of renal tuberculosis is miliary and is common as a part of disseminated miliary tuberculosis. The miliary tubercles, sometimes minute but sometimes attaining a diameter of 2 mm. or more, as a rule are distributed in the cortex and are visible both upon the outer surface and in cross section.

Tubercle bacilli may pass through the capillary loops of the glomerulus and lodge in the collecting tubules to produce an excretion form of tuberculosis of the kidney. In these cases the tubercles appear as elongated streaks, which, when they have attained a certain size, may show daughter tubercles in the neighborhood. It is sometimes possible microscopically to find shadows of original tubules in the center of such tuberculous masses, and

in the lumina of these tubules collections of tubercle bacilli. This form is of especial importance since it may lead to tuberculous infection of the renal pelvis and lower genito-urinary tract. If such a tuberculosis of the renal pelvis cause occlusion of the orifice of the ureter, there may be damming back of urine and of caseous material in the pelvis with subsequent distention and an extension of the infection into the kidney itself, producing a form of tuberculosis resembling very closely the ascending variety. Nevertheless, extensive involvement may occur without obstruction, and in some of these cases there may be a polyuria which is believed to be due to the destruction of the concentrating activity of the tubules of the medulla.

Ascending tuberculous infection of the kidney, or tuberculous pyelonephritis, may originate in the seminal vesicles or the epididymis and then spread to the prostate, bladder, ureter, and renal pelvis. As a rule, it produces obstruction in the ureter with distention of the renal pelvis. The tuberculous process then extends through the pyramids in radiating lines into the cortex. In massive involvement, the neighborhood of the greater tuberculous areas shows daughter tubercles. More particularly when there is obstruction of urinary outflow, the kidney may be converted into a large caseous mass. Thus, the pyramids are partially or completely destroyed by the tuberculosis and only a thin rim of the cortex may remain. Before obstruction is complete, there may be excavation of the mass so that the kidney is made up of a connective tissue shell with a small part of parenchymatous substance, and the pelvis is connected with numerous large tuberculous cavities. The presence of neighboring daughter tubercles is helpful in the diagnosis. This form of the disease, sometimes called renal phthisis, is almost invariably chronic in nature and associated with a good deal of fibrosis. Hematogenous or miliary tuberculosis is usually acute in character as is true also of the excretion form, but as a rule the ascending variety of renal tuberculosis is subacute or chronic. Rarely, vascular involvement by tubercles may produce infarction of the kidney with subsequent spread of the tuberculous infection, leading to a tuberculous infarct. Neighboring daughter tubercles assure the diagnosis.

Syphilis. Gummata of the kidney occur, but are rare, both in acquired and congenital syphilis. In congenital syphilis, defective development and degenerations and inflammations in the kidney, may occur, but a large majority of syphilitic fetuses show no lesions of the kidneys. In congenital syphilis, Falci has demonstrated such changes

litic, but there is no final proof of this. In the interstitial spaces there is an infiltration of lymphocytes, large mononuclear phagocytes, plasma cells and an occasional eosinophil. This mass encroaches on the tubules and may penetrate into them. Cholesterol crystals, sometimes within foreign body giant cells, may be found in the tubules. Cicatrization may be extensive. There are no clear cut clinical manifestations.

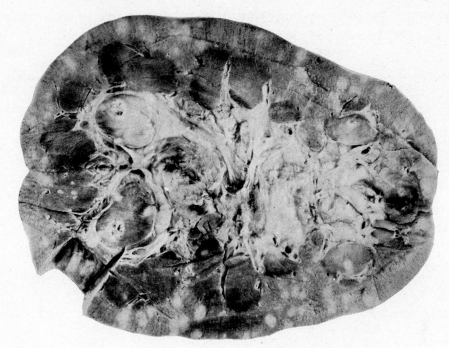

Cross section of kidney with numerous hematogenous tubercles.

as slight diffuse fibrosis, foci of mononuclear cells which are apparently mesoblastic remnants, underdevelopment of tubules and of malpighian bodies with areas of hyalinization of glomerular loops, outspoken focal glomerulonephritis and small collections of cells suggesting multiple miliary gummata. Syphilis may lead to interstitial edema and focal accumulations of mononuclear cells, in both congenital and acquired forms. Warthin reported the presence of *Treponema pallidum*, but this requires confirmation. Florid syphilis may show the clinical signs of a nephrosis, but this has not been shown to be specific and in some instances may be due to therapy.

Rich describes an occasional lesion of the kidneys which he believes to be syphi-

Actinomycosis of the urinary tract is rare and is probably secondary to intestinal infection (see Cecil and Hill).

Regeneration

Evidences of epithelial regeneration in the kidney are not uncommon. More particularly in diffuse diseases of the kidney, multinucleated cells, new epithelium identified by hyperchromatic nuclei and poorly stained cytoplasm, and occasional mitotic figures are observed. The tubular arrangement of newly formed epithelium may occur around focal lesions but is rare in diffuse lesions. Epithelial growth has been observed in tissue culture by Fleischer and Loeb; with tubule formation by Drew. Oliver found that following experimental nephrosis, epithelial repair, both anatomic and functional, may occur, with new formation of Heidenhain rods and rich urea content. Glomeruli do not regenerate after destruction, but hypertrophy may occur in the remaining intact glomeruli.

Tumors

Benign Tumors. The most common benign tumor of the kidney is the fibroma, observed as one or several nodules in the

bryonal derivation are usually single and in the cortex, but may be multiple. They are usually several millimeters in size, well defined and of pale or bright yellow color. Microscopically, three forms are recognized by Dunn. The tumor mass may show a definite capsule both grossly and microscopically. In one form the cells are believed to represent displaced remnants of adrenal cortical substance, and show parallel rows of

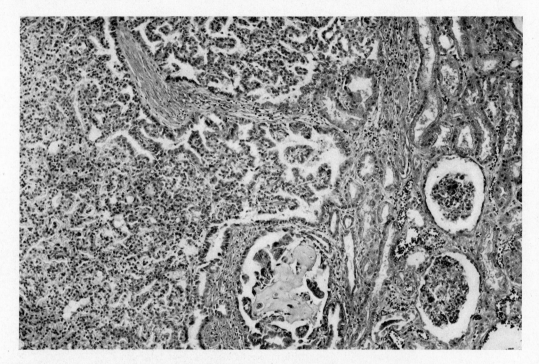

Adenoma of the kidney.

pyramids rarely exceeding 3 mm. in diameter; smooth muscle may be intermingled to constitute a leiomyofibroma. Lipoma may also occur in the same position but is said to be somewhat more frequent in the cortex.

Adenoma is of two general orders. One form is believed to be the result of regeneration following chronic fibrotic diseases of the organ. In such instances they appear as minute, pale yellow, well defined, slightly bulging areas and are found in small scarred spaces of the kidney. Microscopically, they are often poorly defined and show many small acini, sometimes with slight papillary ingrowth. The cells are small and cuboidal in shape.

The adenoma is believed to be of embryonal—

large vesiculated cells resembling adrenal cortex in cell form and in arrangement. Another form shows simple acini lined with small cuboidal cells or, what is more frequent, papillary ingrowth in the acini. The third form is the papilliferous cyst, lined by cuboidal cells; numerous papillary outgrowths spring from the walls to fill the cavity. Practically all of these tumors are benign, but rarely metastasis may arise without there being any microscopic evidence of malignancy in the original tumor.

Malignant Tumors. THE RENAL CARCINOMA, sometimes called the malignant nephroma, is the most frequent tumor of the kidney in adult life. It is most often observed in the sixth decade and affects the two sexes about equally. Geschickter and Widenhorn found that in nearly one-third the cases the duration is in terms of years rather than months and that the younger age groups have the more malignant tumors.

The tumor arises in upper or lower pole, but somewhat more often in the mid-portion of the kidney. It begins near the

tion by fibrous trabeculae, and numerous areas of necrosis and hemorrhage. The mass of tumor often compresses and distorts the renal pelvis and may eventually invade it.

Microscopically these tumors may show notable differences. The most common form is made up of large cuboidal or polyhedral cells with clear vesicular cytoplasm,

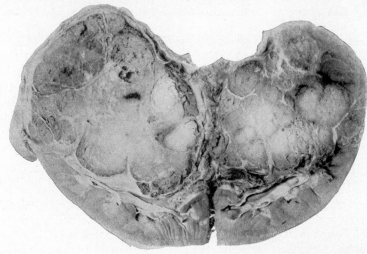

A kidney bisected open to show extensive primary carcinoma of upper pole.

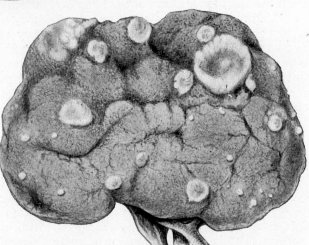

Metastases of carcinoma in a kidney the seat of chronic pyelonephritis.

capsule and enlarges to form a generally globular mass. Fibrous tissue, as a sort of capsule, may partly surround the tumor, kidney substance may be in direct contact and somewhat compressed, and regions of definite invasion are often demonstrated. The tumor is soft and in the cross section is bulging, of yellow color or mottled yellow and red, bleeds freely, often shows a lobula-

which may contain fat and glycogen. The nuclei are small, fairly dense and often situated eccentrically in the cell. Mitotic figures are infrequent. These cells grow in bands and papillary projections from a delicate fibrous reticulum, containing many capillaries, which may give an alveolated character to the tumor. Necrosis, hemorrhage and blood pigment are common. Other tumors are made up of smaller cells with granular cytoplasm and dense centrally disposed nuclei. In these the "combing" away from the supporting framework is less apparent and the cells are commonly in large nests and sheets. Either of these forms may show acinus formation and sometimes papillary arrangement of the lining cells. These carcinomas usually show the preponderance of either the clear-cell or the granular-cell type, but examination of many sections will disclose that they are mixtures with predominance, often great, of one cell type. The fact that vascularization is rich and that many vessels of considerable size are present, explains the usual metastasis by way of the blood stream. In addition, growth into veins, as far as the renal vein and well up into the vena cava, also serves for dissemination by the blood stream. The rich vascularization probably accounts for the hematuria of many of these patients. Fetter states that metastases are most frequent in lungs, liver, adrenals and bones, and less frequent in kidney, spleen, heart and brain. Pathologic fracture of involved bone may be the first sign of the presence of the tumor.

THE HYPERNEPHROMA is a tumor which grossly is like the carcinoma and microscopically is like the clear-cell type. It is probably derived from adrenal remnants in the renal cortex. These remnants are uncommon, and so is the hypernephroma. The clear cells are like those of the adrenal cortex, but in order to identify the tumor as hypernephroma it seems necessary to find tumorous elements such as may arise from adrenal medulla, the ganglioneuroma, the sympathicoblastoma, or the phaeochromocytoma.

THE CONGENITAL MIXED TUMOR, or as it is sometimes called, the embryonal adenosarcoma, or Wilms' tumor, occurs principally in early life. It is usually unilateral, may involve the whole kidney and may become huge. Grossly, it is a firm, fairly well encapsulated, lobulated mass. The cross section usually shows a variegated appearance in which pale and dark red areas, sometimes intermingled with areas of necrosis, are scattered irregularly.

Microscopically, there is a mixture of elements. There are regions of mature and immature connective-tissue, as well as sheets of small round cells which may show acinic or tubular differentiation. Structures suggestive of glomeruli, as well as small cysts, may be found. Cartilage, bone, embryonal type of striated and smooth muscle, and tissues of nervous system also may be encountered. The tumors originate from mesoblast and in small part from the neural crest; thus they are embryomas rather than teratomas. (See Masson.) They may grow to enormous size and are frequently malignant; metastases occur by blood and lymph stream, with involvement especially of lungs or brain (Ladd and White).

THE SECONDARY TUMORS, both carcinoma and sarcoma, are usually carried to the kidney by the blood stream, with the production of numerous metastases.

LYMPHOSARCOMA may involve the kidney, and in lymphoid leukemia there are often lymphomas in the kidney.

Cysts

These may be acquired or congenital. The most frequent acquired cysts are multiple, small, thin-walled retention cysts, situated in the outer part of the cortex. These may occur in any chronic disease of the kidney and are due to obstruction of tubules by fibrous tissue. Large cysts, measuring up to several centimeters in diameter, usually but not invariably occur at one of the poles of the kidney. The wall is thin and fibrous, the lining smooth, and the content thin limpid watery fluid of the chemical character of dilute urine. This form of cyst is usually solitary and unilocular, but may be multiple or sometimes loculated. It may be due to retention in connection with fibrosis of the kidney or due to obstruction the result of disease of a minor calyx, the so-called hydrocalicosis (Watkins). It is possible that in some instances these large cysts are of congenital origin. (See Gutierrez.)

Congenital cysts include the rather rare dermoid cyst and fairly frequent congenital cystadenoma of the kidney or multiple cystic kidney. Congenital cystadenoma may be encountered at practically any age. About a third of these patients die in early life, but many survive to late middle and some to advanced years. There is clear evidence of a hereditary influence.

The condition is usually bilateral, occasionally associated with similar cyst forma-

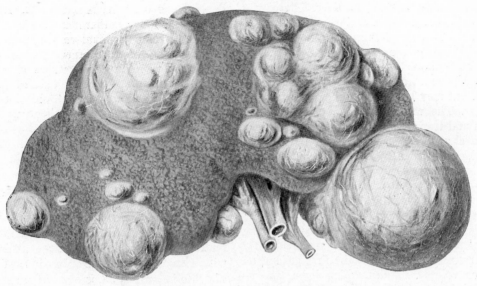

Multiple retention cysts in arteriolar nephrosclerosis.

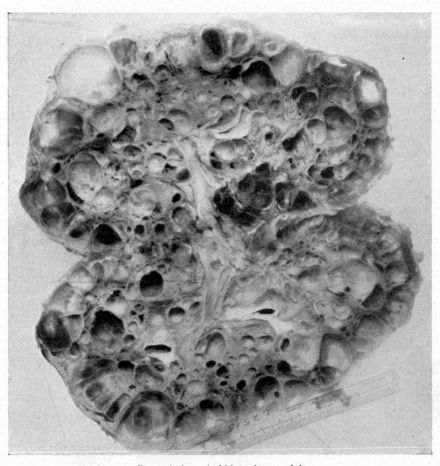

Congenital cystic kidney in an adult.

tion in the surface of the liver. The organs are enlarged, sometimes markedly so, weighing as much as 1000 grams each, or more.

Grossly, the surface of the kidney is markedly lobulated by the projecting cysts. These have an average diameter of 6 to 10 mm. but may be much smaller or somewhat larger. The walls of the cysts are usually thin and transparent. The cyst content may be a clear, limpid, colorless, or pale yellow fluid, or a hyaline, firm, jelly-like mass either of light yellow or brown color. Microscopically, the cysts have thin fibrous walls, lined with flat or cuboidal cells and may show tiny glomerular structures. As the cysts expand there is progressive atrophy of surrounding renal parenchyma. The cysts are apparently the result of isolation of the first generation of convoluted tubules which have the capacity, in association with mesoblast, to form glomeruli. Filtration takes place but ultimately resorption is inadequate and cysts form; when they reach a certain size, the glomeruli disappear evidently because of compression atrophy. The fluid in the cysts has a composition as to urea and creatinine like that of tubular urine (Lambert and Muller).

Pseudocysts may be due to healing and encapsulation of such lesions as abscess, hemorrhage, tuberculosis, etc. Hemangiomas and aneurysms may be cystic. The only parasitic cyst is the echinococcus cyst.

Parasites

These are rare in the kidney. The most frequent is *Taenia echinococcus*. The cyst grows in the kidney usually as the simple cyst of this sort described in the chapter on Liver and Pancreas. Rupture into the pelvis may result in the discharge of hooklets in the urine. *Distomum hematobium* sometimes invades the renal pelvis. *Eustrongylus gigas,* observed in the kidneys of lower animals, occurs only rarely in man.

RENAL PELVIS AND URETER

Congenital Anomalies

One or both ureters may be double, in which instance the renal pelvis usually shows greater or lesser division into two corresponding parts. If the orifice into the bladder be double, one occupies the usual position in the trigone and the other may empty into the colliculus, vas or seminal vesicle. Congenital narrowing or stricture of the ureter occurs particularly at the points where it is normally narrow, namely, at the outlet from the renal pelvis and at the entrance into the bladder (see Meyer). If sufficiently marked, such congenital stricture may lead to a congenital form of hydronephrosis. The ureters may show numerous variations in their course.

Circulatory Disturbances

Passive hyperemia of ureter and of renal pelvis is not uncommon and shows distention of the veins, sometimes associated with edema. Hemorrhage occurs in the course of acute inflammation, is one of the manifestations of diseases of the blood and of certain poisons, and may be due to erosion by calculi, or to the presence of tumors. The blood may coagulate in the ureter and be discharged, sometimes with colic, in the form of long narrow cast-like clots.

Inflammations

Inflammation of the renal pelvis, pyelitis, is usually combined with ureteritis. Such inflammations may be descending, caused by passage of organisms through the kidney, or may originate in renal infections. The ascending form has been discussed in connection with pyelonephritis. Infections of ureter and pelvis appear to be favored by urinary stagnation. Pyelitis is common in female children and adults. It is thought that in these instances the inflammation is slight and confined to the pelvis, but probably there is often extension into the kidney (Griffin). In severe pyelitis the kidney is usually involved to constitute a pyelonephritis.

Pyelitis and Ureteritis. It may be catarrhal, purulent or fibrinous. It may be due to bacterial invasion, the use of drugs and catheters, or to the presence of calculi. Purulent inflammations are due to the colon bacillus and to the pyogenic cocci. Rarely, such inflammations may be pseudomembranous in character and, particularly when calculi are present, the inflammation may be ulcerative. If obstruction to the outflow of urine does not occur before the onset of inflammation, the more severe inflammations almost invariably lead to obstruction with damming back of urine. Thus, the pelvis becomes filled with pus to constitute a pyonephrosis. Hinman and Lee-Brown claim that pressure in the pelvis may cause backflow of bacteria and their products into

merous minute cysts are encountered, apparently arising from misplaced or aberrant epithelium in the wall of the ureter, pelvis and bladder (Morse). In the renal pelvis chronic inflammation and the presence of calculi may produce a thickening of the epithelial layers or a leukoplakia (see Richey). Of great importance is the fact that the

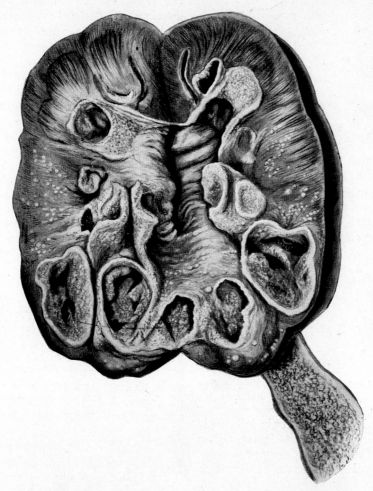

Ascending variety of renal tuberculosis, showing tuberculous ureteritis, pyelonephrosis and tuberculous nephritis.

the veins, but Bird and Moise are convinced that this is due to rupture from tubules into the veins.

Chronic Pyelitis and Ureteritis. Mild infection, or repeated acute attacks of inflammation, may produce a chronic pyelitis and ureteritis, with thickening of the mucosa and fibrosis of the underlying stroma. The epithelium may be thickened to produce numerous small polypi; in other instances nu-

healing of acute inflammations, or prolonged chronic inflammations, may lead to single or multiple strictures of the ureters.

Tuberculosis of the pelvis may be the result of a downward extension of tuberculosis from the kidney, more especially the excretion form, or upward extension from tuberculosis of the bladder. The lesion of the pelvis has been described with tuberculosis of the kidney.

Hydronephrosis

Distention of the renal pelvis by damming back of urine may be due to a variety of causes including stricture of the urethra, which may be congenital in origin or acquired

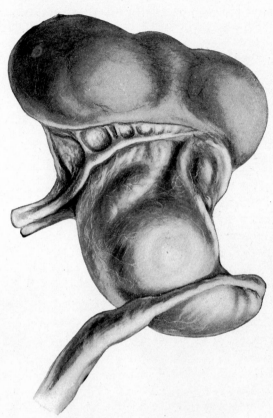

Marked hydronephrosis as a result of obstruction to the ureter by carcinoma of the uterus.

as the result of acute or chronic inflammation; it may be due to kinks in the ureter from misplaced or floating kidney or to pressure by an anomalous renal artery; the ureter may be occluded by accidental ligation in surgical operations, by calculi, by acute, chronic or tuberculous inflammations and by tumors. Other causes include compression by tumors in the abdominal cavity, megalocolon especially with stasis of intestinal content, tumors of the female genitalia, tumors of the rectum, and pregnancy.

Obstruction of the outlet of the bladder because of inflammations, calculi within the bladder, enlarged prostate and stricture of the urethra may lead to bilateral hydronephrosis. As the result of these causes the

hydronephrosis is of the so-called closed variety, or it may be partial. The explanation of open hydronephrosis is more difficult. The passage of urine through the ureters is due in large part to muscular activity, and it is highly probable that atony of the muscle as the result of involvement of the sympathetic or central nervous system, or of the muscle as the direct result of inflammation, may so interfere with ureteral movement of the urine as to cause dilatation of ureter and renal pelvis (see Scott). In those cases where obstruction is in the urethra, the dilatation of ureter and pelvis may be in part due to atony of the muscle and in part to reflux of urine into the ureters from the bladder (see Auer and Seager).

The condition develops slowly, and varies in degree from a simple dilatation of the pelvis with little or no change in the kidney, to enormous dilatation of the pelvis with partial or complete disappearance of kidney substance. In the more severe cases the size of the kidney is considerably increased and the outer surface may be smooth or distinctly lobulated. The lobular projections correspond to the distention of the pelvis between the pyramids; the kidney substance being thicker at the pyramids, is more resistant to the distention than is the cortical substance. The renal substance itself is firm, pale and fibrous. The cross section is pale, usually retracts and bleeds very little. It is materially but irregularly thinned, the pyramids representing the thicker parts. The pelvic wall is thick and fibrous. In the most advanced cases the renal substance cannot be identified grossly and the entire mass is a large sac with dense fibrous wall which, in some instances, is calcified and even ossified.

Microscopically, the renal epithelium shows varying degrees of cloudy swelling, fatty degeneration and atrophy, going on finally to complete disappearance. The atrophy may be marked before there are noteworthy changes in the glomeruli, so that in the microscopic section they are relatively numerous. The atrophy is probably in large part a disuse atrophy (Joelson, Beck and Moritz). Ultimately the capsule of Bowman and glomerular tuft undergo fibrosis and may be converted into fibrous balls. Fibrosis is progressive in the interstitial connective tissue and there is often an accompanying atrophy and fibrosis of the blood vessels.

Experimentally, hydronephrosis is reversible up to about 10 days, but after that the changes are permanent. At first renal function is only slightly impaired, but ultimately it becomes more inadequate and if the disease be bilateral, death results from uremia.

Strong's studies of the pathogenesis of hydronephrosis indicate that the first effect is a slight inflammation of the renal

smaller ones often have a rough, jagged surface but the larger ones are likely to be smooth.

The smaller calculi are made up of products of protein disintegration such as cystine, xanthine or uric acid. Evidently there is supersaturation in the urine leading to precipitation but just why the calculi form is uncertain unless there be a nidus of some sort. The large stones are composed of calcium in combination with magnesium, phosphorus or oxalate. General conditions

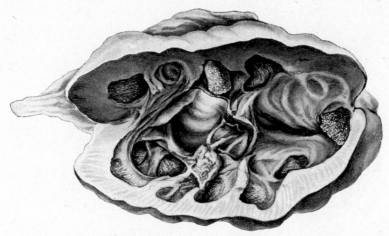

Cross section of kidney, the seat of hydronephrosis and multiple calculi.

papillae which extends into the interstitial tissues and leads to fibrosis. The collecting and distal convoluted tubules become distended and distorted. Atrophy of the proximal convoluted tubules occurs early in the process, with fairly long continued preservation of the loops of Henle. Ultimately atrophy becomes widespread and glomerular changes are a late manifestation.

Calculi

The presence of calculi in the renal pelvis is spoken of as nephrolithiasis. Their composition has been discussed in the chapter on Mineral Infiltrates and Concrements. In newborn infants it is not uncommon to find many small sand-like particles of urates in the renal pelvis, especially when "uric acid infarcts" occur. Discharge of such "sand" in the urine is not uncommon in childhood and in later life. The particles may coalesce to form larger calculi. More especially in adults, calculi may be of considerable size. The

favoring stone formation include hyperparathyroidism and deficiency of vitamin A, but these would account for but few of the cases. Local conditions may include inflammation. Stasis, however, is a result rather than a cause, and this is probably true of inflammation. Careful studies indicate that in the renal papillae there may be deposits of calcium near the tips. Erosion leads to deposits of other salts, furnishing the basis for formation of a calculus. Concrements may rarely be composed of fibrin, in which salts of calcium may be deposited. (See Berke; Quinby; Allen and Ragsdale; Randall et al.)

Tumors

Benign Tumors. Papilloma, covered by the transitional epithelium of the part, sometimes occurs in the renal pelvis but is extremely rare in the ureter. Myoma very rarely occurs in the ureter.

Malignant Tumors. Carcinoma of the renal pelvis, usually a papillary carcinoma made up of cells like those in the papilloma, constitutes a large, spongy, bleeding mass in the pelvis, may invade and destroy a large part of the kidney and may lead to distant metastases. Squamous-cell carcinoma is extremely rare, and results either from prosoplasia of the lining epithelium of the pelvis or of the cells during tumor growth (see Saltzstein and Beaver). The frequent association of calculi and carcinoma suggests irritation as a cause of the tumor, but in some instances the calculus may be a result of the presence of the tumor. Primary carcinoma of the ureter is also rare (Lindner, D'Aunoy and Mailhes).

mucosa, which, if the patient reach adult life, may be the seat of extensive new gland formation. The condition is commoner in male than in female children. It is frequently associated with failure of closure not only of the anterior abdominal wall but also of the pubis, with anteriorly cleft penis or clitoris and often with complete inguinal hernia. Infection may extend to the kidneys and become generalized.

Failure of septum formation may cause congenital vesicorectal or vesicovaginal fistula. The bladder is rarely absent. Septation of the bladder or multiple bladder has been reported. The urachus may remain

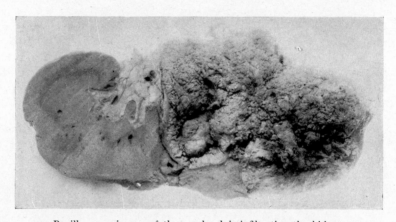

Papillary carcinoma of the renal pelvis infiltrating the kidney.

Teratoid tumors sometimes occur in pelvis and ureter.

Secondary tumors may be transported by the blood or lymph vessels. Direct extension may occur from malignant tumors of rectum, bladder and female genitalia, and from metastases in lymph nodes and in peritoneum. Hematuria is a frequent symptom. Hydronephrosis, sometimes with bloody fluid (hematonephrosis), is a common sequel of both primary and secondary tumors of the ureter.

THE URINARY BLADDER

Congenital Anomalies

The most important of these is exstrophy of the bladder (see Von Geldern). This is due to failure of union of the lateral parts of the urogenital cleft. The bladder is an open sac communicating with the lower abdominal wall, usually with red and swollen

completely or partially patent and in the latter condition sometimes becomes cystic. Cullen describes carcinoma, sarcoma, and tuberculosis of the persistent urachus.

Circulatory Disturbances

Passive hyperemia, more especially in women with displacements of the bladder, may produce varices of the veins near the urethral outlet. Varices may also result from thrombosis of pelvic veins, especially in the aged. Hemorrhage is due to acute inflammations, calculi, tumors, parasites, direct trauma as by introduction of foreign bodies, or indirect trauma especially with fracture of the pelvis.

Inflammations

Although it is probable that slight and evanescent acute catarrhal inflammation of the bladder may occur as the result of introduction of irritant chemicals and other substances, nevertheless the important forms of acute cystitis are due to bacteria. Inflammation may result from the presence of foreign bodies, calculi, animal parasites, etc., but even in these circumstances bacteria are likely to play an important part as secondary invaders. The organisms concerned in cystitis are especially the colon bacillus, various forms of streptococci and staphylococci, the typhoid bacillus and others. Apparently those which produce ammoniacal decomposition of the urine lead to more serious inflammations than those which do not.

The most common route of infection is through the urethra, particularly from introduction of instruments, but apparently organisms are also carried into the bladder from the kidney, through the blood stream, and perhaps also through the lymphatic communications. In the vast majority of instances a most important predisposing cause of bladder inflammation is prolonged hindrance to the outflow of urine. Thus, inflammations and stricture of the urethra, enlargement of the prostate gland, especially the middle lobe, due either to inflammation, hyperplasia or tumor formation, cystocele, calculi in the bladder, tumors of the bladder, and paralysis of the bladder are likely to be complicated by cystitis. Sometimes the inflammation is local, as around the neck of the bladder in case of cystocele in women, or in and about acquired or congenital diverticula of the bladder.

Acute catarrhal cystitis exhibits slight or marked swelling of the mucosa, with hyperemia and sometimes adherent mucus upon the surface. Microscopically there is hyperemia, edema, cloudy swelling of the epithelium with desquamation and slight infiltration of lymphoid cells and leukocytes. The urine contains desquamated epithelium, lymphoid cells and leukocytes and stringy mucus in the form of cylindroids. It may or may not be alkaline, depending upon the type of organism concerned.

Acute purulent cystitis shows pronounced hyperemia and swelling of the mucosa and usually a covering of purulent material. Abscesses in the mucosa and ulceration are not uncommon. Microscopically, there are found hyperemia, edema and diffuse infiltration of inflammatory cells, particularly polymorphonuclear leukocytes, asso-

ciated with necrosis, desquamation and ulceration of the epithelium. As time goes on the process may involve the deeper structures of the bladder to produce an acute phlegmonous cystitis. This may be followed by penetration of the suppurative process into the surrounding tissues, especially where there are diverticula of the bladder. The bladder wall may become so soft as to be ruptured by a catheter or other instrument. We have observed one case in which penetration through a diverticulum resulted in extensive perivesical inflammation and death from pyemia. Penetration into the peritoneum may lead to local or generalized peritonitis.

Since the pyogenic organisms can and do produce ammonia, the urine in purulent cystitis is likely to be alkaline. It contains desquamated epithelium and large numbers of leukocytes and pus cells, which may be so abundant as to form a large bulk of urinary sediment. The alkalinity of the urine may lead to such swelling of the cells that they become indistinguishable. Bacteria are usually present in large numbers. Hemorrhage is distinctly more common than in the catarrhal form. The precipitation of phosphates and carbonates in the urine may produce a certain amount of encrustation of the bladder walls.

Acute fibrinous or fibrinopurulent cystitis usually represents an extremely severe local infection, an infection brought by the blood stream, or an infection complicating corrosive chemical action. The signs of inflammation are pronounced, and in addition there is likely to be not only extensive necrosis and greater or less degree of hemorrhage, but also a deposition of a fibrinous or fibrinopurulent mass, especially along the crests of the contracted muscle bands. The necrotic part and the fibrinous membrane are often of dark brown color and the bladder lining encrusted as in the purulent form (see Carson).

Chronic cystitis may be the sequence of one or repeated attacks of any of the above forms, but is more likely to follow the catarrhal than the purulent or fibrinous variety. Usually the entire bladder wall is thickened and fibrotic but occasionally atrophic forms may be observed. Because of the obstruction which leads to inflammation or which is secondary to prolonged inflammation, there is likely to be hypertrophy of the muscle. Associated with the hypertrophy there is almost always interstitial fibrosis between the muscle bands. The mucosa may show a simple thickening of catarrhal character with fibrosis and infiltration of lymphoid cells, or may be the seat of chronic ulceration. Sometimes the lining epithelium becomes transformed from the transitional form to a stratified squamous epithelium. Chronic cystitis may occur occasionally in peculiar forms. Thus, tiny epithelial cysts may occur to produce CYSTITIS CYSTICA. Granular forms may be found, in which the tiny projections may be made up of nodules of proliferated epithelium. In CYSTITIS FOLLICULARIS, the nodules are composed of lymphoid nodules or of masses of lymphoid cells. In CYSTITIS EMPHYSEMATOSA, cystic spaces are filled with gas. Rarely there may be a bullous emphysema of the bladder. Some of these conditions may be induced by instrumentation. Gas may be produced by fermentation of urine rich in sugar, as in diabetes or following administration of glucose. (See Hinman, Johnson and McCorkle; Wells; Stirling.)

An infrequent chronic ulcerative cystitis is called Hunner's ulcer. This occurs more often in women than in men and is especially a disease of middle life. There is dysuria and reduced capacity of the bladder. More often near the vertex, is an ulcer of variable size associated with a diffuse chronic interstitial cystitis. (See Higgins.)

Leukoplakia may occur in the bladder especially when calculi are present.

MALAKOPLAKIA is uncommon, affects women more often than men, and occurs especially in older people but may be seen in infancy and childhood. The lining of the bladder shows numerous, firm, well-defined plaques, from a few millimeters to a centimeter or more in diameter, usually with a depressed center and a surrounding zone of hyperemia. Microscopically most of the exudative cells are large mononuclear cells with finely granular cytoplasm often containing phagocytosed nuclear and cellular fragments, erythrocytes and bacteria. There are a few lymphocytes, plasma cells and an occasional neutrophilic (rarely eosinophilic) leukocyte. Delicate capillaries penetrate from the base and the connective tissue fibrils are thin and sparse. There are also, especially in older cases, Michaelis-Gutmann bodies, about the size of a large cell, usually basophilic and often concentrically laminated, intracytoplasmic but sometimes free; they may contain iron and calcium. Their nature is not known. The middle of the surface is devoid of epithelium, but otherwise the bladder is not diseased except for rich lymphocytic infiltration at the base of the plaques. Rarely the ureters and renal pelvis and even the kidney may be affected. The condition is without symptoms and the cause is unknown. (See McDonald and Sewall.)

Infectious Granulomata

Tuberculosis. Although in generalized miliary tuberculosis, miliary tubercles may be observed in the bladder wall, and although occasionally tuberculosis may extend from the prostate and seminal vesicles in massive form into the bladder, nevertheless, the most important form clinically and pathologically is that which originates as miliary tuberculosis around the orifice of the ureters, apparently as the result of transmission of bacteria from the upper urinary tract into the bladder. Tubercles may form more widely in the trigone and even further along the posterior bladder wall. They are likely to break down and produce small, shallow, caseous ulcers which may fuse to form large ulcerated areas. The surrounding mucosa is usually distinctly hyperemic, but the bladder as a whole is the seat only of a mild catarrhal cystitis. The margins of larger ulcers may show numerous daughter tubercles. In uncomplicated cases the urine is clear and acid, occasionally blood tinged, but when secondary infection supervenes, the urine may take on all the characters of any of the acute forms of cystitis and the bladder itself may show widespread secondary inflammation.

Syphilis. In the secondary stages of syphilis, mucous patches similar to those observed in other mucous membranes may occur. Gumma is not common but is seen more frequently in the trigone than in other parts of the bladder.

Alterations of Size and Form

Dilatation of the bladder occurs as the result either of paralysis of the muscle or as the result of obstruction to the urethral orifice. If the obstruction be of short duration, as is observed in those spasmodic forms of retention of urine which occur after operations in the region of the pelvis, recovery may be rapid and complete. If the obstruction be prolonged, as in enlarged prostate, a hypertrophy accompanies the dilatation. In uncomplicated dilatation the amount of urine may be very large, and sometimes the bladder is palpated as high as the umbilicus.

least conceivable that in some instances there is a congenital weakness of muscle in these parts. Inasmuch as urine is likely to stagnate in the diverticula they become favored parts for inflammation, with a possibility on the one hand of extension through the wall or rupture of the diverticulum, or on the other hand, extension of the inflammation throughout the bladder. Diverticula also appear to be favorable points for the deposition of calculi.

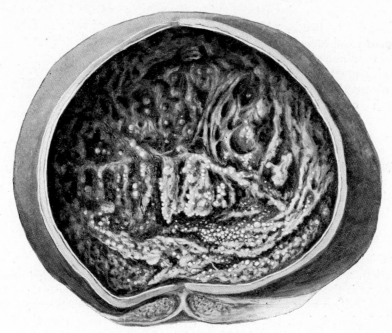

Extensive tuberculosis of the bladder, showing the most marked involvement near the urethral orifice.

LOCALIZED DILATATIONS OR DIVERTICULA of the bladder may be single or multiple, and usually are observed in the posterior wall about the orifices of the ureter or near the insertion of the urachus. Two varieties are distinguishable, although sometimes with difficulty. The true diverticulum is usually of congenital origin and all the coats of the wall of the bladder, somewhat attenuated, take part in the dilatation.

FALSE DIVERTICULA, which in our experience are much more common, appear as dilated areas pouching out between bundles of muscle, usually in a hypertrophic bladder. These are presumably due to increased pressure within the bladder, so that the outpouching occurs at the point where the musculature is thinner than elsewhere. It is at

Malposition. The bladder may rarely take part in hernias, but the most important malposition of the bladder is that due to relaxation of the pelvic floor in women. The support of the posterior wall of the bladder, furnished by proper position of uterus and vagina, may thus give way so that the bladder is displaced posteriorly and bulges into the vagina in the form of the so-called cystocele. The urine may stagnate in the outpouched portion of the bladder and inflammation ensue, but it is rare that such severe inflammation is observed as is true in diverticula. Prolapse of the uterus may cause inversion of the trigone, which may result in kinking of the ureters as they enter the bladder. The upper part of the bladder may pouch downward into the cavity of the bladder, the so-called inversion, or it may even project through the urethral orifice, constituting prolapse of the bladder.

Hypertrophy of the bladder is practically always accompanied by a variable degree of dilatation. It may be caused by any of the conditions mentioned in discussing the etiology of inflammation, which produce prolonged obstruction to outflow of urine. The bladder wall is variably thickened and fibrotic. The outstanding feature is the fact that the muscle undergoes hypertrophy in interlacing bundles or bands, which constitute the so-called trabeculae of the bladder, producing the condition spoken of as trabeculation. There is a great variety of lesions that may cause obstruction to the neck of the bladder, both congenital and acquired (Young).

Rupture

Rupture of the bladder, or perforation, occurs as the result of fractures of the pelvis whereby fragments of bone penetrate the organ. In labor, prolonged pressure of the fetal head upon the bladder and vagina may cause necrosis of the tissue and subsequent perforation. Instrumentation may produce perforation, more especially, however, when the bladder is the seat of inflammation or necrosis. Perforation may also be caused by wounds of bullets, knives, etc. Considerable external pressure upon a distended bladder may produce rupture. Malignant tumors of the bladder, vagina, uterus, and other neighboring structures may lead to perforation of the bladder.

Depending upon the site of perforation, urine may enter the peritoneum or infiltrate the pelvic tissues. If sterile urine be poured into the peritoneum because of rupture, and little or none discharged through the urethra, uremia may occur. If it be infected, peritonitis follows. Infiltration of the pelvic tissues may be followed by extension into the skin of the lower abdomen and thighs; if infected, suppuration ensues. As the result of birth injuries or the presence of malignant tumors, ruptures may lead to the establishment of fistulae between neighboring organs such as vesicovaginal, vesicorectal and vesicouterine fistulae.

Calculi

These occur principally in males in later middle life but are not rare in women and children. They vary in size from a fraction of a millimeter to several centimeters. The larger calculi are usually single and if multiple may be faceted. The smaller ones may be so numerous as to justify the term sand or gravel. Calculi may be primary in the bladder or may pass into the bladder after originating in renal pelvis or ureter. Inflammations of the bladder may be a cause or a sequence of calculus formation. Calculi may be of noninflammatory and of inflammatory origin.

Of the primary calculi of noninflammatory origin, the urate calculus is probably the most important. It is made up principally of ammonium urate, mixed also with sodium urate and sometimes uric acid. Such calculi occur especially where there is undue excretion of uric acid as in leukemias, the puerperium, lobar pneumonia, rheumatic fever, etc. The calculus is usually small, firm, angular, yellowish-brown, and in multiple form usually constitutes gravel or sand. The oxalate calculi, apparently the most common urinary calculi, usually originate in the renal pelvis and are small, hard, of irregular contour and of light or dark brown color. The cystine calculi are unusual; they are small, smooth, round, translucent, waxy, white or pale yellow, sometimes lamellated, bodies. The xanthine calculi are smooth and of brownish-red color. Phosphate calculi, round with slightly granular surface and chalky character, are more often secondary than primary.

Such primary noninflammatory calculi may be discharged with the urine, but if they remain they may act as physical foci for further precipitation and show secondary encrustations in the form of lamellae. In a general way if the urine be acid, the encrustation is of urates, if neutral, of oxalates, and if alkaline, of phosphates. The last occurs principally after bladder infection is established.

The occurrence of inflammation may cause the deposit of phosphates or other salts upon a noninflammatory calculus. Primary inflammatory calculi are due to the presence of urea-splitting bacteria, including the pyogenic cocci, colon bacillus and others, with resultant ammoniacal urine (Chute and Suby). They may be composed of ammonium magnesium phosphate, calcium phosphate, calcium oxalate and ammonium urate (Wells).

The centra for calculus deposition, most especially those of inflammatory nature, include foreign bodies introduced from without, desquamated cells and tissue masses, parasites and their ova, bacteria, mucus, etc., but sometimes, even although organic matter may constitute a part of the calculus, a nidus cannot be found.

Foreign Bodies and Parasites

The foreign bodies include those introduced through the urethra such as instruments or their fragments, and a wide variety of substances such as needles, pins, pencils, etc., introduced as the result of sexual perversion or other mental disturbance, mineral encrustation especially due to inflammation, epithelial cells, tissue masses especially from tumors, solid materials gaining access through fistulae. The parasites include *Distomum hematobium*, the ova of which are often found in the urine, echinococcus, *Filaria bancrofti. Oxyuris vermicularis*, trichomonas and similar organisms may gain access to the urinary bladder presumably through the urethra.

Tumors

Benign Tumors. Except for the papilloma, benign tumors of the bladder are rare. Fibroma, adenoma, hemangioma, leiomyoma, rhabdomyoma, and mixtures of these forms have been reported. Dermoid cysts and other types supposedly originating in embryonal rests are rare; the same is true of those presumably due to failure of obliteration of the urachus. The most frequent tumor of the bladder is the papilloma or papillary fibroepithelioma. This is usually pedunculated but may be sessile.

Grossly, the papilloma is a pale red, shaggy, rough, cauliflower-like growth, a few millimeters to several centimeters in diameter, which bleeds readily. Microscopically, there are numerous delicate papillae of mature connective tissue, richly supplied with small blood vessels. Surmounting the papillae is a regular mass of epithelium like the natural transitional epithelium of the bladder.

Minor changes such as elongation or flattening of the cells, or prosoplastic formation of squamous cells may occur.

Noteworthy is the fact that when a papilloma is removed, another may subsequently develop. Whether this is recurrence or development of a new papilloma in the circumstances which led to growth of the first one is not certain. With or without recurrence, the papilloma has a striking tendency to become a carcinoma. This has led some authorities to group it as grade-I carcinoma. Nevertheless, at least half the cases are cured by operation and in our opinion it is not just to call a tumor a carcinoma because it might become one. It is admitted, however, that microscopic examination often gives no clue as to the potentialities of the papilloma. The papillomas and carcinomas are situated most often in or near the trigone, less often in the neck of the bladder and are unusual in the vault or anterior surface of the bladder.

Malignant Tumors. THE CARCINOMAS may be of papillary infiltrating form, with preservation of papillary growth but with considerable pleomorphism of the epithelial cells and definite invasion of the surrounding tissue. Another form is nonpapillary. It is invasive, shows squamous epithelium with pearl formation but with little pleomorphism. These two carcinomas have been classified as group II. In group III are nonpapillary infiltrating carcinomas without squamous-cell formation but with great pleomorphism, the cells lacking uniformity in size, shape and polarity. These grades do not represent clear differences in degree of malignancy. Adenocarcinomas are rare and must not be confused with extensions from uterus and rectum. Carcinomas of the bladder do not metastasize with any great frequency, and the metastases are usually limited to the pelvic lymph nodes, the pelvic bones and lower vertebrae. Death is usually due to infection of bladder, ureters, renal pelvis and kidneys.

EPITHELIAL TUMORS of the bladder are three times as frequent in males as in females, are rare before the fourth decade and have their highest incidence between the ages of 50 and 70 years. The principal symptoms are dysuria and hematuria. Causes are not well known except for the fact that they are frequent in aniline workers and occur in *Bilharzia* infestation. (See Ash.)

PRIMARY SARCOMA is rare. Grossly, it may be nodular or diffusely infiltrating. Microscopically it may be a lymphosarcoma, a spindle-cell sarcoma or one of the differentiated forms of sarcoma. Care must be taken to distinguish a sarcoma-like proliferation of connective tissue of papillary tumors or spindle-cell carcinoma derived from papillomas.

SECONDARY CARCINOMA of the bladder is most commonly an extension from carcinoma of the cervix uteri, but also may be from prostate and from rectum. It is only rarely that carcinoma in other situations shows metastasis to the bladder. Sarcoma may extend from any of the pelvic viscera or may be metastatic.

Cysts

Cysts of the bladder include dermoid cysts, echinococcus cysts and rarely small serous cysts in the posterior inferior wall. The last occur particularly in men and are believed to represent cystic dilatation of remnants of Müller's duct.

THE URETHRA

Congenital Anomalies

These are distinctly more frequent in the male than in the female. They include atresias of various degrees, folds of various kinds, double urethra, epispadias, hypospadias, and diverticula. In epispadias the urethra opens on the upper surface of the glans or of the penis, and in hypospadias on the lower surface.

Inflammations

Although acute urethritis may be due to various organisms, more especially in the female by introduction from vagina and vulva, or the result of infection of wounds, the most common is that due to the gonococcus introduced by sexual contact.

In the male, gonorrhea is a disease primarily of the anterior urethra. The clinical signs of the disease usually begin about nine days after infection. The gonococci proliferate in the urethral epithelium, especially in the lacunae and excite acute suppurative inflammation, with hyperemia, edema, infiltration of leukocytes, desquamation of epithelium and ulceration. The bacteria enter the connective tissues under the ulcers for a short distance only. Many of the leukocytes contain phagocytosed gonococci, but the organisms are also seen between epithelial cells and elsewhere in the inflamed tissues. Pus discharged from the anterior meatus, often in large amounts, is viscid, yellow or greenish yellow and microscopically shows numerous pus cells, epithelial cells, gonococci both intracellular and extracellular and sometimes other organisms.

The disease is often limited to the anterior urethra but may extend to the posterior portion, to the epididymis, seminal vesicles, prostate, bladder and by so-called metastasis may involve joints, tendon sheaths, endocardium and other structures. In the female, the uterine cervix, fallopian tubes and pelvic peritoneum, and sometimes endometrium, are affected, as described in the chapter on Genital System. Gonococcal conjunctivitis may occur in infants by infection in passage through the birth canal. This is usually less serious than is true of gonococcal conjunctivitis in the adult, the result of transfer of infection by the hands or otherwise from an infected urethra; opacities of the cornea, iritis, iridocyclitis and panophthalmitis may result.

Chronic urethritis is usually gonorrheal and affects especially the posterior urethra as a chronic catarrhal process, sometimes associated with metaplasia to squamous epithelium, a leukoplakia, and ulceration.

Stricture. Stricture of the urethra is common in males but infrequent in females. It is almost invariably the late sequel of urethral gonorrhea, although rarely it may apparently be due to other types of inflammation and to traumatic injury. It is most commonly observed in the posterior parts of the urethra but may occasionally occur nearer the anterior meatus. Although gonococcal urethritis is principally an inflammation of the mucosal surface, there is often an inflammation of the underlying lymphatics and hence in the later stages there may be an interstitial fibrosis. The subsequent contraction of the fibrous tissue may be the contraction of a scar or that of a genuine chronic inflammation. Clinical evidence indicates that the latter is true of most cases.

The urethral lumen becomes narrowed, the urinary stream small and weak and ultimately there may be complete stoppage. If of sufficient degree and duration, urethral stricture may cause dilatation and hypertrophy of the bladder. It may even lead to dilatation of the ureters and hydronephrosis. The urethra behind the stricture may become dilated and there may be associated saccular or elongated outpouchings. These are called false passages, but the same type of condition may be produced anterior to the stricture by rough instrumentation with catheters and sounds. Instrumentation may produce infection and the resultant inflammation may affect bladder, ureters, renal pelvis and kidneys, especially if these structures be dilated. As a sequence of false passages or unskillful instrumentation, the urine dammed behind the stricture may infiltrate into surrounding tissues with extension to scrotum, perineum and adjacent superficial parts of thighs and lower abdomen. This infiltration usually becomes infected, with resultant inflammation and sometimes gangrene.

Infectious Granulomata

Chancre and gumma may affect the urethra. Tuberculosis is usually an extension from a tuberculous prostate or from a lupus of the vulva.

Tumors

Benign tumors such as papilloma, adenoma, fibroma, etc., are rarely encountered. Fairly common in women is the urethral caruncle, which is included here for convenience. That it is a tumor is doubtful. It is situated at or near the internal urethral orifice and is usually a more or less pedunculated mass a few millimeters in diameter. Covered by urethral epithelium, the mass may be granulomatous but is usually either a richly vascularized connective tissue or has a telangiectatic structure; acinic structures may be found presumably originating in the glands of Skene (Olcott).

Malignant Tumors. Primary carcinoma is usually in the form of squamous-cell carcinoma, or rarely adenocarcinoma, probably originating from the glands of Cowper.

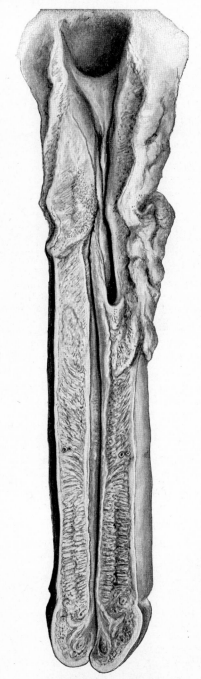

Longitudinal section of penis, showing stricture of membranous urethra, dilatation of the proximal portion and false passage extending distally.

Sarcoma, including lymphosarcoma, rhabdomyosarcoma, spindle cell sarcoma and other forms, is extremely rare. Secondary tumors are also rare.

REFERENCES

Addis, T., and J. Oliver: The Renal Lesion in Bright's Disease, New York, 1931.

Allen, C. D., and J. W. Ragsdale: Fibrin Stones: Report of Four Cases, Arch. Surg., 37: 546, 1938.

Altnow, H. O., C. C. Van Winkle, H. W. Maly, and L. E. Williams: Renal Amyloidosis: Clinical Course and Pathologic Lesions in Sixteen Cases, Arch. Int. Med., 56: 944, 1935.

Anderson, H. C.: The Relation of Blood Pressure to the Amount of Renal Tissue, Jour. Exper. Med., 39: 707, 1924.

Aschoff, L.: Renal Secretion and Renal Diseases, Lectures on Pathology, New York, 1924, p. 340.

——: Pathologische Anatomie, 6th ed., Jena, 1923.

Ash, J. E.: Epithelial Tumors of the Bladder, Jour. Urol., 44: 135, 1940; see also Report of the Registry of the American Urological Association, Grading of Epithelial Tumors of the Urinary Bladder, Ibid., 36: 651, 1936.

Atchley, D. W., and E. M. Benedict: The Distribution of Electrolytes in Dogs Following Ligation of Both Ureters, Jour. Biol. Chem., 73: 1, 1927.

Auer, J., and L. D. Seager: Experimental Local Bladder Edema Causing Urine Reflux into Ureter and Kidney, Jour. Exper. Med., 66: 741, 1937.

Ayer, G. D., and A. G. Gauld: Uremia Following Blood Transfusion: The Nature and the Significance of the Renal Changes, Arch. Path., 33: 513, 1942.

Baehr, G.: Glomerular Lesions of Subacute Bacterial Endocarditis, Ibid., 15: 330, 1912.

Barber, W. H., and J. W. Draper: Renal Infection. A Further Experimental Study of Its Relation to Impaired Renal Function, Jour. Amer. Med. Asso., 64: 205, 1915.

Bell, E. T.: Lipoid Nephrosis, Amer. Jour. Path., 5: 587, 1929.

——: Cystic Disease of the Kidneys, Ibid., 11: 373, 1935.

——, B. J. Clawson, and T. B. Hartzell: Experimental Glomerulonephritis, Amer. Jour. Path., 1: 247, 1925.

——, and T. B. Hartzell: The Etiology and Development of Glomerulonephritis, Arch. Int. Med., 29: 768, 1922.

——, and B. J. Clawson: Primary (Essential) Hypertension, A Study of 420 Cases, Arch. Path., 5: 939, 1928.

Berg, S.: Urinary Protein Partitions in Amyloid Nephrosis, Arch. Int. Med. 67: 1050, 1941.

Berke, J. D.: Nature of Urinary Calculi, Jour. Urol., 38: 118, 1937.

Bird, C. E., and T. S. Moise: Pyelovenous Backflow, Jour. Amer. Med. Asso., 86: 661, 1926.

Blackman, S. S., Jr.: On the Pathogenesis of Lipoid Nephrosis and Progressive Glomerulonephritis, Bull. Johns Hopkins Hosp., 57: 70, 1935.

Brown, G. E., and G. M. Roth: The Anemia of Chronic Nephritis, Arch. Int. Med., 30: 817, 1922.

Burch, G. E.: Formation of Edema in the Eyelids of Man, etc., Ibid., 65: 477, 1940.

Carson, W. J.: Gangrene of the Bladder, Jour. Urol., 13: 205, 1925.

Cash, J. R.: Further Studies on Arterial Hypertension, Proc. Soc. Exper. Biol. and Med., 23: 609, 1925-26.

Cecil, H. J., and J. H. Hill: Actinomycosis of the Urinary Organs, Jour. Amer. Med. Asso., 78: 575, 1922.

Chute, R., and H. I. Suby: Prevalence and Importance of Urea-Splitting Bacterial Infections of the Urinary Tract in the Formation of Calculi, Jour. Urol., 44: 590, 1940.

Councilman, W. T.: Anatomical and Bacteriological Study of Acute Diffuse Nephritis, Amer. Jour. Med. Sci., 114: 23, 1897.

——: The Pathology of the Kidney, Jour. Amer. Med. Asso., 46: 81, 1906.

Croftan, A. C.: The Rôle of the Alloxuric Bases in the Production of Cardiovascular Changes of Nephritis, Amer. Jour. Med. Sci., 120: 592, 1900.

Cullen, T. S.: The Umbilicus and Its Diseases, Philadelphia, 1916.

DeNavasquez, S.: Experimental Symmetrical Cortical Necrosis of the Kidneys Produced by Staphylococcus Toxin: A Study of the Morbid Anatomy and Associated Circulatory and Biochemical Changes, Jour. Path. and Bact., 46: 47, 1938.

Dible, J. H., and J. D. Hay: The Nature of Fatty Change in the Kidneys, Ibid., 51: 1, 1940.

Dickes, R.: Relation Between the Symptoms of Uremia and the Blood Levels of the Phenols, Arch. Int. Med., 69: 446, 1942.

Downey, H.: The Occurrence and Significance of the "Myeloblast" under Normal and Pathologic Conditions, Arch. Int. Med., 33: 301, 1924.

Drew, A. H.: Growth and Differentiation in Tissue Cultures, Brit. Jour. Exper. Path., 4: 46, 1923.

Duff, G. L., and E. D. G. Murray: Bilateral Cortical Necrosis of the Kidneys, Amer. Jour. Med. Sci., 201: 429, 1941.

Dunn, J. S.: The Fundamental Lesion in Acute Diffuse Intracapillary Glomerulonephritis, Jour. Path. and Bact., 51: 169, 1940.

——: Aberrant Epithelial Structures Found in the Renal Cortex, etc., Ibid., 17: 515, 1912-13.

Edwards, J. G.: The Vascular Pole of Glomerulus in Kidney of Vertebrates, Anat. Rec., 76: 381, 1940.

Eisendrath, D. N., and O. T. Schultz: Lymphogenous Ascending Infection of the Urinary Tract, Jour. Amer. Med. Asso., 68: 540, 1917.

——, H. Katz, and J. M. Glasser: Bladder Reflux, Ibid., 85: 1121, 1925.

Evans, G.: A Contribution to the Study of Arteriosclerosis, with Special Reference to Its Relation to Chronic Renal Disease, Quart. Jour. Med., 14: 215, 1920-21.

Fahr, T.: Pathologische Anatomie des Morbus Brightii, in Henke, F., and Lubarsch, O.: Handbuch der speziellen pathologischen Anatomie und Histologie, Berlin, 1925, 6^1: 156.

Fahr, Th.: Zur Frage der Gichtniere, Centralbl. Allg. Path. u. Path. Anat., 57: 49, 1933.

Falci, E.: Ueber die angeborene Syphilisniere und ueber das Treponema Pallidum, Virchow's Arch. Path. Anat., 247: 164, 1923.

Fetter, T. R.: Renal Carcinoma, Jour. Amer. Med. Asso., 110: 190, 1938.

Fishberg, A. M.: Hypertension and Nephritis, Philadelphia, 1930.

Fleischer, M. S., and L. Loeb: The Relative Importance of Stroma and Parenchyma in Culture Media, Proc. Soc. Exper. Biol. and Med., 8: 133, 1911.

Foster, G. S.: Excessive Physical Exertion and Its Effect on the Kidneys, Jour. Amer. Med. Asso., **112**: 891, 1939.

Foster, N. B.: Uremia. Cecil's Textbook of Medicine, Philadelphia, 1927, p. 879.

Fuller, R. H.: Lipoids in the Kidney, Arch. Path., **32**: 556, 1941.

Gaskell, J. F.: On the Changes in Glomeruli and Arteries in Inflammatory and Arteriosclerotic Kidney Disease, Jour. Path. and Bact., **16**: 287, 1911-12.

Geschickter, C. F., and Widenhorn, H.: Nephrogenic Tumors, Amer. Jour. Cancer, **22**: 620, 1934.

Goldblatt, H.: Studies on Experimental Hypertension. VII. The Production of the Malignant Phase of Hypertension, Jour. Exper., Med., **67**: 809, 1938.

Goldstein, A. E., and B. S. Abeshouse: Urinary Calculi in Bone Diseases: Review of the Literature and Report of Cases, Arch. Surg., **31**: 943, 1935.

Goormaghtigh, N.: Histological Changes in the Ischemic Kidney with Special Reference to the Juxtaglomerular Apparatus, Amer. Jour. Path., **16**: 409, 1940.

Griffin, M. A.: Investigation into Pyuria in Infancy and Childhood, Glasgow Med. Jour., **114**: 21, 1930.

Gutierrez, R.: Large Solitary Cysts of the Kidney: Types, Differential Diagnosis and Surgical Treatment, Arch. Surg., **44**: 279, 1942.

Harrison, T. R., and M. F. Mason: The Pathogenesis of the Uremic Syndrome, Medicine, **16**: 1, 1937.

Hartman, F. W., A. Bolliger, and H. P. Doub: Experimental Nephritis Produced by Irradiation, Amer. Jour. Med. Sci., **172**: 487, 1926; *see also* Jour. Amer. Med. Asso., **88**: 139, 1927, and **89**: 1936, 1927.

Hartz, P. H., A. Van der Sar, and A. van Meeteren: The Occurrence of Mitotic Divisions in Glomeruli in Glomerulonephritis and Malignant Sclerosis, Amer. Jour. Path., **17**: 563, 1941.

Hayman, J. M., Jr., N. P. Shumway, P. Dumke, and M. Miller: Experimental Hyposthenuria, Jour. Clin. Invest., **18**: 195, 1939.

——, and J. W. Martin: Acute Nephritis. Review of 77 Cases, Amer. Jour. Med. Sci., **200**: 505, 1940.

——: Experiments on the Patency of the Blood Vessels of Nephritic Kidneys Obtained at Autopsy, Jour. Clin. Invest., **8**: 89, 1929-30.

——, and Bender, J. A.: Nephritic Albuminuria, Arch. Int. Med., **51**: 447, 1933.

Herbert, F. K., H. G. Miller, and G. O. Richardson: Chronic Renal Disease, Secondary Parathyroid Hyperplasia, Decalcification of Bone and Metastatic Calcification, Jour. Path. and Bact., **53**: 161, 1941.

Hewlett, A. W.: Pathological Physiology of Internal Diseases, New York and London, Appleton, 3d Ed., 1928.

Higgins, C. C.: Hunner Ulcer of the Bladder; Review of 100 Cases, Ann. Int. Med., **15**: 708, 1941.

Hinman, F., C. M. Johnson, and J. H. McCorkle: Pyelitis and Ureteritis Cystica, Jour. Urol., **35**: 174, 1936.

——, and T. E. Gibson: Tumors of the Epididymis, Spermatic Cord and Testicular Tunics, Arch. Surg., **8**: 100, 1924.

——, and R. K. Lee-Brown: Pyelovenous Backflow, Jour. Amer. Med. Asso., **82**: 607, 1924; *see also* Lee-Brown, R. K., and J. W. S. Laidley: Ibid., **89**: 2094, 1927.

Hooker, D. R.: Postural or Orthostatic Albuminuria, Arch. Int. Med., **5**: 491, 1910.

Horn, H.: The Experimental Nephropathies, Arch. Path., **23**: 71, 241, 1937.

Horn, R. C., and H. Smetana: Intercapillary Glomerulosclerosis, Amer. Jour. Path., **18**: 93, 1942.

Hueper, W.: Cystitis Emphysematosa, Amer. Jour. Path., **2**: 159, 1926.

Hueper, W. C.: "Aniline Tumors" of the Bladder, Arch. Path., **25**: 856, 1938.

Huffman, L. F.: Congenital Displacements of the Kidney, Jour. Urol., **12**: 363, 1924.

——: Unilateral Renal Aplasia, Ureter Opening into Vas., Ibid., **12**: 379, 1924.

Huntington, G. S.: The Genetic Interpretation and Surgical Significance of Some Variations of the Genito-urinary Tract, Harvey Lectures, 1906-07, p. 222, Philadelphia, 1908.

Jackson, H.: The Histogenesis of Urinary Casts, Amer. Jour. Path., **3**: 285, 1927.

Jacobson, V. C., and E. W. Goodpasture: Occlusion of the Entire Inferior Vena Cava by Hypernephroma, etc., Arch. Int. Med., **22**: 86, 1918.

Joelson, J. J., C. S. Beck, and A. R. Moritz: Renal Counterbalance, Arch. Surg., **19**: 673, 1929.

Kannerstein, M.: Histologic Kidney Changes in the Common Acute Infectious Diseases, Amer. Jour. Med., Sci., **203**: 65, 1942.

Karsner, H. T., S. P. Reimann, and S. C. Brooks: Studies of Uranium Poisoning: IV. The Relation of Acid Intoxication to Nephritis, Jour. Med. Res., **39**: 177, 1918-19.

Kay, C. F.: The Mechanism by Which Experimental Nephritis Is Produced in Rabbits Injected with Nephrotoxic Duck Serum, Jour. Exper. Med., **72**: 559, 1940.

——, P. F. Lucchesi, and R. B. Rutherford: An Experimental Investigation of an Immunologic Mechanism as the Cause of Glomerulonephritis, Jour. Immunol., **42**: 369, 1941.

Kellaway, C. H., C. J. O. Brown, and F. E. Williams: Paths of Renal Infection, Brit. Jour. Exper. Path., **7**: 337, 1926.

Keyes, E. L.: Urology, New York, Appleton, 1923.

Kimmelstiel, P.: Acute Hematogenous Interstitial Nephritis, Amer. Jour. Path., **14**: 737, 1938.

Kitani, Y.: Hydronephrotische Atrophie oder hydronephrotische Schrumpfniere, Virchow's Arch. Path. Anat., **254**: 115, 1925.

Klemperer, P., and S. Otani: "Malignant Nephrosclerosis" (Fahr), Arch. Path., **11**: 60, 1931.

Kretschmer, H. L.: Solitary Cyst of the Kidney: Report of Five Cases, Jour. Amer. Med. Asso., **95**: 179, 1930.

Ladd, W. E., and R. R. White: Embryoma of the Kidney, (Wilm's Tumor) Jour. Amer. Med. Asso., **117**: 1858, 1941.

Lambert, P. P., and P. Muller: Contribution à l'interprétation physiopathologique du rein polykystique, Acta Med. Scandinav., **101**: 338, 1939.

Leiter, L.: Observations on the Relation of Urea to Uremia, Arch. Int. Med., **28**: 331, 1921.

Linder, H. J., R. d'Auncy, and R. J. Mailhes: Primary Carcinoma of the Ureter, Med Jour. and Rec., **132**: 290, 1930; *see also* Rousselot, L. M. and J. D. Lamon: Surg., Gynec. and Obst., **50**: 17, 1930; McCown, P. E., Jour. Amer. Med. Asso., **4**: 468, 1930.

Loeb, L.: Edema, Medicine, **2:** 171, 1923.

Löhlein, M.: Ueber Nephritis nach dem heutigen Stand der pathologisch-anatomischen Forschung, Ergeb. Inner. Med. u. Kinderheilk., **5:** 411, 1910.

———: Zur Pathogenese der vaskulären Schrumpfniere, Med. Klin., **12:** 741, 1916.

Mackay, E. M., E. M. Hall, and F. M. Smith: A Renal Lesion Occurring in Rats Maintained at Low Environmental Temperatures, Proc. Soc. Exper. Biol. and Med., **32:** 320, 1934.

MacMahon, H. E., and J. H. Pratt: Malignant Nephrosclerosis (Malignant Hypertension), Amer. Jour. Med. Sci., **189:** 221, 1935.

Major, R. H.: Renal Function and Arterial Hypertension, Amer. Jour. Med. Sci., **176:** 637, 1928.

Mark, M. F., and H. O. Mosenthal: Kidney Function and Uremia in Renal Amyloidosis, Amer. Jour. Med. Sci., **196:** 529, 1938.

Masson, P.: The Rôle of the Neural Crests in the Embryonal Adenosarcomas of the Kidney, Amer. Jour. Cancer, **33:** 1, 1938.

Matthews, E.: Glomerulonephritis, Amer. Jour. Med. Sci., **203:** 134, 1942.

McCann, W. S., and M. J. Romanowsky: The Effect of Ptosis of the Kidney on Blood Pressure, Renal Blood Flow and Glomerular Filtration, Trans. Asso. Amer. Phys., **55:** 240, 1940.

McDonald, S., and W. T. Sewell: Malakoplakia of the Bladder and Kidneys, Jour. Path. and Bact., **18:** 306, 1913-14.

McElroy, J. B.: Nephroses, Jour. Amer. Med. Asso., **89:** 940, 1927.

McGregor, L.: The Cytological Changes Occurring in the Glomerulus of Clinical Glomerulonephritis, Amer. Jour. Path., **5:** 559, 1929.

———: Histological Changes in the Renal Glomerulus in Essential (Primary) Hypertension. A Study of Fifty-one Cases, Ibid., **6:** 347, 1930.

Meyer, J. M.: Congenital Atresia of the Vesical Extremities of Both Ureters, Proc. New York Path. Soc., **24:** 115, 1924.

Mills, R. G.: Cystitis Emphysematosa, Jour. Urol., **24:** 217, 1930; Surg., Gynec. and Obst., **51:** 545, 1930; Amer. Jour. Obst. and Gynec., **20:** 688, 1930.

Mitchell, A. G.: Nephrosclerosis (Chronic Interstitial Nephritis) in Childhood, with Special Reference to Renal Rickets, Amer. Jour. Dis. Child., **40:** 101, 1930.

Mitchell, A. G., and G. M. Guest: Certain Phases of Nephrosclerosis in Childhood, Jour. Amer. Med. Asso., **97:** 1045, 1931.

Moise, T. S., and A. H. Smith: The Effect of High Protein Diet on the Kidneys, Arch. Path. and Lab. Med., **4:** 530, 1927.

Moore, R. A., and L. M. Hellman: The Number of Open Glomeruli in Acute Mercuric Chloride Nephrosis, Jour. Exper. Med., **53:** 303, 1931.

Moritz, A. R., and J. M. Hayman, Jr.: The Disappearance of Glomeruli in Chronic Renal Disease, Amer. Jour. Path., **10:** 505, 1934.

———, and M. R. Oldt: Arteriolar Sclerosis in Hypertensive and Non-Hypertensive Individuals, Amer. Jour. Path., **13:** 679, 1937.

Morse, H. D.: Etiology and Pathology of Pyelitis cystica, Ureteritis cystica and Cystitis cystica, Amer. Jour. Path., **4:** 33, 1928.

Murphy, F. D., L. M. Warfield, J. Grill, and E. R. Annis: Lipoid Nephrosis: A Study of Nine Patients, with Special Reference to Those Observed Over a Long Period, Arch. Int. Med., **62:** 355, 1938.

Myers, V. C., and E. Muntwyler: Chemical Changes in the Blood and Their Clinical Significance, Physiol. Rev., **20:** 1, 1940.

Nakano, H.: Atlas der Harnsteine, zugleich eine krystallographisch-chemische Studie über deren Entstehung, Leipzig and Vienna, 1925.

De Navasquez, S.: The Excretion of Haemoglobin, with Special Reference to the "Transfusion" Kidney, Jour. Path. and Bact., **51:** 413, 1940.

Nye, L. J. J.: Chronic Nephritis and Lead Poisoning, Sydney (Australia), 1933.

O'Connor, V. J.: Perirenal Sclerosis (Chronic Cicatrizing Perinephritis), Jour. Amer. Med. Asso., **85:** 1118, 1925.

O'Hare, J. P., and W. G. Walker: Observations on Salt in Vascular Hypertension, Arch. Int. Med., **32:** 283, 1923.

Olcott, C. T.: Urethral Caruncle in the Female, Surg. Gynec. and Obst., **51:** 61, 1930.

Oliver, J.: The Architecture of the Kidney in Chronic Bright's Disease, New York, Hoeber, 1939.

Peabody, F. W.: Clinical Studies on Respiration, II. The Acidosis of Chronic Nephritis, Arch. Int. Med., **16:** 955, 1915.

Quinby, W. C.: Urinary Stone. Some Present Day Concepts, Trans. Cong. Amer. Phys. and Surg., **16:** 45, 1938.

Randall, A.: The Initiating Lesions of Renal Calculus, Surg., Gynec. and Obst., **64:** 201, 1937.

———, J. Eiman, and P. R. Leberman: Studies of the Pathology of the Renal Papilla. Relationship to Renal Calculus, Jour. Amer. Med. Asso., **109:** 1698, 1937.

Rich, A. R.: The Pathology of 19 Cases of Peculiar and Specific Form of Nephritis Associated with Acquired Syphilis, Bull. Johns Hopkins Hosp., **50:** 357, 1932.

Richards, A. N.: Methods and Results of Direct Investigation of the Function of the Kidney, Baltimore, 1929.

Richey, DeW. G.: Leukoplakia of the Pelvis of the Kidney—A Study in Metaplasia, Jour. Lab. and Clin. Med., **5:** 635, 1920.

Rolnick, H. C.: A Pathway of Infection in Perinephritis, Arch. Surg., **26:** 41, 1933; *see also* Eisendrath, D. N., and H. C. Rolnick: Urology, Philadelphia, 1930.

Saltzstein, H. C., and D. C. Beaver: Papillary Carcinoma of the Pelvis of the Kidney, Arch. Surg., **40:** 949, 1940.

Schürman, P., and H. E. MacMahon: Die maligne Nephrosklerose, zugleich ein Beitrag zur Frage der Bedeutung der Blutgewebsschranke, Virchow's Arch. Path. Anat., **291:** 47, 1933.

Schwentker, F. F., and F. C. Comploier: The Production of Kidney Antibodies by Injection of Homologous Kidney plus Bacterial Toxins, Jour. Exper. Med., **70:** 223, 1939.

Scott, D. E.: The Part Played by Ureteral Inflammation in Dilatation of the Ureter, Arch. Surg., **28:** 296, 1934.

Seegal, B. C.: Chronic Acidosis in Rabbits and in Dogs, with Relation to Kidney Pathologic Change, Arch. Int. Med., **39:** 550, 1927.

Smadel, J. E.: Nephrotoxic Nephritis, The Year Book of Pathology and Immunology, Chicago, Year Book Publishers, 1940, p. 229.

———, and H. F. Swift: Experimental Nephritis in Rats Induced by Injection of Antikidney Serum. V. Chronic Nephritis of Insidious Development following Apparent Recovery from Acute Nephrotoxic Nephritis, Jour. Exper. Med., **74:** 345, 1941.

Smith, H.: The Physiology of the Kidney, New York, Oxford Univ. Press, 1937.

Stirling, W. C.: Cystitis Follicularis, Jour. Amer. Med. Asso., **112:** 1326, 1939.

Strong, K. C.: Plastic Studies in Abnormal Renal Architecture: V. The Parenchymal Alterations in Experimental Hydronephrosis, Arch. Path., **29:** 77, 1940.

Volhard, F., and T. Fahr: Die Bright'sche Nierenkrankheit, Berlin, 1914.

Von Geldern, C. E.: The Etiology of Exstrophy of the Bladder, Arch. Surg., **8:** 61, 1924.

Warthin, A. S.: The Excretion of Spirocheta Pallida Through the Kidneys, Jour. Infect. Dis., **30:** 569, 1922.

Watkins, K. H.: Cysts of Kidney Due to Hydrocalycosis, Brit. Jour. Urol., **11:** 207, 1939.

Weiss, S., and F. Parker, Jr.: Pyelonephritis: Its Relation to Vascular Lesions and to Arterial Hypertension, Medicine, **18:** 221, 1939.

Wells, H. G.: Report of Seven Cases of Cystitis Emphysematosa, Jour. Urol., **39:** 391, 1938.

———: Chemical Pathology, 5 ed., Philadelphia, Saunders, 1925.

Widdowson, E. M.: A Comparative Investigation of Urine and Serum Proteins in Nephritis, Biochem. Jour., **27:** 1321, 1933.

Wolbach, S. B., and K. D. Blackfan: Clinical and Pathological Studies on So-called Tubular Nephritis (Nephrosis), Amer. Jour. Med. Sci., **180:** 453, 1930.

Young, H. H.: The Pathology and Treatment of Obstructions at Vesical Neck in Women, Jour. Amer. Med. Asso., **115:** 2133, 1940.

Zimmerman, H. M., and J. P. Peters: Pathology of Pregnancy Toxemias, Jour. Clin. Invest., **16:** 397, 1937.

19

The Genital System

THE MALE GENITALIA

CONGENITAL ANOMALIES

The penis may be absent, the urethra opening into perineum or rectum. The organ may be unusually small (micropenis) or large (megalopenis). It may be cleft, double, or may be adherent to the scrotum. Epispadias and hypospadias have been mentioned in discussing the urethra. "The foreskin may be absent, incompletely developed, redundant, or adherent to the glans; the preputial orifice may be absent or extremely small; the frenum may be abnormally short" (White and Martin). Phimosis, a condition in which the preputial orifice is too small to permit retraction of the prepuce is a common congenital defect.

The anomalies of the testes include those of number, size and position. It is doubtful that supernumerary testes, or polyorchism, occurs. Anorchism may be unilateral or bilateral, associated usually with absence of the epididymis and scrotal vas. Fusion or synorchism is reported in the fetus. Testes vary in size normally. Congenital aplasia or hypoplasia is referred to as micro-orchism and if severe may be associated with the eunuchoid state, in which certain feminine secondary sex characters are exhibited.

Alterations in position include ectopy, or position outside the normal sites, as in the groin or perineum, inversion or retroversion in the scrotum, but the most important is undescended testis. This last is due to incomplete descent of the testis through the inguinal canal to the scrotum. If unilateral it is usually called undescended testis, but if bilateral the term cryptorchism or cryptorchidism is employed. The terms abdominal nondescent and inguinal nondescent are employed to indicate the position; the latter is more frequent than the former. The testis may be essentially normal up to about 24 years of age, but thereafter spermatozoa are not likely to be formed (Rea). The undescended testis is especially susceptible to inflammation following traumatic injury, and is more likely to be the seat of malignant tumors than if normally situated, as will be discussed later. Hernia is a common accompaniment of undescended testis.

HERMAPHRODISM

True hermaphrodism occurs when there is present, in one individual, functioning testicular and ovarian tissue. It is rare in higher mammals and man. This usually is in the form of unilateral or bilateral ovotestis, an organ containing both testicular and ovarian tissue. To be conclusive there should be evidence of function on the part of both components.

Malformations of genitalia give rise to the condition called pseudohermaphrodism in which the external genitalia may resemble one sex and the general body make up be that of the other, the latter being determined by the character of the sex glands. In males undescended testes and bifid scrotum may look like labia majora, which when associated with aplastic penis, with perineal hypospadias and sometimes a perineal pouch, give the appearance of female genitalia. Females may exhibit a large clitoris, absence of, or small vagina (with small uterus and ovaries), thus giving the external appearance of male genitalia. (See Young.)

THE PENIS

Phimosis

Congenital phimosis has been referred to. Acquired phimosis may result from acute inflammations with so much swelling that the foreskin cannot be retracted, or from cicatricial contraction of the preputial orifice. Paraphimosis, a condition in which a retracted prepuce cannot be brought forward by ordinary means, results from inflammatory or edematous swelling of a retracted

foreskin, from swelling which produces a rolling back of the foreskin, or from forcible retraction of a phimotic foreskin. The frenum may be short congenitally or as the result of cicatricial contraction, and this may interfere with erection and coitus.

Circulatory Disturbances

Marked passive hyperemia and edema of the glans accompany paraphimosis. The penis may be the seat of passive hyperemia and edema as the result of general diseases such as myocardial insufficiency. Local edema may result from blocking of lymphatics by scar tissue or by *Filaria bancrofti*. Thrombosis of veins as the result of wounds, or sometimes as the result of leukemia, may lead to priapism.

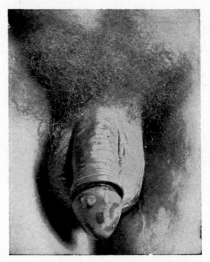

Balanitis, from Genito-Urinary Surgery, by Martin, Thomas and Moorhead.

Inflammations

Balanitis and Balanoposthitis. The more common acute inflammations include balanitis or inflammation of the glans, balanoposthitis in which the inflammation involves also the prepuce, chancroid, and herpes. Balanitis and balanoposthitis are favored by redundant or phimotic prepuce with accumulation of the secretion of Tyson's glands, desquamated epithelium and urine. Although smegma bacilli may be abundant, the exciting organisms are usually colon bacilli or pyogenic cocci. The inflammation may be slight, but may become ulcerative.

and in the presence of phimosis may become gangrenous. Involvement of the inguinal lymph nodes is not common. Balanitis may also be due to irritant urethral discharges, particularly of gonorrhea.

HERPES PROGENITALIS is characterized by the abrupt appearance, usually in the coronary sulcus, of vesicles with a slightly inflamed base. The surface of the vesicles quickly macerates, leaving small discrete or confluent ulcers. The lesion may be due to balanitis, to immoderate coitus, to contact with irritating discharges from vagina or uterus, or to some of the general causes of herpes.

Acute inflammations may extend into and produce acute lesions of the substance of the penis. The condylomata which may follow prolonged superficial inflammations will be discussed with tumors. Leukoplakia is sometimes observed.

Chancroid or soft chancre is defined admirably by Keyes as "a specific, local, contagious, auto-infectious venereal ulcer." It

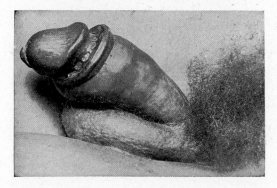

Multiple chancroids of coronary sulcus, from Genito-Urinary Surgery, by Martin, Thomas and Moorhead.

occurs in single or multiple form, usually in the coronary sulcus near the frenum, and in females about the introitus, but it may spread to neighboring regions or may be primary in other situations. It is caused by the *Haemophilus ducreyi* which in the hands of Davis and others has fulfilled the postulates of Koch. It is a gram-negative, short, relatively thick bacterium with rounded ends and a narrow median portion which gives the "dumb bell" shape. The pus from the lesions shows intra- and more especially extracellular organisms, single, in pairs, and in short chains, grouped in parallel or fan-like rows.

The lesion appears after a variable but short incubation period, which in auto-inoculation lesions is about 24 hours. An interruption of surface continuity is essential for the implantation of the causative organism. It is primarily a seropurulent lesion in and immediately under the epiderm. The surface sloughs in a few hours leaving the ulcer. As usually seen the ulcer is rounded, has soft, sharply defined, sometimes undermined edges, a surrounding zone of hyperemia and a necrotic, smooth or irregular base covered with pus. Microscopically, the ulcer shows the necrotic base infiltrated with leukocytes. The surrounding zone shows a similar infiltration combined with plasma cells, lymphoid and endothelial cells. In addition to the dilatation of the blood vessels there is an acute peri- and endovasculitis. The organisms can be demonstrated in the sections.

Secondary infections often occur, and organisms other than the Ducrey-Unna bacillus may predominate. This may produce a spreading destructive phagedenic ulcer or even gangrene. Although lymphangitis is not common, suppuration of the inguinal lymph nodes is frequent and rarely the iliac nodes may be involved. The inguinal "bubo," if not incised, often breaks through the skin of the groin to produce purulent deep ulcers which may become gangrenous.

Infection with syphilis may occur at the same time as that with chancroid. The latter lesion with its shorter incubation period appears first and is followed by the indurated inactive ulcer of hard chancre. This combination is often called mixed chancre.

Chronic inflammations of the penis with deposition of fibrous tissue are sometimes observed in older men, and usually cannot be ascribed to definite cause. The fibrosis appears especially in the corpora cavernosa and tunica albuginea testis, as small or extensive nodules which may be calcified or even ossified.

Infectious Granulomata

Syphilis. The primary lesion of syphilis, the chancre or hard chancre, is seen usually upon the glans, near the frenum or upon the prepuce. Its character has been described in the chapter on Infectious Granulomata. In the secondary stage, mucous patches or flat condylomata may be observed upon glans, prepuce, or skin near the scrotum. In late syphilis gumma may occur in the glans and the corpora cavernosa; the scars may produce much deformity.

Tuberculosis may involve the penis following the tuberculous urethritis of extensive urogenital tuberculosis. Rarely a tuberculous infection occurs by coitus, or by sputum in perversion or in ritual circumcision. Lupus is also rare.

Granuloma inguinale described in the chapter on Infectious Granulomata may affect the skin of the penis. Actinomycosis and leprosy are rare.

Tumors

Benign tumors include lipoma, adenoma, angioma and papilloma. The papillo-

or uncleanliness. It is possible that cutaneous horns may occur.

Malignant Tumors. Although sarcoma, usually with rapid regional metastasis, may occur in the penis, the most important malignant tumor is the squamous cell carcinoma. This originates most frequently on the glans and somewhat less so on the prepuce, and in contrast to the acuminate condyloma is not often primary in the coronary sulcus. It usually occurs after fifty years of age but cases in much earlier life have been reported. It is likely to have a history of wart, prolonged balanitis or phimosis. It is exceedingly rare among those who have been circumcised. The commoner form, grossly, is a destructive infiltrative papillary or cauliflower-like tumor, but there is also a form which occurs as an indurated sluggish ulcer. It invades the penile structures slowly, and

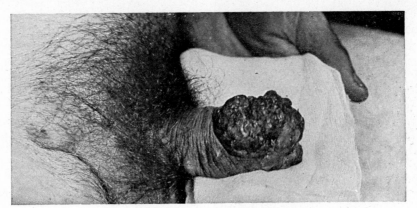

Carcinoma of penis with early lymphatic involvement, from Genito-Urinary Surgery, by Martin, Thomas and Moorhead.

mata include the common wart and also the acuminate condyloma, which latter although not necessarily of venereal origin is sometimes called venereal wart. The acuminate condyloma, sometimes single but usually multiple, occurs in the coronary sulcus, but may be seen upon glans, foreskin or even in the urethra. The cauliflower-like mass may be sessile or pedunculated, shows numerous villi covered by stratified squamous epithelium, is usually pink in color and bathed in a thin mucoserous or seropurulent discharge. As noted in the chapter on tumors, such growths may be regarded as either inflammatory hyperplasias or as tumors. They follow irritations of the part resulting from the various forms of balanoposthitis, urethritis

shows metastasis to inguinal lymph nodes in about a third of the cases, but seldom extends to the pelvis or beyond (Jorstad). Inflammatory reaction and keratinization of epithelium are usually pronounced in the histologic section. Owing to the infection of the superficial tumor, inflammatory enlargement of the inguinal lymph nodes is common and should not be confused with metastasis.

Cysts and Concrements

Cysts about the raphe are usually congenital epidermoid cysts or dermoid cysts. Cystic dilatations of sebaceous glands or of Tyson's glands are sometimes observed.

Concrements in the preputial sac are either waxy masses of inspissated smegma, sometimes infiltrated with phosphates, or calculi made up of urinary salts which may be primary or secondary from small calculi originating in bladder or renal pelvis.

THE URETHRA

Lesions of the urethra including gonorrhea have been discussed in the chapter on Urinary System.

THE SCROTUM

The scrotum is subject to a wide variety of skin diseases of which eczema and dermatitis venenata may lead to great swelling. Intertrigo is a mild dermatitis resulting

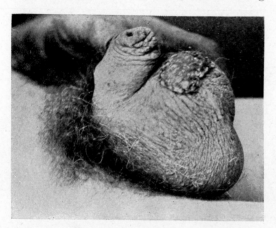

Epithelioma of scrotum, from Genito-Urinary Surgery, by Martin, Thomas and Moorhead.

from moisture and uncleanliness in obese individuals or in children. Pityriasis is sometimes severe. Pediculosis is due to *Pediculus pubis* which differs slightly from the body louse. Inflammations of all kinds, originating from wounds, from urinary infiltrations, from extensions of neighboring inflammation, are likely to show marked edema. Phlegmon, cellulitis or abscess are most often the result of urinary infiltration from ruptured urethra.

Elephantiasis is a prolonged lymph stasis accompanied by chronic lymphangitis and fibrosis of the interstitial tissue. Moderate grades may occur following cicatricial closure of lymphatics or excision of inguinal lymph nodes. The most severe grades are due to occlusion of the lymphatics by the adult *Filaria bancrofti*, and the associated chronic inflammatory change which the parasite sets

up. The microfilaria may be found in the circulating blood. Mosquitoes take up the microfilaria and serve as intermediate hosts for the development of the larval prefilarial phases, which are transmitted to a new human host by the mosquito bite. The scrotum may attain enormous size; rupture of the dilated lymphatics into the urinary tract may cause chyluria or hematochyluria.

Tumors

Numerous benign tumors such as affect the skin may occur. Sebaceous cysts, epidermoid and dermoid cysts, and small blood cysts may also occur. The most important tumor is the squamous-cell carcinoma of the scrotum or "chimney-sweep's cancer" which is a squamous-cell carcinoma appearing grossly either as a papillary or ulcerative form. It is seen also in workers in coal-tar products. It grows slowly and metastasizes late.

TUNICA VAGINALIS

Only the commoner lesions of this sac will be considered. Acute inflammations may be of traumatic origin, most commonly result from extensions from testis and epididymis, or may rarely be blood borne as in a septicemia. The exudate may be serous, serofibrinous or purulent. Tuberculous or syphilitic involvement is usually by extension from epididymis or testis. Chronic inflammations may represent a continuation or sequel of acute lesions. There may be considerable accumulation of fluid, or adhesions, or both with the formation of loculi.

Hydrocele is the accumulation of fluid in the tunica vaginalis. In the congenital form the fluid is peritoneal and due to failure of closure of the funicular process. In the infantile form the process is closed and fluid is found both in the tunica and in the process. Congenital and infantile forms are often accompanied by hernia. The lesion found in adults is a gradual, or less often rapid, accumulation of fluid, usually 100 to 300 cc. in amount but sometimes more than two liters. The cause is unknown but it is more common in middle life and in the tropics. The fluid is clear, colorless, slightly viscid and contains from 6 to 10 per cent of solids, including proteins, fibrin, salts and sometimes grossly visible cholesterol. It contains desquamated epithelium, leukocytes and sometimes erythrocytes and also bacteria. Wells suggests that its character simulates both exudate and transudate. Usually repeated drainage by puncture leads to a character more closely resembling exudate.

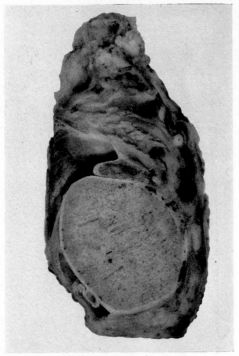

Loculated hydrocele and fibrosis of tail of epididymis.

Hematocele indicates the presence of blood in the tunica vaginalis. It may be due to trauma, to hemorrhagic diseases or secondary to hydrocele.

Chylocele occurs in connection with elephantiasis in which lymphatics rupture into the tunica.

Spermatocele is a cystic dilatation of ducts in the head of the epididymis or in the rete testis. It may rupture into the tunica vaginalis to produce spermatic hydrocele.

Varicocele is included here for convenience. It is a varicose dilatation of the veins of the pampiniform plexus. Usually without known cause, the condition may sometimes be due to venous stasis from pressure of tumors in the abdomen. It is frequent in young men and affects the left side especially. General passive hyperemia is only rarely a cause. The lesion is of little or no significance.

Hernia has been discussed in the section on peritoneum in the chapter on alimentary system.

TESTIS AND EPIDIDYMIS

These organs may share to a moderate degree in general passive hyperemia. Hemorrhage may result from trauma, hemorrhagic disease or torsion of the spermatic cord. Fatty degeneration of epithelium may be seen in atrophy and in chronic inflammations. Iron-bearing pigment is observed in severe anemias, hemochromatosis and in atrophy. Hyalin occurs in various atrophic and fibrotic lesions of the testis; secondary amyloid may be observed in association with amyloid of other viscera.

Inflammation

Acute Inflammations. Both acute orchitis and epididymitis are most commonly caused by extensions from the urinary tract. Therefore the epididymis is affected first, more severely and sometimes solely. The most frequent cause is gonorrhea, which may first affect seminal vesicles and vasa, but often attacks the epididymis directly. Rarely the testis is attacked independently of the epididymis. The lesion begins as a rule in the tail of the epididymis, extends to involve the whole organ, becomes associated with a serous or serofibrinous vaginalitis and may involve, presumably by lymphatic extension rather than by continuity, the neighboring parts of the testis. Suppuration begins in the tubules and extends to the interstitial tissues, where following a preliminary infiltration of lymphocytes and plasma cells, an abscess forms. Only rarely does the abscess become large or rupture. Practically all cases show regression of the acute lesion followed by cicatrization. If sufficiently extensive no discharge of spermatozoa can occur, but sexual activity is undisturbed and atrophy of the testis does not necessarily follow.

Nongonorrheal acute epididymis and orchitis are usually due to staphylococci or colon bacillus, much more rarely to other organisms. It may rarely follow nongonorrheal urethritis, but is most commonly secondary to cystitis complicating enlarged prostate or urethral stricture. Often a seminal vesiculitis intervenes. The involvement of epididymis and testis has much the same situation and histologic features as the gonococcal form. The onset may be rapid or may be so slow as to resemble that of tuberculosis. Spontaneous retrogression and cicatrization occur, but not infrequently the suppuration extends and is either incised or ruptures. Extension into the abdominal cavity is rare. Rare cases of fulminant epididymitis and orchitis are reported, and the process may also be gangrenous.

Metastatic acute infections are observed in the epididymis, more especially in septicemias and pyemias, in typhoid fever, cerebrospinal meningitis, etc. The same is true of orchitis, which also occurs in smallpox and typhus fever. Of particular interest is the so-called metastatic orchitis of mumps, occurring usually in patients at the time of puberty. The lesion is apparently nonsuppurative but in a considerable number of cases leads to fibrosis and atrophy of the testis. Orchitis usually appears at the end of the first week of the epidemic parotitis, but may rarely occur without parotid involvement (Stengel).

Chronic Inflammations. Fibrosis of the testis may be visible in gross cross section or may only be inferred by difficulty in stripping out the tubules by a forceps. Microscopically, there is a form that can only be called *fibrosis testis*, in which there is partial or complete disappearance of epithelium with increase of interstitial connective tissue, often hyalinized where it surrounds the tubules. On the other hand, there may be a similar lesion with extensive infiltration of lymphoid and plasma cells, an indication of a progressive chronic orchitis. The lesions may be local or diffuse, unilateral or bilateral. The cause is not known except that certain cases are due to syphilis and others accompany passive hyperemia and wasting diseases. As a rule, the epididymis is not involved. Fibrosis, however, is usually the cicatrix of a preceding acute inflammation.

Infectious Granulomata

Tuberculosis. The development of conglomerate tubercles is the more common mode of tuberculous affection of the epididymis and testis. The lesions may occur at any time of life. It is secondary to tuberculosis elsewhere in the body, as lungs and other parts of the urogenital tract, even though clinically these other lesions may be inconspicuous and difficult to detect. In some instances it seems probable that a preceding gonococcal epididymis predisposes to tuberculous epididymitis.

The lesion is ordinarily first observed in the globus minor of the epididymis. It is stated that early in the lesion there may be simply a small yellow mass of necrotic material visible grossly, which microscopically shows desquamated epithelium, leukocytes, fat globules, and large numbers of tubercle

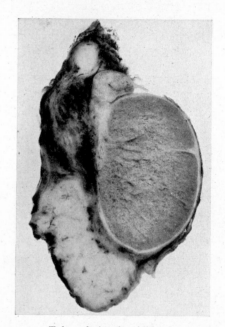

Tuberculosis of epididymis.

bacilli. At any rate, a small tubercle with typical characters develops, and subsequently extends by the formation of daughter tubercles with fusion. This may retrogress and become calcified. More commonly it progresses and may ultimately involve the tunica vaginalis and the testis. The resulting inflammation in the tunica vaginalis may produce either serous or serofibrinous exudate, and occasionally a purulent or caseous and purulent exudate. This may extend further, involve and penetrate through the skin with the establishment of tuberculous fistula.

Involvement of the testis is usually by direct extension and may ultimately destroy the entire organ. More especially in the later stages, the vas deferens and surrounding tissue are involved by the formation of a number of relatively small tubercles. The lesion primarily is unilateral and when the other testis becomes involved it is usually by way of a tuberculosis of the seminal vesicles and prostate. Although sexual activity is undisturbed, the patient is usually sterile even although only one testis is involved, a fact that is not satisfactorily explained. Sometimes the disease extends through the cord to the seminal vesicles and prostate and thence into the urinary tract, from which it can be widely disseminated. The lesion is only rarely observed first in the testis, except in case of disseminated miliary tuberculosis of infants and children. Here the lesion is usually primary in the interstitial tissue. Sometimes, however, a diffuse tuberculous granulation tissue is produced which renders diagnosis difficult. These lesions may also regress and undergo cicatrization, sometimes with small foci of calcification.

Syphilis. In contrast to tuberculosis, acquired syphilis affects the testis first rather than the epididymis. Only infrequently does it extend beyond testis to the epididymis and other structures. There are two forms of acquired syphilis, namely, gumma and diffuse fibrosis. The latter occurs independently of gumma, but gumma is usually accompanied by diffuse fibrosis. The gumma may be single or multiple, and variable in size. It shows the usual elastic consistency and the cross section bulges.

Microscopically, there is the usual picture of gumma with complete necrosis of the testicular tissues surrounded by round-cell infiltration. Not uncommonly the tunica vaginalis is involved, with the production of a moderate amount of serous exudate; after cure of the lesion there may be extensive adhesions in the tunica vaginalis. Rarely the gummatous process may extend and involve the epididymis, but it is almost never primary in and confined to the epididymis. The diffuse fibrosis is likely to lead grossly to an increase in density in the organ and difficulty in stripping the tubules with a forceps. It may be diffuse or somewhat localized.

The earlier and more active diffuse lesions show an infiltration of plasma and lymphoid cells in the interstitial connective tissue, fibroblasts, diminution of spermatogenesis, thickening of the basement membrane, and the presence of spirochetes. In the later lesions there is diffuse fibrosis of the interstitial tissue, with preservation and sometimes enlargement of the interstitial cells, fibrosis and hyaline transformation of the tissue immediately around the tubules, degeneration, necrosis and even disappearance of the epithelium with reduction in size of the tubules. In this stage it is extremely difficult to demonstrate *Treponema pallidum*. In the late cases there may be loss of sexual power and of fertility, but the gummatous process may be fairly extensive without loss of either.

Leprosy. Involvement of the testis in leprosy is not at all frequent, but when it occurs usually results in a diffuse fibrosis, subsequently with destruction of the epithelial cells of the tubules. Typical lepra cells, rich in bacilli, are to be found both within the tubules and in the interstitial tissues.

Tumors

The epididymis is only infrequently the seat of primary or secondary tumors. Lipoma, fibroma, myxoma, leiomyoma, dermoids, and adenomas have been reported. Sarcoma, carcinoma and malignant teratoid tumors also occur. Similar tumors may be encountered in the spermatic cord.

Tumors of the testis are common. They include those derived from connective tissues, from the interstitial cells of Leydig, from the epithelium, and those of embryonal teratoid character. Connective-tissue tumors are infrequent. The same is true of interstitial-cell tumors. These are usually of small or moderate size and microscopically show sheets of cells with all the morphologic characters of Leydig cells. Furthermore they may apparently produce excess of androgenic substance so that hypergenitalism, pseudo-hermaphrodism, hirsutism and other changes of secondary sex characters occur (Stewart, Bell and Roehlke). Somewhat similar, grossly and microscopically, are tumors which are derived presumably from embryonally displaced adrenal cortical cells. These may be accompanied by "feminization" and probably also by hypergenitalism.

The teratoid tumors include benign and malignant forms. The benign teratoma

See arch Path, 41 : 580

Gonadotropin = 2 types "chronic" = luteinizing
"Castrate" (pituitary) = follicularizing
"castrate" in castrates ♂♀ & elderly people

is usually a solid tumor which contains representatives of all three embryonal layers, although in a given section not all these may be present. Any cell group may become malignant, but carcinoma is more frequent than sarcoma. Dermoid cysts, common in the ovary, are rare in the testis.

There is a group of malignant tumors of the testis, which are probably derivatives of teratoma, but show such a preponderance of one cell type that others may be found only after search of many sections (Ewing). Although others think some of these tumors do not originate in teratoma, we agree with Ewing. In a series of 85 cases studied by Herger and Thibaudeau, 80 per cent occurred between 20 and 40 years of age, and 95 per cent occurred before 50 years of age. As observed clinically, the tumor is usually unilateral, but there is a definite tendency to bilateral involvement. The incidence is higher in undescended than in scrotal testes. If the nondescent be abdominal, the proportional incidence of malignant tumor is much higher than if inguinal, and the chance of bilateral involvement is greater the higher the site of the testes. (See Hamilton and Gilbert; Campbell.) The tumor may grow rapidly or slowly and there may be periods of remission.

Grossly, the tumor is usually more or less globular in form and may attain a diameter of several centimeters. Encapsulation may be almost complete. The cross section shows a soft, bulging, pallid tumor with foci of necrosis and occasionally of hemorrhage. Five microscopic forms are distinguished. 1. The malignant teratoma of mature or adult type shows areas carcinomatous in character, associated with which are mature cell types such as cartilage, muscle, glandular epithelium, etc. 2. The embryonal carcinoma is made up of sheets of large round or polyhedral cells with vesicular but deeply stained nuclei, and alveolated by more or less dense bands of connective tissue. It is also called seminoma (and disgerminoma) because of the resemblance of the cells to testicular epithelium. These two forms constitute half or more of this general order of tumor. 3. The embryonal carcinoma with lymphoid stroma differs from the foregoing principally in the presence of many lymphocytes in the stroma. 4. The embryonal adenocarcinoma is often alveolated and in addition to solid masses of cells shows the formation of acini lined by cuboidal or low columnar cells. This tumor may be encapsulated. 5. The chorionepithelioma has the same microscopic characters as the chorionepithelioma of the uterus. It is a rare tumor in the testis. Experience has shown that these tumors, from 1 to 5, represent increasing orders of malignancy, but the embryonal carcinoma with lymphoid stroma responds best to irradiation therapy, the others less so and the chorionepithelioma least so (Barringer and Earl).

The urine of patients with these tumors contains variable amounts of gonadotropic substance. The amount varies in different cases, but with a controlled Aschheim-Zondek test, is not found to be correlated with the microscopic character of the tumor or the course of the disease (Twomby et al.). After removal or irradiation therapy, the gonadotropic substance often disappears but may be found in cases of recurrence or metastasis even before these are evident otherwise.

There may be related changes in other organs. The pituitary may show hyperplasia of basophils such as occurs in pregnancy. Gynecomastia is seen in connection with the chorionepithelioma and sometimes with the other forms. The prostate and seminal vesicles may show epithelial hyperplasia and the opposite testis may show hyperplasia of the interstitial cells. Hyperplasia may also occur in the adrenal cortex.

Metastasis from malignant tumors of the testis is usually by way of lymphatics. The tumor occurs in the rete and then involves the whole testis. By direct extension it involves the epididymis and may grow along the spermatic cord. Metastases are found in pelvic lymph nodes and then in retroperitoneal lymph nodes. Huge metastatic masses may be found in the retroperitoneal region. Occasionally directly, but more especially after lymphatic metastasis, dissemination may occur through the blood stream. The lungs are thus involved and metastasis may be widespread in other parts of the body. More especially with chorionepithelioma, the original tumor may be small and unnoticed, but metastasis extensive. Microscopically the metastases of the 5 forms noted above are like the original tumor.

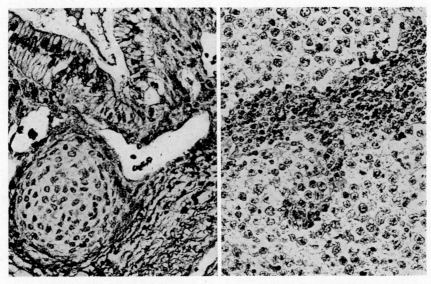

Adult type of teratoma of testis.

Embryonal carcinoma with lymphoid stroma—testis.

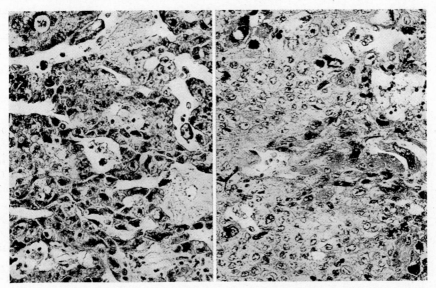

Adenocarcinoma of testis.

Chorionepithelioma of testis.

Those the result of malignant change in the mature teratoma are usually of one cell type but may be complex.

Metastatic tumors are exceedingly rare in the testis, but the organ may be involved in lymphosarcoma.

SEMINAL VESICLES

The general retrogressive changes include especially atrophy and fibrosis in old age and following chronic inflammations. Severe arteriosclerosis may lead to hemorrhages into the vesicles. Acute seminal vesiculitis may be an extension from neighboring structures, as urethra, bladder and prostate, or may be hematogenous as in septicemia and pyemia. The extension forms begin as a catarrhal inflammation and may become purulent. Cicatrization following the vesiculitis and the commonly associated perivesiculitis, may result in marked atrophy or complete disappearance of the vesicle. Cicatricial obstruction may result in cyst formation.

Tuberculosis occurs more often in the seminal vesicle than in any other part of the genital tract. It may be unilateral or bilateral. It begins as miliary tubercles of the wall, which fuse, involve the mucous membrane and produce a caseous purulent inflammation. Tubercles are usually found in the neighboring peritoneum. Extensions to prostate and bladder are common. Tuberculous abscess of the perirectal tissues may be followed by perineal fistula.

The commonest tumor involvement is by extension from malignant tumors of prostate, bladder and rectum. Fibroma, primary carcinoma and sarcoma are reported. (See Thompson.)

THE PROSTATE GLAND

Retrogressive Changes

Degenerations of the epithelium occur in connection with those of systemic diseases causing such changes elsewhere. There may be amyloid in the vessel walls, hemosiderin deposits, or extensive pigmentation in hemochromatosis. Corpora amylacea have been discussed in the chapter on degenerations and infiltrations. These concentrically laminated, sometimes radially striated, acidophilic bodies are common in the acini of the glands after adult life has been reached, and may increase in number and size in various pathologic conditions. Sometimes small calcareous concrements are observed in the acini and these rarely may lead to secondary inflammatory changes. The changes of development and of aging involution, apparently due to hormonal influence of the pituitary, are described by Moore.

Inflammations

Acute prostatitis may be hematogenous, or be due to extension from neighboring inflammations. Hematogenous infection occurs in septicemia and pyemia, especially staphylococcal, and is manifested in the form of numerous small abscesses; rarely an abscess of this sort may be large. There is usually an associated seminal vesiculitis and often an acute epididymitis. Acute prostatitis most commonly arises as the result of extension from neighboring foci of inflammation. By far the commonest cause is gonorrhea. Inflammations of the bladder may involve the prostate by extension along the mucous surfaces. Trauma and infection of the urethra by catheterization are common causes. Although cocci of various kinds may be found, the colon bacillus is the most common organism.

Acute prostatitis may be catarrhal, follicular or suppurative, and diffuse. Acute catarrhal prostatitis is a common accompaniment of gonorrhea and produces catarrhal inflammation of the prostatic acini and ducts. This may clear up, may at times become chronic, or because of obstruction to outlets there may be an accumulation of desquamated cells and exudate within acini, finally leading to suppuration. It is then called a follicular prostatitis because the suppuration is confined within the acini, but there may be extension into the supporting tissue in the prostate with abscess formation. Less frequent than these is acute diffuse prostatitis in which there is extensive hyperemia, edema and moderate cellular infiltration of the entire prostatic substance.

Chronic prostatitis is most often confined to the region of the caput gallinaginis where there is a chronic catarrhal inflammation, sometimes associated with small papillary outgrowths of epithelium. (See Moore.)

Infectious Granulomata

Tuberculosis. Although leprosy and syphilis may exhibit prostatic involvement the nature of the lesions is not well known. Tuberculosis is the most frequent and most important of the infectious granulomata in the prostate. The disease is secondary to tuberculosis elsewhere in the body but the prostate may be the first or only organ of the genito-urinary system involved. Only rarely is a prostate, the seat of benign enlargement, affected. The lesions appear grossly as yellow caseous masses in the peripheral portions of the gland. The microscopic appearance is that of tuberculosis in other organs. The tubercle begins in periacinic tissues, extends into the acini and ducts to excite a tuberculous inflammation, with fusion and caseation. In most cases, the bacilli appear to be carried in the blood stream and lodge in the periacinic capillaries, often without other evidence of hematogenous tuberculosis. In only about one-fifth of the cases is the involvement secondary to tuberculosis elsewhere in the genito-urinary system, with extension from the urethra or epididymis. (See Moore.)

Enlarged Prostate

This is the most common lesion of the adult prostate gland. It is often called hypertrophy, but even although the nature of the lesion is not fully understood, the functional implications of this term render it incorrect. Microscopically the changes are hyperplastic and the division between hyperplasia and tumorous characters is often difficult. The enlargement is usually moderate but may exceed a weight of 200 grams. There are, however, forms in which the organ, showing all the characteristic microscopic changes, may be somewhat reduced in size.

Sometimes the organ is a large, smooth, and dense, but elastic body. More often, however, it is nodular and the nodularity may be diffuse or involve either the lateral lobes, the middle lobe or the anterior lobe, which last represents the glandular tissue about the verumontanum. As a rule, the enlargements involving the middle lobe are due almost entirely to hyperplasia of the glandular acini. In cross section the character depends upon the important elements contributing to the enlargement. Thus, if the stroma be the

important part, the cross section is glossy, firm, elastic and pallid. If the hyperplasia be glandular, the cross section usually shows well-defined, somewhat spongy, projecting, yellowish-gray nodules of variable size.

Microscopically, there are variable degrees of hyperplasia of glands, hyperplasia of

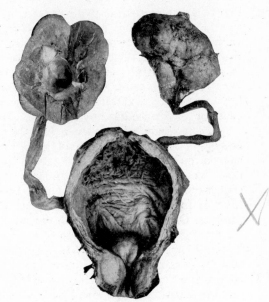

Enlargement of prostate, especially medial lobe, dilatation and hypertrophy of bladder, hydro-ureter and hydro-nephrosis. Army Medical Museum 30614.

connective tissue and increase in the amount of muscular tissue which also is probably to be regarded as a hyperplasia. The hyperplasia usually affects both epithelial and connective tissue elements, the epithelial often predominating. It is rare to find the change in one without some participation by the other. It is only with extreme rarity that the muscle elements proliferate to constitute a true leiomyoma. The glandular hyperplasia not infrequently simulates very closely a nodular variety of adenoma, but may also be a diffuse adenomatous hyperplasia. The acini are increased in number, irregular in outline and sometimes distinctly dilated. The epithelium may be in the form of a single layer of cells, multiple layers of cells, and not infrequently shows papillary growth into the lumina. These acini may contain granular material or desquamated cells and a considerable number of corpora amylacea. The supporting tissue may be more or less distinctly infiltrated with lymphoid cells.

Various theories have been offered to explain benign enlargement of the prostate. It has been thought that infection, principally gonococcal, is the cause, but the evidence is not convincing and many patients have no history of gonorrhea. The supposition that arteriosclerosis is the cause is difficult to support and it is evident that more victims of arteriosclerosis escape prostatism than are afflicted. The idea that it is tumorous, like the fibromyoma of the uterus, has as much against as for it. There is nothing to indicate that either sexual incontinence or abstinence has any influence.

The study of hormones has thrown new light on the problem. Hypophyseal gonadotropic hormones stimulate the production of the testicular male hormone which controls growth of the prostate. Hypophysectomy is followed by atrophy of testes and prostate. Orchidectomy leads to atrophy of the prostate, and administration of male sex hormone causes enlargement. It is supposed that with reduction of spermatogenesis, gonadotropic hormones excite excessive production of male sex hormone by the interstitial cells of Leydig and enlargement of the prostate. Variations in site and type of hyperplasia may be influenced by the action of theelin, which persists in older life. The mechanisms are not altogether clear, but some sort of hormonal imbalance evidently is significant in the cause of prostatic enlargement. (See MacCallum; Moore.)

Most of the patients are 50 years of age or more, but occurrence in somewhat earlier life is not rare. The symptoms are due to obstruction near the internal urethral meatus and include burning on urination, small stream, difficulty in starting or stopping and ultimately complete retention. The obstruction to urinary outflow leads ultimately to hypertrophy of the bladder. In numerous cases a small sac may form behind the enlarged prostate and may contain the so-called residual urine, namely that which cannot be expelled during urination. Infection of the bladder is likely to occur especially because of catheterization, and may be followed by extension of the infection along the ureters into the renal pelvis and into the kidney. Prostatics also suffer from diminution of renal function. Although this may be due to damming back of urine through the ureters into the renal pelvis, as has already been discussed, it is also possible that it is due to reflex inhibition of urinary secretion, because the autonomic nerve supply through the sympathetic system is common to both the kidney and the base of the bladder.

Tumors

Benign tumors of the prostate are distinctly rare. Although adenoma occurs independently, it is usually a part of general prostatic hyperplasia. Leiomyoma may also occur (Dial and Halpert). Benign prostatic tumors are found mainly in adult life but may rarely occur in childhood (Sysak).

Malignant Tumors. CARCINOMA of the prostate occurs in two forms. In the one, the disease is clinically manifest because of urinary obstruction. Indeed, it constitutes about 15 per cent of cases of obstructive prostatic lesions. In the other form, there are no symptoms and the carcinoma is discovered only on microscopic examination; it is said to be an occult carcinoma. Carcinoma is infrequent before the fifth decade, but thereafter is fairly common both as to manifest and occult forms. The latter are from two to four times as frequent as the former. Both forms increase in incidence as age advances. Moore found that in men over 80 years of age, the prostate showed carcinoma in 29 per cent. On the basis of a smaller material, Baron and Angrist report occult carcinoma in 46 per cent of men over 50 years of age. Differences of percentage are bound to occur because of the determination of what constitutes occult carcinoma. Carcinoma is situated most frequently in the posterior lobe, although it is almost as common in lateral lobes. Benign enlargement is a frequent accompaniment, but is an incident rather than a cause or predisposing factor.

Grossly, the manifest lesion is a firm, pallid, poorly defined, irregularly nodular mass which may advance through the capsule and anchor the gland to neighboring structures. Microscopically, it differs from the adenoma in that the acini are more numerous, more irregular, more constantly filled with multiple layers of epithelium, and show invasion of the surrounding tissue in the form of solid cords. The epithelium becomes less typical as the process extends. Although it is possible to distinguish adenocarcinoma and carcinoma simplex, the former practically always has some of the elements of the latter type.

Sometimes, however, a pure carcinoma simplex is observed. In this case there are solid nests and bands of epithelial cells, usually in rounded form and extending widely through the supporting tissue. Uncommonly, scirrhous carcinoma may be observed, and in such cases the prostate is likely to be hard and small. Rare cases of squamous-cell carcinoma of the prostate are attributed to remnants of the embryonal and fetal stratified squamous epithelium of the glands or to metaplasia of adult epithelium.

Metastasis occurs frequently in the pelvis and vertebrae probably because of the venous drainage demonstrated by Batson; less often, in other bones such as femur, skull, ribs, sternum, humerus and tibia. The bony metastases show both osteolytic and osteoplastic changes but the latter predominate (Sharpe and McDonald). Metastasis to soft tissues is seen especially in the pelvic and para-aortic lymph nodes. Other lymph nodes, including the inguinal nodes, and the internal viscera are much less frequently affected.

Normal prostatic tissue contains acid phosphatase and, in the presence of large tumor masses, there is increased output of this in the urine. Evidently androgenic activity favors the production of acid phosphatase (Huggins and Hodges). The presence of acid phosphatase in urine and blood aids in distinguishing metastases of prostatic carcinoma from other lesions of the bone. Death from prostatic carcinoma is due to urinary infections more than to any other complication.

Sarcoma of the prostate is distinctly unusual. Herrick's analysis of the cases reported shows that one-third of the cases occur before 10 years of age, three-fourths occur before 40 years and that four-fifths occur before the age when prostatic cancer is likely to be observed. The round-cell sarcoma is usually a lymphosarcoma. Ewing has found, however, that at least one such case was really a carcinoma. Nevertheless, the fact that lymphomata of lymphoid leukemia may

be found in the prostate makes it seem possible that lymphosarcoma may also occur there. Spindle-cell sarcoma also occurs in the prostate but should not be confused with the tumors of spindle forms of epithelium. These tumors may be in the form of a pure spindle-cell sarcoma or they may be myxomatous or angiomatous. Sarcoma of more differentiated cells also occurs and among them rhabdomyosarcoma of the prostate is reported. The sarcoma usually is a large, rapidly growing tumor, which invades widely in the region and may produce distant metastases.

Secondary tumors in the prostate arise usually by direct or lymphatic extension from malignant tumors of the bladder and rectum. It is only rarely that metastasis from more remote situations is observed.

THE FEMALE GENITALIA

CONGENITAL ANOMALIES

There are numerous malformations of the uterus, which depend upon anomalous development and fusion of the müllerian ducts. Perhaps the simplest classification is that into four groups. Anomalies arising in earliest embryonal life are rare and include absence of uterus and vagina and completely separated double uterus. Graves states, however, that complete absence of uterus does not occur even though the vagina be absent. Anomalies of the second group arise after the formation of the müllerian ducts and include UTERUS DUPLEX BICORNIS CUM VAGINA SEPTA, partial duplication with normal vagina but with a septum at the fundus (UTERUS SUBSEPTUS UNIFORIS), or a septum in the cervix (UTERUS SUBSEPTUS BIFORIS). This group includes also aplasia of one-half of the uterus with production of UTERUS UNICORNIS, and aplasia of the entire uterus with atresia of the vagina.

The third group arises during fusion of the müllerian ducts and includes UTERUS BICORNIS UNICOLLIS, UTERUS ARCUATUS (with lateral prolongations of the fundus and cavity toward the tubes) and UTERUS SUBSEPTUS UNICOLLIS. The fourth group includes those anomalies which arise after formation of the uterus, such as the fetal and infantile types of uterus and imperforate cervix. Pregnancy may be impossible or complicated in the anomalous uterus. It is said that tumors of uterus and adnexa are more frequent in anomalous than in normal uteri.

The ovaries may fail to descend to normal position. Apparent absence may be due to detachment or misplacement in fetal life. Complete absence of the ovaries occurs almost solely in the nonviable fetus. Nevertheless, it is probable that this condition can be followed by survival, with absence of ovarian hormones and failure of growth to reach full stature (Albright et al.). Most cases of what appear to be accessory ovary are due to separation of a small part of ovarian tissue by torsion at a late period of fetal life, or inflammations or tumor pressure in postfetal life. True accessory ovary occurs rarely and, to be identified, must have an accessory tube. Hypoplasia of the ovary may be found in infantilism, and sterility is often the result. Grossly, it is usually small but may be large and is identified microscopically by the incomplete development of the follicles. The most important anomaly of the tubes is a torsion of the distal portions, which may cause sterility.

Anomalies of the vagina include developmental defects and those probably due to inflammations in late fetal life. To the former probably belong all cases of absence of the vagina, septation and complete doubling of the tube. Extensive atresia may be due to a failure of hollowing of the primary vaginal cord. Imperforate hymen may also be developmental. Other local atresias, or even complete atresia, as well as transverse membranes, are probably due to fetal inflammations.

The vulva may be absent but only in the nonviable fetus. Vulvar hypoplasia is seen in infantilism. Hypoplasia of various parts of the vulva may be encountered. Complete duplication of uterus and vagina may be accompanied by double vulva. In hypospadias the urethra opens into the vagina. Epispadias is rare; the urethra may open above the clitoris; increasing degrees of epispadias result in exstrophy of the bladder. Hermaphrodism has been discussed with male genitalia.

THE VULVA

Circulatory Disturbances

The labia are often involved in general edema. Local causes of edema include inflammations, pregnancy and pelvic tumors. Dilatation of the veins, or vulvar varices, may occur in general passive hyperemias but is most common in pregnancy. The straining of labor may rupture the veins with the production of vulvar hematoma. Exclusive of labor, such hematoma may rarely be due to direct trauma. The lesions of skin and muscle during labor are fully discussed in the texts on obstetrics.

Elephantiasis affects the labia majora and sometimes the labia minora with chronic swelling, increased firmness, irregularity of cutaneous surface. Ulceration and lymphorrhea may occur. Prolonged interruption of drainage as by chronic inflammations, extensive removal of inguinal lymph nodes or filariasis explain most cases. Others are unexplained.

Inflammations

Acute vulvitis of adults may be either catarrhal, mucopurulent or ulcerative. It is not common because of the resistance of the surface epithelium to injury. It may be caused by the irritation of scratching, masturbation, excessive or violent coitus, and more especially by the irritation of discharges from vagina and uterus, and by the irritation of urine, especially that in diabetes. The vulva may be involved in such infectious diseases as smallpox, scarlatina, diphtheria, dysentery and typhoid fever. Gonorrhea is rarely a cause of vulvitis in adults. In children both gonococcal and nongonococcal vulvitis are common. Inflammation of the glands of Bartholin is a frequent complication. The parts are red, swollen and covered with mucus or exudate. Tenderness, pain and pruritis may be present with edema of the labia minora. Ulceration is more common in postpartum streptococcal infections and may be followed by gangrene. Gangrene may also be due to serious infectious diseases or to trauma, and may be a manifestation of noma. Chancroidal ulcers, similar in appearance to those of the penis and often accompanied by inguinal lymphadenitis, are usually multiple and situated especially about the frenulum.

Catarrhal, gonococcal and other acute inflammations may become chronic.

Kraurosis vulvae is a disease which appears at or after the menopause, rarely earlier. Leukoplakia and kraurosis represent early and late stages of the same disease (Graves and Smith). Irritant discharges and pruritis are associated, perhaps in some causative relation. The disease affects the labia minora, frenulum, prepuce and inner surfaces of the labia majora. These areas in the leukoplakic stage are red, swollen and partly covered by white, firm, thick superficial epiderm.

Microscopically there is marked surface keratinization, hyperplasia of the epiderm and prolongation of interpapillary epithelium, with subacute inflammation of the dermis. In later stages atrophy leads to obliteration of labial and preputial folds with a thin pallid translucent surface. Microscopically the hyperkeratinization is not marked, the epidermis is thin and the papillae flattened. The dermis is sclerotic and hair follicles, sebaceous and sweat glands atrophic. In both stages the vessel walls are thickened and the cutaneous elastica reduced in amount. Carcinoma sometimes develops in kraurosis, but the frequency of this change is not fully established.

Esthiomène, also called ELEPHANTIASIS VULVAE CHRONICA ULCEROSA, is a chronic enlargement and ulceration of the vulva, usually but not always anterior or posterior to the vaginal orifice. It is accompanied by marked chronic swelling, especially of the labia minora, upon which the ulcers may be symmetrical. Microscopically, in addition to surface ulceration, there is a rich infiltration of lymphoid and plasma cells together with a few giant cells of Langhans type and of foreign-body type containing fat. Although various causes have been suspected, it is now known that the lesion is one of the manifestations of lymphogranuloma venereum.

Infectious Granulomata

Tuberculosis is uncommon. It may occur as a lupus, rarely as miliary tubercles, or as a conglomerate tuberculosis with a disposition to marked and irregular enlargement of the labia with ulceration.

Syphilis. Chancre is rare on the vulva, but when it occurs is usually found on the labia majora. Mucous patches on vulva and neighboring skin are common and may occasionally be converted into deep ulcers. Gumma may rarely attack any part of the vulva.

Tumors

Benign Tumors. Approximately in descending order of frequency, the benign tumors include fibroma, lipoma, hemangioma, neurofibroma, leiomyoma, ganglioneuroma and lymphangioma (Lovelady et al.). Pigmented nevi frequently occur on the labia majora and may become malignant. For convenience the acuminate condyloma is mentioned here. As in the male, it is due principally to irritant discharges. It occurs often in multiple form and may be found at the vaginal orifice or about the labia minora.

Of interest is the fact that the labia majora may contain fibroma, fibromyoma and adenofibroma of the pre-inguinal part of the round ligament. The sweat glands and the glands of Bartholin rarely give origin to adenomas.

Malignant Tumors. SQUAMOUS-CELL CARCINOMA of the vulva originates in the clitoris, at the orifice of urethra or in the sulcus between the labia. Grossly, it may be a flat, ulcerative, firm mass, a rapidly progressing ulcer, or a cauliflower-like growth. In contrast to carcinoma of the penis, metastasis to the inguinal and iliac lymph nodes occurs early in the disease. The rare adenocarcinoma probably originates in the glands of Bartholin. Melanoblastoma of the vulva may produce early and widespread metastasis.

SARCOMA is rare, usually diagnosed only upon microscopic examination and may be of round-cell, spindle-cell or more highly differentiated types.

TERATOID tumors including the dermoid cysts are rare.

Cysts

Cysts include those of Bartholin's glands, cysts of the hymen, cysts of sebaceous and other glands. Echinococcus cyst has been reported. (See Hunt.)

THE VAGINA

Circulatory Disturbances

Local and general passive hyperemia may produce varices in the vaginal wall. Hemorrhage may be due to ruptured varices, to trauma by instruments and foreign bodies introduced for various purposes, to labor, to violent coitus. Large clots may form in the vagina and be discharged. Hemorrhage into the vaginal tissues (HEMATOMA VAGINAE) may infiltrate widely in the pelvic and retroperitoneal tissues. Accumulation of menstrual or other blood in the vagina behind zones of atresia is called hematocolpos.

Inflammations

The commoner forms of vaginitis or colpitis run a somewhat prolonged course and are subacute rather than acute. The mucous membrane is hyperemic and swollen, especially at the crests of the folds. The exudate is mucous, mucopurulent or purulent, but may be fibrinous or hemorrhagic. Ulceration is not uncommon. Gonorrhea is a common cause in children but not in adults. In the latter when present it affects the upper part of the vagina in continuity with the cervix.

Other organisms which may cause vaginitis include staphylococci, streptococci, colon bacilli, etc., present in, or introduced into, the vagina but exhibiting virulence only when the vaginal surface is abraded or wounded. Various fungi may produce low-grade vaginitis. Animal parasites may irritate, especially the *Oxyuris vermicularis*. Graves speaks of an ameba urogenitalis as pathogenic. Vaginitis of moderate degree may be due to *Trichomonas vaginalis*. *Distomum hematobium* may invade from the bladder. Numerous nonpathogenic spirochetes are described (Noguchi and Kaliski). The presence of foreign bodies, such as neglected pessaries, may produce vaginitis, sometimes ulcerative in character. Most important are irritative or corrosive douches. Discharges from endocervicitis or from putrefying tumors of the cervix or fundus of the uterus, may be extremely irritant.

Various forms of vaginitis are described. In addition to the catarrhal and suppurative forms, there is a nodular vaginitis in which small projecting nodules are made up of focal accumulations of lymphoid and plasma cells, a papillomatous vaginitis in which minute papillary projections of epithelium are thrown up, and a macular form in which there are numerous small foci of hemorrhage or blood pigment in healed or still existent minute erosions. Pseudomembranous vaginitis may be a true diphtheria, may be an accompaniment of other infections such as variola, cholera, dysentery, etc., or may be a part of puerperal infection. Emphysematous vaginitis is a condition, usually postpartum, in which small gas-containing vesicles occur in the vaginal wall, of little significance and probably due to slight invasion of gas-forming bacteria. Exfoliative vaginitis is rare; casts of vaginal mucosa are separated and discharged. It is usually due to corrosive chemical but may be a part of membranous dysmenorrhea. The more severe inflammations may lead to involvement of the surrounding parts, a paravaginitis, usually suppurative or phlegmonous. Extensive gangrenous vaginitis may occur, and rarely noma involves the vagina.

Infectious Granulomata

Tuberculosis of the vagina, without neighboring involvement, is rare and occurs practically only as hematogenous miliary tuberculosis. Infection by coitus is doubtful. Ulcerative lesions may extend from the vulva as in lupus or from the uterus or other organs in extensive urogenital tuberculosis.

Syphilis. Primary lesions of syphilis are rarely seen and secondary mucous patches are probably often overlooked. Gumma is more likely to extend from neighboring structures than to originate in the vagina. The cicatrization of syphilitic lesions may result in marked deformity of the vagina.

Tumors

The benign tumors are rare and include the fibromyoma and myoma. The papillae of papillomatous vaginitis may become tumor-like in character. The accuminate condyloma also occurs in the vagina. An important tumor is the adenomyoma of the rectovaginal tissues. This may attain considerable size and is difficult to remove. It is supposed to originate from uterine mucosa or remnants of the müllerian duct, but it is probable that the lesion is one of the manifestations of endometriosis, to be discussed with diseases of the ovary.

Malignant Tumors. CARCINOMA of the vagina is usually a squamous-cell carcinoma. Although an uncommon lesion it is seen most often in the upper posterior wall. It is an eroding ulcerative mass with metastasis to the regional nodes. Adenocarcinoma is extremely rare and is supposed to arise from embryonal remnants. Carcinoma of the cervix often extends to the vault of the vagina.

SARCOMA of the vagina in the adult is infrequent, but any of the mature and immature forms may occur. In infancy and childhood the vault of the vagina may be the point of origin for the mesoblastic mixed tumor called sarcoma botryoides, which is described later in the section on sarcoma of the uterus.

METASTATIC TUMORS, other than the direct extensions of neighboring malignant tumors, are rare. Of interest is the chorionepithelioma which often leads to metastatic growths in the vagina, nodular, dark red, rapidly growing, bleeding tumor masses, with the typical microscopic character. The original uterine tumor may be small and difficult to find.

Cysts

Cysts of the vaginal wall are fairly common. They may vary in size from a diameter of a few millimeters to several centimeters, are lined by low cuboidal or flattened epithelium, and are filled with a clear or cloudy mucinous fluid containing desquamated cells and often cholesterol. They may originate from glandular embryonal inclusions in the vaginal wall, from remnants of Gärtner's duct, or in case of double anomalies of vagina and uterus, may be cystic dilatations of a remaining müllerian duct or rudimentary vagina.

Fistulae

Fistulae may exist between vagina and urethra, bladder or rectum. Thus, urine or feces may be discharged through the vagina. Fistulae are most often caused by tissue necrosis due to birth injuries, although their incidence is being reduced by improved obstetric practice. They may result from infections in operations, from abscesses of various kinds and from the invasion and necrosis of malignant tumors.

Alterations of Size and Position

The most important dilatations are those due to retention of fluids behind an atresia. Pyocolpos is usually due to accumulation of pus in inflammations. The congenital atresias and alterations of form have been noted. Acquired atresias are usually the result of acute inflammations, wounds, or syphilis.

The most important alterations of position are those due to failure of support. The pelvic viscera are maintained in position principally by the integrity of the muscles and fascias of the pelvic floor. Failure of support is usually due to lacerations of the muscles and fascias from injuries in labor, although wounds, other injuries and tumors may produce the same effect. As a rule, the loss of support affects the anterior vaginal wall first; this sags backward and downward and may project through the vaginal orifice, producing partial prolapse of the anterior vaginal wall. With it goes the floor of the bladder, producing cystocele.

In the more severe lacerations the posterior wall may also be involved and sags downward and forward, as a partial prolapse of the posterior vaginal wall. Bulging of the rectum is rectocele. Protrusion of the vaginal wall through the introitus constitutes prolapse of the vagina. Uncomplicated vaginal prolapse is uncommon, for as a rule when this degree of failure of support is reached, the uterus has become more vertical by retroversion, the isthmus elongated, the whole uterus displaced downward in a partial prolapse of the uterus, which is associated with the vaginal prolapse. The cervix or indeed the entire uterus may project through the vaginal orifice to constitute procidentia, usually associated with eversion of the vagina and partial or complete inversion of the uterus. The surface epithelium of the vagina becomes keratinized and the lining membrane of the uterus transformed to squamous epithelium. Genital prolapse may permit of hernial projection of intestinal loops to constitute enterocele or vaginal hernia. Much the same condition may be produced by congenital anomaly of the pouch of Douglas, permitting the intestinal loops to descend as far as the perineal floor.

THE UTERUS

Circulatory Disturbances

Passive hyperemia of the uterus may be due to general causes such as chronic heart disease, to local causes which produce pressure upon the pelvic veins as, for example, the presence of tumors in the pelvis, or damming back of blood in the uterus itself because of alterations in form or position. Thus, retroversion, retroflexion, marked anteflexion or prolapse may interfere with venous drainage. Secondary to all these conditions there may be edema of the uterus which is most evident in the endometrium. Edema of the cervix may be due to passive hyperemia, to inflammation in that region, or may be the result of pregnancy.

Hemorrhage from the uterus is normal in the menstrual period. The various disturbances of the physiologic function of menstruation are discussed adequately in the textbooks on gynecology. Severe or prolonged menstruation is referred to as menorrhagia. In contrast to this is metrorrhagia or hemorrhage not incident to menstruation. This is a common clinical phenomenon and may be due to a wide variety of causes. It sometimes occurs in the passive hyperemia of heart disease. Hyperplasia of the endometrium may produce either menorrhagia or metrorrhagia. Metrorrhagia may also be due to traumatism, to local inflammations, to poisons such as phosphorus, to malignant tumors, or may be a local manifestation of general acute infectious diseases.

Benign tumors, either growing in the wall of the uterus or growing into the cavity as polyps, may produce only menorrhagia, but occasionally they produce metrorrhagia. One of the most important causes of metrorrhagia, especially in women past the menopause, is carcinoma of cervix or fundus. The so-called feminizing tumors of the ovary, such as the granulosa-cell tumor, may be accompanied by metrorrhagia or menorrhagia. In some cases of metrorrhagia in advanced life, the only lesions found are medial and intimal arteriosclerosis of the intramural arteries, and atrophy and fibrosis of the myometrium. Why bleeding is associated is not known, for it is not due to rupture of the diseased arteries (Baker). Hemorrhage during pregnancy is usually due to the detachment of the placenta, as a rule because of the development of the placenta near the cervix instead of in the fundus.

Inflammations

Inflammations of the uterus may involve the endometrium, endometritis, the wall of the uterus, myometritis, the peritoneum covering the uterus, perimetritis, and the broad ligaments, parametritis. These are all more or less interrelated and begin as a rule in the endometrium. Endometritis may affect the lining of the fundus in a somewhat different way from that of the cervix; in other words, true endometritis may differ somewhat from endocervicitis. There is also a great difference in susceptibility to inflammation on the part of the nonpregnant uterus and the pregnant uterus. With the exception of gonorrhea, inflammations of the nonpregnant uterus are unusual.

In acute gonorrhea the lining of the cervix is more markedly affected than is that of the fundus. Gonococcal endocervicitis is in the earliest stage an acute catarrhal inflammation with a large amount of mucous secretion in addition to the exudate. Subsequently, it becomes more distinctly purulent and quantities of greenish-yellow pus are discharged. In this stage the mucosa resembles very much that of the male urethra as regards the pathologic changes. There is rich infiltration of leukocytes throughout the endometrium and the glands are likely to show an excess of mucus.

As the disease decreases in severity, a chronic catarrh of the cervical mucosa with the discharge of a thick, glairy mucus containing relatively few pus cells or gonococci is likely to develop. Although the endometrium of the body of the uterus may harbor gonococci for long periods of time, it is unusual for acute inflammations to develop in the nonpregnant uterus. The organisms live and grow and pass on into the fallopian tubes with little or no involvement of the fundal endometrium. Nevertheless, the changes incident to pregnancy or to puerperium may serve to excite a severe gonococcal endometritis which may go on to involvement of the muscle, a true gonococcal myometritis. In this condition there are large numbers of gonococci and a rich infiltration of leukocytes, with mucoid degeneration, desquamation and necrosis of the glands.

Acute, subacute and chronic catarrhal endocervicitis is not uncommonly due to causes other than gonorrhea. In the condition spoken of as leukorrhea, there is a discharge of mucous secretion from the cervix. It may be found at almost any period of life, and is often without definite cause other than malposition of the uterus or exposure to cold. It is not confined to parous women and may even occur in virgins. In the subacute and chronic forms the cervix,

tion may be catarrhal or purulent. It may progress so as to involve the wall of the uterus and the surrounding structures, although such an extension is rare.

Occasionally, due to the more violent methods of treatment such as cauterization of the cavity of the uterus, infection of tumors, more especially carcinoma, and accompanying acute infectious diseases, acute fibrinous or fibrinopurulent endometritis with extensive necrosis of the endometrium occurs. This, of course, is more likely to be followed by invasion of the wall of the uterus

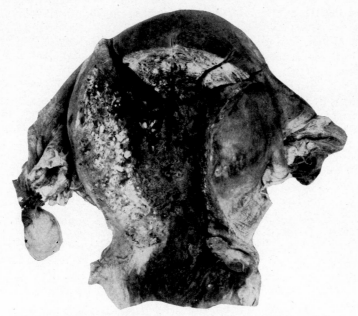

Acute suppurative endometritis and metritis, in the puerperium. Staphylococcus aureus septicemia. Army Medical Museum 30792.

in addition to the rich secretion of mucus, may show retention cysts of the mucous glands, the so-called nabothian cysts. The cylindrical cells may become squamous in type.

Acute endometritis, not of gonococcal origin, is unusual in the nonpregnant uterus. It may be caused by retained products of pregnancy such as fragments of placenta, necrosis of polyps and endometrial tumors, retention of menstrual blood and irritation by instrumentation and various therapeutic washes. It is generally thought that when inflammation occurs in these circumstances it is due to infectious organisms ascending from the vagina. The inflamma-

and the surrounding structures than are the simpler forms. The condition must not be confused with MEMBRANOUS DYSMENORRHEA. The latter occurs more especially at the menstrual period and in infantile forms of uterus, and is characterized by the discharge of the lining of the uterus in the form of a cast. Microscopic examination of the material shows that it is made up in most cases of the compact and spongy layers of the endometrium, the basal layer remaining in the uterus. Occasionally all three layers are discharged. The cells of the tunica propria are often swollen and resemble very closely those of decidua. If necrosis has preceded the desquamation of the membrane, there may be a considerable infiltration of leukocytes, but many cases are observed without any leukocyte infiltration whatever.

The puerperal uterus, whether following full-term pregnancy, miscarriage or abortion, is especially susceptible to infection because of the open cervix and the raw surface left by the placental detachment. The organisms most frequently encountered are the streptococcus, staphylococcus, and sometimes the gonococcus latent in the endometrium. Occasionally, low-grade infection of the puerperal uterus occurs because of saprophytic invasion of retained placenta. This really constitutes a gangrene of the retained placenta and the victim may suffer from absorption of the products of decomposition, the so-called sapremia.

Independently of this, or following it, there may occur a serious infection. The pyogenic organisms readily gain access to the dilated veins of the endometrium and myometrium and set up the most profound inflammation. There may be a violent purulent endometritis, or a fibrinopurulent endometritis, either of which may be accompanied by extensive necrosis of endometrium and underlying layers of myometrium. This process may extend by continuity into the fallopian tubes and thence to the peritoneum, or by contiguity into the walls of the uterus, and thence into the parametrial tissues and peritoneum. Usually, the condition develops into a septicemia or even pyemia.

The healing of acute endometritis may lead to extensive cicatrization of the endometrium, sometimes with adhesions. It is also probable that the inflammation may result in the so-called chronic atrophic endometritis, in which there is thinning of the endometrium with atrophy of the glands and overgrowth of interstitial tissue of the tunica propria. The inflammatory nature of such an atrophic state is indicated by infiltration of plasma cells and lymphoid cells and the presence of blood pigment. This must not be confused, however, with the simple noninflammatory atrophy and fibrous overgrowth of the senile uterus.

Endometrial Hyperplasia. In the normal menstrual cycle, approximately the first half of the period following menstruation is under the control of ovarian hormone and the newly formed glands are simple, practically straight tubes. In the second half, or progestational stage, the follicular hormone stimulates a more complex glandular form with elongation, tortuosity and papilla-like infolding of the lining cells.

In hyperplasia, these patterns are altered, elongation and tortuosity become more marked so that the glands are coiled, the cells may be heaped up in multiple layers and various degrees of cystic dilatation may occur. The tunica propria may be hyperemic and richly cellular; foci of hemorrhage may be found. In prolonged cases, fibrosis may take place. Grossly, the endometrium is usually thick and may be thrown up into polypoid folds. The functional disturbance is usually menorrhagia, but some cases have metrorrhagia and some dysmenorrhea; sterility is common.

In some instances, no cause can be discovered although it is safe to say that there is a disturbance of ovarian or follicular hormone. Some are due to displacement of the uterus and some to tumors, both of which may lead to prolonged passive hyperemia of the uterus. The same effect may be produced by other pelvic disease. Hyperplasia, often cystic, is a common accompaniment of granulosa-cell tumors of the ovary.

Infectious Granulomata

Tuberculosis. In generalized miliary tuberculosis, the endometrium or more rarely the myometrium may be affected. The usual manifestation, however, is an extension from tuberculous salpingitis. The tubercles form under or in the mucosa and may enlarge, fuse and slough to constitute caseous tuberculous endometritis. The process may extend into the myometrium by way of lymph or blood channels. It may also affect the cervix (Douglass and Ridlon). Tuberculous perimetritis accompanies pelvic peritoneal tuberculosis.

Syphilis affects the cervix more often than the fundus. Chancre may occur upon the cervix. Mucous patches or papules occur, and by cicatrization may produce stenosis. Gummata in the cervix are usually small. Sometimes in the course of syphilis, a catarrhal endometritis occurs, but this has not been proved to be due to syphilis.

Actinomycosis sometimes extends

from the neighborhood, especially the intestinal tract, to involve the uterus.

Tumors

Benign Tumors. The most common benign tumor of the uterus is the fibromyoma. Adenofibromyoma is distinctly less frequent. Only rarely are other benign tumors, such as lipoma, lipomyoma, angioma, and hemangio-

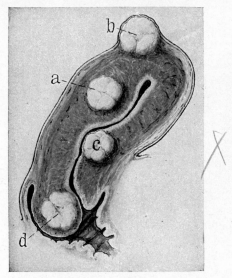

Schematic longitudinal sagittal section of uterus, showing various positions of fibromyomata; a, intramural; b, subperitoneal; c, submucous; d, cervical. From Gynecology, by B. M. Anspach.

endothelioma reported. The most important malignant tumors are the squamous-cell carcinoma of the cervix, the adenocarcinoma of the fundus, and the chorionepithelioma. Rarely, however, sarcoma of the uterus is observed.

FIBROMYOMA. This is the commonest tumor of the uterus and one of the most frequent in the entire body. Graves states that 20 per cent of all women have fibromyoma, and that nearly all unmarried women after middle life have them. They are more frequent in the black than in the white race. They are frequently multiple, and there may be a diffuse fibromyomatosis of the uterus. According to their situation within the uterus they are spoken of as subserous, intramural, and submucous. The subserous or submucous fibromyomata may become pedunculated. In the order of frequency these tumors may be found in the posterior, anterior or lateral

walls, and in about 10 per cent of the cases in the cervix. Similar tumors are encountered in the fallopian tubes, the broad ligaments, the round ligaments, the ovary, the vagina and other parts of the urogenital tract.

The fibromyoma is either a smooth, spheroidal or an irregular, nodular mass. In the earlier stages it is not sharply defined from the surrounding tissue, but as it grows older it becomes definitely encapsulated and may be easily shelled out. It is ordinarily firmer in consistency than the uterine muscle, and with increasing growth of connective tissue may become very dense and hard, the FIBROMYOMA DURUM. Secondary changes, particularly edema, may give it a soft consistency, the FIBROMYOMA MOLLE. It is usually a pale pink color but with increasing fibrous tissue becomes a glossy, light gray color. It cuts with considerable resistance and usually bulges markedly above the softer surrounding uterine tissue. The cross section is moderately moist but may be edematous, and shows a characteristic whorling of muscle and connective tissue bands, which gives it the so-called "watered silk" appearance.

Microscopically, the essential cell is the smooth muscle cell with its long spindle form body and long nucleus with rounded ends. In the earlier stages this constitutes practically the entire tumor, but subsequently connective-tissue cells and fibrils appear in greater number until finally they constitute the larger part of the tumor. Supporting the whorled muscle and connective-tissue cells, which may be cut longitudinally, obliquely and transversely, there are trabeculae of connective tissue with blood and lymph vessels. The blood vessels ramify through the tumor mass and in their finer divisions may have extremely thin walls. In addition, there may be gland spaces and acini, often tubular in character and sometimes dilated to form small cysts. This constitutes the so-called adenofibromyoma. About 6 or 7 per cent of the fibromyomas are of this sort. Grossly they do not differ in appearance from the usual fibromyoma unless the glandular masses are large enough to produce small spongy foci in the cross section.

The factors that lead to the development of the fibromyoma are unknown. Suggestions as to irregular or abnormal action of estrogens have yet to be established. The glandular part of adenomyoma is thought to be due to embryonal misplacement of müllerian duct or to infolding of endometrium. Some think it may be implantation of endometrium by lymphatic transport, i.e., one of the manifestations of endometriosis, discussed in the section on ovary.

The uterine fibromyoma is subject to a variety of secondary changes. Thus, owing to vascular disturbance which may occur,

Sterility is frequent in women with uterine fibromyomas, although conception often occurs. Abortion and miscarriage may ensue, but pregnancy and labor may be normal. Nevertheless, complications may be due to position and size of the tumors. Fibromyomas may enlarge during pregnancy and recede after its termination. The cause of sterility is not known, but it does not appear to be related to alterations of ovarian func-

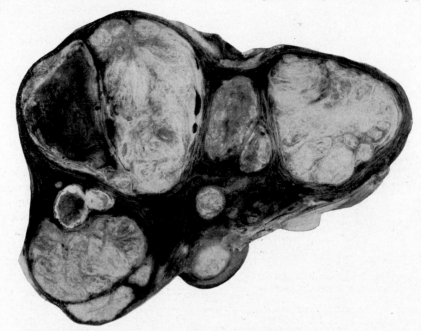

Interstitial fibromyomata. Note whorling in cut surface, necrosis and calcification.
Army Medical Museum 46830.

especially from malposition of the uterus, there may be edema which sometimes is so great as to produce cysts within the tumor. As a sequence of edema, or perhaps independently, mucoid may accumulate and lend a myxomatous character. Fatty degeneration is common in the smooth muscle and may affect other parts as well. If the circulation be obliterated, necrosis may produce softening of the entire tumor but more commonly it is present in small foci. Calcification may occur in foci within the tumor and may also form within the denser part in and near the capsule. More especially in the submucous tumors, inflammation is likely to occur and in the same situation gangrene sometimes ensues. Dilatation of lymphatics and of blood vessels may give rise to lymphangiectatic or hemangiectatic fibromyoma.

tion or to endometrial changes (Brewer and Jones).

Malignant Tumors. LEIOMYOSARCOMA. Occasionally, the fibromyoma may be transformed into a sarcoma. The incidence of malignant change varies with different pathologists. If the criterion be the presence of many mitotic figures, the incidence is 1 per cent or more. We require more definite indications of malignancy and in our experience the incidence is about 0.1 per cent of patients with fibromyomas removed surgically. Rarely fibromyoma may metastasize without any morphologic change to indicate malignancy. The metastases may not show microscopic features of malignancy (see Steiner).

The grossly invasive tumors extend through the wall of the uterus to neighboring structures, involve lymphatics and ultimately metastasize by the blood stream to lungs and other viscera. The microscopic changes include an increased vascularity of the tumor, variation in size and staining character of cells and nuclei, multinucleated cells, irregular mitoses, and more or less characteristic vascularization in which the wall of the vessel is made up of tumor cells. When malignancy is established, it is impossible to say whether the cells originated from the smooth muscle to constitute a leiomyosarcoma, or from connective tissue to constitute a spindle-cell sarcoma, or are derived from both.

The most common functional changes incident to leiomyofibroma are menorrhagia ing particularly multiparae and those who have had cervical lacerations or erosions. It may originate as a small, firm lump in the cervix, or as an ulcer, which may extend by erosion or by infiltration. It extends into the cervix fairly rapidly and produces early lymphatic metastasis in the parametrial tissues. Extension to the body of the uterus is not frequent.

Grossly, the tumor may appear as an indurated infiltrating ulcer with a somewhat necrotic base, as an extensive ulceration with shaggy, gray necrotic or bleeding base and everted edges, and only rarely as a fungating or projecting polypoid or cauliflower-like mass. In the more advanced cases, infection

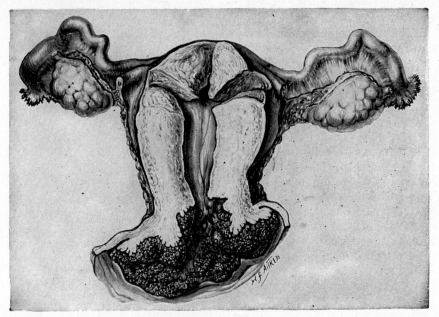

Advanced squamous cell carcinoma of the cervix. The vaginal cervix has been destroyed by the tumor which has reached the internal os. From Gynecology, by B. M. Anspach.

and metrorrhagia. The condition apparently predisposes to, if it does not actually excite, uterine endometrial hyperplasia. Uterine malposition, especially retroversion, and even prolapse, may be caused by fibromyoma. Impaction of large masses of tumor in the pelvis may produce pressure symptoms, particularly of the rectum, with constipation, and of the ureters, with damming back of the urine into ureters and renal pelvis.

SQUAMOUS-CELL CARCINOMA. One of the most common of all carcinomas, this may occur at any time of life but is most frequently a disease of the fifth decade, affect- may play a prominent part, and often saprophytic invasion produces a foul-smelling discolored mass. Discharge from the vagina may be mucous, mucopurulent, bloody or gangrenous. Cross section of the uterus usually shows the tumor to be a fairly firm, gray mass with or without foci of hemorrhage and necrosis. Its margins as a rule are irregular but fairly well delimited.

Microscopically, the picture is usually that of fairly large nests of cells, the outer members being of basal character and the inner members somewhat differentiated toward intermediate cells. The central parts often consist of more or less necrotic cells with pyknotic and fragmented nuclei. Lymphoid infiltration is extremely common and in many cases there are considerable numbers of eosinophils. Not infrequently polymorphonuclears infiltrate in considerable quantities and there may be small foci resembling abscesses. In some cases there is actual differentiation of cells to form prickle cells and squamous cells, but keratinization and pearl formation are not especially frequent. Metastasis occurs early into the parametrial tissues and thence may be widespread through the lymphatic system. It is unusual, however, for the superficial lymph nodes of the groin to be involved. (See Warren.)

The cervix is one of the places in which noninvasive intra-epithelial carcinoma may occur. The microscopic section shows a region, usually well demarcated from neighboring mucosa, in which the basement membrane is preserved but the epithelial cells show marked variations in size and shape with such loss of polarity that there is no regular progression from basal to squamous cells. Experience indicates that this may subsequently become invasive in the form of squamous cell carcinoma.

Occasionally parts of an adenocarcinoma of the fundus show squamous epithelium. Usually this is a metaplasia and the condition is called adeno-acanthoma. It is said that a squamous-cell carcinoma can originate in the fundus from misplaced squamous epithelium.

ADENOCARCINOMA arises especially in the endometrium of the fundus. It may develop upon a pre-existing endometrial hyperplasia or without any preceding history of disturbance. Fibromyomas are often associated, but they are common anyway and there is no clear indication of causative relation. The adenocarcinoma of the fundus occurs in somewhat later life than does the carcinoma of the cervix, grows less rapidly and metastasizes later. In the 44 tumors studied by Meigs only four showed metastasis. It may be a focal area usually high in the fundus or a diffuse adenocarcinomatosis of the endometrium. Its first growth is apparently into the cavity of the uterus in the form either of a somewhat roughened, solid mass of soft, proliferated mucosa, or as multiple papillae. It then slowly infiltrates the

muscle and may eventually occupy a large area in the muscle and penetrate through into the peritoneum.

Microscopically, the carcinoma may vary from carcinoma simplex to different degrees of differentiation of adenocarcinoma. The latter often show multiplication of layers

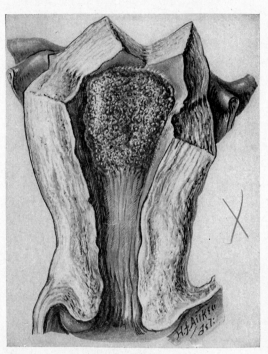

Early adenocarcinoma of fundus. From Gynecology, by B. M. Anspach.

of lining cells together with loss of polarity, pleomorphism and mitotic figures. There are often solid masses of undifferentiated epithelial cells. Inflammation is not so common in adenocarcinoma of the fundus as in the carcinoma of the cervix, and the tumor may attain considerable size with relatively little necrosis. As has been mentioned above, a small number of cases may show metaplasia with the formation of stratified squamous epithelium and pearls. Lymphatic extension, when it occurs, is along the lymphatics accompanying the tubes, and the tumor is not so likely to show early parametrial metastases as is the carcinoma of the cervix. In some cases, however, blood-stream metastasis occurs to the liver and other organs.

Adenocarcinoma of the uterine cervix is much less common than is squamous-cell carcinoma. It appears first in the cervical canal and originates in the cervical glands, although it is possible that rare cases may arise in the columnar epithelium covering erosions. The microscopic picture shows much variation in the degree of differentiation, the poorly differentiated tumors being the most malignant. Mucinous carcinoma is rare. Metastasis and extension are like the same phenomena in squamous cell carcinoma. (See Norris.) Opinion is drifting away from the view that inflammation of the cervix and endometrium are common precursors of uterine carcinoma and the suggestion is made that estrogens have much to do with it in patients who are susceptible to the disease.

CHORIONEPITHELIOMA. Although this may occur at any time after sexual maturity, it is usually a tumor of multipara after the fortieth year. The tumor develops three or four months after delivery of a hydatidiform mole, or less frequently after abortion, miscarriage or normal pregnancy. It may, however, occur very soon after any of these events or be much delayed. The tumor usually begins as a relatively small nodule in the fundus of the uterus, and enlarges by growth into the cavity and extension through the endometrium into the uterine wall. It is a soft, bulging, irregular mass, only rarely papillary in character. It is usually red because of rich vascularization, and undergoes necrosis early in its course. Cross section shows definite penetration of the mass into the uterine wall.

Microscopically, it shows irregular masses of cuboidal cells with small vesicular or solid nuclei and finely granular or somewhat vesicular edematous cytoplasm which contains glycogen. Intermingled with these cells are multinucleated cell masses representing the chorionic syncytium. The cytoplasm of the multinucleated cell masses is usually vesicular and may contain much fat, but the nuclei are usually dense rather than vesicular. Mitotic figures are more common in the cuboidal than in the multinucleated cells. The blood vessels are numerous and often cavernous, and the larger spaces often contain masses of tumor cells. The rich vascularization is responsible for bleeding, which occurs comparatively early in the course of the disease, so that early diagnosis is made, and cure by excision of the uterus is by no means

infrequent. On the other hand, invasion of the vessels is early so that secondary nodules appear in various parts of the body. As has been mentioned, cell masses of chorion or of tumor may be transported to the vagina. Metastasis, or vascular permeation from a uterine chorionepithelioma may occur in the vagina. Distant metastasis is more commonly to the lungs but may appear in other viscera including the heart.

The chorionepithelioma is to be distinguished from the malignant hydatidiform mole or chorio-adenoma. The majority of the hydatidiform moles are strictly benign and after they are delivered no further consequences occur. Nevertheless, the mole as a whole may become invasive, in which case penetration of the endometrium and of the muscularis occurs, participated in by the connective tissue of the mole as well as the covering epithelium. The degree of epithelial proliferation, however, is distinctly less marked than in the case of chorionepithelioma. The uterine wall may be invaded, but distant metastasis is rare (see Schmitz and Hueper). The urine of patients with chorionepithelioma may contain gonadotropic substances, in greater amounts than in patients with hydatidiform mole.

SARCOMA of the myometrium is usually the leiomyosarcoma derived from leiomyoma, described above. Sarcoma of the endometrium is rare; it usually is a polypoid or sessile projecting mass which grows rapidly and bleeds freely. Microscopically, it may be a characteristic spindle-cell sarcoma or a tumor with marked pleomorphism of the cells. Recurrence after removal is common, but metastases are not frequent.

SARCOMA BOTRYOIDES. In addition, the uterus may rarely be the seat of a mesodermal mixed tumor, often referred to as sarcoma botryoides. This occurs in vagina or cervix of children, as mentioned above. In adults, it is usually a polypoid lesion which originates either high in the fundus or in the cervix. The disease occurs in women between 45 and 65 years of age or more. Microscopically, the tumor is a mixture of connective tissue, usually myxomatous, smooth-muscle, embryonal type of striated muscle, and cartilage; one or more may predominate. The tumor is probably derived from rests of multipotential cells of the müllerian duct.

Although there is a tendency to recurrence after removal, metastases are usually local. (See Amolsch; Liebow and Tennant.)

Alterations of Position

The uterus normally lies almost horizontally over the bladder and practically at right angles to the vaginal axis. When the uterine axis is angulated within the uterus beyond the normal degree, it is the seat of various forms of flexion. When the whole uterine axis is out of normal position it exhibits various forms of version. Retroversion occurs in three degrees, the first in which there is a backward elevation of the axis so that the uterus assumes a more verti-

procidentia. This may be accompanied by partial or complete inversion. The most common cause of uterine displacements, more particularly retroversion and prolapse or procidentia, is injury to the supporting muscles and fascias in labor. Retroversion, however, may occur in nullipara because of failure of support due to the so-called lax habitus. Other causes include specially the action of tumors, either by weight or destruction of tissues, and the traction of adhesions.

The lumen may be narrowed or occluded by tumors, cicatrices, internal adhesions or by congenital faults. Behind obstructions, fluids may accumulate; if blood, to constitute hematometra; if pus, to consti-

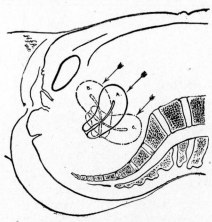

The normal position of the uterus, A; extreme anteversion, B; and retroversion, C. The uterus remains anteflexed in all. The directions of intra-abdominal pressure is indicated by the arrows.

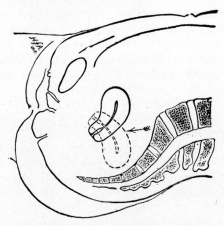

Retroversion and retroflexion of uterus in the figure with broken lines.

From Gynecology, by B. M. Anspach.

cal position, the second in which the uterine axis is in line with that of the vagina, and the third in which the axis is posterior to that of the vagina and usually bent to have a retroflexion.

The uterus is normally in a position of anteversion and anteflexion and it is only rarely that the former exceeds the normal degree. Hyperanteflexion, however, is sometimes observed. Lateroversion and lateroflexion are not common except in marked lesions of the pelvis. Anteposition and retrocession indicate that the whole uterus is either forward of, or posterior to, the normal situation. Prolapse indicates descent of the uterus as far as the vaginal outlet; when it projects beyond the outlet it is the seat of

tute pyometra; if uterine secretion, which frequently becomes serous in character, to constitute hydrometra.

THE PLACENTA

Anomalies and Retrogressive Processes

Anomalies of the placenta include placenta diparita, triparita, etc., in which the placenta shows segmentation, placenta duplex, triplex, etc., in which the placenta is completely divided into two or more parts, placenta arcuata, the horseshoe form, and other variations from the normal. Eccentric attachment of the cord is not uncommon.

Retrogressive Processes. These include cloudy swelling, fatty degeneration, hyaline necrosis and calcification. The last occurs in smaller or larger areas of necrosis and is often of no significance.

Circulatory Disturbances

Various forms of interruption of venous drainage may produce passive hyperemia which is usually present only in foci. Edema is not uncommon. Many cases are without known cause but some are due to maternal nephritis. Thrombosis may occur in maternal or fetal circulation.

The so-called infarcts of the placenta may be well-circumscribed red masses of coagulated blood with slight tissue necrosis, or pale yellow, decolorized masses of necrotic blood and placental tissue. They are somewhat more frequent in toxic than in nontoxic pregnancies but are probably a sequence rather than a cause of toxemia. That they are due to vascular occlusion is not necessarily true of all cases. Whether they are due to disturbance of either the fetal or the maternal circulation, without involvement of the other, is not known. Frazer's injection experiments indicate that occlusion of fetal circulation would be sufficient to produce such a lesion. Adair summarizes the causes as endarteritis, periarteritis, and thrombosis and localized hemorrhages, which may result from static, traumatic or toxic conditions. It is probable that infection and inflammation play a part in only a small number of the cases. Hemorrhage or uteroplacental apoplexy is referred to in discussing abnormal attachment of the placenta.

Inflammation

With the exception of that due to infection of the placenta retained after birth, inflammation is unusual. Infection, however, may be transmitted from decidua to placenta, or rarely there may be metastatic abscess in the placenta.

Infectious Granulomata

Tuberculosis of the placenta is not common. The bacilli are deposited from the maternal blood in the intervillous spaces from which, probably subsequent to thrombosis, the process penetrates the villi to set up miliary tubercles, often poor in giant cells, or larger conglomerate tuberculosis masses.

Syphilis. In many cases where syphilitic fetuses are born, the placenta shows no abnormality. The most significant finding is a large hyperplastic placenta and a small fetus. The large, pale placenta shows enlarged villi in which there is overgrowth of connective tissue and moderate edema. Gumma is extremely rare and it is unusual to find any marked lymphoid infiltration. Peri- and endovasculitis are common but by no means diagnostic. Infarcts occur in about one-third of the cases. In fact any of the changes described may occur in nonsyphilitic, chronic inflammations of the placenta. Spirochetes are not often found. Apparently, the placenta permits free passage of spirochetes but is not a favorable place for their growth. Practically identical changes are observed in the placenta in cases of erythroblastosis fetalis, referred to in the chapters on Hematopoietic System, and are not related to syphilis.

Hydatidiform Mole

This occurs in older multipara more often than in primipara. It is to be regarded as a hyperplasia rather than a tumor. The villi are enlarged to constitute pale, soft, translucent, more or less pedunculated, grapelike masses varying in size from a few millimeters to a centimeter or more. Microscopically, the villi are the seat of marked edema, often with compression or disappearance of capillaries. The trophoblastic epithelium may be normal or more often shows focal increases in the number of cuboidal cells and increase in mass of the syncytium with vacuolization of the cytoplasm. Probably most moles originate from the chorion frondosum but a few may originate from the chorion laeve. The relation to chorio-adenoma and chorionepithelioma has been discussed with uterus.

Tumors

Aside from those just mentioned, there remains principally the angioma which may be localized or extensive in the form of angioma, fibroangioma or cavernous angioma (see Siddall).

Cysts may originate in amnion, vitelline duct, allantois, chorionic villi or may occur as hemorrhagic pseudocysts in the placenta.

Abnormalities of Attachment

Ordinarily the placenta is attached in or near the fundus, but may be attached at the side near the cervical portion or completely cover the internal os, PLACENTA PREVIA. Sometimes the placenta is of ring form or crescent form and is attached to the

THE FALLOPIAN TUBES

Circulatory Disturbances

Passive hyperemia occurs as the result of general diseases such as heart disease, or of local conditions which may obstruct outflow of blood, such as malposition of the uterus or torsion of the tubes. Hemorrhagic infarcts may also result from torsion. Hemorrhage may be due to passive hyperemia,

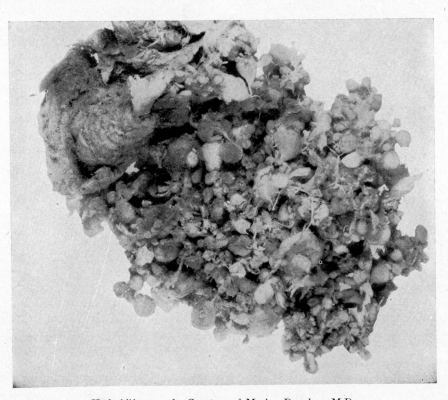

Hydatidiform mole. Courtesy of Marion Douglass, M.D.

uterine wall without intervening decidua; this is probably due to absence of endometrium at the site because of previous inflammation and cicatrization.

More especially when the placenta is abnormally placed, but also when in normal position, it may be detached (ablatio) with accompanying hemorrhage. In placenta previa, this uteroplacental apoplexy is due to mechanical causes, but in placenta previa as well as in normally situated placentae it may be due to traumatism, to pathologic changes in the uteroplacental junction such as infarction or inflammation, or to toxemia of renal or eclamptic nature.

inflammations and extra-uterine pregnancy. The tube may take part in menstruation. Hematosalpinx occurs in tubes obstructed at the fimbriated or at both ends and is principally due to menstrual blood originating in the tube or infiltrating from the uterus.

Inflammation

Exposure to cold or other vague causes may bring about acute hyperemia of the tubes which may be painful, but such things do not cause inflammation. It is now believed that acute salpingitis is invariably due to bacteria. In the majority of instances the infection travels by way of the uterine mucosa and is nearly always due to the gono-coccus. In a number of cases of puerperal acute endometritis the tubes are also involved, but the infection is spread by way of the lymphatics from uterus to tubes. Infection may enter the fimbriated end from a peritonitis, may attack the peritoneal surface when invading from appendicitis or may be blood borne in septicemias or pyemias.

Acute Salpingitis. Acute gonococcal salpingitis is usually catarrhal at first and then becomes more or less purulent. The tubes are hyperemic, swollen, elongated, tense, tender and painful. The mucosa is swollen and is covered with catarrhal or mucopurulent exudate, which may leak through the fimbriated extremity and produce a mild fibrinous peritonitis, practically always confined to the pelvis. Microscopically, the epithelium is swollen, degenerate and nonciliated. Often there is extensive desquamation and ulceration, the ulcers sometimes covered with a small amount of fibrin. The underlying connective tissues are infiltrated with lymphoid, endothelial and eosinophilic cells and, in most cases but not always, enormous numbers of plasma cells. If the case be recent, the pus shows the usual intracellular gram-negative diplococci, but in later stages the pus is sterile. The inflammation may extend through the entire wall of the tube and even into the parametrial tissues.

Acute suppurative or septic salpingitis most commonly is secondary to puerperal endometritis and metritis. Because of lymphatic transmission of the infection the lesion begins within the tubal wall and then involves the entire structure. Hyperemia, edema, suppuration, necrosis and ulceration constitute the changes. Mild cases may show less cellular infiltration; more severe cases may become phlegmonous.

Acute salpingitis of any form may become quiescent and heal. The septic forms, however, are likely to be fatal because of the accompanying widespread infection. Gonococcal salpingitis is likely to become converted into a chronic inflammation, although some cases cease to progress and the fibrosis is then to be regarded as cicatrization. Within the tube the diffuse inflammation is followed by fibrosis, the destroyed

epithelium is only partly replaced, the villi are short and adherent, the internal adhesions may be so constituted as to produce cysts, the epithelium may grow into the surrounding tissues to produce small papillary cysts, and the lymphoid and plasma cell infiltrates may remain over long periods of time. The local peritonitis produces adhesions between tubes and ovaries, bladder, rectum, intestine and appendix, and may lead to a dense matting together of all the pelvic viscera. Contraction of adhesions about the tubes may produce tortuosity and marked deformity.

TUBAL OCCLUSIONS. The adhesion of plicae within the tubes may produce com-

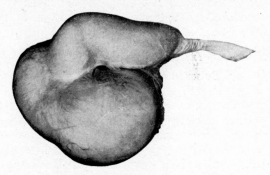

Hydrosalpinx.

plete occlusion, especially at the uterine end; the adhesions of fimbriae may close the fimbriated extremity. If the acute inflammation persist, pus accumulates in the tube, dilates it and forms PYOSALPINX. The ampulla is most widely dilated. Adhesions of the peritoneum, scar-like bands of tissue on the outer surface, or adhesions within the tube may divide the accumulated contents into saccular areas, a pyosalpinx saccata. The pus may become inspissated into a cheesy mass, not to be confused with tuberculosis, or may become calcified. It probably only rarely liquefies to form a limpid serous fluid. Provided suppuration subside, the accumulation of secretion may dilate the tube in even greater degree to form HYDROSALPINX or in the sacculated forms SACTOSALPINX SEROSA.

The pyosalpinx is usually lined by more or less chronic granulation tissue; the hydrosalpinx is lined by flattened columnar epithelium without cilia. The walls show the changes noted above, but in hydrosalpinx extreme dilatation may thin the walls so that they are merely a mass of dense connective tissue from which muscle has disappeared. Occasionally gonococcal salpingitis may heal and leave only a mass of chronic inflammatory or cicatricial connective tissue at the uterine end, SALPINGITIS ISTHMICA NODOSA. Similar multiple nodules give rise to the name SALPINGITIS NODOSA.

The fimbriae may become adherent to the ovary instead of fusing together. Accumulations of pus in this situation form the TUBO-OVARIAN ABSCESS. The inflammation may finally penetrate through the albuginea into the ovarian tissue. The nature of tubo-ovarian cyst is the subject of some question. It may possibly be like a localized hydrosalpinx but is probably more commonly produced by rupture of an ovarian cyst into the area of adhesion.

Infectious Granulomata

Tuberculosis is common and is usually bilateral. It may be a tuberculous perisalpingitis, as a part of tuberculous peritonitis, in which the wall is studded with miliary or small conglomerate tubercles. The process may extend thence into the substance of the tubes. In our experience, it also occurs frequently as miliary tubercles in the mucous and muscular coats in association with a chronic salpingitis. It may affect principally the mucosa. Involving muscularis or mucosa, the process may advance with extensive caseation, not infrequently complicated by mixed infection.

Syphilis is only rarely observed and then in the form of gumma.

Actinomycosis is usually an extension from the neighborhood, especially from the intestine.

Tumors

These are unusual in the tubes. Fibroma, fibromyoma, and angioma are reported. Adenoma may occur but should not be confused with hyperplasia of epithelium such as occurs in chronic salpingitis. Adenofibroma is probably in most cases a form of endometrioma. Although adenocarcinoma may occur, the usual carcinoma is a papillary carcinoma which may penetrate into and widely invade the peritoneum. Lymphatic metastasis may occur in lymph nodes, ovaries and uterus. Sarcoma is extremely rare. Secondary tumors originate in ovary, uterus and neighboring organs or may extend from the peritoneum.

Extra-uterine Pregnancy

Although impregnation of the ovum occurs normally in the fallopian tube, the ovum descends into the uterus before it embeds itself and pregnancy proceeds. Nevertheless, it is not rare for the ovum to implant itself within the fallopian tube and indeed this may occur in the tubo-ovarian junction, in the ovary and in the peritoneum. Pre-existing chronic disease of the tubes with tortuosity, elongation and sacculation, presumably delaying passage of the ovum, favors extra-uterine pregnancy. The frequent association of uterine anteflexion suggests that genital hypoplasia may be important (Behney). The condition sometimes occurs in an otherwise normal tube. Chronic inflammation often produces tubo-ovarian adhesion which may account for ovarian pregnancy, but it is also supposed that impregnation may occur in the mature graafian follicle. Implantation in the peritoneum may be primary, but is usually due to dislodgment of an ovum implanted near or in the fimbriated extremity of the tube. Decidua may be formed at the site of extra-uterine pregnancies, but is much less common in the endometrium than is usually supposed (Moritz and Douglass).

Tubal pregnancy usually occurs in the outer third of the tube. The ovum penetrates the epithelium, attaches itself to the underlying connective tissue and often burrows into the muscular layer. The trophoblast and the earlier stages of the embryo develop normally. The blood vessels of the parts undergo marked dilatation and supply blood for the developing ovum. The patient exhibits all the signs of pregnancy except the gradually enlarging uterus. The tube enlarges at the site of implantation, becomes tense and hyperemic.

Usually the pregnancy is interrupted before the third month. In about one-fourth of the cases the tube ruptures, hemorrhage occurs, which may be profound and even fatal, and the embryo is dislodged into the peritoneum and dies. More often, however, the membranes rupture within the tube and tubal abortion is said to have occurred. The hemorrhage may be confined to that segment of the tube and constitute hematocele. If the blood does not clot, hemorrhage, sometimes severe, may occur through the fimbriated extremities. Most cases are terminated by surgical intervention because of pain, hemorrhage or both. In others, however, the embryo dies and the whole mass of membrane, embryo and hemorrhage, if it has occurred, is organized and cicatrized.

THE OVARY

Circulatory Disturbances

Passive hyperemia may be due to general circulatory diseases or may be the result of local interference with drainage of the blood such as occurs in malposition of the ovary, malposition of the pelvic viscera, or torsion of the ovary upon a pedicle. Edema is usually associated with the passive hyperemia. The ovary may be distinctly anemic because of pressure upon it by tumors in the pelvis. Usually prolongation of the anemia and pressure is followed by atrophy.

Hemorrhage in the ovary is fairly common, originating in the graafian follicle or at some stage following its rupture. The hemorrhage incident to rupture may be severe and lead to collapse. Bleeding may occur into a corpus luteum, more frequently that of pregnancy than the ordinary menstrual corpus luteum, and produce ovarian hematocele. Diffuse hemorrhage is much less frequent than focal hemorrhage. It may be due to rupture of vessels in the margin of a corpus luteum, to general hemorrhagic infections, or to twisting of the pedicle of an enlarged ovary. These hemorrhages, as well as those due to general passive hyperemia, are found upon microscopic examination to be in the stroma rather than in the follicles.

Inflammation

Acute inflammations of the ovary are not frequent. Many of the conditions formerly supposed to represent chronic inflammation are now looked upon as either cystic disease of noninflammatory origin, the cicatrization of an old inflammatory process, or are merely atrophy due either to pre-existing disease or to age. Acute oophoritis may be due to infection either through the lymphatics or by direct invasion from primary suppurative processes in the uterus, the fallopian tubes, the parametrium, the appendix or the peritoneum. It may be hematogenous in cases of pyemia and septicemia. Acute inflammation, presumably of metastatic character, occurs in the course of mumps but this is less frequent in the ovary than in the testis. Similar lesions may accompany diphtheria and measles, scarlet fever and typhoid fever. Gonococcal infection may spread from the tube and affect the surface of the ovary in an acute perioophoritis. Occasionally, the organisms may enter the ovary to produce diffuse inflammation. If, however, an abscess be formed it is probably due to the ascent of other organisms through the uterus, the tubes and the parametrium.

Acute oophoritis may be present as a diffuse acute seropurulent process or as abscess. The organ is enlarged, tense, somewhat fluctuant and of pink color. It cuts easily and the cross section is smooth, usually quite moist, and from it may be expressed a seropurulent exudate. Microscopically, there is severe hyperemia, marked edema and infiltration of lymphoid and plasma cells and polymorphonuclear leukocytes. In those forms accompanying such conditions as puerperal sepsis, the polymorphonuclear leukocytes are in abundance. In the form due to gonococcus there are usually many plasma cells. If abscess supervene, the features are grossly and microscopically about the same as those observed elsewhere, except that as the abscess becomes older the marginal zone of granulation tissue may show a distinct yellow line. Microscopically, this appearance is found to be due to large, finely vacuolated cells resembling those of the corpus luteum. They are, however, macrophages, probably phagocytic for fatty and lipoid materials rather than true cells of the corpus luteum. As acute inflammation subsides, there is a proliferation of granulation tissue with subsequent cicatrization and marked atrophy of the organ.

Infectious Granulomata

Tuberculosis may affect the ovary. It may extend from tuberculous peritonitis in the neighborhood or may be transmitted by blood or lymphatic stream. When extending from tuberculous peritonitis the process rapidly involves the ovary itself. The lesions may be miliary or may be conglomerate with extensive caseation. Diseased and cystic ovaries are not exempt from tuberculous infection. The only important manifestation of syphilis is the gumma. Actinomycosis may spread to the ovary from lesions in the neighborhood.

Cysts

Retention Cysts. The ovary is subject to cystic disease in various forms. Some cysts are proliferative in nature and are justifiably classed with tumors. The others included in this section are not proliferative, although the ovary may be riddled with them. The fluid is formed as the result perhaps of passive hyperemia, irritation, secretion by lining cells, or attraction on the part of necrotic material within the space, but the mechanism is not clearly understood. In some of the cysts, both retention and proliferative, estrogenic substance is occasionally found in amounts indicative of its formation in the cyst rather than mere storage (Adair and Watts). Such cysts may be formed at any stage of development of the graafian follicle, the corpus luteum or the corpus fibrosum.

Follicular cysts are those which originate in the graafian follicles. It is well known that many follicles do not mature. Ordinarily they undergo complete organization and atresia. Even normally some become small cysts. The conditions which cause large numbers to become cystic are not known, although passive and repeated active hyperemia and fibrosis of the capsule appear to have some influence. In the less severe instances, the ovary is moderately enlarged and shows on both the outer surface and cross section large numbers of thin walled monolocular cysts containing clear, colorless or amber fluid. The fluid may become viscid by inspissation or be converted into a semisolid hyaline mass. Microscopically, the small cysts are lined by remnants of the stratum granulosum. In the course of the disease one or two cysts may enlarge to diameters of 20 or 30 cm. or more. They are usually also monolocular and contain the same type of fluid, but the lining cells have disappeared or may occasionally be represented by small wart-like excrescences.

Corpus-luteum cysts are usually single and only occasionally attain large size. The cyst wall shows a fairly thick convoluted yellow line resembling that of the corpus luteum. Microscopically, the convoluted masses of lutein cells are found. The fluid is usually cloudy, limpid, but of dark or reddish-yellow color. When the cyst enlarges the lining layer becomes less distinct and may disappear. Then the distinction between this type and follicular cyst cannot be certain. If the cyst originate during the hemorrhagic stage of the corpus, the lutein cells may be covered by a layer of connective tissue with a few granules of blood pigment.

Theca-lutein cysts are usually small and may be multiple. They probably originate in follicles. The lining is of connective-tissue cells of the theca interna, which undergo hyperplasia and take up lutein pigment. The cell mass, however, does not show the convolutions of the corpus luteum. Theca-lutein cysts are the especial accompaniment of hydatidiform mole and chorionepithelioma. Frankl states that in from 50 to 63 per cent of the cases of chorionepithelioma, cystic disease of the ovary was present, and that in practically all of the instances the cysts were theca-lutein cysts.

Tumors

Many of the benign tumors of the ovary tend to become malignant and to show stages in which diagnosis is difficult. Fibroma, fibromyoma and solid adenoma occur. Of greater frequency, however, are the forms of cystadenoma, a proliferative cystic disease, progressive in course and capable of malignant change. Although by the names employed for the two forms, pseudomucinous cystadenoma and serous cystadenoma, the cyst content would seem to be a differential feature, there are other points of difference.

Benign Tumors. PSEUDOMUCINOUS CYSTADENOMA. This is the most frequent tumor of the ovary. The tumor almost or completely replaces the ovary. It is more commonly unilateral and as a rule is pedunculated but may grow in the broad ligament (intraligamentary). The cystic mass is encapsulated, oval in shape, with a smooth, glossy, somewhat lobulated surface and is multilocular. The loculi are variable in size and more especially with the larger ones have thin walls.

The content is primarily a viscid fluid, principally pseudomucin. This differs from mucin in that it takes acid stains and although soluble in dilute alkalies is not precipitated by weak acids. It contains a copper reducing body, probably mucoitin-sulfuric acid. It is a pale yellow fluid which may be discolored by hemorrhage. The pseudomucin may by inspissation become semisolid or solid and when brown in color resembles colloid but does not contain iodin. Old cysts may contain cholesterol crystals.

Microscopically, the material, whether viscid or solid, takes the acid stain and is either granular, thready or homogenous. The cysts are lined with a single layer of nonciliated columnar cells with dense basal nuclei, and are often goblet cells because of accumulation of the pseudomucin which they secrete. They are supported on a connective tissue framework only moderately well vascularized. They may be flattened by pressure of fluid in the cyst. Epithelial proliferation into the cyst cavity forms papillae which may be large and extensive. Proliferation into the connective tissue produces acinic spaces or adenoma. Either type of proliferation may become malignant.

Rupture into the peritoneum may lead to PSEUDOMYXOMA PERITONEI. The pseudomucin is taken up by peritoneal lymphatics and may accumulate to form grapelike cystic projections from the peritoneum. These are lymphatic cysts, lined by endothelium. In addition, however, are similar cysts lined by cylindrical epithelium probably representing implants of cells with tumorous or carcinomatous character. A similar lesion may be due to mucinous carcinoma of the appendix. The disease may cause extensive fibrous adhesions sometimes leading to intestinal obstruction.

The origin of this tumor is not definitely established. Some believe that it originates in follicles and others regard it as a one-sided development of a teratoma.

SEROUS CYSTADENOMA. This is not so common but is more frequently bilateral than the pseudomucinous form. It usually does not exceed a diameter of 18 or 20 cm. It is more often intraligamentary than pedunculated. Upon gross examination it is often apparently monolocular with thick walls, but as a rule, further examination shows numerous minute additional cysts in the walls. It contains a thin serous fluid rich in protein but devoid of pseudomucin. It is lined by low columnar epithelium covered with cilia and with centrally placed nuclei. The cilia are best seen by examining cells scraped off the fresh surface and placed in warm salt solution.

Proliferation may occur into the wall to produce adenoma, but much more frequent and striking is the disposition to proliferate internally and produce extensive papillary growth. The tumor is almost constantly a papilliferous cystadenoma. The papillae are intricately branched, are covered by the ciliated columnar cells and may fill the entire cavity. In large cysts under pressure or in peritoneal growths the cilia often disappear. It is not uncommon for the epithelial masses to grow through the cyst wall and produce papilloma on the peritoneal surface. Either from rupture of the cyst, accidental spilling of the contents during operation, or most frequently by detachment of cells from the extracystic papilloma, the process may be implanted widely upon the peritoneum. The secretion continues and marked ascites is produced. Even extensive papillary growth may not be microscopically invasive, but ultimately in many cases carcinoma develops. Nevertheless, the removal of the primary ovarian tumor may be followed by disappearance of the peritoneal implants (Pfannenstiel). It is practically agreed that this type of tumor is derived from germinal epithelium.

Endometrioma. Sampson maintains that these tumors which he calls "ovarian hematomas (hemorrhagic cysts) of endometrial (müllerian) type," probably are the most frequent pelvic lesions found at operation in women between 30 years of age and the menopause. Polster found records of 1000 instances in the ovary, tubes and broad ligaments, 34 in the inguinal region, 56 in laparotomy scars, 90 in the rectovaginal septum, 5 in the vesicovaginal septum, 30 in the umbilicus and 90 in intestinal peritoneum.

When in the ovary the lesion is bilateral in about one-third the cases. The masses vary in size from a millimeter to 9 cm., are of cystic character, either monolocular or

15931 (CA)

multilocular, have moderately thick, often friable walls, and contain viscid, granular or solid chocolate colored material. Microscopically the cyst walls are lined by cylindrical epithelium, sometimes with acinus formation, and tunica propria like that of the endometrium. The cysts undergo menstrual

deeply situated lesions are due to lymphatic or venous transmission. We are of the opinion that the peritoneal and ovarian lesions result from implantation of endometrial fragments and that the more deeply situated cysts are probably due to embryonal faults. (See Block.)

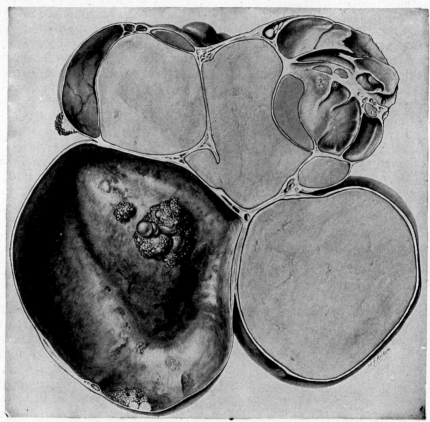

Serous cystadenoma of ovary with papilla formation. From Gynecology, by B. M. Anspach.

changes, and become filled with blood, which inspissates to form the chocolate mass. They may show a decidual reaction in pregnancy (Oberling) and undergo atrophy at menopause.

There are three theories as to the origin of this lesion. It has been supposed that it is due to misplacement of rudiments of the müllerian duct. It has been suggested that due to inflammation and the associated action of ovarian hormones, peritoneal cells may proliferate and undergo metaplasia to produce the cysts. The most widely accepted view is that of Sampson who explains them as due to transportation of endometrial fragments through the fallopian tubes; the more

Malignant Tumors. CARCINOMA is fairly frequent in the ovary and usually affects women in late middle life, although it may occur earlier. It may be solid or cystic. Although the cystic form of primary carcinoma of the ovary may originate as a carcinoma, most of the cases represent a secondary malignant degeneration in cystadenoma, and of the two varieties, the serous papilliferous cystadenoma is the more common point of origin. Not infrequently, the invasiveness of this type of tumor, which distinguishes it from the benign cystadenoma, can be seen with the naked eye. Microscopic examination shows the invasive character either in the form of adenomatous groups of epithelial cells or as solid bands of cells traversing the tissues.

The solid primary carcinoma only rarely exceeds a diameter of 18 to 20 cm. Bilateral involvement is by no means rare, but it is usually difficult to determine whether there are two primary carcinomas or whether this distribution is due to early metastasis

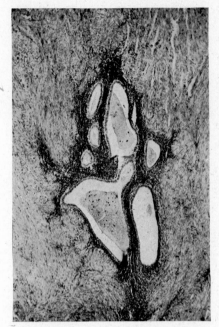

Endometrioma of recto-vaginal septum.
Army Medical Museum 43134.

from one ovary to the other. The tumor constitutes a nodular mass which in the earlier stages is encapsulated and covered with smooth, glossy peritoneal surface. Subsequently the tumor breaks through and shows rough, irregular areas in the surface. The consistency varies with the amount of connective tissue, for these tumors may be medullary or scirrhous or intermediate in variety. The cross section is yellowish-gray or gray, and both its color and consistency depend in part upon the amount of connective tissue present. Necrosis is fairly common and not infrequently small foci of hemorrhage are observed. Many of these carcinomas are adenomatous in type and may show numerous cystic areas.

Microscopically, it is usually an adenocarcinoma with considerable irregularity in size and shape of the acini and atypi-

cal epithelial cells sometimes in multiple layers. Small solid bands of epithelium invade from the acinic spaces. Carcinoma simplex usually shows more or less interlacing bands of epithelial cells running throughout the tissue. In either form it is not uncommon to find small calcareous balls, the so-called psammoma bodies. These may be so numerous as to justify the term psammomatous carcinoma. Squamous-cell carcinoma is sometimes observed but this, in all likelihood, is a manifestation of teratoma. Metastasis from primary carcinoma of the ovary is not frequently observed in distant viscera. Metastasis is usually in the lymph nodes of the region and through the lymphatic spaces into the uterus and into the opposite ovary. (See Taylor.)

Chorionepithelioma is sometimes observed in the ovary but it is more unusual here than in the testis.

Secondary carcinoma of the ovary is frequently bilateral and is usually derived from tumors of the stomach, intestinal tract or organs of the urogenital system. The exact mode of transfer from the primary site is not clear, but it may be by way of retrograde lymphatic transmission or perhaps also by implantation of small bits of tissue from the primary tumor upon the peritoneum of the ovary. The so-called KRUKENBERG TUMOR of the ovary is usually bilateral, with moderate or marked symmetrical and nodular enlargement of the ovaries.

Microscopically, there are numerous epithelial cells of signet-ring form containing mucin, arranged as carcinoma simplex, occasionally with acinic differentiation. These are metastatic carcinoma, the primary tumor being more often in the stomach than elsewhere. Nevertheless, carcinoma with mucin containing signet-rings may rarely be primary in the ovary (Schiller and Kozoll).

SARCOMA. This is an uncommon tumor of the ovary. It is usually unilateral, grows to only moderate size, rarely exceeding a diameter of 18 to 20 cm., may or may not be pedunculated, is usually solid but occasionally shows small cysts. It may be a smooth tumor or distinctly nodular in character, sometimes with glistening outer surface and sometimes with growth of tumor tissue through the capsule. It is usually soft, cuts easily and shows a fleshy, bulging cross section with areas of hemorrhage or necrosis. Microscopically, it is usually an immature type of sarcoma, only uncommonly showing differentiation to myxosarcoma, chondrosarcoma or angiosarcoma. The fibroma and fibromyoma may become sarcomatous. Ovarian sarcoma is likely to metastasize to regional lymph nodes before blood vascular dissemination occurs. Secondary sarcoma in the ovary is infrequent.

Upon cutting the warm specimen the cyst is found filled with an oily material, but when cooling occurs this has the consistency of soft soap or wax. This material is probably secreted by sebaceous glands, is fluid at temperatures of 34° C. to 39° C., and solidifies at temperatures of 20° C. to 25° C. (Wells). It is made up principally of glycerides of fatty acids, cholesterol and other alcohols. A tangled mass of hair is almost always mixed with the oily material.

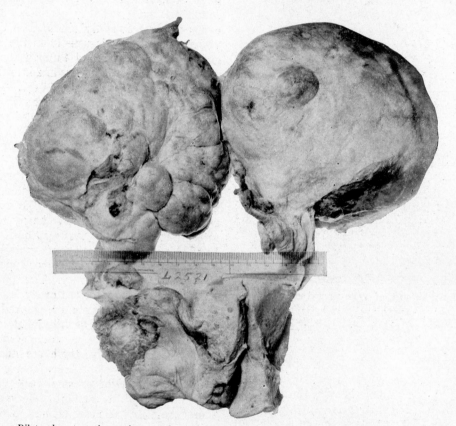

Bilateral metastatic carcinoma of ovaries secondary to mucinous carcinoma of stomach.

TERATOMA. The ovarian teratoma occurs in two forms, the DERMOID CYST which is fairly common and the solid teratoma which is rare. The complex dermoid cyst is most frequent in adult life but may occur any time. It is usually a unilateral pedunculated tumor which may vary greatly in size. The outline may be smooth or somewhat nodular and the cyst wall is either thick, or thin with local areas of thickening. In the body it is somewhat fluctuant, but after cooling it is semisolid in consistency.

Most of the hair grows from a knob-like projection from one part of the cyst wall. This presumably represents the anlage of the anterior part of the body and sometimes shows, teeth and structures resembling jaw bone in addition to the hair.

Microscopically, a wide variety of tissues may be identified. Ectoblast is represented by skin and its associated structures, mucous glands, teeth and nerve tissue. Mesoblast may be represented by bone, muscle, etc. Entoblast may be represented by various glands and mucosa of alimentary canal. These are relatively mature tissues and malignant change is rare. Occasionally true EPIDERMOID CYSTS are found.

The solid teratoma of the ovary is like that of the testis and may be small or grow to large size. It is rare (Graves). The tumor may be smooth or nodular, solid or spongy due to the presence of small cysts. Microscopically, cell masses of immature or organoid form can be traced to all three embryonal layers. Sarcomatous or carcino-

quent near or shortly after the menopause. In childhood it is associated with precocious development of secondary sex characters and irregularly periodic uterine bleeding, probably nonovulatory. During sexual life, there may be menorrhagia, metrorrhagia or shortened periods. After the menopause there may be irregularly periodic bleeding, or continuous metrorrhagia. Usually unilateral but sometimes bilateral, the tumor is most often about 15 or 20 cm. in diameter, but may be much smaller and sometimes is enormous.

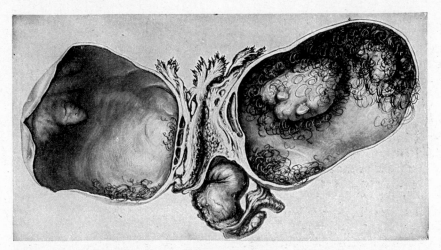

Dermoid cyst of ovary cut open to show interior. From Gynecology, by B. M. Anspach.

matous change may occur, to form the teratoblastoma. It is probable that struma ovarii which contains true colloid, chorionepithelioma and melanoma are a one-sided development of such tumors. (Winternitz; Emge.)

Special Tumors of Ovary. In addition to the tumors discussed above are certain tumors which are more or less peculiar to the ovary. In one group are tumors which may have endocrine functions and in the other are the Brenner tumor, the dysgerminoma and the so-called mesonephroma.

The functioning tumors include those that are said to be feminizing and those that are virilizing. In the former group are the granulosa-cell tumor, its subvariety the luteinizing granulosa-cell tumor, and the theca-cell tumor. The virilizing tumors are the arrhenoblastoma and a tumor that tentatively is classed as a tumor derived from adrenal cortex inclusion.

THE GRANULOSA-CELL TUMOR occurs at almost any time of life, but is most fre-

Microscopically, the tumor is moderately well vascularized and is composed of cells morphologically like those of granulosa. These may be arranged as diffuse masses, or as trabeculae, or are folliculoid with small acinus-like spaces. Some contain Call-Exner spaces which resemble immature graafian follicles, but the central ovum-like material is made up of degenerate tumor cells. We have not encountered malignant change, but others report it in as high as 38 per cent. Metastasis occurs in the peritoneum and rarely elsewhere. Luteinization may occur in some or most of the cells of the tumor, but in our opinion, this does not justify a separate classification. Endometrial hyperplasia, often cystic, is common with granulosa-cell tumors.

THECA-CELL TUMORS, or thecomas, usually occur in postmenopausal life. The tumor is usually unilateral and does not grow to large size. Grossly, it looks like a fibroma but usually has a yellow tinge. Mi-

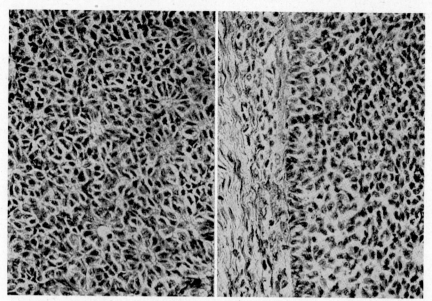

Granulosa-cell tumor of ovary.   Granulosa-cell tumor of ovary.

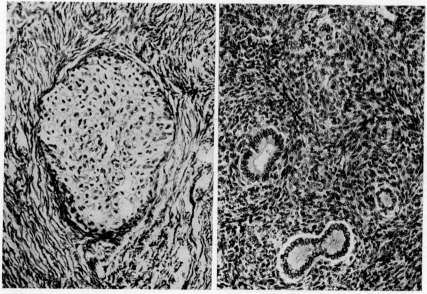

Fibroepithelioma (Brenner tumor) of   Arrhenoblastoma of ovary.
ovary.

croscopically, the cells are of long spindle form; special stains show small groups enclosed in a reticulum. The cytoplasm contains numerous fine droplets of lipid material. Sheets of hyalinized connective tissue, the so-called hyaline plaques, are a distinguishing feature. "Feminization" may occur and sometimes hirsutism is associated, but often there are no functional manifestations.

THE ARRHENOBLASTOMA is grossly much like the granulosa-cell tumor, but is likely to be somewhat nodular. Microscopically it may show a cellular arrangement suggesting tubules of the testis; this is called the testicular tubular adenoma. It is usually nonfunctioning. The sarcomatoid form is the most active functionally. It is composed of short spindle cells arranged in irregular coarse whorls and is moderately well vascularized. The mixed form has components of both the tubular and sarcomatoid types and occupies a mid-position as to function. The effects include amenorrhea, hirsutism, atrophy of breasts, enlarged clitoris and deep voice. This tumor occurs usually in early adult life and is seldom malignant.

THE ADRENAL INCLUSION TUMORS are relatively small, unilateral, soft and of yellow or brown color. Microscopically, the cells are large and the cytoplasm is vesicular because of lipid content. They are arranged in clusters and cords, after the fashion of adrenal cortex. That they are derived from adrenal inclusion is only assumption; their exact nature is not known. They occur at almost any time of life and are not likely to be malignant. They may have the same virilizing effect as the adrenal cortical tumors and the arrhenoblastoma.

Hormone Production. The evidence strongly favors the view that the granulosa-cell tumor produces estrogenic substance and that the arrhenoblastoma produces androgenic substance. The situation is not altogether clear as concerns the adrenal tumor, but it is probable that it also produces androgenic substance.

THE BRENNER TUMOR has no endocrine manifestations. It may be solid or cystic and grossly resembles the fibroma. Microscopically it is characterized by the appearance of nests of epithelial cells, cuboidal or rounded, sometimes with formation of acini. It is a disease of older women and is not malignant. (See Fox.)

THE DYSGERMINOMA is the counterpart in the ovary of the embryonal carcinoma or seminoma of the testis. (See Sailer.)

THE SO-CALLED MESONEPHROMA is a rare tumor, usually small, and usually malignant. Microscopically there are structures which have a certain resemblance to the primitive glomeruli of the mesonephros. There is dispute as to their exact nature. (See Schiller; Jones and Jones; Kazancigil et al.)

THE EMBRYOGENESIS of these various tumors is not altogether clear. It seems probable that the granulosa-cell and theca-cell tumors are derived from mesenchymal cells of the primitive sex gland. Similarly, the arrhenoblastoma probably originates in remaining primitive cells which are "male-directed." The adrenal-type tumors may be derived from misplaced cells of the adrenal cortical anlage. The origin of the Brenner tumor is vague but probably it develops from Walthard rests. The dysgerminoma is probably derived from primitive mesenchymal cells. (See Karsner.)

TORSION OF PEDUNCULATED TUMORS. Slight twisting of the pedicle of ovarian tumors is common, but is not significant unless it obstructs circulation. Torsion through 90° is not effective, but beyond 180° is usually obstructive. The weight of tumors may lead to sinking into the pelvis, and the resistance of the pelvic and abdominal walls as well as intestinal movement may cause the torsion. In general, tumors of the left side show a right spiral and those of the right side a left spiral twist.

Ordinarily, the torsion occurs slowly, but in women with relaxed muscles, and in the puerperium, blows, falls or sudden stresses may lead to rapid torsion. Rarely the twist may be reversed upon itself and is then called retorsion. If the tumor be adherent to the gut, torsion may produce intestinal obstruction. As a rule, the more rapid the rate of torsion the more serious are the results. Interference with venous drainage leads to hyperemia, edema, cellular degenerations and hemorrhage. Arterial occlusion causes necrosis and the tumor, especially if cystic, ruptures. If adhesion to the intestine has been established, bacteria may enter the tumor and, if there be the changes secondary to torsion, suppuration may occur.

Pregnancy and Ovarian Tumors. Pregnancy may occur in spite of the presence of ovarian tumors both benign and malignant. Nevertheless the interference with ovulation, as well as the malposition of the uterus which is often associated, probably diminishes the incidence of pregnancy. The increased abdominal pressure of labor may be sufficient to rupture the tumorous and other cysts. Pregnancy favors torsion of pedunculated tumors and this is also particularly true in the puerperium.

Parovarium

Parovarian Cysts. These are retention cysts in the same sense as those of the ovary. They represent cystic dilatation of the tubules of the parovarium. They therefore originate in the broad ligament near the fimbriated end of the tube and may be either pedunculated or intraligamentary. They are usually only a few millimeters in diameter and multiple, but may be solitary and may attain great size. They are thin walled, monolocular and contain thin, clear, serous fluid of low specific gravity, containing very little protein and no pseudomucin.

In the earlier stages the cyst wall and peritoneum are easily separable and the blood vessels of each can be seen coursing in different directions. Subsequently, however, these two membranes may fuse. Usually the lining is smooth but may show small nodular outgrowths or papillary structures. Microscopically, the cyst wall is made up principally of vascularized connective tissue with small amounts of elastica and smooth muscle. The lining is a single layer of ciliated low columnar, cuboidal or flattened epithelium. The pedunculated cysts may undergo torsion with its consequences as described in ovarian tumors.

Tumors of the parovarium are rare but include fibro-adenoma, papilliferous cystadenoma, teratoma, carcinoma and sarcoma. They should always be carefully distinguished from tumors of an accessory or third ovary.

THE BREAST

Congenital Anomalies

CONGENITAL ABSENCE OF THE BREAST, amastia, may be unilateral or bilateral, and although more frequent and noticeable in females, occurs also in males. The underlying embryonal fault in the "milk-line" or breast anlage often affects nearby structures, since amastia is frequently associated with anomalies of the pectoral muscles, chest and arm. Concomitant anomalies of the genital organs and amastia in female pseudohermaphrodites indicate an influence of the sex glands.

ATHELIA or absence of the nipple is rare. It occurs in amastia but may also be observed with a well-developed breast.

MICROMASTIA AND MICROTHELIA are usually associated but may be independent of each other and are looked upon as congenital hypoplasias. Other deformities are flattened nipples and inverted nipples.

POLYMASTIA, or excessive number of breasts, is not infrequent. The milk-line of the embryo extends from the axilla to the inguinal region and the supernumerary breasts may occur at any corresponding situation. With extreme rarity they may appear upon the thigh. They are most frequent in females and in the axilla. They usually enlarge in periods of lactation and may secrete milk. If there be no nipple the swelling of lactation is often painful and may lead to inflammation. It is probable that supernumerary breasts are more susceptible to malignant tumors than normal breasts.

POLYTHELIA, or supernumerary nipples, is rare. The extra nipples may be in the areola or on other parts of the breast. When extra nipples occur elsewhere than on the normally situated breast they have underlying breast tissue and are a part of polymastia.

Acquired Anomalies. Abnormal enlargement of the breast in females is called hypertrophy and in males gynecomastia.

HYPERTROPHY OF THE BREAST is usually bilateral but in occasional cases only one breast is affected. Although hypertrophy may rarely be congenital or occur in early life, it usually arises at the period of puberty and less commonly in pregnancy or lactation.

The enlargement is usually uniform and may reach enormous proportions.

Microscopically, the breast shows increase in amount of gland tissue and supporting tissue, but in some cases there may be dilatation of ducts or even adenoma-like hyperplasia of glands. The cause is unknown. Familial incidence is unusual; morphologic disease of sex glands is not common; and hormonal influence, although perhaps of importance, is difficult to apply in cases of unilateral hypertrophy. Diffuse lipomatosis of the breast or large nodular lipoma should not be confused with hypertrophy. If destruction of the breast tissue by various pathologic processes be sufficiently extensive, a hypertrophy of the remainder of the breast tissue may occur.

GYNECOMASTIA, in which the male breast is enlarged, is uncommon, usually but not always bilateral, and is sometimes familial. It is observed in connection with tumors of the testis, especially the chorionepithelioma, but some of the cases are unexplained. It is a glandular hypertrophy and in a few instances adenofibroma may develop.

ATROPHY, except that of age, is uncommon. Rarely postlactation involution may progress to atrophy. Local atrophy may occur as the result of pressure from tumors.

Circulatory Disturbances

The breast may be somewhat enlarged and hyperemic in the premenstrual phase, and a few drops of blood may be discharged from the nipples. Bleeding from the nipples may be due both to benign tumors, especially the papilliferous adenoma, and to malignant tumors. Small or large hemorrhage into the breast may be due to trauma or may be without known cause. The larger hemorrhages have been given the name apoplexy of the breast.

Inflammation

Nonsuppurative diffuse inflammations are seen in the newborn. In the adult they are due to retained secretion dammed back either by fibrous occlusion of ducts, inspissation of secretion in the nipple ducts, or by athelia.

The suppurative inflammations usually occur during lactation, presumably because of infection extending along the ducts. With or without retention of secretion, suppuration begins in the ducts or glands and involves the supporting tissues. Sometimes the inflammation is found only in and under the nipple; it forms a subareolar abscess. The abscess may be intramammary, subcu-

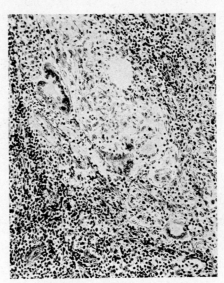

An area in chronic abscess of the breast with multinucleated giant cells.

taneous or, when it occurs beneath the breast and on the chest wall, submammary. The more extensive forms may become phlegmonous. Abscesses of the breast may occur in pyemia or may extend from suppuration in the chest wall or thorax. It is conceivable that in septicemia the excretion of bacteria in the milk may excite inflammation and suppuration. This is a possible explanation of the acute mastitis which sometimes complicates typhoid fever. In mumps there may be a so-called metastatic acute diffuse mastitis. Trauma may cause acute mastitis and in the male is the commonest causative factor. Acute suppurative mastitis is usually due to the staphylococcus, but other pyogens may also be causative.

The abscess may result in complete cicatrization following evacuation, or the granulation tissue may become dense and form a chronic abscess. Occasionally, the contents are completely liquefied, become serous in character by removal of solid material, and the wall condenses to form a pseudocyst. The chronic abscesses may be mistaken clinically for tumor. Microscopically, it is not uncommon to find in the abscess pseudo-tubercles with foreign-body giant cells surrounding small particles of tissue detritus or cholesterol crystals.

Chronic mastitis may follow the acute forms or be a chronic fibrosing process from the start. The chronic hyperplastic mastitis, seen especially in the male breast, is often without history of preceding acute inflammation. It is a progressive connective tissue hyperplasia which may produce moderate enlargement of the breast. In the female, chronic mastitis usually follows some form of acute mastitis. In the majority of cases it is merely a cicatrization of the old process and not progressive. In other cases, however, the firm area may enlarge somewhat and show microscopically a sufficient infiltration of lymphoid and plasma cells, together with epithelial proliferation, to justify the assumption that it is a chronic inflammation. The so-called chronic cystic mastitis will be discussed under the heading of abnormal involution.

Infectious Granulomata

Tuberculosis may affect the skin of the breast in the form of lupus. In rare cases, tubercle bacilli may enter the breast through abrasions of nipple and skin. Tuberculous mastitis, however, is usually secondary to tuberculosis elsewhere, especially of the lungs and of the lymph nodes. Deaver and McFarland accept as authentic the reports of 90 cases, of which only 10 were in the male breast. It does not occur before puberty, may be seen in advanced years, but is most frequent in the third and fourth decades of life. Since the early stage is usually found in ducts or glands, it seems possible that the lesion is due to excretion of tubercle bacilli into the lumen and subsequent tubercle formation. It is also probable that infection may occur from retrograde lymph transport from lymph nodes of mediastinum or axilla, but it is difficult in such cases to decide that the lymph-node involvement is not secondary to the breast lesion.

According to Deaver and McFarland the tuberculosis may be (1) miliary, (2) conglomerate with large single or multiple nodular masses, (3) sclerosing tuberculous mastitis, comparable to chronic fibroid tu-berculosis of the lungs, (4) mastitis tuberculosa obliterans in which chronic periacinar and periductal tuberculosis leads to obliteration of the breast epithelium, and (5), various atypical forms. In the more extensive lesions, sinuses may discharge through the skin. Tuberculosis may be associated with benign or malignant tumors or with other lesions of the breast, but should always be distinguished from pseudotubercles as mentioned in reference to chronic abscess. The diagnosis depends not only upon the presence of histologically demonstrable tubercles, but must be supported by bacteriological evidence.

Syphilis may affect the breast as chancre, as mucous patches or other secondary cutaneous lesions, as gumma, and as a diffuse chronic inflammation with diffuse and perivascular lymphoid cell infiltration associated with endovasculitis.

Actinomycosis and sporotrichosis may be primary in the breast.

Cysts

Cysts of the breast may be the result of a wide variety of conditions including retention of secretion, accumulation of serous fluid, inflammation, hyperplasia, abnormal involution, tumor growth. In addition there are pseudocysts resulting from encapsulation of abscess or hemorrhage.

Galactocele is a retention cyst of the ducts, usually single but sometimes multiple, whose origin is often without explanation. The content may be milky, may be like butter or may be thin and serous, with or without casein flakes.

Simple cysts usually appear as fairly large single cysts, often with associated cystic dilatation of neighboring ducts, with chronic inflammation or with abnormal involution. The wall is thin and when approached surgically in the living breast has a blue color, the blue-dome cyst of Bloodgood. As soon as the cyst is cut the blue color disappears. The fluid is thin, serous, clear or turbid, sometimes viscid but never milky. The lining is smooth. The papilliferous cyst, often called papilloma of the breast, may be a cyst of the order just discussed, or the cystic nature may be caused by papillary growth within a duct or ducts. Thus the papilloma may constitute a tumor mass. In itself, the lesion is benign, but there is a definite tendency for it to become a carcinoma.

Abnormal Involution of the Breast. In this category we include conditions characterized by the formation of multiple small cysts of the mammary gland. They are probably all closely related and have been given various names including chronic cystic mastitis, fibrocystic disease of the breast, mastopathia cystica, Schimmelbusch's disease and others. McFarland found that all the changes observed, including lymphocytic infiltration, occur in the course of normal involution of the breast. In abnormal involution these changes vary in degree and in proportion. Attempts are made to distinguish varieties of the disorder.

The condition may occur in relatively early life but is most common at about the time of menopause. It is most frequent in women who have lactated but occurs in the nulliparous. Early symptoms include pain and discharge of secretion or even blood from the nipple. Usually both breasts are affected, but the condition may be unilateral.

Grossly, the breast is usually not enlarged and the condition is not circumscribed or encapsulated. The organ is dense and firm and in cross section shows usually a variable number of small cysts, or even a single "blue dome" cyst.

Microscopically, the connective tissue is densely fibrillar but not notably increased in amount and may show a rich infiltration of lymphoid cells. The cysts are found to be

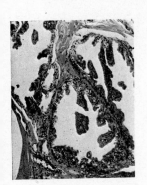 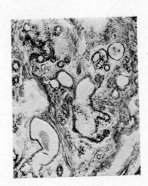 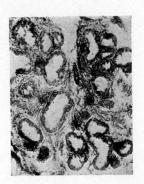

Three photomicrographs from abnormal involution of the breast to show various types of epithelial change and cyst formation.

Thus Cheatle and Cutler describe mazoplasia in which there is proliferation of cells in terminal ducts and acini, with desquamation and also fibrous-tissue growth in the neighborhood. The more marked abnormality, they call cystophorous desquamative hyperplasia. Geschickter distinguishes (a) the painful breasts of women in the thirties, called mastodynia, (b) the diffusely nodular breasts of slightly later life, adenosis, and (c) cystic disease of the breast with larger cysts occurring in women near or after the menopause. We think that these various distinctions are somewhat artificial separations of what is fundamentally the same process. It is probable that the condition is due to some abnormality of action of ovarian and perhaps pituitary hormones upon the nonlactating breast, but the exact mechanism is not clear (see Goodman).

dilated ducts, but microscopically the glands also may show irregular cystic dilatation, apparently an adenomatous hyperplasia. Some of the acini show papilla-like spurs which are probably due to fusion of adjacent acini and rupture of their walls. The epithelium may be piled up in several layers. The epithelium of many acini shows a markedly eosinophilic cytoplasm. Other acini show cells resembling those of sweat glands, especially those of apocrine type.

There is much difference of opinion as to whether or not abnormal involution predisposes to the development of carcinoma. Warren has analyzed the question statistically and concludes that carcinoma occurs on an average of 4.5 times as often in women with cystic disease and chronic mastitis as in those with otherwise normal breasts.

Tumors

Benign Tumors. The simpler benign tumors such as pure adenoma, fibroma and myxoma are rare. Fibromyoma is a great rarity (see Lebowich and Lenz). Lipoma is infrequent and may be bilateral. The most frequent benign tumorous lesion is adeno-fibroma. (See de Cholnoky.)

ADENOFIBROMA. Also called fibroadenoma and periductal fibroma, this lesion constitutes nearly one-fourth of the tumorous lesions of the female breast and may occur occasionally in the male breast (McFarland).

mingled. The intercanalicular variety shows diffuse connective-tissue proliferation with a relatively small number of tubular epithelial spaces. In the pericanalicular variety the connective tissue shows dense and often concentrically arranged connective tissue masses immediately around the epithelial areas. In the intracanalicular adenofibroma there is a considerable proliferation of epithelium arranged in more or less stellate figures. This peculiar configuration is presumably due to ingrowth into the canal of blunt projections or papillae of connective tissue. The lumina

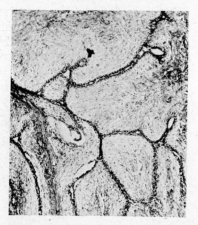

Intracanalicular fibroadenoma of the breast.

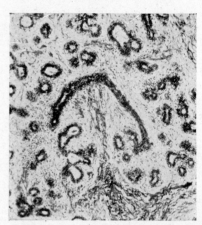

Adenoma of the breast with edema of supporting tissue.

It occurs at various ages, the average being 32 years. Of these women, 75 per cent are nullipara and 95 per cent have not reached the menopause. Although the nodules are usually single they may be multiple. They are slow-growing, dense, usually painless masses, which ordinarily are brought to the attention of the surgeon when they have attained a diameter of about 3 to 6 cm. The nodule is firm, dense, smooth in outline or slightly nodulated, well defined and shells out easily from the surrounding tissue. It usually cuts with considerable resistance and shows a gray or grayish-pink, firm, fibrillated cross section, although it may be soft, or gelatinous in character. Sometimes the cross section shows clefts or small cysts but is practically never lobated.

Microscopically, proliferation of connective tissue and of epithelium is found. It is possible to distinguish three general types although often enough these are inter-

of the epithelial spaces are likely to be obliterated, and the epithelium is disposed in parallel rows of cells. In all the varieties of adenofibroma the epithelial spaces usually are lined with only a single layer of cuboidal epithelium, resembling that of the finer ducts. Occasionally, the epithelium is in double layers resembling more closely that of the glandular acini. As a rule, the connective tissue is moderately cellular but may be of a densely fibrillar character. Edema is not infrequent especially in those parts of the connective tissue immediately around the epithelial acini. Mucoid degeneration is also common and occasionally fat infiltration is observed.

Careful reconstruction studies of this lesion show that it is directly connected with, and is an outgrowth from normal mammary tissue. Experimentally the repeated injection of large quantities of estrogenic substance into animals produces proliferation of ducts and to a lesser degree of acini, which resembles the epithelial component of the lesion. Question has been raised as to its being only a hyperplasia but in our opinion the nodular character justifies the assumption that it is a tumor, even though it may be initiated by some alteration of estrogenic stimulation.

A lesion of the same general order is the so-called CYSTOSARCOMA PHALLYDES, in which there is connective tissue in large nodular masses, with only relatively little epithelial proliferation. There is no indication that it is a true sarcoma. Owens and Adams view it as a giant manifestation of adenofibroma.

ADENOMA in pure form is rare in the breast (Pavie). Grossly, except in density of consistence, it resembles the adenofibroma, but microscopically it shows extensive multiplication of glandular acini which may be uniform, regular and small, or may be very irregular in outline and with multiple layers of cells. This is referred to as the solid adenoma in contrast to the cystadenoma. Usually, however, the cystadenoma is classified as an adenofibroma with cystic dilatation of the epithelial spaces. It is probable that many of the cysts discussed in the preceding section are of this character.

Malignant Tumors. CARCINOMA. According to McFarland, carcinoma of the breast constitutes about three-fourths of the breast tumors. It may occur in early life or in late life but is especially frequent between 40 and 60 years of age, occurring in the upper outer quadrant of the breast in about half the cases. It is at least one hundred times more common in the female than in the male breast. It is usually first observed as a lump in the breast which may grow rapidly or slowly, is firm, poorly defined and adherent to the surrounding breast tissue.

The commoner forms include the soft, medullary, or encephaloid carcinoma and the firm, scirrhous carcinoma. Either form may grow up to and into the skin and penetrate through it to produce a small or large ulcerated area, but this is more especially true of the medullary carcinoma. Contraction of connective tissue may produce depression or actual inversion of the nipple, more especially in the scirrhous carcinomas. Some-

times the retraction is seen particularly in the connective-tissue columns of the skin, producing the so-called pigskin, or the skin may be flat and glossy. Rarely, the tumor may extend laterally underneath the skin to form a dense mass over the thoracic wall, the "cancer en cuirasse."

Microscopically, the tumor may appear as a carcinoma simplex or an adeno-

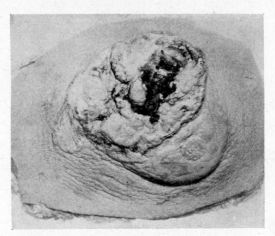

Medullary carcinoma of breast with penetration of skin.

carcinoma. Most of the true cases of carcinoma leave no reasonable doubt as to the diagnosis. The greatest difficulty is encountered in diagnosticating malignant change in abnormal involution of the breast or in adenofibroma of the breast. In the scirrhous carcinoma, carcinoma simplex is more common than adenocarcinoma although the latter is sometimes observed. Carcinoma may be largely intraductal, in which case plugs of partly necrotic tumor can be expressed from the ducts in the gross cross section; this has been called comedo carcinoma. Mucin may be produced in any of the forms of mammary carcinoma, but the true mucinous carcinoma is rare (Saphir). Occasionally a noninvasive or pre-invasive stage of carcinoma occurs called "carcinoma in situ," in which one or several lobules show microscopically a well-defined mass of cells which have lost their polarity and exhibit pleomorphism in moderate degree (Foote and Stewart). Squamous-cell metaplasia may occur in mammary carcinoma, but the true squamous-cell carcinoma originates in the skin.

Estimation of degrees of malignancy

of mammary carcinoma is sometimes made on the basis of grading, but there are so many variables, including variations in the

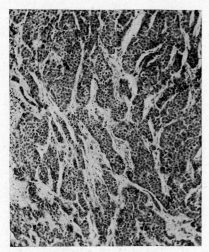

Medullary carcinoma of breast (carcinoma simplex). Army Medical Museum 46847.

picture in different sections, that it is often misleading.

As indicated in the chapter on Tumors, mammary carcinoma follows the ex-

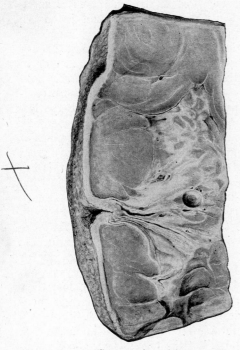

Cross section of breast with scirrhous carcinoma, small cysts, and marked retraction of nipple.

perimental injection of estrogenic substances into mice and rats. The dosage must be far beyond what could be produced naturally in the animal and the administration long continued. Smaller doses may increase the susceptibility to the large doses (see Geschickter and Byrnes). The application of these observations to women is not clear. Although estrogenic substances are used therapeutically, the dosage is not large enough to be dangerous (Allen).

The metastasis of carcinoma of the breast is most frequently observed in the lymph nodes of the axilla, but in microscopic diagnosis care should always be exercised to differentiate between tumor metastasis and endothelial hyperplasia which is extremely

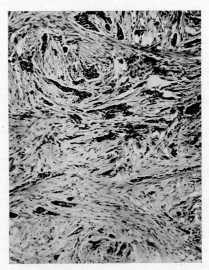

Fibrous carcinoma simplex of breast.

common. The hyperplasia of the lymph nodes is regarded by some as preparing the soil for metastasis. This hypothesis, however, is not certainly established. Many cases of carcinoma of both breasts represent metastasis from one breast to the other, but occasionally carcinoma may develop simultaneously in the two organs.

The pectoral muscles, the lymph nodes of the thorax and the lymphatic tracts and lymph nodes of the abdominal cavity may be involved by lymphatic metastasis. Metastases are fairly frequent in lungs, liver and adrenal, may occur in spleen and ovaries, and sometimes are seen in more remote sites. (See Saphir and Parker.) Metastasis to bones is frequent and may be so extensive as to lead to profound myelophthisic anemia. The metastases are usually osteolytic and not associated with increase of acid phosphatase (see Sharpe and McDonald).

SARCOMA of the breast is relatively infrequent but occurs far more often in the female than in the male breast. It may be seen at any period of life but is most frequent between 30 and 50 years of age. Those that develop in the periductal tissue are said to be indigenous, and those that develop in the outlying supporting tissues are said to be nonindigenous sarcomas. Sarcoma often grows and develops as does the adenofibroma, may be removed with this diagnosis and only upon microscopic examination is found to be malignant. Some sarcomas show a sudden increase in rate of growth, whereas others appear to grow rapidly from the beginning. When the tumor has attained considerable size, the superficial veins of the breast are distended. Erosion of the skin is common. Microscopically, the most frequent sarcoma is a fibrosarcoma. Lymphosarcoma, liposarcoma, myxosarcoma and malignant hemangiosarcoma occur (see Hill and Stout). There is difference of opinion about the nature of more mature forms such as osteosarcoma and chondrosarcoma. Some think they are derivatives of epithelial tumors; others think they are of mesoblastic origin; and others believe them to be derivatives of teratoid tumors (see D'Aunoy and Wright.) Rare cases of combined sarcoma and carcinoma are recorded.

Paget's Disease of the Nipple. The nipple may be the seat of inflammations, often eczematous. Paget's disease of the nipple, however, is not simply an inflammation. It occurs in women, usually between about 40 to 60 years of age. It begins as a reddening of the nipple which goes on to shallow erosion and ulceration with discharge of a small amount of slightly viscid colorless or pink fluid. The disease may extend to involve the areola and sometimes spreads to the skin. The nipple may shrink to the level of the areola.

Microscopically, the epidermis is usually thickened especially by growth of intermediate cells. The interpapillary epithelium extends slightly or deeply into the corium where there is usually an infiltration of lymphocytes and plasma cells. The ducts of the nipple show proliferation of the lining cells in the form of a noninvasive carcinoma simplex. In the intermediate layer of the epidermis and sometimes in the ducts there are the "Paget cells," larger than the surrounding cells with poorly stained cytoplasm and small but vesicular nuclei. Carcinoma of duct-cell type is frequent in the underlying mammary gland, but not invariably present.

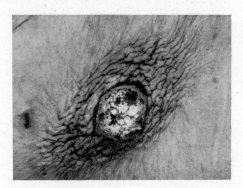

Paget's disease of the nipple.

In our opinion, Paget's disease of the nipple is a carcinoma of ducts of the nipple, or epidermis, or both. Some think that the disease of the nipple is secondary to carcinoma of the breast, but cases are observed without carcinoma of the breast. The carcinoma of the breast is of duct-cell type and is usually scirrhous. It is probable that the ducts of the mammary gland become carcinomatous because of extension from the ducts of the nipple. This extension may be due to intra-epithelial invasion along the ducts or to a gradual progressive transformation of the duct lining to carcinoma. (See Muir.)

REFERENCES

Adair, F. L.: Some Observations on Placental Infarcts, Amer. Jour. Obst. and Gynec., 6: 552, 1923.

Adair, F. L., and R. M. Watts: A Study of the Hormonal Content of Ovarian Cyst Fluids, Ibid., 34: 799, 1937.

Albright, F., P. H. Smith, and R. Fraser: Syndrome Characterized by Primary Ovarian Insufficiency and Decreased Stature: Report of Eleven Cases, with a Digression on Hormonal Control of Axillary and Pubic Hair, Trans. Asso. Amer. Phys., Vol. 56, 1942, in press.

Allen, E.: Ovarian Hormones and Female Genital Cancer, Jour. Amer. Med. Asso., 114: 2107, 1940.

——: Regurgitation of Endometrial Tissue Through Fallopian Tube, etc., Ibid., 90: 507, 1928.

——, and E. A. Doisy: Ovarian and Placental Hormones, Physiol. Rev., 7: 600, 1927.

Amolsch, A. L.: Mixed Mesodermal Tumors of the Uterus and Vagina; with Report of Six Cases, Amer. Jour. Cancer, 37: 435, 1939.

Baker, A. B.: Fibrosis Uteri, Amer. Jour. Path., 9: 369, 1933.

Baron, E., and A. Angrist: Incidence of Occult Adenocarcinoma of the Prostate after Fifty Years of Age, Arch. Path., 32: 787, 1941.

Barringer, B. S., and D. Earl: Teratoma Testis. Survey of Thirty-seven Autopsy Records, Surg., Gynec., and Obst., 72: 591, 1941.

Bartlett, E. I.: Breast Hypertrophy, etc., Ibid., 38: 798, 1924.

Batson, O. V.: The Function of the Vertebral Veins and Their Role in the Spread of Metastases, Ann. Surg., 112: 138, 1940.

Behney, C. A.: Extra-Uterine Pregnancy—A Study of 167 Consecutive Cases, Jour. Amer. Med. Asso., 95: 1557, 1930.

Block, F. B.: Endometriosis, Amer. Jour. Med. Sci., 199: 579, 1940.

Bloodgood, J. C.: Lesions of the Female Breast, Binnie's Regional Surgery, Vol. 1, Section 23, Philadelphia, 1917.

——: The Pathology of Chronic Cystic Mastitis of the Female Breast with Special Consideration of the Blue-domed Cyst, Arch. Surg., 3: 445, 1921.

——: Cancer Cysts of the Breast and Their Relation to Non-malignant Cysts, Jour. Amer. Med. Asso., 53: 1475, 1909.

——: Benign Tumors of the Breast, etc., Ann. Surg., 79: 172, 1924.

Brewer, J. I., and H. O. Jones: A Study of the Corpora Luteum and the Endometriums in Patients with Uterine Fibroids, Amer. Jour. Obst. and Gynec., 41: 733, 1941.

Campbell, H. E.: Incidence of Malignant Growth of the Undescended Testicle: A Critical and Statistical Study, Arch. Surg., 44: 353, 1942.

de Cholnoky, T.: Benign Tumors of Breast, Ibid., 38: 79, 1939.

Cullen, T. S.: Cysts of Bartholin's Glands, Jour. Amer. Med. Asso., 44: 204, 1905.

D'Aunoy, R., and R. W. Wright: Sarcoma of the Breast, Ann. Surg., 92: 1059, 1930.

Davis, L.: Observations on the Distribution and Culture of the Chancroid Bacillus, Jour. Med. Res., 9: 401, 1903.

Deaver, J. B., and J. McFarland: The Breast: Its Anomalies, Its Diseases and Their Treatment, Philadelphia, 1917.

Dial, D. L., and B. Halpert: Leiomyoma of the Prostate. Report of Three Cases, Arch. Path., 16: 332, 1933.

Douglass, M., and M. Ridlon: Tuberculosis of the Cervix Uteri, with a Report of Two Cases, One Probably Primary in the Cervix, Surg., Gynec. and Obst., 48: 408, 1929.

Emge, L. A.: Functional and Growth Characteristics of Struma Ovarii, Amer. Jour. Obst. and Gynec., 40: 738, 1940.

Ewing, J.: Neoplastic Diseases, Philadelphia and London, 4th ed., 1940.

Foote, F. W., Jr., and F. W. Stewart: Lobular Carcinoma in Situ. A Rare Form of Mammary Cancer, Amer. Jour. Path., 17: 491, 1941.

Fox, R. A.: Brenner Tumor of the Ovary. Case Reports, Discussion and Bibliography, Ibid., 18: 223, 1942.

Fraenkel, A.: Ist das Fibroadenom der Mamma ein Blastom?, Franfürt. Zeitschr. Path., 46: 195, 1933.

Fraser, J.: Placental Circulation, Amer. Jour. Obst. and Gynec., 6: 645, 1923.

Geschickter, C. F.: The Endocrine Aspects of Chronic Cystic Mastitis, South. Surgeon, 10: 457, 1941.

——, and E. W. Byrnes: Factors Influencing the Development and Time of Appearance of Mammary Cancer in the Rat in Response to Estrogen, Arch. Path., 33: 334, 1942.

Goodman, B. A.: Fibrocystic Disease of the Breast, Arch. Surg., 38: 917, 1939.

Graves, W. P.: Gynecology, 3d ed., Philadelphia and London, 1923.

——, and G. Van S. Smith: Kraurosis Vulvae, Jour. Amer. Med. Asso., 92: 1244, 1929.

Hamilton, J. B., and J. B. Gilbert: Studies in Malignant Tumors of the Testis. IV. Bilateral Testicular Cancer. Incidence, Nature and Bearing upon Management of the Patient with a Single Testicular Cancer, Cancer Res., 2: 125, 1942.

Herger, C. C., and A. A. Thibeaudau: Teratoma of Testis, Amer. Jour. Cancer, 22: 525, 1934.

Herrick, F. C.: Sarcoma of the Prostate, Ann. Surg., 71: 168, 1920.

Hertig, A. T., and H. W. Edmunds: Genesis of Hydatidiform Mole, Arch. Path., 30: 260, 1940.

Hill, R. P., and A. P. Stout: Sarcoma of the Breast, Arch. Surg., 44: 473, 1942.

Hinman, F., and T. E. Gibson: Tumors of the Epididymis, Spermatic Cord and Testicular Tunics, etc., Arch. Surg., 8: 100, 1924.

Huggins, C., and C. V. Hodges: Studies on Prostatic Cancer. I. The Effect of Castration, of Estrogen and of Androgen Injection on Serum Phosphatases in Metastatic Carcinoma of the Prostate, Cancer Res., 1: 293, 1941.

Hunt, E.: Disease Affecting the Vulva, St. Louis, Mosby, 1940.

Jacobson, V. C.: The Intraperitoneal Transplantation of Endometrial Tissue: An Experimental Study, Arch. Path., 1: 169, 1926.

Jones, H. W., Jr., and G. E. S. Jones: Mesonephroma of the Ovary, Arch. Path., 33: 18, 1942.

Jorstad, L. H.: Carcinoma of the Penis, Amer. Jour. Roentgenol., 46: 232, 1941.

Karsner, H. T.: Certain Ovarian Tumors Associated with Sexual Endocrine Dysfunction, Trans. and Stud., Coll. Phys., Philadelphia, 7: 301, 1940.

Kazancigil, T. R., W. Laqueur, and P. Ladewig: Papillo-Endothelioma Ovarii. Report of Three Cases and a Discussion of Schiller's "Mesonephroma Ovarii," Amer. Jour. Cancer, 40: 199, 1940.

Kwartin, B., and J. A. Hyams: True Hermaphroditism in Man, etc., Jour. Urol., 18: 363, 1927.

Lebowich, R. J., and G. Lenz: Primary Fibromyoma of the Breast. Report of a Case and Review of the Literature, Amer. Jour. Cancer, 38: 73, 1940.

Liebow, A. A., and R. Tennant: Mesodermal Mixed Tumors of the Body of the Uterus, Amer. Jour. Path., 17: 1, 1941.

Lipschütz, A.: The Internal Secretions of the Sex Glands, Baltimore, 1925.

Lovelady, S. B., J. R. McDonald, and J. M. Waugh: Benign Tumors of Vulva, Amer. Jour. Obst. and Gynec., 42: 309, 1941.

MacCallum, W. G.: Pathological Physiology of the Prostate, Physiol, Rev., **17**: 73, 1937.

McFarland, J.: Surgical Pathology, Philadelphia, 1924.

——: Residual Lactation Acini in the Female Breast and Their Relation to Chronic Cystic Mastitis and Malignant Disease, Arch. Surg., **5**: 1, 1922.

——: Adenofibroma and Fibro-adenoma of Female Breast, Surg., Gynec. and Obstet., **45**: 729, 1927.

Meigs, J. V.: A Study of Adenocarcinoma of the Fundus of the Uterus, Amer. Jour. Obst. and Gynec., **4**: 241, 1922.

Moore, R. A.: The Morphology of Small Prostatic Carcinoma, Jour. Urol., **33**: 224, 1935.

——: The Evolution and Involution of the Prostate Gland, Amer. Jour. Path., **12**: 599, 1936.

——: Tuberculosis of the Prostate Gland, Jour. Urol., **37**: 372, 1937.

——: Inflammation of the Prostate Gland, Ibid., **38**: 173, 1937.

——: The Physiological Response of Prostatic and Vesicular Transplants in the Anterior Chamber of the Eye, Jour. Exper. Med., **66**: 281, 1937.

——: Experimental Genital Tuberculosis in the Rabbit, Jour. Urol., **39**: 367, 1938.

Moritz, A. R., and M. Douglass: A Study of Uterine and Tubal Decidual Reaction in Tubal Pregnancy, Surg., Gynec. and Obst., **47**: 785, 1928.

Muir, R.: Further Observations on Paget's Disease of the Nipple, Jour. Path. and Bact., **49**: 299, 1939.

Noguchi, H., and D. J. Kaliski: The Spirochetal Flora of the Normal Female Genitalia, Jour. Exper. Med., **28**: 559, 1918.

Norris, C. C.: Adenocarcinoma of the Cervix. A Study of Forty-three Cases, Amer. Jour. Cancer, **27**: 653, 1936.

Oberling, C.: Les Endometriomes, Ann. d'Anat. Path. Med. Chir., **1**: 541, 1924.

Owens, F. M., Jr., and W. E. Adams: Giant Intracanalicular Fibroadenoma of the Breast, Arch. Surg., **43**: 588, 1941.

Pavie, P.: Adénomes purs de la Glande Mammaire, Ann. Anat. Path., **7**: 449, 1930.

Pfannenstiel, J.: Die Erkrankungen des Eierstockes und des Nebeneirerstockes, Veit's Handbuch der Gynaekologie, IV¹, p. 1, Weisbaden, 1908.

Polster, K. O.: Beiträge zur Kenntnis der heterotopen Wucherungen vom Bau der Uterusschleimhaut, Virchow's Arch. Path. Anat., **259**: 96, 1926.

Popoff, N. W.: Testicular Tubular Adenoma of the Ovary, etc., Arch. Path., **9**: 31, 1930.

Rea, C. E.: Histologic Character of the Undescended Testis after Puberty: Its Significance with Reference to the Performance of Orchioplexy, Arch. Surg., **44**: 27, 1942.

Sailer, S.: Ovarian Dysgerminoma, Amer. Jour. Cancer, **38**: 473, 1940.

Sampson, J. A.: Metastatic or Embolic Endometriosis due to the Menstrual Dissemination of Endometrial Tissue into the Venous Circulation, Amer. Jour. Path., **3**: 93, 1927.

——: Implantation Peritoneal Carcinomatosis of Ovarian Origin, Ibid., **7**: 423, 1931.

——: Carcinoma of the Tubes and Ovaries Secondary to Carcinoma of the Body of the Uterus, Ibid., **10**: 1, 1934.

Saphir, O.: Mucinous Carcinoma of the Breast, Surg., Gynec. and Obst., **72**: 908, 1941.

——, and M. L. Parker: Metastasis of Primary Carcinoma of the Breast, with Special Reference to Spleen, Adrenal Glands and Ovaries, Arch. Surg., **42**: 1003, 1941.

Schiller, W.: The Histogenesis of Ovarian Mesonephroma, Arch. Path., **33**: 443, 1942.

——, and D. D. Kozoll: Primary Signet-Ring Cell Carcinoma of Ovary, with Case Report, Amer. Jour. Obst. and Gynec., **41**: 70, 1941.

Schmitz, H., and W. Hueper: Malignant Chorionepithelioma Uteri, Jour. Amer. Med. Asso., **95**: 1413, 1930.

Sharpe, W. S., and J. R. McDonald: Reaction of Bone to Metastasis from Carcinoma of the Breast and Prostate, Arch. Path., **33**: 312, 1942.

Siddall, R. S.: The Occurrence of Chorioangiofibroma (chorioangioma). A Study of 600 Placentas, Bull. Johns Hopkins Hosp., **38**: 355, 1926.

Stein, A.: Syphiloma Vulvae, Surg., Gynec. and Obst., **31**: 227, 1920.

Steiner, P. E.: Metastasizing Fibroleiomyoma of the Uterus. Report of a Case with Review of the Literature, Amer. Jour. Path., **15**: 89, 1939.

Stengel, A., Jr.: Mumps Orchitis, Amer. Jour. Med. Sci., **191**: 340, 1936.

Stewart, C. A., E. T. Bell, and A. B. Roehlke: An Interstitial-cell Tumor of the Testis with Hypergenitalism in a Child of Five Years, Amer. Jour. Cancer, **26**: 144, 1936.

Sysak, N.: Ein Beitrag zu den Tumoren der Prostata in Kindesalter, Virchow's Arch. Path. Anat., **247**: 604, 1924.

Taylor, H. C., Jr.: Malignant and Semimalignant Tumors of the Ovary, Surg., Gynec. and Obst., **48**: 204, 1929.

Thompson, G. J.: Tumors of the Spermatic Cord, Epididymis and Testicular Tunics, Surg., Gynec. and Obst., **62**: 712, 1936.

Thompson, J. E., and V. H. Keiller: Multiple Skeletal Metastases from Cancer of the Breast, Surg., Gynec. and Obst., **38**: 367, 1924.

Thornton, H. C.: Granulosa-Cell Tumors of the Ovary, Amer. Jour. Cancer, **23**: 522, 1935.

Twombly, G. H., H. M. Temple, and A. L. Dean: Clinical Value of the Aschheim-Zondek Test in the Diagnosis of Testicular Tumors, Jour. Amer. Med. Asso., **118**: 106, 1942.

Walz, K.: Zur Frage der Entstehung der heterotopen Wucherungen vom Bau der Uterusschleimhaut, Centralbl. Allg. Path., **37**: 290, 1926.

Warren, S.: Relation of "Chronic Mastitis" to Carcinoma of Breast, Surg., Gynec., and Obst., **71**: 257, 1940.

——: The Grading of Carcinoma of the Cervix Uteri as Checked at Autopsy, Arch. Path., **12**: 783, 1931.

Wells, H. G.: Chemical Pathology, 4th ed., Philadelphia and London, 1920.

Winternitz, M. C.: Primary Melanotic Sarcoma of the Ovary, Bull. Johns Hopkins Hosp., **20**: 314, 1909.

Wood, F. C.: Delafield and Prudden's Text Book of Pathology, New York, 1922.

Young, H. H.: Genital Abnormalities, Hermaphroditism and Related Adrenal Diseases, Baltimore, Williams and Wilkins, 1937.

20

The Ductless Glands

INTRODUCTION

The glands of internal secretion include the hypophysis, pineal, thyroid, parathyroids, thymus, adrenals, pancreatic islets and gonads. The pancreatic islets and the gonads have been discussed in preceding chapters and attention has been paid to certain of the endocrine aspects. The others are grouped in this chapter. They are characterized by the production of chemical substances called hormones. These circulate in the blood and body fluids, influencing growth, metabolic, sexual and other activities and are interchangeable between species. They have been studied biologically by use of extracts of the particular gland under investigation and also by noting the effects of extirpation.

Certain of the hormones have been identified chemically, including especially the steroids which make up the sex hormones, thyroxin of the thyroid and a few others. There is a close interrelation between the various glands, both synergistic and antagonistic. Thus disease of one gland often is reflected in disturbance of other glands, either in the form of stimulation or depression. In some instances these secondary effects are not notable, but in others the patient is the subject of pluriglandular disease. Afunction exists when production of hormones is completely suppressed, hypofunction when secretion is reduced either by disease of the gland or by action of antagonistic hormones, and hyperfunction when there is increased amount of secretion due to lesions in the gland or to action of synergistic hormones. The term "dysfunction" implies an alteration in quality of the hormone or a change of proportion of hormones in cases where more than one hormone is produced. Comparable is the possibility of loss of balance between a hormone and its degradation products or metabolites. Dysfunction probably exists, but as yet has not been finally proved. In the following sections, the presentation of morphologic disturbances will be followed by a brief discussion of functional alterations.

THE HYPOPHYSIS

Congenital Anomalies

The hypophysis is formed by the junction of an entodermal pouch from the roof of the buccopharyngeal junction, which ultimately constitutes the pituitary gland, and a bud from the anterior cerebral vesicle which constitutes the infundibular process. A remnant is practically constant under the pharyngeal mucosa, the pharyngeal hypophysis or "Rachendachhypophyse." Accessory hypophyses may be found in the pharynx, the sphenoid bone and the sella turcica. Dandy and Goetsch describe a parahypophysis in the dog and cat made up of chromophobe cells in the floor of the sella. Congenital hypoplasia of the pituitary gland is common in cretins and other types of dwarfism.

Retrogressive Changes

Atrophy usually affects principally the pituitary gland and shows decrease in chromophile cells with fibrosis. It occurs in old age, may be the result of pressure, and sometimes is seen in myxedema, exophthalmic goiter, arteriosclerosis, alcoholism, diabetes mellitus and other diseases.

Pigmentations, calcification, cloudy swelling, amyloid and necrosis are occasionally observed. The colloid of the pars tuberalis or intermedia may be much increased. In infectious diseases, so-called toxic necroses are sometimes observed, but that these are of toxic nature is not established. Circulatory disturbances include passive hyperemia, dilatation of veins, various forms of arterial disease, embolism and infarction. Any of these may be followed by necrosis. Necrosis is probably not rare as a sequel of pregnancy, but the cause is not certain (see Gotshalk and Tilden). It may ultimately lead to Simmonds' disease, discussed later.

Inflammations

Inflammations of meninges and of neighboring bone may extend to the hypophysis. Metastatic abscesses and infarcts may occur in septic diseases but are unusual in such diseases as scarlatina, diphtheria, measles, typhoid, etc. (Plaut). Tuberculosis may affect the hypophysis by direct extension or by blood transport. Syphilis, both acquired and congenital, may be present as diffuse mononuclear-cell infiltration, foci of necrosis, gumma formation, or fibrosis (Schmitt).

Progressive Tissue Changes

Hyperplasias affect the pituitary gland rather than the neural infundibular process. The cells concerned are usually the chromophobe or chief cells, which normally are situated in the middle of the cell columns. Acidophile cells may be solely involved in the hyperplasia. Hyperplasias of pregnancy (see Erdheim) are to be regarded as part of a normal cycle in the gland but may readily be confused with and perhaps change into pathologic states. The distinction between hyperplasia and diffuse adenomatous struma is difficult in many cases. Even focal adenomas may apparently occur and disappear in the course of hyperplasia.

Tumors

Tumors may arise from various parts of the hypophysis: (1) the pars distalis or the pituitary gland and the pars tuberalis (pars intermedia), (2) the pouch of Rathke and its derivatives, (3) the infundibular process (pars nervosa). (See Erdheim.) The order of frequency of tumors of this region is: adenomatous tumors of the pituitary, tumors of Rathke pouch derivatives, suprasellar meningiomas and gliomas of the chiasm (Davidoff). The angioma is rare. Chordoma, which is not infrequent at the base of the skull, may rarely involve the hypophysis.

Adenoma of the pituitary may be diffuse or nodular. In the latter case, it is often difficult to say whether it is hyperplasia or neoplasia, but in those few instances where it becomes invasive, it is obviously a carcinoma. The nodular growths are generally regarded as tumors and called adenomas. These may be single or multiple and may vary from microscopic size to large masses several centimeters in diameter. Microscopically, they are usually well vascularized and composed of sheets and cords of pituitary cells; only rarely is there any tendency to form acini. Those made up of chromophobe cells are the most common and manifest themselves by the local pressure effects of brain tumor rather than by endocrine manifestations. Less frequent are tumors composed of acidophilic or basophilic cells, usually with endocrine changes as indicated below.

As with other tumors of the endocrine glands, various microscopic changes such as pleomorphism, loss of polarity, etc., are not certain guides to identification of malignant change. Invasion of surrounding structures is the only safe guide to distinguish between adenoma and carcinoma.

Any of the epithelial tumors may become cystic by necrosis, or because of secre-

tions, colloid, calcification and ossification may be observed. When large amounts of cholesterol are present, the tumor is the cholesteatoma. Complex teratomas are derived from embryonal rests. The adamantinoma of this region may be a Rathke's duct tumor or part of a teratoma.

Physiologic Considerations

Although extracts of the pars nervosa have cardiovascular, metabolic and oxytocic effects, it is difficult to assess any definite

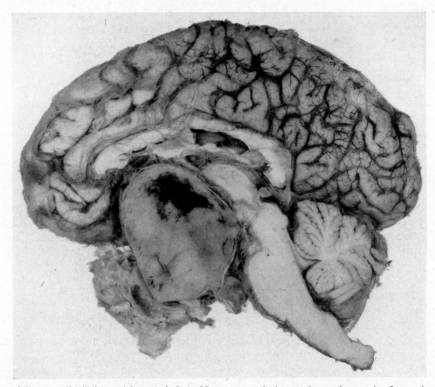

Adenoma of pituitary (chromophobe). Note encapsulation and attachment in floor of sella.

tions such as colloid. Sarcomas are rare and often are really atypical epithelial tumors.

Following the embryonal development of the pituitary, remnants of Rathke's pouch may be found in the position of the stalk or as clefts near the pars intermedia. Tumors arise from the stalk and are often called CRANIOPHARYNGIOMA. They are more common than cleft tumors (see Frazier and Alpers). The tumors are usually cystic and are lined by cuboidal or columnar epithelium, often ciliated, but stratified intermediate or squamous epithelium may be found. Fluid secre-

part played by this structure in the animal economy and no disease can be definitely ascribed to it (Geiling). The pars anterior produces numerous hormones, whose number increases as investigation advances. Thus there are hormones which have to do with growth, those which stimulate and control the gonads, lactogenic, thyrotropic, interrenotropic and metabolic hormones, each having a special function and some interrelated with the action of other endocrine glands (see Evans). The specific cells may be altered in quantity and quality in various

PLATE XV

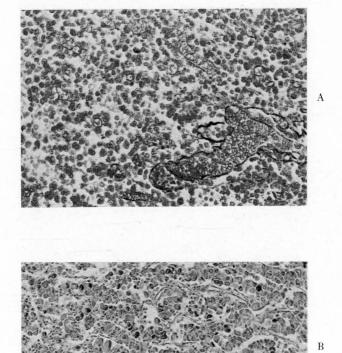

A

B

A. Acidophilic adenoma of pituitary, stained by azan carmine
method. Case of acromegaly.

B. Basophilic adenoma of pituitary, stained by azan carmine
method. Case of Cushing's syndrome.

states; the growth function appears to reside in the acidophils and the sexual functions in the basophils (see Severinghaus).

The pars anterior is intimately connected with sexual activity. Sexual cycles, pregnancy and gonadectomy have functional and morphologic effects. The gonadotropic hormones stimulate the production of the

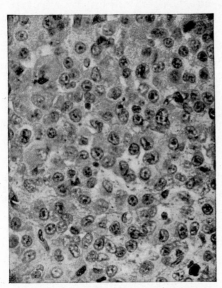

Chromophobe adenoma of pituitary gland. From Cushing, H., The Pituitary Body and Its Disorders.

male and female sex hormones and include the follicle stimulating and luteinizing principles. Overproduction is found in pregnancy, hydatidiform mole, chorionepithelioma and testicular tumors, etc. Underproduction accompanies infantilism, amenorrhea and Schroeder's disease with its hyperplasia of uterine glands and menorrhagia.

Simmonds' Disease. The disease most clearly associated with decreased activity is Simmonds' disease or cachexia hypophyseopriva. This occurs principally in women of middle life and is characterized by loss of sexual function, loss of axillary and pubic hair, atrophy of breasts and progressive emaciation. It is due to destruction of the pituitary, by tumors such as craniopharyngioma (Farber et al.), to puerperal necrosis (Sheehan) and other destructive disease (Farquharson, et al.), including rare cases of tuberculosis (Kirschbaum and Levy). There is associated atrophy of the other ductless glands. The disease is rare in

males. Somewhat similar clinically is the condition called anorexia nervosa, but this is not related to any special disease of the endocrine glands (see Brosin and Apfelbach).

Fröhlich's Syndrome. Less clearly related to decreased function of the pituitary

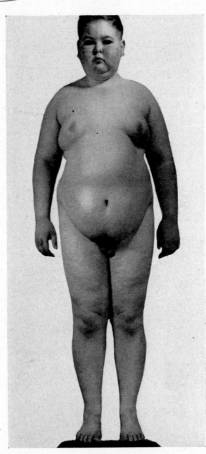

Adiposogenital syndrome (Fröhlich) in a boy 16 years of age.

is Fröhlich's syndrome, or adiposogenital dystrophy. In the male, there is a feminine body type. In either sex there is moderate obesity, of girdle type, genital hypoplasia and scanty growth of hair on pubis, on face and in the axillae. The condition is usually manifest in early life, but mental development is not disturbed. There is no constant pathologic picture and the condition is probably due to various lesions that affect the hypothalamic region. (See Kunstadter.)

The Lawrence-Moon-Biedl syndrome may also show adiposogenital dystrophy, but is accompanied by mental retardation, pigmentation of retina, polydactylism or syndactylism and is hereditary. It is probably due to congenital defects in the diencephalon. (See Anderson.)

In contrast are states of hyperpituitarism. These vary from minor disturbances, which are suspected of being due to increased activity, to outspoken manifestations.

Gigantism and Acromegaly. If the increased function occurs in early life, the chief sign is gigantism. Originating in later life, acromegaly develops. This syndrome includes enlargement of the skeleton, espe-

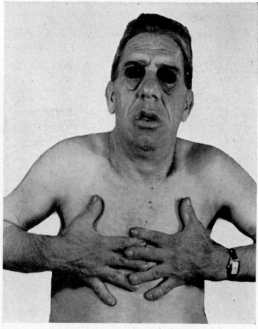

Acromegaly, to show prognathism, heavy lips, and "spade" hands.

cially of the extremities, mandibular prognathism, large hands and feet, polyuria, glycosuria, together with changes due to the presence of intracranial tumor such as headache, vomiting, hemianopsia and even blindness. The polyuria is probably due in large part to secondary effects of the pituitary tumor on the hypothalamic region. Other signs are due to production of pituitary hormones; the reduced sugar tolerance and diabetes are associated with disturbance of the interrelated activities of pituitary, pancreas and adrenal.

Patients with acromegaly show disease of the pituitary in the form of hyperplasia, adenoma or carcinoma. Usually these lesions are made up principally of acidophilic cells, but this is not invariably the case. Tumors may be large enough to compress neighboring parts of the brain and the optic commissure or tracts. The thoracic and abdominal viscera are usually enlarged, this being called macrosomia.

Cushing's syndrome occurs in middle life and exhibits obesity especially about the trunk, "moon face," cutaneous striae, amenorrhea and hirsutism in women and impotence in men, hypertension, diabetes or diabetic type of glucose tolerance curve, osteoporosis and sometimes signs of intracranial tumor. Of 67 autopsied cases, Eisenhardt and Thompson reported that 48 had basophilic adenomas of the pituitary and that 10 had other lesions of the pituitary including acidophilic and chromophobe adenoma as well as other forms of tumor. In most of the cases of basophilic adenoma, the basophils showed the peculiar Crooke change, namely degranulation of the cytoplasm of the basophilic cells. Identical clinical manifestations were associated with tumors of the adrenal cortex, carcinoma of thymus and virilizing tumors of the ovary. Kepler and Keating would reserve the term Cushing's disease for those cases with pituitary lesions and Cushing's syndrome for those in which the pituitary is not affected. Albright and associates attribute the principal manifestations of the condition to hyperactivity of the adrenal cortex. Arteriosclerosis is well marked, cardiac hypertrophy is present and some cases show malignant nephrosclerosis (MacMahon et al.).

Cushing has extended his conception of "pituitary basophilism" with the assumption that basophilic infiltration of the pars nervosa is related to eclampsia and other hypertensive states, but the lesion is not constant in these conditions and is observed without them, thus throwing doubt upon the validity of the hypothesis.

Intermedin. In fish and amphibia a hormone designated intermedin regulates pigment metabolism, and the same or a closely similar substance is found in the urine of human patients with melanoma and neurogenic tumors. It may be that cloasma and vitiligo in man are related to deficiency of this hormone. Clinically it appears to decrease urinary output in diabetes insipidus better than pituitrin. (See Zondek.)

Diabetes insipidus with its polyuria and thirst, without functional disease of the kidney, is thought to be due to disease of the pars posterior or the hypothalamus, but only rarely are definite lesions found. Piney and Coates found a metastatic carcinoma of the hypophysis and Moore and Cushing a local inflammation of the hypothalamus.

THE PINEAL GLAND

General Pathology

In the course of involution of the gland, multiple small cysts of the acini may occur. Much more common are fairly diffuse or focalized, microscopically laminated, sand-like deposits of phosphates and carbonates of lime, which may give a shadow in x-ray plates. In infectious diseases small hemorrhages may occur and in meningitis the gland may be the seat of suppuration. Tubercles and gummata are rare; the gland may show a diffuse round cell infiltration in congenital syphilis.

Tumors

Tumors of the pineal gland are infrequent and attain only moderate size. They produce symptoms and signs principally because of obstruction to the aqueduct of Sylvius with consequent bilateral internal hydrocephalus. Some are encapsulated and theoretically benign, but most are somewhat invasive. Microscopically they contain large round "parenchymal" cells and small dense cells of the stroma. Either may predominate; often clusters of the large cells are separated into an alveolar arrangement by the small dense cells. (See Globus.) Teratoid and other tumors of diverse origin may involve the pineal, with clinical manifestations like those of the pinealoma (Haldeman). The pressure of fluid may distend the recessus of the infundibular process with marked compression of the hypophysis in the sella.

Physiologic Considerations

The pineal is apparently not essential to life. Immediate effects of extracts have not been clearly demonstrated. McCord, however, claims that prolonged administration of extracts to young animals increases the rate of growth and produces early sexual maturity. Whereas Dandy's experiments with total extirpation of the pineal failed to induce noteworthy change in growth, sexual development or metabolism, the experiments of Horrax Izawa and others, show excessive growth of gonads and early development of secondary sex characters. The results of Davis and Martin are not so definite, but suggest that in immature life the pineal, in some way not yet explained, has an influence on sexual and somatic development. Thus administration of extracts and extirpation of the gland apparently produce much the same changes.

Clinically, lesions of the pineal, more especially tumors, may produce definite signs and symptoms. Tumors developing before puberty may produce signs of brain tumor only or may lead, practically solely in males, to precocious sexual and mental development, early development of secondary sex characters and increased body growth (Horrax, Izawa). In both experimental and clinical observations, it is difficult to determine whether the changes are due to the pineal lesion or to associated change in the hypophysis. There may be involvement of other glands such as atrophy of the hypophysis from pressure, hyperplasia of the adrenal cortex and of the interstitial cells of the testis, and persistence of the thymus.

THE THYROID GLAND

Congenital Anomalies

The thyroid may be absent. In some such cases a small nodule of thyroid tissue may be found at the lingual end of the thyroglossal duct, and may exhibit the various pathologic changes which affect the normally situated gland. Accessory nodules of thyroid may appear in the upper thorax but are most frequent in the neck, especially under the sterno-mastoid muscle. Remnants of the thyroglossal duct may persist and give rise to cyst formation or to tumor growth. Cell masses of parathyroid and thymus may be included in the thyroid.

Thyroidits vs strumitis (handwritten annotation at top)

Retrogressive Changes

In a wide variety of infectious diseases, swelling and increased granularity of the epithelial cells, often with vague cell outline, justify the assumption that cloudy swelling occurs. Desquamation and necrosis are common in the same circumstances. The cells normally contain fat and it is therefore difficult or impossible to distinguish fatty degeneration. Hyalin affects the stroma of the gland especially in atrophy, long standing goiters and scars. Amyloid occurs in the vascular walls as a local process or as a part of generalized amyloidosis, and may sometimes produce notable enlargement (Hunter and Seabrook). Calcification and ossification are common in old goiters, cyst walls, scars and sites of old hemorrhages. The voluminous colloid in colloid goiters is regarded by some as a sort of colloid degeneration, but is probably only a residuum of cyclic changes in activity.

Arteriosclerosis is common in goiters, often quite independent of arteriosclerosis elsewhere. Transitory hyperemia is likely to accompany menstruation and pregnancy. Prolonged hyperemia is seen in hyperplasias and various forms of goiter and may produce tortuosity of the vessels. Passive hyperemia may accompany general passive hyperemia. Hemorrhages are extremely common either into the acini, staining the colloid, or into the interstitial tissues, sometimes with subsequent encapsulation and cyst formation. They are seen much more often in goitrous than in normal thyroids.

Atrophy occurs in advanced life. It often accompanies wasting diseases, particularly tuberculosis, may be due to local pressure from tumors either within or outside the thyroid gland, and may be of unknown cause, especially in connection with such clinical conditions as adiposis dolorosa, endemic cretinism and myxedema. Grossly, the organ is usually small and underweight, and even although it may be of normal size or slightly larger, the connective tissue growth is extensive. The organ is firm and the capsule thickened. It cuts with increased resistance and shows a firm cross section which may or may not show lobular arrangement and contains little or no colloid.

Microscopically, there is more or less dense fibrosis of the capsule and of the stroma. In the atrophic thyroid of comparatively young individuals there may be a considerable vascularization, but in the atrophy of old age there is likely to be no increase of vascularization and considerable arteriosclerosis. Colloid is reduced or absent. Acini are small and irregular in size. The cells show a lack of uniformity in size and shape and occasionally, more particularly in young individuals, may be in several layers. The nuclei show lack of uniformity in size and some irregularity in shape, often with increased density of staining.

Inflammation

Gierke distinguishes between thyroiditis, if the gland be otherwise normal, and strumitis, if the gland be the seat of goiter.

Acute diffuse thyroiditis occurs especially in relation to infectious and septicemic diseases but may rarely occur without known cause. The gland is likely to be swollen, hyperemic and tender or painful. Microscopically, there is a variable amount of exudation into the interstitial tissue, which may be largely fluid or largely cellular in character, and is accompanied by degeneration, desquamation and necrosis of the epithelium. This inflammatory lesion is not to be confused with the acute hyperplasias which also are likely to occur as an accompaniment of infectious disease. Acute focal thyroiditis is usually in the form of single or more commonly multiple abscesses, occurring in connection especially with septicopyemias. Abscess may also arise by extension from the neighborhood of the thyroid or from the thyroglossal duct.

It is often difficult to determine objectively whether fibrosis in the thyroid is inflammatory or cicatricial. Atrophies may be accompanied by fibrosis but it is not certain that this is more than a replacement process. The presence of accumulations of lymphoid cells may be constitutional or dependent on factors other than inflammation.

There is little doubt that RIEDEL'S STRUMA, the "eisenhartes struma" or ligneous thyroid, is a chronic progressive thyroiditis. The gland is irregularly involved in the process or the lesion may be largely unilateral; it may be small, or enlarged, is markedly firm and often adherent to neighboring tissues. Microscopically, there is diffuse fibrosis, with infiltration of lymphoid and plasma cells and eosinophils. Atrophy and partial disappearance of epithelium are usual, although adenomatous foci of hyperplasia may be found.

THAT HASHIMOTO'S "STRUMA LYMPHOMATOSA" is inflammatory is doubtful. The gland is diffusely enlarged, fairly firm but not usually adherent. The fibrosis is delicate and diffuse and the cellular infiltration of lymphocytes extensive. The epithelium is hyperplastic. (See Graham and McCullagh.) Riedel's struma is more frequent in women than men, occurs at almost any age and is not likely to be associated with functional disturbance of the thyroid, except that after removal myxedema may develop. Struma lymphomatosa is a disease principally of elderly women and is without functional alteration.

In fibrosis of the thyroid as a sequel of hyperplasias and exhaustion, or as a part of Riedel's struma, there may be foci of necrosis associated with granulomatous inflammation and giant cell formation. This should not be confused with tuberculosis. (See Goetsch; German.)

Infectious Granulomata

Tuberculosis of the thyroid is uncommon, is most frequently miliary and associated with acute generalized miliary tuberculosis. Microscopically, the tubercles are situated especially in the connective tissue. Conglomerate tuberculosis usually develops as the result of extension from a neighboring focus, particularly the cervical lymph nodes. Occasionally, cases are encountered in which the primary focus of tuberculosis cannot be identified. Care must be taken to differentiate between tubercles and pseudotubercles. As the result of destructive lesions in the thyroid, pseudotubercles may be encountered with foreign-body giant cells formed in response to the presence of dead cells and free colloid. In acquired syphilis, gumma of the thyroid may be observed, or there may be a diffuse fibrosis. In congenital syphilis there may be a diffuse mononuclear infiltration or gumma formation.

Hypertrophy and Hyperplasia

The thyroid apparently is susceptible to a cyclic series of changes which are initiated by various stimuli. The immediate result, really the first change in the cycle, is hypertrophy, which is closely followed by, or associated with, hyperplasia. In practical experience these two conditions go hand in hand. When the gland returns to the resting state it is no longer structurally normal, but contains an increased amount of colloid, larger acini and low cuboidal epithelium. It is a colloid goiter. While the term goiter means enlargement of the thyroid, it is usu-

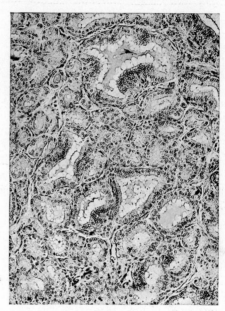

Hypertrophy and hyperplasia of thyroid in a case of exophthalmic goiter.

ally restricted to changes occurring in this cycle. With repeated cycles of hypertrophy and hyperplasia, fibrosis is likely to become more and more marked. Physiologically, there may be an enlargement of the thyroid at puberty, in the menstrual period, during pregnancy and sometimes at the menopause. Other than this, the examples of thyroid hypertrophy and hyperplasia, or goiter, are commoner in comparatively early life and in females, but may occur at any period of life and in both sexes.

Much study has been given to the cause of goiter. In endemic form it is likely to exist in certain regions of the earth, as for example in and around Switzerland and around the Great Lakes in the north American continent. There are, however, numerous other areas, usually small in extent, in which the lesion may be very frequent. Many theories have been advanced to account for the condition. It has long been held that goiter is a deficiency disease due to inadequate intake of iodine. It is now known that there are agents which induce goiter, spoken of as positive goitrogenic substances. Experimentally, these agents include cabbage, calcium salts, cyanides and perhaps others. Hellwig, for example, found that a diet rich in calcium and deficient in iodine produced hypertrophy and hyperplasia in the thyroid of white rats. If the diet were rich in calcium and adequate in iodine, the result was colloid goiter. In man, it is likely that a combination of iodine deficiency and goitrogenic factor or factors is responsible for the disease. In geographic regions where goiter is endemic, the waters are usually poor in iodine and rich in lime salts, but an adequate supply of iodine alone will prevent the disease. Neither infection nor vitamin deficiencies are causative. The influence of the thyrotropic hormone of the pituitary is evident in the fact that administration of anterior pituitary extracts produces the lesion (see Thurston).

The first stage of the process which leads eventually to the formation of a hyperplastic gland is simple hypertrophy, which, however, is rarely observed in practical experience (Graham). It is stated that the enlarged thyroid of puberty, that of menstruation and of pregnancy, and of the menopause, are examples of simple hypertrophy. The gland is enlarged and heavier than normal, but much of this increase in size and weight may be due to hyperemia. Microscopically, the gland follicles are larger than normal and the lining epithelial cells become high cuboidal and then columnar in type.

Hypertrophy and hyperplasia are characterized by changes which vary considerably in degree, and no strict correspondence is to be found between the clinical symptoms and the degree of hypertrophy and hyperplasia. In fact extensive hyperplasia may exist without clinical signs other than the enlargement of the gland. Marine and Lenhart distinguish two groups of hyperplasia, namely the primary and secondary types. The primary hyperplasias arise in a gland which previous to the time has been normal, whereas the secondary hyperplasias

arise in the glands which have other pathologic lesions, particularly those due to the cycle of hyperplasia and involution.

Grossly, the hyperplastic gland is large, heavy but of normal shape. It is soft and richly vascularized. It cuts with increased resistance and shows a slightly bulging, soft,

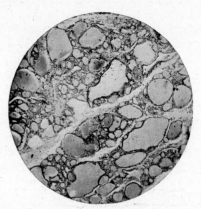

Colloid goiter in the resting stage.

red, cross section whose translucency depends materially upon the degree of hypertrophy and hyperplasia and the degree of disappearance of colloid. The capsule and supporting connective tissue are overgrown. All these changes, however, depend for their manifestations upon the degree and duration of the lesion.

Microscopically, the changes are usually diffuse in the primary hyperplasias, but

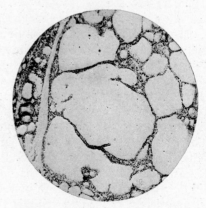

Colloid goiter in the resting stage, showing spur formation.

may be more circumscribed and accompanied by various secondary changes such as calcification, hemorrhage, cyst formation and increase in colloid, in the secondary hyper-plasias. There is usually a connective-tissue increase with a variable infiltration of lymphoid cells. Although this is sometimes interpreted as an indication of chronic inflammation, it is more probably a part of a general lymphoid hyperplasia which frequently accompanies the disease. The blood vessels are enlarged, hyperemic, elongated and tortuous. The acini are large and the lining cells thrown into more or less prominent plications depending upon the severity of the process. The cells in the early stages are high cuboidal but finally become cylindrical. The colloid in the stained sections is at first pale, then vacuolated and then disappears.

The colloid gland, or colloid goiter, represents the quiescent or resting state of the thyroid after it has undergone hypertrophy and hyperplasia one or more times. Grossly, it resembles a normal gland in many respects but is usually larger, heavier and contains a greater quantity of colloid. It is likely to be firm and have a somewhat thickened capsule. It cuts with increased resistance and shows a brownish-red, glossy, translucent cross section, due to the increased amount of colloid. As a rule the acini can be discerned with the naked eye as tiny, round, translucent, light brown gelatinous beads.

Microscopically, the capsule and connective tissue show variable degrees of fibrosis. The arteries and frequently also the veins show residual thickening of the walls, often with calcification, and there is likely to be an obliterating endarteritis. Most of the acini are considerably larger than in the normal gland, and spurs, which are the end result of the infolding which took place during the stage of hyperplasia, project into the acini. The cells have returned to the normal cuboidal state, the acini are filled with colloid which stains well and contains considerable quantities of iodine. The colloid may, in this condition as in others, and indeed in normal thyroid, show a scalloping of its edges near the cells, a condition demonstrated by De Robertis to be artefact.

Recognizing the fact that these cyclic changes are likely to be repeated, it is not to be wondered at that the same gland may show various stages of the entire process. In the thyroid, as in other glands, there is often difficulty in distinguishing between hyper-

plasia and adenoma. In fact, glands occur in which the acini may be very large and there may be irregularity in form and disposition, sometimes associated with the formation of numerous small adenoma-like masses. Such glands are frequently referred to as the diffuse adenomatous goiter or DIFFUSE NODULAR GOITER. This lesion occurs practically only in adult life. It appears to start in one or both lateral lobes near the trachea, as a clump of adenoma-like masses, and may finally involve the whole gland. This is the type of lesion which gives rise to very large goiters and is the one which most commonly causes symptoms of pressure on the trachea. Microscopically, one usually finds considerable fibrosis, various vascular changes, areas of colloid goiter, areas of hypertrophy and hyperplasia, minute adenomas often poorly defined, and larger similar masses well defined, with compression atrophy of neighboring thyroid tissue. Hemorrhagic or glandular cysts may occur.

Regeneration

When portions of the thyroid are destroyed by disease or are removed surgically, there is little or no anatomic regeneration. Nevertheless, the remaining glandular tissue is subject to various stimuli and may exhibit hypertrophy and hyperplasia representing increased function, a sort of functional regeneration.

Tumors

In the consideration of this subject it must be borne in mind that the material presented here is a mere outline of the outstanding tumorous conditions. Fairly typical pictures may be given but departures from these are frequent. Furthermore, the anatomic character of the thyroid is such that considerable difficulty is often encountered in diagnosing tumors. Indeed, even metastases of malignant epithelial tumors of the thyroid may so resemble normal thyroid as to make distinction extremely difficult. As Marine and Lenhart point out, the tumorous growths do not respond in the same way to iodine as does the thyroid gland, and this fact may aid materially in differentiating between hyperplasia which, in the course of a few weeks undergoes regression by the administration of iodine, and adenoma which does not.

Various forms of adenoma are encountered.

Microfollicular Adenoma. That which is most clearly a tumor is the one called microfollicular adenoma. This tumor usually appears in early adult life. It may be single but is not infrequently multiple. It may be situated in any part of the gland. When it attains a sufficient size it produces a nodular outgrowth in the thyroid and by pressure may lead to atrophy of the neighboring gland substance. It is an encapsulated, sharply defined, relatively soft, reddish-gray mass which projects slightly in the cross section and is practically free of colloid. Some forms of this tumor, however, show moderate amounts of colloid.

Microscopically, it is made up of a large number of very small acini, free of col-

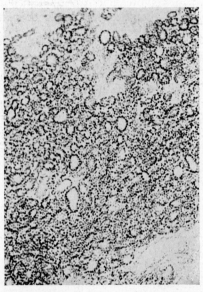

Microfollicular adenoma with slight differentiation to small colloid acini.

loid and lined with either cuboidal, high cuboidal or low columnar cells. There are minute fibrous septa running through the tumor, which support numerous blood vessels. Hemorrhage is a common complication and the blood may be absorbed and replaced by connective tissue which rapidly undergoes hyalinization. New alveoli grow into the hyaline mass. Quite similar tumors may show larger alveoli with lower epithelium and a stainable colloid content. It is still an open

question as to whether the adenomas of this type which contain colloid represent a resting stage of a cycle which takes place in the adenoma, similar to that in the thyroid gland as a whole, or whether they represent a further differentiation, both morphologically and functionally, of the cells composing the primary strictly microfollicular type of adenoma.

Simple Adenoma. In addition to the microfollicular adenoma is the type called by

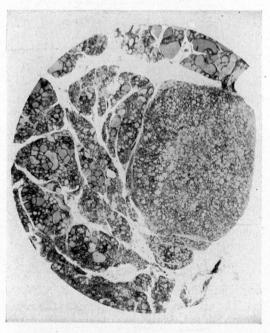

Low power photomicrograph of a simple adenoma of the thyroid.

Marine and Lenhart the simple adenoma which, we believe, corresponds with that adenomatous hyperplasia discussed in connection with diffuse adenomatous goiter. Usually there are multiple nodules made up of irregularly sized and shaped acini with low cuboidal epithelium and colloid content.

In either of these instances it appears necessary that some form of hyperplasia affects the gland before the adenoma develops (Kline). This inference is reached by the fact that it is only rarely that microfollicular adenoma occurs in a gland otherwise normal, and practically never does the simple adenoma occur in a normal gland. The microfollicular adenoma does not respond to the administration of iodine, but in occasional instances the administration of iodine may bring about involution of the simple adenoma. The origin of new acini in adenoma, nodular goiter and hyperplasias has been ascribed to embryonal epithelial rests. Moritz has shown that the interfollicular islands are detached buds of follicular epithelium, that in the pathologic lesions new acini are the result of proliferation of follicular epithelium and that the new masses, originally part of an intricate follicular pattern, may be detached.

Other adenomatous masses may be encountered in the thyroid. Thus, an adenoma composed of large cells and small

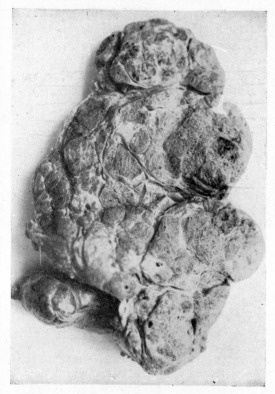

Cross section of diffuse adenomatous goiter.

alveoli is supposed to be derived from the postbranchial body, and constitutes the struma postbranchialis of Getsowa. Apparently this is disposed to undergo malignant transformation in its course (Richardson). Somewhat similar are small adenoma-like masses of tissue resembling the parathyroid gland, usually spoken of as parastruma. Adenomas may be made up of large cells with clear cytoplasm and small nuclei. These

are often called Hürthle cell adenomas; they resemble parastruma (Wilensky and Kaufman) but may be degenerations due to poor fixation.

Carcinoma. Any attempt at classification of carcinoma of the thyroid encounters many difficulties because of the wide varia-

15937
(adenoma
c̄
met)

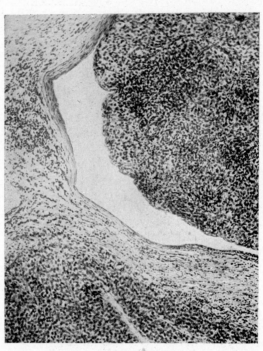

Carcinoma simplex of the thyroid with a tumor mass in a vein.

tion in microscopic picture, and also because of the fact that tumors which microscopically give no indication of malignancy may metastasize widely. Grossly, the carcinoma is usually a fleshy, relatively soft, richly vascularized, invasive tumor with adhesions to surrounding parts.

Microscopically, there is usually no difficulty in distinguishing the papilliferous adenocarcinoma and the scirrhous carcinoma, and the same is true of most cases of carcinoma simplex or as it is often called, carcinoma solidum. There is, however, a group of carcinomas of the thyroid which we may call, for simplification, the adenocarcinoma. This includes the outspoken adenocarcinoma, the malignant adenoma, and a variety of other adenomatous lesions in which the microscopic picture may be extremely varied. Thus, thyroid glands may be removed which microscopically may show the picture of microfollicular adenoma, the more highly differentiated or simple adenoma, hyperplasia and hypertrophy, as well as atrophy, but which show nothing clearly indicative of malignancy; yet in such cases tumors may recur after removal, or distant metastases may develop. The metastases often show nothing indicative of malignancy other than their situation. Graham has found that although the original thyroid tumor is not characteristic of carcinoma, microscopically or grossly, yet careful search will demonstrate invasion of blood vessels upon microscopic and often upon gross examination. It is possible that surgical removal of such thyroids, which do not show associated metastasis, may result in cure, but vascular invasion justifies guarded prognosis (Warren).

The metastasis of malignant thyroid tumors is often to bone, lung, and other similar situations where blood transport seems the most likely method. The papillary adenocarcinoma and the scirrhous carcinoma, and in many instances also the carcinoma simplex, metastasize through the lymphatics to the regional lymph nodes.

Most of the patients with carcinoma give a history which indicates that they have had some preceding lesions of the thyroid, either in the form of adenoma or of hyperplasia and hypertrophy. This was found to be true in 92.6 per cent of the malignant tumors reported by Smith, Pool and Olcott. Furthermore, carcinoma of the thyroid is more frequent in goitrous districts than elsewhere (Coller). Graham thought the microfollicular adenoma to be the principal preexistent lesion. It is conceivable, however, that carcinoma may originate in glands which show no previously existent pathologic change.

The connective-tissue tumors of the thyroid are much less frequent than are the epithelial tumors. Occasional cases of fibroma and osteochondroma are reported. Sarcoma may occur as a spindle-cell sarcoma or as a lymphosarcoma. Ewing, however, points out that in the growth of carcinoma the relationship between epithelium and stroma may be such that the epithelial cells become elongated and of spindle form. It is probable that a careful study of many cases heretofore called spindle-cell sarcoma will show that they belong to the group of carcinomas. Care must always be exercised to distinguish lymphosarcoma, or lymphomas of leukemia, from small-cell carcinomas. More highly differentiated sarcomas, such as the osteochondrosarcoma, are rare.

Mixed tumors of any kind are rare and it is probable that reported cases of carcinosarcoma are carcinomas with spindle-cell forms of epithelium.

Tumors, particularly papilliferous adenoma, may develop in aberrant thyroid tissue situated lateral to the main gland. What may seem to be recurrence after operation is often a new tumor in another aberrant gland. Nevertheless some of these tumors are true carcinomas (see Moritz and Bayless).

Metastatic tumors occur in the thyroid secondary to bronchiogenic carcinoma, tumors of kidney, pancreas, breast and various other situations (Mayo and Schlicke).

Cysts

Although the acini of the thyroid may be much enlarged, they rarely if ever constitute large cysts. Follicular cysts are due to hemorrhage into the follicles. They are usually small but may attain a diameter of 6 or 8 cm. They contain more or less colloid, mixed with blood in various stages of degeneration, and often cholesterol. The capsule is made up of the wall of the follicle to which, in the larger cysts, are added connective tissue stroma of gland and gland capsule, with new connective tissue produced in response to pressure and irritation.

Adenomatous cysts are due to necrosis in the center of an adenoma, usually followed by softening and hemorrhage. They contain a granular fluid material stained with blood or brown hematogenous pigment and little or no colloid. Later the fluid may be clear and of yellow or pale green color. The wall is made up of the peripheral parts of the adenoma and its capsule, or the latter alone, and the neighboring gland is compressed and atrophic. The walls of both varieties often contain foci of calcification. Echinococcus cysts have been reported.

Physiologic Considerations

The thyroid is not necessary for life, but if absent, cretinism or myxedema occur.

Marine, Lenhart, Kimball and others have demonstrated the significance of iodine for thyroid activity. Apparently thyroid hypertrophy and hyperplasia are due in part to iodine deficiency, and if iodine be administered the glands undergo involution. Similarly, in districts where goiter is prevalent, the administration of iodine prevents its occurrence. Kendall isolated an iodine-bearing complex from the thyroid, thyroxin, analyzed and synthesized by Harington and Barger. Its administration relieves the symptoms of athyreosis and in normal individuals may produce many of the symptoms associated with excessive thyroid activity.

Hypothyroidism produces cretinism of the young or myxedema of the adult. The term hyperthyroidism is applied to a state of increased nervous excitability and metabolism, as well as to exophthalmic goiter. In both of these, however, it is difficult to be sure that the thyroid is either primarily or solely at fault. In both hypothyroidism and hyperthyroidism there are important changes in the autonomic mechanism, in metabolism, in muscular and mental activity. Admitting that all may be due to increased thyroid activity, it is also possible that this activity is due to alterations in the autonomic nervous system or that it is but part of, and secondary to, a widespread disturbance of the nervous system and ductless glands. In adults it is not uncommon to find, coincidentally, changes indicative of both decreased and increased thyroid function.

Cretinism. This is a condition of early life characterized by delay in the development of bones, often with dwarfism, delayed dentition, reduced metabolism, retarded mental development which may be a state of idiocy, so-called cretinistic facies and myxedematous skin. It is presumably due to deficient thyroid hormone and may occur as sporadic cretinism, often called congenital myxedema, and endemic cretinism.

The sporadic form may be encountered anywhere and is usually due to congenital aplasia or hypoplasia of the thyroid. Endemic cretinism occurs principally in goitrous districts, develops as late as the fifth year, is less amenable to relief by administration of thyroid and often shows a large thyroid, although aplastic or hypoplastic or-

gans may be found. The large thyroids may show hypertrophy and hyperplasia, colloid goiter, adenoma, and diffuse adenomatous goiter. Nevertheless, it seems probable that in spite of the anatomic conditions, the thyroid is deficient in function. The bones often show a persistence of epiphyseal cartilage for long periods after maturity. Gonads and pituitary are often atrophic in cretinism and also may occur thus in hypothyroidism of adults.

Myxedema. This term is usually applied to adult cases of thyroid hypofunction, although some authors refer to sporadic cretinism as congenital myxedema. In the adult, the bony changes of cretinism do not occur and the curious non-pitting swelling of the skin is often a most prominent feature. This type of edema is due principally to the deposit of mucoid in the corium and subcutaneous tissues. There are dryness of skin, loss of hair, dull heavy facies, "spade hands," chilliness, decreased metabolism, dull mentality sometimes with dementia, secondary anemia, leukopenia with relative lymphocytosis and other signs and symptoms in variable degree. Occasionally, the entire thyroid is removed surgically, and myxedema follows.

Characteristically, the thyroid is the seat of atrophy and fibrosis, but grossly may be of considerable size. Late in the course of exophthalmic goiter or other similar conditions the gland apparently reaches a stage of exhaustion, and the patient while still suffering from many symptoms of hyperthyroidism shows also signs of myxedema. The gland in such instances is often the seat of interlobular and interacinic fibrosis, and the parenchyma shows lack of uniformity in size of cells and of nuclei, some of the latter being large and deeply chromatic. Mitotic figures and multinucleated cells are not infrequent. Both cretinism and myxedema are benefited by administration of thyroid substance.

Exophthalmic Goiter. This syndrome, often spoken of as Parry's disease, Graves' disease or Basedow's disease, is one of early adult life and confined to the human race, especially women. Enlarged thyroid, exophthalmos, tachycardia and muscular tremor are present. The exophthalmos is associated with other more or less characteristic signs, such as lagging of the upper lid, infrequent winking and decreased power of convergence. The skin is warm and moist and may show areas of depigmentation, the pa-

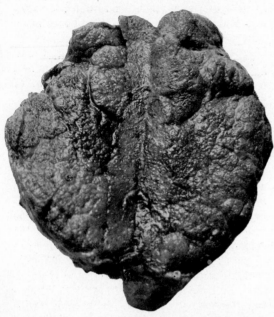

Cross section of a hyperplastic thyroid of exophthalmic goiter.

tients often feel warm, the basal metabolic rate is increased, the patients are mentally excitable and may become delirious, blood pressure is normal or slightly elevated, micturition is frequent, hyperglycemia and glycosuria are common, there is muscular weakness and usually decrease in sexual excitement and power. In addition to tachycardia, other cardiovascular disturbances occur. The thyroid is almost certainly not the primary source of the widespread bodily disturbances, but appears to exhibit constant involvement. The disease is regarded by Kessel and Hyman as due to imbalance of the autonomic nervous system. Warthin considers it the manifestation of an abnormality of constitution.

The pathologic changes in the thyroid are by no means constant. The majority of cases, as in the studies of Marine and Lenhart and others, show hypertrophy and hyperplasia of the thyroid. The gland is large, soft or firm, hyperemic, with the usual microscopic picture of mild or slight fibrosis and often outspoken lymphoid hyperplasia. The picture varies, depending upon whether the

hyperplasia is primary or recurrent (secondary). Some patients, however, show pure colloid goiter, some show premature atrophy, and others show fetal or simple adenoma. In a few cases the gland may be normal as regards gross and microscopic structure and iodine content. In these, however, the patients are likely to have all the signs and symptoms of exophthalmic goiter except exophthalmos.

The hyperplastic glands characteristically show decrease of iodine content. The thymus, especially the cortical part, spleen and lymph nodes are often the seat of hyperplasia. The heart is often the seat of hypertrophy, but microscopically there may be foci of necrosis as observed by Goodpasture and produced experimentally by him with thyroxin, or areas of fibrosis, presumably scars of the acute lesions (see Weller et al.). The liver may be the seat of foci of necrosis and acute or chronic hepatitis; accompanying functional alterations sometimes occur (see Weller; Shaffer). Skeletal muscle may be atrophic and bones may be the seat of imperfect calcification or osteomalacia.

Exophthalmos appears to be due to the action of thyrotropic hormone of the pituitary. The retrobulbar tissues show an increased amount of fat together with marked edema of the connective tissue and muscles (Smelser). There may be a pseudohypertrophy of muscles with degeneration and lymphocytic infiltration (Aird).

Hyperthyroidism. Numerous patients with or without goiter exhibit groups of symptoms mentioned under exophthalmic goiter. Such patients are usually older than those with exophthalmic goiter and may have had simple goiter for years. The symptoms may be severe, moderate or slight, and are ordinarily ascribed to increase of thyroid function and may closely resemble the symptoms following injections of thyroxin. If, however, exophthalmic goiter be regarded as a syndrome with its origin in the autonomic nervous system, it is possible that these less marked symptoms are manifestations of the same disturbance.

As in exophthalmic goiter, the thyroid may exhibit hypertrophy and hyperplasia or a variety of other changes. Adenoma may be found in the gland, and removal of the adenoma or the entire gland may be followed by

Hyperplasia parath - water clear cells
Adenomas — chief cells
Degenerated chief - or oxyphil (acidophile cells)

THE DUCTLESS GLANDS 699

relief of symptoms, hence the name "toxic adenoma" has been given. There is, however, some question as to the functional properties of the adenoma. Goetsch is of the opinion that even although the cells may be low cuboidal and without any indication of increased activity in the ordinary microscopic picture, yet the presence of large numbers of mitochondria indicates increased activity. It is somewhat doubtful that the number of mitochondria is an index of the secretion of hormones. The fact that Nicholson finds them increased in experimental compensatory hypertrophy suggests that they might be related to cell size as well as to function or perhaps to size alone. Graham's experiments with tadpoles show that the microscopic picture of the adenomata bears no relation to their content of iodine. Convincing evidence that these adenomas are toxic has not been offered (see Enzer).

Hyperthyroidism may occur in patients with carcinoma of the thyroid, but that increased function is to be found on the part of the tumor is not certain; the surrounding gland may account for the disturbance. (See Frisdell.)

Role of Other Ductless Glands. Clinically other ductless glands are probably involved in producing some of the symptoms and signs which may complicate the picture of thyroid disease. These include hypophysis, parathyroid, adrenals and gonads. Anatomically, the thymus is enlarged and presumably the seat of hyperplasia in 75 per cent of exophthalmic goiter patients and lymphoid hyperplasia is almost as frequent. Changes in the other ductless glands are less regular in incidence and in anatomic form.

THE PARATHYROID GLANDS

General Pathology

The congenital anomalies of the parathyroids are not well known. Their absence is incompatible with life. Their position may vary widely and glands or cell clumps can be included in the thyroid. Congenital aplasia of the thyroid is not associated with absence of the parathyroids. Congenital syphilis may be accompanied by parathyroid hypoplasia. Atrophy may be the result of pressure, as by an enlarged thyroid, or the result of age.

The infant's gland may contain only chief cells, but as life advances there may be an increase in oxyphil cells and increase of interstitial fatty tissue. In generalized amyloidosis the vessels of the parathyroids may be affected. Hydropic infiltration and also necrosis occur.

Hemorrhage, induced especially by difficult labor, is fairly frequent. The blood is soon encapsulated and may be entirely absorbed.

Metastatic abscess may occur in pyemia, miliary tubercles in a generalized tuberculosis.

Hyperplasia

Hyperplasia usually affects all the parathyroids in about equal degree. The total weight is considerably increased above the normal total of about 130 mg. but the shape is not altered. Microscopically, the architecture is not materially altered but there is a proliferation of the large cells with poorly stained rich cytoplasm, the so-called water clear cells, sometimes with acinic arrangement. Only occasionally is the hyperplastic gland made up of the small chief cells with moderate or scanty well-stained cytoplasm. Clumps of large or small cells with deeply acidophilic cytoplasm, the oxyphils, may be present but these are probably degenerate cells (Castleman and Mallory). Hyperplasia is due principally to low levels of inorganic calcium in the blood such as occur in rickets, osteomalacia, prolonged renal insufficiency, low calcium in the diet, and in the disturbances of calcium metabolism such as may be observed in sprue. (See Ham et al.)

compensatory

Tumors

The principal tumor is the adenoma, which occurs in one gland or a part of it. The adenoma is a nodular well-defined growth, which may attain a diameter of several centimeters. Microscopically, it is usually made up of masses and nests of chief cells, often with acini of considerable size. Sometimes the adenoma contains many water-clear cells, and may also show foci of oxyphils. In a few instances, the tumor has occurred in aberrant parathyroid in neck or thorax. Rarely, invasion and metastasis occur. The microscopic character of the malignant tumor may be little altered from that of the adenoma or there may be marked pleomorphism with many mitotic figures. (See Hall and Chaffin.) Occasionally metastases of other tumors are found in the parathyroids.

Physiologic Considerations

These include the phenomena incident to decreased and to increased functional activity. Abrupt removal of all parathyroid tissue usually results in death in a few days, although older animals may survive longer. Death is delayed by the presence of pregnancy and of rickets, the use of meat in the diet and by administration of calcium and of parathormone. Death follows the convulsions of marked tetany or profound general alteration of metabolism. (See Dragstedt.)

Tetany is a condition in which there are muscular tremors or spasms, and in which minor stimuli may set up local or widespread convulsions. The increase in irritability of nerves is due principally to low levels of serum calcium and to alkalosis. Although phosphates and chlorides are increased when the calcium is decreased, this is not responsible for the tetany. Various conditions may give rise to tetany, but the form due to destruction of the parathyroids, or reduction in secretion of their hormone, is especially severe, and it is particularly in this form that the serum calcium is decreased. Occasionally cases of idiopathic hypoparathyroidism are reported in which tetany, with low serum calcium and high phosphate, normal bones and normal kidneys, are observed. In one autopsy, atrophy of the parathyroids was found. (See Drake et al.)

Hyperparathyroidism occurs in hyperplasia, in adenoma and in carcinoma of the parathyroids. It may be produced experimentally by the use of the parathormone of Collip. In this state, the serum calcium is high and the phosphate low, there is loss of calcium from the bones and a progressive fibrosis of the marrow, osteitis fibrosa cystica, discussed further in the chapter on Organs of Locomotion. Renal calculi are often found. Parathormone stimulates calcification of osteoid tissue and may bring about metastatic calcification.

Of interest is the probable sequence of events in chronic renal insufficiency referred to in the chapter on the Urinary System. The retention of phosphate leads to a reduction of serum calcium, which in turn stimulates hyperplasia of the parathyroids. Ultimately this may cause a state of hyperparathyroidism with resultant elevation of serum calcium, the decalcification of bone of osteitis fibrosa cystica and metastatic calcification (see Herbert et al.).

THE THYMUS

Congenital Anomalies

The thymus may be congenitally absent in otherwise normal or in malformed fetuses. Accessory thymic nodules may be found in the mediastinum or in the thyroid. Congenital hypoplasia may occur in cases of myxedema. Hyperplasias may be congenital. Inclusions of thyroid and of parathyroid may be found.

Retrogressive Changes

At birth the thymus is well developed, and although the body as a whole grows at a more rapid rate, the thymus continues slowly to enlarge until puberty, when involution begins. Boyd's studies show that the maximum weight is attained at from 10 to 15 years of age, with a median of 11 years. At about 4 years, involution of the cortex begins, but there is an increase in amount of fatty and connective tissues. The weight of the medulla follows that of the whole gland and involution begins at the time the total weight begins to decrease. The gland does not fully disappear in adult life and traces remain indefinitely. Accelerated involution and atrophy are essentially the same and may be due to general inanition, irradiation, vaccinations and a wide variety of acute and chronic infections, although the same conditions may sometimes produce hyperplasias. In normal involution there is a gradual reduction in the number of cells and of Hassall's corpuscles and a replacement growth of fatty tissue. In atrophy the cortical cells show reduction in number and fatty degeneration, followed by reduction of the medullary cells, which leaves the Hassall's corpuscles closer together. As the process goes on, connective tissue increases in amount and this may be so great as to produce the so-called sclerotic atrophy.

Cloudy swelling, fatty degeneration and foci of necrosis may occur in the thymus in acute infectious diseases. Calcification of Hassall's corpuscles is common and of no real significance.

Circulatory Disturbances

Passive hyperemia is associated with general passive hyperemia and is prominent in birth asphyxia. Petechiae occur in infectious diseases and in hemorrhagic diseases of the new born. Large hemorrhage, or "thymic apoplexy," is uncommon, occurs especially in infants and may sometimes be associated with sudden death. Wahl and Walthall believe that syphilis is a most important factor in its etiology but that other factors such as hemorrhagic disease, passive hyperemia, trauma and infections may cause the lesion.

Inflammation

Swelling, hyperemia and cellular infiltration with degeneration or necrosis of the parenchyma, apparently an acute parenchymatous thymitis, may occur in acute infectious diseases. Abscess may result from infections of the new born or in later life and by direct extension from neighboring suppurative processes. The thymus may be so enlarged as to produce pressure upon the trachea. Chronic inflammations result in the progressive fibrosis of sclerotic atrophy.

Infectious Granulomata

Tuberculosis of the thymus occurs in disseminated miliary tuberculosis and sometimes appears to follow caseous pneumonia. The mediastinal lymph nodes are also often extensively involved.

Syphilis. In acquired syphilis, gumma formation is rare. In congenital syphilis an interstitial fibrosis may be observed, sometimes with a diffuse lymphoid-cell infiltration. Occasionally, syphilitic infants show the so-called Dubois abscesses of the thymus. These are single or multiple, smooth-walled, well-defined cavities, a few millimeters in diameter, which contain a puriform material. Spirochetes have been found in several such cases. These are regarded by many as an inflammatory dilatation of Hassall's corpuscles, which Hammar speaks of as luetic sequestral cysts. Other authors consider the lesions as softened gummata.

Progressive Changes

A distinction is to be made between persistence of the thymus and hyperplasia. Both may be associated with the condition known as status lymphaticus. The thymus involutes at or about puberty, if not earlier. A gland of normal size for a ten-year-old child if found in later life may represent a persistence or may be a hyperplasia of a gland which had undergone some degree of involution. Grossly, only those glands markedly overweight can be regarded as hyperplastic. Microscopically, the persistent gland shows a normal ratio of size of cortex and medulla. The hyperplastic gland may show increase in number of cells of cortex and medulla, of medulla alone, usually with reduction of cortex, or of cortex alone, usually with reduction of medulla. Hyperplasia is common in exophthalmic goiter and occurs in a variety of other conditions including status lymphaticus.

The thymus may be involved in lymphoid leukemia and in Hodgkin's disease.

Status Lymphaticus

Status lymphaticus, thymolymphaticus or thymicolymphaticus, or probably more correctly, the lymphatic diathesis, occurs in early life, and is more common in males than in females and in whites than in negroes. There are enlargement of lymph nodes and other lymphoid tissues, hypoplasia of chromaffin, genital and cardiovascular systems and feminine type of secondary sex characters. The thymus may be merely persistent, may be markedly hyperplastic with a weight of 70 or 80 grams or more, or may be partly involuted. The hyperplasia may affect the medulla or the cortex. The corpuscles of Hassall are often necrotic. The spleen may or may not be enlarged. The lymph nodes are usually hyperplastic. Thus, the systemic and superficial lymph nodes, the lymphoid follicles of the entire alimentary canal, and those of the liver, lung and bone marrow may show hyperplasia.

Microscopically, the secondary nodules of the follicles of spleen and lymph nodes show marked hyperplasia which is rapidly followed by necrosis with disappearance of cytoplasm and conspicuous karyorrhexis. The necrotic foci undergo fibrosis and it is probable that necrosis may recur, for the same follicle may show both necrosis and fibrosis (see Symmers). The condition is probably a constitutional defect and the disturbance in the thymus is only one part of the whole disorder. Certain investigators do not believe in the existence of the condition (see Young and Turnbull) but we hold the view, with others, that it is an entity. As the children grow up, the disorder usually disappears.

What is called thymic death may occur abruptly in victims of status lymphaticus, and is usually cardiac. Explanations include pressure of thymus upon neighboring structures; deficiency of chromaffin tissue and autonomic imbalance; hypersusceptibility to incitants of shock; anaphylaxis; and intoxication of thymolymphoid origin. Pressure cannot be marked enough to cause death. The conception of autonomic imbalance is not sufficiently concrete to justify drawing conclusions. There are few, if any, exact observations tending to support the idea of vagal lesion. The hypothesis offered by Symmers, that the body is sensitized by germinal center necrosis and is shocked by a subsequent necrosis, is not borne out by studies of the phenomenon of anaphylaxis, for this would be an iso-anaphylaxis, the existence of which has not been demonstrated. The lesions of the lymph nodes probably are the result of some general intoxication, the origin of which is not known, but which may be responsible for death. It is probable that patients with status lymphaticus are highly susceptible to intoxications, since it is well known that in them infectious diseases run a severe course and are often fatal.

Pressure by enlarged thymus, whether a part of status lymphaticus or due to some other condition may produce inspiratory and expiratory stridor, dyspnea, cyanosis and even dysphagia, but these are in no sense a part of status lymphaticus itself (Mitchell and Warkany).

Tumors

Tumors of the thymus are infrequent. Lipoma, myxoma and thymic cysts are reported. Tumors of thymic tissue proper are said to be benign and malignant. The former are usually localized masses of hyperplastic thymic cells, sometimes practically all small cells but also sometimes containing all the structures of thymus. Malignant tumors are more frequent and may extend widely in the mediastinum, into the pericardium and into the sternum. Metatasis is often widespread.

Three microscopic varieties are recognized. The malignant thymoma or lymphosarcoma is made up of small round and polyhedral cells and multinucleated giant cells, often also with islets of cells of epithelial appearance sometimes arranged as duct-like structures. The so-called carcinomas are made up principally of the large cells of epithelial type, presumably derived from cells of Hassall's corpuscles. The spindle-cell sarcomas and myxosarcomas are derived from the stroma. The lymphosarcomas and carcinomas may be mixed.

The terminology obviously depends upon the nature of the thymic cells. If the small cells be lymphoid, the term lymphosarcoma is justified, but Foot inclines to the view that all these tumors are epithelial. Jaffe and Plavska regard the cells of Hassall's corpuscles as reticular and not related to the duct of Remak. If this be correct, the large cell tumors are sarcomas rather than carcinomas. Thus the classification of the round cell tumors is doubtful and the term malignant lymphoma the most acceptable (Crosby). The thymic tumor may be part of a pluriglandular disease (Leyton et al.). Thymic tumors occur at widely different age periods and are more frequent in males than females (Margolis). Metastatic tumors in the thymus are rare.

Dermoid cysts and simple cysts lined by ciliated columnar epithelium are probably derived from thymus anlage, but this is probably not true of the complex mediastinal teratomas.

Physiologic Considerations

Experimental work on the thymus has led to conflicting results. The organ is not essential to life. Although alterations in bones have been described as the result of thymectomy, Park and McClure, working under carefully controlled conditions, found no observable effects following excision of the thymus. Feeding thymus to tadpoles caused no alteration of metamorphosis. Uhlenhuth observed tetany in salamander larvae when fed thymus before the parathyroids developed, and assumed that thymus contains a tetany-producing toxic body which may be neutralized by the parathyroids. Hammar fed thymus to rats, and found that in young animals there is a delayed development of the testes and in adults degeneration of the testes.

tion in mammals may be merely vestigial. The gland is often hyperplastic in exophthalmic goiter, and in such cases its partial removal may be followed by improvement of symptoms and decrease of relative lymphocytosis. Myasthenia gravis, discussed in the chapter on Organs of Locomotion, is often accompanied by persistence of, or tumor of, the thymus. Blalock and associates suggest that the thymus liberates a hormone which

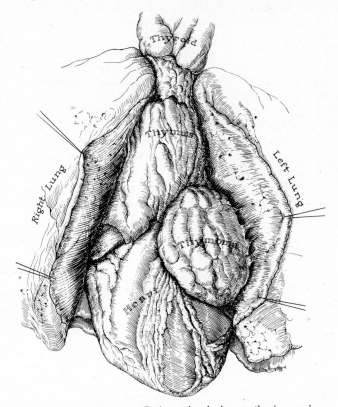

Drawing of thymoma. Patient also had myasthenia gravis.

This is in keeping with the fact that puberty and thymic involution are ordinarily concurrent. Marine, Manley and Baumann found that thyroidectomy hastens, while gonadectomy delays, involution of the thymus. Jaffe observed thymic hyperplasia in young and mature animals as a sequel of double adrenalectomy, which he believes is a manifestation of disturbed interrelation between gonads, thymus and adrenal cortex.

Riddle states that in pigeons thymectomy is followed by the production of eggs without shells, and feeding thymus to these birds is followed by development of shells. The organ in as far as it deals with calcifica-

acts at the neuromuscular junction to destroy acetylcholine.

In summary, it seems probable that the thymus may have some influence on calcium metabolism, may be responsible for toxic manifestations in thyroid and parathyroid disease and may be of importance in muscular activity, but in general its functions are not yet clearly demonstrated.

THE ADRENALS

Congenital Anomalies

Severe malformations or absence of adrenals occur almost solely in monsters, es-

Riboflavin feeding

pecially in anencephaly. In cases where they are apparently absent, careful search will disclose adrenal substance in other situations. In renal dystopia or aplasia, the adrenal usually retains the normal situation but may be of generally spherical form. The adrenals may be within the renal capsule. Heterotopia may also occur in the liver (Weller).

Accessory adrenals may be found in various parts of the urogenital tract, as for example, the broad ligament, in the lower surface of the liver or in the retroperitoneal tissues. These are usually made up principally of cortical substance. They are not uncommon, usually as single nodules, in the renal cortex near the upper pole. Hypoplasia of the chromaffin system is often associated with status lymphaticus. To be regarded as congenital anomalies are adenoma-like masses of cortical cells in the gland capsule.

Retrogressive Changes

In infectious diseases there is a reduction of the lipoid content. This may be widespread, leaving only fatty substance in the glomerulosa or islands in the reticularis or fasciculata. Edema is also commonly present. Petechiae sometimes occur. In guinea pigs, inoculation with virulent diphtheria bacilli, or with toxin, produces characteristic changes in the adrenals, especially hyperemia, hemorrhage, reduction in lipoid content and degeneration or necrosis of the cells.

Amyloid occurs in cases of secondary amyloidosis. The organ is firm and gray. Microscopically, it shows the amyloid in the capillary walls between the cortical cells. The amyloid may involve the medulla and may lead to atrophy of the cortical cells, in addition to the atrophy of the cells of the medulla. Cases of Addison's disease on the basis of amyloid adrenals have been reported. Atrophy of the adrenals affects the cortex much more markedly than the medulla. It occurs in cases of destructive lesions of the pituitary, as in Simmonds' disease, and sometimes in cases of functioning tumors of the gonads. Atrophy of the opposite adrenal occurs in cases of adrenal cortical tumors and is called compensatory atrophy (Selye). Atrophy can be produced experimentally by injections of androgenic substance, progesterone and desoxycorticosterone, by hypophysectomy and by gonadectomy.

Necrosis may occur in connection with certain dietary deficiencies, especially of members of the vitamin-B complex. Cytotoxic suprarenal contraction is a necrosis limited almost selectively to the cortex and is discussed subsequently in connection with Addison's syndrome.

Frequently, at autopsy, the adrenals show more or less wide slits deep in the cortex, so that the cortex appears to be separated from the medulla. The line of cleavage is in the region of the zona reticularis and the condition is called corticorrhexis. Its exact significance is not clear, but it probably is due to degeneration or necrosis, especially marked in the reticularis.

Circulatory Disturbances

The adrenals are affected in generalized passive hyperemia. Active hyperemia may occur in acute infectious diseases. Hemorrhage, usually minor but sometimes extensive, may be observed in the newborn as a part of hemorrhagic disease, birth trauma, asphyxia and in infants born of eclamptic mothers. Thrombosis of blood vessels and infarction may occur; either can be responsible for acute adrenal insufficiency.

In infancy and childhood, the so-called Waterhouse-Friedrichsen syndrome may occur. In patients who have been previously well, there is sudden onset of headache, fever, vomiting, abdominal pain and sometimes diarrhea. In a few hours there is profound cyanosis, punctate hemorrhagic cutaneous eruption, collapse and death. The blood sugar is usually low and leukocytosis is frequent. The condition is apparently due to fulminant bacterial infection; hemolytic streptococci, pneumococci, influenza bacilli, meningococci, and others have been recovered in different cases. In the chapter on General Phenomena of Disease there is mention of the possibility of a relation to deficiency of vitamin C or E. There is bilateral hemorrhage in the adrenals, varying from petechiae to such massive hemorrhage that the organs are practically blood-cysts. (See Lindsay, et al.)

Inflammations

In septicemias and pyemias, abscesses may be found in the adrenals, sometimes followed by extensive cicatrization. An apparently progressive chronic fibrosis with contraction of the organ may be observed, especially in cases of similar disease in the kidneys.

Acute miliary tuberculosis as a part of disseminated tuberculosis is frequent and of no demonstrable functional significance. Massive caseous tuberculosis, usually with more or less prominent fibrosis is less common but is the most frequent cause of Addison's syndrome. The lesion is usually bilateral and the organs are enlarged, nodular or smooth, may retain their general shape, and are often adherent to neighboring structures. They cut with increased resistance and show a gray, firm, cross section with extensive, irregularly disposed caseation, the necrotic material being firm, dry and granular rather than soft or diffluent. Remnants of adrenal substance may be found. Occasionally, the fibrosis may produce contraction of the organ.

In congenital syphilis, spirochetes may be present in large numbers without microscopic lesion. There may, however, be diffuse round-cell infiltration, cortical necroses, or gumma formation. In late, acquired syphilis, there may be diffuse fibrosis or gumma.

Progressive Changes

Hyperplasia of the adrenals affects the cortex and is usually most pronounced in the zona fasciculata. It may occur in prolonged infections, is reported in experimental animals following orchidectomy and following injection of extracts of pituitary, may occur in pregnancy and may be marked in Cushing's syndrome. Indeed, Albright and his associates attribute the principal manifestations of Cushing's syndrome to hyperadrenocorticism, whether hyperplasia is present or not. Infants may exhibit an adrenal hyperplasia syndrome, with protracted vomiting resembling that of pyloric stenosis, and death; the only important observation at autopsy is cortical hyperplasia of the adrenals but its relation to the clinical manifestations is not clear (Kepler and Keating). Various investigators have maintained that patients with persistent hypertension have an associated cortical hyperplasia, diffuse or focalized as adenomas (see Rinehart et al.). Although

this is sometimes true, our observations show that it is not especially frequent.

Tumors

Tumors may occur in cortex or medulla, may be silent or may be accompanied by hormonal disturbances. The most frequent tumorous lesion of the cortex is the adenoma. This is often referred to as a focalized hyperplasia. It is usually only a few millimeters in diameter, well defined, is often multiple and may be situated in cortex, capsule or medulla. Occasionally, a large adenoma several centimeters in diameter is

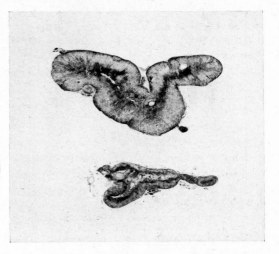

Photographs of microscopic sections of adrenals. Above is an adrenal, the seat of cortical hyperplasia in a case of Cushing's syndrome. Below is a normal adrenal for comparison.

found. Microscopically, adenomas are made up of vesicular cells like those of the cortex but arranged irregularly and sometimes with acinic structure; vascularization is variable.

Malignant tumors of the adrenal cortex are usually called carcinomas even though the cortex is mesenchymal in origin. The tumor is clearly invasive and may metastasize widely. Microscopically, pleomorphism may be marked or slight, and it may be impossible to determine the malignant character except by gross signs of invasion. Females are affected more often than males and although the carcinoma may occur in early life, is more frequent in later adult life.

Functioning tumors of the adrenal cortex are not rare. They are accompanied

[handwritten annotations at top: "Functioning tumors adrenal— cortex" "adenoma vascular—also α cortex Vascular" "CA Invasion is only sign" "" "medulla — Pheochromocytoma 15% malignant" "about half = no special signs"]

by the adrenogenital syndrome, which Groll-man divides into a juvenile form occurring in childhood and adrenal virilism occurring usually in early adult life. Both occur more

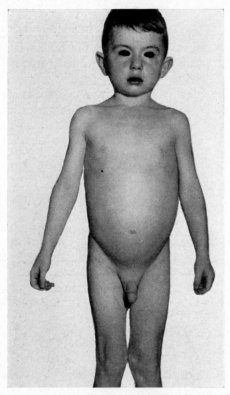

Hypergenitalism in a boy 3 years of age who had malignant tumor of adrenal cortex.

often in females than in males. In girls, there is virilism, with growth of hair on pubis and in axillae, often acne, enlargement of the clitoris, advancement of bone age and other phenomena. In boys, there is hypergenitalism, sometimes but not always with emissions and spermatogenesis; acne may occur and bone age is advanced. In women, there are the signs of virilism with amenorrhea, hirsutism, flat breasts, male distribution of pubic hair, enlarged clitoris, abdominal striae, deep voice, frontal baldness, sometimes loss of libido and rarely homosexual manifestations. In men, there may be loss of pubic and axillary hair, impotence, reduction in size of genitalia and an increased output of estrogenic substance in the urine.

THE VIRILIZING TUMORS may contain considerable quantities of androgenic substance. There is likely to be a considerable increase in output of androgenic substance, particularly the intermediate product dehydroisoandrosterone rather than testosterone; indeed the latter may be decreased. When hypertension occurs, it is likely to be persistent rather than spasmodic.

Grossly, these tumors may be benign or malignant. The former attain only moderate size, are of brownish-yellow color, well encapsulated and replace most of the adrenal, although remnants of adrenal substance are stretched over the capsule. Microscopically, the tumor is made up of vesicular cells like those of cortex arranged like one or another layer of the cortex; vascularization is usually rich. Pleomorphism may be marked in parts of the adenoma.

MALIGNANT ADENOMAS. The proportion between benign and malignant functioning cortical tumors is not yet established. The malignant adenomas may attain great size. They are soft, brownish yellow or yellow, often show foci of necrosis and hemorrhage, are friable and only partly if at all encapsulated. Microscopically, they resemble the adenoma, but pleomorphism may be marked. Vascularization is rich and metastasis, first to the lungs, may be widespread and massive.

The tumors of the medulla are principally those of the sympathetic system. As discussed in the chapter on Tumors, they include the sympathogonioma, the sympathoblastoma, the ganglioneuroma and the pheochromocytoma or paraganglioma. The ganglioneuroma may appear at any time of life and is usually benign.

THE SYMPATHOGONIOMA and the sympathoblastoma are usually grouped together as neuroblastoma. This occurs most often in childhood, is highly malignant and is often first recognized by metastasis to the head. The original tumor is of moderate size, well defined but poorly or not at all encapsulated; it is pale gray or yellow in color, soft and exhibits foci of necrosis and hemorrhage. Microscopically, it is made up of masses of small cells with dense nuclei and scanty cytoplasm; associated are bundles of delicate fibrils, probably neurofibrils. Pseudorosettes are frequent. Metastasis may be widespread. Although it was formerly thought that metastases from tumors of the left adrenal are most frequent in skull and other bones and

[handwritten note in left margin: "all malignant except in men."]

PLATE XVI

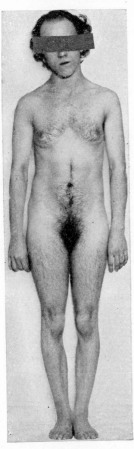

Female patient, 22 years old, with cortical adenoma of adrenal. Patient of Drs. Hudson and Joelson.

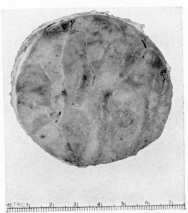

Gross photograph of cortical adenoma of adrenal.

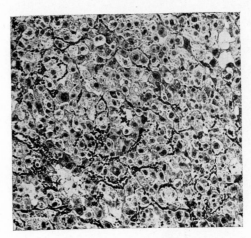

Cellular arrangement of cortical adenoma of adrenal, resembling zona glomerulosa.

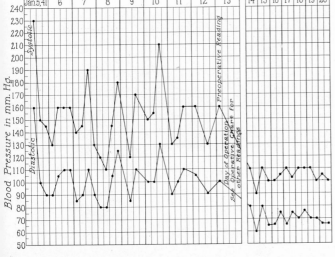

Chart of blood pressures before operative removal of pheochromocytoma of adrenal. Readings after operation are in section of chart at right.

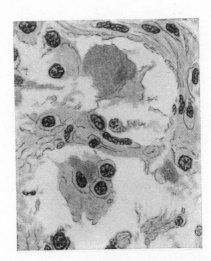

Micro-drawing of pheochromocytoma of adrenal to show brown coloration of chromaffin cells.

those from tumors of the right adrenal are found especially in the liver, this distinction is not valid.

THE PHEOCHROMOCYTOMA is the functioning tumor of the adrenal medulla, but probably about half are not accompanied by any special symptoms. It may occur at almost any time of life, but is most frequent between 20 and 40 years of age. Females are affected about twice as often as males. The symptoms occur in attacks that last a few hours or longer with free periods that may extend for several weeks. In the attacks there are giddiness, weakness, blanching, sweating, headache, vomiting, tachycardia, precordial pain, faintness and coma. Associated are hyperglycemia and spasmodic hypertension which may be marked. In some cases the hypertension may be persistent, but it is likely to vary considerably from time to time. Death may occur in the attack. These symptoms and signs are like those of an overdose of adrenalin and it is probable but not finally proved that there is an excess of epinephrine in the blood. In a few cases that have been assayed, the tumor has contained a great quantity of epinephrine.

Grossly, the benign pheochromocytoma is rarely more than a few centimeters in diameter, is well defined, encapsulated, of dark brown color, fleshy consistency and although sometimes cystic, shows little or no necrosis or hemorrhage. Microscopically, the characteristic cell is polygonal, fairly large, with a relatively small nucleus and slightly granular cytoplasm which takes up chrome salts from appropriate fixatives; it is a chromaffin cell. These cells may become elongated into large spindle cells. Pleomorphism may be marked in tumors clearly benign. In addition there are often clusters of cells with vesicular cytoplasm, resembling cortical cells. Vascularization is usually rich.

Malignant pheochromocytomas or pheochromoblastomas may attain large size, are partly or not at all encapsulated, locally invasive, and may metastasize widely. Microscopically, this form does not differ significantly from the benign form. About 15 per cent of pheochromocytomas are malignant.

Occasionally cortical tumors arise in aberrant adrenal tissue. Pheochromocytomas may arise wherever there is sympathetic tissue. Thus they may be found in the thorax, in the carotid gland and in the region of Zuckerkandl's organ.

Benign tumors, such as fibroma, occasionally occur. Lipoma-like nodules are not infrequent, but most if not all are heterotopic fatty bone marrow.

Metastases from carcinoma of lung, breast, stomach and other situations are fairly common, as are metastases from sarcomas. The adrenals may be markedly involved in lymphoid leukemia, lymphosarcoma and occasionally in Hodgkin's disease. General references are to Grollman, to Goldzieher and to Geschickter.

Physiologic Considerations

Complete removal of the adrenals in experimental animals leads to death in from a few days to as much as three weeks. Survival varies in different species, is longer in older than in young animals and is determined in part by operative technic and care of the animals. Life is prolonged in pregnant females probably because of secretion from fetal adrenals, and may be prolonged in estrus because of storage of hormone. Prolonged survival is usually due to the presence of accessory cortical tissue which undergoes hypertrophy. Survival can be somewhat prolonged by administration of salt and considerably by the use of cortical extracts and of desoxycorticosterone. The effects of adrenalectomy are much the same as those which will be described in connection with Addison's syndrome.

Studies of output of epinephrine are difficult because of available methods of assay. Cannon and his associates have maintained that in emotional states, asphyxia, stimulation of sensory nerves, etc., the output of epinephrine is increased and glucose mobilized. Although confirmed by others, Rogoff and also Stewart maintain that output of epinephrine in sufficient amounts to cause hyperglycemia has never been demonstrated.

The part played by epinephrine in maintenance of blood pressure is not altogether clear. Administration of adrenalin is temporarily effective in elevating the pressure of adrenalectomized animals. Cortical extract is much more effective and lasting, as is true in connection with shock. Excess output with production of hypertension probably

Cortex important in B. P. maintenance

occurs with pheochromocytomas but as indicated above, there are serious by-effects. The presence of cortex is necessary for the production of the experimental hypertension of renal circulatory disturbance, but the mechanism is not understood.

The adrenal cortex is closely related to sexual characters. Pseudohermaphroditism may be associated with cortical hyperplasia or tumors. The adrenogenital syndrome, adrenal virilism in females, hypergenitalism in young males and feminization of mature males, and the various manifestations of Cushing's syndrome, all have alterations of secondary sex characters as well as increased output of sex hormones or their metabolites. The suggestion that certain cells of the cortex are related to its sexual functions has not been established.

The adrenals play an important part in metabolism. Although injections of adrenalin cause hyperglycemia, the hypoglycemia of adrenal insufficiency is attributed to absence of cortical activity. Adrenalectomy leads to marked fall in basal metabolic rate and in body temperature, phenomena dependent upon the cortex rather than the medulla. Adrenalectomy is usually followed by increase of cholesterol in the blood. There is usually hemoconcentration and associated with that is decreased renal excretory function and accumulation of nitrogenous metabolites. Both sodium and chloride are much reduced in the blood, with excess secretion in the urine and a negative balance. Potassium and magnesium may be considerably increased in the blood.

The effects of adrenalectomy on resistance have been widely studied. Adrenalectomized animals do not produce antibodies as well as normals, probably because of disturbance of water balance. There is a temporary sensitivity to various drugs, diphtheria toxin, histamine and to certain infections. While natural resistance is depressed by adrenalectomy, an acquired resistance due to immunization before operation is not altered. The cortex is apparently important in all these phenomena, because administration of cortical extracts prevents the changes. Perla and Marmorston are of the opinion that there is a disturbance of general cellular metabolism, possibly in the oxidation-reduction systems.

Cortex important in sugar level maintenance phosphorylation ?

Addison's Disease. The clinical manifestations of Addison's disease include asthenia, gastro-intestinal disturbances and pigmentation. Asthenia is first shown by lassitude and weakness, which ultimately may become marked. Even mental effort may lead to great fatigue. Low blood pressure may become profound. Loss of weight is usually moderate but may be marked. Low basal metabolic rate and low temperature are probably part of the asthenia. The gastro-intestinal symptoms include anorexia, nausea, vomiting, diarrhea, often alternating with constipation, and abdominal pain. The pigmentation has been referred to in the chapter on Pathologic Pigmentation. It occurs in skin, especially those parts exposed to light and to pressure. It frequently occurs in the buccal mucosa and under surface of the tongue; these situations are of diagnostic importance in the negro. It is said to occur in the vagina and the serous membranes. Pigmentation is not constantly present and remissions may occur.

There may be a moderate normochromic anemia. The leukocytes are about normal in number but there is often a relative lymphocytosis. One of the most important changes chemically, is the reduction of sodium and chloride in the blood, associated with decrease of bicarbonate ion and increase of potassium. Loeb has shown that many of the manifestations of the disease may be relieved by adequate administration of sodium chloride. There is hemoconcentration and an increase in nitrogenous metabolites. The sugar tolerance curve may be altered, and adrenalin does not produce the usual rise of blood sugar.

Addison's disease is not common. It occurs far more often in whites than in negroes and is twice as frequent in males as in females. It is a disease of middle life, especially the third and fourth decades, but may be observed earlier or later. There is no convincing evidence of heredity as a factor. Addison's disease occasionally runs a short course of days or weeks, but usually is prolonged and may show marked remissions. Gutman found that when the adrenal disease was tuberculosis, there was an average duration of 13 months but in cases of cytotoxic contraction the average was 34 months.

Nevertheless rare cases may survive 10 years or more.

Of the 566 cases collected by Gutman, tuberculosis of the adrenals was found in 281 (68.3 per cent), cytotoxic contraction in 65 (19.4 per cent) and 40 cases showed other lesions of the adrenals including amyloidosis, fatty degeneration, secondary and primary tumors, venous thrombosis, arterial embolism, infarction, pyogenic infection and gumma. Four cases were reported without adrenal disease, but there is serious doubt as to the clinical diagnosis. Experimental and anatomic observations point to the cortex as the significant factor, but involvement of the medulla is a frequent accompaniment. The effectiveness of cortical extracts and of desoxycorticosterone acetate lend support to this view.

Tuberculosis is secondary to tuberculosis elsewhere, but the primary disease may not be conspicuous. The lesion in the adrenal is an extensive caseous or fibrocaseous tuberculosis.

The gland in cytotoxic contraction is usually much reduced in size, firm and in the cross section is diffusely gray. Microscopically, the cortex is present as only a few clusters of enlarged cells; most of it is lost even though remnants of cells and fragmented nuclei are present. The cortex is the seat of extensive lymphocytic infiltration and fibrosis. There may also be destruction of small parts of the medulla followed by fibrosis and lymphocytic infiltration (Saphir and Binswanger). The cause is unknown, but Wells likens the microscopic appearance to that of the liver in acute diffuse necrosis (yellow atrophy), and necrosis of adrenal occurs experimentally in some of the dietary deficiencies that lead to hepatic necrosis (see Nelson).

At autopsy on a case of Addison's disease there is usually some wasting of flesh but only rarely emaciation. Occasionally there is active pulmonary tuberculosis. There is often a considerable degree of atrophy of the heart as well as of gastric mucosa and other organs. The aorta and other arteries are sometimes hypoplastic. The lymph nodes and spleen are often enlarged, and the thymus may be persistent. The kidneys show cloudy swelling of the tubules and often atrophy of the cells. Chronic pyelonephritis and also renal tuberculosis may be found. (See Grollman; Goldzieher.)

THE CAROTID BODY

The only pathologic lesion of significance that is now known is tumor of the carotid body, gland or glomus. The embryology is not settled, but it is highly probable that the body arises as part of the sympathico-chromaffin system. Thus the tumors are of the same order as those described in the adrenal medulla. Most of them appear to be pheochromocytomas, but as is usual in tumors of this type, immature cells are encountered and sometimes nerve fibrils.

The fact that these tumors are occasionally bilateral and in one instance a similar tumor of Zuckerkandl's organ was found associated with a carotid-body tumor, suggests that a system disease may play a part. Generally these tumors are benign. Chromaffin cells are often abundant but it is doubtful that epinephrine has ever been demonstrated in the tumors. (See Chase; Cragg; Engelbreth-Holm.)

REFERENCES

Aird, R. B.: Experimental Exophthalmos and Associated Myopathy Induced by the Thyrotropic Hormone, Ann. Int. Med., 15: 564, 1941.

Albright, F., W. Parsons, and E. Bloomberg: Therapy in Cushing's Syndrome Interpreted as Hyperadrenocorticism Leading to Hypergluconeogenesis: Results of Treatment with Testosterone Propionate, Jour. Clin. Endocrinol., 1: 375, 1941.

——, J. C. Aub, and W. Bauer: Hyperparathyroidism, etc., Jour. Amer. Med. Asso., 102: 1276, 1934; see also Arch. Int. Med., 54: 315, 1934.

Anderson, N. L.: The Lawrence-Moon-Biedl Syndrome, Jour. Clin. Endocrinol., 1: 905, 1941.

Aub, J. C.: The Relation of the Internal Secretions to Metabolism, Jour. Amer. Med. Asso., 79: 95, 1922.

Bailey, P., and F. Bremer: Experimental Diabetes Insipidus, Arch. Int. Med., 28: 772, 1921.

Blalock, A., M. F. Mason, H. J. Morgan, and S. S. Riven: Myasthenia Gravis and Tumors of the Thymic Region. Report of a Case in which the Tumor Was Removed, Ann. Surg., 110: 544, 1940; see also B. Gillespie: Thymoma in Myasthenia Gravis, Arch. Path., 32: 659, 1941.

Boycott, A. E., and C. H. Kellaway: Compensatory Hypertrophy of the Suprarenals, Jour. Path. and Bact., 27: 171, 1924.

Boyd, E.: Weight of the Thymus and Its Component Parts and Number of Hassall's Corpuscles in Health and in Disease, Amer. Jour. Dis. Child., 51: 313, 1936.

Brannan, D.: Carcinoma of Thymus and Occlusion of the Superior Vena Cava, Arch. Path., 1: 569, 1926.

Brosin, H. W., and C. Apfelbach: Anorexia Nervosa. Case Report with Autopsy Findings, Jour. Clin. Endocrinol., 1: 272, 1941.

Cannon, W. B.: Bodily Changes in Pain, Hunger, Fear and Rage, New York, 1915.

——, and D. de la Paz: Emotional Stimulation of Adrenal Secretion, Amer. Jour. Physiol., 28: 64, 1911.

——, and R. G. Hoskins: The Effects of Asphyxia, Hyperpnoea and Sensory Stimulation on Adrenal Secretion, Ibid., 29: 274, 1911.

Castleman, B., and T. B. Mallory: The Pathology of the Parathyroid Gland in Hyperparathyroidism, Amer. Jour. Path., 11: 1, 1935.

——: Parathyroid Hyperplasia in Chronic Renal Insufficiency, Ibid., 13: 553, 1937.

Chase, W. H.: Familial and Bilateral Tumours of the Carotid Body, Jour. Path. and Bact., 36: 1, 1933.

Christie, C. D., and G. N. Stewart: Study of a Case of Diabetes Insipidus with Special Reference to the Mechanism of the Diuresis and of the Action of Pituitary Extract on It, Arch. Int. Med., 20: 10, 1917.

——: Study of Some Cases of Diabetes Insipidus with Special Reference to the Detection of Changes in the Blood When Water Is Taken or Withheld, Ibid., 29: 555, 1922.

Coller, F. A.: Adenoma and Cancer of the Thyroid: A Study of Their Relation in Ninety Epithelial Neoplasms of the Thyroid, Jour. Amer. Med. Asso., 92: 457, 1929.

Coller, F. A., H. Field, Jr., and T. M. Durant: Chromaffin Cell Tumor Causing Paroxysmal Hypertension, Relieved by Operation, Arch. Surg., 28: 1136, 1934.

Collip, J. B.: The Parathyroid Glands, Medicine, 5: 1, 1926.

Cragg, R. W.: Concurrent Tumors of the Left Carotid Body and Both Zuckerkandl Bodies, Arch. Path., 18: 635, 1934.

Crosby, E. H.: Malignant Tumors of the Thymus Gland, Amer. Jour. Cancer, 16: 461, 1932.

Curtis, G. M.: The Production of Experimental Diabetes Insipidus, Arch. Int. Med., 34: 801, 1924.

Cushing, H.: The Pituitary Body and Its Disorders, Philadelphia and London, Lippincott, 1912.

Cushing, H.: Pituitary Body, Hypothalamus, and Parasympathetic Nervous System, Springfield, Ill. Thomas, 1932.

——: "Dispituitarism": Twenty Years Later, with Special Consideration of the Pituitary Adenomas, Arch. Int. Med., 51: 487, 1933.

——: Hyperactivation of the Neurohypophysis as the Pathological Basis of Eclampsia and Other Hypertensive States, Amer. Jour. Path., 10: 145, 1934.

——, and L. M. Davidoff: The Pathological Findings in Four Autopsied Cases of Acromegaly with a Discussion of Their Significance. Monographs Rock. Inst. for Med. Research, No. 22, New York, 1927.

Dandy, W. E.: Extirpation of the Pineal Body, Jour. Exper. Med., 22: 237, 1915.

——, and E. Goetsch: The Blood Supply of the Pituitary Body, Amer. Jour. Anat., 11: 137, 1911.

Davidoff, L. M.: Tumors of the Pituitary Gland and Its Neighboring Structures, Psychiatr. Quart., 7: 72, 1933.

Davis, L., and J. Martin: Results of Experimental Removal of Pineal Gland in Young Mammals, Arch. Neurol. and Psychiatr., 43: 23, 1940.

Dragstedt, L. R.: The Physiology of the Parathyroid Gland, Physiol. Rev., 7: 499, 1927.

Drake, T. G., F. Albright, W. Bauer, and B. Castleman: Chronic Idiopathic Hypoparathyroidism: Report of Six Cases with Autopsy Findings in One, Ann. Int. Med., 12: 1751, 1939.

Eisenhardt, L., and K. W. Thompson: A Brief Consideration of the Present Status of So-called Pituitary Basophilism, Yale Jour. Biol. and Med., 11: 507, 1939.

Engelbreth-Holm, J.: Vier Fälle von Carotisdrüsentumor, Acta Pathologica et Microbiol. Scandinav., 17: 32, 1940.

Enzer, N.: The Pathology of the Nodular Goiter, Ann. Int. Med., 3: 1241, 1929-30.

Erdheim, J.: Ueber den Kalkgehalt des wachsenden Knochens und des Callus nach der Epithelkörperchenextirpation, Frank. Zeitschr. Path., 7: 175, 1911.

——: Pathologie der Hypophysengeschwülste, Ergebn. Allg. Path. u. Path. Anat., 21: 482, 1926.

Evans, H. M.: Clinical Manifestations of Dysfunction of the Anterior Pituitary, in Glandular Physiology and Therapy, Chicago, Amer. Med. Asso., 1935, p. 1.

——: The Growth Hormone of the Anterior Pituitary, ibid., p. 45.

Ewing, J.: Neoplastic Diseases, 4th ed., Philadelphia and London, 1940.

Farber, J. E., K. Goldstein, and W. F. Beswick: Simmonds' Disease with a Cranio-Pharyngioma, Jour. Clin. Endocrinol., 1: 688, 1941.

Farquharson, R. F., T. H. Belt, and G. L. Duff: Simmonds' Disease: Clinical and Pathological Observations on Four Cases, Trans. Amer. Clin. and Climatolog. Asso., 54: 106, 1938.

Foot, N. C.: Concerning "Malignant Thymoma" with a Report of a Case of Primary Carcinoma of the Thymus, Amer. Jour. Path., 2: 33, 1926.

Frazier, C. H., and B. J. Alpers: Tumors of Rathke's Cleft (Hitherto Called Tumors of Rathke's Pouch), Arch. Neurol. and Psychiat., 32: 973, 1934.

Friedell, M. T.: Hyperthyroidism and Adenocarcinoma of the Thyroid Gland, Arch. Surg., 43: 386, 1941.

Friedlander, A., and N. C. Foot: Report of a Case of Malignant Small-celled Thymoma with Acute Lymphoid Leukemia, Amer. Jour. Med. Sci., 169: 161, 1925.

Geiling, E. M. K.: The Posterior Hypophysis, in Glandular Physiology and Therapy, Chicago, Amer. Med. Asso., 1935, p. 139.

——, and F. K. Oldham: The Site of Formation of the Posterior Lobe Hormones, Trans. Asso. Amer. Phys., 52: 132, 1937.

German, W. M.: Granulomas in Struma Fibrosa of Thyroid, West. Jour. Surg., 49: 120, 1941.

Geschickter, C. F.: Suprarenal Tumors, Amer. Jour. Cancer, 23: 104, 1935.

Globus, J. H.: Pinealoma, Arch. Path., 31: 533, 1941.

Goetsch, E.: Origin, Evolution and Significance of Giant Cells in Riedel's Struma, Arch. Surg., **41**: 308, 1940.

———: Functional Significance of Mitochondria in Toxic Thyroid Adenomata, Bull. Johns Hopkins Hosp., **27**: 129, 1916.

Goldzieher, M. A.: The Adrenals, New York, Macmillan, 1929.

Goodpasture, E. W.: Myocardial Necrosis in Hyperthyroidism, Jour. Amer. Med. Asso., **76**: 1545, 1921.

———: The Influence of Thyroid Products on Production of Myocardial Necrosis, Jour. Exper. Med., **34**: 407, 1921.

Gotshalk, H. C., and I. L. Tilden: Necrosis of the Anterior Pituitary Following Parturition, Jour. Amer. Med. Asso., **114**: 33, 1940.

Graham, A.: Malignant Epithelial Tumors of the Thyroid, Surg., Gynec. and Obst., **39**: 781, 1924.

———: Diseases and Pathology of the Thyroid Gland, The Thyroid Gland Clinics of G. W. Crile and Associates, Philadelphia and London, 1922; p. 35.

———: Physiological Activity of Adenomata of the Thyroid Gland, etc., as Evidenced by Feeding Experiments on Tadpoles, Jour. Exper. Med., **24**: 345, 1916.

———: Malignant Tumors of the Thyroid, Ann. Surg., **82**: 30, 1925.

———, and E. P. McCullagh: Atrophy and Fibrosis Associated with Lymphoid Tissue in the Thyroid: Struma Lymphomatosa (Hashimoto), Arch. Surg., **22**: 548, 1931.

Grollman, A.: The Adrenals, Baltimore, Williams and Wilkins, 1936.

Guttman, P. H.: Addison's Disease: A Statistical Analysis of Five Hundred and Sixty-six Cases and a Study of the Pathology, Arch. Path., **10**: 742, 895, 1930.

Haldeman, K. O.: Tumors of the Pineal Gland, Arch. Neurol. and Psychiat., **18**: 724, 1927.

Hall, E. M., and L. Chaffin: Final Report of a Case of Malignant Adenoma of the Parathyroid Glands, West Jour. Surg., **48**: 685, 1940.

Ham, A. W., N. Littner, T. G. H. Drake, E. C. Robertson, and F. F. Tisdall: Physiological Hypertrophy of the Parathyroids, Its Cause and Its Relation to Rickets, Amer. Jour. Path., **16**: 277, 1940.

Hammar, J. A.: The New Views as to the Morphology of the Thymus Gland and Their Bearing upon the Function of the Thymus, Endocrinol., **5**: 543; 731, 1921.

Harington, C. R., and G. Barger: Chemistry of Thyroxine; Constitution and Synthesis of Thyroxine, Biochem. Jour., **21**: 169, 1927.

Hellwig, A. C.: Experimental Goiter Due to Calcium, Arch. Surg., **40**: 98, 1940.

Herbert, F. K., H. G. Miller, and G. O. Richardson: Chronic Renal Disease, Secondary Parathyroid Hyperplasia, Decalcification of Bone and Metastatic Calcification, Jour. Path. and Bact., **53**: 161, 1941.

Hertzler, A. E.: Diseases of the Thyroid Gland, New York, Hoeber, 1941.

Hirsch, M.: Handbuch der Inneren Sekretion. Eine umfassende Darstellung der Anatomie, Physiologie und Pathologie der endokrinen Drusen, Leipsig, 1928.

Hofbauer, J.: Concerning the Etiology of Hyperplasia of the Endometrium, Surg., Gynec. and Obst., **52**: 222, 1931.

Horrax, G.: Studies on the Pineal Gland, I, II, Arch. Int. Med., **17**: 607, 627, 1916.

Hunter, W. C., and D. B. Seabrook: Goitrous Enlargement of the Thyroid Gland Due to Amyloidosis, Arch. Surg., **20**: 762, 1930.

Izawa, Y.: A Contribution to the Physiology of the Pineal Body, Amer. Jour. Med. Sci., **166**: 185, 1923.

Jaffe, H. L.: The Influence of the Suprarenal Gland on the Thymus, Jour. Exper. Med., **40**: 325, 619, 753, 1924.

———, and A. Plavska: Experimental Studies on the Formation of Hassall's Corpuscles, Proc. Soc. Exper. Biol. and Med., **23**: 91, 1925; see also Popoff, N. W.: The Histogenesis of the Thymus as Shown by Tissue Cultures, Transplantation and Regeneration, Ibid., **24**: 148, 1926.

Janney, N. W.: Concerning the Pathogenesis of Thyrotoxicosis, Endocrinol., **6**: 795, 1922.

Kendall, E. C.: Physiological Action of the Thyroid Hormone, Amer. Jour. Physiol., **49**: 136, 1919.

———: Isolation of the Iodine Compound Which Occurs in the Thyroid, Jour. Biol. Chem., **39**: 125, 1919.

Kepler, E. J., and F. R. Keating: Diseases of the Adrenal Glands. II. Tumors of the Adrenal Cortex, Diseases of the Adrenal Medulla and Allied Disturbances, Arch. Int. Med., **68**: 1010, 1941.

Kessel, L., and H. T. Hyman: Studies of Exophthalmic Goiter and the Involuntary Nervous System: XV. The Diagnosis of Exophthalmic Goiter, Jour. Amer. Med. Asso., **88**: 1478, 1927.

Kimball, O. P., and D. Marine: The Prevention of Simple Goitre in Man, Arch. Int. Med., **22**: 41, 1918.

Kirschbaum, J. D., and H. A. Levy: Tuberculoma of Hypophysis with Insufficiency of Anterior Lobe. A Clinical and Pathological Study, Ibid., **68**: 1095, 1941.

Kline, B. S.: The Origin of Adenomatous Goitre, Amer. Jour. Path., **1**: 235, 1925.

Krabbe, K. H.: The Pineal Gland, Especially in Relation to the Problem on Its Supposed Significance in Sexual Development, Endocrinol., **7**: 379, 1923.

Kunstadter, R. H.: Adiposogenital Dystrophy, Jour. Amer. Med. Asso., **117**: 1947, 1941.

Lenhart, C. H.: The Influence upon Tadpoles of Feeding Desiccated Thyroid Gland, etc., Jour. Exper. Med., **22**: 739, 1915.

Leyton, O., H. M. Turnbull, and A. B. Bratton: Primary Cancer of the Thymus with Pluriglandular Disturbance, Jour. Path. and Bact., **34**: 635, 1931.

Lindsay, J. W., E. C. Rice, M. A. Selinger, and L. Robins: The Waterhouse-Friderichsen Syndrome, Amer. Jour. Med. Sci., **201**: 263, 1941.

Loeb, R. F., D. W. Atchley, E. B. Gutman, and R. Jillson: On the Mechanism of Sodium Depletion in Addison's Disease, Proc. Soc. Exper. Biol. and Med., **31**: 130, 1933-34.

Long, C. N. H.: The Influence of the Pituitary and Adrenal Glands upon Pancreatic Diabetes, Harvey Lectures, Baltimore, Williams and Wilkins, **32**: 194, 1937.

MacMahon, H. E., H. G. Close, and G. Hass: Cardiovascular Renal Changes Associated with Basophile Adenoma of the Anterior Lobe of the Pituitary (Cushing's Syndrome), Amer. Jour. Path., **10**: 177, 1934.

Margolis, H. M.: Tumors of the Thymus: Pathology, Classification and Report of Cases, Amer. Jour. Cancer, **15**: 2106, 1931.

Marine, D.: The Present Status of the Functions of the Thyroid Gland, Physiol. Rev., **2**: 521, 1922.

———: The Importance of Our Knowledge of Thyroid Physiology in the Control of Thyroid Disease, Arch. Int. Med., **32**: 811, 1923.

———, and E. J. Baumann: Influence of Glands with Internal Secretion on Respiratory Exchange. V. Further Observations on the Effect of Suprarenal Insufficiency (by removal) in Thyroidectomized Rabbits, Jour. Metab. Res., **1**: 777, 1922.

———, and C. H. Lenhart: The Pathological Anatomy of the Human Thyroid Gland, Arch. Int. Med., **7**: 506, 1911.

———, and ———: Pathological Anatomy of Exophthalmic Goitre, etc., Ibid., **8**: 265, 1911

———, O. T. Manley, and E. J. Baumann: The Influence of Thyroidectomy, Gonadectomy, Suprarenalectomy, and Splenectomy on the Thymus Gland of Rabbits, Jour. Exper. Med., **40**: 429, 1924.

Mayo, C. W., and C. P. Schlicke: Exogenous Tumors of the Thyroid Gland, Amer. Jour. Path., **17**: 283, 1941.

McCord, C. P.: The Pineal Gland in Relation to Somatic, Sexual and Mental Development, Jour. Amer. Med. Asso., **63**: 232, 1914.

Miloslavich, E.: Ueber Bildungsanomalien der Nebenniere, Virchow's Arch. Path. Anat., **218**: 131, 1914.

Mitchell, A. G., and J. Warkany: The Problem of the Thymus in Children, Jour. Amer. Med. Asso., **112**: 283, 1939.

Moehlig, R. C.: Pituitary Tumor Associated with Gynecomastia, Endocrinol., **13**: 529, 1929.

Moore, R. A., and E. H. Cushing: Diabetes Insipidus and Fröhlich's Syndrome Associated with Encephalitis of the Hypothalamic Region, Arch. Neurol. and Psychiat., **34**: 828, 1935.

Moritz, A. R.: Interacinar Epithelium of the Thyroid Gland, Amer. Jour. Path., **7**: 37, 1931.

———, and F. Bayless: Lateral Cervical Tumors of Aberrant Thyroid Tissue, Arch. Surg., **24**: 1028, 1932.

Nelson, A. A.: Hemorrhagic Cortical Necrosis of Adrenals in Rats on Deficient Diets, Publ. Health Rep., **54**: 2250, 1939.

Nicholson, F. M.: An Experimental Study of Mitochondrial Changes in the Thyroid Gland, Jour. Exper. Med., **39**: 63, 1924.

Oppenheimer, B. S., and A. M. Fishberg: The Association of Hypertension with Suprarenal Tumors, Arch. Int. Med., **34**: 631, 1924.

Ornsteen, A. M.: A Contribution to the Pathogenesis and Heredity of the Laurence-Biedl Syndrome (Dystrophia Adiposogenitalis, Retinitis Pigmentosa, Mental Deficiency and Polydactylism). Report of Three Cases in One Family, Amer. Jour. Med. Sci., **183**: 256, 1932.

Park, E. A., and R. D. McClure: The Results of Thymus Extirpation in the Dog. With a Review of the Experimental Literature on Thymus Extirpation, Amer. Jour. Dis. Child., **18**: 317, 1919.

Pearce, L., and C. M. Van Allen: Effect of Thyroidectomy and Thymectomy in Experimental Syphilis in the Rabbit, Jour. Exper. Med., **43**: 297, 1926.

Perla, D., and J. Marmorston: Relation of Suprarenal Glands to Resistance, Arch. Path., **16**: 379, 1933.

Piney, A., and I. Coates: Metastatic Carcinoma of the Pituitary Gland and Diabetes Insipidus, Jour. Path. and Bact., **27**: 211, 1924.

Plaut, A.: Hypophysenbefunde bei akuten Infektionskrankheiten, Virchow's Arch. Path. Anat., **237**: 165, 1922.

Reinhart, H. L., and E. Scott: The Hormone Test for Pregnancy, Amer. Jour. Clin. Path., **1**: 113, 1931.

Riddle, O.: Studies on the Physiology of Reproduction in Birds. XIX. A Hitherto Unknown Function of the Thymus, Amer. Jour. Physiol., **68**: 557, 1924.

———: Factors in the Development of Sex and Secondary Sexual Characters, Physiol. Rev., **11**: 63, 1931.

Rinehart, J. F., O. O. Williams, and W. S. Cappeller: Adenomatous Hyperplasia of the Adrenal Cortex Associated with Essential Hypertension, Arch. Path., **32**: 169, 1941.

de Robertis, E.: Intracellular Colloid of Normal and Activated Thyroid Gland of the Rat Studied by the Freezing-Drying Method, Amer. Jour. Anat., **68**: 317, 1941.

Robertson, T. B.: The Influence of Tethelin. The Growth-controlling Principle of the Anterior Lobe of the Pituitary Body, upon the Growth of the White Mouse, Jour. Biol. Chem., **24**: 397, 1916.

Rogoff, J. M.: On the Liberation of Epinephrin from the Adrenal Glands, Jour. Lab. and Clin. Med., **3**: 209, 1917-18.

———, and G. N. Stewart: Studies on Adrenal Insufficiency in Dogs: V. The Influence of Adrenal Extracts on the Survival Period of Adrenalectomized Dogs, Amer. Jour. Physiol., **84**: 660, 1928.

———, and ———: VI. The Influence of "Heat" on the Survival Period of Dogs after Adrenalectomy, Ibid., **86**: 20, 1928.

Sachs, E., and M. E. MacDonald: Blood Sugar Studies in Experimental Pituitary and Hypothalamic Lesions, Arch. Neurol. and Psychiatr., **13**: 335, 1925.

Saphir, O., and H. F. Binswanger: Suprarenal Cortical Insufficiency and Cytotoxic Contraction of the Suprarenals, Jour. Amer. Med. Asso., **95**: 1007, 1930.

Schmitt, P.: Hypophysenuntersuchungen bei kongenitaler Lues, Centralbl. Allg. Path., **34**: 466, 1924.

Scott, W. J. M.: Effect of Suprarenal Insufficiency in Cats, Jour. Exper. Med., **36**: 199, 1922.

———: The Influence of Adrenal Glands on Resistance. I. The Susceptibility of Adrenalectomized Rats to Morphine, Ibid., **38**: 543, 1923.

———: II. The Toxic Effect of Killed Bacteria in Adrenalectomized Rats, Ibid., **39**: 457, 1924.

Selye, H.: Compensatory Atrophy of the Adrenal, Jour. Amer. Med. Asso., **115**: 2246, 1940.

Severinghaus, A. E.: Cellular Changes in the Anterior Hypophysis with Special Reference to Its Secretory Activities, Physiol. Rev., **17**: 556, 1937.

Shaffer, J. M.: Disease of the Liver in Hyperthyroidism, Arch. Path., **29**: 20, 1940.

Sheehan, H. L.: Post-partum Necrosis of the Anterior Pituitary, Jour. Path. and Bact., **45**: 189, 1937.

Simmonds, M.: Ueber Kachexie hypophysaren Ursprungs, Deutsche Med. Wochenschr., **43**: 190, 1916.

Smelser, G. K.: The Histology of Orbital and Other Fat Tissue Deposits in Animals with Experimentally Produced Exophthalmos, Amer. Jour. Path., **15**: 341, 1939.

Smith, L. W., E. H. Pool, and C. T. Olcott: Malignant Disease of the Thyroid Gland. A Clinico-Pathological Analysis of 54 Cases of Thyroid Malignancy, Amer. Jour. Cancer, **20**: 1, 1934.

Smith, P. E.: The Disabilities Caused by Hypophysectomy and Their Repair, etc., Jour. Amer. Med. Asso., **88**: 158, 1928.

Steinbiss, W.: Ueber eine eigenartige Degeneration der Nebennieren bei Addisonscher Krankheit, Virchow's Arch. Path. Anat., **262**: 286, 1926.

Stewart, G. N.: Adrenalectomy and the Relation of the Adrenal Bodies to Metabolism, Physiol. Rev., **4**: 163, 1924.

Symmers, D.: Status Lymphaticus, Amer. Jour. Med. Sci., **156**: 40, 1918.

Thurston, E. W.: A Comparison of Hypertrophic Changes in Thyroid Caused in Different Species by Acid Extract of the Anterior Lobe of the Bovine Pituitary Gland, Arch. Path., **15**: 67, 1933.

Tierney, J. L.: Classification and Treatment of Hypophyseal Disorders, Endocrinol., **7**: 536, 1923.

Uhlenhuth, E.: The Effect of Iodine and of Iodothyrine on the Larvae of Salamanders, etc., Ibid., **6**: 102, 1922.

Vincent, S.: Current Views on "Internal Secretion," Physiol. Rev., **7**: 288, 1927.

Wahl, H. R.: Neuroblastomata, Jour. Med. Res., **30**: 205, 1914.

——: Malformation of Adrenal Glands with the Clinical Picture of Addison's Disease, Med. Clin. N. Amer., **7**: 1357, 1923-24.

Wahl, H. R., and D. Walthall: Thymus Apoplexy, Amer. Jour. Dis. Child., **24**: 27, 1922.

Warren, S.: The Significance of Invasion of Blood Vessels in Adenomas of the Thyroid Gland, Arch. Path., **11**: 255, 1931.

Warthin, A. S.: The Constitutional Entity of Exophthalmic Goiter and So-Called Toxic Adenoma, Ann. Int. Med., **2**: 553, 1928-29; *see also* C. H. Fortune: A Clinical Study of the Graves' Constitution and Its Relation to Thyroid Disease, Ibid., **6**: 869, 1933.

——, W. A. Crane, and J. B. Jackson: Pigmentation of the Skin (Addison's Disease) Associated with Lymphosarcoma, etc., Arch. Derm. and Syphil., **10**: 139, 1924.

Wegelin, C.: Zur Kenntniss der Kachexia thyreopriva, Virchow's Arch. Path. Anat., **254**: 689, 1925.

Weller, C. V.: Heterotopia of Adrenal in Liver and Kidney, Amer. Jour. Med. Sci., **169**: 696, 1925.

——: Hepatic Pathology in Exophthalmic Goiter, Ann. Int. Med., **7**: 543, 1933.

——, R. C. Wanstrom, H. Gordon, and J. C. Bugher: Cardiac Histopathology in Thyroid Disease, Amer. Heart Jour., **8**: 8, 1932.

Wells, H. G.: Addison's Disease with Selective Destruction of the Suprarenal Cortex ("Suprarenal Cortex Atrophy"), Arch. Path., **10**: 499, 1930.

Wilensky, A. O., and P. A. Kaufman: Hurthle Cell Tumor of the Thyroid Gland, Surg., Gynec. and Obst., **66**: 1, 1938.

Young, M., and H. M. Turnbull: An Analysis of the Data Collected by the Status Lymphaticus Investigation Committee, Jour. Path. and Bact., **34**: 213, 1931.

Zondek, B.: Chromatophorotropic Principle of the Pars Intermedia of the Pituitary, in Glandular Physiology and Therapy, Chicago, Amer. Med. Asso., 1935, p. 133.

21

Organs of Locomotion

BONES

Local Deficiencies of Growth

Most of the anomalies of bone are referable to faulty growth rather than to defects originating in embryonal life. In rare instances aplasia of bones, more especially those of the extremities, may be attributed to embryonal faults; these are true aplasias and represent congenital anomalies. Aplasia may also account for skull defects in monsters. The pressure of the growing brain may presumably be responsible for fibrosis and failure of ossification, especially in the parietal bones near the interparietal suture. Defective fusion of the lateral halves of the vertebral bodies may be due to persistence of the notochord (Krause). Defective bone formation occurs in many varieties of monsters.

Single bones, for example, the clavicle, may be absent. Entire limbs may be absent (amelus), or hands and feet may be directly attached to the trunk (phocomelus).

Injuries to or defects of the central nervous system in fetal life are responsible for the hypoplasias of bone in which the bones of an entire extremity are small. Local disturbances of growth may be due to defects in epiphyseal or symphysis cartilage, or the connective tissue of cranial sutures. Similarly, premature calcification and fusion of these within the neighboring bone may inhibit development. In this general category are probably the cases of cleidocranial dysostosis, in which, often on a familial or perhaps hereditary basis, the membranous cranial bones and the clavicles fail to ossify (McCurdy and Baer). In fetal and postfetal life, inflammations and trauma to epiphyseal cartilage may lead to inhibition of growth and short diaphyses. Contractures of skin, following burns in early life, may prevent full development of bones, especially of the extremities.

General Deficiencies of Growth

These include especially dwarfism, chondrodystrophia fetalis, osteogenesis imperfecta, cretinism and myxedema. Rickets and osteomalacia are classified as metabolic disturbances.

Dwarfism. True dwarfism, independent of endocrine disturbances, is rare. The individual is small in stature, with proportionately developed trunk and extremities but with large head. The epiphyses ossify later than normal, and according to M. B. Schmidt growth may continue slowly to the thirtieth year or later. Development of the brain and mentality are usually normal. In some instances heredity appears to play a part (Kraft).

As indicated in the chapter on Ductless Glands, dwarfism may be due to disturbances of the pituitary and the thyroid. Dwarfism is part of the picture of cretinism. It also occurs in rickets and sometimes in chondrodystrophia fetalis. In the chapter on Ductless Glands, reference is made to the disturbances of phosphate and calcium metabolism due to renal disease in early life, which may produce renal dwarfism.

Chondrodystrophia Fetalis. This condition has been variously called achondroplasia, micromelia chondromalacia, hereditary deforming chondrodysplasia, multiple cartilaginous exostoses. Different cases show variations and are sometimes separated into different categories, but in our opinion there is an essential unity to all.

The condition affects males far more often than females and although there is a hereditary basis, it is not sex-linked. The cause is unknown; it is not due to rickets or other vitamin deficiency, to infection nor to any identified disturbance of the endocrines. It may be present at birth, but usually develops at about 5 or 6 years of age, the first sign being "round shoulders." Associated with this there is flattening or wedge-shaped deformity of the vertebrae. There is defect in the formation of bone from cartilage, called endochondral bone formation, so that the extremities become short and irregularly bowed, and the bridge of the nose often depressed. The trunk may be of full length.

The early classification of Kaufmann into three types is still used for anatomic distinctions.

IN CHONDRODYSTROPHIA HYPOPLASTICA, the cartilage is underdeveloped and seems incapable of proliferation, but is otherwise normal.

IN CHONDRODYSTROPHIA MALACIA or chondromalacia fetalis, similarly underdeveloped cartilage is soft in consistency.

IN CHONDRODYSTROPHIA HYPERPLASTICA the cartilage is larger than normal and may form massive nodular, irregularly ossified projections about the bone ends. In this condition the term multiple cartilaginous exostoses is often employed. The principal change in the cartilage is loss of the arrangement of cells in regular rows. At the ends of long bones, cartilage may be deficient. Sometimes irregularly disposed masses of cartilage are found in the marrow cavity. Periosteal bone formation proceeds so that as a rule the bones

are normally thick or may appear to be thickened. Curving of the extremities may be due to a greater longitudinal growth along one side of the bone than the other or, in forearm and leg, may be due to greater effect upon one bone than the other. Sometimes there is an unexplained internal hydrocephalus with enlarged head and optic atrophy.

The studies of Underhill, Honeij and Bogert indicate that in the progressive stage of the disease there is a tendency to loss of calcium from the body, and that in both progressive and stabilized stages the magnesium output is increased. (See Graney; Jacobsen.)

Osteogenesis Imperfecta. The manifestations of this disease include fragility of the bones, blue sclerae and otosclerosis. The fault is not in endochondral bone formation, as in chondrodystrophia fetalis, but in periosteum, endosteum and the fibrous osteoplastic tissues of the flat bones of the cranium (Knaggs). Thus there is deficient osteogenesis, which is regarded as due to an inherent hypoplasia of the mesenchyme. The flat bones of the skull show deficient ossification, are soft and rubbery with only a few islands of bone formation. In the long bones the cancellous tissue is delicate, the cortex is thin or absent and the periosteum thick. Osteoblasts are present in small numbers or absent.

There are various types of the disease. The hereditary form may occur in utero, infancy, childhood, or later, and appears to depend upon a dominant mendelian factor (Hills and McLanahan). The fragility and blue sclerae are conspicuous but the deafness may not occur until late. The nonhereditary form may be congenital or may occur in later life as osteopsathyrosis. The blue sclerae are not always present in this form. The teeth may show faults of development (Rushton). There are no clear-cut alterations of mineral or nitrogen metabolism. In a small number of cases, the phosphatase may be increased (Smith and Mitchell).

Fragility of bones is also observed in OSTEOPETROSIS, also called marble-bone disease, osteopathia condensans disseminata, Albers-Schönberg disease, etc. There are two forms, infantile and postpubertal, the former being more frequent. The first manifestation is fracture of bones, with but little or no trauma. The anatomic changes, well shown in the roentgenogram, include marked increase in density of the spongiosa, and more or less marked increase in thickness and density of the cortex of the shafts. Microscopically, there are many trabeculae of dense bone arranged irregularly, and also marked endochondral bone formation. Fractures may heal with excessive callus, and when they occur in fetal life and infancy, healing may be accompanied by deformity and shortening of long bones. The occurrence of myelophthisic anemia is referred to in the chapter on Hematopoietic System. The disease is evidently due to a constitutional fault in differentiation of osseous and hematopoietic tissues. It is familial, but the exact mode of hereditary transmission is not known. (See Clifton, et al.; Baker and Jones; Vidgoff and Brocher.)

Cretinism. Myxedema. These conditions have been referred to in the chapter on Ductless Glands. Cretinism often is associated with a peculiar type of dwarfism. The face is broad, round, with little expression, the forehead low, the lips thick and the bridge of the nose sunken. The fontanelles remain open for a long time; the sphenooccipital synchondrosis persists, leads to little ossification and thus produces the sunken nose.

There is delay of endochondral bone formation throughout, and the epiphyseal disks are clearly visible up to the fifth or sixth year. Periosteal bone formation continues but the bones are either normal in width or more slender. Kaufmann describes cross striations at the diaphyseal border, often visible in roentgenograms, which are probably due to a failure of osteoblasts to grow into the cartilage with a resultant transverse arrangement. When myxedema develops in early life, bone changes similar to those of cretinism may occur.

Increases of Growth

These occur in gigantism and in acromegaly. Local forms accompany hypertrophic osteo-arthropathy, leontiasis ossea and other diseases.

Gigantism. The difference between tallness and gigantism is not entirely an arbitrary measure of stature, although two meters (about 6 feet 6 inches) is set by Schmidt as the point beyond which gigantism may be said to occur. Occasionally, well-proportioned individuals may be seen in excess of this height. As a rule, however, giants are distinguished not only by height, but also by disproportionate growth, in which arms and legs are long and skull small; in some cases the small head may be the only evidence of lack of proportion.

The change is apparently due to excessive endochondral bone formation, which may first be apparent at about the tenth year, and be complete at or somewhere later than the physiologic period of growth. Muscles may be poorly developed and bone formation may be imperfect, with spinal curvature and genu valgum. Gigantism may be the sequence of castration in early life, and is attributed by some to removal of gonadal antagonism to the activity of the pituitary gland. Acromegaly usually affects adults and is different in several characters from true gigantism.

Partial gigantism may affect individual long bones as the result of irritation or hyperemia of the cartilage due to inflammations of bones or joints either pyogenic or tuberculous in nature, or to partial separation of the epiphysis (see Speed). If the process destroy the cartilage the reverse effect occurs.

Acromegaly. Although acromegalics are often spoken of as giants, the condition of the skeleton is more in the nature of a hypertrophy or hyperplasia of some of the bones than it is a uniform overgrowth. The conformation of the face with its sloping forehead and overhanging eyebrows is due to an increase in size of the air sinuses, especially the frontals. The prognathism results from an increase in size of the mandible due principally to periosteal bone formation. The same process is found in the long bones of the extremities, together with bony growth at the points of attachment of muscles and fasciae. The general nature of the condition is discussed in the chapter on Ductless Glands.

Hypertrophic Pulmonary Osteoarthropathy. In patients with various chronic diseases of the lungs, inflammatory, noninflammatory and tumorous, prolonged cardiac decompensation, diseases of liver, diseases of lymph nodes, malignant tumors and syphilis, the ends of fingers and toes may be enlarged and bulbous, the nails rounded in both diameters, the skin thickened and sometimes cyanotic. In some cases there is osteophytosis of the terminal phalanges and of other bones (Crump) but in others, there is only increased vascularity of the subcutaneous tissues of the phalanges.

Leontiasis Ossea. Owing to a widely distributed thickening of the bones of the face, jaws and skull, patients with this disease have the leonine face. The cause is unknown. Knaggs describes two types of bone involvement. One begins as a chronic periostitis in the region of the nose and spreads slowly to the bones of face and skull. The other is a chronic osteitis with great thickening and ivory-hardness of the bones.

Alterations of Nutrition

Atrophy of bones may take place by any of three mechanisms. The most frequent form of atrophy is seen in osteoporosis. This is due to enlargement of the haversian system producing a spongy character of the cortex of bones, often accompanied by thinning of the cortex and enlargement of the marrow cavity. There is evidently a loss of balance between the activity of the osteoblasts and osteoclasts, so that bone destruction proceeds more rapidly than bone formation. Occasionally, atrophy is due to the penetration through the bone lamellae, either from periosteum or marrow, of perforating canals which contain newly formed blood vessels. Whether the canal formation or blood-vessel formation is primary is not known. The condition may heal completely.

In the third form of atrophy there is an osteoid tissue poorly calcified and sometimes fibrous in character. This is said by some to be due to withdrawal of calcium salts from the bones, halisteresis, although others maintain that it is due to excessive activity of the osteoclasts. Atrophy may be eccentric or concentric. Eccentric atrophy begins in the marrow cavity and extends outward. Concentric atrophy begins at the periosteal side and extends inward.

Atrophy may be general or local. The former is said to be endogenous and affects practically all the bones as in the osteoporosis of advanced years and of malnutrition. Local atrophy is said to be exogenous. It affects bones of extremities which are immobilized because of ankylosis of joints, prolonged splinting, or paralysis. More sharply localized is pressure atrophy from compression by tumors, aneurysms and other causes.

The general atrophy or osteoporosis of old age is probably a part of nutritional disturbances, contributed to by arteriosclerosis and inactivity. It occurs as the result of prolonged inanition as in famines, diets deficient in lime and phosphorus, and occurs in experimental animals with biliary fistulae. The changes are probably due principally to decrease in function of osteoblasts. The long bones and vertebrae become porous and fragile, chiefly as the result of lacunar resorption. The bones of the face, the flat bones of the skull and the scapulae show much the same change together with decreased vascularity.

The atrophy of inactivity is manifested as osteoporosis. In an amputation stump the bone ultimately becomes tapered at the end as the result of porous atrophy, concentric in type. The atrophy of lesions of the nervous system is exemplified in bones of the lower extremities in tabes dorsalis and in upper extremities in syringomyelia. Anterior poliomyelitis, occurring in early life, usually results in decrease of growth, but atrophy may ensue. These forms of atrophy are often called neurotrophic, but whether the condition is actually trophic or due to inactivity is not settled.

Pressure atrophy usually shows lacunar resorption accompanied by fibrosis and probably is attributable to increased osteoclastic activity. This is seen in compression by tumors and in the local atrophy about enlarged pacchionian bodies of the dura. Atrophy may occur as the result of compression by aneurysms, but this soon goes on to actual erosion as described in the chapter on the Cardiovascular System.

Rickets. Rickets or rachitis is a disease of early life characterized by disturbance of salt metabolism, especially of calcium and phosphorus, and by deficient deposit of lime salts in the bones due to deficiency of vitamin D. As concerns the bones, the disease affects the growing rather than the mature skeleton. Its first manifestations usually occur at about the fourth month of life, but the time of its beginning is unknown. There is much doubt, however, that it begins in utero. It may develop at about the time of puberty, or somewhat later, when it is designated *rachitis tarda*. It is a disease of urban civilization, principally of Europe and North America, and is more frequent in the winter than in the summer. It appears among animals subjected to the artificial conditions of urban civilization but practically never when they are in the free state.

In children, even though they may be well nourished, the chief manifestations are square head with soft bones (craniotabes), corrugated teeth, enlarged costochondral junctions of the ribs (rachitic rosary), bow-

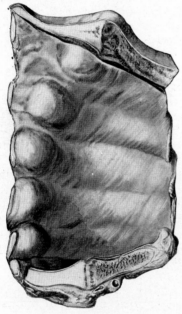

Rachitic rosary, viewed from inside the thorax. A costochondral junction is cut longitudinally to show the rachitic metaphysis.

ing of the long bones and enlargement of the epiphysodiaphyseal junctions. Tetany is frequent. Infantile scurvy is said to be often accompanied by rickets, but in some cases this may be due to confusion of rachitic rosary with somewhat similar enlargement of the rib ends in infantile scurvy.

Although all the bones are softer than normal the striking changes are seen in the long bones. Those of the extremities are likely to be bowed. The ends are large and cartilaginous. A longitudinal section shows a large, poorly ossified epiphysis. The epiphysodiaphyseal junction is broad, poorly

defined, with irregular margins and has a pale blue color. A large amount of spongy osteoid tissue is found near the ends, and sometimes throughout the shaft. The periosteum may be thick. The cortical bone is often thickened, but much less firmly calcified than normal. In ill-nourished children the epiphyseal enlargement may be absent.

For the sake of clarity the microscopic changes are described as they affect the epiphysis and the shaft, although they progress coincidently. In the shaft the principal changes are poor calcification and the presence of an excess of osteoid tissue, especially near the ends of the shaft. The osteoid tissue contains the bone cells and a fibrous matrix without calcification. Osteoporosis and its rarefaction of bone near the periosteum and bone marrow, and enlargement of haversian canals, is common but is not a necessary feature of rickets. The enlargement of the epiphysis is not due to increased cellular proliferation but rather to a failure of absorption as bone formation proceeds. The parallel columns of cartilage cells near the diaphysis are disorganized and irregular, and the blood vessels growing in from the marrow are long and tortuous. The zone of provisional calcification in this area shows a striking decrease or complete absence of deposit of lime salts, although immediately under the perichondrium there may be distinct calcification.

Following the fracture of rachitic bones, the amount of callus is greatly increased and, instead of normal ossification, osteoid tissue is found in large quantities.

Chemically the bones in rickets are deficient in calcium and phosphorus and contain an increased amount of water. No conclusions can be drawn as to the amount of these salts in the soft tissues. In the blood the calcium may be low and the inorganic phosphorus at or near normal; the inorganic phosphorus may be low and the calcium at or near normal; or both may be low. The deposit of salts in the bones, especially calcium, is not necessarily dependent upon the amount in the blood.

Most investigators regard the state of the bones as due to inadequate deposit of salts rather than removal of lime from the bones, halisteresis. A deficiency of calcium or of phosphorus associated with a deficiency of antirachitic vitamin in the diet can induce rickets in animals that are not directly exposed to ultraviolet rays. Whether rickets can result from a deficiency of antirachitic vitamin alone with adequate calcium and phosphorus in the diet and in the absence of direct exposure to ultraviolet rays, is still a matter of controversy.

The basis of vitamin D is ergosterol, a sterol found in the oils of fish and other animals and present in various foods such as egg yolk and butter. Ergosterol is activated by irradiation and the most active component so produced is calciferol. This is synthesized in the skin by the action of ultraviolet rays of sunlight. The influence of sunlight is seen in the frequent absence of rickets in the tropics, seasonal variation of incidence of the disease elsewhere, and the cure of the disease by sunlight or ultraviolet irradiation. (See Park.)

Osteomalacia. In osteoporosis, the matrix of the bone is insufficient in amount or destroyed. In osteomalacia, the matrix is present but is not calcified. It is essentially a form of rickets in adult life, which may affect man, certain mammals and birds. The principal changes are softening of the bones, bowing of the extremities, scoliosis of the spine and deformity of the pelvis.

The disease occurs in three main forms. In the later stages of pregnancy, sometimes also in early puerperium, a form occurs which is usually mild. It is apparently due to a reduced intake of vitamin D and calcium inadequate for both mother and fetus. The growing bone of the fetus utilizes the available calcium and consequently demineralization of the mother's skeleton follows (see Liu et al.). Somewhat similar is the osteomalacia of prolonged malnutrition such as occurs in famines, but often there is a good deal of osteoporosis as well. A mild form, affecting especially spine and pelvis occurs in advanced life, but in this also, osteoporosis may dominate the picture. These forms tend to recovery with institution of proper dietary measures, but permanent deformity often results.

The third form is more severe, progressive and less amenable to dietary treatment. It may result from repeated attacks of the disease in pregnancy, but occurs more often after natural or artificial menopause. In this form, osteoporosis is usually far more marked than is the osteomalacia. The spine and pelvis are the most markedly affected. Administration of estrogenic substance favors positive calcium and phosphorus balance and is of aid in treatment. The interrelationship of mineral metabolism and estrogenic hormones is not clear. (See Albright, Smith and Richardson.) The disease occasionally affects men.

Grossly, the spongy bones show increased porosity. The shafts show an enlarged cavity, and thinning and softening of the cortical parts. The red marrow is often hyperplastic. Fractures are not uncommon. Microscopically, there is a marked increase in osteoid tissue, in spongy bone and in the inner layers of the cortical bone. The bones give the appearance of rickets as the latter might be expected to involve adult bone. Variable degrees of osteoporosis may also be present.

Experimentally, osteomalacia may be produced in mature animals under much the same conditions that induce rickets. Both calcium deficiency and absence of the antirachitic factor appear to be highly important. The bones show much the same chemical changes as in rickets. The blood calcium is about normal in human osteomalacia and the phosphorus low but there is a marked negative calcium balance, both with and without excess of dietary calcium. Gargill, Gilligan and Blumgart found that adequate dosage of vitamins A and D associated with ultraviolet irradiation restores the calcium balance and that retained calcium is deposited as bone.

Scurvy, or Möller-Barlow disease, is a general disease which attacks infants and children more commonly than adults. Its principal manifestations are multiple small hemorrhages and lesions of the bones. It is due to a dietary deficiency of vitamin C, a thermolabile substance found in fresh milk, fruits, especially the orange, and certain vegetables, particularly the potato. Secondary anemia is common, sometimes of chlorotic type and although perhaps contributed to by the hemorrhages, which are probably due to increased capillary permeability as demonstrated by the "capillary resistance test," is principally the result of vitamin C deficiency (Mettier, Minot and Townsend). The small hemorrhages occur in subcutaneous tissue, dentulous gums, and sometimes in the internal viscera, the alimentary canal and frequently under the periosteum of the bones. There is a striking disposition to edema of the skin and certain of the serous cavities; the process in the latter may become exudative in character and lead to adhesions. Rapid heart rate is often observed and at autopsy many cases show hypertrophy of the heart, particularly on the right side. Human scurvy is fully discussed by Hess and the experimental form by Meyer and McCormick.

In infants and children the bones show striking changes. The costochondral junctions are enlarged to resemble closely the rachitic rosary, but in many instances the enlargements are angular and irregular. Similar enlargement may be palpated at the ends of the bones of the extremities, but as a rule the pathologic alteration is more striking in the ribs than in other bones. The lesion involves the junction of diaphysis and cartilage and grossly appears as a curved, transverse, pale yellow bar, the convexity of the curve being toward the bone.

Microscopically, the junction is a field of disorganization in which fragmented trabeculae of spongy bone, recent or old hemorrhage and detritus lie in a confused mass. The number of osteoblasts is reduced. The proliferating columns of cartilage cells are somewhat irregularly arranged and toward the center of the bone are reduced in number. The intervening bony trabeculae are irregular in shape and size. The marrow may be fibrous and may also show the slight hyperplasia of secondary anemia.

In the human marrow the bony trabeculae are usually poorly calcified, but in animals, although very slender, they are well calcified. The corticalis is thin and often the seat of osteoporosis. There is frequently a disjunction of the diaphysis and epiphysis and sometimes the epiphysis is displaced into the poorly calcified diaphyseal end. Fractures of the shaft are not uncommon and are followed by the production of large amounts of callus. Hemorrhage into the periosteum is associated with edema, subsequently organizes and becomes calcified.

In adults the bony lesions are not so marked and the anemia, edema and hemorrhages are prominent. The hemorrhage of the gums only occurs when teeth are present and

appears in the connective tissue immediately under the mucosa. In an experimental analysis of the disease, Wolbach and Howe conclude that it is characterized by an "inability of the supporting tissues to produce and maintain intercellular substances."

Necrosis. Necrosis of bone occurs in inflammations and is often called septic necrosis. In contrast is aseptic necrosis, which is essentially infarction of bone. The necrosis in fractures is due to interference with nutrition. Furthermore, blood supply may be interrupted by dislocations in which nutrient arteries are severed, and as a sequel of occlusive arterial disease such as arteriosclerosis and embolism. It is reported also in caisson disease. When near joints, it may lead to a deforming arthritis. The bony trabeculae in the necrotic focus become fragmented and resorbed. Fibrosis occurs in the region or may encapsulate it. Calcification occurs in the dense fibrous mass, which if encircling may give a roentgen-ray picture of bone cyst. (See Hirsch; Phemister.)

Inflammations

Inflammations of bone usually begin either in the periosteum or in the marrow. Periostitis may be entirely confined to the periosteum and not involve the bone. Osteomyelitis, or inflammation of the marrow, usually involves the bone. The term "osteitis" is usually restricted to those cases where spongy bone is involved without extension to the marrow cavity of the shaft. Inflammation of any of these origins may extend so as to involve marrow, bone and periosteum and is then called panosteitis.

Acute Periostitis. Simple periostitis occurs in children and poorly nourished adults as a result of direct trauma or without known cause. The periosteum is swollen, soft and tender. Microscopically, there are hyperemia, marked edema and infiltration of a few leukocytes. The lesion may heal, sometimes with the formation of small masses of bone, osteophytes, or may progress to more severe forms. It is usually abacterial, but may occasionally contain organisms of low virulence, especially *Staphylococcus aureus*.

Purulent periostitis may be due to infected wounds, to extension from neighboring infections, may be hematogenous or may be secondary to acute infectious diseases. It usually begins in the deeper layers as an exudative inflammation, which rapidly results in the accumulation of pus between the bone and the outer layers of the periosteum. In the more favorable cases the bone is not involved, and the abscess points through the soft tissues and skin with discharge of the contents, and cure. In other cases, the pus may remain and become inspissated to form a cheesy mass, which is finally organized. In less favorable cases the inflammation involves the soft parts, with extensive suppuration, or leads to necrosis of bone and involvement of the marrow.

Occasionally acute purulent periostitis becomes transformed to a so-called albuminous periostitis or "periostitis albuminosa." This is probably due to a reduction of virulence of the bacteria or an incomplete development of resistance of the host. The lesion may also be primary. It runs a subacute or chronic course, and shows in the deeper layers of the periosteum a viscid cloudy fluid which is rich in albumin and contains fibrin, degenerated cells and a few leukocytes; rarely it contains mucoid.

Acute Osteomyelitis and Osteitis. Acute purulent osteomyelitis is most common in early life, affects in order of frequency the femur, tibia, humerus, and is unusual in other bones. It begins usually in the spongy diaphyseal end. Rarely the process may be confined to the epiphysis. In the large majority of cases it is hematogenous in origin and is secondary to pyemia or other acute infectious disease. In a few cases it appears to be primary but is probably secondary to some hidden focus of infection elsewhere. It may be caused by infected wounds, by compound fractures, or result from direct extension from neighboring inflammations. The organisms most commonly found are the pyogenic staphylococci and streptococci, but typhoid bacilli, pneumococcus and other bacteria are occasionally recovered. In the spongy bone or marrow there is a diffuse exudative inflammation with focal abscesses which tend to become confluent. The process extends into the denser bone through the haversian system and may involve periosteum. It may also extend to diaphyseal cartilage, sometimes with diaphyso-epiphyseal separation, to the epiphysis and to the joint.

SEQUESTRUM FORMATION. Necrosis of the bone occurs especially in osteomyelitis, but also in periostitis. This does not necessarily correspond in extent with the severity of the lesion. Experimentally, it has been found that the necrosis is due in part to the products of bacteria and in part to the pressure exerted by the exudate (Cressman and Blalock). The dead bone becomes separated from the living tissue to form a sequestrum. Sequestra may be made up of the central part of the bone, central sequestra, or the peripheral parts, cortical sequestra, or of the entire thickness, total sequestra. Granulation tissue or the inflammatory process may lead to partial or complete destruction of sequestra. When new bone surrounds a sequestrum it is then called an involucrum. The dead bone may be identified by its white color when washed free of blood, or, microscopically, by its entire lack of cellular elements (see Phemister).

COURSE AND SEQUELS. Acute osteomyelitis may have a short or a prolonged course. It may rapidly, or slowly lead to a general septicemia or pyemia. It may be complicated by more or less distant foci in other bones, which are sometimes almost symptomless (silent foci of Phemister). It may regress and remain quiescent, only to become active as the result of accidental or surgical trauma, or local loss of resistance. When it heals, restitution of bone occurs, or there may be residual masses of dense or porous bone.

Chronic fibrous periostitis may occur as a result of acute simple periostitis or accompany chronic lesions of bone or neighboring soft tissues. The periosteum is thick, dense, fibrous and adherent to the bone. It is often difficult to distinguish this lesion from a cicatrization of an acute process.

Chronic Ossifying Periostitis. This differs from the fibrous form in the deposition of new bone. Similarly, it occurs in connection with chronic inflammations and tumors of bone, chronic inflammations of neighboring soft parts, around fractures and foci of necrosis, may occur in rickets and syphilis, and may rarely be primary. The new bone is formed in the deep layers of the periosteum, is of porous, spongy character, with the main trabeculae vertical to the bone surface, and is sometimes covered with compact bone. The nodules or osteophytes may be single, or multiple over a large area. Small

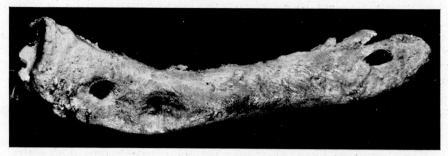

Chronic suppurative osteomyelitis of tibia with two sinuses. Hamann Museum.

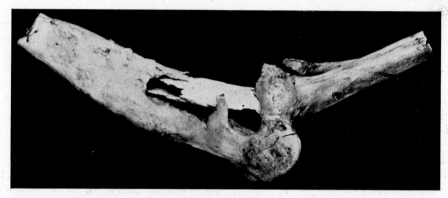

Chronic suppurative osteomyelitis of humerus with sequestrum formation. Hamann Museum.

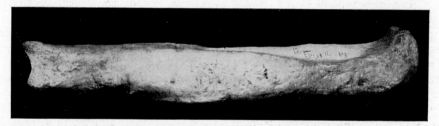

Chronic ossifying periostitis of the tibia. Hamann Museum.

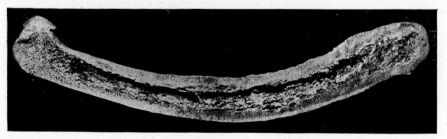

Osteitis deformans of femur. Hamann Museum.

osteophytes may be absorbed. The larger areas may fuse with the underlying bone to constitute a hyperostosis.

Metabolic Craniopathy. Included here for convenience, this is a condition in which the notable lesion is the production of bony masses projecting into the cranial cavity from the frontal bone, or HYPEROSTOSIS FRONTALIS INTERNA. It occurs most often in women past the menopause but may be found in younger women and even in men. There is some indication of hereditary transmission. Endocrine changes such as obesity, hirsutism and virilism, and rarely acromegaly, may be associated, probably because of functional alteration in the pituitary. The condition is often called Morgagni's syndrome. (See Knies and LeFevre.)

Chronic Osteomyelitis and Osteitis. Under a variety of conditions, including prolonged acute osteomyelitis, tumors, fractures, tuberculosis, syphilis, necrosis and other lesions, chronic inflammation occurs. Two forms occur. In rarefying osteitis, there is resorption of bone, a sort of inflammatory osteoporosis. In condensing or ossifying osteitis, there is condensation of bone. Both forms may be combined.

Rarefying osteitis is essentially a formation of granulation tissue from the marrow, and a consequent absorption of bone either as lacunar resorption by enlargement of the haversian system, or by the formation of perforating canals as described in discussing atrophy. The process is of importance in providing for the separation of sequestra.

Caries is a local manifestation of essentially the same process, which leads to a complete breaking down of the bone. It may proceed from the outside as peripheral caries or from the inside as central caries. The soft necrotic bone is usually moist because of exudation of fluid and leukocytes from the granulation tissue, and true pus formation may occur. Less commonly exudation is absent and the lesion is spoken of as dry caries or "caries sicca."

Condensing Osteitis. This proceeds in the outer layers of the marrow and in the haversian system. The marrow becomes dense and fibrous (chronic fibrous osteomyelitis) and new spongy bone is formed which gradually increases in density. Pre-existing spongy bone becomes more and more compact.

The original compact bone increases in density due to deposition of bone in the haversian system. The bone may become extremely dense and of ivory-like hardness, the so-called eburnation of bone. The disease is not common but is seen most often in males younger than thirty years.

The term OSTEOSCLEROSIS is often regarded as synonymous with condensing osteitis but osteosclerosis may present essentially the same changes without any clear sign of inflammation, as for example, in acromegaly. Condensing osteitis is usually limited to one or a few bones, but an osteosclerosis may be widely distributed, for example in osteopetrosis, described above.

Chronic Sclerosing Nonsuppurative Osteomyelitis. This lesion, sometimes called Garré's disease, is usually observed in the lower extremity and presents a fusiform, firm swelling of the shafts of the bone, with reduction in the size of the marrow cavity and a thickened but only slightly adherent periosteum. The cortical bone is eburnated. The marrow may show considerable fibrosis. In some cases there may be necrosis of part of the bone with the formation of a sequestrum. The lesion probably originates in some preceding general infectious disease.

Osteitis Deformans. Paget's Disease of Bone. This, and osteitis fibrosa cystica, are really dystrophies rather than true inflammations, but the name osteitis is so widely used that they are discussed in this section.

Paget's disease of bone, osteitis deformans, or osteodystrophia deformans, is a disease of late life which may be monostotic, polyostotic, or, when it affects only a portion of a bone, merostotic. It is not widely distributed in the skeleton. There is no known cause, but the lesion is found in bones subject to stress, as sacrum, vertebrae and femur. Other bones may also be affected. The trabeculae of spongy bones become prominent and irregular, and the compacta of long bones thick and dense. Microscopically, there are fibrosis and irregularly disposed trabeculae made up of intercalated segments of bone to give a mosaic-like appearance, due apparently to repeated destruction and new formation of bone. Sarcoma may arise more especially in the polyostotic form. (See Jaffe.)

Osteitis Fibrosa Cystica. Von Recklinghausen's Disease of Bone. Also called osteodystrophia fibrosa cystica, this is a general disease due to hyperparathyroidism, discussed in the chapter on Ductless Glands. It occurs in earlier age periods than Paget's disease and is said to affect women more often than men. It is less common than Paget's disease. The condition is accompanied by pain, fractures, and deformities. Parathyroid hyperplasias or adenomas are associated, and the blood shows the high calcium and low phosphorus of hyperparathyroidism.

The bones that are likely to be affected are long bones such as tibia and femur, flat bones of the skull and spongy bones of the vertebrae. The long bones may be curved, sometimes with bulging of the shaft and healed or new fractures. The spongy bones often collapse. Short bones usually escape the disease. Cysts are common and brown nodules may be seen, but the picture is essentially that of rarefaction and fibrosis. There is resorption by the lacunar process and perhaps by perforating canals and a replacement of pre-existing bone and of marrow by cellular fibrous tissue. The "brown tumors" are largely the result of hemorrhage with organization and the production of masses of multinucleated cells, to suggest benign giant cell tumor, but the process is not neoplastic. The origin of the cysts is not clear. Removal of diseased parathyroids results in improvement or cure. (See Jaffe; Hunter; Pick; Gutman and Kasabach, Albright, Sulkowich and Bloomberg.)

OSTEITIS FIBROSA CYSTICA OF ALBRIGHT is a different disease. It is rare and occurs principally in children, especially females. It is characterized by irregularly distributed foci of a fibrotic type of osteitis, areas of cutaneous pigmentation and in females precocious puberty. The bone shows fibrosis, vascularization and infiltration of lymphocytes and large mononuclears. Pathologic fractures may occur. There is no constant disturbance of levels of calcium and phosphorus in the blood, but the blood phosphatase is increased, probably because of osteoblastic activity. (See Neller.)

Osteochondritis of Growth Centers. Harbin and Zollinger classify this lesion as primary or secondary, depending upon whether a primary or secondary center of ossification is first involved. It is usually confined to one center, or, as in the spine, one group of centers. It occurs in childhood and youth and may exhibit tenderness, pain and deformity. Manifestations in particular centers have been given many eponymic terms such as Legg-Perthes disease at the head of the femur, Koehler's disease of the tarsal navicular bone, Osgood-Schlatter disease of the tibial tubercle, etc.

The center shows necrosis, sometimes infiltration of leukocytes, and a fixed-tissue reaction with fibroblasts and mature connective tissue, sometimes with osteoid and islands of cartilage. Neighboring joints may show turbid fluid and villous synovia. Theories of origin include infection, direct and indirect trauma and vascular disturbance. Phemister implicates streptococcal infection, but whether primary or secondary is uncertain. Some are forms of aseptic necrosis, or infarction, due to vascular interruption or occlusion, as discussed above. Harbin and Zollinger believe that direct or indirect trauma is of great significance, but cannot exclude other factors.

Infectious Granulomata

Tuberculosis. Tuberculosis is usually hematogenous, but occasionally may be due to direct extension from neighboring regions, as for example tuberculous lymph nodes. In disseminated miliary tuberculosis, small tubercles are often found in the marrow and sometimes in the periosteum, but the bone remains unaffected. Tuberculous periostitis not uncommonly involves ribs and bones of the face. It may be due to direct extension or may be blood borne. The lesion begins in the deeper layers of the periosteum, becomes caseous and may extend widely along the long bones. The underlying bone may show tuberculous caries.

Tuberculosis of the bone may begin as a tuberculous osteitis or tuberculous osteomyelitis. It is common in childhood and early life but also occurs in adults. Although formerly bovine bacilli were responsible for cases in childhood, at the present time the lesion is practically always due to the human form in children and adults (Amberson). In childhood the bone lesion is often secondary to lymph node tuberculosis and in adults to pulmonary tuberculosis.

The disease tends to attack spongy bone such as vertebrae, ends of long bones, short bones of hand and foot, skull and pelvis, probably because of the rich vascularization with greater likelihood of lodgment of bacilli (see Kolodny). A history of trauma is common, but it is probable that any significance of trauma is in the awakening of latent disease rather than in the establishment of a

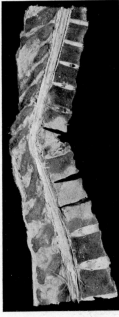

Active tuberculosis of lower thoracic vertebrae. Cross section to show tuberculosis in bodies of vertebrae, destruction of intervertebral disks, compression of ninth thoracic vertebra and angulation of spine with compression of spinal cord.

point of lowered resistance for the lodgment of organisms.

Tuberculous osteomyelitis begins as a small tuberculous mass which gradually enlarges, involves the bone and destroys it. The destruction is usually in the form of a tuberculous rarefying osteitis, but there may also be condensing osteitis. There is little disposition to new bone formation. At times, granulation tissue, with only few bacilli and few tubercles, predominates; the lesion shows little caseation and is called granulating or fungous tuberculosis. The destruction of bone is limited and the process may continue for a long time with little or no deformity. It may, however, become caseous or the process may be caseous from the onset.

Caseous osteomyelitis may produce extensive destruction of bone with sequestrum formation, or sequestration may be due to extensive vascular obstruction by the lesion in the marrow. In contrast to the sequestra of acute osteomyelitis, those of caseous tuberculosis are the seat of rarefaction and are often carious. Sometimes the lesions appear to be cystic in the roentgenogram (Martin). Secondary infection, with suppuration, may be carried in by the blood stream, or enter through fistulae. As the disease penetrates through the bone, it involves the soft parts to produce caseous tuberculosis (cold abscess) which proceeds directly to the surface or along fasciae, as for example, from tuberculous Pott's disease of the vertebrae along the psoas fascias to the groin or buttock.

Syphilis. In congenital syphilis, the usual lesion of the bones is osteochondritis syphilitica. On longitudinal section of the long bones of the newly born congenital syphilitic, the diaphyso-epiphyseal junction shows a more or less broad, irregular, chalky or light yellow zone, instead of the normal straight narrow gray line. Microscopically, M. B. Schmidt distinguished two forms. The one appears to be principally an abnormality of development with a broad zone between diaphysis and epiphysis, in which there is a network of broad bands of calcified cartilage containing marrow. The other, more truly inflammatory, shows in addition to the calcified cartilage, a mass of granulation tissue derived probably from the perichondrial tissue, which projects irregularly into the cartilage. The fragile calcified cartilage permits epiphyseal separation upon slight trauma. *Treponema pallidum* is present in variable numbers. Much less common is progressive ossifying periostitis. Rarely the periosteum shows gumma formation. (Freund.)

The bone lesions of acquired secondary syphilis are found in the periosteum in the form of localized or fairly extensive swellings. The periosteum is the seat of hyperemia, slight edema and infiltration of cells, especially lymphocytes. In later stages of the disease there may be an ossifying chronic periostitis, especially likely to affect the anterior tibial borders and the vertex of the skull. The osteophytes fuse to form more or less extensive hyperostosis, often associated with a similar process in the endosteum and extensive enostosis. Gumma occurs in the periosteum and usually causes destruction of the underlying bone, sometimes with extension into the marrow.

Gummatous osteomyelitis begins either in the marrow or spongy bone as circumscribed, usually multiple nodules, with the characteristic gross and microscopic features of gumma. The enlargement of the lesions causes destruction of bone and formation of sequestra. Whereas in tuberculosis, new bone

of the nose, "saddle nose," is due to destruction of the bones of the septum and bridge, but the gummatous process usually starts in the mucosa and involves the bone secondarily.

Actinomycosis, owing to its common situation near bones, for example the jaw, involves the neighboring bone in a superficial rarefying osteitis and peripheral caries, with underlying granulation tissue.

Leprosy of bones begins as osteomyelitis with the cellular make-up of the lepra nodule, which leads gradually to partial or complete resorption of the affected bone without necrosis or sequestrum formation. It is possible that leprous neuritis produces a trophic atrophy, either with or without leprous osteomyelitis. The loss of distal

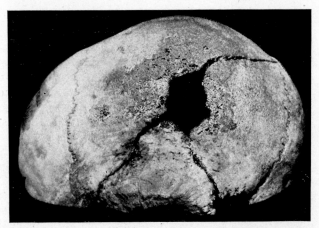

Syphilitic caries of skull. From collection of Dr. Dudley P. Allen.

formation is uncommon, in syphilis it occurs in the immediate neighborhood of the lesion, often with the production of overlying osteophytes and hyperostosis.

Syphilitic caries is especially likely to occur in the flat bones of the skull. It apparently begins as a gummatous periostitis which extends widely into the tables, more particularly as perforating canals, and produces a worm-eaten appearance. It is usually a caries sicca with the formation of large, fragile and spongy sequestra, which remain under the intact fascias and skin. The neighboring bone shows condensing osteitis and the margins are elevated by production of new bone. The destruction is usually confined to the external and superficial part of the middle tables, but may extend through the entire thickness of the skull. Falling of the bridge

phalanges in anesthetic leprosy is due to repeated unsensed trauma and secondary infection with resultant local osteomyelitis.

Hodgkin's Disease frequently shows involvement of the marrow but only rarely is there any destruction of cortex. The involvement of bones in the various lipidoses, such as Gaucher's disease, Niemann-Pick disease and Schüller-Christian syndrome, is discussed in the section on reticulo-endothelial system in the chapter on Hematopoietic System.

Fractures and Their Repair

Fractures, interruptions of continuity of bone or cartilage, may be due to direct violence or to muscular contraction. They are most frequent in the second, third and fourth decades of life and much more common in males than females. Among other predisposing causes, destructive disease of bones is conspicuous, particularly tumors, osteomyelitis, erosion by aneurysms, and such diseases as osteomalacia, osteogenesis imperfecta, etc.

Fractures may be partial, in the form of fissures and "green stick" fractures in children, or complete when the fracture involves the entire thickness. Closed fractures do not communicate with body surfaces; compound fractures either show penetration of bony fragments upon surfaces or are due to injuries, such as gunshot wounds, in which the surface is injured at the same time as the bone. In relation to the line or lines of break, fractures may be longitudinal, transverse, oblique, spiral, V-, T-, or Y-shaped, or com-

from the endosteum and periosteum and is converted into a fibrocartilaginous mass around the fractured ends, i.e., callus. A fusiform enlargement is produced by the periosteal or ring callus. Callus between the fractured ends is called intermediary callus and that which extends for a short distance in the marrow cavity is the internal callus.

This whole mass of provisional callus is gradually reduced as repair proceeds. Bone matrix is formed by endosteum and periosteum, beginning a short distance from the fracture and then penetrating into the callus, especially the intermediary part. This matrix is almost immediately converted into bone with little or no formation of osteoid tissue. As this process continues, the cartilage of the

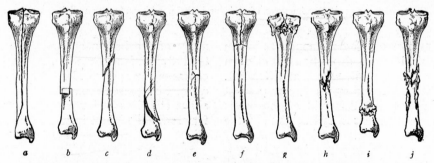

Fractures considered in relation to the character and line of fracture: (a) longitudinal fracture; (b) transverse; (c) oblique; (d) spiral; (e) subperiosteal; (f) V-, T-, or Y-shaped; (g) compression; (h) comminuted; (i) impacted; and (j) crushing.

minuted. Compact shaft may be pushed into the spongy bone at the end to produce impacted fractures. Subperiosteal fractures occur without rupture of periosteum. Fragments may or may not be displaced.

The term pathologic fracture is applied to those in which there is antecedent disease of the bones, such as tumors, primary or secondary, osteoporosis, the forms of osteogenesis imperfecta, chondrodystrophia fetalis, etc. The fracture takes place with only minimal injury, or simply as the result of weight-bearing without any injury noticed by the patient.

Fracture results in hemorrhage in the immediate neighborhood, with hyperemia and often edema. The necrotic bone undergoes decalcification and then destruction of the matrix; fragments are removed by macrophages and foreign-body giant cells rather than by osteoclasts. Granulation tissue grows

callus disappears but osteoblasts may form bone from some of the connective tissue. (See Urist and McLean.)

The regeneration of bone is principally in the intermediate callus. The ring callus is reduced and ultimately disappears almost if not quite completely. The resorption of the internal callus re-establishes the marrow cavity. The new cortex is of about the same thickness as the normal but may be somewhat denser. The strength of healing fractures increases until the medullary cavity begins to form; it then falls, to rise again as the cortex becomes thickened (McKeown et al.).

Physiologically, phosphatase activity is low at the start of healing but rises with active proliferation of bone; the rate of healing seems to depend upon the degree of activity of phosphatase (Tollman et al.). Calcium and phosphorus must be present in adequate amounts in the blood, and there must be an adequate supply of vitamin D as well as of A and C (Hertz).

Union is favored by good apposition of fragments and immobilization, as well as by diets adequate as to minerals and vita-

Tumors

Primary tumors of bone may arise from periosteum, endosteum, perhaps from bone cells, and from marrow. With the exception of marrow tumors and certain others,

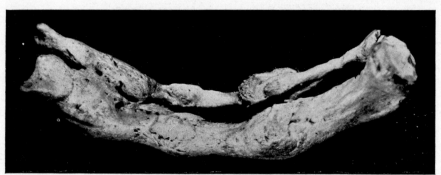

Faulty union of multiple fractures of tibia and fibula, with malposition and excess bone formation. Hamann Museum.

mins. Parathormone does not appear to hasten final repair but the deposition of calcium may be accelerated (Dragstedt and Kearns).

Various factors may delay or prevent union. Thus repair is delayed by osteoporosis of old age or other cause, by infection, by the

many of the benign and malignant tumors tend to produce bone or cartilage in the course of their growth. In an analysis of 1000 cases, Christensen found bone tumors to be about equally distributed among males and females. The highest incidence is in the sec-

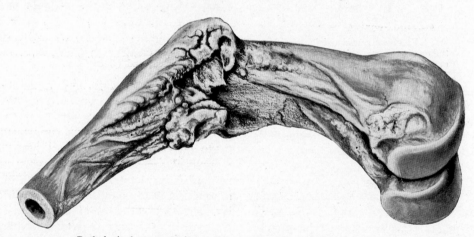

Pathologic fracture of femur due to osteogenic sarcoma of the shaft.

presence of tumors, by poor apposition or incomplete immobilization, by dietary deficiencies, etc. Experimentally, parathyroidectomy delays union, but when calcium is administered, repair proceeds at a normal rate. It is said that thyroidectomy, ovariectomy and perhaps other endocrine disturbances delay repair (Kolodny). In delay or nonunion, the fractured ends are held together by fibrous tissue and are freely movable so as to constitute a "mobile joint" or PSEUDARTHROSIS.

ond decade, but about one third the cases occur after the thirtieth year. The following classification is that proposed by Ewing and adopted by the American College of Surgeons in 1939.[1]

Benign Tumors. FIBROMA is much more frequently periosteal (peripheral) than endosteal (central) in origin and, although

[1] By permission from Ewing: Neoplastic Diseases, 4th ed., W. B. Saunders and Co., 1940; p. 295.

	Malignant	*Benign*
1. Osteogenic series	a. Medullary and subperiosteal b. Telangiectatic c. Sclerosing d. Periosteal e. Fibrosarcoma, medullary, subperiosteal	Exostosis Osteoma
2. Chondroma series	a. Chondrosarcoma b. Myxosarcoma	Chondroma
3. Giant-cell series	a. Benign, malignant	Epiphyseal giant-cell tumor
4. Angioma series	a. Angio-endothelioma b. Diffuse endothelioma	Cavernous angioma Plexiform angioma
5. Myeloma series	a. Plasma-cell b. Myelocytoma c. Erythroblastoma d. Lymphocytoma	

6. Reticulum-cell sarcoma

7. Liposarcoma

uncommon, affects the bones of the face more often than other bones. Fibromas may grow in the bony air sacs and are sometimes found in the tooth sockets or jaw as fibrous epulis. They may calcify, ossify, or become cystic. They should not be confused with old granulation tissue. Rarely fibroma arises from the connective tissue of the marrow, is benign and cured by thorough curettage (Jaffe and Lichtenstein).

MYXOMA, as a pure tumor, is rare and arises in periosteum more often than in endosteum. Usually the tumor is a myxochondroma. In either case there is a decided tendency to recur after removal.

ANGIOMA, originating from either blood or lymph vessels, is rare, usually central and shows telangiectases. Situated in vertebrae, hemangioma may sometimes produce signs of compression of the cord (Kelly). Rarely hemangiosarcoma occurs as a multiple lesion (Hauser).

OSTEOCHONDROMA in this classification includes osteoma and chondroma, neither of which is likely to occur in pure form, as well as various combinations of these with each other and with fibrous and mucoid tissue. The combination may be so complex as to be spoken of as fibro-osteomyxochondroma or may show fewer elements.

OSTEOMA. The principal members of this group are the exostoses and enostoses. It is difficult and often impossible to distinguish these tumor forms from the osteophytes of inflammatory origin. The exostoses and enostoses grow from bone and may be spongy, medullary if they contain marrow, compact or eburnated. Two subvarieties are discussed by Schmidt as cartilaginous and fibrous exostoses, both of which are likely to be multiple. The cartilaginous exostoses begin in the cartilaginous part of the diaphyso-epiphyseal junction, show bone centrally and cartilage peripherally, extend down the metaphysis and shaft as the bone grows and cease to grow when the bone is mature. The fibrous exostoses originate in periosteum, tendons or fascias. The periosteal forms are seen most often on the flat bones of the skull; the tendinous and fascial forms represent excessive growth of normal tuberosities and bony crests.

CHONDROMA. This may be single or multiple and usually appears in the interior of the bone as enchondroma. Ecchondroma is rare. The enchondroma affects the phalanges of the hand and may be bilateral. Less often it occurs in the foot, the pelvis, the scapula and other bones of endochondral type of growth. The tumor presumably originates in remnants of growth cartilage.

The microscopic examination shows irregularity in arrangement and often of size of the cells and lacunae. The intercellular tissue may be osteoid in character, producing the osteoid chondroma. Bone formation, producing the osteochondroma, is frequent. The tumor, even though neither microscopically nor grossly malignant, shows a striking tendency to recur after removal. This is true also of the more complex tumors.

Chondrosarcoma is likely to be central rather than peripheral, extends through marrow cavity and through bone cortex. Curable by early amputation, nevertheless it may metastasize and produce death. It deserves separation from the group of osteogenic sarcoma because of somewhat lesser degree of malignancy (Phemister).

GIANT-CELL TUMOR OF BONE. This is a disease which occurs principally in early

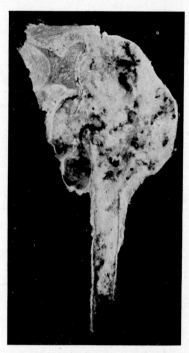

Chondrosarcoma of head of humerus. Cross section. Note thinning of and penetration through cortex, extension through marrow and upper margin of a pathological fracture.

adult life. It affects the spongy ends of long bones, but may rarely occur in the shaft. Grossly, it is a somewhat poorly defined, dark red, bleeding, soft, friable mass. Microscopically, it is well vascularized and composed of a stroma of short spindle cells with little collagen formation. Intermingled are variable numbers of multinucleated giant cells. These have a rich cytoplasm and contain a few or many fairly dense nuclei. The nature of these cells is not clear; some think they are foreign-body giant cells and others that they are giant osteoclasts. As a general rule, these tumors are benign but there are occasional instances of metastasis.

Jaffe and his associates classify the tumors into three grades of increasing invasiveness, according to the character of the stroma. In grade I, the stromal cells are uniform in appearance, abundant and compact. In grade II, the stromal cells are not so compact and often disposed in whorls; tumors of this order may recur and become malignant. The grade III tumors are frankly invasive and metastasize. The stroma is loosely arranged, there is much pleomorphism of cells and many mitotic figures. Although the cortex may be thinned in any of the giant-cell tumors and new bone formation is not evident, these authors maintain that there are no characteristic or diagnostic roentgenographic features. The tumors are usually cured by thorough curettage or excision; irradiation by roentgen rays is useful in surgically inaccessible tumors.

Malignant Tumors. Osteogenic Sarcoma. The cells of the osteogenic sarcomas are principally spindle cells, variable in size and outline and often so short and rounded as to look like round cells. Ewing, however, maintains that round cells arise only from the marrow. The nuclei show great variability in chromatin arrangement and content. The intercellular substance varies much in amount, may be fibrous or hyaline, osteoid or osseous. The vascular supply is also variable in amount, almost always sarcomatous in character with close apposition of tumor cells, and the vessels not infrequently contain tumor thrombi. The more cellular, rapidly growing tumors are likely to invade the neighboring soft parts, and to metastasize early and widely by way of the blood stream.

The fibrocellular osteogenic sarcoma is best exemplified by the PERIOSTEAL SPINDLE-CELL SARCOMA. This originates in the deeper layers of the membrane, attacks long bones, especially of the extremities, and nearly always develops near the ends of the shaft. Its growth is often rapid, extends around the shaft as a dense spindle-formed enlargement and, while it may not penetrate into the bone, often does so with the formation of a smaller mass within the spongy bone or marrow cavity. Bone formation is usually moderate in amount, as spongy masses, but may be extensive and lead to a bony hardness of the entire tumor. Lines of bone formation radiate out from the shaft. Although usually of large spindle type, the cells may be small and rounded or large and polyhedral. The larger polyhedral cell tumors may show much cartilage with little bone or may be almost entirely devoid of both.

THE TELANGIECTATIC SARCOMA may arise in any part of the bone, but is somewhat more often central than peripheral. It invades so rapidly as a rule, that the periosteum does not form a new layer of bone. Microscopically, the cells are usually rounded or polyhedral, lack uniformity in size, and many of the nuclei are hyperchromatic. It is characterized by the presence of many large vascular spaces, from which hemorrhage is not infrequent. Foreign body giant cells may be so numerous as to suggest benign giant-cell sarcoma, but the vascularization and the types of tumor cell are usually sufficiently characteristic.

THE SCLEROSING OSTEOGENIC SARCOMA is not common and is central more often than peripheral. It is characterized by slow growth and the formation of new bone in the tumor, which may become extremely dense. It invades pre-existing bone, the shaft of which may be much enlarged, to form a solid spindle form swelling. The cellular parts show the usual arrangement of sarcoma. In spite of the slow growth, metastasis is frequent.

Occasionally, what appear to be osteogenic sarcomas originate in soft tissues, but these are probably originally carcinomas, in which the connective tissue undergoes hyalinization, vascularization and bone formation of neoplastic character (Binkley and Stewart).

BONE ANEURYSMS. In discussing the bone sarcomas, mention of the so-called aneurysms of bone is necessary. These are usually situated near the ends of long bones, are more or less invasive, often pulsate and sometimes a bruit is audible. Ewing expresses the view that most of these are telangiectatic osteogenic sarcomas, in which the vessels are extremely large and the cellular content much reduced in amount. Others may be due to softening of a giant-cell tumor, so that blood flows directly through the large central space. They are not aneurysms in the strict sense of the word.

MYELOMA SERIES. The tumors of this general group and the reticulum-cell sarcoma are discussed in the chapter on Hematopoietic System. The myeloma is almost always multicentric in origin and is derived from the marrow of ribs, sternum, skull and other bones. There is usually an associated Bence-Jones albumosuria. The tumor invades the bone and may extend into the soft parts. Metastases to the viscera are not rare. New tumors in other bones are probably a manifestation of system disease rather than metastases. The tumors are soft, gray, poorly defined, well vascularized and may be made up of plasma cells, or their derivatives. They do not form bone. (See Geschickter and Copeland.)

ENDOTHELIOMA. These tumors are included in the angioma series in the classification given above, indicating that the cells of the tumors probably arise from vascular endothelium, although this cannot be established for all forms. The tumors of this order usually occur in one bone, but rarely may involve several. They are richly cellular, well vascularized, invade the bone and soft parts but do not metastasize readily. They may be accompanied by severe anemia. They are readily susceptible to treatment by roentgen rays, but are not permanently cured and recur.

There are three principal forms. The solitary cystic telangiectatic angio-endothelioma affects the ends of long bones as a large, invasive, highly vascular mass which sometimes has the character of bone aneurysm. The multiple endothelioma affects a large number of bones, especially spongy bone, as small tumor nodules. The solitary diffuse endothelioma is the form often referred to as "Ewing's tumor" and as endothelial myeloma. It occurs in the shaft of a long bone with absorption of the bone and thickening of the organ as a whole. Other bones may be involved subsequently, and metastasis to the viscera is not uncommon.

Microscopically, the telangiectatic form shows a pseudo-alveolar arrangement of large polyhedral cells with loosely arranged cytoplasm and relatively small nuclei. The tumor is richly vascularized and shows wide, cavernous blood spaces. The multiple endothelioma shows cells of the same type, arranged in sheets, sometimes multinucleated, but the large vascular spaces are infrequent or absent. These tumors often resemble carcinoma metastases. The solitary, diffuse form shows broad sheets of cells similar to those in the other forms, but usually smaller, and

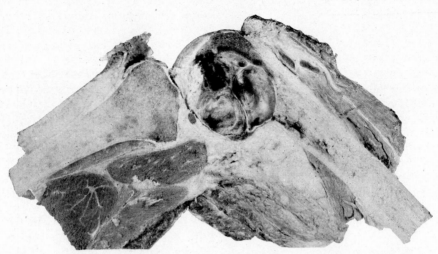

Osteogenic sarcoma of the lower end of the femur, telangiectatic in type. Army Medical Museum, 17904.

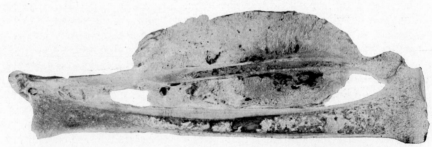

Osteogenic sarcoma of fibula and tibia, periosteal in origin. Army Medical Museum, 17872.

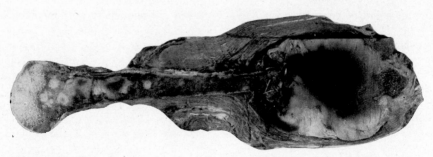

Multiple myeloma of humerus, which at one end has become invasive. Army Medical Museum, 17871.

the picture may suggest lymphosarcoma. (See Geschickter and Copeland.)

LIPOSARCOMA. This is derived from the fat of the marrow. There is a tendency to multiplicity of lesions and probably some of these are metastases into bone from the original bone tumor. Ultimately metastasis occurs to soft tissues, especially the lungs. Grossly, the tumor is soft, grayish yellow and often lobulated. Microscopically, the appearance varies greatly. Usually there are interlacing large spindle cells with blunted ends. Intermingled are small round cells like those of embryonal fat. In some cases the cells are large with vesicular cytoplasm, so that the lesion may be confused with metastasis from adrenal or renal carcinoma. (See Ewing; Duffy and Stewart.)

Metastatic Tumors. Practically any carcinoma may metastasize to bones but metastasis is most common with carcinomas of prostate, breast, thyroid and kidney. The metastasis is usually by blood vascular routes, but may occur through the lymphatics. The establishment of metastases is especially frequent in the spongy red marrow and is not dependent on proximity to the original tumor except in metastasis from carcinoma of the prostate or thyroid. The situation of the metastases is variable, but as a rule they are found most often in vertebrae, pelvis, femur, skull, ribs and humerus. Metastases from sarcomas are secondary to soft-tissue sarcomas; only exceptionally, as with the liposarcoma, do bone sarcomas metastasize to bone.

The metastases of most tumors destroy bone and are said to be osteoclastic. More especially with metastases from the prostate, the metastases may stimulate bone production and are osteoplastic. The manifestations of phosphatase activity are generally proportional to the osteoplastic properties of primary and secondary tumors, except that in metastases from prostatic carcinoma the tumor itself appears to be responsible for the production of acid phosphatase. (See Willis; Geschickter and Copeland.)

Cysts

Cysts of the bones may be monolocular or multilocular. They may result from the breakdown of benign or malignant tumors, or from hemorrhages, and are common in osteitis fibrosa, where, according to Bloodgood, they occur principally in the shafts of long bones. Cysts of the jaw have been discussed in the chapter on alimentary canal.

Parasites

Echinococcus cyst of the bones affects spongy bones especially, and produces atrophy of bone by pressure. Sequestra may result from necrosis due to loss of blood supply. Penetration of the bone leads to thickening of the periosteum and hyperostosis. Fractures may result from destruction of the bone.

JOINTS

Congenital Anomalies

The most important of these is congenital dislocation of the hip. This occurs much more frequently in females than males and in about one-third the cases is bilateral. It is due in most cases to a hypoplasia of the acetabulum, so that the socket is flattened, associated with which the head of the femur is often of somewhat conical shape. In contrast to traumatic dislocations, the joint capsule and ligaments are not ruptured, but are stretched and thickened. The head of the femur is displaced upward toward the dorsum ilii, usually posterior, sometimes anterior. Malposition of extremities in utero may lead to partial dislocation of joints. Traumatic dislocations may occur during labor.

Probably of congenital origin is the so-called herniation of the nucleus pulposus of the intervertebral disc, in which this portion of the disc projects into the spongiosa of the vertebral body. (See Donohue.)

Circulatory Disturbances

Hemorrhage is usually due to injury. The blood may remain fluid for a long time and apparently may be completely absorbed. If clots form they undergo organization, sometimes with slight fibrous adhesion of joint surfaces. In either event the synovial membrane is likely to show hemosiderin pigmentation. Pigmentation of this membrane also occurs in hemochromatosis and in hemorrhagic diseases.

Joint Lesions in Hemorrhagic Diseases. Lesions of the joints, which should not be confused with those of infectious or rheumatic origin, may occur, especially in hemophilia but also in other hemorrhagic diseases, particularly purpura. Hemorrhage into the cartilage and joint may be followed by fibrosis and pigmentation of the synovial membrane, as well as some calcification. The cartilage may show degeneration and erosion as far as the bone (see Freund).

Inflammation

Acute Inflammations. ACUTE ARTHRITIS may be primary or secondary, monarticular or polyarticular. Primary arthritis may be due to trauma, especially penetrating injuries. Included also are those forms in which, even although the infectious agent be blood borne, the lesion is found especially in the joints with minor or no lesion at the portal of entry. Secondary arthritis may be due to direct extension of inflammation from the neighboring bone or soft parts, or may be hematogenous.

The hematogenous forms occur in infectious diseases, notably in pyemia, also in many others such as typhoid fever, erysipelas and the acute exanthemata, pneumococcal infections and gonorrhea. These are often spoken of as metastatic arthritides, and in certain diseases such as typhoid, erysipelas, pneumococcal and gonococcal infections the organisms can be recovered from the joints, but in the exanthemata it is difficult to say whether the joint lesions are truly metastatic, or are due to poisonous products of the disease. In the latter case, the condition is often called toxic arthritis.

ACUTE SEROUS ARTHRITIS is usually monarticular, may be due to trauma, to infection, or may occur without known cause. The inflammation affects mainly the synovial membrane and shows hyperemia, edema and serous exudation into the joint cavity. The disease either heals or may become chronic with fibrosis of the membrane. If bacterial in origin it may progress to suppuration.

ACUTE SEROFIBRINOUS ARTHRITIS is usually of bacterial origin, the organisms gaining entrance either by direct infection or by blood transport. It is usually polyarticular. The inflammation is confined to the synovial membrane, but the surrounding parts may be the seat of hyperemia and edema. The membrane is covered with a thin film of fibrin, and flocculi are present in the fluid.

The cavity is filled and somewhat distended with cloudy limpid fluid, which contains in addition to the fibrin a moderate number of leukocytes and mononuclear cells. The lesion may heal completely or there may be slight residual fibrous adhesion. This is the kind of lesion seen in acute rheumatic fever.

Acute suppurative arthritis is due principally to direct extension from neighboring foci of suppuration, when it is usually monarticular; or due to blood transport, as in pyemia or other infectious disease, when it may be either monarticular or polyarticular. The pus in the cavity may be small in amount or may be mixed with serum to fill the sac. Usually the inflammation involves the periarticular structures and is especially serious because of destruction of cartilage. Suppurative osteitis may then ensue. If the cartilage be spared, the lesion may heal with contraction of the capsule and fibrous adhesion of joint surfaces (false ankylosis). If the bone be laid bare and the lesion heal, the apposed bony surfaces organize and ossify to form a permanent union (true or bony ankylosis). The destruction of cartilage is greatest at the points of closest contact between the articular surfaces (Phemister).

Rheumatic Fever. The general manifestations of this disease have been discussed in the chapter on Infectious Diseases. The character of the lesion in the joints is one of the features that points toward the allergic nature of rheumatic fever. The arthritis is usually polyarticular and migratory. The joints are swollen, red, painful and tender, and as one clears up, another may become involved. The synovial membrane shows hyperemia, proliferation of lining cells and sometimes small areas of necrosis. The joint contains serous or fibrinoserous exudate. The periarticular structures are hyperemic and edematous, and show diffuse and focal cellular infiltrations, the latter resembling Aschoff bodies. (See Sacks.)

Gonococcal Arthritis. Cases with monarticular and polyarticular involvement are about equally distributed. It complicates genital and occasionally other gonococcal infections of long standing and deep situation. The monarticular form involves especially the knee, but other joints may be affected. The acute disease may persist for a long period with amelioration of symptoms. The joint may show simply a serofibrinous inflammation, or it may become purulent with suppurative involvement of the periarticular structures. The polyarticular form may be like the monarticular, but may also be migratory and resemble rheumatic fever. Gonococci may be grown in pure culture, especially if the lesion be suppurative and monarticular. Failure of cultivation from some of the polyarticular cases, suggests that they are part of a general infectious process, or perhaps represent allergic phenomena similar to those of rheumatic fever. (See Keefer and Spink.)

Chronic Arthritis. This term includes a variety of chronic lesions of the joints, difficult of classification because of combinations of lesions. The involvements of synovial membrane, of cartilage, of bone and of joint capsule are usually sufficiently distinctive to permit of a fair degree of differentiation. Included as a chronic arthritis is the dry ulcerative form, which has little or no inflammatory reaction. Arthritis deformans constitutes the great group of chronic non-tuberculous inflammations of the joints.

CHRONIC DRY ULCERATIVE ARTHRITIS occurs in the aged and is usually monarticular with involvement of the hip joint, but may affect knee, shoulder, elbow or fingers. The lesion is probably of nutritional origin. The principal findings are degeneration, atrophy and fibrosis of the cartilage. The ulceration is usually superficial but may lay bare the bone; reaction in cartilage or bone is slight or absent. The synovial membrane may become thickened and fibrous.

Arthritis Deformans. This is generally divided into two forms, (a) the chronic adhesive, proliferative or synovial type, and (b) osteo-arthritis, degenerative arthritis or chondro-osseous arthritis. The causes are not known and the distinctions are based on anatomical and clinical manifestations. We employ the terms chronic adhesive arthritis and osteo-arthritis because they have wider usage.

CHRONIC ADHESIVE ARTHRITIS, the proliferative type of Nichols and Richardson, the synovial type of Fisher, is also spoken of as rheumatoid arthritis or chronic rheumatism. It is a progressive disease, often polyarticular in distribution. The lesion begins in the synovial membrane, usually at the margins of the cartilage, as a growth of vascularized connective tissue, granulomatous in type, which gradually extends over the articular surface. With the thickened synovial surface, or articular pannus, the deeper connective tissues of the synovia and of the perichondrium are involved. This may result simply in fibrous adhesions between the joint surfaces, but frequently the underlying cartilage disintegrates and the bone may be irregularly denuded of cartilage and covered only by the granulation, or denser fibrous, tissue. The connective tissue of the marrow proliferates in the form of granulations and there follows a new formation of osteoid, and then of bony trabeculae. Bony union between the joint surfaces, bony ankylosis, may be brought about by ossification of fibrous adhesions, or by ossification of proliferating cartilage, or by endosteal bone formation in the epiphyses. In some cases synovial tags, like those of osteo-arthritis, are formed. Subluxations are not uncommon and ankylosis may fix the joints in abnormal position.

OSTEO-ARTHRITIS, the degenerative form of Nichols and Richardson, the chondro-osseous form of Fisher, the great second type of Ely, is regarded by many as the lesion included in the term arthritis deformans, or chronic deforming arthritis. The primary change is in the cartilage, usually in the center, in the form of fibrillation associated with softening of the hyaline matrix and a disappearance of the fibrous part of the perichondrium. Many of the cartilage cells disappear, but others show multiplication. The erosion of the cartilage is irregularly distributed and the opposite articular surface may show proliferation of cartilage or bone. Thus, the cross section of the joint surfaces may be markedly irregular. This may produce interlocking with limitation of motion, but no true ankylosis is likely to occur.

Loss of cartilage may expose a fairly large part of the end of the bone, which undergoes osteosclerosis, and as the result of joint motion gains a porcelain-like polish, eburnation. There is also a bony proliferation which produces the so-called lipping of the joint, an irregular marginal projection of bone. This is probably due to a proliferation of perichondrium at its junction with the capsule, which ossifies, and the process may be contributed to by periosteal bone formation from the margin of the epiphysis. It should not be confused with slight lipping that is common in persons of more than thirty-five years of age, without joint lesions. The synovial membrane and the capsule may be markedly fibrotic.

From the synovial membrane, especially at the joint margins, numerous sessile

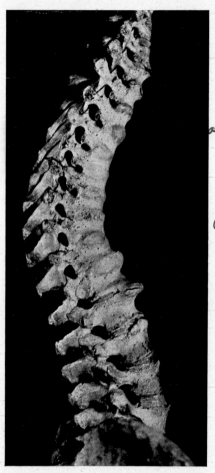

Osteo-arthritis of spinal column, showing lipping of the joint borders and bony bridges between adjacent vertebral bodies. Hamann Museum.

or pedunculated masses of connective tissue may grow, in villous arrangement. These may be of vascularized connective tissue or edematous fibrous tissue. The tissue may differentiate to form cartilage, bone or fat, "lipoma arborescens." The little masses may break loose from their peduncles and appear free in the cavity as "joint mice." Subcutaneous nodules occur, principally on the dorsum of

the forearm, which show foci of necrosis surrounded by large mononuclear cells, marked dense fibrosis and peripheral subacute arteritis (Dawson and Boots). Similar are the so-called Heberden's nodes, which occur near the finger joints and appear to have a hereditary basis (Stecher).

CHRONIC INFECTIVE ARTHRITIS may be monarticular, but is usually polyarticular, and may involve spine, wrists, knees, ankles, tarsal joints and finger joints. It appears to be associated with foci of infection, for example in the tonsils, the alveolar processes and the deeper genitalia. Pathologically, it is the milder form of synovial chronic arthritis, often with villus formation, but may become *i. e. adhesive* more severe. Its tendency is toward recovery, especially after removal of the focus of infection, in contrast to the progressive character of both forms of arthritis deformans. Similar lesions have been produced experimentally by the injection of various cocci (Nathan).

Chronic adhesive The cause of arthritis deformans is unknown. Rheumatoid arthritis usually begins before 50 years of age, may be associated with trauma and various infectious diseases. By some it is thought to be of infectious origin (see Cecil), but this is contradicted by others (see Blair and Hallman). Pemberton believes the joint lesions to be due to decreased oxidation, the result of vasoconstriction. Osteo-arthritis is usually found in patients over 50 years of age and may be associated with trauma, dislocations, bone tumors and nervous diseases. Identical changes in the joints are found as the result of advancing age. (See Parker et al.)

STILL'S DISEASE is a chronic polyarthritis in children, probably of infectious origin, with synovial hyperplasia, with peripheral involvement of the cartilage, thinning and perforation of the central parts of the cartilage, and rarefaction of the bone. This is usually thought to be a juvenile form of rheumatoid arthritis. The systemic nature of the disease is indicated by enlargement of spleen and lymph nodes the result of a chronic hyperplasia. Secondary amyloidosis may occur. (See Portis.)

chr adhesive In adults, rheumatoid arthritis may be accompanied by enlargement of spleen and lymph nodes, with anemia and leukopenia. Although often called *Felty's syndrome*, Cur-

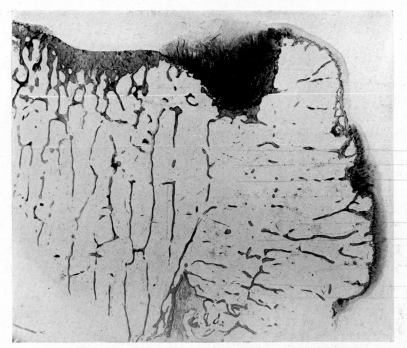

End of tibia in osteo-arthritis to show fibrillation of marginal cartilage and central loss of cartilage with osteosclerosis. Lower part of field under the cartilage shows remains of cortex and to the right is bone formation as part of lipping of the joint.

tis and Pollard consider these additional changes as incidental and variable; they recommend abandoning the term.

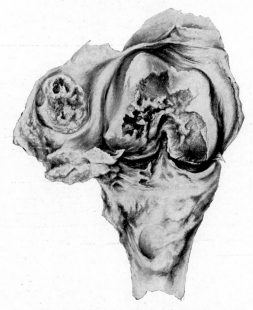

Chronic infective arthritis of the knee. The central parts of the cartilage are eroded and the peripheral parts preserved.

Infectious Granulomata

Tuberculosis. As with bones, tuberculosis may affect the joints at any period of life, but is especially common in childhood. In childhood, bovine bacilli are sometimes the cause. Most cases are secondary to obvious tuberculosis elsewhere and due to hematogenous transport. Nichols expresses the view that the bacilli always lodge first in the bone marrow, although most agree (Ely) that the lesion may originate either in the marrow or in the synovial membrane. As with bones, trauma probably excites a pre-existent lesion instead of furnishing a point of diminished resistance. The spine is most frequently affected, and next in order the hip, knee, and tarsus, elbow, wrist, and shoulder.

Primary synovial involvement, less common pathologically than the primary diaphyseal form, usually affects the knee. The membrane is the seat of an acute or subacute inflammation, shows numerous small tubercles, and the cavity becomes filled with a fibrinoserous exudate. As a rule, the periarticular structures, the cartilage and the bone are not involved.

Beginning in the marrow of the diaphysis, rather than in the epiphysis, tuberculosis extends to the joint and invades along the capsule and the margins of the cartilages. Phemister points out that in contrast to pyogenic infections, the articular surfaces of the cartilages may remain free for a long time. Indeed the lesion may remain in the capsule and periarticular tissues as a tuberculous granulation tissue, producing "white swelling," for a considerable period before the joint is invaded.

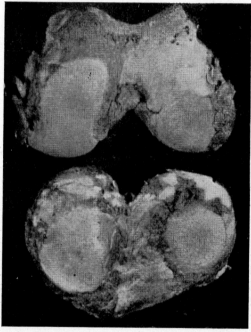

Tuberculosis of knee. Cartilage preserved where patella and tuberosities come in contact with femur, and partly destroyed along unopposed surfaces of tibia and femur. From Phemister, D.B., Annals of Surgery.

Involvement of the joint is usually in the form of a villous arthritis. Tuberculous granulation tissue grows from the capsule and synovia and destroys cartilages, especially at the margins. The cavity contains a cloudy, thick, semipurulent fluid which contains leukocytes, fibrin, desquamated fatty degenerated cells from synovial membrane, and tubercles, but only a small number of bacilli. The formation of villi, like those of osteo-arthritis, may be extensive. In severe cases, the granulation tissue may destroy all or nearly all the cartilage by growth over the surface as pannus, or extension between cartilage and bone. This is followed by tuberculous caries of the bone end. Tuberculosis does not ordinarily stimulate new bone formation, and therefore ankylosis does not occur.

Frequently the exudate of tuberculous arthritis contains the so-called "rice bodies," small, flat or oval, pale yellow, firm masses a few millimeters in diameter. They are made up of fibrotic or hyaline fibrin, or may be derived from small masses of granulation tissue broken off by the joint movements.

Syphilis. Joint manifestations occur, in congenital syphilis and in early acquired syphilis, but little is known of their exact nature. In late acquired syphilis, gummatous involvement of the joint may be secondary to lesions in the synovial membrane or the bone end. The cartilage may be destroyed and the joint surface nodular. The synovial membrane may become markedly fibrotic and adherent. Living spirochetes have been recovered (Chesney et al.).

Leprosy may be accompanied by a joint lesion like osteo-arthritis, or in the neural form may exhibit neuropathic arthropathy.

Coccidioidal granuloma occurs in bones and joints, in characteristic form, and may be confused clinically with tuberculosis (Ely).

Special Lesions

Gout. Although many lesions of joints are suspected of being metabolic in origin, this conception is unqualifiedly applicable to gouty arthritis. It may be monarticular or polyarticular and is especially prone to occur in the metatarsophalangeal articulation of the great toe, and also in the fingers and hand. The lesion may be entirely periarticular, or may involve capsule, synovia, cartilage and bone. Wells accepts the view that the deposit of urates, especially sodium mono-urate, is the primary event. If the deposit be rapid, hyperemia, edema and inflammation occur. If the deposit be slow, there is only little reaction and ultimately slight fibrosis. Necrosis occurs secondarily in the area of deposition. The destruction of cartilage may be merely an ulceration with fibrillation of the hyaline matrix, or adhesion with fibrous ankylosis may result.

Neuropathic Arthropathies. More especially in tabes dorsalis and syringomyelia, but also in other diseases of the cord, lesions of peripheral nerves and of the cerebrum (Shands), the joints may be involved. This is usually monarticular in larger joints such as knee, hip, shoulder or elbow. The onset is often abrupt with a considerable exudation of fluid into the joint. It may for a time closely resemble osteo-arthritis, but is different clinically in that it is painless. It usually progresses to, or may be primarily, the destructive lesion of joint structures and bone referred to as Charcot's joint.

ferred to above as joint mice. According to Ely three classes are recognized, those which result from intra-articular fracture, those due to disease, especially osteo-arthritis, and those of uncertain origin spoken of as "essential joint mice." As to whether this last group is caused by loss of nutrition and sloughing (osteochondritis dissecans of Koenig), to embolism of bacteria or fat, or to fracture has not been finally established. Phemister states that after detachment, degenerative and proliferative processes take place, in that the

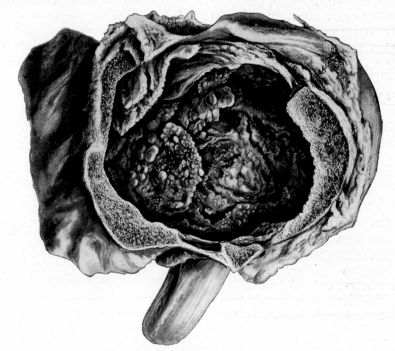

Neuropathic arthropathy (Charcot joint) of knee.

The destruction involves synovia, cartilage and often a considerable extent of bone, leaving a large joint cavity filled with clear or slightly cloudy fluid. With the destruction of articular surface and bone, the capsule becomes fibrotic, the joint becomes flail-like and subject to subluxations and dislocations. In some cases there is, in addition to the destruction, a proliferation of cartilage and bone to form irregular, projecting masses in the joint, which may become free bodies. Often there occurs marked lipping, sometimes with bony and cartilaginous masses in the capsule and periarticular structures. (See Moritz.)

Loose Bodies. These have been re-

original cartilage and bone undergo gradual necrosis, and there is a subsequent proliferation of fibrocartilage which becomes calcified or ossified.

Tumors

Lipoma, fibroma and various types of sarcoma occasionally occur.

Synovioma. Peculiar to synovia of joints, bursae and tendon sheaths is a group of tumorous lesions called synovioma or syovial sarcoma. This is a disease of early middle life, but not exclusively so. It affects males more often than females and although it may occur in various situations, is most frequent in the region of the knee and elbow. It usually grows slowly over the course of several years. De Santo, Tennant and Rosahn describe three forms, encapsulated, circumscribed and diffuse. The encapsulated form usually arises in a para-articular bursa, the circumscribed form in a bursa or tendon sheath and the diffuse form in the knee, where it may involve the joint, the suprapatellar pouch and may invade adjacent bone.

Grossly, the tumors are usually firm, pale or mottled with red. Encapsulation, as indicated above, may be complete, partial or absent. Microscopically, two types of cells participate. The lining synovial cells multiply in solid masses, may form structures like synovial villi, and sometimes acinic spaces are present. In these spaces and also inter-

dle cells and xanthomatous cells occur (see Jaffe, Lichtenstein and Sutro).

Malignant tumors may metastasize to joints or may invade directly from surrounding structures.

SKELETAL MUSCLE

Rigor mortis has been discussed in the chapter on Necrosis and Somatic Death.

Congenital Anomalies

These represent complete or partial defects in the development of muscles or groups of muscles. The condition affects especially the muscles of the shoulder girdle, although others may be involved. The chief manifestation in addition to the obvious defi-

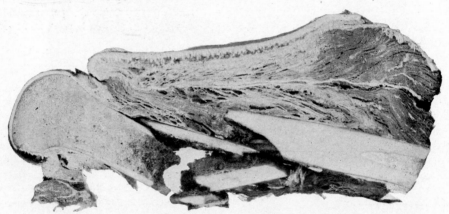

Gas gangrene of muscles and compound comminuted fracture of femur due to shell wound. Army Medical Museum, 2879.

stitially, mucin may be found. The mesenchymal cells multiply in much the same way as in reticulum-cell sarcoma and it is this growth which gives rise to the polymorphocellular tumors, with large mononuclear or multinucleated giant cells, often phagocytic for blood pigment; xanthomatous cells also occur. Calcification may occur and rarely cartilage and bone are formed.

Often considered to be benign, these tumors tend to recur after removal and are potentially if not actually malignant. The diffuse forms and those made up largely of reticulum cell types are especially likely to be malignant. The lesion should not be confused with proliferative forms of synovitis, bursitis and tenosynovitis, in which villous masses may form and proliferations of spin-

ciency of muscle is elevation of the scapula. Small remaining bundles of muscle are microscopically normal. The condition is probably due to fault of embryonal development of the muscle, since examination of the spinal cord shows no lesion that can be held responsible.

Retrogressive Changes

Cloudy swelling and fatty degeneration have much the same characters as in cardiac muscle. In the former, the muscle substance is granular and shows diminution or loss of transverse striation. In the latter there are, in addition, fat globules in longitudinal rows, which soon occupy the entire width of the fiber. These conditions occur as the result of infectious diseases, inflammation in the muscle and intoxications, especially by phosphorus and poisonous fungi. Fat infiltration occurs sometimes as a replacement process consequent upon atrophy.

Hyaline necrosis, waxy degeneration or Zenker's hyalin, has been described in the chapter on Degenerations and Infiltrations. It affects especially the recti abdominis, but may be seen in other muscles, as the result of infectious diseases, notably typhoid fever, influenza and avitaminosis C or E. Grossly, the muscle is pallid, glassy and fish-like, and often shows hemorrhage. Microscopically, the fibers lose transverse and longitudinal striations, become structureless, often show fracture and retraction within the sarcolemma. Subsequently, there may be infiltration of monocytes and lymphocytes and proliferation of sarcolemma nuclei. Since the sarcolemma is not destroyed, regeneration may occur.

Necrosis due to direct injury or vascular occlusion may show hyaline or granular necrosis, or both, of the muscle fibers. The reaction otherwise is the same as in other tissues. Gas gangrene, due to invasion of saprophytic anaerobes, has been discussed in the chapter on Necrosis and Somatic Death. The muscle is at first pallid and fish-like, loses its contractility, is usually foul smelling, and subsequently becomes dark brown in color and finally filled with gas bubbles. Microscopically, the muscle necrosis is usually granular and the large bacilli numerous and easily recognizable.

Circulatory Disturbances

Passive hyperemia occurs as the result of general or local disturbances. Hemorrhage occurs as the result of wounds and in the course of acute infectious diseases, hemorrhagic diseases and intoxications. Unless the collateral circulation is much reduced, for example by arteriosclerosis, small emboli do not produce infarction. The occlusion of large vessels, whose terminals show little anastomosis, by ligation, thrombosis, embolism, and the reduction of large areas of circulation by tight bandages, lead to granular necrosis with resultant partial or complete loss of function.

Atrophy

Atrophy may be widespread, due to general exhausting diseases such as chronic tuberculosis and malignant tumors, and to the nutritional deficiencies of advanced age. Atrophy also affects local groups of muscle

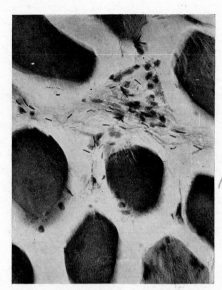

Muscle, the seat of gas gangrene, stained by MacCallum's method for bacteria. Army Medical Museum, 31044.

due to inactivity such as occurs in ankylosis of joints and in paralysis. Paralysis may be due to lesions of central neurones, and the atrophy due to inactivity. When paralysis is caused by interruption of peripheral neurones, there is a factor of trophic disturbance.

Grossly, atrophic muscle may be soft or firm, normal in color, pallid or dark brown, and reduced in bulk. The microscopic appearance differs in atrophy of inactivity and in neurotrophic atrophy. In the former, there is simply reduction in the size of fibers and if of long duration slight fibrous or fatty replacement. Full recovery follows removal of the cause.

In neurotrophic atrophy, there is disintegration of sarcoplasm and sarcostylic elements followed by death of some but not all of the fibers. Nuclei of sarcolemma and muscle proliferate but there is no true regeneration. The intramuscular nerves and their endings degenerate. Fibrosis and fatty replacement may ensue. If activity is restored, the function is assumed by the remaining undestroyed fibers.

Chemically, muscle the seat of atrophy of inactivity shows no change but in neurotrophic atrophy there is an early decrease of phosphorus. (See Chor et al.) The alterations of electric reactions are described in the texts on physiology.

Special Forms of Atrophy. The muscle atrophy of progressive spinal muscular atrophy, type Duchenne-Aran, belongs in the group of neurotrophic atrophy, since the peripheral neuron shows an associated atrophy.

JUVENILE PROGRESSIVE MUSCULAR ATROPHY of Erb or progressive pseudohypertrophic muscular dystrophy, which is familial and occurs usually in early life, is in part an atrophy and in part a hypertrophy. It is essentially a muscle disease although there may be paucity of cells in the anterior horns of the cord. Not only is there atrophy of many fibers, but many others show marked hypertrophy, and numerous fibers are vacuolated. Fat infiltration of the perimysium is frequent. Although there are said to be decreased ability to transform creatine and hypoglycemia with deficient glycogenesis, these changes are not regularly present (see Scheman et al.).

In other forms of muscular atrophy, the perimysium is fibrotic and may become so infiltrated with fat, that grossly the muscle is of normal size or somewhat enlarged; this is also called pseudohypertrophy.

MYASTHENIA GRAVIS is included here for convenience, even although atrophy of the muscles is not constant. It occurs at almost any period of life but is most frequent in the third decade, and affects the sexes about equally.

It is characterized clinically by the ready fatigue of muscles and the long period necessary for recovery from fatigue. Ultimately the muscular weakness is so great that it is practically a paralysis and death may be due to paralysis of the diaphragm. As indicated in the chapter on Ductless Glands, there is probably an exhaustion of acetylcholine. Persistence of or tumors of the thymus occur in about half the cases, but it is doubtful that the disease is due to thymic disorder (see Campbell et al.).

The muscle may be of normal size or somewhat reduced in bulk and is likely to be flabby. Microscopically, the fibers may be normal or the seat of cloudy swelling or hyaline necrosis; the sarcolemma nuclei may multiply. Occasionally atrophy is observed. Most characteristic is the presence of focal collections of lymphoid cells, so-called lymphorrhages, near which the muscle changes may be pronounced. Lymphorrhages may be present in the heart and other viscera. Except for the observation of lymphorrhages in the spinal ganglia the nervous system shows no important lesions. There is no constant departure from normal of any of the chemical constituents of the blood (Adams, Power and Boothby).

MYOTONIA. This is a condition in

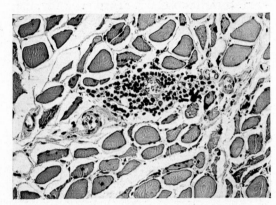

Lymphorrhage in skeletal muscle of myasthenia gravis.

which, as the result of nerve impulse, electrical stimulus or mechanical percussion, the muscular contraction persists for an abnormally long time and relaxation is slow. Myotonia occurs in several forms.

Myotonia congenita is hereditary through a single dominant factor and usually begins in the first or second decade of life. It affects various groups of muscles, which undergo hypertrophy. Strength is not in proportion to the size of the muscle and is often reduced. Microscopically, the muscle fibers are considerably increased in size and there may be a proliferation of nuclei. The use of quinine greatly reduces the disability. Lesions of anterior horn cells and anterior nerve roots are described, but there is no assurance that this is constant (see Forbus and Wolf).

Dystrophia myotonica or myotonic atrophy is similarly hereditary, but the disease becomes progressively more severe in succeeding generations. The disease also appears in early life, but may occur later. Myotonia is first evident in hand grasps but may involve muscles of mastication, of legs and of other situations. There is progressive weakness and atrophy of muscles. Heidenhain describes transversely arranged fibrils in the outer part of the sarcoplasm, which encircle the fiber in ring or spiral fashion.

Myotonia congenita intermittens or paramyotonia is inherited in the same way and is exhibited by myotonia on exposure to cold, usually on voluntary movement but occasionally spontaneous.

Myotonia acquisita is exceedingly rare and is said to occur as a sequel of trauma or acute infectious disease. Myotonia also occasionally occurs in myxedema. (See Ravin.)

Hypertrophy

Hypertrophy is due to increased work, as for example, that of the blacksmith and athlete. The increase in bulk and weight is due to an increase in the transverse diameters of pre-existent fibers and is not a hyperplasia.

Regeneration

Regeneration of skeletal muscle, aside from the usual factors controlling regeneration, depends upon the extent of the injury and the degree of involvement of the perimysium. A clean wound with extremely little destruction may be followed by practically complete regeneration. The sarcoplasm forms processes or muscle buds which usually contain numerous nuclei. The buds from the adjacent fibers meet, fuse and form longitudinal fibrils with transverse striations, while the nuclei decrease in number and assume the natural lateral position. If destruction be somewhat more extensive, the muscle buds cannot bridge the gap, and the area is filled with scar tissue. If only the contractile substance be injured, for example, in Zenker's hyalin, the dead muscle is removed by phagocytosis and the defect filled by regeneration of the sarcoplasm.

Inflammation

Acute myositis may be suppurative or nonsuppurative. The suppurative form may be due to direct extension from neighboring abscess or from superficial ulcers. Pyemia does not frequently produce abscesses in muscle, perhaps because of relatively decreased circulation while the muscles are at rest. Pyemic abscesses are usually small, elongated collections of pus, but if the condition continue they may attain a diameter of a centimeter or more. Abscess of the muscle may complicate typhoid fever and be due either to the typhoid bacillus or to pyogenic cocci. Rarely suppuration may occur without a determinable portal of entry. Microscopically, the pus is made up in part of leukocytes and in part of tissue cells and muscle. The muscle nuclei in the neighborhood show multiplication and increase in chromatin content.

Nonsuppurative inflammations are rare. ACUTE POLYMYOSITIS may follow acute infectious diseases or may apparently be primary. It involves many muscles in the form of localized painful swellings, runs a febrile course of a few weeks and may lead either to complete recovery, sometimes with residual atrophy, or to death, especially when respiratory muscles are involved. Microscopically, there are edema, slight fibrin formation, infiltration of lymphoid cells and sometimes small areas of hemorrhage. The muscle substance shows cloudy swelling and vacuolization.

ACUTE CREPITATING PERIMYOSITIS is also extremely rare, and is due to a fibrinous edema of the perimysium and the inner surfaces of the muscle fascias. Rarely a polymyositis may be associated with output of dark brown urine which contains myoglobin, myositis myoglobinurica.

DERMATOMYOSITIS is a systemic disease with inflammations in skin and muscles. It occurs at almost any age, with insidious onset. Lassitude and fever are followed by tenderness and pain in muscles and cutaneous lesions. The skin may show areas of erythema, followed by atrophy and loss of hair. The urine may show an increase in amount of creatine and decrease of creatinine.

Microscopically, the late lesion shows atrophy of the epidermis, flattening of the papillae and a peculiar balloon-like vacuolization of the basal cells; the corium shows edema, dilatation of blood vessels, fibrosis and lymphocytic infiltration which may be perivascular. The muscle shows atrophic fibers intermingled with normal fibers. Inflammation is present in the form of diffuse infiltration of lymphocytes. There may be perivascular infiltration of lymphocytes and leukocytes sometimes with necrosis of vascular walls and focal hemorrhages. In some instances the inflammatory lesions appear around and in nerves. (See Kinney and

Maher; Guy, Grauer and Jacob.) The inflammatory reaction in trichinosis will be discussed under the heading of parasites.

Chronic Fibrous Myositis. In this lesion there is a productive overgrowth of connective tissue between the muscle fibers, which varies from a young cellular type to the older fibrillar or even hyaline form. Atrophy of the muscle may accompany the lesion, in which case it is often difficult to say that the fibrosis is inflammatory, because it may be a replacement fibrosis subsequent to atrophy. Fibrosis of the sternocleidomastoid muscle is found in congenital wry neck or caput obstipum. There is question in these cases as to whether the fibrosis is inflammatory, or a cicatrization following rupture during labor, or fibrosis secondary to some fault in intrauterine growth of the muscle.

Myositis Ossificans. There are two varieties of the disorder, a local form and a generalized form of progressive multiple ossifying myositis. The local or circumscribed form is of traumatic origin and is common in young men. The condition is usually due to tears of tendon or muscle due to athletics, occurs in the adductors of the thigh as "rider's bone" and in the shoulders of soldiers as the result of repeated trauma in rifle drill. It may follow a variety of accidental injuries.

The lesion may or may not be continuous with periosteum. In the early stages there is much fibrocartilage, then the development of hyaline cartilage and the formation of bone. Later there is much lamellar bone, irregularly arranged with little or no remaining cartilage. Thus the process is similar to endochondral bone formation. (See Hirsch and Morgan; Thorndike.)

Progressive multiple ossifying myositis is a disease which begins in early life, affects boys more often than girls and ends in death after a course of one or two decades. Numerous muscles are affected, with painful swellings, edema of the overlying skin, and evanescent fever. Ossification ensues and progressively increases, but finally may lead to reduced function and atrophy, and may extend from one bone to another so as to immobilize the joint, usually in a position of flexion. The lesion is primary in the aponeuroses, tendons, sometimes the ligaments, especially those of the spinal column, and may extend from the periosteum. From these regions the fibrosis and ossification extend into the connective tissues of the muscles.

Microscopically, the muscle fibers lose their cross striations, undergo complete atrophy and are replaced by the growing connective tissue. Ossification proceeds from the connective tissue or may follow cartilage deposition. Various hypotheses have been offered as to the cause of the disease, but, as Opie points out, it is probably a progressive anomaly of osteogenesis. This supposition is based on the early age of incidence, the rarefaction of skeletal bone as revealed by the x-ray, and various associated anomalies, especially microdactylism of the great toes, from which one phalanx may be missing. (See Koontz.)

Infectious Granulomata

Tuberculosis. The most common form of tuberculosis of the muscle is conglomerate tuberculosis, or tuberculous abscess, due either to direct extension or lymphatic transmission from some neighboring focus such as bones, joints, or lymph nodes. Muscles are rarely involved in a disseminated miliary tuberculosis. The reason for the infrequency of miliary tuberculosis is unexplained. The tubercles are made up from the connective tissues; the muscle cells play no part in their formation.

Syphilis. The characteristic lesion is the gumma, which may attain great size. Multiple small gummata may also occur. In addition, skeletal muscle may show a chronic interstitial inflammation with consequent fibrosis and atrophy of the muscle fibers, similar to that observed in the myocardium in syphilis (Busse).

Tumors

The supporting tissues of muscle may give rise to fibroma, myxoma, hemangioma, lipoma and sarcomas including liposarcoma. Tumors of striated muscle are rare. Myoblastomas occur especially in mouth and neck, as slowly growing fleshy tumors. Microscopically, the typical cell is a large round cell with relatively small nucleus and tiny rods or nodules in the cytoplasm. Unless removal is complete, recurrence is frequent; occasionally the tumor is malignant. Benign rhabdomyoma is rare, and is made up of fairly uniform striated fibers. Less rare is rhabdomyosarcoma, composed of cells like myoblasts, spindle cells, large syncytial multinucleated masses and embryonal forms of striated muscle. The muscle surrounding any of these tumors may be atrophic, there may be lymphocytic infiltration and multiplication of sarcolemma nuclei. (See Geschickter; De and Tribedi.) Metastasis of other tumors to muscle is infrequent, but direct extension is common (Willis).

Parasites

Trichinosis. Aside from the occasional occurrence of echinococcus cysts and other cysticerci, the most important parasite of muscles is the *Trichinella spiralis*. This nematode is introduced into man usually by ingestion of infested pork, which is not cooked sufficiently to kill the parasite. The encapsulated larvae are liberated in the duodenum and mature in about 48 hours. Nausea, diarrhea and fever may occur about 24 hours after ingestion, probably because of absorption of poisonous products released by digestion of the cyst wall of the larvae. Sexual reproduction occurs and the females, in two or three weeks, give birth viviparously to embryos, which gain access to the blood stream and are deposited within the sarcolemma sheaths, where they assume a coil form and are encysted by connective tissue. The involvement of the muscles may be almost symptomless or may produce fever, and pain, stiffness and swelling of the muscle.

Microscopically, practically all the larvae are in the same stage of encystment. This is followed by swelling and proliferation of the sarcolemma which results in fibrous encystment. In the meantime the involved muscle fibers have undergone cloudy swelling, fatty degeneration and necrosis. The neighboring fibers may show hydropic or fatty degeneration or hyaline necrosis. Attempts at regeneration may be observed as minute muscle buds, but more especially in multiplication of the muscle nuclei principally by mitosis. Human muscle may show minute, white or gray, firm specks, which microscopically are found to be the coiled larvae. In some cases inflammation may still be present, and in others the encystment may be complete with little or no remaining reaction other than the cyst wall. Ultimately, the parasite dies and may become calcified. The examination of diaphragm and skeletal muscle at autopsy discloses the fact that the disease probably affects about one-fifth the adult population. (See Most and Helpern.)

REFERENCES

Adams, M., M. H. Power, and W. M. Boothby: Chemical Studies in Myasthenia Gravis, Ann. Int. Med., 9: 823, 1936. Boothby, W. M.: Myasthenia Gravis: Eighth Report, Trans. Asso. Amer. Phys., 51: 188, 1936.

Albright, F., P. H. Smith, and A. M. Richardson: Postmenopausal Osteoporosis: Its Clinical Features, Jour. Amer. Med. Asso., 116: 2465, 1941.

——, H. W. Sulkowitch, and E. Bloomberg: Further Experience in the Diagnosis of Hyperparathyroidism, Including a Discussion of Cases with a Minimal Degree of Hyperparathyroidism, Amer. Jour. Med. Sci., 193: 800, 1937.

Amberson, J. B., Jr.: Pathogenesis and Medical Treatment of Tuberculosis of the Vertebrae, Jour. Bone and Joint Surg., 22: 807, 1940.

Baker, L. D., and H. A. Jones: Osteopathia Condensans Disseminata, etc., Jour. Bone and Joint Surg., 23: 164, 1941.

Binkley, J. S., and F. W. Stewart: Morphogenesis of Extraskeletal Osteogenic Sarcoma and Pseudo-Osteosarcoma, Arch. Path., 29: 42, 1940.

Blair, J. E., and F. A. Hallman: Rheumatoid (Atrophic) Arthritis: Bacteriologic Cultures of Synovial Fluid and of Tissues, Arch. Int. Med., 53: 87, 1934.

Bloodgood, J. C.: Bone Tumors: Benign Bone Cysts and Osteitis Fibrosa, Southern Med. Jour., 13: 888, 1920.

——: The Diagnosis and Treatment of Benign and Malignant Tumors of Bone, Jour. Radiol., 1: 147, 1920.

Blount, W. P.: Hodgkin's Disease: An Orthopaedic Problem, Jour. Bone and Joint Surg., 11: 761, 1929.

Busse, O.: Pathologie der Willkürlichen Muskulatur, Lubarsch-Ostertag Ergebnisse Allg. Path., 9 (1): 1203, 1903.

Campbell, E., N. F. Fradkin, and B. Lipetz: Myasthenia Gravis Treated by Excision of Thymic Tumor: Report of Two Cases, Arch. Neurol. and Psychiatr., 47: 645, 1942.

Cecil, R. L.: Rheumatoid Arthritis: A New Method of Approach to the Disease, Jour. Amer. Med. Asso., 100: 1220, 1933.

Chesney, A. M., J. E. Kemp, and F. H. Baetjer: An Experimental Study of the Synovial Fluid of Patients with Arthritis and Syphilis, Jour. Clin. Invest., 3: 131, 1926.

Chor, H., and R. E. Dolkart: A Study of "Simple Disuse Atrophy" in the Monkey, Amer. Jour. Physiol., 117: 626, 1936.

——, ——, and H. A. Davenport: Chemical and Histological Changes in Denervated Skeletal Muscle in the Monkey and Cat, Ibid., 118: 580, 1937.

Christensen, F. C.: Bone Tumors. An Analysis of 1000 Cases with Special Reference to Location, Age and Sex, Ann. Surg., 81: 1074, 1925.

Clawson, B. J.: Studies on the Etiology of Acute Rheumatic Fever, Jour. Infect. Dis., 36: 444, 1925.

Clifton, W. M., A. Frank, and S. Freeman: Osteopetrosis (Marble Bones), Amer. Jour. Dis. Child., **56**: 1020, 1938.

Codman, E. A.: The Method of Procedure of the Registry of Bone Sarcoma, Surg., Gynec. and Obst., **38**: 712, 1924.

——: The Registry of Cases of Bone Sarcoma, Ibid., **34**: 335, 1922.

——: The Nomenclature Used by the Registry of Bone Sarcoma, Amer. Jour. Roentgenol. and Rad. Ther., **13**: 105, 1925.

——: Bone Sarcoma, Hoeber, New York, 1925.

Cressman, R. D., and A. Blalock: Experimental Osteomyelitis: Effects on Ribs of Increased Intra-medullary Pressure and of Toxin- and Nontoxin-producing Strains of Staphylococci, Surgery, **6**: 535, 1939.

Crump, C.: Histologie der allgemeinen Osteophytose (Ostéoarthropathie hypertrophiante pneumique), Virchow's Arch. Path. Anat., **271**: 467, 1929.

Curtis, A. C., and H. M. Pollard: Felty's Syndrome; Its Several Features, including Tissue Changes, Compared with Other Forms of Rheumatoid Arthritis, Ann. Int. Med., **13**: 2265, 1940.

Dandy, W. E.: Hydrocephalus in Chondro-dystrophy, Bull. Johns Hopkins Hosp., **32**: 5, 1921.

Dawson, M. H., and R. H. Boots: Subcutaneous Nodules in Rheumatoid (Chronic Infectious) Arthritis, Jour. Amer. Med. Asso., **95**: 1894, 1930.

De, M. N., and B. P. Tribedi: Skeletal Muscle Tissue Tumour, Brit. Jour. Surg., **28**: 17, 1940-41.

De Santo, D., R. Tennant, and P. D. Rosahn: Synovial Sarcomas in Joints, Bursae and Tendon Sheaths, Surg., Gynec. and Obst., **72**: 951, 1941.

Dickman, A.: Trichinosis: Distribution of Trichinella Spiralis in Pork Products Sold in Philadelphia, Jour. Lab. and Clin. Med., **23**: 671, 1937-38.

Donohue, W. L.: Pathology of the Intervertebral Disc, Amer. Jour. Med. Sci., **198**: 419, 1939.

Dragstedt, C. A., and J. E. Kearns, Jr.: Experimental Study of Bone Repair: Effect of Thyro-parathyroidectomy and of the Administration of Parathormone, Arch. Surg., **24**: 893, 1932.

Duffy, J., and F. W. Stewart: Primary Liposarcoma of Bone, Amer. Jour. Path., **14**: 621, 1938.

Ely, L. W.: Inflammation in Bones and Joints, Philadelphia and London, 1923.

——: Joint Tuberculosis, New York, Wood, 1911.

Ewing, J.: Neoplastic Diseases, 4th Ed., Philadelphia and London, Saunders, 1940.

Faulkner, J. M., and P. D. White: The Incidence of Rheumatic Fever, Chorea and Rheumatic Heart Disease, etc., Jour. Amer. Med. Asso., **83**: 425, 1924.

Fisher, A. G. T.: The Nature of the So-called Rheumatoid Arthritis and Osteo-arthritis, etc., Brit. Med. Jour., **2**: 102, 1923.

Forbus, W. D., and F. S. Wolf: Amyotonia Congenita (Oppenheim's Disease) in Identical Twins, Bull. Johns Hopkins Hosp., **47**: 309, 1930.

Freund, E.: Die Gelenkerkrankung der Bluter, Virchow's Arch. Path. Anat., **256**: 158, 1925.

——: Ueber Knochensyphilis, Ibid., **288**: 146, 1933.

Gargill, S. L., D. R. Gilligan, and H. L. Blumgart: Metabolism and Treatment of Osteomalacia. Its Relation to Rickets, Arch. Int. Med., **45**: 879, 1930.

Geschickter, C. F.: Osteogenic Sarcoma, Arch. Surg., **24**: 602, 798, 1932.

——: Tumors of Muscle, Amer. Jour. Cancer, **22**: 378, 1934.

——: and M. M. Copeland: Tumors of Bone, 2d ed., New York, 1936.

Graney, C. M.: Hereditary Deforming Chondro-dysplasia: Report of Ten Cases in One Family, Jour. Amer. Med. Asso., **112**: 2026, 1939.

Gutman, A. B., and H. Kasabach: Paget's Disease (Osteitis Deformans). Analysis of 116 Cases, Amer. Jour. Med. Sci., **191**: 361, 1936.

Guy, W. H., R. C. Grauer, and F. M. Jacob: Poikilodermatomyositis, Arch. Derm. and Syphilol., **40**: 867, 1939.

Harbin, M., and R. Zollinger: Osteochondritis of the Growth Centers, Surg., Gynec. and Obst., **51**: 145, 1930.

Hauser, H.: Angiosarcoma of Bone, Amer. Jour. Roent. and Radium Ther., **42**: 656, 1939.

Heidenhain, M.: Ueber progressive Veränderungen der Muskulatur bei Myotonia atrophica, Ziegler's Beitr. Path. Anat., **64**: 198, 1918.

Hertz, J.: Studies on the Healing of Fractures, with Special Reference to the Significance of the Vitamin Content of the Diet, Acta Path. et Microbiol. Scandinav., Suppl. 28, 1936.

Hess, A. F.: Scurvy, Past and Present, Philadelphia and London, Lippincott, 1920.

Heyman, C. H.: Charcot Joint Following Trauma, Ohio State Med. Jour., **19**: 496, 1923.

Hills, R. G., and S. McLanahan: Brittle Bones and Blue Scleras in Five Generations, Arch. Int. Med., **59**: 41, 1937.

Hirsch, E. F.: Arterial Occlusion with Aseptic Necrosis of Bone, Arch. Surg., **37**: 926, 1938.

——, and R. H. Morgan: Causal Significance to Traumatic Ossification of the Fibrocartilage in Tendon Insertions, Arch. Surg., **39**: 824, 1939.

Honeij, J. A.: A Study of Multiple Cartilaginous Exostosis, etc., Arch. Int. Med., **25**: 584, 1920.

Hunter, D.: The Significance to Clinical Medicine of Studies in Calcium and Phosphorus Metabolism, Lancet, **1**: 897; 947; 999, 1930.

——, and H. M. Turnbull: Hyperparathyroidism: Generalized Osteitis Fibrosa, etc., Brit. Jour. Surg., **19**: 203, 1931-32.

Jacobsen, A. W.: Hereditary Osteochondrodystrophia Deformans: A Family with Twenty Members Affected in Five Generations, Jour. Amer. Med. Asso., **113**: 121, 1939.

Jaffe, H. L., L. Lichtenstein, and R. B. Portis: Giant Cell Tumor of Bone: Its Pathologic Appearance, Grading, Supposed Variants and Treatment, Arch. Path., **30**: 993, 1940.

——, ——, and C. J. Sutro: Pigmented Villonodular Synovitis, Bursitis and Tenosynovitis: A Discussion of the Synovial and Bursal Equivalents of the Tenosynovial Lesion Commonly Denoted as Xanthoma, Xanthogranuloma, Giant Cell Tumor of Myeloplaxoma of the Tendon Sheath, with Some Consideration of this Tendon Sheath Lesion Itself, Arch. Path., **31**: 731, 1941.

——, and L. Lichtenstein: Non-osteogenic Fibroma of Bone, Amer. Jour. Path., **18**: 205, 1942.

Jaffe, H. L.: Paget's Disease of Bone, Arch. Path., **15**: 83, 1933; Hyperparathyroidism (Recklinghausen's Disease of Bone), Arch. Path., **16**: 63, 236, 1933.

Kaufmann, E.: Lehrbuch der speziellen pathologischen Anatomie, Berlin and Leipzig, 1922, Vol. 1, p. 816.

Keefer, C. S., and W. W. Spink: Gonococcic Arthritis, etc., Jour. Amer. Med. Asso., 109: 1448, 1937.

Kelly, L. C.: Vertebral Hemangioma with Neurologic Symptoms, New York State Jour. Med., 40: 1607, 1940.

Kinney, T. D., and M. M. Maher: Dermatomyositis. A Study of Five Cases, Amer. Jour. Path., 16: 561, 1940.

——: Leontiasis Ossea, Brit. Jour. Surg., 11: 347, 1923.

——: Osteogenesis Imperfecta, Brit. Jour. Surg., 11: 737, 1924.

Knies, P. T., and H. E. LeFevre: Metabolic Craniopathy: Hyperostosis Frontalis Interna, Ann. Int. Med., 14: 1858, 1941.

Kolodny, A.: A Contribution to the Knowledge of Pathogenesis of Skeletal Tuberculosis, Jour. Bone and Joint Surg., 7: 53, 1925.

——: Endocrine Disturbances and Non-union of Fractures, Surg., Gynec. and Obst., 38: 793, 1924.

——: The Periosteal Blood Supply and Healing of Fractures. Experimental Study, Jour. Bone and Joint Surg., 5: 698, 1923.

——: A Case of Primary Multiple Endothelioma of Bone, Arch. Surg., 9: 636, 1924.

——: Diagnosis and Prognosis of Bone Sarcoma, Jour. Bone and Joint Surg., 7: 911, 1925.

Koontz, A. R.: Myositis Ossificans Progressiva, Amer. Jour. Med. Sci., 174: 406, 1927.

Kraft, A.: Ein Beiträg zum Erbgang des Zwergwuchses (Nanosomia Infantilis), Münch. Med. Wochenschr., 71: 788, 1924.

Krause, G. R.: Persistence of the Notochord, Amer. Jour. Roentgenol. and Rad. Ther., 44: 719, 1940.

Kugel, M. A., and E. Z. Epstein: Lesions in the Pulmonary Artery and Valve Associated with Rheumatic Cardiac Disease, Arch. Path., 6: 247, 1928.

Lee, W. E.: Surgery of the Extremities. Shock, Anesthesia, Infections, Fractures, Dislocations and Tumors, Progressive Medicine, 4: 157, 1930.

Liu, S. H., H. I. Chu, H. C. Hsu, H. C. Chao, and S. H. Cheu: Calcium and Phosphorus Metabolism in Osteomalacia. XI. The Pathogenetic Role of Pregnancy and Relative Importance of Calcium and Vitamin D Supply, Jour. Clin. Invest., 20: 255, 1941.

Martin, D. W.: Multiple Cystic Tuberculosis of the Bones: Report of Case, Jour. Pediatr., 15: 254, 1939.

McCurdy, I. J., and R. W. Baer: Hereditary Cleidocranial Dysostosis, Jour. Amer. Med. Asso., 81: 9, 1923.

McKeown, R. M., S. C. Harvey, and R. W. Lumsden: The Breaking Strength of Healing Fractured Fibulæ of Rats. IV. Observations on the Influence of Bilateral Ovariectomy, Arch. Surg., 26: 430, 1933; see also II. Observations and Standard Diet, Ibid., 24: 458, 1932.

Melnick, P. J.: Histogenesis of Ewing's Sarcoma of Bone, with Post-mortem Report of a Case, Amer. Jour. Cancer, 19: 353, 1933.

Mettier, S. R., G. R. Minot, and W. C. Townsend: Scurvy in Adults., etc., Jour. Amer. Med. Asso., 95: 1089, 1930.

Meyer, A. W., and L. M. McCormick: Studies on Scurvy, Stanford University Press, 1928.

Moritz, A. R.: Tabische Arthropathie, Virchow's Arch. Path. Anat., 267: 746, 1928.

Most, H., and M. Helpern: The Incidence of Trichinosis in New York City, Amer. Jour. Med. Sci., 202: 251, 1941.

Myers, C. S.: Myasthenia Gravis, J. Path. and Bact., 8: 306, 1903.

Nathan, P. W.: Arthritis Deformans as an Infectious Disease, Jour. Med. Research, 36: 187, 1917.

Neller, J. L.: Osteitis Fibrosa Cystica (Albright), Amer. Jour. Dis. Child., 61: 590, 1941.

Nichols, E. H., and F. L. Richardson: Arthritis Deformans, Jour. Med. Research, 21: 149, 1909.

——: Tuberculosis of the Bones and Joints, Trans. Amer. Orthop. Asso., 11: 353, 1898.

Nussbaum, A.: Ueber die Gefässe des unteren Femurendes und ihre Beziehungen zur Pathologie, Beitr. Klin. Chir., 129: 245, 1923.

Opie, E. L.: Progressive Muscular Ossification (Progressive Ossifying Myositis)—A Progressive Anomaly of Osteogenesis, Jour. Med. Res., 36: 267, 1917.

Pappenheimer, A. M., and W. C. von Glahn: Studies in the Pathology of Rheumatic Fever, etc., Amer. Jour. Path., 3: 583, 1927.

Park, E. A.: Observations on the Pathology of Rickets with Particular Reference to the Changes at the Cartilage-Shaft Junctions of the Growing Bones, Harvey Lectures, Baltimore, Williams and Wilkins, 34: 157, 1939.

——: The Etiology of Rickets, Physiol. Rev., 3: 106, 1923.

Parker, F., Jr., C. S. Keefer, W. K. Myers, and R. L. Irwin: Histologic Changes in the Knee Joint with Advancing Age; Relation to Degenerative Arthritis, Arch. Path., 17: 516, 1934.

——, and W. K. Myers. The Incidence and Pathogenesis of Degenerative Arthritis, Jour. Amer. Med. Asso., 102: 811, 1934.

——, and C. S. Keefer: Gross and Histologic Changes in the Knee Joint in Rheumatoid Arthritis, Arch. Path., 20: 507, 1935.

Pemberton, R.: Arthritis and Rheumatoid Conditions, Philadelphia, Lea & Febiger, 1929; A. D. Goldhaft, L. M. Wright and R. Pemberton: The Production of Hypertrophic Arthritis by Interference with the Blood Supply, Amer. Jour. Med. Sci., 180: 386, 1930.

Phemister, D. B.: Changes in Bones and Joints Resulting from Interruption of Circulation: I. General Considerations and Changes Resulting from Injuries, Arch. Surg., 41: 436, 1940.

——: The Recognition of Dead Bone Based on Pathological and X-ray Studies, Ann. Surg., 72: 466, 1920.

——: Silent Foci of Localized Osteomyelitis, Jour. Amer. Med. Asso., 82: 1311, 1924.

——: The Effect of Pressure on Articular Surfaces in Pyogenic and Tuberculous Arthritides and Its Bearing on Treatment, Ann. Surg., 80: 481, 1924.

——: Changes in the Articular Surfaces in Tuberculous and in Pyogenic Infections of Joints, Amer. Jour. Roentgenol. and Rad. Therap., 12: 1, 1924.

——: Changes in the Articular Surfaces in Tuberculous Arthritis, Jour. Bone and Joint Surg., 7: 835, 1925.

——: The Causes of and Changes in Loose Bodies Arising from the Articular Surface of the Joint, Jour. Bone and Joint Surg., 6: 278, 1924.

Phemister, D. B.: Chondrosarcoma of Bone, Surg., Gynec. and Obst., **50**: 216, 1930.

——, A. Brunschwig, and L. Day: Streptococcal Infections of Epiphyses and Short Bones: Their Relation to Köhler's Disease of the Tarsal Navicular, Legg-Perthes' Disease and Kienbock's Disease of the Os Lunatum, Jour. Amer. Med. Asso., **95**: 995, 1930.

Pick, L.: Pathologic, Anatomic and Clinical Considerations Concerning the Malacic Diseases of the Bones, Harvey Lectures, **27**: 179, 1931-32, Baltimore, 1932.

Portis, R. B.: Pathology of Chronic Arthritis of Children (Still's Disease), Amer. Jour. Dis. Child., **55**: 1000, 1938.

Ravin, A.: Myotonia, Medicine, **18**: 443, 1939.

——, and J. J. Waring: Studies in Dystrophia Myotonica. IV. Myotonia: Its Nature and Occurrence, Ann. Int. Med., **13**: 1174, 1940.

Rosenheim, O., and T. A. Webster: The Parent Substance of Vitamin D, Biochem. Jour., **21**: 389, 1927.

Rushton, M. A.: The Structure of the Teeth in a Late Case of Osteogenesis Imperfecta, Jour. Path. and Bact., **48**: 591, 1939.

Sacks, B.: The Pathology of Rheumatic Fever. A Critical Review, Amer. Heart Jour., **1**: 750, 1926.

Scheman, L., P. Lewin, and S. Soskin: Pseudohypertrophic Muscular Dystrophy, Jour. Amer. Med. Asso., **111**: 2265, 1938.

Schmidt, M. B.: Die Bewegungsapparat, Aschoff's Pathologische Anatomie, Vol. II, p. 190, Jena, 1921.

——: Allgemeine Pathologie und Pathologische Anatomie der Knochen, Lubarsch-Ostertag, Ergeb. Allg. Path., **4**: 531, 1897; **5**: 895, 1898; **7**: 221, 1900-1901.

Shands, A. R., Jr.: Neuropathies of the Bones and Joints: Report of a Case of an Arthropathy of the Ankle due to a Peripheral Nerve Lesion, Arch. Surg., **20**: 614, 1930.

Small, J. C.: Rheumatic Fever, etc., Amer. Jour. Med. Sci., **175**: 638, 650, 1928.

Smith, O. N., and J. McK. Mitchell: Serum Phosphatase in Osteogenesis Imperfecta, Amer. Jour. Med. Sci., **190**: 765, 1935.

Speed, K.: Longitudinal Overgrowth of Long Bones, Surg., Gyn. and Obst., **36**: 787, 1923.

Stecher, R. M.: Heberden's Nodes. Heredity in Hypertrophic Arthritis of the Finger Joints, Amer. Jour. Med. Sci., **201**: 801, 1941.

Swift, H. F., C. L. Derick, and C. H. Hitchcock: Bacterial Allergy (Hyperergy) to Nonhemolytic Streptococci in its Relation to Rheumatic Fever, Jour. Amer. Med. Asso., **90**: 906, 1928.

Thorndike, A., Jr.: Myositis Ossificans Traumatica, Jour. Bone and Joint Surg., **22**: 315, 1940.

Tollman, J. P., D. H. Drummond, A. R. McIntyre, and J. D. Bisgard: Tissue Metabolism and Phosphatase Activity in Early Callus, Arch. Surg., **40**: 43, 1940.

Underhill, F. P., J. A. Honeij, and L. J. Bogert: Studies on Calcium and Magnesium Metabolism in Disease. II. Calcium and Magnesium Metabolism in Multiple Cartilaginous Exostosis, Jour. Exper. Med., **32**: 65, 1920.

Urist, M. R., and F. C. McLean: Calcification and Ossification; I. Calcification in Callus in Healing Fractures in Normal Rats, Jour. Bone and Joint Surg., **23**: 1, 1941.

Vidgoff, B., and G. J. Bracher: Osteopetrosis: Report of Case, Amer. Jour. Roentgenol. and Rad. Ther., **44**: 197, 1940.

Weber, M.: Osteogenesis Imperfecta Congenita: A Study of its Histopathogenesis, Arch. Path., **9**: 984, 1930.

Wells, H. G.: Chemical Pathology, Philadelphia and London, 1925.

Wheeler, P. H., and M. Harbin: Dermatomyositis, Arch. Derm. and Syphilol., **26**: 1039, 1932.

Willis, R. A.: The Spread of Tumours in the Human Body, London, 1934.

Wolbach, S. B., and P. Howe: Intercellular Substances in Experimental Scorbutus, Arch. Path. and Lab. Med., **1**: 1, 1926.

Wolf, A., and S. L. Wilens: Dermatomyositis. A Report of Two Cases with Complete Autopsy, Amer. Jour. Path., **12**: 235, 1936; *see also* Marcus, I. H., and J. Weinstein: Dermatomyositis: Report of a Case with a Review of the Literature, Ann. Int. Med., **9**: 406, 1935.

22.

The Nervous System

INTRODUCTION

It must be recognized that the subject of neuropathology is so extensive that the material in a general text book can represent only the most important lesions. Furthermore, the disturbances of function are in many instances so intricate that their correlation with alterations of structure can only be indicated in the briefest fashion. The various parts of the nervous system, the meninges, brain, spinal cord, peripheral nerves and sympathetic system are so closely interrelated in pathologic changes, that a consideration of each part separately may readily lead to much duplication and perhaps to an incorrect conception of the various special diseases. Textbooks such as those of Weil, of Freeman and of Hassin give more extensive discussions.

CONGENITAL ANOMALIES

These are most frequently due to defective closure of the neural groove.

Anencephaly, with complete absence of the brain including cerebrum and cerebellum, is accompanied by absence of the flat bones of the skull, and rudimentary basal bones.

Hemicephaly is a less marked degree of the same anomaly, in which rudimentary basal ganglia and cerebellum are found and the skull defect, hemicrania, is less marked. Moderate or slight defects in the skull may be accompanied by a bulging of the brain substance, exencephaly, or merely of the meninges, meningocele.

Spina bifida, rachischisis, or spinal dysraphism, exhibits lesions varying in severity from those which are incompatible with life to those which give no symptoms whatever. In complete or total spina bifida, which is usually associated with anencephaly, the vertebral processes are incomplete, the posterior part of the cord does not fuse and the incomplete central canal lies exposed or covered only by meninges and skin.

INCOMPLETE OR PARTIAL SPINA BIFIDA shows a defect in the lumbosacral region accompanied by external bulging. The bulge may be due to meningocele, a combination of meninges and cord, myelomeningocele, or by local dilatation of the central canal, myelocystocele. In the simpler forms, the medullary groove is closed, but the cord may be rudimentary.

IN SPINA BIFIDA OCCULTA, there is a defect in the transverse processes of the vertebrae, but no bulging. The overlying skin

sulci shallow. The condition is usually associated with other anomalies such as microcephaly. A pseudomicrogyria may be produced by fetal inflammations of meninges and cortex.

Cyclencephaly is a failure of separation, or fusion, of the cerebral hemispheres, which is usually associated with cyclopia.

In porencephaly there is a failure of development of cortical white and gray mat-

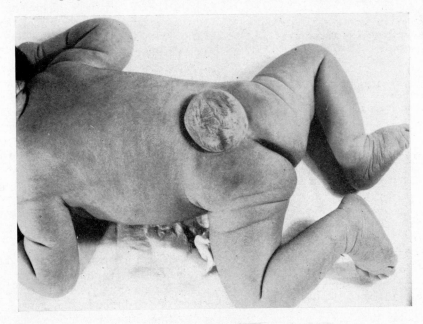

Infant with spina bifida.

is often pigmented and hairy. Tumors, such as lipoma, neurofibroma and fibromyomas may occur in the cord. Spina bifida is often accompanied by other abnormalities such as hydrocephalus, stenosis of the aqueduct of Sylvius and other lesions (Lichtenstein).

Other developmental defects occur with a completely formed bony case.

Microcephaly is a hypoplasia of the cerebrum, associated with abnormal thickness of the skull and early closure of sutures and fontanelles. The cerebrum may be of adult or embryonal type, or resemble that of lower animals, but the cerebellum is usually well developed. Occasionally, as in amaurotic familial idiocy, there may be partial or complete agenesis of the cortex, often associated with other anomalies of brain development.

In microgyria the gyri are small, narrow and increased in number, and the

ter, so that the ventricles communicate with the surface of the brain. The cavities are lined by a continuation of the pia arachnoid. If bilateral, the lesions are usually symmetrical and may be so severe that there is almost no cortex, but even in these cases the basal ganglia persist. There may also be dystrophy and agenesia in remote parts of the brain, in the cord and pons.

Pseudoporencephaly shows a cyst surrounded by a thick cicatricial wall, and blood pigment and scavenger cells presumably the remains of destructive lesions of the brain.

Pneumocephalus, the presence of air or gas in the brain, may be traumatic, as in association with ruptured air sinuses, or of bacterial origin (Dandy; Rand). Rarely cells may be found in abnormal positions, a sort of heterotopic misplacement.

Tuberous sclerosis is usually listed as a nervous disease, but the lesions in the nervous system are only part of a more widespread disorder and may not even be a major part. Included in the complex are mental retardation, sebaceous adenomas of the skin, tumor-like nodules in the retina and tumors in organs such as kidney and liver and sometimes in peripheral nerves. The disease becomes manifest in early life and in some cases there is a background of heredity.

In the brain there are globular nodules, a few millimeters to 1 or 2 cm. in diameter,

The cutaneous lesions and the tumors of viscera and nerves are of a congenital mixed type and evidently developmental faults. We agree with Moolton that the lesions are all of the same basic order and are the result of faults in tissue combination or balance during development, much as is true of hamartomas. Thus, the disease would be a disseminated hamartial disturbance.

Hydrocephalus may be congenital or acquired. External hydrocephalus, a distention of the arachnoid space by fluid, may be congenital and of unknown cause; the

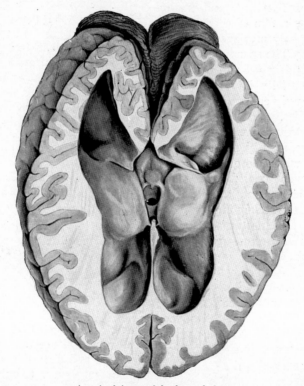

Acquired internal hydrocephalus.

usually in the cortex and accompanied by distortion and pallor of the affected convolutions. Nodules may also occur in the walls of the ventricles and less often in the white matter. Microscopically, the nodules are made up largely of irregularly disposed glia fibrils; there are atypical cells some of which are altered ganglion cells and others of which appear to be glial cells. An atrophic form is described, in which there are small cavities surrounded by fibrillar gliosis.

The lesion appears to be due to faulty development of tissue from the neural groove.

same condition may be acquired as the result of cicatrization or inflammation of the large lymph cisterns at the base of the brain. This form of hydrocephalus is rare. Internal hydrocephalus is a distention of the ventricles by accumulation of fluid produced by the choroid plexuses. In either congenital or acquired forms, it is due to interference with drainage of the fluid. The distention in the congenital form is usually greater than in the acquired forms.

CONGENITAL HYDROCEPHALUS may be due to anomalous occlusion of the foramen of

Monroe or aqueduct of Sylvius or to occlusion of foramina of Luschke and Magendie; sometimes the cause of the obstruction is not demonstrable. The distention is not usually severe before birth but often progresses markedly after birth. Moderate grades are consistent with normal bodily and mental development, but the more severe progressive forms lead ultimately to death. The pressure has little effect on the basal ganglia but the white matter and subsequently the cortical gray matter undergo pressure atrophy. As the pressure continues, distention increases, the convolutions become flattened, and finally there may be merely a film of cortical substance, or in places, only meninges, covering the dilated ventricles. The ependyma may be locally or diffusely thickened and adhesions may divide the ventricles into loculi. The head may be enormously enlarged, with open sutures and fontanelles.

ACQUIRED HYDROCEPHALUS, considered here for convenience, may be due to meningeal inflammations which close off drainage, to blockage by cysts or tumors, and to intracerebral pressure which pushes the pons and inferior parts of the cerebellum into the foramen magnum and thus prevents drainage. Sometimes there is no demonstrable cause. The distention leads to enlargement of the ventricles, flattening of the convolutions and pallor of the brain substance, but unless the lesion occur in very early life, the skull is not deformed. The fluid is clear, unless clouded by inflammatory exudate. The ependyma may be normal, inflamed, or as in the congenital form, hyperplastic.

HYDROCEPHALUS EX VACUO is common when the ventricles are widened as the result of shrinkage of the cortex in agenesis, or disease such as cerebral atrophy and arteriosclerosis.

Hydromyelia is a dilatation of the central canal of the cord. In the congenital form the dilatation may be diffuse, is at the expense principally of the gray matter and in cross section has a key-hole or shield outline. There may be destruction of the ependyma, gliosis and hemorrhage, and the condition merges into a syringomyelia. Acquired hydromyelia may be due to compression injuries of the cord or to tumors of the cerebellum.

FAMILIAL AND CONGENITAL DISEASES

In addition to those diseases in which involvement of muscle is the dominant feature, such as have been discussed in the chapter on organs of locomotion, other somewhat similar diseases occur with lesions principally in the nervous system. Some of these attack several members of one generation while others may be traced through two or more generations. Because of variations in manifestations, the actual mechanisms of hereditary transmission are not altogether clear. Furthermore, it is probable that certain parts of the nervous system are especially vulnerable to conditions that cause degeneration. This state of abiotrophy is evidently inherent in the tissue and may possibly be hereditary. Thus, in Friedreich's ataxia certain columns of the cord undergo degeneration without observable cause, and in progressive lenticular degeneration, the lenticular nucleus seems to be susceptible to some vague poison.

Amaurotic Idiocy

This disease occurs in several forms. The infantile form of Tay and Sachs, most common in Jews, begins at the age of a few months and usually terminates fatally by the age of eighteen months. The child develops weakness, spastic paralysis and optic atrophy. The "cherry red spot" in the macula is diagnostic and occurs only in the infantile form. The brain is large, leathery, the convolutions atrophic. The ganglion cells of the retina and entire central nervous system show marked swelling and distortion and are filled with a lipoid substance. Gliosis, phagocytosis and demyelinization are widespread. In the retina, atrophy of the fovea centralis and marginal edema produce a light red fovea and pale macula. The late infantile form of Jansky, Schob and Bielschowsky begins at the age of three and one-half years and lasts about four years. The juvenile form of Spielmeyer and the adult form of Kufs begin later in life and last longer. The late infantile and juvenile forms are more frequent in non-Jews than in Jews.

It has been suggested that the disease is a manifestation of Niemann-Pick disease, discussed in the chapter on Hematopoietic System. Epstein, however, indicates that the proportions of lipids are different in the two and that in amaurotic idiocy there is a sugar-containing lipid not present in Niemann-Pick disease. Thannhauser holds that in the two diseases there are different deviations of phospholipid metabolism.

Friedreich's Ataxia

This disease begins in childhood or adolescence, often affects several members of the same family, may appear in more than one generation or may show no family relationship. Usually ataxia begins in the lower extremities and progresses upward; muscles of the extremities and trunk are weak but not atrophic, and reflexes depressed or absent; speech may be defective, and there is often nystagmus. Spinal curvatures and flat foot may occur apparently due to the muscular weakness.

Grossly, the principal lesion is of the cord, which is moderately or markedly reduced in size. Degeneration accompanied by secondary gliosis is well marked in the posterior columns, more especially the column of Goll, and less marked in the direct cerebellar and crossed pyramidal tracts. This is a disease of tracts in contrast to Marie's hereditary cerebellar ataxia, in which there is atrophy of the ganglion cells of the cerebellum and pons.

Progressive Lenticular Degeneration

This condition, often called Wilson's disease, is usually familial, occurs during puberty or early adult life and is associated as a rule, but not invariably, with a cirrhosis of the liver. The chief symptoms are rhythmic tremors, progressive muscular spasm followed by contractures, difficulty in speech and a highly emotional state. Grossly, there is degeneration of the lenticular nucleus, varying from numerous small cavities to a single large cavity, symmetrical, affecting chiefly the putamen, to a less extent the globus pallidus and occasionally in slight degree the caudate nucleus and internal capsule. Microscopically, there is degeneration of nerve fibers and cells, together with gliosis which also is subject to degeneration. The liver is the seat of cirrhosis identical with Laennec's cirrhosis. Although Wilson supposed that the lenticular degeneration is due to some poison generated in the liver, this has not been proved. It seems more likely that there is some cause which is common to the disease in the liver and in the brain.

Chronic Progressive Chorea

This disease, often referred to as Huntington's chorea, is familial in incidence, may occur in two generations, begins in middle life and is characterized at first by jerky movements, followed slowly by paralysis and mental deterioration. Grossly the cerebral dura is fibrotic and thickened, adherent to a thickened pia arachnoid, and sometimes associated with a chronic hemorrhagic pachymeningitis. There is generalized atrophy of the brain, especially of the frontal lobes and insular cortex. The caudate nucleus and putamen are often much shrunken and may show a yellow discoloration. As a rule the ventricles are dilated. Microscopically, the cells of the neostriatum are greatly reduced in number and there is considerable replacement gliosis. The dentate nucleus may show a loss of ganglion cells. In the cortex, the lower three layers of ganglion cells are often atrophic, and there is slight or marked gliosis.

RETROGRESSIVE CHANGES

Degenerations. Essential to the understanding of the degenerations in nerve tissue is the conception of the neuron with its cell and nerve fiber. Degeneration results when a nerve fiber is divided or its cell body destroyed. Degenerative changes in the cell may be primary, or they may be secondary to lesions of the nerve fiber. Thus the term degeneration as here employed, covers a variety of changes from minor deterioration to necrosis. When a nerve fiber is divided, the distal part undergoes the so-called wallerian degeneration. The entire distal part of the axis cylinder becomes fibrillated and exhibits a nodular or varicose swelling. The myelin is converted into droplets of unsaturated fats, positive by Marchi stain, and are further broken down and disappear. The cells of the sheath of Schwann proliferate, phagocytose the destroyed axis and myelin, fill in the defect and extend toward the proximal segment.

The changes in the proximal portion are of signficance in reference to the regeneration of nerve. Although the myelin degenerates up to the first or second node of Ranvier, the axis cylinder remains intact. In a few hours the terminal part forms a bulb-like swelling and fibrillates in an intricate fashion, and numerous fibrils grow out in all directions. These again may produce bulbs which resemble the pseudopodia of the embryonal nerve cell, as described by Harrison. Together with this change the cells of the sheath of Schwann multiply and accompany the growing fibrils. If the distance to be transversed be not too great, or the intervening granulation or connective tissue not too dense, a certain number of the fibrils grow into the original fiber path beyond the injury, and the proliferating sheath cells from both cut ends meet.

The sheath cells become arranged in tubular fashion as the new axis cylinder grows and finally, after several months, the latter replaces all the destroyed axis. Apparently, the reproduction of new myelin is the result of the combined action of axis cylinder and sheath cells, since without the presence of the axis no myelin is formed. The participation of sheath cells in regeneration has been discussed in the chapter on Inflammation. According to Harrison, they have nothing to do with the formation of the new axon.

The nerve cells may degenerate as a result of direct injury, action of poisonous substances, passive hyperemia and hyperpyrexia. In a general way it may be said that the cell swells, becomes rounded and the cytoplasm becomes vacuolated. The chromatic granules of Nissl are broken into small fragments, chromatolysis or tigrolysis, and may lose their affinity for dyes, achromatosis. The nucleus is displaced to one side of the cell and may be swollen and pale. Occasionally, it may be extruded, with death of the cell. After the extrusion or lysis of the nucleus, chromatolysis and achromatosis proceed, the cell becomes a mere shadow and ultimately disappears by solution and by the action of glial and endothelial phagocytes (neuronophagia).

The central part of the intracellular neurofibrillar network disappears at the time of chromatolysis, and this probably initiates the degeneration of the axis cylinders. Those peripheral fibrils which communicate between processes may remain until degeneration of the cell is advanced. Recovery, however, may ensue if the destructive influence abate before actual cell death occurs. Whereas passive hyperemia produces these changes, interruption of circulation is more likely to produce shrinkage and condensation of cell and nucleus, so that nuclear chromatin and Nissl substance form a homogeneous mass of basophilic substance. Following hyperpyrexia (42-43° C.), the cell swells, loses the basophilic character of nucleus and Nissl granules and becomes a more or less homogeneous acidophilic mass. (See Spielmeyer.)

Those changes in cells, which are secondary to lesions of the axons, vary in the motor and peripheral sensory neurons, and may be divided into a deteriorative or reactive stage and a reparative stage. In the deteriorative stage the cell shows changes similar to those described as occurring in response to poisons. Some cells may die and disappear, especially if repair of the axon be impossible. Repair may follow any stage short of necrosis. The Nissl granules are restored and assume normal arrangement, the nucleus resumes its normal position and the swelling of the cell gradually subsides. In the bipolar cells of the peripheral sensory axon in the posterior root ganglia, division of the peripheral axon leads to changes similar to those observed in the motor cells. Division of the central axon may be followed by no change in the cells or by slight atrophy. Nevertheless, division of the central axon may be followed by degeneration of the myelin in the peripheral axon and vice versa.

Corpora amylacea occur in various parts of the brain and cord, secondary to softening, to inflammations, to atrophy and to scar formation. They are round, vaguely laminated, rarely exceed 50 micra in diameter, are acidophilic, iodophilic, and contain glycogen.

Pigmentation. Nerve cells contain two types of pigment, which differ chemically and morphologically. In the substantia nigra, the locus caeruleus and dorsal vagus nucleus, a brown melanotic type of pigment is found, which may disappear especially in late stages of epidemic encephalitis. Lipochromes are found in many cells of the brain and increase in amount with age. As pointed out in the section on hemorrhage, blood pigments may occur free in the tissues and within phagocytic cells.

Reactions in Interstitial Tissues

In response to injuries of the nervous system the cells of the interstitium play an important rôle. The older confusion in regard to the part played by certain cells has been much clarified by modern special staining methods. The cells of epiblastic origin found normally are the protoplasmic neuroglia and

has long been known as the typical neuroglia cell or astrocyte, with small, fairly dense nucleus, well-stained finely granular cytoplasm from which fibrils, often branched, ramify into the surrounding spaces. One of the cell processes, from which most of the fibrils are supposed to originate, has a foot-like terminal in apposition to a small blood

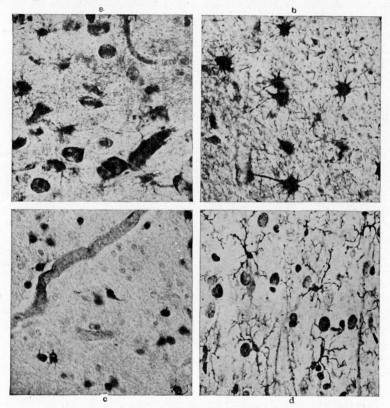

a, Protoplasmic astrocytes, human cerebral cortex. Gold-sublimate method. × 300. b, Fibrillary astrocytes. Human cerebral subcortex. Gold-sublimate method. × 300. c, Oligodendroglia. Cerebral cortex ot dog. Robertson's platinum chloride method. × 300. d, Microglia. Cerebral cortex of rabbit. Hortega's silver carbonate method. × 300. From Bailey, P., and Cushing, H., A Classification of the Tumors of the Glioma Group, etc., Philadelphia, Lippincott, 1926.

the fibrillary neuroglia. The protoplasmic neuroglia cell has a large oval nucleus with chromatin massed near the nuclear membrane. The large cytoplasmic mass is granular and is prolonged in numerous wide processes, one of which is likely to be attached by a foot-like expansion to a small blood vessel. These cells are not normally fibrillar. In response to inflammation they were supposed by Alzheimer to become ameboid, but it is now known that such an appearance is due to degeneration. The fibrillary neuroglia cell

vessel. Either of these cells may occur with only a small number of processes or fibrils. In the replacement of defects in the central nervous system, the scar is made up of neuroglia of astrocytic type, contributed to principally by the fibrillary neuroglia but also sometimes by transformation of protoplasmic neuroglia with enlargement and production of fibrils.

Two other cell types are observed which Bailey classifies under the heading of "mesoglia (?)," namely, the microglia and oligodendroglia cells. Although some doubt exists as to their origin, it seems probable at the present time that they are of mesoblastic origin. The nucleus of the microglia is small, oval and has heavy bands of chromatin. The cytoplasm is scanty and from it extend a few long processes, not fibrillae, which branch dichotomously and show minute spine-like projections at right angles to the stems of the processes and their branches.

Under pathologic conditions, where debris is to be removed, these cells become phagocytic. The destruction of tissue liberates cell and fiber detritus, neutral fats, fatty

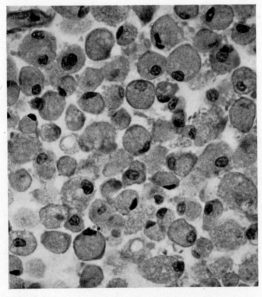

Scavenger cells, or compound granule cells, in the margin of a cerebral infarct (encephalomalacia).

acids, soaps, lecithin, cerebrosides and phosphatides (Spielmeyer). The microglia cells multiply by mitotic division, show swelling of the cell body, thickening, shortening and disappearance of the processes, and increase further in size as the debris is ingested. The result is a large cell the cytoplasm of which is filled with small lipoidal and fat globules and minor amounts of other debris, which has been given various names including compound granule cells, "gitterzellen" and scavenger cells. They accumulate about wounds and later stages of inflammatory and other destructive areas, and in response to destruction of tissues by gliomas (Penfield). They transport the ingested material to neighboring

capillaries or perivascular spaces. Opinion now places these cells in the group of reticuloendothelial cells, which means that they are mesoblastic rather than glial.

Also derived from the microglia cells are the rod cells, or "stäbchenzellen," elongated cells found in the cortex under various pathologic conditions, especially paresis, parallel to vessels, vertical to the cortical surface, with granular cytoplasm projecting from the long ellipsoidal nucleus. These appear to be special forms of phagocytes.

The oligodendroglia cells, or cells with few dentrites, are probably of mesoblastic origin, although some believe them to be epiblastic. The nucleus is somewhat larger than that of the microglia. The cytoplasm is clear or reticulated, extremely scanty, and is prolonged in a small number of nonfibrillar processes which show little branching and no lateral spines, but with occasional points of nodular enlargement. The part played by these cells in reaction to injury is not clear, but some consider that they may act as phagocytes.

TRAUMATIC INJURY

Brain

Tissue Injury. The brain may be wounded by foreign bodies such as knives, shell fragments or bullets, which penetrate the skull, or by fractures of the skull with displacement inward of fragments of the inner or all tables of the skull. There is destruction of tissues accompanied by hemorrhage and edema of the neighboring tissues. The edema may produce moderate, marked, or even fatal increase of intracranial pressure. Death may be almost immediate, due to shock, or may be delayed for several days or weeks. Recovery and scar formation may result, or infection may produce meningitis and encephalitis. Injuries to the skull at one point may produce hemorrhage or contusion of the brain at the opposite pole, or fractures of the skull from within outward, the so-called lesions by *contrecoup*. Hemorrhage near the roof of the fourth ventricle with subsequent fibrosis may rarely lead to internal hydrocephalus (Moritz and Wartman). Direct injuries of the skull or indirect injuries as by falling heavily on feet or buttocks, may, without fracture of the skull, lead to meningeal hemorrhage or to the condition spoken of as concussion.

In concussion, there is coma, which may be prolonged, usually followed by recovery, but sometimes having an intervening period of headache, amnesia and mental confusion. In fatal cases, the cortex and gray matter may show swelling of ganglion cells or actual foci of necrosis, which Helfand attributes to vascular spasm. There are tiny hemorrhages in meninges and cortex as well as in white matter, in basal ganglia and brain stem (Neugebauer). The clinical manifestations of concussion may be produced by meningeal hemorrhage or the lesions of *contrecoup*.

The Spinal Cord

Partial or complete transverse lesions of the cord may be due to penetrating injuries, to fractures or fracture dislocations of the spine the result of trauma or disease, to tumors, to parasitic cysts and to suppurative lesions. Hemorrhage, or hematomyelia, may be local in meninges or cord or both, but occasionally, starting at the point of injury, the hemorrhage may extend longitudinally, especially in the gray matter, produce acute symptoms like those of syringomyelia, and, if organized, absorbed and cicatrized by gliosis, produce a lesion apparently identical with that of syringomyelia.

Interruptions of the cord by either trauma or disease may produce spinal shock with its prolonged depression of reflexes, which is due presumably to a defect in transmission at the synapse of the reflex arc. Degenerations of descending tracts below and of ascending tracts above the point of interruption ensue. The paralysis affects the bladder, and cystitis, inflammation of renal pelvis and kidney, septicemia or pyemia, and death may follow. At the site of injury, more especially when the cord is crushed, there is swelling, hyperemia and softening of the cord, degeneration and finally necrosis of the gray and white matter, with or without petechiae, sometimes acute inflammation and reactive gliosis. This lesion is referred to as compression myelitis and appears to be due rather to the severe passive hyperemia from compression of the veins than to the direct pressure upon the cord.

Concussion of the spinal cord may be due to direct or indirect trauma to the spine. The cord may show practically no lesion or may be the seat of edema, of petechiae and particularly of small areas of softening, either in white or gray matter, and subsequent gliosis. More severe injuries may produce contusion, show more marked lesions with degeneration of nerve cells and fibers at the site of injury and the changes of concussion in more remote areas (Hassin).

"War neuroses," which are neurasthenias, hysterias, psychasthenias, due to exhaustion and emotional stress, have been incorrectly ascribed to the general bodily compression effects of explosions (Hurst).

Birth Injuries

Birth hemorrhages are those which occur in the meninges during or shortly after birth. Symptoms and signs may be slight or death ensue in the first few days. The vessels ruptured are small tributaries of large sinuses, and the hemorrhage is usually subtentorial. Although the trauma of forceps and of prolonged labor may be sufficient to cause the hemorrhage (Chase), it may well be that the hemorrhagic tendency of vitamin-K deficiency can be of significance.

The Nerves

Injuries to peripheral nerves may be indirect and the lesion in the nerve like that of a bruise. There are edema and variable degrees of hemorrhage. The myelin may be damaged, with resultant transitory loss of motor or sensory function, or the axis cylinders may also be involved and wallerian degeneration occur. Division of nerves may be due to knife and projectile wounds, laceration by fragments of fractured bones, or interruption of continuity by abscess, tumors, etc. The resultant changes have been described in the section on degeneration. If a wound be infected, a neuritis may progress along the course of the nerve.

Obstetric paralysis affects especially the arm and is the result of injury during birth. As pointed out by Sever, the injury varies from stretching of the nerve trunks with hemorrhage and edema, to tearing of perineural sheath and of nerve fibers. In the more common upper-arm type, the lesion involves the fifth and sixth cervical roots and the suprascapular nerve. In the whole-arm type there is additional involvement of the seventh and eighth cervical and sometimes the first thoracic roots. Injury to the spinal cord with resultant paraplegia or death is an occasional sequel of labor; this is true of breech extractions more than other mechanisms of labor (Crothers).

Caisson disease, or diver's palsy, in its general aspects, is discussed in the chapter on General Disturbances of Circulation. As indicated there, the decompression of caisson workers and divers may be so rapid as to release bubbles of nitrogen. This is especially injurious in the central and peripheral nervous system, with resultant pain of the "bends," as well as motor and other sensory disturbances. Under compression, the lipids of the nervous system absorb considerable quantities of nitrogen and with too rapid decompression the gas is released as bubbles in the white matter especially. These bubbles compress the surrounding tissues so that foci of softening occur in which there is degeneration of myelin sheaths associated at first with swelling and later with destruction of axis cylinders; the gas may also bring about these effects by lodgment in blood vessels as gas emboli. The ultimate change is a gliosis of the injured parts. (See Thorne.)

The rapid reduction of barometric pressure, such as occurs when aviators are compelled by military needs to ascend quickly to great heights, may have much the same effects (Fulton).

CIRCULATORY DISTURBANCES

Hyperemia

Localized active hyperemia occurs in inflammations, but a generalized cerebral active hyperemia, in the sense of a notably increased bulk of blood, is unusual because of the large area of venous drainage and of drainage of cerebrospinal fluid. Mental activity presumably is accompanied by an increased rate of blood flow rather than by a true hyperemia. If active hyperemia occur in such conditions as sunstroke and acute alcoholism, it is not demonstrable at autopsy. Passive hyperemia may be due to local conditions such as compression of veins by tumors and occlusion by thrombosis, or to general conditions such as heart failure. The brain may be somewhat enlarged, shows dilated meningeal veins, may have a purple tinge and in the cross section shows numerous fine red or purple points in the position of the vessels in the white matter. This must not be confused with a passive hyperemia of the dependent parts of the brain which often occurs after death.

Anemia

Temporary general anemia of the brain is usually due to vasomotor disturbances and may cause fainting. Emotional shock or injury to the splanchnic plexus may so dilate the splanchnic vessels that the amount of blood supplied to the head is insufficient. High-grade anemias and profuse general hemorrhage may produce cerebral anemia. Local anemia may be due to compression of vessels, for example, by tumors. The principal feature grossly is the extreme pallor of white and gray matter and the absence of red punctae in the cross section. Complete interruption of the circulation for as little as eight minutes may produce necrosis in the gray matter (Weinberger, et al.).

Edema

Edema of the brain may be secondary to prolonged passive hyperemia and may occur in uremia and in acute and chronic alcoholism. Local forms of edema may be seen about tumors, abscesses, hemorrhages, and foci of softening of the brain. When the brain is extensively edematous, it is increased in weight, shows flattening of the convolutions and sometimes a bulging of the brain stem and neighboring cerebellum into the foramen magnum, the so-called pressure cone. There is often an increase of fluid in the pia arachnoid and sometimes in the ventricles. The cross section is pale and moist. Microscopically, the changes are often inconspicuous, but dilatation of perivascular spaces, loose arrangement of tissues and swelling of glial cells may be present. Chemically, there is a definite increase in water content.

Thrombosis and Embolism

Thrombosis is usually superimposed on arteriosclerosis, commonly in the middle cerebral artery or its branches. It may, however, be due to acute infectious diseases, more especially in childhood, or to blood diseases such as leukemia. Syphilis may produce a gummatous arteritis with secondary thrombosis. Rarely trauma is a cause of thrombosis. If the lumen of the artery be reduced slowly, the region supplied becomes the seat of atrophy with degeneration and disappearance first of cells and then of nerves, and a replacement gliosis and fibrosis. In this way, numerous large and small areas of the cerebral cortex may be the seat of the so-called arteriosclerotic atrophy. If the vessel be occluded, necrosis results in the same manner as following embolism.

Embolism may be due to the lodging of a fragment of vegetation of acute endocarditis, thrombi in cardiac chambers, on arteriosclerotic plaques or in aneurysms, fragments of diseased aorta, or destructive lesions of the lungs. Emboli lodge most frequently in the middle cerebral artery or its branches, but other arteries may be affected. Fat embolism is often widespread in the brain and may be the cause of convulsive symptoms, but usually is fatal before secondary changes occur. Both thrombosis and embolism may produce the clinical syndrome called apoplexy, thrombosis with gradual onset, embolism with abrupt onset. The onset of symptoms is abrupt in cerebral embolism, less so in hemorrhage and usually gradual in thrombosis; hemorrhage, however, is the most frequent lesion. Cerebral infarction follows thrombosis or embolism, the process being essentially the same as in infarction elsewhere (Cobb). It is often called softening of the brain, or encephalomalacia. Rarely, but more especially in childhood, occlusion of veins may produce softening.

Encephalomalacia. Fresh foci of softening may not be demonstrable grossly until after the brain is properly hardened in a fixative. They are then found to be softer and more friable than the surrounding tissue. The conical shape of the infarct with base toward the cortex may be apparent if a large artery be occluded, but often the vessel is of small size and centrally situated so that the involved region is generally globular. If several days have elapsed, the softened region may be swollen and, if peripheral, the convolutions may be flattened and pale. The necrotic tissue is moist, soft, friable and bulges in the cross surface.

Microscopically, all stages of degener-ation to complete necrosis of nerve cells and fibers are found, with cell detritus and fragments of myelin, but the striking feature is the appearance of the compound granule or scavenger cells described above. Hemorrhage occurs in the early stages of cerebral infarction as is true of other organs and may be slight or marked. Furthermore, after the softening has occurred there may be hemorrhage into it. Subsequently, as the blood degenerates, the area becomes yellow. By this time, the necrotic mass has liquefied and the glial reaction has become so marked that a cyst is formed. In minute foci no such cystic stage occurs because organization fills the defect, but if the infarct have a diameter of about 1 cm. or more, cyst formation results. The cyst content may be cloudy and granular or may be almost clear, of brown or yellow tinge or nearly colorless. If the small focus be organized, the residual granular and crystalline blood pigment gives it a brown color. The cyst wall is similarly pigmented. Scavenger cells may be observed for a long period after the original softening, but in diminishing numbers. In small foci the neuroglia may be preserved but in larger foci it undergoes necrosis. The scar or cyst wall is built up by fibrillary neuroglia and by the growth of mesoblastic tissue which accompanies the blood vessels. The tract degenerations will be discussed with those which follow hemorrhage.

Hemorrhage

Hemorrhage may take place in the meninges, the brain substance or the ventricles. Traumatic hemorrhage may be extradural, subdural, into the pia arachnoid, and into the brain substance. Extradural hemorrhage is usually secondary to skull fracture. That into the brain substance is due to penetration of missiles, of fragments of fractured skull or is indirect in the lesion of *contrecoup*.

Subdural hemorrhage leads to the production of subdural hematoma. It is usually due to direct or indirect trauma, but may occur without injury in local inflammations, infectious diseases and hemorrhagic diseases. It is usually situated over the parietofrontal region and in about 30 per cent of the cases is bilateral. Seen early, there is a flat, dark red or black clot apparently between dura and pia arachnoid, from a few to several centimeters in diameter, compressing the underlying brain. Granulation tissue grows, organization takes place in the periphery and a membrane of richly vascularized connective tissue forms around the hematoma. This becomes firmer as time goes on. In the meantime the clot changes to a coffee colored and later a greenish-yellow fluid which contains small remnants of clot. Often, however, the hemorrhage is extensive and covers a large part of the surface of the brain; when this is true death usually occurs, and thus the sequence of events described in the smaller subdural hematoma does not take place.

The hemorrhage is due, according to most investigators, to tearing of the tiny bridging veins between dura and pia, but some think that the bleeding is really into the deeper layers of the dura from the intradural vessels, with resultant splitting of the dura. Secondary hemorrhage may occur from the vessels of the new membrane. Clinically, there are signs and symptoms due to the local compression of the brain and to a general increase of intracranial pressure. (See Baker.)

Subarachnoid hemorrhage may be slight or extensive. Although it is often called spontaneous it is usually due to aneurysms of arteries at the base of the brain and may be caused by inflammatory or other disease of the vessels.

Aneurysms are considered here because of the possibility of rupture and hemorrhage. Aneurysm may be due to acute arteritis occurring in the course of acute infectious disease or it may be a mycotic aneurysm. Syphilitic arteritis can also lead to aneurysm. Arteriosclerosis is a cause. Aneurysm at the branching of arteries and at the junctions in the circle of Willis may be due to structural weakness of the wall in these situations and in the circle are often accompanied by anomalies especially of the communicating arteries. This is the form of aneurysm referred to as congenital. Such an aneurysm because it is a saccule with a narrow neck at the attachment is often called a "berry aneurysm." In many of these there is also accompanying disease of the artery. Only rarely are fusiform aneurysms encountered.

Most aneurysms are in or near the circle of Willis. They vary in size from a few millimeters to several centimeters. The larger sacs may produce signs and symptoms of local pressure, but often the first indication of their presence is due to rupture. As a rule they project into the subarachnoid space and the hemorrhage is more or less widespread in the subarachnoid space. Sometimes they project into the brain substance and the hemorrhage is into the brain and this may be accompanied by subdural or even intraventricular hemorrhage. Intraventricular hemorrhage, however, is more often due to extension from rupture of an intracerebral artery. (See Richardson and Hyland.)

Within the brain there are often tiny hemorrhagic foci referred to as miliary aneurysms. There is dispute as to the nature of these. They are probably not true aneurysms but rather small hematomas which may or may not be encapsulated. If encapsulated, they are in the category of false aneurysms. Arteriosclerosis and other diseases of the vessel walls are responsible for these minute hemorrhages.

Cerebral Hemorrhage. Although trauma may cause hemorrhage into the brain substance, the term cerebral hemorrhage is usually applied to nontraumatic forms, unless specifically designated as traumatic. Hemorrhage into cerebrum as well as into cerebellum and brain stem may occur as the result of acute infectious disease, especially the hemorrhagic forms, diseases of the blood with purpuric manifestations, leukemia and acute inflammations of arteries such as periarteritis nodosa. These hemorrhages are usually multiple and relatively small.

The large solitary, or rarely multiple, hemorrhage of apoplexy with its resultant hemiplegia is usually due to rupture of one or more of the small lenticulo-striate or lenticulo-optic arteries which branch off at right angles from the middle cerebral artery. Because of this structural arrangement, it is probable that these small arteries at their points of origin are subjected to somewhat higher intravascular pressure than if they were the usual dichotomous branches. Normal arteries can withstand enormous increases of intravascular pressure without rupture. Thus there is a factor of disease that determines rupture. With marked disease, normal or only slightly elevated blood pressure may cause rupture. The disease is

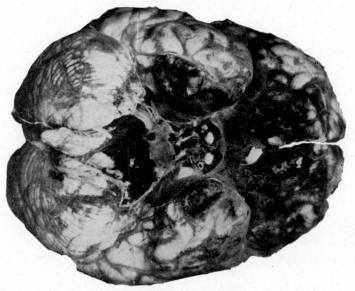

Meningeal hemorrhage, the result of falling on buttocks.

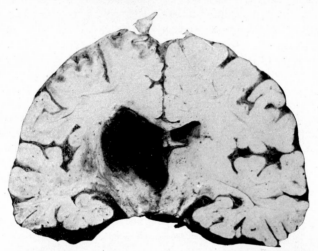

Hemorrhage in cerebrum involving internal capsule.

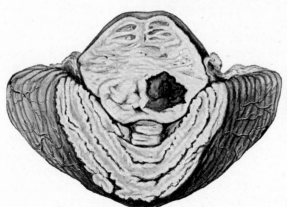

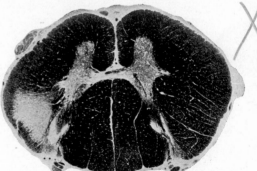

Hemorrhage in pons.

Cross section of cord, showing degeneration of crossed pyramidal tract secondary to cerebral hemorrhage. Weigert-Pal stain for myelin sheaths. Courtesy of Stanley Cobb, M.D.

usually arteriosclerosis, but acute arterial disease, syphilitic arteritis and aneurysms may decrease resistance to internal pressure and lead to rupture. Cerebral hemorrhage is a disease of late middle and advanced life, just as is arteriosclerosis.

When cerebral hemorrhage occurs in earlier life, it is usually caused by persistent hypertension. In these cases the disease of the artery is only slight, but the wall lacks resistance to the high blood pressure. In older and younger subjects, a sudden increase of pressure due to physical stress or emotional excitement may decide the time of rupture.

The larger hemorrhages into the brain occur, in diminishing order of frequency, in the basal ganglia, the external and internal capsule, corona radiata, cortex, pons, cerebellum and rarely in crura and brain stem. Although small aneurysms may be found in the affected vessels, the studies of Lindermann indicate that the actual hemorrhage is from several minute ruptures of the vessel walls rather than rupture of these aneurysmal dilatations. As the blood extravasates, it destroys nerve substance and compresses the surrounding structures.

The hemorrhage may be minute, or may vary from a centimeter in diameter to a mass so large as to occupy almost an entire hemisphere. It is usually fairly well defined and may be surrounded by a zone of edema or by a number of small punctate hemorrhages, the latter probably due to rupture of capillaries from the sudden increase in pressure (Bouman). The blood rapidly clots and the cross section is dark red and relatively dry. Recent hemorrhages may bulge in the cross section, but in the course of time the clot contracts, the serum is drained away and the surface retracts.

Microscopically, the neighborhood of recent hemorrhages shows an infiltration of mononuclear cells and a few leukocytes. Scavenger cells appear and phagocytose the debris of tissue and myelin. The breakdown of blood furnishes both hemosiderin and hematoidin, which for a time are within phagocytic cells. There is a reactive gliosis and fibrosis and the hemorrhage becomes cicatrized if small, or encysted if large. The cyst is filled with limpid or thick fluid, usually brown or yellow in color and the cyst

wall is of similar but usually deeper color, due to the pigment which now lies free between cells and fibers. Persistent blood vessels which have undergone thrombosis and organization may remain as bands in the cavity of the cyst.

The usual hemorrhage interrupts the anterior part of the internal capsule either by pressure or by destruction. The extent of interruption is reduced as edema decreases and the clot contracts. Nevertheless, in the more extensive lesions there is a consequent degeneration of the upper motor neuron, extending through pons, medulla and cord, which involves direct and crossed pyramidal tracts. The partial or complete coma of the apoplectic seizure is presumably due either to the general increase of intracranial pressure, or to pressure upon the healthy side by the swollen diseased side. The conjugate deviation of head and eyes toward the side of the lesion is probably due either to involvement of the laterogyric center of Horsley or to hemianopsia. The early flaccid paralysis and decreased reflexes are probably due to cerebral and spinal shock, but as this is recovered from, the interruption of the inhibitory influence of the upper neuron results in spastic paralysis and contractures. Disturbances of sensation may occur when the posterior part of the internal capsule is involved.

Decubitus ulcers commonly occur, but their exact cause is subject to discussion. Pressure anemia and trophic disturbances are thought to play an important part, but certain observers think that they are due principally to infection of the buttocks as the result of incontinence of urine and feces.

The same general train of events accompanies encephalomalacia due to thrombosis or embolism.

Sinus Thrombosis. Severe acute and chronic infectious diseases, prolonged exhausting diseases, and blood diseases may be complicated by thrombosis of the large venous sinuses of the cerebrum and meninges. The primary or marantic form occurs especially in infants and the aged. In contrast is the secondary form in which the venous thrombosis is secondary to some other lesion, for example, compression by tumors or, more often, inflammations in the neighborhood. Inflammations of the bones of the skull, embolic or secondary to inflammations of the face, mouth, nose or air sinuses, inflammations of the meninges or abscesses within the skull cavity, may produce sinus thrombosis. Probably the most common cause is suppurative otitis media which extends to the mastoid air cells and thence to the lateral venous sinus.

CAVERNOUS SINUS THROMBOSIS may be caused by inflammations of the face or neck, presumably because of retrograde thrombosis of veins. The primary cases show more or less organized, mixed clots, which often extend into tributary veins. In some instances a hyperemic focus of encephalo-

probably because it is more richly vascular than the white matter, and extends longitudinally as noted in the section on traumatic injuries.

Hematorrhachis, or hemorrhage into the spinal canal, may be extradural or subdural. The former may be traumatic or may be the result of rupture of an aneurysm or due to violent convulsions. Subdural hemorrhage may originate in the head, it may be due to direct or indirect injury of the spine, or it may complicate any of the various hemorrhagic diseases. The extrameningeal hemorrhages rarely produce pressure symptoms because of the ready escape of the

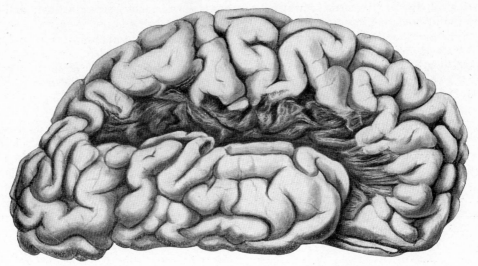

Large area of cortical atrophy due to arteriosclerosis.

malacia occurs. In the secondary cases the thrombus may be simple or may suppurate, and as a result brain abscesses or purulent meningitis may occur.

Circulatory Disturbances of the Spinal Cord

Hyperemia may occur in the spinal cord under the same conditions as in the brain. Passive hyperemia may also be induced by the compression of traumatic lesions or tumors. Small foci of myelomalacia are not rare, and result from minute arterial emboli.

Hemorrhage into the cord or hematomyelia, is usually traumatic in origin and only rarely due to rupture of diseased vessels by high blood pressure. The hemorrhage is usually in the gray matter,

blood outward. Subdural hemorrhages may occasionally lead to compression of the cord. Edema of the cord may result from inflammations and from passive hyperemia. Edema of the meninges is usually secondary to excess drainage of fluid from cerebral ventricles or meninges.

Atrophy

Atrophy of the brain may be local or widespread. Local atrophy may be due to compression by tumors and by hemorrhage as well as to arteriosclerosis in an artery or small group of arteries. Widespread atrophy may occur in chronic poisonings, prolonged exhausting diseases and in paresis. It may also be due to generalized cerebral arteriosclerosis. It occurs in senility, but in our opinion arteriosclerosis is the principal cause of this form of atrophy.

Grossly, the brain is reduced in size and weight and is firm. The convolutions are narrow and shrunken and the sulci correspondingly wide. The meninges may be slightly thickened. Often there is an increase of fluid in meninges and in ventricles. On cross section the cortical gray matter is reduced in thickness and the basal ganglia may be of decreased size. Microscopically, the ganglion cells are atrophic and may show degeneration, chromatolysis, pigmentation, nuclear displacement and may ultimately disappear. The myelin of the sheaths is often reduced in amount. There is a proliferation of fibrillary neuroglia which replaces the atrophic substance.

These are the changes observed in so-called senile dementia as well as in that presenile dementia known as Alzheimer's disease. A circumscribed widespread atrophy, without known cause, occurs in middle and later life and is called Pick's disease; in this the gliosis is especially pronounced.

INFLAMMATIONS

Meningitis

Meningitis may be acute or chronic and may affect either the pia arachnoid as leptomeningitis, or the dura as pachymeningitis.

Suppurative external pachymeningitis is secondary to lesions of the bones of the skull, as osteomyelitis or more especially inflammation of air sinuses. It may spread laterally but is more often confined in the form of an extradural abscess. It may extend through the dura and produce leptomeningitis, brain abscess or sinus thrombosis.

Internal hemorrhagic pachymeningitis is said to be inflammatory but we have not found that to be true, at least in so far as concerns infectious origin. It may be secondary to atrophy of the brain and occurs in general paralysis, chronic progressive chorea and chronic poisonings. The lesion is usually on the vertex and may be bilateral or unilateral. Attached with variable degrees of firmness to the inner surface of the dura is a thin laminated film of red, brown or yellow color. The inner layer of the dura is rich in capillaries which bleed easily. A layer of blood spreads over the inner surface, sometimes with and sometimes without leukocyte infiltration, and with fibrin deposit. This undergoes organization by fibroblasts and blood vessels, and blood pigment is deposited. A second layer is formed and the process repeats itself, each succeeding layer more recent in appearance than its predecessor. The process may be arrested and remain as a dense, adherent, brown or yellow layer of fibrous tissue.

Pachymeningitis cervicalis hypertrophica is a rare lesion, in which the dura and pia arachnoid surrounding the cervical enlargement of the cord become the seat of dense fibrosis, may become calcified and even ossified. Its cause is unknown.

Acute leptomeningitis may be serous, fibrinous, purulent or hemorrhagic. Serous meningitis is not often seen at autopsy but the clinical examination of spinal fluid shows that it frequently precedes the purulent form. Fibrinous meningitis is most often seen in acute tuberculous infection of the membrane. Purulent meningitis is common. Hemorrhagic meningitis is often fulminant clinically. It is due to infection by hemolytic bacteria or to coincidental blood diseases. Except in epidemics of meningococcal cerebrospinal meningitis, the most common organisms are the pyogenic cocci, especially streptococcus, staphylococcus and pneumococcus. A wide variety of other organisms may cause the disease including typhoid, influenza and colon bacilli. Streptococcal meningitis may be apparently primary or may complicate measles, influenza, pneumonia, septicemia, etc. Neither pneumonia nor typhoid fever necessarily precedes meningitis due to the pneumococcus or typhoid bacillus. Intrathecal injections of foreign serum may produce an acute evanescent meningitis.

Acute meningitis may follow surgical or accidental trauma and is usually unilateral. The same is true of meningitis due to inflammations of the air sinuses, particularly those of the mastoid process. The mode of transfer of infection from inflamed accessory air sacs is variable. The disease may cause an osteomyelitis, with transfer of organisms to the meninges. The inflammation may extend into venous channels and to venous sinuses, or extend through the lymphatics surrounding the blood vessels and the nerves (see Kramer and Som). Fractures of the skull may break the air sacs and permit entry of infection to the meninges. Meningitis may also occur in septicemia and pyemia.

SPINAL MENINGES. Inflammations of the spinal meninges may be due to extension from the cerebral meninges or may be caused directly by penetrating wounds or by lymphatic and hematogenous transport of infective organisms.

Grossly, the distribution of the exudate in meningitis depends somewhat on the mode of origin. In epidemic meningitis,

only hyperemia in the underlying nerve substance, but in certain forms, especially suppurative, there may be extension into the surface of the brain, meningo-encephalitis, or into the cord, meningomyelitis.

Hyperemia is marked and there may be petechiae. The exudate may be serous in character, limpid but cloudy, containing numerous leukocytes, desquamated meningeal cells, fibrin threads and bacteria. The purulent exudate is made up largely of leukocytes, normal and in various degrees of degeneration, and contains also mononuclear cells, tissue debris and bacteria, but usually little fibrin. In hemorrhagic meningitis, the

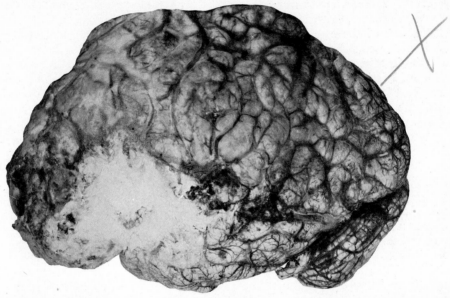

Abscess of temporal lobe of brain, with associated acute purulent meningitis. Army Medical Museum, 30804.

the exudate is usually at the base; in pneumococcal meningitis, it is usually over the vertex; in that due to extension from disease of the middle ear it is on the lateral aspect and in other forms due to direct extension it is likely to be localized. In any of these forms, the exudate may extend widely over the brain and into the spinal meninges. The color of the exudate differs somewhat in different conditions. Usually it is pale yellow, but in pneumococcal meningitis it is pale green and in pyocyaneous meningitis it is darker green. Hyperemia is usually marked and there may be petechiae. Usually the inflammation is confined to the meninges with

hemorrhage may be punctate or widespread and may be massive. Most such cases are fulminant and both grossly and microscopically the inflammation may be masked by the hemorrhage.

In addition to inflammatory irritation, there may be an increase of intracranial pressure. This may be due to the mass of exudate or adhesions in the cisterna magna, to occlusion of the ventricular outlets in similar fashion, or to interference with drainage by the arachnoidal villi. In some instances edema of the brain itself may obstruct the flow of fluid.

The clinical manifestations of acute

meningitis include fever, headache, vomiting, stiff neck, positive Kernig and Brudzinski signs and leukocytosis. The spinal fluid contains many cells, most of which are polymorphonuclear leukocytes. Organisms may be demonstrated on smear and culture.

Clinical manifestations like those of meningitis may occur in acute infectious disease, but the spinal fluid shows little or no change. This is called MENINGISMUS. Autopsy in such cases rarely shows meningeal inflammation and the condition is probably due to products of the infection.

Epidemic Cerebrospinal Meningitis. This disease may be sporadic, endemic or epidemic. It is due to the *Neisseria intracellularis* of Weichselbaum, a small gramnegative diplococcus, often phagocytosed by the leukocytes of the exudate. Its mode of entry into the meninges is not clear, although the fact that it is present in the nasopharynx of victims and carriers, suggests strongly that it enters through the cribriform plate of the ethmoid. It is probably transmitted by droplet infection.

The inflammation usually begins at the base of the brain, whence it extends anteriorly to the temporal and frontal lobes, posteriorly over the cerebellum, laterally over the sylvian fissure and vertex, and inferiorly along the brain stem and cord. The exudate is richly purulent, thick and of yellow or greenish-yellow color. The brain proper is not frequently involved. Microscopically, the exudate is purulent and the polymorphonuclears are likely to contain phagocytosed organisms. As the process becomes subacute and chronic, more and more lymphocytes and large mononuclear cells are found. If recovery ensue, there may be a residual fibrosis, often called chronic posterior basic meningitis, with thickening of the meninges over the pons, medulla and inferior surface of the cerebellum. Here it may involve the cisterna magna and prevent drainage of the ventricles. Thus internal hydrocephalus may more or less abruptly kill patients who seem to have survived the acute disease.

Lymphocytic Choriomeningitis. This is a febrile disease of short duration, caused by a virus. Clinically it may resemble influenza, but without nervous or marked respiratory disturbance, or it may be like acute meningitis. In the meningeal cases, the spinal fluid contains many cells, practically all of which are lymphocytes. Sometimes the presence of somnolence, disturbance of deep reflexes, paralysis and anesthesia suggest that the brain is involved in the form of a meningo-encephalitis. The disease is so rarely fatal that little is known of its anatomic features.

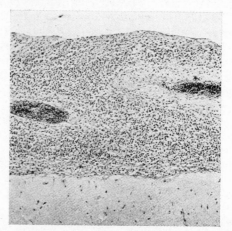

Meningeal exudate in acute suppurative meningitis.

Based on the few observations of human material and the experimental disease in monkeys, it may be said that there is patchy or diffuse infiltration of lymphocytes into the meninges and into the choroid plexuses. The brain may show perivascular collections of lymphocytes and nodular gliosis, especially in the midbrain. The lymph nodes and spleen may be hyperplastic and the liver may show focal necrosis. Healing of the meningeal lesions may result in cicatricial adhesions in the meninges and interference with the movement of cerebrospinal fluid. (See Armstrong; Farmer and Janeway.)

Chronic leptomeningitis may occur upon any part of the brain and cord, in the course of chronic alcoholism, lead poisoning, chronic nephritis and heart disease, or over lesions of the nervous substance. It may be simply a fibrosis which produces a thick, white, dense, adherent area in the meninges, or may also show an associated serous exudate containing a few lymphocytes. Syphilis may produce a condition similar grossly, but with special features microscopically. Cicatrization of a preceding acute meningitis may give much the same appearance as a chronic meningitis.

Meningitis Due to Higher Organisms. Occasionally the meninges are the seat of infection by higher vegetable organisms. Of these, infection by *Torula histolytica* is the most frequent, as indicated in the chapter on Infectious Granulomata. *Toxoplasma* may also infect the meninges, as described in the chapter on Principles of Infectious Disease. Both these forms of disease show involvement of the underlying brain substance and the condition is a meningoencephalitis. Infection by other higher forms such as may occur in oidiomycosis, sporotrichosis, coccidiomycosis, etc., are rare.

Encephalitis

This may be suppurative or nonsuppurative and is to be distinguished from encephalomalacia.

Suppurative encephalitis, or abscess of the brain, is due to infection which may enter in various ways. Infected surgical wounds, compound fractures, and the entry of infected missiles may be followed by abscess. The suppuration, however, may be delayed several days after the trauma. In civil life, suppuration of middle ear and mastoid process is the most common cause of abscess. The abscess may be in continuity with the ear disease, may be separate, lying in the temporosphenoidal region or cerebellum of the same side, or may occur in the opposite side, probably due to lymphatic transmission of the organisms.

Other forms of suppurative bone disease of the skull may produce abscess. Suppurative sinus thrombosis and, rarely, suppurative meningitis may produce abscess, although in the latter instance it is often difficult to determine which is primary, for an abscess rupturing on the surface may produce a widespread meningitis.

Multiple abscess of the brain may complicate almost any of the acute infectious diseases, including the exanthemata, diphtheria, rheumatic fever, typhoid and typhus fevers, anthrax, glanders, and the pyogenic septicemias and pyemias. In many instances the abscesses are microscopic in size and perivascular in arrangement. In pyemia, however, they may be numerous and large.

Destructive diseases of the lung such as purulent bronchitis and bronchiectasis, pulmonary abscess or gangrene may be complicated by abscess of the brain, usually single and in the left side. A very few cases are without demonstrable origin and are called idiopathic. In certain cases trauma, not sufficient to break the skin, may precede brain abscess and there may be no other apparent cause, but it is difficult to understand the relation between the injury and the abscess, and for the present such cases might well be included in the idiopathic group. In addition to various aerobic and anaerobic bacteria, the lesion may be caused by streptothrices.

The gross appearance depends somewhat upon the cause. Traumatic abscess shows the hemorrhage due to the injury. In certain infectious diseases, the abscess may be hemorrhagic, for example, in scarlatina, pertussis, influenza, anthrax and streptococcal endocarditis. The pus is usually creamy and yellow but may show other characters and colors when caused by special organisms. With the more recent abscesses, the surrounding brain substance is edematous and the seat of encephalomalacia. Later there is a wall of organization made up principally of mesoblastic reaction rather than of glial proliferation. Surrounding hyperemia may or may not be present. Ultimately a cyst or scar may result. Depending upon the extent and severity of the abscess or abscesses, the brain may be large and edematous.

Microscopically, the course of the abscess is much the same as elsewhere, with primary hyperemia and necrosis of brain substance, followed by exudation and the processes which lead to encapsulation or cicatrization. The nerve cells and fibers show the ordinary degenerative changes, which progress to necrosis. Three more or less distinct layers can ordinarily be made out in the larger abscesses. The center of the abscess is made up of necrotic brain substance, leukocytes, both normal and degenerate, bacteria and sometimes blood or blood pigment. The second zone is provided principally by mesoblastic granulation tissue derived from the blood vessels. Intermingled with the fibroblasts are tissue debris, lymphoid and large mononuclear cells and scavenger or compound granule cells. The third zone is that of glial reaction, where, in the earlier stages, various degenerative forms may be encountered including the "ameboid" form. Multiplication of glia cells is by mitosis, and multinucleated forms may result. Ultimately, the proliferation of fibrillary neuroglia produces a fairly dense zone of fibrillar gliosis. The surrounding blood vessels may show perivascular infiltration, at first of leukocytes and later of lymphoid cells. Surrounding nerve cells may degenerate. (See Carmichael, et al.)

Nonsuppurative Encephalitis. This occurs in two principal forms, a toxic encephalitis or encephalopathy and various forms of nonsuppurative nonhemorrhagic encephalitis. Acute toxic encephalopathy occurs as the result of poisoning by arsenic, lead, guanidine, and may occur in children without demonstrable cause (Low). There is degeneration of cells of the gray matter, but

sionally also in the cord. Minute hemorrhages may occur in both brain and cord. Microscopically, various changes may be found in the same brain, usually most marked in basal ganglia, pons and medulla. Hyperemia and a few small hemorrhages are present, but the most striking feature is a perivascular infiltration, especially about the venules of the gray matter, of lymphocytes and plasma cells. This infiltration may be preceded by perivascular hemorrhage or even fibrin formation, but polymorphonuclear leukocytes play practically no part. Small foci of encephalomalacia may follow vascular thrombosis. The nerve cells may show chromatolysis, which may proceed to recovery or to cell degeneration and death, the fragments being removed by phagocytes. The meninges may escape or may show slight diffuse and perivascular lymphoid infiltra-

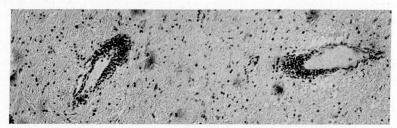

Perivascular infiltration of lymphoid cells in epidemic encephalitis.

no inflammatory reaction except for hyperplasia of connective tissue and formation of new capillaries in the meninges. Essentially degenerative is SCHILDER'S DISEASE or encephalitis periaxialis diffusa, in which there is symmetrical demyelinization of subcortical nerve fibers, widespread edema of white matter and sometimes degeneration of axis cylinders.

Acute nonsuppurative encephalitis occurs as epidemic encephalitis, also called lethargic encephalitis and von Economo's disease, as viral forms of encephalitis, and as postvaccinal and postinfectious encephalitis.

EPIDEMIC ENCEPHALITIS. The cause has not been discovered but the disease is evidently infectious and the demonstration of intranuclear inclusion bodies in degenerate nerve and glial cells by Dawson suggests a viral cause. Grossly, the brain shows swelling hyperemia and pink color of the gray matter especially at the base and occa-

tion, especially at the base of the brain and sometimes about the cord.

The viral forms of epidemic encephalitis include St. Louis encephalitis, Japanese B encephalitis, equine encephalitis, all of which may occur at almost any time of life and X disease, described in Australia as affecting children. The encephalitis of rabies and of acute poliomyelitis are also viral. Laboratory workers have been infected by the virus of louping ill of sheep and the B virus of monkeys. The viruses of St. Louis encephalitis and Japanese B encephalitis are similar, but have immunologic differences. The virus of equine encephalitis has a Western and an Eastern form, of which the latter is more pathogenic for man. The virus of herpes simplex and virus III have produced encephalitis experimentally but this has not been proved for man. (See Webster.)

POSTVACCINAL ENCEPHALITIS may follow vaccination against smallpox and rabies. The cerebral lesion has been ascribed to the vaccine virus itself, to activation of some other virus latent in the body and to allergy, but none of these has been proved (Thompson).

POSTINFECTIOUS ENCEPHALITIS may follow influenza, pertussis, measles, smallpox, chicken pox (Waring, et al.) and perhaps other infections. The mechanism of development is no more clear than is true of the postvaccinal form.

The pathologic anatomy of these various forms does not differ materially from that of epidemic encephalitis. In some the demyelinization is especially marked and in others there are varying degrees of perivascular infiltration and there may be numerous polymorphonuclear leukocytes, meningeal reaction may be conspicuous as may degenerative and proliferative lesions of blood vessels. In the Western variety of equine encephalitis there may even be small abcesses (Baker and Noran).

Epidemic encephalitis and sometimes other forms may leave residual destruction of nerve tissue, and the development of a parkinsonian syndrome is not rare.

Myelitis

As with encephalitis, the term "myelitis" is used to cover various truly inflammatory lesions and also degenerations and necroses without inflammation. For the latter group the term myelopathy is now preferred. Since the term myelitis is widely used, the discussion is placed under this heading.

The inflammatory forms may be simply exudative or definitely suppurative. Suppuration and abscess formation are less frequent in the cord than in the brain. Bacteria may gain access by direct extension from suppurative lesions of vertebrae and meninges, or occasionally by blood transport as in pyemia. Lymphatic transport is more important in cord lesions than in those of the brain. Abscesses of thorax, abdomen and pelvis may extend to the cord by way of the perineural lymphatics of the spinal nerves. Abscess in the cord is likely to extend longitudinally. The neighboring cord tissue is softened, degenerate, and the neuroglia reaction usually slight. The meninges may or may not share in the inflammation.

According to distribution, myelitis and myelopathy may be transverse, diffuse, focal, or disseminated. The transverse form extends through the substance of several segments, usually in the thoracic region. The diffuse form extends irregularly throughout the cord. The disseminated form shows numerous foci in disconnected areas.

Nonsuppurative acute myelitis is usually of infectious origin. Acute infectious fevers play a part, but some cases may be without ascertainable cause. The entry is by way of blood stream or lymphatics, but even with suppurations of meninges and vertebrae nonsuppurative myelitis may occur.

Grossly, in nonsuppurative myelitis and in myelopathy, the cord is swollen, soft, and pale or white. On section, the distinction between white and gray matter is lost and the pale gray or white pulp mass bulges over the cut margin. In the exudative disease, minute punctae of hemorrhage may be seen, which are larger in the hemorrhagic forms. Secondary tract degenerations may occur below and above the major points of destruction. In late lesions the cord may be shrunken and firm. (See Davison and Keschner.)

Microscopically, the cord shows hyperemia, degeneration and necrosis, more evident in white matter than in gray matter. In some instances there is infiltration of polymorphonuclears but the more common cells are lymphocytes and plasma cells. The infiltration may be diffuse, but perivascular arrangement is usually prominent. The meninges are often but not always affected. Occasionally the inflammation is of hemorrhagic type and in the later stages blood pigmentation is present.

Degenerative or parenchymatous acute myelitis, or preferably acute myelopathy may be of toxic form, or secondary to circulatory interference. The nature of the toxic material is uncertain, but includes various drugs and the toxemias of pregnancy. Circulatory disturbances may be due to arteritis of cord or meninges or to pressure from nodules of Hodgkin's disease or leukemia, tumors and kyphosis. Microscopically, there is marked degeneration of myelin sheaths and axis cylinders, with little or no proliferation of glia, found especially in the margins of the cord. The gray matter usually shows no change. Hyperemia may be marked but if exudative cells be present they constitute only a minor part of the picture. The meninges are not often affected.

Acute anterior poliomyelitis is often called infantile paralysis and Heine-Medin disease. The disease is infectious and occurs in what appear to be epidemic forms especially in the late summer and early autumn. It is due to a virus, one of the smallest known, which is highly neurotopic. It can be recovered only from the nervous system and from the alimentary canal, especially pharynx and intestine. It can be transmitted to rhesus monkeys by pharyngeal and intracerebral inoculation, but to cynomolgous monkeys also by feeding. The chimpanzee is susceptible and can be infected by feeding, and it is claimed that the virus can be adapted to rats, mice, guinea pigs and cotton mice. The virus has been cultivated in tissue culture of embryonal nerve tissue. (See Sabin.)

The mode of transmission is not known. The presence of the virus in the stools and in sewage suggests that it may be transmitted as are typhoid fever and dysentery, but this is not proved. Although flies may contain virus there is no good reason to believe that they are vectors (Toomey et al.). Experimentally, infection has been shown to be carried in the air, but this is not proved for man (see Faber and Silverberg). There is a general disposition to the belief that the virus is widespread in man and exists in a certain state of balance between virulence and resistance (Jungeblut). Various conditions may lead to breakdown of resistance such as unfavorable environmental conditions, various stresses of life, injury and nutritional factors. There is an indication of familial incidence which suggests constitutional susceptibility (Aycock).

The disease affects children especially, but may occur in adults. The mode of transmission in the body is through the neurones (Bodian and Howe). Sabin suggests that transfer from the pharynx is along the olfactory tract and this produces the bulbar form of the disease. The transmission from the intestine is probably along the sympathetic nerves and thus the spinal cord is especially affected. The lesions are principally in the cord, not infrequently also in the medulla, pons and dentate nucleus of the cerebellum and sometimes in other parts of the brain.

Grossly, in the earlier stages the cord is swollen, edematous and on cross section shows a bulging surface with pink gray matter. The gray matter of the brain is also likely to be pink. Gross hemorrhages are unusual. The meninges may be hyperemic, but show no grossly visible exudate.

Microscopically, hyperemia is conspicuous, small hemorrhages may be seen and

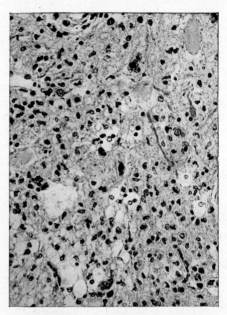

Destruction of cells of the anterior horn and cellular exudation in acute anterior poliomyelitis.

there may be perivascular infiltration of small mononuclear cells in cord and meninges. In the cord, especially in the gray matter, and in the spinal meninges there may be a diffuse infiltration of small mononuclear cells and a few large mononuclears, occasionally arranged in clumps and in rings around nerve cells. Polymorphonuclear leukocytes are found in the anterior horns early in the disease, but later are present only when there are small foci of necrosis. The nerve cells, especially of the ventral horns, but also of Clark's column and the dorsal horn, show various degrees of degeneration and some undergo necrosis. Phagocytosis of the cells by large mononuclear cells may be prominent; this is called neuronophagia. These so-called scavenger cells or compound granule cells may persist for a long time. The white matter is much less affected than the gray matter but wallerian degeneration can be found in some of the fibers. As healing progresses, the acute reaction becomes less marked and the only change observable grossly is reduction in size of the anterior horns. Cicatrization is almost solely by gliosis, which replaces destroyed ganglion cells and foci of necrosis, and surrounds degenerate nerve tracts.

In the acute stage there is often well-marked lymphoid hyperplasia of intestine, spleen and lymph nodes, sometimes with necrosis, cloudy swelling of parenchymatous viscera and rarely focal necrosis of the liver.

Clinically and pathologically, the condition is clearly an acute infectious disease. The resultant flaccid paralysis and muscle atrophy are due to the destruction of motor ganglion cells of the ventral horns. Acute poliomyelitis and epidemic encephalitis may be confused both clinically and pathologically. Poliomyelitis, however, is usually of more rapid onset and resembles more closely an acute infection. It is more likely to show the pathologic signs of acute infection in the viscera but if, as sometimes happens, the case of epidemic encephalitis has an associated infection, especially pneumonia of influenzal type, the organs may show cloudy swelling and lymphoid hyperplasia. Hassin points out that both degeneration of cells and fibers and inflammatory reaction are more profound in poliomyelitis, and that, whereas in both diseases the lesions may involve the entire central nervous system, they decrease in intensity toward the brain in poliomyelitis and toward the cord in encephalitis.

CHRONIC POLIOMYELITIS follows the acute disease as a progressive degeneration rather than as an inflammation (Steegmann).

Neuritis

This term is applied to lesions of the peripheral nerves, which may be either predominantly degenerative or inflammatory. A single nerve may be affected, mononeuritis, or several may be involved, polyneuritis or multiple neuritis. Anatomically, parenchymatous or degenerative, and interstitial forms occur. Predisposing causes seem to be present in many cases of both types, and include prolonged exhausting diseases and the rheumatic or gouty diatheses. Degenerative forms of neuritis are usually multiple and may be caused by poisons such as arsenic, mercury, lead and alcohol. The neuritis of beriberi is evidently due to deficiency of vitamin B_1 and it is suspected that minor degrees of B_1 deficiency may produce multiple neuritis. It is suspected that viruses may play a part in some forms of the disease.

Infectious polyneuritis is also a degenerative form. Synonyms include infectious neuronitis, acute febrile neuritis, acute infective polyneuritis, and the Guillain-Barré syndrome. Acute ascending paralysis, or Landry's disease, appears to be a form of infectious polyneuritis, in which the signs progress from the lower to upper extremities and cranial nerves (see Brown).

Infectious polyneuritis may occur at any time of life, affects the sexes about equally and usually begins during convalescence from acute infections, especially those of the upper respiratory tract. The onset is usually with numbness of hands and feet, paresthesias, pain in back and legs, progressing to anesthesia and paralysis of various muscle groups. It may begin in and be limited to cranial nerves, including auditory with dizziness, or optics with visual disturbances and even blindness. Spinal fluid often shows increased protein content, without an increase in the number of cells. After several months, recovery, either complete or partial, ensues. Death is infrequent.

Grossly, the nervous system shows no change. Microscopically, the principal lesions are in peripheral nerves. The bundles show hyperemia and edema, with swelling and beading of myelin sheaths, as well as fragmentation of axis cylinders and disappearance of some; there may be proliferation of cells of neurilemma and an occasional lymphocyte. The cells of the anterior and posterior horns of the cord may be degenerate and some may disappear. Spinal ganglia may also show disease of cells and lymphocytic infiltration. The brain shows edema with hyperemia of the meninges. It is probable that in those cases which recover these changes are less marked. (See Roseman and Aring; Fox and O'Connor.)

Localized Neuritis. The local nerve changes following diphtheria which involve the nerves of the palate and sometimes other nerves are degenerative. In neural leprosy, as described in the chapter on Infectious Granulomata, they are localized and specific forms of neuritis. Localized neuritis may be the result of pressure of tumors, scars and various injuries.

Interstitial neuritis is the truly inflammatory form of the disease. It usually involves only one nerve. Grossly, the nerve may be hyperemic and exhibit diffuse or nodular swelling. Microscopically, there is hyperemia and often edema, together with infiltration of small and large mononuclear cells, some of which may contain cellular debris and products of myelin degeneration. As the result of pressure, the myelin sheaths may degenerate but the axis cylinders are rarely affected. Healing is accompanied by fibrous tissue growth and restoration of myelin sheaths. Many neuralgias show no anatomic basis in the nerves, in others there is neuritis, and in trigeminal neuralgia, or tic douloureux, the gasserian ganglion may show fibrosis.

INFECTIOUS GRANULOMATA

Tuberculosis

Tubercle bacilli gain entrance to the central nervous system through the blood stream, or by direct extension of tuberculosis from neighboring lesions, particularly those in bones such as the parietal, or the vertebrae. Lymphatic transmission probably occurs, especially from perirenal tuberculosis and retropharyngeal tuberculosis.

Tuberculous cerebral meningitis is probably hematogenous. The suggestion that the meningitis is due to tuberculous foci in the cortex has been denied by various investigators (Beres and Meltzer). Perhaps allergic states in the meninges have to do with the exudative type of reaction (Burn and Finley). The lesion is most frequent in childhood, with a source in tuberculosis of mediastinal lymph nodes, lungs, cervical lymph nodes, retropharyngeal region, and bones. In adults it is usually secondary to pulmonary tuberculosis, but other lesions may be the source, especially those of the urogenital tract.

The lesion is usually at the base of the brain, covers the brain stem and extends forward to the optic commissure. Owing to the loose arrangement of pia arachnoid, it tends to spread. Thus, it passes laterally in the sylvian fissures, also over the upper surface of the cerebellum and into the great longitudinal fissure, sometimes along the olfactory bulbs, downward into the spinal canal, and may ultimately be generalized over the entire brain. Not infrequently, it extends into the ventricles. The lesion affects the pia arachnoid but, as a rule, affects the dura only when bony involvement is present. In some

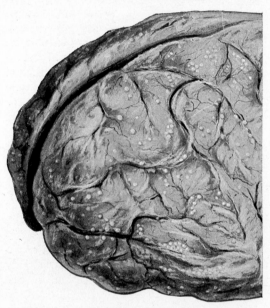

Miliary tubercles in pia-arachnoid of the cerebrum.

of the earlier cases the lesion is a miliary tuberculosis of the meninges, hidden in the sulci and fissures and more clearly visible when the pia is stripped and held up to the light. Usually, however, in the fresh specimen the tubercles are clearly visible. Frequently, there is in these cases a small amount of fibrinous exudate which may merely cloud the membranes or may be easily seen. Sometimes the disease, especially at the base of the brain, appears as a fibrinous or fibrinoserous inflammation with only little tendency to form tubercles. The exudate sometimes becomes purulent. In some cases the process extends a short distance into the brain substance to produce a tuberculous meningo-encephalitis. Microscopically, the lesion may be predominantly an acute inflammation. Tubercles identify it, as a rule, but sometimes only foci of necrosis give the clue. Special stains usually show numerous tubercle bacilli.

Tuberculous spinal meningitis is often found in the upper parts of the cord as a result of extension from cerebral meningitis. A most important form is that due to tuberculosis of the vertebrae. This may result in a subacute or chronic tuberculous pachymeningitis, usually localized, conglomerate, and sometimes so massive as to produce pressure. The more acute forms invade also the pia arachnoid and may remain local or extend along the cord, even to the brain. This may be a miliary tuberculosis of the meninges with little acute inflammation, or may be an acute fibrinous tuberculous inflammation, or may become purulent. Tuberculous meningitis of the cord, especially near bone lesions from which it takes origin, is more likely to involve nerve substance than is tuberculous cerebral meningitis. This tuberculous meningomyelitis may become a complete transverse myelitis.

Tuberculosis of the Ependyma. The ependyma of the ventricles may be involved as a result of extension from meningitis or occasionally may be attacked without involvement of the meninges. The lesion may be miliary tuberculosis or a fibrinous or purulent inflammation. Interference with drainage may produce internal hydrocephalus. This may be due to the exudate, or may result from large tuberculous masses in cerebellum or brain stem. In the former case the fluid contains exudate; in the latter it is usually clear.

Tuberculosis of the brain usually occurs as a conglomerate tubercle, or tuberculoma. Sometimes, these lesions may be multiple. The condition is much more frequent in childhood and adolescence than in later life. It occurs most frequently in the cerebellar cortex, next in the cerebral hemispheres and least often in the brain stem (Weil). The bacilli evidently lodge in a small blood vessel immediately under the meninges and produce a small tubercle which enlarges by the formation of daughter tubercles. Even in tuberculomas with a diameter of a centimeter or more, daughter tubercles are to be found, but sometimes the lesion seems to become quiescent and daughter tubercles, fusing with the parent mass, are no longer present as such.

Grossly, the mass is well defined, with slight or no marginal hyperemia, but sometimes with a surrounding zone of softening of the nerve substance. The firm caseous mass, sometimes gelatinous to gross inspection, only rarely undergoes softening or liquefaction. As such tubercles reach the outer surface, the infection may extend to produce a more or less widespread tuberculous meningitis. Pressure of the tuberculous mass may interfere with drainage from the ventricles and cause internal hydrocephalus.

Microscopically, the margins of the tuberculoma show the characteristic cell forms, and if daughter tubercles be present the diagnosis is easily established. Usually in older lesions, the tubercle bacilli cannot be demonstrated microscopically, and the final diagnosis is made by exclusion or by animal inoculation. Miliary tuberculosis of the brain is rare.

Tuberculosis of the spinal cord is not infrequent. The miliary form is rare. A solitary conglomerate tubercle has much the same appearance as in the brain, but is less common in the cord. Secondary tract degenerations may be prominent. Such a tubercle may be metastatic or result from direct extension of lesions of meninges or vertebrae. Extensive disease of the vertebrae may lead merely to compression of the cord or to a tuberculous transverse myelitis. Tuberculous spinal meningitis may be secondary to tuberculosis within the cord.

Peripheral nerves may be involved and destroyed in tuberculous foci. Sometimes tuberculous meningitis may involve cranial and spinal nerves as they pass through the meninges and lead to degeneration beyond the lesion.

Syphilis

This disease may affect the nervous system in many ways, including subacute inflammations of the meninges, gumma formation, vascular lesions and the progressive glial overgrowths and degenerations of tabes dorsalis and of paresis. For many years, it was thought that there are certain strains of the *Treponema pallidum* which have an especial affinity for the central nervous system, but more recent investigations indicate that this is not true. Lesions may appear fairly soon after the chancre and there is little doubt that in the septicemic period the nervous system is infiltrated with spirochetes. Other lesions may not occur for many years after the chancre.

Congenital syphilis may manifest itself in gummatous and nongummatous meningitis, gummata in various parts of the central nervous system, areas of softening and atrophic changes. It is considered possible that various developmental defects, various paralyses of infancy, areas of softening and porencephaly are due to congenital syphilis.

Gumma may rarely occur in any part of the central nervous system and peripheral

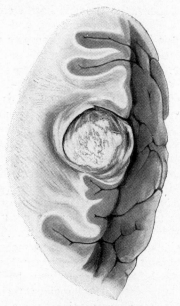

Gumma of cerebral cortex.

nerves. The gumma of these regions has the same characters as elsewhere. It originates either in meninges or nerve sheaths or in the adventitia of blood vessels. In the brain and cord it is most often superficial but penetrates into the nerve substance and may induce severe symptoms. As contrasted with the tubercle, it occurs more often in adult life than in childhood, is more superficial, more irregular in outline, has a broader surrounding zone of fibrous growth, often hyperemic and sometimes hemorrhagic, and is less likely to caseate. The neighboring meninges may show subacute or chronic inflammation and the surrounding nerve substance may show edema, encephalitis or myelitis. The

symptoms are like those of tumor (D'Aunoy, et al.).

Gummatous Meningitis. In order to be positively identified as syphilitic, meningitis must be gummatous in type. Nevertheless, a nongummatous form is described, which, while not microscopically characteristic, seems to be due to syphilis. If gummatous meningitis affect the pia arachnoid alone, it is usually confined to the base of the brain. The membrane is thickened, sometimes edematous and exhibits small white plaques. More frequently, however, the soft meninges and dura are involved together, especially over the vertex, but sometimes extending over the entire cerebral surface so as to form a thick, dense, opaque sheet adherent to skull and brain. A similar condition may occur in the cord. This accounts for some of the cases of chronic cervical pachymeningitis described above, but most of these cases are not syphilitic.

The lesion of syphilitic meningitis is essentially a gummatous granulation tissue. The tissues are infiltrated with cells of lym-

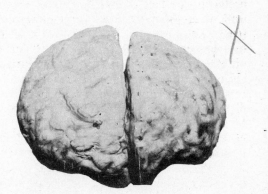

Chronic leptomeningitis of syphilitic origin.
Note opacity of the thickened meninges.

phoid type but, as the process gets older, large mononuclears may predominate. Small gumma-like foci occur and often show necrosis. These may organize to form fibrous plaques. Fibroblastic proliferation, principally from the vascular adventitia, ultimately produces the dense thickening of the meninges. The blood vessels are frequently involved in one or other form of syphilitic vasculitis. The underlying brain or cord substance often shows degeneration of the parenchyma, with intact or proliferated glia. The nerves, especially the cranial nerves, the oculomotor, abducens and optic, may become involved in an interstitial or gummatous neuritis.

Syphilitic arteritis only rarely occurs independently of a syphilitic meningitis. Most cases are therefore meningo-arteritis. The disease begins in the adventitia. There may be a granulation tissue with focal collections of epithelioid cells, lymphocytes and plasma cells, suggestive of miliary gumma formation, the condition called gummatous granulation tissue, or there may be only fibrosis. This involves not only the adventitia but gradually extends into the media, with atrophy and disappearance of muscle. The elastica may show multiple laminae, but this is probably due to splitting rather than multiplication. The intima then takes part in the fibrosis and becomes thickened.

Grossly, the vessels are thick and inelastic and may show minute gray perivascular nodules. The extension of fibrosis into the media may so weaken the wall that an aneurysm forms, which may subsequently rupture; if vasa vasorum be present and become occluded, a comparable weakening of the wall, with aneurysm and rupture may take place. The gradual reduction of the lumen by the intimal thickening may cause atrophy of the area supplied. The vessel may become obliterated with consequent encephalomalacia or myelomalacia, either by advance of the intimal thickening or by thrombosis. Syphilitic arterial disease as it affects smaller arteries in the brain substance may produce irregularly distributed small foci of encephalomalacia.

Syphilitic Myelitis. According to Buzzard and Greenfield, syphilis is the most common cause of myelitis, which as a rule, takes the form of a meningomyelitis of transverse form. The cervical region is usually affected. The meninges are thickened and adherent. The soft meninges are infiltrated with small round cells and show changes in the blood vessels. The vascular lesions of meninges and cord usually are in the form of perivascular infiltration by small lymphoid cells with no alteration of the vessel lumen. With only moderate perivascular infiltration there may be marked dilatation, presumably paralytic, and thrombosis of the finer vessels. There may also be the syphilitic arteritis described above. Degeneration occurs in the nerve cells and fibers as a result of the vascular lesions, and perhaps also due to the effects of products of the spirochetes. Scavenger cells may be numerous. The glia may be well preserved and ultimately proliferates to constitute most of the scar. The infiltration may take on the characters of gummatous granulation and true gumma may be formed.

Paresis, also called general paralysis of the insane and dementia paralytica, is most common in the fourth and fifth decades but may occur in earlier life; it affects males more often than females. The positive serologic tests of blood and spinal fluid and the demonstration of living spirochetes in the brain leave no doubt that the disease is syphilitic.

Grossly, the skull bones may be thick and dense, the dura may be fibrous and adherent, chronic internal hemorrhagic pachymeningitis is common, and the leptomeninges are often thick and opaque, especially over the frontoparietal region. Fluid, sometimes cloudy, may be in excess in the meninges and the ventricles, and the ependyma of the latter is often the seat of hyperplasia and slight roughening. Usually but not invariably the brain is reduced in size and weight, a change due especially to involvement of the cerebrum. The white matter may be soft and edematous. The gyri are reduced in size, especially in the frontoparietal region, and the sulci wide. Cross section shows thinning of the cortical gray matter and prominent blood vessels. The cord may show grossly visible degeneration of the descending tracts. Obvious syphilitic meningitis, myelitis and gumma formation may be found.

Microscopically, the cortex shows perivascular infiltration of lymphoid and plasma cells, dilatation of vessels and sometimes new capillaries. Neuroglia proliferation is prominent and many astrocytes are found. Rod cells are numerous and often contain iron pigment (Spatz). The cortical nerve cells, especially the pyramidal cells, are in disorderly arrangement; various degrees of degeneration, going on to destruction, are observed. Neuronal degeneration affects particularly the association fibers of the brain and the pyramidal tracts of brain, brain stem and cord. Cells of the ventral horns of the cord, of the dorsal root ganglia, and even the Purkinje cells of the cerebellum, may show slight degeneration in the form of chromatolysis. Disease of the posterior columns, similar to that of tabes, may be associated.

Tabes dorsalis, or locomotor ataxia, is a disease of middle and later life, which, like dementia paretica, attacks males more often than females. Many cases give a history of syphilis and the serologic tests of blood and spinal fluid are positive in most

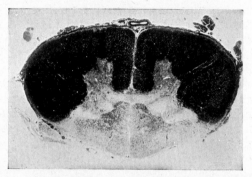

Cross section of cord showing lesion of the posterior columns in tabes dorsalis. Weigert-Pal stain for myelin sheaths. Courtesy of Stanley Cobb, M.D.

cases. It can now be stated with assurance that tabes is due to syphilis, even though spirochetes have not been demonstrated. The lesion probably originates as a syphilitic inflammation of epidural and intradural spaces, causing circulatory disturbances in the perineurial root spaces with consequent degeneration and sclerosis of the posterior columns (Hassin).

Grossly, in the advanced lesion, the posterior columns are shrunken, and on cross section are of pale gray color and retracted. The pia arachnoid, and also the dura, are usually thickened and dense, especially in the posterior aspects.

Microscopically, the posterior root ganglia may be the seat of slight fibrosis but the cells are normal. The peripheral neurons may be the seat of slight atrophy. The central neurons are the seat of degeneration with disintegration and loss of myelin and destruction of axis cylinders. This change affects the nerves as they pass into the cord but is primary in the posterior roots. Thus, the short fibers which pass directly to the

dorsal horns are affected. So also are the medium fibers, which pass upward to enter the column of Clark. The long fibers, similarly affected, pass upward to the nuclei gracilis and cuneatus, gradually assuming a position toward the septum to constitute the column of Goll. Thus, depending upon the level examined, the columns of Burdach and Goll may be variously affected.

The lesion usually begins in the lumbar regions and shows changes as it ascends. If, however, thoracic roots are affected, the change in the upper cord is more extensive. Associated with the degeneration there is a gliosis, the fibrous septa are increased in bulk and the blood-vessel walls become thick and hyalinized. The posterior horns and the column of Clark may be reduced in size by the destruction of the entering fibers. The intersegmental association fibers are usually not affected. The tract of Lissauer, being made up of descending radicals of the entering fibers is usually degenerated. The optic nerve is sometimes the seat of degeneration which begins near the eye and extends toward the commissure. The trigeminal and glossopharyngeal nerves are sometimes affected and accordingly the trigeminal root fibers and those of the fasciculus solitarius in the medulla degenerate and disappear. As with paresis, more distinctive syphilitic lesions, such as syphilitic meningitis, vascular lesions and gumma, may occur.

Leprosy

Leprosy, in its neural form has been described in the chapter on Infectious Granulomata. Aside from its effects on peripheral nerves, the posterior columns of the cord are sometimes degenerated.

Hodgkin's Disease

Hodgkin's disease of the central nervous system affects particularly the cord. The granuloma may extend into the spinal canal from surrounding structures, or be formed in the meninges. Secondary changes in the cord may be due to pressure, or to a transverse myelitis resulting from interference with nutrition. Subacute combined degeneration, diffuse myelitis, and syringomyelia-like gliosis may occur in Hodgkin's disease. (See Shapiro.)

Actinomycosis

Actinomycosis may penetrate the brain or cord from bone lesions or perhaps the organisms may be transported to brain or spinal nerves by the blood stream. Trichinosis may also affect the central nervous system.

SPECIAL INFECTIOUS DISEASES

In addition to those infectious diseases whose manifestations are inflammatory, such as epidemic encephalitis, acute poliomyelitis and the infectious granulomata, certain others require discussion, especially tetanus, herpes, chorea, rabies and trypanosomiasis.

Tetanus

Tetanus is produced by the toxin of *Clostridium tetani*. The organisms, sporebearing anaerobes, are found in the intestine of the horse, sometimes of man and perhaps of other animals. They produce the disease by entry through wounds contaminated by infected soil. The infection is especially favored by wounds of such character as to permit anaerobic growth and to a certain degree by pyogenic infection in the wound. Although toxin can be found in the blood it does not appear to pass the blood-brain barrier, and is transferred from the site of infection to the nervous system through the peripheral nerves along both perineural lymphatics and axis cylinders (see Friedemann et al.). The incubation period is variable but usually is about eight days. In man, as a rule, the first symptom to appear is trismus of the jaw muscles, but in experimental animals, when the toxin has been given subcutaneously or intramuscularly, the first spasms are near the injection site. There follows a period of excitable reflexes, clonic and then tonic spasms, more and more widespread, terminating in death.

The pathologic anatomy of tetanus has no features to distinguish it from infectious disease in general. Petechiae may be found in muscles and other places. Zenker's hyaline necrosis has been observed in skeletal muscle. Although the toxin can produce demyelinization in experimental animals, no such change is observed in man. Various degenerative changes have been described in nerve cells but they are not specific and probably due to postmortem degeneration. Death is usually due to myocardial failure, caused partly by toxemia and partly by asphyxia; some patients die of bronchopneumonia and some of pyogenic infection.

Herpes

The external manifestation of herpes is the appearance of an erythema, followed by a multilocular vesicular eruption which encrusts and the crusts drop off. HERPES FEBRILIS SIMPLEX usually occurs on the face and ordinarily leaves no scar. It accompanies a variety of acute infectious diseases, is frequent following the common cold, or may be spontaneous. Herpes genitalis follows irritation about glans penis or labia. Herpes cornealis resembles herpes febrilis except as to situation. HERPES ZOSTER, or zona, is most frequent on the trunk but may occur over the course of any cutaneous sensory nerves. It is unilateral, often leaves shallow scars and apparently produces a local immunity in the affected region.

The forms of herpes, other than zoster, are due to a virus which is polytropic in experimentally inoculated rabbits, although in man its effects are principally in skin and nervous system. The virus is transmissible to the rabbit, especially upon inoculation into the cornea. With certain strains, the virus extends along the optic tracts and produces an encephalitis. Peripheral inoculation may produce a myelitis. Intranuclear inclusion bodies have been identified in various tissues of the rabbit.

Although experiments have been performed suggestive of the viral nature of herpes zoster, no virus has been conclusively demonstrated. (See Goodpasture.)

Although lesions of ganglia may be observed in herpes simplex (Howard), they are practically constant in zoster. In the usual case of herpes zoster, that affected is a posterior root ganglion of the thoracic region. It is swollen, soft and hyperemic. Microscopically, there are hyperemia, sometimes with small foci of hemorrhage, edema, and infiltration by lymphoid cells, especially around the capillaries. The nerve cells are variously affected. Some are destroyed and others are normal. Some are swollen and stain diffusely but do not show chromatolysis. Some show invasion by mononuclear cells, neuronophagy. The inflammation may extend into nerve or dorsal root. As a result of destruction of cells, degeneration affects the nerve fibers with enormous swelling of the axons and may extend through the roots into the cord. Healing results in cicatrization, sometimes with cyst formation. The lesion in the ganglion is of much the same nature as that observed in other parts of the central nervous system in epidemic encephalitis and acute poliomyelitis.

Herpes zoster may also be secondary to organic diseases of the cord such as tabes, to disease of the vertebrae such as tuberculosis and tumor, or to severe trauma of the spine. This is due to involvement of the spinal root ganglion and is etiologically different from the so-called idiopathic form discussed above.

Chorea

This disease, often called Sydenham's chorea, occurs principally in children but may attack adults, affects females more often

Rabies

This is an acute specific infectious disease to which practically all mammals are susceptible and to which birds and reptiles seem resistant. The virus acts principally upon the central nervous system and is excreted especially through the salivary glands. It is transmitted by bites or by contamination of open wounds by infected saliva. Laboratory infections in man are rare, and it is possible that the saliva exercises some function, other than carriage of the virus, in establishing the infection. The virus seems to travel by way of the axis cylinders (Goodpasture), and head and face bites are followed by a shorter incubation period and more severe brain lesions than those upon the extremities. The average incubation is about 72 days but may vary from 19 days to more than a year. After prodromal symptoms there is spasm of muscles of deglutition, followed by hyperexcitability, convulsions and death either from asphyxia or exhaustion.

The gross examination of the central nervous system usually shows no change, ex-

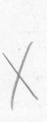

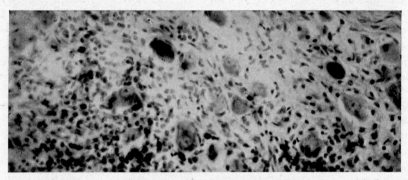

Gasserian ganglion of rabies, showing marked lymphoid cell infiltration, and in lower right hand corner, neuronophagia.

than males and is rare in races other than whites. It is characterized by irregular purposeless movements and may exhibit psychic manifestations, but it is not often fatal. It is generally agreed that it is one of the manifestations of rheumatic fever.

Examinations of the central nervous system have shown hyperemia, minute hemorrhages, thrombi in small blood vessels, small foci of necrosis and sometimes inflammatory exudate, especially in the basal ganglia (Castren). The changes are by no means constant, are not characteristic and do not explain the symptoms.

cept sometimes hyperemia and minute hemorrhages. Microscopically, there is perivascular infiltration of lymphoid cells. The affected nerve cells show degeneration and the dendrites may be swollen and granular. They may be surrounded by a rim of phagocytic cells. The neuroglia may show proliferation. The lesions are encephalitic in character and occur especially in medulla, brain stem and substantia nigra (Freeman). Characteristic of the disease are Negri bodies and lyssa bodies which are found in the cytoplasm of the nerve cells of brain, cord and ganglia, but are especially numerous in the hippocampus major and the Purkinje cells of the cerebellum. The Negri bodies are round, stellate or of spindle form, with acidophilic cytoplasm and a nucleus-like basophilic central body. The lyssa bodies are similar but have no central basophilic mass. Both these are of the order of inclusion bodies of viral diseases. Goodpasture's studies indicate that the acidophilic substance is a fused mass of degenerate intracellular neurofibrils and the central basophilic mass is composed of degenerate products of mitochondria.

The ganglia, including gasserian, plexiform, and spinal, usually show a subacute inflammation, with reticulo-endothelial proliferation and lymphocyte infiltration. The ganglion cells may be degenerate and the seat of neuronophagia. Peripheral nerves, especially those related to the diseased ganglia, may show degeneration. The salivary glands may be acutely inflamed. (See Webster.)

Trypanosomiasis

In African sleeping sickness, caused by *Trypanosoma gambiense* and *Trypanosoma rhodesiense*, the brain and cord show thickening and often adhesion of pia arachnoid. Slight or moderate hydrocephalus may occur and the cerebrospinal fluid may be yellow. There is extensive lymphoid infiltration of the pia arachnoid and perivascular spaces. The cerebral cortex may show degeneration of the pyramidal cells and the cord may show diffuse sclerosis.

In CHAGAS' DISEASE, an infectious disease seen especially in South America, due to the *Trypanosoma cruzi*, the acute form may show marked involvement of the central nervous system. There may be acute inflammation of both cerebral and spinal meninges. In regions of the cord, in relation to lodgment of the parasites, there are areas of marked degeneration of cells and fibers (Chagas).

DISEASES OF OBSCURE ORIGIN

There are certain diseases of the central nervous system whose exciting cause is unknown, and which therefore cannot be classified in the groups which have been discussed. The description of these is given in the following paragraphs.

Amyotrophic Lateral Sclerosis

Amyotrophic Lateral Sclerosis is a disease of middle life characterized by degeneration of the motor neurons and atrophy of voluntary muscles. Clinically, the usual case shows spastic paraplegia or tetraplegia followed by atrophy of the muscles. Although three types are described, the distinction is not always clear. The bulbar type begins in the nerves and muscles supplied from the medulla and usually progresses to involve the extremities. In the amyotrophic type there is marked atrophy and weakness of the muscles, out of proportion to the spasticity. In the spastic type, spasticity is marked and the atrophy is delayed.

The cause is unknown. Possibly there is an inherent susceptibility or abiotrophy of the affected neurons. The suggestion that the disease is due to deficiency or poor absorption of vitamin E, gastro-intestinal disturbance or hepatic disorder, has not been established.

Although thought of as a disease of both upper and lower motor neurons, the studies of Davison point strongly to primary involvement of the upper neurons. In some instances the lesion appears to originate in the giant pyramidal cells of Betz, but usually it starts in the upper neurons, affecting them in the pons, medulla or spinal cord. Subsequently, the anterior horn cells and the peripheral neurons are affected.

Gross examination, in the advanced case, may show atrophy of the precentral convolutions of the brain and reduction in size of the ventrolateral columns of the cord. Microscopically, the effects in the cerebral cortex and the cells of the anterior horns of the cord are much the same. There is degeneration, with chromatolysis, displacement of nucleus, sometimes pigmentation, followed by atrophy and complete disappearance. These changes may be seen in the precentral and sometimes postcentral gyri, and in the various nuclei of the medulla. The changes in the upper motor neurons are observed particularly in the ventrolateral columns of the cord and in the lower neurons especially in the ventral roots and peripheral nerves. The larger nerve fibers show fragmentation and degeneration of medullary sheaths and of axis cylinders, but the smaller fibers are less markedly diseased (Wohlfart and Swank).

The posterior spinal roots and the posterior horn cells are unaffected, but occasionally there is gliosis in the upper parts of the column of Goll. In most of the cases, gliosis in the diseased parts is slight, but occasionally it may be marked.

The skeletal muscles show marked atrophy without fat replacement, and the same is true of the tongue in the bulbar cases. Microscopically, some of the muscle fibers are normal, but others show more or less marked atrophy with preserved transverse striations. The atrophy may go on to complete disappearance of some of the fibers and proliferation of their sarcolemma nuclei. Fibrosis may be marked.

Subacute Combined Degeneration of the Cord

This is a tract degeneration which affects the posterior and posterolateral col-

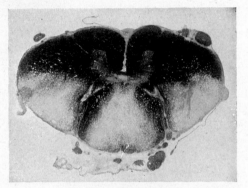

Cross section of cord in subacute combined degeneration, showing degeneration of posterior and posterolateral columns. Weigert-Pal stain for myelin sheaths. Courtesy of Stanley Cobb, M.D.

umns. It is sometimes referred to as a sclerosis, but since gliosis is slight or absent, the term is not justified. It is a part of the general disturbance of pernicious anemia, although it is said that it may rarely occur in other profound anemias. The manifestations occur in a high proportion of cases of pernicious anemia and it is probably present in variable degrees in all. Although it has been suggested that vitamin deficiency or inadequate gastric function is responsible, the available evidence points strongly to its cause by deficiency of the same maturation factor which leads to the anemia (Davison). Subacute combined degeneration occurs principally in the fourth and fifth decades, and

about equally in both sexes. Starting as a mild spastic or ataxic paraplegia, it may progress through a stage of complete spastic paraplegia to one of flaccid paraplegia. Grossly, the cord may be slightly or markedly reduced in transverse diameter. Rarely the white matter of the brain may be affected so as to show foci of slight atrophy. Cross section of the cord may show an opaque pallor in the affected columns. In rare cases the posterior tracts may be much more affected than the lateral.

Microscopically, the degeneration is found in the same situation as seen grossly, but the column of Goll is more diseased than that of Burdach. The degeneration affects the long tracts of fibers especially, but ultimately both exogenous and endogenous fibers are involved. There is swelling and disintegration of myelin sheath so that it disappears. The axis cylinders may remain naked but soon become fragmented and dissolved. Large spaces appear, giving the tissue a spongy appearance. Phagocytes, some of great size, are abundant. The blood vessels are usually unaffected, but there may be some hyalinization of the walls. Such slight glial proliferation as may be present is around the degenerate fibers and does not penetrate between them.

Multiple Sclerosis

This disease, also called disseminated sclerosis, insular sclerosis and "sclerose en placque," is of common occurrence, begins in early adult life and seems to attack both sexes about equally. It is a progressive disease, with periods of remission of symptoms. Easy fatigue and weakness may be followed by paralyses, tremors, ataxia, spasticity, disturbances of speech, vision, hearing and mental changes. Symptoms may appear abruptly, regress or disappear, and after recurrences, become permanent.

Fundamentally, the disease is characterized by foci of demyelinization of nerve fibers scattered in various parts of brain and cord, the lesions predominating in one or the other, or affecting both about equally. Gliosis accompanies the degeneration. There is much discussion as to whether the disease is primarily degenerative or inflammatory, but the majority opinion favors the former. The cause is unknown. There is no reason to believe that it is due to infective agents. Some think that a specific myelinolytic substance is formed in the body (Weil and Heilbrun), but this is not established. Putnam believes the lesions to be due to occlusion of small

tered, may show varicose swelling or may completely disappear. Tract degenerations are irregular and often absent. Ganglion cells are usually unaffected but may rarely be degenerate. The gliosis is largely fibrillar and

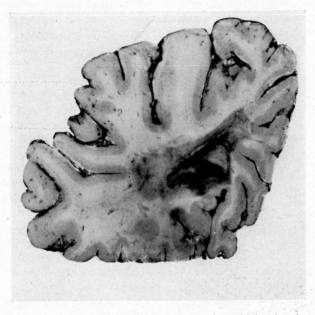

Cross section of cerebral hemisphere in multiple sclerosis. Note focus of sclerosis in lower part of white matter and sclerosis at margin of ventricle.

vessels because of disease of their walls and occlusive thrombosis, with resultant degeneration in the immediate neighborhood. Dow and Berglung find no reason to support this view but cannot say that it is entirely unrelated. They suggest that the thrombi may be due to local absorption of thromboplastic substance from the destroyed tissue.

Gross inspection may disclose more or less firm, translucent gray patches irregular in outline and varying in size from a millimeter or less to several centimeters. Patches may be found in any part of the cord, the pons, the medulla, the basal ganglia and even in the cerebral cortex, but only rarely in the cerebellum.

Microscopically, the medullary sheaths may show granular degeneration, swelling and partial lysis or there may be complete demyelinization. In the earlier stages myelin fragments are seen but later disappear. They are either free or contained in phagocytes which have been called myeloclasts and myelophages. The axis cylinders may be unal-

in comparison the mesoblastic changes are relatively slight. The blood vessels may be normal or fibrotic often with complete occlusion, suggesting that thrombi have become

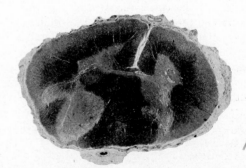

Cross section of cord of multiple sclerosis, showing an area of sclerosis in left posterior columns—not a tract degeneration. Weigert-Pal stain for myelin sheaths. Courtesy of Stanley Cobb, M.D.

organized; recent thrombi also may occur. In earlier stages the perivascular cells may contain lymphocytes and macrophages. The vessels of the choroid plexuses may be fibrotic and the surface cells may contain fatty droplets.

Syringomyelia

Although many cases of syringomyelia represent a tumor-like growth, certain others are not of this nature and for that reason the disease is discussed here instead of under the heading of tumors. It is a disease of early adult life, but may occur in infancy. It affects both sexes about equally. Clinically, there are dissociated anesthesia in which pain and temperature sense are affected without loss of tactile sense, progressive muscular atrophy with twitchings, and trophic and vasomotor disturbances. The bones may be atrophic and

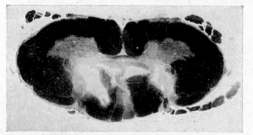

Cross section of cord of syringomyelia, showing irregular, generally central, cavitation. Weigert-Pal stain for myelin sheaths. Courtesy of Stanley Cobb, M.D.

disposed to fractures; the joints may be the seat of arthropathies like those of tabes. The lesion is a cavitation extending along the center of the cord; rarely it affects the medulla and then bulbar symptoms occur.

Grossly, the central cavitation may be so small as to be detected only on transverse section, but it may be so large that the cord is like a tube whose lumen may show irregularity in its caliber. Usually, the cavitation is more marked in the cervical and upper thoracic cord. In the cross section, the cavity is usually central, but may be slightly eccentric. Its outline is circular, elliptical or stellate. The fluid in the cavity may be limpid or gelatinous, is usually clear and varies from colorless to some shade of yellow or brown. Microscopically, the cavity is posterior to the central canal, although at various levels it may fuse with the canal. Thus, the gray commissure is practically always interrupted. The cavity itself is lined by a layer of gliosis varying in thickness. Where it fuses with the

central canal, it is partly lined by ependyma. The glial proliferation is of fibrillary neuroglia, and may be vascularized and show small hemorrhages or foci of blood pigment. The enlargement of the cavity and to a variable degree the gliosis results in compression of the horns of the gray matter and may also cause degenerations of pyramidal, ventrolateral and dorsal columns.

Because of the character of its vascular supply, the central part of the cord seems to be a place of lowered resistance, and offers a path of progress for suppuration, hemorrhage and tumor growth. Occasional cases of syringomyelia seem to originate as the result of these lesions. The formation of the canal may be somewhat irregular and furthermore small islands of ependyma may be found separated from the central canal. This leads to the suggestion that in most cases, syringomyelia is the result of anomalous development of the primitive medullary epithelium. The gliosis may originate in the cell rests. Thus the condition would be hamartial. (See Tamaki and Lubin.)

It is likely that the dissociated anesthesia is due to interruption of the pain and temperature fibers of the gray commissure, whereas the tactile sense fibers ascend directly in the lateral and dorsal tracts and are less subject to interference. The paralyses are due to interruption of motor tracts. The muscular atrophy is due to lesion of the ventral horns.

Paralysis Agitans

This condition, also called shaking palsy and Parkinson's disease or syndrome, occurs most often in advanced middle life and affects males about twice as often as females. Clinically, it usually begins with tremor of head and upper extremities, with rigidity of muscles and mask-like face, followed by weakness affecting at first one extremity and then becoming more extensive.

Pathologically, the most important lesion is degeneration of the large cells of the striatum, the pallidum cells being less involved. Similar symptoms may be produced by lesions in this situation such as tumor, hemorrhage, encephalomalacia, or residual lesions of encephalitis. The cord shows no significant changes. The muscles may be normal or may show areas of atrophy, swollen

See Assoc. for research in Nervous & Mental Disease
Vol. XVI of a series of research publications
Williams & Wilkins
1937

THE NERVOUS SYSTEM   783

hyaloid fibers with diminished transverse striation and prominent longitudinal striation sometimes with splitting.

TUMORS

In the category of brain tumors are included all tumors which occur within the cranial cavity, even although some of them may originate in meninges, nerves, bones or other structures. They are somewhat more common in males than in females. Although they may be found at almost any age, Cushing states that more than half the tumors occur between 20 and 40 years of age. This low age incidence is probably due to the fact that more than 40 per cent of all intracranial tumors are gliomas. Injury to the head may draw attention to the existence of a tumor, but as indicated in the chapter on Tumors, probably plays no part in its cause. Brain tumors are malignant in effect by virtue of their position. Pathologically, some of them are not invasive and most of them show no disposition to metastasize.

The symptoms and signs are the result principally of local pressure or invasion, and of disturbance of the circulation of blood, lymph and cerebrospinal fluid. The brain is almost noncompressible and the skull resistant, so that increase in intracranial pressure is a most important phenomenon in brain tumors. The increase in pressure may be due to the bulk of the tumor, to edema around it, to obstruction to drainage of the great lymph sacs, and principally to obstruction of flow of cerebrospinal fluid. It varies, however, with the type of tumor growth, and some may be so invasive and destructive as not to lead to increased pressure. Situation is also important and the greatest pressures are produced by tumors of the posterior fossa. Multiple minute herniations of brain substance into the dura, particularly where local thinness is due to the presence of arachnoid villi, occur as the result of pressure. The increased brain volume may be seen in flattening of the convolutions and in the formation of the so-called pressure cone on the inferior surface of the cerebellum, due to compression into the foramen magnum. There may be an osteoporotic pressure atrophy of the bones of the skull.

The alleviation of such symptoms as headache, vertigo, drowsiness, vomiting, psychic disturbances, and alterations of respiration, circulation and temperature, by decompression craniotomy, makes it evident that these are due to increased pressure. The bulging optic disc, papilledema, or choked disc, revealed by opthalmoscopic examination, are also due to the pressure. The cranial nerves tend to be pushed into their foramina, and this affects the optic nerve. Of further importance is the hypothesis that the condition is due also to compression of the central vein as it crosses the optic sheath to enter the cavernous sinus.

Convulsions may be due to general increase of pressure or to focal pressure or irritation. Brain tumors may exhibit various focal manifestations in relation to motor, sensory or co-ordinating functions and psychic disturbances, or may be situated in "silent" areas, without the production of focalizing sensory or motor disturbances.

Glioma

Gliomas are tumors originating in cells of the neuroglia or their antecedents, thought by some to be derived from embryonal cell rests (Courville). There are various types of glioma and the following description is a composite generalization. In most forms the tumor is single, but in others, especially the astrocytoma, multiplicity is frequent; some of these nodules may represent metastasis. The size varies from an extremely small mass to that of an entire cerebral hemisphere. The shape is generally spheroidal but may vary much with the situation, and is influenced by the usual, but not invariable, limitation by the pia mater. The glioma is most common in the brain but may occur in the cord and roots of cranial nerves. The situation in the brain varies with the type of tumor, for example, the involvement of cerebellum by the medulloblastoma, of the ventricles by the ependymoma and of the cerebral hemispheres by the astrocytoma.

The outline of gliomas also varies with the type of tumor. The ependymoma is a sharply defined tumor with little tendency to invade surrounding brain. The glioblastoma multiforme is well defined, but actually extends into brain substance somewhat further than would be suspected grossly. The astrocytoma, as it occurs in the cerebrum, is poorly defined and extends microscopically far beyond what would be indicated grossly. Encapsulation does not occur in gliomas. (See Scherer.) The consistency is about that of gray matter. The color, usually pale reddish-gray, may be darker red in a highly vascularized or a telangiectatic tumor, or it may be almost white in a poorly vascularized mass.

Small hemorrhages are common, but large extravasations with apoplectic symptoms may occur. Necrosis may be slight or marked. Cysts occur, filled with pale gray

the spongioblasts produce the astrocyte, and the medulloblasts, in addition to producing oligodendroglia may apparently produce some spongioblasts and neuroblasts. These various cells take part in the production of tumors, and the tumors are named according to the predominant cell.

Types. The work of Cushing and Bailey, of Bailey, of Penfield and others has led to classification into not less than thirteen types of glioma. As a rule, the individual tumor is composed of several types of cell,

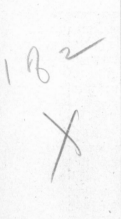
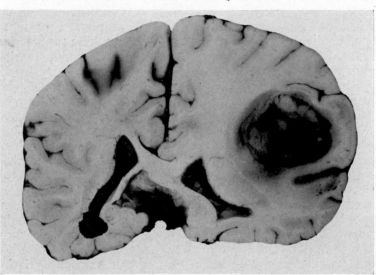

Glioma of cerebral hemisphere, microscopically a glioblastoma multiforme. Note enlargement of the hemisphere and distortion of the lateral ventricle.

cloudy fluid which on fixation often solidifies into a gelatinous mass. Psammoma bodies may be found, calcification may be extensive, and even ossification is said to occur. Extension may be in the form of general enlargement, the tumor may break through the meninges and extend over the surface, or additional discrete masses, presumably metastatic, may be found.

Microscopically, the glioma may be uniform in cell type or show some variations. In the differentiation of the primary neurectodermal cells there are formed medulloblasts, spongioblasts, and neuroblasts, in addition to the precursors of pineal, choroidal and ependymal cells. Through stages of further differentiation the neuroblasts produce the neurone,

but as stated above the diagnosis is made in accord with the preponderant cell. The tumors remain true to type, except that the astrocytoma often contains elements of glioblastoma, which Scherer regards as indicative of increase in malignancy. Occasionally, following operation, the cell type seems to change. The following discussion of the microscopic types of glioma is based largely on the books of Cushing and Bailey and of Bailey.

The tumors which are made up of cells of the low order of differentiation are the neuroepithelioma, the primitive spongioblastoma, the medulloblastoma and the tumors of ependyma.

THE NEURO-EPITHELIOMA is rare in the

brain but fairly frequent among tumors of the retina. It is made up of undifferentiated cells with a tendency to be arranged in rosettes, in which the cells are radially distributed around a central space.

THE PRIMITIVE SPONGIOBLASTOMA or spongioblastoma polare is found about the optic commissure and the brain stem. It is made up of slightly more mature cells, elongated, arranged in parallel rows and with tail-like processes rarely if ever forming glia fibrils.

THE MEDULLOBLASTOMA occurs as a tumor of the cerebellum of children. It is a

nate in or near the ependyma of the ventricles. Two forms of ependymal tumors are distinguished. The ependymoblastoma shows an arrangement of cells into communicating masses. The cells are ependymoblasts with blepharoplasts and long tails differentiated into neuroglia fibrils. The cells of the ependymoma are polygonal, without tails, but also contain blepharoplasts. Both types of tumor have a supporting connective tissue stroma.

THE OLIGODENDROGLIOMA is an exceedingly rare tumor which occurs in the cerebral hemispheres. It grows slowly in the white matter, often becoming calcified. It is com-

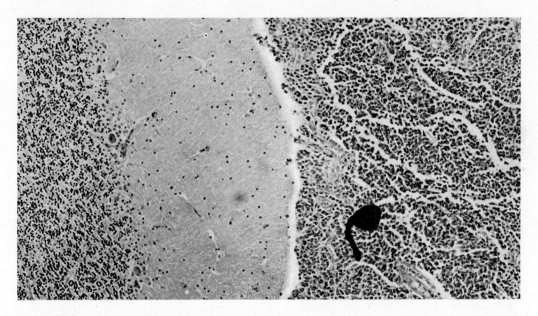

Medulloblastoma of cerebellum. Note situation of the tumor in the meninges, at right, with absence of membrane between tumor and cerebellar cortex but with no invasion of the cerebellum in this field.

globular well-defined mass which may encroach on the fourth ventricle but is not likely to invade it. It is likely to be disseminated along the cerebellar meninges and may extend into the meninges of the cord. There may be slight invasion of the underlying tissue and occasionally metastases are found in the ventricles and other parts of the brain. It is made up of rounded or somewhat polygonal cells with scanty cytoplasm and deeply chromatic nuclei, with many mitotic figures. The cells sometimes have short processes; occasionally pseudorosettes are found.

EPENDYMOBLASTOMA AND EPENDYMOMA. Tumors of the ependymal group originate

posed of round cells with sharp cell borders and well-staining nuclei, the cells resembling somewhat those of the medulloblastoma, but distinguished by having an areola around the nucleus.

THE GLIOBLASTOMA MULTIFORME, formerly called spongioblastoma multiforme, is a pleomorphic-celled tumor made up of cells more mature than those of the neuroepithelioma. About half the gliomas of adults belong to this group. It may be found anywhere in the central nervous system, but occurs most often in or near the cerebral cortex. Usually single, it may infrequently be multiple. It is usually moderately well defined, but microscopic study shows that it invades somewhat further than the gross appearance indicates. The cells are usually without any regularity of arrangement, or are multiform as to outline and nuclei. The cytoplasm varies in amount and the cells may be spindle, polygonal or of other forms, including that of rather imperfect astrocytes. The nuclei vary in size, shape and chromatin content; the mitotic figures show numerous abnormalities. Multinucleated tumor cells are not infrequent. The blood vessels usually have thin walls but endothelial and fibrous proliferation occurs, the walls may be hyalin

rarely invades the gray matter, and the converse is true (Scherer). It is vaguely defined and extends far more widely than the gross picture indicates. When it occurs in the cerebrum it is often multiple, but in the cerebellum it is single.

Microscopically, tumors made up of astrocytes can be divided into fibrillary and protoplasmic types. The fibrillary type is the more frequent. It is usually only moderately vascularized and is made up of glia cells with numerous interlacing glia fibrils. The protoplasmic type differs in that the cells are rich in cytoplasm and the glia fibrils scanty or absent.

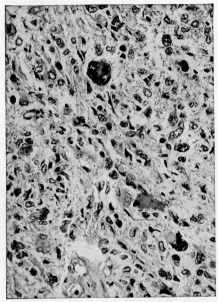

Glioblastoma multiforme, showing variation in cellular morphology. Hematoxylin and eosin.

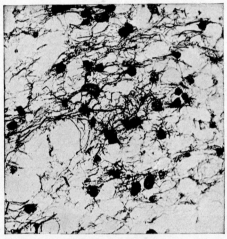

Astrocytoma, showing cells and fibrils. Holzer stain.

and both thrombosis and rupture are common. Necrosis may occur in large masses and liquefaction may produce cysts sometimes lined by pseudo-epithelium made up of tumor cells. In foci of necrosis, the cells around blood vessels may be preserved, so as to resemble perithelioma. Occasionally, the necrotic foci are partly organized my mesoblastic granulation tissue, but adult stroma is scanty. The invaded tissue shows various degenerations in nerve and glia cells.

THE ASTROCYTOMA may be found anywhere in the central nervous system but is most frequent in the cerebral hemispheres. When it originates in the white matter, it

THE ASTROBLASTOMA is less differentiated and is made up of loosely arranged large cells, rich in cytoplasm, sometimes triangular and often multinucleated. There may be dendritic-like processes, but glia fibrils are not formed.

NEUROBLASTOMA. As indicated in the chapter on tumors, the term neuroblastoma is now restricted to those rare tumors made up of neuroblasts. These tumors are practically confined to the sympathetic system, occurring in the adrenal, as well as thorax and other situations. As indicated in the chapter on Tumors, distinction should be made between the sympathogonioma, sympathoblastoma and pheochromocytoma.

THE GANGLIONEUROMA rarely, if ever, occurs in the brain. It is found principally in connection with cranial or spinal nerves. The type cell is a large, practically mature, ganglion cell, from which pass fibers with or without myelin sheath. The cells often contain Nissl granules and may be multinucleated.

PINEALOMA. Tumors of the pineal gland, pinealoma, are discussed in the chapter on Ductless Glands.

TUMORS OF THE CHOROID PLEXUS arise from either the surface cells or from the stroma. The former type is called choroid papilloma or "papilloma chorioideum." This may reduplicate the structure of the choroid plexus or may be less differentiated when it becomes invasive, and may metastasize. Tumors of the stroma which have all the characters of meningioma occur, as well as xanthomatous tumors. The choroid plexus may show cysts that are apparently ependymal in origin. Nodular hyperplasia may occur and calcific masses may be found. (See Liber and Lisa.)

Tumors of the Meninges

These include fibroma, lipoma, angioma and melanoma. The most frequent, however, is the tumor called *meningioma* which was formerly incorrectly called dural endothelioma.

Meningioma. The exact origin of this tumor has been much discussed but opinion favors the ultimate derivation from undifferentiated cells of the meningeal primordium (Globus). In the growth of the tumors, these cells differentiate to form the microscopic types described below.

The meningioma is usually single but may be multiple. It arises in the cerebral meninges at points where arachnoidal villi are encountered and probably arises in the villi. Nevertheless, meningiomas are encountered in the choroid plexus, velum interpositum and elsewhere, without meningeal attachment. The intraspinal tumors, which are less frequent than the intracranial tumors, arise from the position in which the nerve roots pass through the meninges.

The following description is of a characteristic tumor of the cerebral meninges, but many variations occur. The tumor may be flat and superficial, but is usually spheroidal, and loosely attached to the dura. It is well defined, pushes the brain away before it, has a thin capsule, is easily shelled out and often

has a lobulated outer and cut surface; only rarely is it invasive. The consistency varies from moderate firmness to great density. The cross section is firm or dense, usually pale, sometimes has a "watered silk" appearance, with moderate or little vascularization,

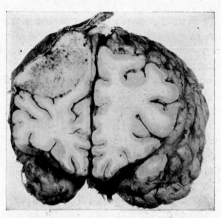

Meningioma of right parietofrontal region, showing compression of cerebral substance.

may be necrotic and may show small hemorrhages. The surrounding brain may show encephalomalacia, and sometimes edema extends for several centimeters beyond the tumor. The overlying bone is usually normal, but there may be hyperostosis both internally and externally. In these cases tumor cells may be found in the lacunae and canaliculi, and these small masses may fuse so that the original tumors extend through the tables.

Microscopically, nine types with variants are described by Cushing and Eisenhardt. The most frequent is type 1, in which cells of endothelial type are arranged in sheets or whorls with little tendency to form reticulin or collagen. In the center of the whorls, the cells may be flat as in pearls of carcinoma; psammoma bodies are not infrequent. Type 2, also frequent, shows whorls, often much smaller than in type 1, and there is moderate formation of both reticulin and collagen. Type 3 shows much greater tendency to formation of collagen and reticulin and may have a fibromatous appearance. In type 4, there is the formation of vascular spaces and the tumor resembles an angioma. In type 5, the cells are arranged in columns and sheets with a suggestion of epithelium. Type 6 is a grossly and microscopically invasive tumor of sarcomatous character, made up either of spindle cells or round cells. Type 7 shows foci of bone formation. It is osteoblastic. Type 8 is chondroblastic and type 9 is lipoblastic. Types 6, 7 and 8 are infrequent and type 9 is rare.

Other Brain Tumors

Primary sarcoma, since the detailed study of gliomas has been made, is now known to be extremely rare. The diffuse meningeal sarcoma is now regarded as an extension from the medulloblastoma or as a primary meningoblastoma. Sarcomas may arise from the mesoblastic tissue of the central nervous system, the meninges or from the bones. (See Hsü.)

Angioma may originate from the mesenchyme of the ependyma, but is principally derived from meninges. According to Cushing and Eisenhardt, this would be type 4 of the meningioma, but Bailey and Ford think the angioma is primary and by a process of sclerosis, the lesion comes to resemble a meningioma. Thus they think that the tumors are not meningiomas but sclerosing angiomas. There are variations from hamartoma to true blastoma. As elsewhere, the angioma may be capillary, cavernous, or richly cellular, is observed in cranial and spinal cavities, and although usually single may be multiple. Especially in the cerebellum the angioma, presumably originating in the roof of the fourth ventricle, may attain considerable size. In some of these instances the condition may be familial and associated with hamartomas and choristomas elsewhere, particularly angioma of the retina, constituting the syndrome known as Lindau's disease. (See Cushing and Bailey; Shapiro; Hosoi.)

Melanoma or melanoblastoma may originate in the meninges or in the choroid plexuses. It is likely to extend widely over the meningeal surfaces, and may invade the underlying nerve substance, but only occasionally shows remote metastases. As in other tumors of the same nature the cells may be round or spindle form and the amount of pigment variable. There is difference of opinion as to whether these tumors arise from meningeal nerves or melanoblasts of the meninges. (See Ray and Foot.)

Lipoma, fibroma, and chondroma are occasionally found in the central nervous system and do not differ in character from similar tumors found elsewhere.

The chordoma is not infrequent at the base of the skull and may compress the brain but is usually quiescent. (See Gardner and Turner.)

Epithelial Tumors

Reference is made, in the chapter on Ductless Glands, to the occurrence of tumors in the region of the hypophysis of tumors derived from remnants of Rathke's pouch. It is probable that most intracranial epithelial tumors originate in this way or from more complex embryonal rests. The adamantinoma of this region may originate from either of these sources. Solid teratoid tumors and dermoid cysts are probably derived from complex rests (Rand; Hosoi).

Cholesteatoma, or pearly tumor, arises from epithelial rests, is usually situated at the base of the brain and is most often in the leptomeninges but may be extradural. Less often, it is near the cerebellum and midbrain. It is also encountered in the middle ear. It may be a spongy mass or may be cystic, and has a pearly luster. It is not invasive but is usually adherent to surrounding structures. It contains fatty material resembling sebum, made up of various lipids, including cholesterol; rarely cholesterol is absent.

Microscopically, it is poorly vascularized and is composed of three layers of growth. The outer layer, or stratum durum, is made up of dense connective tissue, the intermediate layer, or stratum granulosum, is made up of rounded or flattened epithelial cells, sometimes partly keratinized, and the innermost layer, stratum granulosum, is made up of markedly swollen, partly necrotic cells (Bailey). Rarely, dermoid features such as hair follicles are observed.

Tumors of the Spinal Canal

These include (a) those of the bones and those which originate outside or inside the spinal dura, and (b) those of the cord itself. Tumors of the bone may be primary or metastatic, and may compress and ultimately invade the cord. The neurofibroma, originating in nerve roots, especially the posterior, may be either extradural or intradural. Nodules of Hodgkin's disease, lymphosarcoma and echinococcus cyst are usually extradural. Chordoma is usually in the lumbo-sacral region and is extradural. The intra-dural tumors are the meningiomas, and any of the nine types described above may occur in the spinal canal. The extension of medul-loblastoma is along the leptomeninges and thus intradural. The tumors originating in the cord itself are forms of glioma, including particularly the ependymoma, glioblastoma multiforme, astrocytoma and rarely the oligo-dendroglioma. (See Kernohan.) Most tumors of the spinal canal are in the thoracic region, but they frequently occur elsewhere. Meta-static tumors are rare in the cord. The symp-toms and neurologic signs of intraspinal tu-mors are due to pressure by or invasion of tumors, and diagnostic localization is usu-ally exact.

Tumors of Cranial Nerves

With the exception of the acoustic nerve, tumors are uncommon, although Cush-ing reports meningiomas of the acoustic, of the trigeminal and of the optic nerves. Great interest has centered about the tumors of the cerebellopontine angle. These may be of al-most any variety but are usually either meningiomas or more especially neurofibro-mas of the acoustic nerve. The latter usually originate in that part of the nerve within the porus acusticus and grow inward to be in relation to the pons, the upper surface of the cerebellum and the lower surface of the cere-brum. They are usually firm, nodular or smooth, pale tumors, small when they are still in the porus, or attaining diameters of several centimeters in the posterior fossa.

Microscopically, they are usually a mixture of fibrous tissue, sometimes with par-allel rows of nuclei (palisade arrangement) and a loose network of vesicular cells. Cells resembling ganglion cells are sometimes found, which are probably fibroblasts. Glia fibrils may be found, which are either rem-nants of, or perhaps a proliferation of, the supporting glia of the nerve to be found nor-mally for several millimeters of its length before a true endoneurium is encountered.

As a rule, tumors of the nervus acus-ticus are single. They may be bilateral and represent a central neurofibromatosis and according to Gardner and Frazier are hered-itary, transmitted as a mendelian dominant. Some may be part of a generalized neuro-fibromatosis. Multiple meningiomas may ac-company tumors of the nervus acusticus, and multiple herniation of the dura is not in-frequent.

Tumors of Peripheral Nerves

Most of these have been described in other parts of this volume, especially in the chapter on Tumors. They are classified into three groups (a) tumors of nerves, (b) tumors of nerve sheaths and (c) tumors of the nerve termini. Those of nerves, or true neuromas, include the tumors of sympathetics referred to above as the sympathogonioma, the sym-pathoblastoma and the pheochromocytoma. There are also the fibrillary neuroma and the false neuromas such as occur in amputa-tion stumps and in the appendix.

Tumors of nerve sheaths may be sim-ple or compound. The former include the tumors presumably derived from the sheath of Schwann, the so-called neurilemoma and its malignant variety, the neurilemosarcoma. The compound sheath tumors include the neurofibroma, the plexiform neurofibroma, multiple fibromatosis of von Recklinghausen, and the neurogenic, or more correctly neurog-enous, sarcoma.

The tumors of nerve terminals include the melanoma, both the nevus and the malig-nant forms as well as the nerve component of the glomangioma. (See Foot.)

Metastatic Tumors

Metastatic tumors may occur in any part of the central nervous system, but are most frequent in the brain, affecting in de-creasing order the cerebrum, the cerebellum, and the brain stem. The cortex and subcor-tical regions are more often the seat of the tumor than is the deeper white matter. The primary tumor may be in any situation, but most commonly the original tumors are car-cinomas of lung, breast and kidney. The metastases are more often multiple than single and may be nodular or diffuse. The latter appear as widely scattered minute masses, often of microscopic dimensions. The meninges may show nodular or diffuse in-volvement. The route of metastasis is through the blood stream. Around the tumors the brain may show edema, encephalomalacia and hemorrhage. The local reaction is prin-cipally by fibrillary astrocytes and the mesoblastic tissues play little part. Nodular infiltrates may occur in the brain in both lymphoid and myeloid leukemia. Metastases may occur in nerves, but their resistance to direct extension has been noted in the chapter on Tumors. Tumor emboli may cause infarction, manifested as encephalomalacia.

Direct extension may rarely take place in the brain from tumors of bone, orbit and other neighboring structures and from the sarcomatous form of meningioma. Direct extension into the cord is referred to in the section on tumors of the spinal canal.

Tumors of the Sympathetic System

The involvements in Addison's disease and in rabies have been described. Tumors have been discussed in this chapter and that on Tumors. Attempts have been made to correlate functional disturbances of the autonomic nervous system, such as the psychoneuroses, exophthalmic goiter, Raynaud's disease, angina pectoris, etc., with morphologic alterations of the sympathetic ganglia. Changes are also described in acute and chronic infectious disease, arteriosclerosis, gastric ulcer and other organic diseases. These changes vary from simple degeneration to actual death of ganglion cells and infiltration of leukocytes and mononuclear cells, and fibrosis. Terplan finds that the changes in ganglion cells are not regular or extensive and are to be found in the ganglia from normal individuals. Even when mesoblastic reactions are found in association with acute and chronic infectious diseases, the ganglion cells do not show distinctive features. It cannot be said that organic changes in the sympathetic ganglia have been satisfactorily correlated with functional alterations of the autonomic system.

REFERENCES

Armstrong, C.: Studies on Choriomeningitis and Poliomyelitis, Harvey Lectures, Baltimore, Williams & Wilkins, 36: 39, 1940-41.

Aycock, W. L. Familial Aggregation in Poliomyelitis, Amer. Jour. Med. Sci., 203: 452, 1942.

——, and H. L. Amoss: Experiments on Local Specific Therapy in Poliomyelitis, Infantile Paralysis in Vermont. Burlington (State Dept. Pub. Health), 1924, p. 355, Bull. Johns Hopkins Hosp., 34: 361, 1923.

Bailey, O. T., and R. Ford: Sclerosing Hemangiomas of the Central Nervous System. Progressive Tissue Changes in Hemangioblastomas of the Brain and in So-called Angioblastic Meningiomas, Amer. Jour. Path., 18: 1, 1942.

Bailey, P.: Intracranial Tumors, Springfield, Ill. and Baltimore, Thomas, 1933.

——: Further Observations on Pearly Tumors, Arch. Surg., 8: 524, 1924.

——, and P. C. Bucy: Oligodendrogliomas of the Brain, Jour. Path. and Bact., 32: 735, 1929.

——, and H. Cushing: A Classification of the Tumors of the Glioma Group on a Histogenetic Basis with a Correlated Study of Prognosis, Philadelphia, Lippincott, 1926.

——, and G. Hiller: The Interstitial Tissues of the Central Nervous System—A Review, Jour. Nerv. and Ment. Dis., 59: 337, 1924.

Baker, A. B.: Subdural Hematoma, Arch. Path., 26: 535, 1938.

——, and H. H. Noran: Western Variety of Equine Encephalitis in Man: A Clinicopathologic Study, Arch. Neurol. and Psychiatr., 47: 565, 1942.

Beres, D., and T. Meltzer: Tuberculous Meningitis and its Relation to Tuberculous Foci in the Brain, Amer. Jour. Path., 14: 59, 1938.

Bielschowsky, M.: Zur Histopathologie und Pathogenese der tuberösen Sklerose (Neue Beiträge) Jour. Psychol. u. Neurol., 30: 167, 1924; see review Arch. Neurol. and Psychiatr., 13: 117, 1925.

Bodian, D., and H. A. Howe: An Experimental Study of the Role of Neurones in the Dissemination of Poliomyelitis Virus in the Nervous System, Brain, 63: 135, 1940.

——, and ——: Experimental Studies on Intraneural Spread of Poliomyelitis Virus, Bull. Johns Hopkins. Hosp., 68: 248, 1941; also Howe, H. A., and D. Bodian: Neuropathological Evidence on the Portal of Entry Problem in Human Poliomyelitis, ibid., 69: 183, 1941; Howe, H. A., and D. Bodian: Neural Mechanisms in Poliomyelitis, New York, Commonwealth Fund, 1942.

Bouman, L.: Hemorrhage of the Brain, Arch. Neurol. and Psychiatr., 25: 255, 1931.

Brannan, D.: Secondary Gliomatosis of Leptomeninges, Amer. Jour. Path., 2: 123, 1926.

Brown, M. R.: Etiological Study of Landry's Original Case of Acute Ascending Paralysis, Arch. Neurol. and Psychiatr., 40: 800, 1938.

Burn, C. G., and K. H. Finley: The Rôle of Hypersensitivity in the Production of Experimental Meningitis, etc., Jour. Exper. Med., 56: 203, 1932.

Buzzard, E. F., and J. G. Greenfield: Pathology of the Nervous System, New York, 1923.

Carmichael, F. A., Jr., J. W. Kernohan, and A. W. Adson: Histopathogenesis of Cerebral Abscess, Arch. Neurol. and Psychiatr., 42: 1001, 1939.

Castren, H.: Zur pathologischen Anatomie der akuten (Sydenhamschen) Chorea, Centralbl. Allg. Path., 36: 557, 1925.

Chagas, C.: Pathogenic Processes of American Trypanosomiasis, Mem. do Instit. Oswaldo Cruz, 8: No. 2, 1916.

Chase, W. H.: An Anatomical Study of Subdural Haemorrhage Associated with Tentorial Splitting in the Newborn, Surg., Gynec. and Obst., 51: 31, 1930.

Cobb, S.: The Cerebral Circulation: XIII. The Question of "End-arteries" of the Brain and the Mechanism of Infarction, Arch. Neurol. and Psychiatr., 25: 273, 1931.

Cole, R., and A. G. Kuttner: The Problem of the Etiology of Herpes Zoster, Jour. Exper. Med., **42**: 799, 1925.

Courville, C. B.: Cell Types in the Gliomas: Their Relationship to Normal Neurohistogenesis, Arch. Path., **10**: 649, 1930.

Crothers, B.: Injury of the Spinal Cord in Breech Extraction as an Important Cause of Fetal Death and of Paraplegia in Childhood, Amer. Jour. Med. Sci., **165**: 94, 1923.

Cushing, H., and P. Bailey: Tumors Arising from the Blood Vessels of the Brain. Angiomatous Malformations and Hemangioblastomas, Springfield, Ill. and Baltimore, Thomas, 1928.

——, and L. Eisenhardt: Meningiomas. Their Classification, Regional Behaviour, Life History and Surgical End Results, Springfield, Ill. and Baltimore, Thomas, 1938.

Dandy, W. E.: Hydrocephalus in Chondrodystrophy, Bull. Johns Hopkins Hosp., **32**: 5, 1921.

——: The Cause of So-Called Idiopathic Hydrocephalus, Ibid., **32**: 67, 1921.

——: Pneumocephalus of Bacterial Origin, Arch. Surg., **15**: 913, 1927.

D'Aunoy, R., A. Friedrichs, and A. Zoeller: Gumma of the Brain, etc., Amer. Jour. Syph., **14**: 175, 1930.

Davison, C.: Effect of Liver Therapy on Pathways of Spinal Cord in Subacute Combined Degeneration, Arch. Int. Med., **67**: 473, 1941.

——: Amyotrophic Lateral Sclerosis: Origin and Extent of the Upper Motor Neuron Lesion, Arch. Neurol. and Psychiatr., **46**: 1039, 1941.

——, and M. Keschner: Myelitic and Myelopathic Lesions, etc., Ibid., **29**: 332, 600, 702, 1933.

——, and W. Schick: Encephalopathia Periaxialis Diffusa (Schilder's Disease), Ibid., **25**: 1063, 1931.

Dawson, J. R., Jr.: Cellular Inclusions in Cerebral Lesions of Epidemic Encephalitis: Second Report, Ibid., **31**: 685, 1934.

Dow, R. S., and G. Berglung: Vascular Pattern of Lesions of Multiple Sclerosis, Ibid., **47**: 1, 1942.

Epstein, E.: Beiträge zur Pathologie der allgemeinen Lipoidosen, Ergeb. Allg. Path. u. Path. Anat., **33**: 280, 1937.

Faber, H. K., and R. J. Silverberg: Experimental Air-borne Infection with Poliomyelitis Virus, Science, **94**: 566, 1941.

Farmer, T. W., and C. A. Janeway: Infections with the Virus of Lymphocytic Choriomeningitis, Medicine, **21**: 1, 1942.

Foot, N. C.: Histology of Tumors of the Peripheral Nerves, Arch. Path., **30**: 772, 1940.

Ford, F. R.: Cerebral Birth Injuries and their Results, Medicine, **5**: 121, 1926.

Fox, M. J., and R. D. O'Connor: Infectious Neuronitis: Review of Literature and Presentation of Four Cases, Arch. Int. Med., **69**: 58, 1942.

Freeman, W.: Neuropathology: The Anatomical Foundation of Nervous Diseases, Philadelphia, 1933.

Friedemann, U., A. Hollander, and I. M. Tarlov: Investigations on the Pathogenesis of Tetanus III, Jour. Immunol., **40**: 325, 1941.

Fulton, J. F.: Physiology and High Altitude Flying: With Particular Reference to Air Embolism and the Effects of Acceleration, Science, **95**: 207, 1942.

Gardner, W. J., and O. Turner: Cranial Chordomas: A Clinical and Pathologic Study, Arch. Surg., **42**: 411, 1941.

——, and C. H. Frazier: Bilateral Acoustic Neurofibromas: A Clinical Study and Field Survey of a Family of Five Generations with Bilateral Deafness in 38 Members, Arch. Neurol. and Psychiatr., **23**: 266, 1930.

Globus, J. H.: Meningiomas: Origin, Divergence in Structure and Relationship to Contiguous Tissues, etc., Ibid., **38**: 667, 1937.

——: Pinealoma, Arch. Path., **31**: 533, 1941.

Goodpasture, E. W.: A Study of Rabies, with Reference to a Neural Transmission of the Virus in Rabbits, and the Structure and Significance of Negri Bodies, Amer. Jour. Path., **1**: 547, 1925.

——: Herpetic Infection, with Especial Reference to Involvement of the Nervous System, Medicine, **8**: 223, 1929.

——, and O. Teague: Transmission of the Virus of Herpes Febrilis Along Nerves in Experimentally Infected Rabbits, Jour. Med. Res., **44**: 139, 1923-24.

Harrison, R. G.: Neuroblast Versus Sheath Cell in the Development of Peripheral Nerves, Jour. Comp. Neurol., **37**: 123, 1924.

Hassin, G. B.: Histopathology of the Peripheral and Central Nervous Systems, 2d ed., New York, Hoeber, 1940.

Helfand, M.: Changes in Vascular Pattern of Brain in Experimental Trauma, Psychiatr. Quart., **15**: 33, 1941.

Hirsch, E. F., and A. R. Elliott: Ependymomas of the Lateral and Fourth Ventricles of the Brain, Amer. Jour. Path., **1**: 627, 1925; see also Bailey, P.: Quelques Nouvelles Observations de Tumeurs Épendymaires, Ann. Anat. Path. Med. Chir., **2**: 481, 1925.

Hosoi, K.: Multiple Intracranial Angiomas, Amer. Jour. Path., **6**: 235, 1930.

——: Teratoma and Teratoid Tumors of the Brain, Arch. Path., **9**: 1207, 1930.

Howard, W. T.: Further Observations on the Relation of Lesions of the Gasserian and Posterior Root Ganglia to Herpes Occurring in Pneumonia and Cerebrospinal Meningitis, Amer. Jour. Med. Sci., **130**: 1012, 1905.

Hsü, Y. K.: Primary Intracranial Sarcomas, Arch. Neurol. and Psychiatr., **43**: 901, 1940.

Hurst, A. F.: War Neuroses, Nelson Loose Leaf Medicine, New York and London, 1920, Vol. VI, p. 655.

Hurst, E. W., and P. E. Hurst: The Aetiology of Hepato-lenticular Degeneration: Experimental Liver Cirrhosis: etc., Jour. Path. and Bacteriol., **31**: 303, 1928.

Kernohan, J. W.: Tumors of the Spinal Cord, Arch. Path., **32**: 843, 1941.

Kramer, R., and M. L. Som: Intracranial Pathways of Infection from Diseases of Sphenoid and Ethmoid Sinuses, Arch. Otolaryngol., **32**: 744, 1940.

Krause, K.: Beiträge zur pathologischen Anatomie der Hirnsyphilis, Jena, 1915.

Liber, A. F., and J. R. Lisa: Stromal Tumors of Choroid Plexus, Amer. Jour. Clin. Path., **10**: 710, 1940.

Lichtenstein, B. W.: Distant Neuroanatomic Complications of Spina Bifida (Spinal Dysraphism): Hydrocephalus, Arnold-Chiari Deformity, Stenosis of the Aqueduct of Sylvius, etc.; Pathogenesis and Pathology, Arch. Neurol. and Psychiatr., **47**: 195, 1942.

Lindemann, H.: Die Hirngefässe in apoplektischen Blutungen, Virchow's Arch. Path. Anat., **253**: 27, 1924.

Low, A. A.: Acute, Toxic (Nonsuppurative) Encephalitis in Children: A Clinicopathologic Study of Five Cases, Arch. Neurol. and Psychiatr., **23**: 696, 1930.

Moolten, S. E.: Hamartial Nature of the Tuberous Sclerosis Complex and its Bearing on the Tumor Problem. Report of a Case with Tumor Anomaly of the Kidney and Adenoma Sebaceum, Arch. Int. Med., **69**: 589, 1942.

Moritz, A. R., and W. B. Wartman: Post-traumatic Internal Hydrocephalus, Amer. Jour. Med. Sci., **195**: 65, 1938.

Neugebauer, W.: Beitrag zur pathologischen Anatomie der Hirnerschütterung, Frank. Zeitschr. Path., **51**: 210, 1937-38.

Penfield, W.: Oligodendroglia and its Relation to Classical Neuroglia, Brain, **47**: 430, 1924.

——: Microglia and the Process of Phagocytosis in Gliomas, Amer. Jour. Path., **1**: 77, 1925.

——: The Encapsulated Tumors of the Nervous System, etc., Surg., Gynec. and Obst., **45**: 178, 1927.

——: Cytology and Cellular Pathology of the Nervous System, New York, 1932.

Putnam, T. J.: The Biological Significance of the Lesions of Multiple Sclerosis, Science, **80**: 295, 1934.

Putnam, T. J.: Lesions of "Encephalomyelitis" and Multiple Sclerosis. Venous Thrombosis as the Primary Alteration, Jour. Amer. Med. Asso., **108**: 1477, 1937.

Rand, C. W.: Intracranial Dermoid Cysts, Arch. Neurol. and Psychiatr., **14**: 346, 1925.

——: Traumatic Pneumocephalus: Report of Eight Cases, Arch. Surg., **20**: 935, 1930.

Rappaport, B. Z., and B. Kaplan: Generalized Torula Mycosis, Arch. Path. and Lab. Med., **1**: 720, 1926.

Ray, B. S., and N. C. Foot: Primary Melanotic Tumors of the Meninges: Resemblance to Meningiomas. Report of Two Cases in which Operation was Performed, Arch. Neurol. and Psychiatr., **44**: 104, 1940.

Richardson, J. C., and H. H. Hyland: Intracranial Aneurysms, Medicine, **20**: 1, 1941.

Roseman, E., and C. D. Aring: Infectious Polyneuritis, Ibid., **20**: 463, 1941.

Sabin, A. B.: Etiology of Poliomyelitis, Jour. Amer. Med. Asso., **117**: 267, 1941.

Sachs, B.: A Treatise on the Nervous Diseases of Children, New York, 2d Ed., 1905.

Schaffer, C.: Pathogenesis of Amaurotic Idiocy, Arch. Neurol. and Psychiatr., **24**: 765, 1930.

Scherer, H. J.: The Forms of Growth in Gliomas and Their Practical Significance, Brain, **43**: 1, 1940.

——: Cerebral Astrocytomas and Their Derivatives, Amer. Jour. Cancer, **40**: 159, 1940.

Sever, J. W.: Obstetric Paralysis, Report of 1100 Cases, Jour. Amer. Med. Asso., **85**: 1862, 1925.

Shapiro, P. F.: Hemangioblastoma of the Cerebellum with Cyst Formation (Lindau's Disease): Report of a Case, Arch. Path., **8**: 915, 1929.

——: Changes of the Spinal Cord in Hodgkin's Disease, etc., Arch. Neurol. and Psychiatr., **24**: 509, 1930.

Sharpe, W., and A. S. Maclaire: Intracranial Hemorrhage in the Newborn, Surg., Gynec. and Obst., **38**: 200, 1924; Jour. Amer. Med. Asso., **86**: 332, 1926.

Spatz, H.: Zur anatomischen Schnelldiagnose der progressiven Paralyse mittels der Eisenreaktion, München. med. Wochenschr., **71**: 1645, 1924.

Spielmeyer, W.: Histopathologie des Nervensystems, Vol. 1, Berlin, 1922.

Steegmann, A. T.: Poliomyelitis (Poliomyelopathia) Chronica, etc., Arch. Neurol. and Psychiatr., **38**: 436, 1937.

Tamaki, K., and A. J. Lubin: Pathogenesis of Syringomyelia: Case Illustrating the Process of Cavity Formation from Embryonic Cell Rests, Ibid., **40**: 748, 1938.

Teague, O., and E. W. Goodpasture: Experimental Herpes Zoster, Jour. Med. Res., **44**: 185, 1923-24.

Terplan, K.: Zur Frage histo-pathologischer Veränderungen in sympathischen Ganglien und deren Bedeutung, Virchow's Arch. Path. Anat., **262**: 431, 1926.

Thannhauser, S.: Lipidoses: Diseases of the Cellular Lipid Metabolism, Oxford Medicine, New York, Oxford Univ. Press; Chapter VII-A, p. 214.

Thompson, R.: The Etiology of Postvaccinal Encephalomyelitis, Arch. Path., **12**: 601, 1931.

Thorne, I. J.: Caisson Disease. A Study Based on Three Hundred Cases Observed at the Queens-Midtown Tunnel Project, 1938, Jour. Amer. Med. Asso., **117**: 585, 1941.

Toomey, J. A., W. S. Takacs, and L. A. Tischer: Poliomyelitis Virus from Flies, Proc. Soc. Exper. Biol. and Med., **48**: 637, 1941.

Tuthill, C. R.: Cerebral Aneurysms, Arch. Path., **16**: 630, 1933.

Van Wagenen, W. P.: Papillomas of the Choroid Plexus: Report of Two Cases, One with Removal of Tumor at Operation and One with "Seeding" of the Tumor in the Ventricular System, Arch. Surg., **20**: 199, 1930.

Waring, J. J., K. Neubuerger, and E. F. Geever: Severe Forms of Chickenpox in Adults with Autopsy Observations in a Case with Associated Pneumonia and Encephalitis, Arch. Int. Med., **69**: 384, 1942.

Webster, L. T.: Classification of Primary Encephalitides of Man According to Virus Etiology: Present Status, Jour. Amer. Med. Asso., **116**: 2840, 1941. Rabies, New York, Macmillan, 1942.

Weed, L. H.: The Cerebrospinal Fluid, Physiol. Reviews, **2**: 171, 1922.

——: Studies on Cerebrospinal Fluid, Jour. Med. Res., **31**: 21, 51, 93, 1914-15.

——: The Experimental Production of Internal Hydrocephalus, Publications Carnegie Inst. of Wash., 272, p. 425, 1920.

Weil, A.: A Text-Book of Neuropathology, Philadelphia, Lea and Febiger, 1933.

——, and G. Heilbrunn: Demonstration of Myelolytic Substances in Disseminated Sclerosis, Proc. Soc. Exper. Biol. and Med., **48**: 233, 1941.

Weinberger, L. M., M. H. Gibbon, and J. H. Gibbon, Jr.: Temporary Arrest of the Circulation to the Central Nervous System. I. Physiologic Effects,

Arch. Neurol. and Psychiatr., **43:** 615, 1940; II. Pathologic Effects, Ibid., **43:** 961, 1940.

Wilson, S. A. K.: Progressive Lenticular Degeneration: A Familial Nervous Disease Associated with Cirrhosis of Liver, Brain, **34:** 295, 1912.

Winestine, F.: The Relation of von Recklinghausen's Disease (Multiple Neurofibromatosis) to Giant Growth and Blastomatosis, Jour. Cancer Res., **8:** 409, 1924.

Wöhrmann, W.: Ueber Poliomyelitis anterior acuta, Virchow's Arch. path. Anat., **259:** 466, 1926.

Wohlfart, G., and R. L. Swank: Pathology of Amyotrophic Lateral Sclerosis: Fiber Analysis of the Ventral Roots and Pyramidal Tracts of the Spinal Cord, Arch. Neurol. and Psychiatr., **46:** 783, 1941.

Zand, N.: La Microglie et les Histiocytes, Ann. Anat. Path., **7:** 565, 1930; *see also* Bourgeois, P.: La Néuroglie et la Microglie, etc., Ibid., **7:** 853, 1930.

Index

Chicken pox 16043

Cavernous sinus, thromb 16072

cellulitis 16072

Cloudy swelling, 37
of arteries, 381
of liver, 547
of myocardium, 367
of skeletal muscle, 740
Coccidioidal granuloma, 240, 738
Coccidioidis immitis, 240
Coccidioidomycosis, 240
Cohnheim theory of tumors, 294
Congenital anomalies, *see* Anomalies
Congenital atresias of, intestines, 516
Congenital disease, 12
of nervous system, 752
Colitis, ulcerative, 522
Colles-Baumes' law, 232
Colloid degeneration, 51
Complications of, acute appendicitis, 536
of gastric ulcer, 510
of lobar pneumonia, 462
Concrements, 77, 82
biliary, 83
mechanism of, 83
corpora amylacea, 86
intestinal, 86
other forms, 86
pancreatic, 86
in penis, 637
phleboliths, 86
prostatic, 87
psammoma bodies, 87
salivary, 86
uric acid, 85
urinary, 84
chemical composition of, 85
Concussion of brain, 757
of spinal cord, 757
Constitution, 13
Contrecoup, 759
Convalescence, 172
Convulsions, 783
Cord, spinal, *see* Spinal cord
Coronary occlusion, functional effects of, 371
Corpora amylacea, 86
in nervous system, 754
Corpus-luteum cysts of ovary, 666
Corrosion, of esophagus, 500
of stomach, 507
Cranial nerves, tumors of, 789
Craniopathy, metabolic, 723
Craniopharyngoma, 686
Cretinism, 697, 716
Crystalline deposits in tissues, 81
Cushing's syndrome, 688
Cyanosis, 378
Cyclencephaly, 750
Cylindroma, 311
Cylindruria, 606
Cyst, of bone, 733
of breast, 677
simple, 676
congenital, 339
corpus-luteum of ovary, 666
dermoid, 337, 670
echinococcus, of liver, 570
epidermoid, 338
of esophagus, 501
congenital, 500
follicular, of ovary, 666
gas, of intestine, 120, 522
glandular, acquired, 339
of kidney, 616
congenital, 616
of liver, 570
neoplastic, 339
of ovary, 666
of pancreas, 581
in penis, 637
of placenta, 661
pseudocysts, of kidneys, 618
of pancreas, 581
retention, of ovary, 666
of pancreas, 581
simple, 338
in solid organs, 339
theca-lutein, of ovary, 666
of teeth, 497
of thyroid, 696
of urinary bladder, 628
of vagina, 651
of vulva, 649
parovarian, 674
Cystadenoma, 322
of ovary, serous, 667
Cystitis, catarrhal, acute, 623
chronic, 623
cystica, 624
fibrinopurulent, 623
fibrinous, acute, 623
follicularis, 624
purulent, acute, 623
ulcerative, 624
Cystoids, of pancreas, 581
Cystosarcoma phallydes of breast, 679
Cysts, 338

D

Death, morphologic changes in, 65
somatic, 61
autolysis in, 64
morphologic changes in, 65
signs of, 62
Decubitus ulcers, 762
Deficiency, of nicotinic acid, 10
of pantothenic acid, 10
of vitamin A, 9
of vitamin B_1, 10
of vitamin B_2 complex, 10
of vitamin C, 10
of vitamin D, 11
of vitamin E, 11
of vitamin K, 11
Degenerations, 37
albuminous, 37
of arteries, 381
of cardiovascular system, 349
cloudy swellings, 37
colloid, 51
of endocardium, 354
fatty, 43
gross appearance of, 44
pathogenesis, 45
hyaline, 47
Zenker's, 49
of kidney,
fatty, 589
hydropic, 39
lenticular,
progressive, 753
of liver,
fatty, 547
mucinous, 50
of myocardium, 367, 368
parenchymatous, 37
of spinal cord, 780
of veins, 394
Dental caries, 495
Dental granuloma, 496
Deposits, mineral,
in kidney, 587
Dermatomyositis, 743
Dermoid cysts, 337
simple, 338
Desiccation, 64
Diabetes mellitus, glycogen in, 53
pancreatic disease in, 582
Diathermy, 7
Dilatation, of esophagus, 503
of heart, 377
of intestine,
congenital, 517
of stomach,
chronic, 516
of lymphatic vessels, 398
of urinary bladder, 625
of veins, 396
Diphtheria, 179, 498
gravis, 180
pathologic effects in, 180

INDEX

manual (Numbers 16069 16166 16107 16228
Puncture 16026

Heredity, 12
  and tuberculosis, 213
  and tumors, 213
Hermaphrodism, 635
  pseudo-, 635
Hernia, 518
  internal, 518
Herpes, 777
  febrilis simplex, 777
  genitalis, 777
  progenitalis, 636
  zoster, 777
Histiocyte, 140
Histoplasmosis, 191
Hodgkin's disease, 244
  clinical manifestations of, 245
  morbid anatomy of, 246
  of bones, 726
  of lung, 480
  in lymph nodes, 428
  of nervous system, 776
  splenomegaly due to, 422
Hormone production, by ovarian tumors, 673
Hormones, 14
Host, factors favoring, 171
  factors unfavorable to, 171
Hunner's ulcer, 624
Hutchinson incisors, 494
Hyalin epithelial, 47
  in liver, 548
  von Recklinghausen's, 47
  Zenker's, 49, 185
Hyaline, casts, 48
  degeneration, 47
  inclusions, 325
Hyalinization, of kidney, 589
Hydatidiform mole, 661
Hydremia, 97
Hydrocele, 638
Hydrocephalus, 751
Hydrocephalus, acquired, 752
  congenital, 751
  ex vacuo, 752
Hydromyelia, 752
Hydronephrosis, 620
  causes of, 620
  nature of, 620
Hydropic degeneration, 39
Hydrosalpinx, 663
Hydrothorax, 480
Hyperemia, active, 100
  arterial, 100
Hyperemia, of brain, 758
  chronic passive, 102
  of intestine, active, 520
  of kidney, active, 590
    passive, 590
  of liver, passive, 552
Hyperemia—(*Continued*)
  of lung, 453
  of pericardium, 349
  of peritoneum, active, 538
    passive, 538
  of spinal cord, 763
  of spinal meninges, 765
  of spleen, active, 417
    passive, 419
  of uterus, passive, 652
  passive, 101
    morphology of, 101
  venous, 101
Hyperergy, 124
Hypernephroma, 333
  of kidney, 616
Hypertension, 375
  and arteriosclerosis, 384
  in glomerulonephritis, 608
Hyperparathyroidism, 700
Hyperplasia, 256
  of adrenals, 705
  of bone marrow, 431
  causes of, 257
  compensatory, 258
  of endometrium, 654
  of lymph nodes, acute, 425
    chronic, 426
  of parathyroid gland, 699
  of spleen, acute, 420
    chronic, 420
  of thyroid, 691
Hyperthyroidism, 698
Hypertrophy, adaptive, 258
  of arteries, 381
  of breast, 674
  of heart, 375
    congenital idiopathic, 376
  kinds of, 257
  of skeletal muscle, 743
  of thyroid, 691
  of urinary bladder, 626
  pseudo-, 260
Hypoergy, 124
Hypothesis, of Ranke, 203
  of kidneys, 586
  of teeth, 494
Hypophysis, acromegaly, 688
  adenoma of, 685
  anomalies of, 685
  atrophy of, 685
  Cushing's syndrome, 688
  diabetes insipidus, 689
  Frölich's syndrome, 687
  gigantism, 688
  inflammation of, 685
  Lawrence-Moon-Biedl syndrome, 687
  physiologic considerations, 686
Hypophysis—(*Continued*)
  progressive tissue, changes in, 685
  retrogressive changes in, 685
  Simmonds' disease, 687
  tumors of, 685
Hypothyroidism, 697
Hypoplasia, of heart, 375

I

Icterus, hemolytic, 34
Idiocy, amaurotic, 752
Ileitis, 522
Immunity in lobar pneumonia, 461
Incisors, Hutchinson, 494
Inclusion bodies, 193
Inclusions, hyaline, 325
Incubation, 171
Infarct, white, 106
  "anemic," 106
Infarction, 104
  hemorrhagic, 105
  of kidney, 591
  of lung, 458
  of myocardium, 368
    clinical manifestation of, 371
  pathogenesis of, 104
  pulmonary, 456
  of spleen, 419
  uric acid, 81
Infection, and avitaminosis, 12
  as cause of anemia, 404
  classification of, 170
  congenital, 213
  diphtheritic, 179
  dissemination of, 169
  general, from tonsils, 499
  moment of, 171
  of paratyphoid, 181
  pyogenic infection, 177
  septicemic, 181
  special types of, 177
  staphylococcal, 177
  streptococcal, 178
  of throat, 499
  toxemia, 179
  types of, 177
  of typhoid, 181
Infectious disease, 168, 169
  allergic in nature, 194
  classification of, 168
  course of, 171
  dissemination, varieties of, 169
  manifestations of, general, 172
    chills, 174
    fever, 172
    leukocytosis, 175
    pathologic effects, 176

Interauricular septal defect 16065
Interventricular " " 16065
" Congenital stricture 16019 See Lagari
Kapri (?) 34356

Kernicterus 15903
abscesses amb 14853
diabetic 16224
Laceration 16043
Leukemia 16065
Sulfa 16140
Leukemia 16065
Ac 14445 14598 15978 16006
Horseshoe 15895 16101
X Perforation 15791 (foreign body)
ulcer 16077
Transverse reaction 15817
Inter capillary glom sclerosis 16224
Thrombosis renal artery 16230
double colon & rectum 16193 ö structo
gangrene 14692 (volvulus)

Handwritten top margin: *Polycythemia 14781* / *Follicular lymphoma 16112* / *anthrax 16084* / *Salivary gland tumors 16243*

Handwritten left margin: *16263 (86?)* / *14853* / *16065* / *16076* / *16106* / *total 16231*

Handwritten bottom margin: *16010 16040* / *Subarachnoid hem 16038* / *Subcutaneous nodule 197*

Leukemia arts 16243 Thyroglossal tract 16079
Tricuspid valve Sten 16155
recanalized 16166

x *ureter* 15979
xx *Seminal vesicle* 15979

Varicella 16043

Vertelia, ervin 14900
     ca prim K 14740

Ulc Colitis + IGV	Polycystic K	Peptic Ulcers
14673 Diverticulitis	15085	15758 "
14673 "	15307	ulcer "Stomach" #
Diverticulosis	15852	Ulcerated leiomyoma stomach
32042 Ibc strict	Solitary Cyst	16032 healed
32042 " "	15592 Hydronep	14705 leiomyoma
16058 Ibc Colitis	hydronephrosis	CA ē met Stomach
15228 Ibc Ilcitis	16215	CA Slate Hosp see Stomach
Amebic dys .		16106
" " " leiv		16214 ham
16056 Amebic n ulc . c .		CA ulcer Stomach
16056 " "		15688 perf
16203 Ulc colitis		15805 "
32193 Mutliple ulc CA		14824
CA Rectum		14882
CA Rectum		
16206 Rectum		
16206 Colon	Subdurals	
16206 Zubicon	15389 chr .	
	15237 Wade	
	15868 chr	
Pyelonephritis	Brain Obs	
16051 Hydro	Brain Surg excis .	
14415 Perinephric abs .	c . 14629 chr months	
16001 Chronic C U scars	b . 15822 Oc . hmo	
Kidney chr pyelo	a . 15602 acute	
16051 acute	16040 ē contum + fracture	
Pyemia Sec Kidny	Brain - Subarachnoid	
16001 hydro pyelo	Fracture - Sping	
16006	Fracture subdural + extradural Spin	
Kidney chr .	Battle Seyn Spin	
Abyp besta 16224	16237 duplicated brain	
	16237 " "	